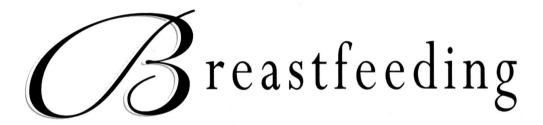

Breastfeeding

A GUIDE FOR THE MEDICAL PROFESSION

Sixth Edition

Ruth A. Lawrence, MD

Professor of Pediatrics, Obstetrics, and Gynecology
Department of Pediatrics
University of Rochester School of Medicine and Dentistry
Rochester, New York

Robert M. Lawrence, MD

Clinical Associate Professor
Pediatric Immunology, Rheumatology, and Infectious Diseases
Department of Pediatrics
University of Florida College of Medicine
Gainesville, Florida

With 190 illustrations

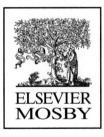

**ELSEVIER
MOSBY**

ELSEVIER
MOSBY

The Curtis Center
170 S Independence Mall W 300E
Philadelphia, Pennsylvania 19106

Breastfeeding: A Guide for the Medical Profession,   ISBN 0-323-02823-3
Sixth Edition
Copyright © 2005, Mosby, Inc. All rights reserved.

No part of this publication may be reproduced or transmitted in any form or by any means, electronic or mechanical, including photocopying, recording, or any information storage and retrieval system, without permission in writing from the publisher. Permissions may be sought directly from Elsevier's Health Sciences Rights Department in Philadelphia, PA, USA: phone: (+1) 215 238 7869, fax: (+1) 215 238 2239, e-mail: healthpermissions@elsevier.com. You may also complete your request on-line via the Elsevier homepage (http://www.elsevier.com), by selecting 'Customer Support' and then 'Obtaining Permissions'.

NOTICE

Pediatrics is an ever-changing field. Standard safety precautions must be followed, but as new research and clinical experience broaden our knowledge, changes in treatment and drug therapy may become necessary or appropriate. Readers are advised to check the most current product information provided by the manufacturer of each drug to be administered to verify the recommended dose, the method and duration of administration, and contraindications. It is the responsibility of the licensed prescriber, relying on experience and knowledge of the patient, to determine dosages and the best treatment for each individual patient. Neither the publisher nor the author assumes any liability for any injury and/or damage to persons or property arising from this publication.

Previous editions copyrighted 1980, 1985, 1989, 1994, 1999

Library of Congress Cataloging-in-Publication Data

Lawrence, Ruth A., 1924-
   Breastfeeding : a guide for the medical profession / Ruth A. Lawrence, Robert M.
Lawrence.–6th ed.
      p. ; cm.
   Includes bibliographical references and index.
   ISBN 0-323-02823-3
   1. Breast feeding. 2. Breast milk. 3. Lactation. I. Lawrence, Robert M. (Robert
Michael), 1951-II. Title.
   [DNLM: 1. Breast Feeding. WS 125 L422b 2005]
   RJ216.L358 2005
   613.2'69–dc22   2004055247

Acquisitions Editor: Todd Hummel
Publishing Services Manager: Joan Sinclair
Project Manager: Mary Stermel
Marketing Manager: Theresa Dudas

Printed in United States of America

Last digit is the print number: 9   8   7   6   5   4   3   2   1

Affectionately dedicated to

Rob, Barbara, Timothy, Kathleen,

David, Mary Alice, Joan, John, and **Stephen** for their love and patient understanding

and to **Bob**

for his boundless faith, trust, and inspiration.

—Ruth A. Lawrence

Sincerely dedicated to

all the health professionals who continue to support women

in their efforts to breastfeed their children.

—Robert M. Lawrence

$\mathcal{F}$oreword

The 6 years since the publication of the fifth edition of this excellent book have been a time of incredible advances in understanding several previously unknown physiologic and behavioral processes directly linked or associated with breastfeeding and beautifully described in this new volume.

These findings change our view of the mother-infant relationship and signal an urgent need to completely review present perinatal care procedures. These new research results include the observation that, when the infant suckles from the breast, there is a large outpouring of 19 different gastrointestinal hormones, including cholecystokinin, gastrin, and insulin, in both the mother and infant. Several of these hormones stimulate the growth of the baby's and the mother's intestinal villi, thus increasing the surface area for the absorption of additional calories with each feeding. The stimuli for these changes are touching the nipple of the mother or the inside of the infant's mouth. The stimuli in both infant and mother result in the release of oxytocin in the periventricular area of the brain, which leads to production of these hormones via the vagus nerve. These pathways were essential for survival thousands of years ago, when periods of famine were common, before the development of modern agriculture and the storage of grain.

The discovery of the additional significance of the mother's breast and chest to the infant comes from the studies of Swedish workers who have shown that the normal infant, when dried, placed on the mother's chest, and covered with a light blanket, will warm or maintain body temperature as well as an infant warmed with elaborate, high-tech heating devices. The same researchers found that, when infants are skin-to-skin with their mothers for the first 90 minutes after birth, they hardly cry at all compared with infants who are dried, wrapped in a towel, and placed in a bassinet. In addition, the researchers demonstrated that if a newborn is left quietly on the mother's abdomen after birth he or she will, after about 30 minutes, crawl gradually up to the mother's breast, find the nipple, self-attach, and start to suckle on his or her own.

It would appear that each of these features—the crawling ability of the infant, the absence of crying when skin-to-skin with the mother, and the warming capabilities of the mother's chest—evolved genetically more than 400,000 years ago to help preserve the infant's life.

Research findings related to the 1991 Baby Friendly Hospital Initiative (BFHI) of WHO and UNICEF provided insight into an additional basic process. After the introduction of the BFHI, which emphasized mother-infant contact with an opportunity for suckling in the first 30 minutes after birth and mother-infant rooming-in throughout the hospital stay, there has been a significant drop in neonatal abandonment reported in maternity hospitals in Thailand, Costa Rica, the Philippines, and St. Petersburg, Russia.

A key to understanding this behavior is the observation that, if the lips of the infant touch the mother's nipple in the first half hour of life, the mother will decide to keep the infant in her room 100 minutes longer on the second and third days of hospitalization than a mother whose infant does not touch her nipple in the first 30 minutes. It appears that these remarkable changes in maternal behavior are probably related to increased brain oxytocin levels shortly after birth. These changes, in conjunction with known sensory, physiologic, immunologic, and behavioral mechanisms, all help attract the mother and infant to each other and start their attachment. As pointed out in the fourth edition, a strong, affectionate bond is most likely to develop successfully with breastfeeding, in which close contact and interaction occur repeatedly when the infant wishes and at a pace that fits the needs and wishes of the mother and the infant, resulting in gratification for both. Thus, breastfeeding plays a central role in the development of a strong mother-infant attachment when begun with contact immediately after birth, which in turn has been shown to be a simple maneuver to significantly increase the success of breastfeeding. All of these exciting findings provide further evidence of why breastfeeding has been so crucial in the past and deserves strong support now.

In addition, these past few years have been associated with fundamental biochemical findings, including the importance of docosahexaenoic acid (DHA) in optimal brain development. All in all, the many new observations described in this sixth edition place milk and the process of breastfeeding in a key position in the development of many critical functions in human infants and their mothers. We salute the author for her special skill in bringing together these many unique and original observations in this new and most valuable book.

SUGGESTED READINGS

1. Christensson K, Cabrera T, Christensson E, et al: Separation distress call in the human neonate in the absence of maternal body contact. In Care of the Newborn Infant: Satisfying the Need for Comfort and Energy Conservation, thesis of Kyllike Christensson. Stockholm, Karolinska Institute, 1994.
2. Christensson K, Siles C, Moreno L, et al: Temperature, metabolic adaptation and crying in healthy newborn cared for skin-to-skin or in a cot. Acta Paediatri Scand 81:488, 1992.
3. Uvnäs-Moberg K: The gastrointestinal tract in growth and reproduction. Sci Am 261(1):78, 1989.
4. Widström AM, Ransjo-Arvidson AB, Christensson K, et al: Gastric suction in healthy newborn infants: effects on circulation and developing feeding behavior. Acta Paediatr Scand 76:566, 1987.
5. Widström AM, Wahlberg V, Matthiesen AS, et al: Short-term effects of early suckling and touch of the nipple on maternal behavior. Early Hum Dev 21:153, 1990.

JOHN H. KENNELL
MARSHALL J. KLAUS

$\mathscr{P}$reface to the sixth edition

Almost 3 decades ago, work began on the first edition of this text. Much has changed in the field of human lactation and in the world at large. The trickle of scientific work on the subject has swollen into a river overflowing its banks. The Lactation Study Center at the University of Rochester has more than 30,000 documents on file that describe peer-reviewed scientific studies and reports, and there are thousands more unfiled documents that recount individual experience and anecdotal reports of events. The field has abandoned the dogma of rules about breastfeeding that demanded rigid scheduling and specific managements to a period in which thoughtful contemplation and recognition of the variability of the human condition are key. Well-trained, skilled clinicians recognize the value of flexibility and the individualization of care. The Baby Friendly approach, whose very being was spawned to set women free from rigid dicta, requires protocols and policies. Mothers tell their doctors that they cannot breastfeed because there are too many rules, an impression created by overzealous teaching of too much detail. Medicine, itself in the era of managed care, has come forth with care guidelines for one disease or circumstance after another. Will breastfeeding be next?

In 1994, the Academy of Breastfeeding Medicine was founded for the promotion and support of breastfeeding. It is designed to provide physicians all over the world and from every discipline a forum for scientific learning and discussion about breastfeeding and human lactation. Its members form a nucleus of medical professionals dedicated to the advancement of breastfeeding. In December 1997, the American Academy of Pediatrics proclaimed with renewed energy that mothers should breastfeed for six months exclusively and then continue breastfeeding while introducing weaning foods through the first year and for as long thereafter as desired by mother and infant. The Section on Breastfeeding of the American Academy of Pediatrics reaffirmed that position in 2004. The health care provider can promote these goals most effectively when armed with information.

The intent of this volume is to provide the basic tools of knowledge and experience that will enable the clinician to provide the thoughtful counseling and guidance to the breastfeeding family that is most applicable to that particular breastfeeding dyad and its circumstances, problems, and lifestyle. No protocol should ever replace thinking, however.

As the field has become more complex, it is clear that one of the most difficult issues centers around infection in the mother or infant and sometimes both. Robert Michael Lawrence, MD, Clinical Associate Professor of Pediatrics and Immunology at the University of Florida College of Medicine, has again produced the chapters on immunology and infectious disease, as well as Appendix E, to bring the most accurate information in these areas to these pages. He has also assisted in the editing of many other chapters. The drug database and Appendix D, Drugs in Breast Milk and the Effect on the Infant, has been thoroughly revamped.

Dr. James Woods, Professor of Obstetrics and Gynecology, provided wise counsel on contraceptive issues. The thousands of queries to the Lactation Study Center at the University of Rochester have served as a basis for new topics and new clinical discussions.

The sixth edition was assembled with the help of many. Carole Sydelnik prepared the typed manuscripts from handwritten, reedited drafts with great skill and precision. The undergraduate students at the Center—Sara, Catey, Meghan, Emily, and Caralyn—have been reference sleuths as well as loyal filers, copiers, and errand runners. Marjorie Waterman, a recent graduate of the University of Rochester and now a medical student, has worked tirelessly this semester as an editorial assistant and general computer wizard to move production from cut-and-paste to CD-ROM.

Ruth A. Lawrence

$\mathscr{P}$reface to the first edition

This book was written in an effort to provide the medical profession with an easily accessible reference for the clinical management of the mother-infant nursing couple. After many decades of championing formula for the newborn and infant, the medical profession has recognized that human milk is preferable for the human infant. The world literature reflects scientists' work on breastfeeding in the fields of nutrition, biochemistry, immunology, psychology, anthropology, and sociology. These researchers have demonstrated what most mothers have long believed: Human milk is specifically designed for human infants.

Although reports in dozens of journals have contributed information valuable in the clinical management of lactation, it has remained difficult for the practitioner to gain access to it when an emergency arises. There are other topics, such as the pharmacokinetics of human milk, on which more knowledge and data are needed. This book is intended to provide the information that is available as well as identify areas of deficient information. The first part of this book is basic data on the anatomical, physiological, biochemical, nutritional, immunological, and psychological aspects of human lactation. The remainder centers on the problems of clinical management and, I hope, maximizes scientific data and minimizes anecdotal information. The goal is to provide practical information for managing individual mothers and their infants. It is also hoped that a balance has been struck between basic science, on which rational management should rest, and advice garnered by experience. Through use of the bibliographies, interested readers may seek out the original works for details and supporting data.

I recognized some years ago that specific data were accumulating rapidly but remained in scattered, sometimes inaccessible, references. The increasing requests for consultation about breastfeeding sparked the idea for a more formal publication to replace the information sheets and brochures that I had been putting together. My interest in breastfeeding started during internship and residency at Yale-New Haven Hospital where Dr. Edith Jackson, Dr. Grover Powers, and Dr. Milton Senn expressed genuine concern for the declining rate of breastfeeding. Dr. Jackson provided excellent training in the art of breastfeeding for families and professionals in the rooming-in project in New Haven.

This book does not speak to world issues or the political issues of nutrition, since they have been eloquently discussed by Derrick and E. P. Patrice Jelliffe in their many works.

Throughout this book, because a nursing mother is a female, the personal pronoun *she* has been used. In referring to the infant, the choice between *he* or *she* has been made, using the male pronoun only to enhance clarity between reference to mother or child. The physician has been referred to as *he*, although I am thoroughly cognizant of the inordinate injustice perpetrated by this historical usage.

I should like to acknowledge the help and support of the many colleagues who encouraged me to investigate this subject and the hosts of nursing mothers who helped me learn what I am sharing here.

Extensive library research was done by Nancy Hess and Cathy Goodfellow, who worked as professional volunteers. Editing and tracking specific data were done by Timothy Lawrence, whom I also wish to thank. No writing is accomplished without diligent preparation of the manuscript. Loretta H. Anderson prepared many of the rough drafts. Carleen Wilenius was invaluable for her many skills with manuscripts, not the least of which were final preparation and typing of many of the lengthy charts and bibliographies. I also wish to thank Rosemary E. Disney, who designed the cover art.

Ruth A. Lawrence

Contents

APPENDICES

$\mathcal{B}$reastfeeding in modern medicine

"There is a reason behind everything in nature."
ARISTOTLE

As the new millennium dawns, breastfeeding has taken a critical role in public health, child survival, maternal health, and national and international strategies. Breastfeeding initiation rates have increased substantially and duration rates have begun to improve.

Scientists have provided the evidence-based data for the clinician to take an aggressive stand in promoting, protecting, and supporting breastfeeding. Women have heard the message and are making informed decisions to breastfeed their children. Peer support is becoming an important element of success in all socioeconomic groups. Programs target high-risk groups who have not been breastfeeding in recent decades.

This movement is not without obstacles. The fear of inducing guilt in those who do not choose to breastfeed is still a major defense some health care providers use for not mentioning it. There is no scientific evidence to support this position, and there is evidence that women do not feel guilty about their informed decisions. Other barriers are being developed by formula manufacturers who have been hastily developing additives for formula in the effort to present cow milk and soy milk formulas as similar to human milk.

Until recently, breastfeeding has been a subject considered too imprecise and nonspecific to justify consideration by scientists and clinicians confronted with questions of infant nutrition. Decades have been spent in the laboratory deciphering the nutritional requirements of the growing neonate. A considerably greater investment in time, talent, and money has been put toward the development of an ideal substitute for human milk. At the same time, artificial feeding has been described as the world's largest experiment without controls.[102] In veterinary medicine, a careful study of the science of lactation in other species, especially bovine, has been made because of the commercial significance of a productive herd.

Advances in technology have allowed the gathering of much data about human milk, which unarguably is best for human infants. Some of the world's finest scientists have turned their attention to human lactation. Time and talent are providing a wealth of resource information about this remarkable fluid—human milk. Old dogmas are being reviewed in the light of new data, and previous data are being reworked with newer methods and technology. An interface for the exchange of scientific information worldwide around issues of human

TABLE 1-1	National health promotion and disease prevention objectives	

Mothers breastfeeding their babies (special population targets)	1998 baseline	2010 target
During early postpartum period		
Low-income mothers (WIC mothers)	56.8	75.0
Black mothers	45.0	75.0
Hispanic mothers	66.0	75.0
American Indian/Alaskan Native mothers	1998 data not collected 1988 baseline—47%	75.0
At age 5–6 months		
Low-income mothers (WIC mothers)	18.9	50.0
Black mothers	19.0	50.0
Hispanic mothers	28.0	50.0
American Indian/Alaskan Native mothers	1998 data not collected 1988 baseline—28%	50.0
At age 12 months		
Low-income mothers (WIC mothers)	12.1 (in 1999)	25.0
Black mothers	9.0	25.0
Hispanic mothers	19.0	25.0
American Indian/Alaskan Native mothers	1998 data not collected	25.0

Healthy People 2010 is a statement of national opportunities. Although the federal government facilitated its development, it is not intended as a statement of federal standards or requirements. It is the product of a national effort, involving 22 expert working groups, a consortium that has grown to include almost 300 national organizations and all the state health departments, and the Institute of Medicine of the National Academy of Sciences, which helped the U.S. Public Health Service to manage the consortium, convene regional and national hearings, and receive testimony from more than 750 individuals and organizations. After extensive public review and comment, involving more than 10,000 people, the objectives were revised and refined to produce this report. (From U.S. Department of Health and Human Services. Heathy People 2010 (Conference Edition, in Two Volumes). Washington, DC, January 2000.)

lactation, breastfeeding, and human milk is developing. The more detail that is deciphered about the specific macro- and micronutrients in human milk, the clearer it becomes that human milk is precisely engineered for the human infant.[50] The clinician should not have to justify the recommendation for breastfeeding; instead, the pediatrician should have to justify the replacement with a cow milk substitute. Harnessing the continuing stream of scientific information into a clinically applicable resource has been encumbered by the need to identify reproducible, peer-reviewed scientific information and to cull the uncontrolled, poorly designed studies and reports appearing in print as a result of the widening interest in the clinical field of lactation.

The Healthy People 2010 goals,* first published in 1978 and restated in 1989 and again in 1999, are that the nation will increase the proportion of mothers who exclusively or partially breastfeed their babies in the early postpartum period to at least 75% and the proportion who continue breastfeeding until their babies are 5 to 6 months old to at least 50%. Furthermore, at least 25% will be breastfed at a year post partum.

The report further states that special populations should be targeted (Table 1-1) because breastfeeding

*Healthy People 2000: National Health Promotion and Disease Prevention Objectives, DHHS Pub. No. (PHS) 91-50213. Washington, DC, U.S. Department of Health and Human Services, Public Health Service, U.S. Government Printing Office, 1990.

is the optimal way of nurturing infants while simultaneously benefiting the lactating mother. Former Surgeon General of the United States C. Everett Koop agreed, noting, "We must identify and reduce the barriers which keep women from beginning or continuing to breastfeed their infants."[72] Former Surgeon General David Satcher developed the Health and Human Services Blueprint for Action on Breastfeeding in 2000 saying, "Breastfeeding is one of the most important contributions to infant health . . . in addition, breastfeeding improves maternal health and contributes economic benefits to the family, health care system, and work place."[20]

In 1984 the surgeon general convened a workshop to address the barriers and devise a plan to reach the breastfeeding goals.[72] One barrier identified was the lack of training and education of health care professionals in human milk and the physiology of lactation. A second workshop was convened[73] to bring together representatives of the professional organizations—(American Academy of Pediatrics, American Academy of Family Practice, American College of Nurse Midwives, American College of Obstetricians and Gynecologists, American Dietetic Association, National Association of Pediatric Nurse Practitioners, and Nurses' Association of American College of Obstetricians and Gynecologists, now called Association of Women's Obstetric Neonatal Nurses) charged with the education and accreditation of their respective members. Through individual action of their boards of trustees, the organizations endorsed a statement supporting breastfeeding and human lactation. They also devised a plan to ensure appropriate education for their members and the inclusion of the material in the certifying examination for their respective specialties (see Appendix N for model curriculum).

Another targeted need for the nation was public education about the subject.[104] Education, in order to put breastfeeding in the mainstream and to classify it as normal behavior, has to start with preschoolers and continue through the educational system. Courses in biology, nutrition, health, and human sexuality should all include the breast and its functions.

New York State has taken a leadership position with respect to education of its youth. In 1994, a curriculum from kindergarten through 12th grade was jointly developed by the Department of Education and the Department of Health* and reviewed by teachers and school districts. The curriculum is not a separate course but provides recommendations about how to include age-appropriate information on breastfeeding and human lactation throughout the school years. The senior high school materials are more detailed and designed to be included in the subject matter regarding reproduction and family life.

The media should include breastfeeding, not always bottle feeding, in reference to young infants. Dolls should not come with bottles. Public policy should facilitate breastfeeding and provide space to breastfeed in public buildings and at the workplace. Of interest were the results of a national survey conducted by professional poll takers for the surgeon general's office to explore ideas and feelings about breastfeeding.[73] The pollsters obtained a statistically representative sample of all age groups from youth to old age, both genders, married and unmarried, and all socioeconomic and ethnic groups. The majority in all age groups knew breastfeeding was best for infants and would want their child breastfed (75%). Very few people were embarrassed by breastfeeding or thought it should not be done in public.

This commitment to policy for breastfeeding has been part of the Code for Infant Feeding of the World Health Assembly (WHA Code) to protect developing countries from being inundated with formula products, which discourage breastfeeding, where infant survival depends on being nourished at the breast.[102]

Although the major countries of the world endorsed the WHA Code in 1981, the United States did not. Finally, on May 9, 1994, President Clinton supported the worldwide policy of WHA's International Code of Marketing of Breast Milk Substitutes by joining with the other member nations at the World Health Assembly in Geneva, signaling a tremendous policy shift. Despite many efforts by the United States, Italy, and Ireland to add weakening amendments, the Swaziland delegation, speaking for the African nations, voted to strengthen the resolution

---

*New York State Health Dept.: Breastfeeding—First step to good health: A breastfeeding education activity package for grades K-12. Albany, NY, NYS Health Research Inc., 1995.

even more, and all amendments were dropped. One by one, all the countries, including the United States, agreed to Resolution 47.5, and it was ratified.[9]

The battle to control formula distribution worldwide has not been won. The pandemic of acquired immunodeficiency syndrome (AIDS) has provided a new reason to distribute formula to developing countries to stop the spread of human immunodeficiency virus (HIV) to infants from their HIV-positive mothers. This requires serious consideration of the risk/benefit ratio for breastfeeding because the death rate for infants from other causes if not breastfed exceeds the possible death rate from HIV via breast milk.[2]

In 1987, the Nutrition Taskforce of the Better Health Commission of Australia[15] set as targets for the year 2000 that 90% of mothers would be breastfeeding on discharge from the hospital and that 80% of babies would still be breastfed at 3 months of age. The rate of breastfeeding in Australia in a survey in 1984 to 1985 was 80% of mothers exclusively breastfeeding on leaving the hospital.[6] The rate at 3 months was 50%. These rates had been achieved without public health intervention. The efforts now target high-risk groups with low rates. Worksite-based programs encompass prenatal care, pregnancy-related nutrition and drug education, and preparation for infant feeding during pregnancy.

In 1991, the rate in Australia was reported as 92% for initiating breastfeeding and 50% for those still breastfeeding at 6 months. The rate of initiating breastfeeding in 2003 was 90.1% with 82.4% exclusively breastfeeding at discharge. At 6 months, 47.7% were still breastfeeding.

The Queensland Anti-Discrimination Act, which took effect in 1992, prohibits discrimination on the grounds of gender, marital status, breastfeeding, lawful sexual activity, age, disability, religion, political belief, or trade-union activity. Under this act, breastfeeding mothers cannot be asked to leave restaurants, cinemas, or other public places. Nursing mothers have fed their infants in places such as pubs, parks, and banks. Any transgressions can be reported to the Anti-Discrimination Tribunal, whose decisions are legally binding.

A similar law has been enacted in Florida to encourage breastfeeding and "authorize" it in public (March 1993). The law provides that breastfeeding a baby does not violate prohibitions against unnatural and lascivious acts; exposure of sexual organs; or lewd, lascivious, or indecent conduct in the presence of a child. Nor is breastfeeding an obscenity, harmful to minors, or unlawful nudity or sexual conduct (Appendix L contains the text of the law). Other states have enacted similar laws, and the list is long (33 states). A state that has no such protection for its mothers and babies is in the minority.

Box 1-1 provides a summary of interventions presented at the surgeon general's workshop.[72] A national conference was held in Washington, DC, again with federal funding and came to the same conclusions in 1994 as in 1984.

Although these recommendations have been promoted since 1984, many hospitals and health care facilities have not achieved them.[102] As a result, UNICEF and the WHO initiated the Baby Friendly Hospital Initiative, which has been implemented in developing countries with considerable success. Box 1-2 lists the 10 steps to becoming a designated Baby Friendly Hospital. A joint WHO/UNICEF statement, *Protecting, Promoting and Supporting Breastfeeding*, describes suggested actions for maternity services.[94]

In 1996, Evergreen Hospital in Kirkland, Washington, was the first Baby Friendly Hospital designated in the United States. This initiative has been reorganized and reestablished through Healthy Children, a not-for-profit organization that created Baby Friendly, USA.* Ten more hospitals were certified in the first 6 months of 1997. The program is slowly expanding, with a total of 40 hospitals certified and 49 with letters of intent as of January 1, 2004. For certification, the hospital must provide evidence that it has met the 10 criteria (see Box 1-2) and must demonstrate its effectiveness to a visiting team of assessors.

---

*The address to contact to initiate the process is Baby Friendly, USA, 327 Quaker Meeting House Road, East Sandwich, MA 02537; (508) 888-8044.

BOX 1-1   Key elements for promotion of breastfeeding in the continuum of maternal and infant health care

1. Primary care settings for women of childbearing age should have:
   - A supportive milieu for lactation
   - Educational opportunities (including availability of literature, personal counseling, and information about community resources) for learning about lactation and its advantages
   - Ready response to requests for further information
   - Continuity allowing for the exposure to and development over time of a positive attitude regarding lactation on the part of the recipient of care
2. Prenatal care settings should have:
   - A specific assessment at the first prenatal visit of the physical capability for and emotional predisposition to lactation. This assessment should include the potential role of the father of the child as well as other significant family members. An educational program about the advantages of and ways of preparing for lactation should continue throughout the pregnancy.
   - Resource personnel—such as nutritionists/dietitians, social workers, public health nurses, La leche League members, childbirth education groups—for assistance in preparing for lactation
   - Availability and utilization of culturally suitable patient education materials
   - An established mechanism for a predelivery visit to the newborn care provide to ensure initiation and maintenance of lactation
   - A means of communicating to the in-hospital team the infant-feeding plans developed during the prenatal course
3. In-hospital settings should have:
   - A policy to determine the patient's infant-feeding plan on admission or during labor
   - A family-centered orientation to childbirth, including the minimum use of intrapartum medications and anesthesia
   - A medical and nursing staff informed about and supportive of ways to facilitate the initiation and continuation of breastfeeding (including early mother-infant contact and ready access by the mother to her baby throughout the hospital stay)
   - The availability of individualized counseling and education by a specially trained breastfeeding coordinator to facilitate lactation for those planning to breastfeed and to counsel those who have not yet decided about their method of infant feeding
   - Ongoing inservice education about lactation and ways to support it. This program should be conducted by the breastfeeding coordinator for all relevant hospital staff.
   - Proper space and equipment for breastfeeding in the postpartum and neonatal units. Attention should be given to the particular needs of women breastfeeding babies with special problems.
   - The elimination of hospital practices/policies that have the effect of inhibiting the lactation process (e.g., rules separating mother and baby)
   - The elimination of standing orders that inhibit lactation (e.g., lactation suppressants, fixed feeding schedules, maternal medications)
   - Discharge planning that includes referral to community agencies to aid in the continuing support of the lactating mother. This referral is especially important for patients discharged early.
   - A policy to limit the distribution of packages of free formula at discharge to only those mothers who are not lactating
   - The development of policies to support lactation throughout the hospital units (e.g., medicine, surgery, pediatrics, emergency room)
   - The provision of continued lactation support for those infants who must remain in the hosptial after the mother's discharge

Continued

BOX 1-1   Key elements for promotion of breastfeeding in the continuum of maternal and infant health care—cont'd

---

4. Postpartum ambulatory settings should have:
   - A capacity for telephone assistance to mothers experiencing problems with breastfeeding
   - A policy for telephone follow-up 1–3 days after discharge
   - A plan for an early follow-up visit (within first week after discharge)
   - The availability of lactation counseling as a means of preventing or solving lactation problems
   - Access to lay support resources for the mother
   - The presence of a supportive attitude by all staff
   - A policy to encourage bringing the infant to postpartum appointments
   - The availability of public-community-health nurse referral for those having problems with lactation
   - A mechanism for the smooth transition to pediatric care of the infant, including good communication between obstetric and pediatric care providers

From Report of the Surgen General's Workshop on Breastfeeding and Human Lactation. Presented by U.S. Department of Health and Human Services. June 1984. DHHS Pub. No. HRS-D-MC 84.2.

THE HISTORY OF BREASTFEEDING

The world scientific literature, predominantly from countries other than the United States, includes many tributes to human milk. Early writings on infant care in the 1800s and early 1900s pointed out the hazards of serious infection in bottle fed infants. Mortality charts were clear in the difference in mortality risk between breastfed and bottle fed infants.[37,38] Only in recent years have the reasons for this phenomenon been identified in terms comparable with those used to define other antiinfective properties. The identification of specific immunoglobulins and determination of the specific influence of the pH and flora in the intestine of the breastfed infant are examples. It became clear that the infant receives systemic protection transplacentally and local intestinal tract

---

BOX 1-2   Toward becoming a Baby Friendly Hospital: 10 steps to successful breastfeeding

---

Every facility providing maternity services and care for newborn infants should:
1. Have a written breastfeeding policy that is routinely communicated to all health care staff.
2. Train all health care staff in skills necessary to implement this policy.
3. Inform all pregnant women about the benefits and management of breastfeeding.
4. Help mothers initiate breastfeeding within a half hour of birth.
5. Show mothers how to breastfeed and how to maintain lactation even if they should be separated from their infants.
6. Give newborn infants no food or drink other than breast milk, unless *medically* indicated.
7. Practice rooming-in—allow mothers and infants to remain together—24 hours a day.
8. Encourage breastfeeding on demand.
9. Give no artificial teats or pacifiers (also called *dummies* or *soothers*) to breastfeeding infants.
10. Foster the establishment of breastfeeding support groups and refer mothers to tham on discharge from the hospital or clinic.

From WHO/UNICEF: Protecting, promoting and supporting breastfeeding: The special role of maternity services, a joint WHO/UNICEF statement. Geneva, World Health Organization, 1989.

protection orally via the colostrum and mature milk. The intestinal tract environment of a breast-fed infant continues to afford protection against infection by influencing the bacterial flora until the infant is weaned. Breastfed infants also have fewer respiratory infections, occurrences of otitis media, gastrointestinal infections, and other illnesses. The immunologic protection afforded by specific antibodies such as respiratory syncytial virus and rotavirus also protects the infant from illness.

Refinement in the biochemistry of nutrition has afforded an opportunity to restudy the constituents of human milk. Attention to brain growth and neurologic development emphasizes the unique constituents of human milk that enhance the growth and development of the exclusively breastfed infant. Because the human brain doubles in size in the first year of life, the nutrients provided for brain growth are critical (see Chapter 7). A closer look at the amino acids in human milk has demonstrated clearly that the array is physiologically suited for the human newborn. Forced by legislation in the 1970s that mandated mass newborn screening for phenylalanine in all hospitals, physicians were faced with the problem of the newborn that had high phenylalanine or tyrosine levels. It became apparent that many traditional formulas provided an overload of these amino acids, which some infants were unable to tolerate even though they did not have phenylketonuria.

The mysteries and taboos about colostrum go back to the dawn of civilization.[96] Most ancient primitive peoples let several days go by before putting the baby to the breast, with exact times and rituals varying from tribe to tribe. Other liquids were provided in the form of herbal teas; some were pharmacologically potent, and others had no nutritional worth. Breastfeeding positions varied as well.[96] Most cultures held their infants while seated; however, Armenians and some Asians would lean over the supine baby, resting on a bar that ran above the cradle for support (Fig. 1-1). These infants were not lifted for the purpose of burping. Many groups carried their infants on their backs and swung them into position frequently for

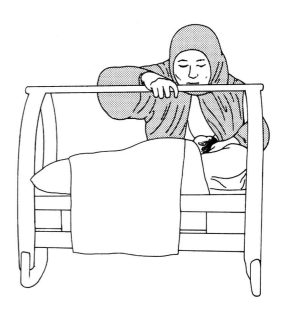

Figure 1-1. Armenian woman suckling her child. (Redrawn from Wickes IG: A history of infant feeding. Arch Dis Child 28:151, 1953.)

feedings, a method that continues today. These infants are not burped either but remain semierect in the swaddling on the mother's back. The ritual of burping is actually a product of necessity in bottle feeding because air is so easily swallowed.

Although the modern woman may be selectively chastised for abandoning breastfeeding because of the ready availability of prepared formulas, paraphernalia of bottles and rubber nipples, and ease of sterilization, this is not a new issue. Meticulous combing of civilized history reveals that almost every generation has had to provide alternatives when the mother could not or would not nurse her infant. Blame cannot be placed solely on an uninformed and unsupportive medical profession or on the formula manufacturers.

Hammurabi's code, from about 1800 BC, contained regulations on the practice of wet nursing, that is, nursing another woman's infant, often for hire. Throughout Europe, spouted feeding cups have been found in the graves of infants dating from about 2000 BC. Although ancient Egyptian feeding flasks are almost unknown, specimens of

Greek origin are fairly common in infant burials. Paralleling the information about ancient feeding techniques is the problem of abandoned infants. Well-known biblical stories report such events, as do accounts from Rome during the time of the early popes. In fact, so many infants were abandoned that foundling homes were started. French foundling homes in the 1700s were staffed by wet nurses who were carefully selected and their lives and activities controlled to ensure adequate nourishment for the foundling.

In Spartan times a woman, even if she was the wife of a king, was required to nurse her eldest son; plebeians were to nurse all their children.[84] Plutarch, an ancient scribe, reported that a second son of King Themistes inherited the kingdom of Sparta only because he was nursed with his mother's milk. The eldest son had been nursed by a stranger and therefore was rejected. Hippocrates is said to have written, "One's own milk is beneficial, others' harmful."

No known written works describe infant feeding from ancient times to the Renaissance.[97] In 1472, the first pediatric incunabulum, written by Paul Bagellardus, was printed in Padua, Italy. It described the characteristics of a good wet nurse and counseled about hiccups, diarrhea, and vomiting. Thomas Muffett (1584) wrote of the medicinal and therapeutic use of human milk for men and women of "riper years, fallen by age or by sickness into compositions." His writings referred to the milk of the ass as being the best substitute for human milk at any age when nourishment was an issue. The milk of an ass is low in solids compared with that of most species, low in fat and protein, and high in lactose:

	Total Solids %	Fat %	Protein %	CHO %	Ash %
Human	12.4	3.8	1.0	7.0	0.2
Ass	11.7	1.4	2.0	7.4	0.5
Cow	12.7	3.7	3.7	4.8	0.7

CHO, carbohydrates; Ash, residual after burning, includes Na, Ca, etc.

From AD 1500 to 1700, wealthy English women did not nurse their infants, according to Fildes,[27] who laboriously and meticulously reviewed infant feeding history in Great Britain. Although breastfeeding was well recognized as a means of delaying another pregnancy, these women preferred to bear anywhere from 12 to 20 babies than to breastfeed them.[104] They had a notion that breastfeeding spoiled their figures and made them old before their time. Husbands had much to say about how the infants were fed. Wet nurses were replaced by feeding cereal or bread gruel from a spoon. The death rate in foundling homes from this practice approached 100%.

The Dowager Countess of Lincoln wrote on "the duty of nursing, due by mothers to their children" in 1662.[97] She had borne 18 children, all fed by wet nurses; only one survived. When her son's wife bore a child and nursed it, the countess saw the error of her ways. She cited the biblical example of Eve, who breastfed Cain, Abel, and Seth. She also noted that Job 39:16 states that to withhold a full breast is to be more savage than dragons and more cruel than ostriches to their little ones. The noblewoman concluded her appeal to women to avoid her mistakes: "Be not so unnatural as to thrust away your own children; be not so hardy as to venture a tender babe to a less tender breast; be not accessory to that disorder of causing a poorer woman to banish her own infant for the entertaining of a richer woman's child, as it were bidding her to unlove her own to love yours."

Toward the end of the 18th century in England, the trend to wet nursing and artificial feeding changed, partially because medical writers drew attention to health and well-being and mothers made more decisions about feeding their young.

In 18th-century France, both before and during the revolution that swept Louis XVI from the throne and brought Napoleon to power, infant feeding included maternal nursing, wet nursing, artificial feeding with the milk of animals, and feeding of pap and panada.[22] *Panada* is from the French *panade,* meaning bread, and means a food consisting of bread, water or other liquid, and seasoning and boiled to the consistency of pulp (Fig. 1-2). The majority of infants born to wealthy and middle-income women, especially in Paris, were placed with wet nurses. The reason given for this

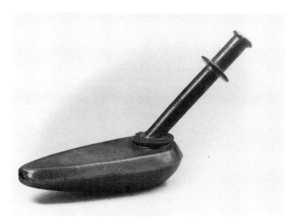

Figure 1-2. Pewter pap spoon, circa AD 1800. Thin pap, a mixture of bread and water, was placed in bowl. Tip of bowl was placed in child's mouth. Flow could be controlled by placing finger over open end of hollow handle. If contents were not taken as rapidly as desired, one could blow down on handle.

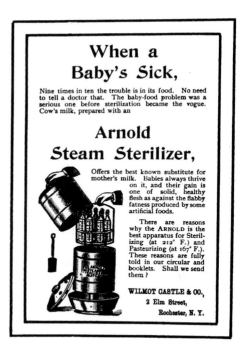

Figure 1-3. Arnold Steam Sterilizer advertisement. (From NY Med J, June 22, 1895.)

widespread practice was that maternal nursing was "not the custom." Mothers wished to "guard their beauty and freshness." In 1718, Dionis wrote, "Today not only ladies of nobility, but yet the rich and the wives of the least of the artisans have lost the custom of nursing their infants." As early as 1705, laws controlling wet nursing required wet nurses to register, forbade them to nurse more than two infants in addition to their own, and stipulated that a crib should be available for each infant, to prevent the nurse from taking a baby to bed and chancing suffocation.[22] On the birth of the Prince of Wales (later George IV) in 1762, it was officially announced: wet nurse, Mrs. Scott; dry nurse, Mrs. Chapman; rockers, Jane Simpson and Catherine Johnson.[97]

A more extensive historical review would reveal other examples of social problems in achieving adequate care of infants. Long before our modern society, some women failed to accept their biologic role as nursing mothers, and society failed to provide adequate support for nursing mothers (Fig. 1-3).* Breastfeeding was

more common and of longer duration in stable eras and rarer in periods of "social dazzle" and lowered moral standards. Urban mothers have had greater access to alternatives, and rural women have had to continue to breastfeed in greater numbers.

A handful of research-oriented physicians sought a substitute for mother's milk to replace wet nursing in the mid-nineteenth century.[97] Most of the solutions were cow milk with added sugar and water. Dr. William H. Cumming of Atlanta recognized that these solutions were low in "butter," creating a "deficiency of nerve food." He added cream and then lime water to bring the pH up and make the solution digestible. In 1884, Dr. A. V. Meigs published a surprisingly accurate comparative analysis of human and bovine milks. He then set about improving bovine milk to match human milk by adding lime water, fat, and sugar. When these preparations were boiled to sterilize them, scurvy became common.

---

*The National Convention of France of 1793, laws were passed to provide relief for infants of indigent families. The provisions are quite similar to those in our present-day welfare programs.[22]

Pierre Budin (1846–1907) is credited with creating perinatal medicine as well as with establishing the first clinics for nurslings.[85] Written when infant mortality rate was 288 per 1000 live births, his book *The Nursling* stated, "Favor breastfeeding by all possible means and provide mothers with advice and help in order to provide the best nutrition for the infant."

Soon, chemists entered the field of infant feeding, which had been previously limited to physicians who had mothers make the profitable mixtures and concoctions.[97] Henri Nestlé, a Swiss merchant, combined sugar and wheat flour with milk from Swiss cows fed Alpine grass. The wheat flour had been cooked with malt. Nestlé advertised his product as "scientifically correct so as to leave nothing to be desired." He directed most of his promotional efforts to mothers, as he insisted that "mothers will do my publicity for me." Most infant food companies, however, advertised in medical as well as nonmedical journals. As industry took over producing human milk substitutes from physicians who had prescribed their own formulas, the mother became the consumer target. Some concoctions contained no milk at all. Little attention was paid to the fact that the product might be reconstituted with contaminated water. In 1888, the American Medical Association (AMA) subcommittee on infant feeding could not reach a consensus as to the best mother's milk substitute, although little enthusiasm existed for wet nursing.

The competition for the nonnursing mother's market was well launched by the end of the 19th century. Science was equated with progress. Infant-feeding concoctions were described as scientifically prepared, although the statements were never supported by any documentation. The popular lay journals of the day, such as *Babyhood* and *Ladies' Home Journal*, were the arena in which mothers could support or condemn various infant-rearing practices in light of their own limited personal experiences. Apple[4] pointed out that "the commercialization and medicalization of infant care established an environment that made artificial feeding not only acceptable to many mothers but also natural and necessary."

Apple[4] further stated that "a combination of the ideology of scientific motherhood, confidence in the medical profession, and shrewd media presentation altered the relationship between mothers and physicians and encouraged mothers to seek out commercial and medical solutions to the problems of infant feeding." Despite a renewed interest in breastfeeding in the mid-20th century among mothers and physicians, the legacy of scientific motherhood lives on.

Sociologists reviewed the reasons for the decrease in breastfeeding in the 20th century.[21] Urbanization and technologic advances have affected social, medical, and dietary trends throughout the world.[30] The social influences include the changing pattern of family life—smaller, isolated families that are separated from the previous generation. The practice of medicine has emphasized disease and its treatment, especially as it relates to laboratory study and hospital care. The science of nutrition has developed a reliance on measurement and technology, which has led to the conclusion that prepared foods are superior because they can be measured and calculated to meet precise dietary requirements.

In the 1920s, women were encouraged to raise their infants scientifically. "Raising by the book" was commonplace. The U.S. government published *Infant Care,* referred to as the "good book," which was the bible of child rearing read by women from all walks of life. It emphasized cod liver oil, orange juice, and artificial feeding. A quote from *Parents* magazine in 1938 reflects the attitude of women's magazines in general, undermining even the staunchest breastfeeders: "You hope to nurse him, but there is an alarming number of young mothers today who are unable to breastfeed their babies and you may be one of them."[13] Apple[4] detailed the transition from breastfeeding to raising children scientifically, by the book, and precisely as the doctor prescribes.

There are encouraging trends, however. The acceptance or rejection of breastfeeding is being influenced in the Western world to a greater degree by the knowledge of the benefits of human milk and breastfeeding. Cultural rejection, negative attitudes, and lack of support from health professionals are being replaced by interest in child rearing and preparation for childbirth. This has created a system that encourages a prospective mother to consider the options for herself and her infant.[79] The attitude in the Western world toward the female breast as a sex object to the exclusion of its ability to nurture has influenced young mothers in particular not to breastfeed. The emancipation of women, which began in the 1920s, was symbolized by short hair, short skirts, contraceptives, cigarettes, and bottle feeding. In the second half of the 20th century, women sought to be well informed, and many wanted the right to choose how they fed their infant.

The great success of the mother-to-mother program of the La Leche League and other women's support groups in helping women breastfeed or, as with International Childbirth Education Association (ICEA), in helping women plan and participate in childbirth, is an example of the power of social relationships. Raphael[70] described the *doula* as a key person for lactation support, especially in the first critical days and weeks after delivery.

Bryant[11] explored the social networks in her study of the impact of kin, friend, and neighbor networks on infant-feeding practices in Cuban, Puerto Rican, and Anglo families in Florida. She found that these networks strongly influenced decisions about breastfeeding, bottle feeding, use of supplements, and introduction of solid foods. Network members' advice and encouragement contributed to a successful lactation experience. The impact of the health care professional is inversely proportional to the distance of the mother from her network. The health care worker must work within the cultural norms for the network. For individuals isolated from their cultural roots, the health care system may have to provide more support and encouragement to ensure lactation success and adherence to health care guidelines.[75]

The trend in infant feeding among mothers who participated in the Women, Infants, and Children (WIC) Program in the late 1970s and early 1980s was analyzed separately by Martinez and Stahl[57] from the data collected by questionnaires mailed quarterly as part of the Ross Laboratories Mother's Survey. The responses represented 4.8% of the total U.S. births in 1977 and 14.1% of the total U.S. births in 1980. WIC participants in 1977, including those who supplemented with formula or cow milk, were breastfeeding in the hospital in 33.6% of cases. A steady and significant increase occurred in the frequency of breastfeeding; it rose to 40.4% in 1980 ($p < 0.5$).

WIC data continue to be collected, and the trends have paralleled other groups (Table 1-2). In 1992, there were 38.4% breastfeeding at birth and 10.7% still breastfeeding at 5 to 6 months. The rate of initiation was 46.6% in 1996, with 12.9% continuing to 5 to 6 months.

In 2001, 58.2% of WIC participants initiated breastfeeding in the hospital and 20.8% were breastfeeding at 6 months. These rates represented a 24.9% and 61.2% increase, respectively, according to the Ross Mother's Survey Report in 2002.

The Food and Consumer Service (FCS) of the U.S. Department of Agriculture (USDA) entered into a cooperative agreement with Best Start, a not-for-profit social marketing organization that promotes breastfeeding to develop a WIC breastfeeding promotion project that is national in scope and being implemented at the state level. The project consists of six components: social marketing research, a media campaign, a staff support kit, a breastfeeding resource guide, a training conference, and continuing education and technical assistance. With an annual $8 million budget for WIC, the project's goals are to increase the initiation and duration of breastfeeding among WIC clients and to expand public acceptance and support of breastfeeding. Breastfeeding women are favored in the WIC priority system when benefits are limited; they can continue in the program for a year, whereas those who do not breastfeed are limited to 6 months. All pregnant WIC participants are encouraged to breastfeed.

Montgomery and Splett[61] reported the economic benefits of breastfeeding infants for mothers enrolled in WIC. Comparing the costs of the WIC program and Medicaid for food and health care in Colorado, administrative and health care costs for a formula-fed infant, minus the rebate for the first 180 days of life, were $273 higher than those for the breastfed infant. These calculations did not include

TABLE 1-2	Percentage of breastfeeding among WIC participants 1977–2002	
Year	In hospital	At 6 months of age
1977	33.6	12.5
1978	34.5	9.7
1979	37.0	11.2
1980	40.4	13.1
1981	39.9	13.7
1982	45.3	16.1
1983	38.9	11.5
1984	39.1	11.9
1985	40.1	11.7
1986	38.0	10.7
1987	37.3	10.6
1988	35.3	9.2
1989	34.2	8.4
1990	33.7	8.2
1991	36.9	9.0
1992	38.8	10.1
1993	41.6	10.8
1994	44.3	11.6
1995	46.6	12.7
1996	46.6	12.9
1997	50.4	16.5
1998	56.8	18.9
1999	56.1	19.9
2000	56.8	20.1
2001	58.2	20.8
2002	58.8	22.1

Data collected from Martinez GA, Stahle DA: The recent trend in milk-feeding among WIC infants. Am J Pub Health 72:68, 1982. Ryan AS, Rush D, Krieger FW: Recent declines in breastfeeding in the United States, 1984 through 1989. Pediatrics 88:719, 1991. Krieger FW: A review of breastfeeding trends. Presented at the Editor's Conference, New York, September 1992; Ross Laboratories Mothers Survey, unpublished data, Columbus, Ohio, 1992; Mothers Survey, Ross Products Division, Abbott Laboratories, unpublished data, 1998; Ryan AS: The resurgence of breastfeeding in the United States. Pediatrics 99:2, 1997 (electronic article). Mothers Survey, Ross Products Division, and Abbott Laboratories—Breastfeeding Trends 2002.

the pharmacy costs for illness. When these figures are translated to large WIC programs in high-cost areas (e.g., New York City, Los Angeles) and multiplied by millions of WIC participants, the savings from breastfeeding are substantial. If the goal of 75% breastfeeding by the year 2010 were realized among WIC recipients, the cost savings could be at least $4 million a month for the WIC program.[61]

Frequency of breastfeeding

Data collected in the 1970s in the Ross Laboratories Mothers Survey MR77-48, which included 10,000 mothers, revealed a general trend toward breastfeeding.[56] In 1975, 33% of the mothers started out breastfeeding, and 15% were still breastfeeding at 5 to 6 months. In 1977, 43% of the mothers left the hospital breastfeeding, and 20% were still breastfeeding at 5 to 6 months. Other studies have shown a regional variation, with a higher percentage of mothers breastfeeding on the West Coast than in the East.

A continuation of the study of milk-feeding patterns in 1981 in the United States by Martinez and Dodd[56] showed a sustained trend toward breastfeeding in 55% of the 51,537 new mothers contacted by mail. Although mothers who breastfeed continue to be more highly educated and have a higher income, the greatest increase in breastfeeding occurred among women with less education. From 1971 to 1981, breastfeeding in the hospital more than doubled (from 24.7% to 57.6%), with an average rate of gain of 8.8%. For infants 2 months old, breastfeeding more than tripled (from 13.9% to 44.2%) in this 10-year period.

The National Natality Surveys (NNS) conducted by the Centers for Disease Control in 1969 and 1980 included questions about infant feeding practices after birth by married women.[29] Questionnaires were mailed at 3 and 6 months post partum. In 1969, 19% of white women and 9% of black women were exclusively breastfeeding. The highest rate was among white women up to 34 years old with three to six children. In 1980, 51% of white women and 25% of black women were exclusively breastfeeding, and they were more highly educated and primiparous.

The Ross Laboratories Mothers Survey remains the only national study that includes sampling of all women who give birth in the 50 states.[76-78] The study has been expanded to monthly mailings, with special efforts to ensure participation of low-income and less-educated mothers; 725,000 surveys are mailed annually. The results have documented the persistent decline in the number of women initially breastfeeding, from a high in 1982 of 61.9% to an apparent low in 1991 of 51%, with the decline finally involving all categories of women, including those with higher socioeconomic status and higher education. The decline in duration of breastfeeding was similar, with a peak in 1982 of 27% and a trough in 1991 at 18.5% at 6 months. The data for 1992 reflected an increase that persisted through the months across all categories. By 1996, the initiation rate had risen in all categories according to 744,000 mailed surveys, averaging 59.2%.[76] Duration showed a steady increase to 21.7% at 6 months. The greatest increase was seen in the groups least likely to breastfeed (e.g., low income, less education).

The Mothers Survey included 1.4 million questionnaires mailed in 2001, and this time two categories of questions were asked: any amount of breastfeeding and exclusive breastfeeding. Record high levels of any breastfeeding were reported: 69.5% initiation rate and 32.5% at 6 months post partum with increases across all sociodemographic groups. The greatest increases were among young mothers (<20 years of age), the less educated, primiparous mothers, and those employed at the time of the survey. Mothers who practiced exclusive breastfeeding at hospital discharge (46.2%) and at 6 months (17.2%) were older and better educated. The authors predicted that if the rate of increase (approximately 2% per year) continues for women at hospital discharge, the goal of at least 75% will be reached by 2010. The 6-month goal of 50% will not be reached, especially among high-risk groups. These data support the position of the Academy of Breastfeeding Medicine's emphasis on extending the duration of all the women who now breastfeed through education, support, and role modeling.

Although the validity of questionnaires requesting mothers to recall their feeding behaviors months later has been questioned, a study of maternal recall of infant-feeding events demonstrated that recall is accurate up to 18 months later when breastfeeding is the mode. Data on formula feeding recall were not as accurate as those for breastfeeding and solid food feeding.[53]

Ethnic factors

The Pediatric Nutrition Surveillance System (PedNSS) is a child-based public health surveillance system that monitors the nutritional status of low-income children in federally funded maternal and child health programs. The process begins in the clinic aggregates of the state level and the data are submitted to the Centers for Disease Control (CDC) for analysis. In 2001, 39 states, the District of Columbia, Puerto Rico, American Samoa, and six tribal governments participated, representing 5 million children from birth to 5 years of age; 37% of findings were from children under 1 year representing the six major ethic groups.

In 2001, PedNSS reported 50.9% of children were ever breastfed, 20.8% were breastfed for at least 6 months, and 13.6% were breastfed for at least 12 months (Fig. 1-4). Breastfeeding rates improved 45% from the 1992 rate of 34.9% across all racial and ethnic groups. Although blacks still maintain the lowest rates (37.8%), the current rates have more than doubled since 1992 (16.6%).

International trends are difficult to summarize because definitions vary and population assessments may be more or less complete. In an effort to improve reporting and implement its global strategy, the WHO has prepared a tool for assessing national practices, policies, and programs entitled, "Infant and Young Child Feeding in 2003." It is detailed and extensive. It is available on its Web site: http://www.who.int/child-adolescent-health/publications/nutrition/IYCF_AT.htm.[93]

Breastfeeding practices in developing countries have been improving since 1990, according to Population Reports. The level of exclusive breastfeeding in the first 3 months increased 10% in 35 countries predominantly because mothers stopped the introduction of nonmilk foods so early. Malawi improved 59% in exclusive breastfeeding. The trend is to delay complementary foods until 6 months as recommended by WHO. Still, exclusive breastfeeding dropped in Jordan, Benin, Turkey, Niger, and Rwanda. Surveys have continued to confirm the impact of breastfeeding on child survival. With other factors accounted for, an infant is

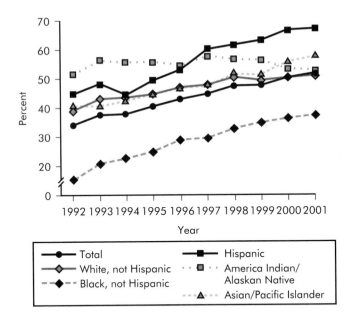

Figure 1-4. Trends in the percentage of infants ever breastfed, by race and ethnicity. (From Polhamus B, Dalenius K, Thompson D, et al: Pediatric Nutrition Surveillance 2001 Report. Atlanta, CDC, 2003.)

four times more likely to die if a mother stops any breastfeeding at 2 to 3 months of age than an infant who continues to breastfeed. At 9 to 12 months, if the infant is not breastfed, the risk of death is 2.3 times greater (Fig. 1-5).

Almost all infants in developing countries are breastfed at least partially in the first 3 months. In 56 countries, one third of infants are exclusively breastfed for 4 months. Breastfeeding up to age 2 years along with appropriate complementary feeding after 6 months contributes to good nutrition and the prevention of diarrhea. At 12 to 15 months, 78% are breastfeeding and by 24 months only 45%. Mothers in sub-Saharan Africa and Asia are almost twice as likely to continue breastfeeding through the second year, as are those in other developing regions (Table 1-3).

Demographic factors

The demographic factors associated with a higher incidence of breastfeeding have remained the same

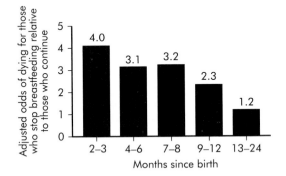

Figure 1-5. Effect of stopping breastfeeding on infant and child mortality. (Zlidar VM, Gardner R, Rutstein SO, et al: New Survey Findings: The Reproductive Revolution Continues. Population Reports, Series M, No. 17, Fig. 2. Baltimore, The Johns Hopkins Bloomberg School of Public Health, The INFO Project, Spring 2003; Rutstein S: Effect of birth intervals on mortality and health. Calverton, Maryland, Measure/DHS+, Macro International, Inc., 65 pp.)

TABLE 1-3   Breastfeeding to 24 Months of Age, 1990–2001

Region, Country and Year	0–3 Months Not BF	0–3 Months Exclusive *	0–3 Months Predominant †	6–9 Months Complemented ‡	12–15 Months Continued BF‖	20–23 Months Continued BF¶
Sub-Saharan Africa						
Benin 2001	2	47	23	64	94	60
Burkina Faso 1998–1999	1	5	88	49	96	86
Cameroon 1998	3	16	55	71	85	30
Cape Verde 1998	2	57	15	64	60	NA
Central African Rep. 1994–95	1	4	63	93	96	54
Chad 1995–96	3	2	82	71	91	63
Comoros 1996	3	5	48	86	80	44
Côte d'Ivoire 1998–1999	2	4	77	63	94	55
Eritrea 1995	1	65	28	45	91	60
Ethiopia 2000	1	62	20	42	94	77
Gabon 2000	13	7	28	62	44	8
Ghana 1998	1	36	48	63	97	57
Guinea 1999	2	12	68	27	95	73
Kenya 1998	1	17	33	88	89	54
Madagascar 1997	2	61	25	88	90	49
Malawi 2000	2	62	15	92	97	72
Mali 2001	2	28	62	32	93	65
Mozambique 1997	4	38	37	83	94	59
Namibia 1992	2	22	52	66	75	27
Niger 1998	2	1	86	71	95	48
Nigeria 1990	4	1	60	51	87	44
Rwanda 2000	2	88	2	75	93	61
South Africa 1998	16	10	15	62	68	33
Senegal 1997	2	14	63	62	90	50
Tanzania 1999	2	40	39	63	90	49
Togo 1998	3	15	54	88	96	77
Uganda 2000–2001	2	74	5	73	88	44
Zambia 1996	3	25	45	93	94	43
Zimbabwe 1999	3	39	26	90	95	37
median	**2**	**22**	**45**	**66**	**93**	**54**
mean (unweighted)	**3**	**29**	**43**	**68**	**88**	**53**
Near East and North Africa						
Egypt 2000	4	66	18	64	79	30
Jordan 1997	6	15	32	63	42	12
Mauritania 2000–2001	1	28	38	62	88	52
Morocco 1992	6	62	15	35	63	19
Turkey 1998	7	9	50	33	51	21
Yemen 1997	8	22	30	51	59	37
median	**6**	**25**	**31**	**57**	**61**	**25**
mean (unweighted)	**5**	**34**	**30**	**51**	**64**	**29**

*Exclusive: breast milk only.
†Predominant: breast milk and water and other non-milk liquids.
‡Complemented: breast milk and solid or semi-solid foods
‖Continued: any breastfeeding, independent of type of supplements.

Continued

TABLE 1-3 Breastfeeding to 24 Months of Age, 1990–2001—cont'd

	% of Infants of Age:					
	0–3 Months			6–9 Months Complemented‡	12–15 Months Continued BF∥	20–23 Months Continued BF¶
Region, Country and Year	Not BF	Exclusive*	Predominant†			
Asia						
Bangladesh 1999–2000	1	53	18	59	94	86
Cambodia 2000	2	14	71	71	87	54
India 1998–1999	2	55	25	34	88	69
Indonesia 1997	3	52	8	81	86	66
Nepal 2001	1	78	10	66	98	85
Pakistan 1990–1991	5	25	41	29	78	51
Philippines 1998	18	48	11	58	48	23
Vietnam 1997	4	25	39	84	80	23
median	**3**	**50**	**22**	**63**	**87**	**60**
mean (unweighted)	**4**	**44**	**28**	**60**	**82**	**57**
Latin America and Caribbean						
Belize 1999	10	24	24	54	NA	23
Bolivia 1998	2	60	10	70	76	31
Brazil 1996	15	40	15	30	33	17
Colombia 2000	6	33	15	60	49	23
Dominican Rep. 1996	12	26	15	38	31	8
Ecuador 1999	6	42	23	70	60	25
El Salvador 1998	7	21	28	77	65	40
Guatemala 1998–1999	5	45	27	61	83	45
Haiti 2000	4	31	26	74	79	27
Honduras 2001	8	43	16	61	76	34
Nicaragua 2001	5	39	15	67	62	36
Paraguay 1995–1996¶	8	7	59	59	40	15
Peru 2000	1	72	9	75	83	46
median	**6**	**39**	**16**	**61**	**64**	**27**
mean (unweighted)	**7**	**37**	**22**	**61**	**61**	**28**
Eastern Europe and Central Asia						
Armenia 2000	6	44	29	51	29	13
Azerbaijan 2001	5	NA	NA	NA	NA	NA
Kazakhstan 1999	1	47	38	64	61	18
Kyrgyz Republic 1995	5	30	45	55	73	18
Turkmenistan 2000	5	16	68	70	76	27
Uzbekistan 1996	5	4	60	57	64	34
median	**5**	**30**	**45**	**57**	**64**	**18**
mean (unweighted)	**4**	**28**	**48**	**59**	**60**	**22**
All Developing Countries						
median	**3**	**29**	**28**	**63**	**87**	**45**
mean (unweighted)	**4**	**34**	**35**	**64**	**79**	**45**

¶Data NA for 1998 survey.

BF, breastfeeding; NA, not available

Breastfeeding is considered exclusive when a child receives no food or liquid other than breast milk. Predominant breastfeeding is defined as infrequent feedings of vitamins, minerals, water, juice, or ritualistic feedings in addition to breast milk. No food-based fluids other than fruit juice or sugar water are allowed under this definition, Labbok[63] and World Health Organization.[141] **Population Reports** since the low point in 1970.[3] The rate for well-educated, higher socioeconomic status families was more than 80% initiation at birth in 2002 (Table 1-4). In 2002, 45.8% of the infants in this group were still breastfeeding at 5 to 6 months of age with an average of all groups at 5 to 6 months of 32.5%. The rate among blacks was 21.9% and among WIC participants only 20.8% at 6 months, an increase in all groups.

Study after study has confirmed the relationship of breastfeeding to education, social status, marriage, and other demographic factors. The well-educated, well-to-do groups of all races breastfeed. In a study by Wright and associates[103] of 1112 healthy infants in a health maintenance organization (HMO) in Arizona,

70% were breastfed, with a mean duration of almost 7 months. Education and marriage were associated with breastfeeding. Maternal employment outside the home and ethnicity (being Hispanic rather than Anglo-American) were related to higher rates of bottle feeding. The authors suggest that effects of ethnicity are independent of those of education. New immigrants who would have breastfed in their homeland tend to bottle feed in the United States because they think this practice is "American."

The impoverished mother is choosing to bottle feed not because she is working; statistics show she is staying home and bottle feeding. When mothers were interviewed about their infant feeding choice at

TABLE 1-4	In-hospital breastfeeding rates: all infants and selected maternal demographics (%)							
Demographic feature	1995	1996	1997	1998	1999	2000	2001	2002
All infants	59.7	59.2	62.4	64.3	67.2	68.4	69.5	70.1
Parity								
Primiparous	61.6	61.0	64.6	66.5	69.6	71.1	72.0	72.5
Multiparous	57.8	57.4	60.1	62.0	64.5	65.4	66.5	67.3
Education								
Any grade school	43.8	46.8	47.0	48.4	52.2	54.5	55.1	55.1
Any high school	49.7	49.2	53.0	55.0	58.5	59.8	61.1	60.7
No college	49.5	49.1	52.8	54.9	58.4	59.7	61.0	60.5
Any college	74.4	73.8	76.3	78.2	80.1	81.2	82.1	81.2
Employment								
Employed full time	60.7	60.2	61.8	63.3	65.6	66.2	67.6	69.0
Employed part time	63.5	63.3	64.8	66.3	69.7	70.7	71.5	72.7
Total employed	61.7	61.3	62.9	64.4	67.0	67.7	68.8	70.2
Not employed	58.0	57.5	60.9	63.1	66.5	68.0	69.0	69.0
Income								
WIC	46.6	46.6	50.4	56.8	56.1	56.8	58.2	58.8
Non-WIC	71.0	70.8	73.4	75.2	76.9	77.8	78.9	79.2
Maternal Age								
Younger than 20 years	42.8	43.3	47.3	50.5	54.4	56.2	57.2	56.2
20–24 years	52.6	52.7	56.2	58.9	62.9	64.1	65.6	66.0
25–29 years	63.1	62.2	65.7	67.5	70.6	71.7	72.8	73.4
30–34 year	68.1	67.5	70.1	71.5	73.9	74.9	75.8	76.4
35+ years	70.0	69.3	71.1	72.6	74.7	75.3	76.1	74.1

From Mothers Survey, Ross Products Division, Abbott Laboratories, Columbus, OH, 2003. Updated breastfeeding trend through 2003.

a prenatal WIC clinic, they knew mother's milk was best.[34] They said it was too difficult to breastfeed and there were too many rules. In the classes on breastfeeding given by lactation experts, the instructions on preparing the breasts and diet rules were overwhelming. The mothers said if their physician would tell them breastfeeding was important, they would do it for as long as the physician said.[34] Similar data in the Ross Laboratories Mothers Survey also indicated the power of the physician's word. Mothers trusted their physician's advice and were more successful at breastfeeding if the physician was supportive and expressed his or her views.[77, 78]

Duration of breastfeeding

Coupled with concerns about the decreasing number of mothers who breastfeed their infants when they leave the hospital is the concern about duration of breastfeeding (Fig. 1-6). A sharp decline occurs by age 6 months; in 1977, this decline was from 43% to 20%. Other studies have noted an appreciable decline shortly after discharge from the hospital.[44]

By 1996, the rate of decline from the first week to 6 months of age had slowed. Overall, 21.7% of infants were breastfed at 6 months in 1996 and 32.5% in 2002 (a 49.8% improvement) (Figs. 1-7 and 1-8).

The two types of breastfeeding, as Newton[63] pointed out, are unrestricted and token. *Unrestricted breastfeeding* usually means that the infant is put to the breast immediately after delivery and breastfed on demand thereafter, without rules or limitations. There may be 10 or 12 feedings a day in the early weeks, with the number gradually decreasing over the first year of life. Breast milk continues to be a major source of nourishment during infancy.

Token breastfeeding, in contrast, is characterized by constant restrictions on the time and duration of nursing. Usually the feedings are scheduled. Even the amount of mother-infant contact is limited initially, and the infant is often offered water or glucose water by bottle. The whole process is inhibited, and a secure milk supply may not be established. The duration of breastfeeding is one of the major differences between unrestricted-feeding and token-feeding groups. Comparative studies have been plagued with problems of definition of breastfeeding.

In 1988, the Interagency Group for Action on Breastfeeding met to develop a set of definitions that could be used as standardized terminology for the collection of information on breastfeeding behavior. The recommendations were then reviewed

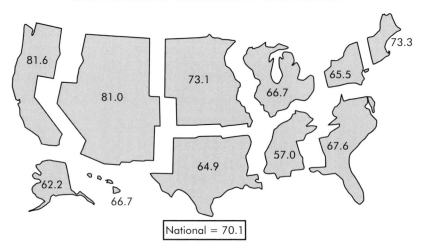

2002 INCIDENCE OF BREASTFEEDING CENSUS REGION

National = 70.1

Figure 1-6.   Census breastfeeding data, 2002. Numbers represent percentage of new mothers per unit population. (Modified from Ross Laboratories, Mothers Survey, Columbus, Ohio.)

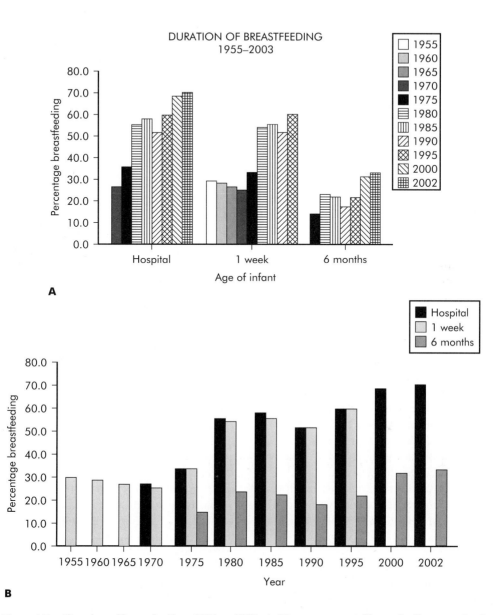

Figure 1-7.   Duration of breastfeeding, 1951 to 2002. **A,** The percentage of breastfeeding at each of three ages in each year, 1995 to 2002. **B,** The percentage of breastfeeding over time, 1955 to 2002. (Data from Woo-lun M, Gussler J, Smith N (eds): The International Breast-feeding Compendium, 3rd ed. Columbus, Ohio, Ross Laboratories, 1984; Kreiger F: A review of breastfeeding trends. Presented at the Editor's Conference, New York, September 1992; and Ryan AS: The resurgence of breastfeeding in the United States. Pediatrics 99(4):2, 1997 [electronic article].)

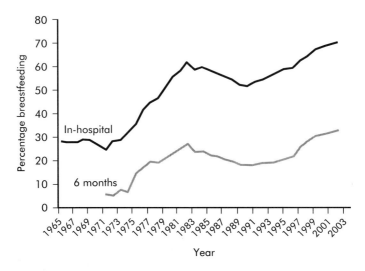

Figure 1-8.   U.S. breastfeeding rates, 1965 through 2003. (Modified from Li R, Zhao Z, Mokdad A, et al: Prevalence of breast-feeding in the United States: The 2001 National Immunization Survey. Pediatrics 111: 1198, 2003; Ryan AS: The resurgence of breastfeeding in the United States. Pediatrics 99:2, 1997 [electronic article]; Ryan AS, personal communication, 2004; Ryan AS, Zhou W, Acosta A: Breastfeeding continues to increase into the new millennium. Pediatrics 110:1103, 2002.)

extensively by researchers and providers, and a schema was finalized, as follows[52]:

1. Acknowledge that the term *breastfeeding* alone is insufficient to describe the numerous types of breastfeeding behavior.
2. Distinguish full from partial breastfeeding.
3. Subdivide full breastfeeding into categories of exclusive and almost-exclusive breastfeeding.
4. Differentiate among levels of partial breastfeeding.
5. Recognize that token breastfeeding has little or no nutritional impact.

The group hoped that the schema and framework would assist researchers and agencies in efforts to describe and interpret breastfeeding practices accurately (Fig. 1-9).

The definition of breastfeeding continues in debate. On behalf of the Breastfeeding Promotion Consortium (BFC) of the USDA and the United States Breastfeeding Committee (USBC), a document has been put forth as final recommendations that these groups support. Different contexts in which breastfeeding is defined include benefit eligibility, surveillance, monitoring, policies, guidelines, and research. The results were a complex report.

Cultural differences also affect duration of breastfeeding. In societies not yet industrialized that maintain ancient cultural patterns of child rearing, the duration is well beyond a year. A study of 46 such societies by Ford[28] revealed that weaning at about 2 to 3 years of age occurred in three fourths of them. One fourth of the groups began weaning at 18 months of age, and one culture started at 6 months. A similar anthropologic investigation of primitive child-rearing practices found a distinct correlation between the time of weaning and the behavior of the tribes.[28] When weaning was delayed, tribes were peaceful. In contrast, tribes that abruptly weaned their infants at 6 months of age and practiced other rigid disciplinary practices were warlike.

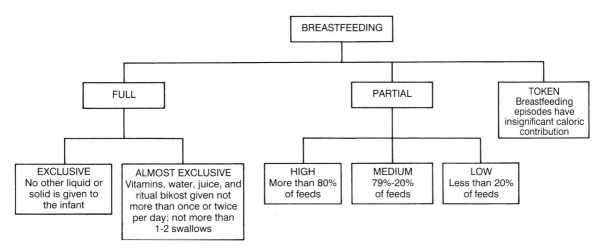

Figure 1-9. Schema for breastfeeding definition. (Modified from Labbok M, Krasovec K: Toward consistency in breastfeeding definitions. Stud Fam Plan 21:226, 1990.)

When weaning practices were evaluated among 945 women in Guinea-Bissau, West Africa, the data revealed that all infants had been breastfed at least 18 months. Among the reasons for terminating breastfeeding were the child became ill, the mother became ill, or the mother became pregnant. By 23 months, weaning occurred because the infant was healthy and old enough.[48] Although there are few studies since the 1980s focusing on the reasons why women wean early, a recent study conducted by Schwartz and associates[81] of women in Michigan and Nebraska revealed that the reasons for weaning are quite similar. They reported a prospective cohort study of 946 women over the first 12 weeks post partum. The demographic features were similar to older studies. Women older than 30 with a bachelor's degree were most likely to continue breastfeeding throughout the study. In the first 3 weeks, "not enough milk" was the most common reason to stop, and after 4 weeks the most common reason was a "return to work" (Table 1-5).[81]

In a study reported by Ramos and Almeida[69] carried out in a Baby Friendly Maternity Hospital in Brazil, 24 mothers who weaned their infants by 4 months were interviewed in depth. The reasons for weaning were similar to studies from decades before: weak or little milk, problems with breasts (sore nipples), lack of experience, disparity between needs of mother and needs of the baby, and work. The investigators described a sense of isolation and solitude on the part of the mother and need for support from health care providers and society in general. They concluded that breastfeeding should be treated as an act to be learned by women and protected by society. These studies point out the pivotal role for the pediatrician in the successful maintenance of lactation, as well as the importance of the postpartum environment[14, 92] (Tables 1-6 and 1-7).

The positive and negative emotional and physical experiences of 152 long-term breastfeeding American and Canadian women were reported by Reamer and Sugarman.[71] This sample of mothers was randomly selected from 1038 women who responded to a request for volunteers in a La Leche League newsletter. They all answered the eight-page questionnaire, which had 51 short-answer and 52 free-response questions. All the respondents were older, better educated, and predominantly white and had belonged to the league at some time. The average age was 29.4 years, age at first child was 25, 77% had more than 1 year of college, and 44% had 4 or more years of college. Far fewer were

TABLE 1-5   Percentage of women citing given reason for termination of breastfeeding

Reason	Week 3 (n = 67)	Week 6 (n = 60)	Week 9 (n = 32)	Week 12 (n = 36)
Insufficient milk supply	37.3	35.0	25.0	13.9
Inconvenient	17.9	25.0	21.9	33.3
Returned to work	4.5	31.7	53.1	58.3
Breast pain or infection	32.9	23.3	0	5.6
Baby stopped nursing	7.5	5.0	3.1	11.1
Other	22.4	18.3	3.1	5.6

Note: Percentages total more than 100% because respondents could cite multiple reasons.

employed than the national average (13% full or part time versus 34% nationally). The average weaning age for the 339 children represented by this study was 18 months, with a range of 3 weeks to 5 years. At the time of the study, 136 children were still being breastfed. Two mothers thought there were no positive effects of prolonged nursing

on their children, but others offered more than one perceived positive consequence (Table 1-8). Emotional security, happiness, mutual love, and future independence were the key positive outcomes of long-term nursing in the mothers' view. Good health was mentioned by 22%.

When asked to list the negative aspects of nursing longer than 6 months, 47% of mothers said there were none at 6 months, but only 26% of mothers had no negative feelings about nursing past 12 months. Perceived social hostility was the major negative effect, reported by 24% of mothers at 6 months and by 42% at 12 months (Table 1-9). Ninety percent felt there were no negative effects for the children. The social stigma has driven many well-educated, caring, dedicated mothers to conceal nursing, called "closet nursing." Unfortunately, this leads physicians and the public alike to think that breastfeeding in the United States terminates by 6 months of age.

Impact of commercial discharge packs

Several studies have evaluated whether commercial discharge packs result in diminished breastfeeding duration. Unfortunately, none of the studies was so

TABLE 1-6   Selected demographic characteristics associated with duration of breastfeeding[*]

	Group 1: never breastfed (n = 12)	Group 2: breastfed ≤ 7 days (n = 22)	Group 3: breastfed > 7 days (n = 153)
Black	9 (75%)	10 (46%)	57 (37%)
		$\chi^2 = 6.81, df = 2; p = .03$	
Mean years of education	11.3	13.5	14.9
		$F = 10.14, df = 2; p = .0001$	
Mean age	23.3	26.7	27.9
		$F = 4.57, df = 2; p = .01$	
Married	2 (17%)	16 (73%)	124 (81%)
		$\chi^2 = 25.37, df = 2; p = .001$	
<$10,000 income	6/10 (60%)	3/19 (16%)	15/143 (10%)
		$\chi^2 = 27.02, df = 6; p = .001$	
First pregnancy	5 (42%)	9 (41%)	53 (35%)
		$\chi^2 = .52, df = 2; p = .77$	

[*]See Table 1–7 for explanation.

TABLE 1-7   Probability of early cessation by selected prenatal and postpartum characteristics among women initiating breastfeeding

	Probability	Odds ratio (95% confidence interval)
Prenatal characteristics		
Confidence in ability		
Low (n = 47)	.28*	5.05 (1.99, 6.42)
High (n = 128)	.07*	
Certainty of decision		
Low (n = 21)	.33†	4.86 (1.68, 14.01)
High (n = 150)	.09†	
Postpartum characteristics		
Timing of first breastfeeding		
Late (n = 92)	.18‡	3.44 (1.21, 9.87)
Early (n = 81)	.06‡	
Baby's daytime location		
Nursery (n = 23)	.26§	3.00 (1.03, 8.71)
Mother's room (n = 152)	.11§	

Early cessation is defined as breastfeeding for 7 days or less. The confidence scale was dichotomized to reflect less confident (raw scores 1–3) and more confident (raw scores 4–6).
*$\chi^2 = 13.31$, $df = 1$; $p < .001$.
†$\chi^2 = 9.85$, $df = 1$; $p < .01$.
‡$\chi^2 = 5.88$, $df = 1$; $p < .02$.
§$\chi^2 = 4.40$, $df = 1$; $p < .05$.
Modified from Buxton KE, Gielen AC, Faden RR, et al: Women intending to breastfeed: Predictors of early infant feeding experiences. Am J Prev Med 7:101, 1991.

TABLE 1-8   Positive consequences of long-term nursing as perceived by the mother

Perceived consequences	Mothers (n = 130)	%*
Positive emotional effect on child—child is more secure	65	50.0
Better physical health (fewer allergies)	29	22.3
Child is loving, friendly, cheerier	27	20.8
Child can separate more easily—relative independence achieved with less stress	22	16.9
Enhanced maternal sensitivity	19	14.6
Close relationship of mother and child	18	13.8
Positive influence or education for older siblings	11	8.5
Child easily comforted during crisis, pain, or teething	10	8.0
Broad, all-encompassing positive effect	6	4.6
Incidental positive consequences	13	10.4
No positive effects perceived	2	1.5

*Mothers could give multiple responses; thus, percentages add to more than 100%.
From Reamer SB, Sugarman M: Breastfeeding beyond six months: Mothers' perceptions of the positive and negative consequences. J Trop Pediatr 33:93, 1987.

TABLE 1-9   Mothers' responses to the question, "What do you think are the negative aspects of nursing past 6 months (past 1 year)?"

Negative aspects listed by mothers	Past 6 months (total responses = 132)		Past 12 months (total responses = 133)	
	No.	%	No.	%
Mother states there are no negative aspects	62	47.1	35	26.4
Social stigma—negative attitudes of others	32	24.3	56	41.9
Mother's activities are restricted	19	14.7	9	6.6
Baby is less discreet—embarrassing in public	3	2.2	13	9.6
Tiredness	7	5.1	3	2.2
Breastfeeding mother has special concerns	1	0.7	5	3.7
Intrudes upon life with husband	1	0.7	4	2.9
Breast discomfort/leaking, soreness	2	1.5	1	0.7
Sex life interrupted—less interest in sex	2	1.5	2	1.5
Mother believes she should ignore negative aspects	2	1.5	1	0.7
Intrudes upon mother's time with siblings	0	—	1	0.7
Baby care, not nursing, causes negative aspects	0	—	1	0.7

From Reamer SB, Sugarman M: Breastfeeding beyond six months: Mothers' perceptions of the positive and negative consequences. J Trop Pediatr 33:93, 1987.

well randomized and controlled that the answer was clear. Those studies that did mention use of bottles in the hospital noted a stronger correlation between bottle use and diminished duration of breastfeeding.[8] What had not been measured is the impact of office prenatal formula advertising on breastfeeding. In a study by Howard and associates[45] of 547 women randomized to receive formula company gift packs or specially designed educational pacts at their first prenatal visit, feeding method was recorded at delivery. The 294 women who chose to breastfeed were interviewed at 2, 6, 12, and 24 weeks post partum. Women who received the commercial pack were more likely to discontinue breastfeeding by 2 weeks. Among women who had indefinite goals of breastfeeding for less than 12 weeks, exclusive, full, and overall breastfeeding duration were shortened.

In New York State, regulations regarding breastfeeding support instituted in July 1984, among other things, disallowed discharge packs to breastfeeding women unless requested by the mother or prescribed by the physician. A mother who

requests such a pack is usually at high risk for early termination of lactation in most investigators' experience. Giving such a packet to a vulnerable mother (young, less educated, single, poor support system) may be a message not unlike *Parents* magazine circa 1938: "You may be one of them . . . " (i.e., those who fail).[71] In a study in Virginia, Hayden and associates[41] reported that most pediatricians did not know and had never been asked if they approved of the discharge packages with samples of powders, creams, baby food, and other baby items that may or may not be appropriate for indiscriminate use. The authors suggest that pediatricians should investigate and review the procedures in their own hospitals.

Controlling discharge packs deflects attention from the real problem: inadequate counseling about breastfeeding and a system to support the mother who needs it. This point is well illustrated in a study by Feinstein and associates,[25] who found that initiating breastfeeding in the first 16 hours and minimizing use of formula in the nursery correlated highly with successful lactation. The negative impact of supplementation could be overcome by frequent breastfeeding at home.

Frank and associates[32] found that a gift packet of breast pads and breastfeeding information of equal monetary value to a formula packet, along with a special counselor who made five home visits in the first 28 days and three more in the next 6 weeks, resulted in longer duration of breastfeeding. Howard and associates[46] showed that discharge packs did not have the same impact on duration as many other factors, including bottle feeding in the hospital and the mother's original plan about how long she would breastfeed.

A force that is difficult to measure is the public advertising of infant formula, a direct violation of the letter and the intent of the WHO Code (see earlier discussion). Some formula companies have television advertisements that include a subliminal message that their product is equal to breastfeeding, so why bother.[36] Furthermore, when the message says, "Just ask your doctor," it implies that physicians agree. Sending free samples and coupons aimed at the vulnerable woman 2 to 4 weeks post partum, when she is fatigued and overwhelmed, can undermine the confidence of even a dedicated breastfeeding mother. In addition to the pregnant woman or new mother, the audience consists of the world of television viewers. The daily repetition of the message that bottle feeding is just as good as breastfeeding is cementing the national image that it is "American" to bottle feed.[54]

Young children, adolescents, and new immigrants all are relentlessly receiving the message. The ads are played during programs that attract low-income, less-educated viewers who are already the least likely to breastfeed. Studies that examine television advertising of breastfeeding have measured the impact of only one viewing of the ad, not the effect of daily repetitions, which, as marketing experts know well, is more important. Greer and Apple[36] note that advertising directly to the public "will once again remove the control of infant feeding from the supervision of the physician and will likely have a negative impact on the incidence and duration of breastfeeding."

Infants in Latin America were less likely to be breastfed than infants in Africa and Asia, and the duration was 6 months compared with 12 months or more in Asia and Africa.[35] A significant increase in the Latin American rates resulted after an aggressive breastfeeding promotion program (PROALMA) was initiated and supported by the various governments.[65,66]

A study of attitudes toward breastfeeding and infant feeding among Iranian, Afghan, and Southeast Asian immigrant women in the United States reported that women discontinue breastfeeding to return to work because (1) economics is important, (2) the workplace is hostile to nursing mothers, and (3) there is little or no maternity leave.[35] The author recommends that (1) health care workers should have greater sensitivity to cultural barriers, (2) adult language school programs coordinate infant nutrition programs with WIC, (3) workplaces encourage breastfeeding, and (4) American social customs recognize breastfeeding as normal.[35]

In an effort to identify the "real" reason women stopped breastfeeding, Ferris and associates[26] followed more than 250 women who delivered in Connecticut. They tried to identify crucial biologic and sociocultural links in the chain of events that precede the change in feeding from breast to bottle.

Hospital routines influenced the early "failures." Successful breastfeeders experienced milk let-down a full day sooner than those who discontinued by 2 weeks. They had also fed their infant 5 hours earlier than those who discontinued. Mothers who nursed early had prepared themselves to insist on early feeding. Mothers who were unsure and lacked confidence turned to supplements. Providing just 1 oz of formula per day led to ultimate discontinuation.[55] A small amount of doubt eroded confidence. The most vulnerable time was the immediate postpartum period. Women who had wanted to lose weight post partum were disappointed that they did not lose more rapidly. The authors also identified the need for close follow-up by the pediatrician in these critical 2 weeks (Table 1-10).[26]

A number of hospital routines were found to be potentially detrimental to breastfeeding in a

TABLE 1-10   Sources of advice on breastfeeding: comparison of intent vs. action

| | Intent: at 1 week post partum, mothers were asked: | | Action: at 10 weeks, mothers were asked: | |
Source of advice	(1) If you have a problem with nursing, whom will you call? (*n* = 113)	(2) If you have already had a problem, whom did you call? (*n* = 19)	(1) If you had a problem with nursing, and continued nursing, whom did you go to for advice? (*n* = 23)	(2) If you stopped nursing, whom did you go to for advice? (*n* = 26)
			%	
Pediatrician	36	32	65	46
Support group	24	32	5	0
Family	12	5	4	0
Friends	10	5	0	0
Obstetrician/gynecologist	6	5	0	4
Nurse/midwife	6	21	9	0
No one	0	0	17	50
Do not know	3	0	—	—

From Ferris AM, McCabe LT, Allen LH, et al: Biological and sociocultural determinants of successful lactation among women in eastern Connecticut. J Am Diet Assoc 87:316, 1987.

literature review of breastfeeding initiation and duration by Dennis.[19] These included interruption of mother-infant contact, supplementation, and restriction feedings.

Attitudes of health care professionals

A 1980 survey of physicians' and nurses' medical and educational practices regarding breastfeeding was published when breastfeeding was at its zenith. A follow-up survey was completed in the summer of 1991, after several years of decline. A comparison of the results of these two surveys showed little change in the current practices of health professionals regarding breastfeeding, their attitudes toward breastfeeding, and who among them they believed to be primarily responsible for managing breastfeeding and supporting the breastfeeding mother.

Regarding responsibility for managing breastfeeding mothers and infants, more than 80% of pediatricians believed that medical encouragement or support of breastfeeding was primarily a responsibility of the infant's physician. Approximately two thirds of family practitioners thought that both the mother's physician and the infant's physician were responsible.

The respondents viewed mother's employment as the main reason for the decline in breastfeeding.[54] Most obstetricians have always supported breastfeeding according to Queenan,[68] an active advocate of breastfeeding, but some have appeared to be neutral. He stated that mothers should be informed of the strikingly valuable health benefits of breastfeeding so the mother can make an informed choice. "It's your gift to the mother and it's her gift to her baby."[68]

Health care professionals can be a negative source of support, reported Dennis in her review of breastfeeding literature from 1990 to 2000, covering almost 200 articles. This is explained by the lack of knowledge that results in inaccurate or inconsistent advice.[19]

MORBIDITY AND MORTALITY STUDIES IN BREASTFED AND ARTIFICIALLY FED INFANTS

Assessing the mortality rate of breastfed infants compared with bottle fed infants is difficult today because many breastfed infants also receive supplements of formula and solid foods. The risk of death in the first year of life diminished in civilized countries in the 20th century since the advent of antibiotics, additional immunizations, and many other advances in pediatric care.[83] Data from previous decades and other nations do show a significant difference, however.[37,38] Knodel[51] presented a complete table, including rates from cities in Germany, France, England, Holland, and the United States (Table 1-11). The mortality rate among breastfed infants is clearly lower than that among bottle fed infants. Knodel pointed out that early neonatal

deaths, in the first week or so of life, were excluded. In the early 20th century, as part of the National Campaign to lower infant mortality rates, posters urging mothers to breastfeed were displayed everywhere by the health department without fear of inducing guilt in mothers. According to Wolf, the language was direct: "To lessen baby death let us have more mothers breastfeed." "For your baby's sake, nurse it." Little has changed in a century.[99]

Woodbury[100] reported the trends in infant feeding (Fig. 1-10) and in another study in 1922 reported mortality rates of infants by type of feeding. Mortality rate is lower at all ages for breastfed infants. Overwhelming evidence of the impact of human milk on mortality rate is displayed in the widely publicized statistics currently available on third world countries, where infant formulas are rapidly replacing human milk. The death rate is higher, malnutrition starts earlier and is more severe, and the incidence of infection is greater in

TABLE 1-11   Mortality rates and survivorship to age 1 year in breastfed and artificially fed infants*

Study area	Date	Mortality rate (per 1000)		Survivors to age 1 yr (per 1000)		
		Breastfed	Artificially fed	Breastfed	Artificially fed	Difference
Berlin, Germany	1895–1896	57	376	943	624	319
Bremen, Germany	1905	68	379	932	621	311
Hanover, Germany	1912	96	296	904	704	200
Boston, Mass.	1911	30	212	970	788	182
Eight U.S. cities[†]	1911–1916	76	255	924	745	179
Paris, France	1900	140	310	860	690	170
Cologne, Germany	1908–1909	73	241	927	759	168
Amsterdam, Holland	1904	144	304	856	696	160
Liverpool, England	1905	84	134	916	866	144
Eight U.S. cities[‡]	1911–1916	76	215	924	785	139
Derby, England	1900–1903	70	198	930	802	128
Chicago, Ill.	1924–1929	2	84	998	916	82
Liverpool, England	1936–1942	10	57	990	943	47
Great Britain	1946–1947	9	18	991	982	9

*Most of these rates do not include deaths in the first few days or weeks of life; mortality rate is therefore underestimated and survival rate overestimated. Only the rates for the eight U.S. cities in 1911–1916 represent mortality rate from birth; deaths that occurred before any feeding are proportionately allocated to the two feeding categories. The rates for Berlin, Bremen, Hanover, Cologne, and the eight U.S. cities were derived by applying life table techniques to mortality rates given by single months of age.
†Comparison of breastfed infants with infants artificially fed from birth.
‡Comparison of breastfed infants with all infants artificially fed in the period of observation.
From Knodel J: Breastfeeding and population growth. Science 198:1111, 1977. Copyright © 1977 by the American Association for the Advancement of Science.

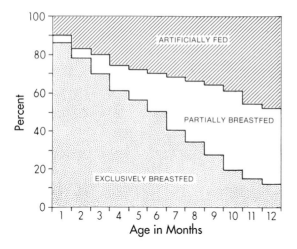

Figure 1-10. Percentage of infants who were breastfed, partially breastfed, and artificially fed by age in months. (Modified from Woodbury RM: The relation between breast and artificial feeding and infant mortality. Am J Hyg 2:668, 1922.)

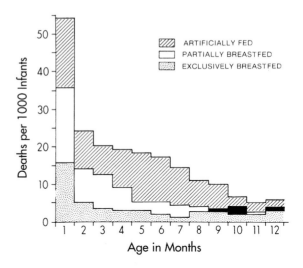

Figure 1-11. Death rate per 100 infants by type of feeding and age in months. (Modified from Woodbury RM: The relation between breast and artificial feeding and infant mortality. Am J Hyg 2:668, 1922.)

formula fed infants (Figs. 1-11 and 1-12). Data from the work of Scrimshaw and associates[82] show a mortality rate of 950 of 1000 live births in artificially fed infants and 120 of 1000 in breastfed infants. The data were collected in Punjab villages from 1955 through 1959. The deaths were predominantly caused by diarrheal disease. The Pan American Health Organization has reported similar correlations among malnutrition, infection, and mortality. In Puffer and Serrano's[67] 1973 work in São Paulo, death rates among breastfed infants and proportions from diarrheal disease and malnutrition were also lower than among bottle fed infants.

The incidence of illness or morbidity among artificially fed infants in third world countries is as dramatic as the mortality rate. Kanaaneh's[49] observations in Arab villages in Israel showed hospitalization rates vary with method of feeding. Only 0.5% of breastfed infants required hospitalization, whereas infants fed more than 3 months but less than 6 months at the breast had a 2.9% hospitalization rate, and infants who were bottle fed had a 24.8% rate. This is a 50-fold difference.

There is a bias against bottle feeding, as sicker, smaller infants are bottle fed. Infants who die are weaned early by death. The benefits of breastfeeding are enhanced by these confounding variables. Habicht and associates[40] point out that had there been no breastfeeding in the sample, twice as many infants would have died after the first week of life. In 1968, Lee Forrest Hill[42] articulated what many physicians have believed: "Formula feeding has become so simple, safe, uniformly successful that breastfeeding no longer seems worth the bother." This statement ignores the protective qualities of human milk, not only in the third world but in industrialized nations as well. It neglects the immunologic protection.

Evidence for protection by breastfeeding against infant death from infectious diseases in Brazil in 1987 is even more persuasive, as noted in a carefully controlled study by Victora and associates.[90,91] Compared with infants who were breastfed without supplementation, those who were completely bottle fed had a relative risk 14.2 times greater of death from diarrhea and a relative risk 3.6 times greater of death from respiratory

THE MESSAGE ON BREAST-FEEDING ISN'T NEW

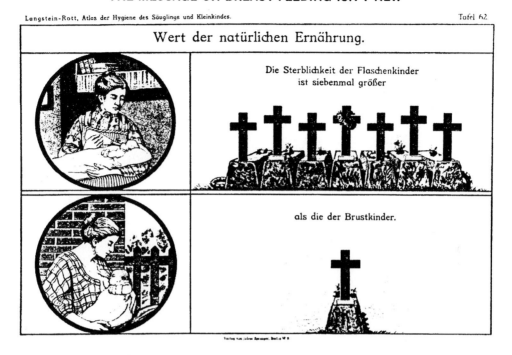

Figure 1-12. "Value of Natural Feeding" poster used in 1918 to educate parents. Text explains that the mortality rate of bottle-fed infants (Flaschenkinder) is seven times higher than that of breastfed infants (Brustkinder). (From Langstein R: Atlas der Hygiene des Sauglings und Kleinkindes. Berlin, Springer-Verlag, 1918.)

infection. Partial breastfeeding was less protective. Formula and cow milk were equally hazardous. The greatest risk from diarrhea was in the first 2 months of life. Barros and associates[7] noted that birth weight influences breastfeeding and that small infants tend to be weaned sooner.

Demonstrating the differences in morbidity between breastfed and bottle fed infants has become even more complex in industrialized countries since the resurgence of breastfeeding. Among the confounding variables are the inherent differences between mothers who choose to breastfeed and those who choose to bottle feed. Although many investigators have recognized the necessity of controlling these variables, none has succeeded totally because an unavoidable factor of self-selection makes random assignment of infants impossi-

ble.[24] There is a one-way flow of infants from the breastfed group to the bottle fed group, because a baby may change from breast to bottle but rarely from bottle to breast. Documenting breastfeeding practices is difficult when the possibility exists that some bottle feedings are included or that solid foods have been introduced.

Investigators[47,65,67,90] have reported differences between breastfed and bottle fed infants in the incidence of morbidity associated with diarrhea, respiratory infections, otitis media, and pneumonia; they have also compared breastfed and bottle fed infants seen in clinics and emergency rooms or hospitalized in the first year of life. This extensive material has been reviewed by Cunningham.[16] The majority of reports demonstrate a significant advantage for the breastfed group. The relationship between breastfeeding or bottle feeding and respiratory illness in the first year of life among nearly 2000 cohort children was reported by Watkins and associates[91] in England. There was a significant advantage to breastfeeding. Mothers who smoked were less likely to breastfeed, but even when smoking was considered, the breast-feeding advantage remained. In the Yale Harvard Research Project, Young and associates[105] reported on 1000 infants in Tunisia who were followed from birth to 26 months and found breastfed infants had fewer infections, illnesses, and allergies.

Victora and associates[89,90] investigated 127 respiratory deaths in the first year of life in Brazil in 1985. Having controlled for prematurity, congenital malformation, and socioeconomic factors, the researchers believed that 82 of the deaths could be attributed to feeding method (i.e., lack of breast-feeding). A number of well-controlled studies of industrialized countries in the past 15 years have shown at least a twofold relative risk of respiratory infection with bottle feeding and that the infections breastfed infants do experience are usually less severe.[47] A meta-analysis by Bachrach and associates in 2003 revealed that "among generally healthy infants in developed nations, more than a tripling in severe respiratory tract illnesses resulting in hospitalizations was noted for infants who were not breastfed compared with those who were exclusively breastfed for 4 months."[5]

When Victora[88] presented his studies of the impact of early weaning on infection and disease at a workshop held by the Pontifical Academy of Sciences and The Royal Society, he stated that a 40% reduction in nonbreastfeeding would prevent up to 15% of diarrhea deaths and 7% of pneumonia deaths. He noted that even the introduction of water or herbal teas to a previously exclusively breastfed infant increases morbidity and mortality rates. Figures 1-13 and 1-14 illustrate the relative risks of pneumonia and otitis media.

Cunningham[17] undertook a study in rural upstate New York to determine the impact of feeding on infant health. Of 326 infants studied, 162 were fed proprietary formula and 164 were breastfed at birth, with only 4% still breastfed at 1 year. Breastfeeding

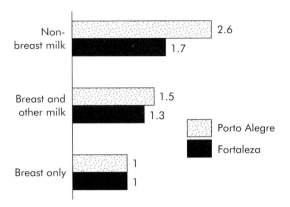

Figure 1-13.   Risk of pneumonia (odds ratio for incidence) in children under 2 years of age at two Brazilian sites, Porto Alegre and Fortaleza, in 1993–1995 according to type of milk. (Modified from Victora CG: Infection and disease: The impact of early weaning. Food Nutr Bull 17:390, 1996.)

was associated with significantly less illness during the first year of life. The protection was greatest during the early months, increased with the duration of breastfeeding, and appeared more striking for serious illness (Table 1-12). Breastfeeding was associated with a higher level of parental education, but controlling for that factor, the difference in the morbidity rate is even more significant.[88]

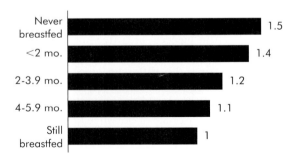

Figure 1-14.   Risk of otitis media (odds ratio for incidence in last month) in infants 6 months of age in Brazil in 1993–1994 according to duration of breastfeeding. (Modified from Victora CG: Infection and disease: The impact of early weaning. Food Nutr Bull 17:390, 1996.)

TABLE 1-12	**Illness, disease, and development, with feeding measure and risk ratio range**		
	Feeding measure	**Risk ratio range**[*]	**Reference(s)**
Common illnesses			
Acute diarrhea	Breastfed <3 months	6.10 (4.1–9.0)	Victoria & Barros, 2000
Lower respiratory tract infections	Breastfed <4 months / sharing bedroom	3.29 (1.8–6.0)	Wright et al, 1989
Pneumonia	No breastfeeding	16.7 (7.7, 36.0)	César et al, 1999
Ear infections (recurring vs. acute)	Breastfed <6 months	1.61 (1.27, 1.79)[*]	Duncan et al, 1993
Asthma	Breastfed <4 months	1.25 (1.02, 1.52)	Oddy et al, 1999
Atopy	Breastfed <4 months	1.30 (1.04, 1.61)	Oddy et al, 1999
Less common illnesses			
Necrotizing enterocolitis	39% formula fed/ 7% breastfed	4.50 (3.00, 6.00)[*]	Lucas & Cole, 1990
Urinary tract infections	Never breastfed	1.62 (1.35, 1.78)[*]	Mårild, Jodal & Hanson, 1990; Mårild, Jodal & Mangelus, 1989; Pisacane et al, 1992
Insulin-dependent diabetes mellitus	Breastfed <4 months	1.63 (1.22, 2.17)	Fort et al, 1986
Acute lymphobastic leukemia	Never breastfed	1.21 (1.09, 1.30)[*]	Shu et al, 1999
Sudden infant death syndrome	Current infant-formula-feeding	1.35 (1.09, 1.54)[*]	Ford et al, 1993
Cholera	Not breastfeeding	1.70 (p <.0001)[*]	Clemens et al, 1990
Immunologic disease			
Celiac disease	Breastfed <3 months	1.63 (1.36, 1.79)[*]	Falth-Magnusson et al, 1996; Peters et al, 1996
Crohn's disease	Lack of breastfeeding	1.90 (1.50, 3.60)	Corrao et al, 1998; Koletzko et al, 1989
Ulcerative colitis	Lack of breastfeeding	1.50 (1.10, 2.10)	Corrao et al, 1998; Koletzko et al, 1991
Juvenile rheumatoid arthritis	Lack of breastfeeding	1.60 (1.19, 1.80)	Mason et al, 1995
Multiple sclerosis	Breastfed <7 months	1.62 (1.26, 1.81)	Pisacane et al, 1994
Development			
Cognitive development in preterm	Lack of breastfeeding	↓mean IQ of 8.3 pts[*]	Lucas et al, 1992
Cardiovascular disease	Lack of breastfeeding	↑mean total cholesterol[*]	Bergstrom et al, 1995
Metabolic development	Lack of breastfeeding	↑ApoB values[*]	Bergstrom et al, 1995
Obesity	Breastfed <6 months	1.25 (1.02, 1.43)	von Kries et al, 1999

[*]The risk ratios have been adjusted to reflect a level of risk of infant formula rather than protection of breast milk. This was done to ensure consistency of results. Some results are given as *p* value or other measurement effect.

ApoB, apoplipoprotein B

From Oddy W: The impact of breastmilk on infant and child health. Breastfeeding Rev 10:5, 2002.

In the United States, diarrheal disease is uncommon in breastfed infants, and the treatment is usually to continue to breastfeed. Similarly, breastfed infants have fewer episodes of respiratory illness and otitis media. When afflicted with such febrile illnesses, the breastfed infant does not become dehydrated and rapidly toxic.[24]

The issue is not as clear in other Western countries because of the associated variables among bottle feeders, that is, young mothers with low socioeconomic status and less education and small, sick infants who are more likely to be bottle fed.

Despite the clear-cut data on mortality and morbidity rates from past generations and from cultures seemingly remote from industrialized and medically sophisticated societies, pediatricians had discounted any but the psychologic advantages of breastfeeding for many years.[8] The current increase in illness in young infants in daycare centers is providing a new study group. To date, breastfeeding appears to be protective for the few children whose mothers continue to nurse them while in daycare.

In a study in Scotland, Forsyth[31] confirmed that breastfeeding during the first 3 months (13 weeks) of life confers protection against gastrointestinal disease that persists beyond the period of breastfeeding (Table 1-13). There was a significant reduction in hospitalization in breastfed infants and a smaller but significant reduction in respiratory illness until 40 to 52 weeks of age. These data parallel the global epidemiologic review by Cunningham and associates[17] that breastfeeding reduces illness in early life. Thus, Forsyth[31] concluded that the answer to the question, "Is it worthwhile breastfeeding?" is a resounding "*yes!*" In the third millennium, adequate consumption of human milk as an infant and toddler is still a powerful guarantor of health and long life. Wolfe stated that to forget the history of the struggle to lower infant mortality and morbidity rates can be equally dangerous as it was in 1900. Pediatricians must recognize that failure to consume sufficient human milk carries vital implications for public health.[99]

The United States Breastfeeding Committee in conjunction with the Office of Women's Health has launched a National Campaign whose tagline is "Babies are born to breastfeed." The messages illustrate the risks of not breastfeeding because clearly it does not work just to reiterate the benefits of breastfeeding.

SUDDEN INFANT DEATH SYNDROME AND OTHER ISSUES

Recent interest in sudden infant death syndrome (SIDS) has generated several studies investigating the position in which the infant is put down in the

TABLE 1-13   Percentage of babies with gastrointestinal illness up to 1 year of age according to duration of breastfeeding*

Age of baby (weeks)	Duration of breastfeeding (full and partial)						χ^2	
	Never (*n* = 246)	1–13 weeks (*n* = 164)	14–26 weeks (*n* = 49)	27–39 weeks (*n* = 71)	40–52 weeks (*n* = 60)	>52 weeks (*n* = 30)	Never vs. 1–13 weeks	Never vs. 14–52 weeks
0–13	15.7	16.6	2.2	3.5	6.3	7.7	0.06	11.02§
14–26	18.0	20.3	8.6	9.1	7.2	3.5	0.32	8.06‡
27–39	21.6	21.0	13.7	13.4	16.0	7.4	0.02	4.03‡
40–52	22.3	12.7	7.9	14.2	11.7	13.4	6.02†	6.70‡

*Adjusted for social class, maternal age, and parental smoking.
†$p < .05$.
‡$p < .01$.
§$p < .001$.
From Forsyth JS: Is it worthwhile breastfeeding? Eur J Clin Nutr 46 (suppl 1):S19, 1992.

crib and SIDS.[23,60] The New Zealand Cot Death Study showed the prone sleeping position to be a greater risk, but not greater than the risk of not being breastfed.[60] Other investigators have shown the importance of breastfeeding as a risk-lowering factor.[23] Although breastfeeding does not eliminate SIDS, its incidence is lower among breastfed infants.

No single consistent factor has been a predictor of SIDS.[23] Prone sleeping has continued to be a cofactor in studies, but maternal smoking is a relative causative factor as well. Breastfeeding has been shown to be the strongest protection. Infants of smokers who breastfeed and sleep supine have a reduced risk of SIDS. Several studies confirmed a reduced risk while breastfeeding, and one study linked the effect to a dose response of the amount of breastfeeding. The National Maternal and Infant Health Survey of 10,000 births and 6000 deaths of infants born in 1988 and 1989 was analyzed using a consistent "dosage definition" of breastfeeding while controlling for major confounding factors. These factors included birth weight; maternal age, race, and education; smoking; prenatal cocaine use; lack of private insurance; household smoking; daycare; and household size. In 7102 control subjects, 499 SIDS deaths and 584 non-SIDS deaths occurred. Fredrickson and associates[33] reported that "the risk of SIDS for black infants increased by 1.19 for every month of not breastfeeding, and 2.13 for every month of not exclusively breastfeeding. Among white infants, the risk increased by 1.19 and 2.0 times, respectively. These associations remained even when deaths within the first month of life were excluded. A similar protective association existed for non-SIDS deaths."

The Nordic Study of sudden infant death syndrome collected cases of SIDS and controls from 1992 to 1995 in Norway, Sweden, and Denmark. The investigators studied 244 cases of SIDS and 869 control children. The study was supportive of a weak relationship between breastfeeding and SIDS reduction. Breastfeeding rates were high, with exclusive breastfeeding rising from 40% to almost 80% at 4 months during the study period.[1]

Sleep patterns of infants have been the subject of much study.[21] In the early weeks of life, infants have REM (rapid eye movement) sleep, active body movements, and rapid, irregular heart and respiratory rates. At about 2 to 3 months of age, they begin to increase the proportion of quiet sleep, which coincides with the peak incidence of SIDS. When breastfeeding decreased, the advantage of co-sleeping seemed to diminish. Child care became very organized and focused on encouraging the infant to sleep alone and through the night. Only in about the last century have Western industrialized societies considered breastfeeding and infant sleep location to be separate issues. McKenna and Bernstraw[58] and Mosko[59] describe the physiologic benefits to infants sleeping in proximity to their caregivers. They have documented the physiologic changes infants experience as they move from a solitary sleep environment to co-sleeping. They monitored a group of mother-infant pairs in the sleep laboratory, using each pair as their own control (i.e., co-sleeping and sleeping separately). Infants moved from one stage of sleep to the other more frequently when co-sleeping than when sleeping alone, even when briefly waking and increasing their heart and respiratory rates. The authors commented that modern technology, including baby monitors, breathing teddy bears, and other gadgets, has replaced traditional co-sleeping.[59]

THE MAMMARY GLAND AND SCIENCE

Newer additions to the laboratory have permitted rapid advances in the understanding of the mammary gland, especially actions of hormones and enzymes. The "knock-out mouse" is a concept using mice whose DNA (deoxyribonucleic acid) has been altered to "knock out" a specific gene that controls a specific hormone, such as one important to lactation. Observations of growth and development in these animals provide new insights into the physiology of the mammary gland. In evolutionary biology, lactogenesis is one of the most important functions for the survival of the species. Advances in molecular biology have provided biologists with a better understanding of the mechanisms that produce milk and its specific nutrient constituents. Mammary epithelial cells secrete milk. In an innovative experimental model, mammary epithelial cells are cultured in a petri dish and form a *mammosphere,* a micromodel of the mammary gland. The advantage of bioengineering the mammary gland, initially focused on the dairy species, is to advance our knowledge and understanding of human lactation in the laboratory so that more women may nurse their infants successfully.[74]

SUPPORT FOR THE BREASTFEEDING WOMEN OF THE WORLD

On May 12, 1995, His Holiness John Paul II granted a Solemn Papal Audience in the Apostolic Palace of the Vatican to the participants of the Working Group on Breastfeeding: Science and Society. In response to the group report, the Holy Father pronounced the following discourse (in part):

> The advantages of breastfeeding for the infant and the mother . . . include two major benefits to the child: protection against disease and proper nourishment. . . . This natural way of feeding can create a bond of love and security between mother and child and enable the child to assert its presence as a person through interaction with the mother. . . . Responsible international agencies are calling on governments to ensure that women are enabled to breastfeed their children for four to six months from birth and to continue this practice, supplemented by other appropriate foods, up to the second year of life and beyond.[64]

A NATIONAL CAMPAIGN TO PROMOTE BREASTFEEDING

In an attempt to capture the attention of the American public and improve the national statistics on breastfeeding initiation and duration, the Office of Women's Health and the United States Breastfeeding Committee initiated a national advertising campaign with the professional expertise of the National Advertising Council in 2002. Considerable effort and study went into the planning and design. It included 36 focus groups in four cities nationwide with an ethnic, gender, and age mix. The Ad Council recom-

mended and designed a risk-focused campaign. For decades, breastfeeding has been promoted based on all of its benefits. It has not worked. Wolf[98] described fully the health issues of the day and their solutions. Of historical significance is the use of a risk-focused campaign by public health groups attempting to stem the tide of higher mortality and morbidity rates in infants and children who were not breastfed, 1890 to 1910 (Fig. 1-15).[103]

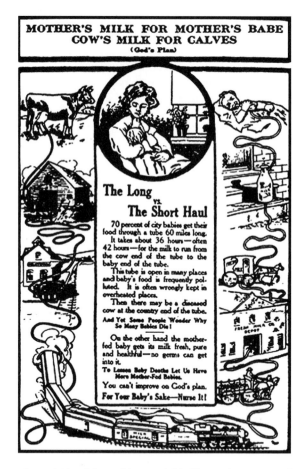

Figure 1-15.   Many cities used this illustration as part of their campaign to increase breastfeeding rates. The wording on the poster, however, changed from city to city. This is Chicago's version. (From Bulletin Chicago School of Sanitary Instruction, 3 June 1911; reprinted in Wolf JH: Don't Kill Your Baby: Public Heath and the Decline of Breastfeeding in the 19th and 20th Centuries. Columbus, The Ohio State University Press, 2001.)

In 2003, as the campaign was about to be released, a massive effort was launched on the part of formula companies to defuse and delay the program. Several of the television spots have been withdrawn at the insistence of the Department of Health and Human Services. Objections to the risk-focused approach were voiced loudly even by some pediatricians who were unaware of the evidence-based research supporting the statements of the risk of not breastfeeding.

REFERENCES

1. Alm B, Wennergren G, Norvenius SG, et al, on behalf of the Nordic Epidemiological SIDS Study: Breast feeding and the sudden infant death syndrome in Scandinavia, 1992–95. Arch Dis Child 86:400, 2002.
2. American Academy of Pediatrics: Red Book, 26th ed. 2003 Report of the Committee on Infectious Diseases. AAP, Elk Grove Ill, 2003, p 63.
3. Andrew EM, Clancy KL, Katz MG: Infant feeding practices of families belonging to a prepaid group practice health care plan. Pediatrics 65:978, 1980.
4. Apple RD: Mothers and medicine: A social history of infant feeding, 1890–1950. Madison, University of Wisconsin Press, 1987.
5. Bachrach VRG, Schwarz E, Bachrach LR: Breastfeeding and the risk of hospitalization for respiratory disease in infancy. Arch Pediatr Adolesc Med 157:237, 2003.
6. Baghurst KI: Infant feeding: Public health perspectives. Med J Aust 148:112, 1988.
7. Barros FC, Victora CG, Vaughn JP, et al: Birthweight and duration of breastfeeding: Are the beneficial effects of human milk being overestimated? Pediatrics 78:656, 1986.
8. Bauchner H, Leventhal JM, Shapiro ED: Studies of breastfeeding and infections: How good is the evidence? JAMA 256:887, 1986.
9. Baumslag N, Michels DL: Milk, money and madness. Westport, CT, Bergin & Garvey, 1995.
10. Bergevin Y, Dougherty C, Kramer MS: Do formula samples shorten the duration of breastfeeding? Lancet 1:1148, 1983.
11. Bryant CA: The impact of kin, friend, and neighbor networks on infant feeding practices. Soc Sci Med 16:1757, 1982.
12. Buxton KE, Gielen AC, Faden RR, et al: Women intending to breastfeed: Predictors of early infant feeding experiences. Am J Prev Med 7:101, 1991.
13. Carroll EGC: Home from the hospital. Parents 13:22, 52, 1938.
14. Cole JP: Breastfeeding in Boston suburbs in relation to personal-social factors. Clin Pediatr 16:352, 1977.
15. Commonwealth Department of Health: Towards better nutrition for Australians. Report of the Nutrition Taskforce of the Better Health Commission. Canberra, AGPS, 1987 (catalogue no 86-1660).
16. Cunningham AS: Breastfeeding and morbidity in industrialized countries: An update. In Jelliffe DB, Jelliffe EFP (eds): Advances in International Maternal and Child Health. Vol 1. Oxford, Oxford University Press, 1981.
17. Cunningham AS, Jelliffe DB, Jelliffe EFP: Breastfeeding and health in the 1980's: A global epidemiologic review. J Pediatr 118:659, 1991.
18. Deem H, McGeorge M: Breastfeeding. NZ Med J 57:539, 1958.
19. Dennis CL: Breastfeeding initiation and duration: A 1990–2000 literature review. J Obstet Gynecol Neonatal Nurse 31:12, 2002.
20. Department of Health and Human Services, Office of Women's Health: HHS Blueprint for Action on Breastfeeding. Washington, Department of Health and Human Services, 2000.
21. Dettwyler KA: Beauty and the breast: The cultural context of breastfeeding in the United States. In Stuart-Macadam P, Dettwyler KA (eds): Breastfeeding: Biocultural Perspectives. Hawthorne, NY, Aldine de Gruyter, 1995.
22. Drake TGH: Infant welfare laws in France in the 18th century. Ann Med Hist 7:49, 1935.
23. Dumas K, Pakter J, Krongrad E, et al: Postnatal medical and epidemiological risk factors for the sudden infant death syndrome. In Harper RM, Hoffman HJ (eds): Sudden infant death syndrome. New York, PMA, 1988.
24. Fallot ME, Boyd JL, Oski FA: Breastfeeding reduces incidence of hospital admissions for infections in infants. Pediatrics 65:1121, 1980.
25. Feinstein JM, Berkelhamer JE, Gruszka ME, et al: Factors related to early termination of breastfeeding in an urban population. Pediatrics 78:210, 1986.
26. Ferris AM, McCabe LT, Allen LH, et al: Biological and sociocultural determinants of successful lactation among women in eastern Connecticut. J Am Diet Assoc 87:316, 1987.
27. Fildes V: Breast, bottles, and babies. Edinburgh, Edinburgh University Press, 1986.
28. Ford CS: A comparative study of human reproduction. Anthropology Pub No 32. New Haven, CT, Yale University Press, 1945.
29. Forman MR, Fetterly K, Graubard BI: Exclusive breastfeeding of newborns among married women in the United States: The National Natality Surveys of 1969 and 1980. Am J Clin Nutr 42:864, 1985.
30. Forman MR, Graubard BI, Hoffmann HJ, et al: The PIMA infant feeding study: Breastfeeding and gastroenteritis in the first year of life. Am J Epidemiol 119:335, 1984.
31. Forsyth JS: It is worthwhile breastfeeding? Eur J Clin Nutr 46(suppl 1):S19, 1992.

32. Frank DA, Wirtz SJ, Sorenson JR, et al: Commercial discharge packs and breastfeeding counseling: Effects on infant-feeding practices in a randomized trial. Pediatrics 80:845, 1987.

33. Fredrickson DD, Sorenson JR, Biddle AK, et al: Relationship of sudden infant death syndrome to breastfeeding duration and intensity. Am J Dis Child 147:460, 1993.

34. Gabriel A, Gabriel KR, Lawrence RA: Cultural values and biomedical knowledge: Choices in infant feeding. Soc Sci Med 23:501, 1986.

35. Ghaemi-Ahmadi S: Attitudes toward breastfeeding and infant feeding among Iranian, Afghan, and South East Asian immigrant women in the United States: Implications for health and nutrition education. J Am Diet Assoc 92:354, 1992.

36. Greer FR, Apple RD: Physicians, formula companies and advertising: A historical perspective. Am J Dis Child 145:282, 1991.

37. Grulee CG, Sanford HN, Herron PH: Breast and artificial feeding. JAMA 103:735, 1934.

38. Grulee CG, Sanford HN, Schwartz H: Breast and artificially fed infants. JAMA 104:1986, 1935.

39. Grummer-Strawn L, on behalf of the Breastfeeding Promotion Consortium and the U.S. Breastfeeding Committee: Defining breastfeeding in the United States. (in press).

40. Habicht JP, DaVanzo J, Butz WP: Does breastfeeding really save lives or are apparent benefits due to biases? Am J Epidemiol 123:279, 1986.

41. Hayden GF, Nowacek GA, Koch W, et al: Providing free samples of baby items to newly delivered parents. Clin Pediatr 26:111, 1987.

42. Hill LF: A salute to La Leche League International. J Pediatr 73:161, 1968.

43. House JS, Landis KR, Umberson D: Social relationships and health. Science 241:540, 1988.

44. Houston MJ, Howie PW, Smart L, et al: Factors affecting the duration of breastfeeding: Early feeding practices and social class. Early Hum Dev 8:55, 1983.

45. Howard C, Howard F, Lawrence R, et al: Office prenatal formula advertising and its effect on breast-feeding patterns. Obst Gynecol 95:296, 2000.

46. Howard CR, Howard FM, Weitzman MD, et al: Antenatal formula advertising: Another potential threat to breastfeeding. Pediatrics 94:102, 1994.

47. Howie PW, Forsyth JS, Ogston SA, et al: Protective effect of breastfeeding against infection. Br Med J 300:11, 1990.

48. Jakobsen MS, Sodemann M, Molbak K, Aaby P: Reason for termination of breastfeeding and the length of breastfeeding. Int J Epidemiol 21:115, 1996.

49. Kanaaneh H: The relationship of bottle feeding to malnutrition and gastroenteritis in a preindustrial setting. J Trop Pediatr 18:302, 1972.

50. Konner M: The nursing knot. Sciences 25:10, 1985.

51. Knodel J: Breastfeeding and population growth. Science 198:1111, 1977.

52. Labbok M, Krasovec K: Toward consistency in breastfeeding definitions. Stud Fam Plan 21:226, 1990.

53. Launer LJ, Forman MR, Hundt GL, et al: Maternal recall of infant feeding events is accurate. J Epidemiol Community Health 46:203, 1992.

54. Lawrence RA: Choosing to breastfeed: A national challenge. Will it become American to breastfeed? Birth 18:226, 1991.

55. Loughlin HH, Clapp-Channing NE, Gehlbach SH, et al: Early termination of breastfeeding: Identifying those at risk. Pediatrics 75:508, 1985.

56. Martinez GA, Dodd DA: 1981 milk feeding patterns in the United States during the first 12 months of life. Pediatrics 71:166, 1983.

57. Martinez GA, Stahle DA: The recent trend in milk feeding among WIC infants. Am J Pub Health 72:68, 1982.

58. McKenna JJ, Bernstraw NJ: Breastfeeding and infant-parent co-sleeping as adaptive strategies: Are they protective against SIDS? In Stuart-Macadam P, Dettwyler KA (eds): Breastfeeding: Biocultural Perspectives. Hawthorne, NY, Aldine De Gruyter, 1995.

59. McKenna JJ, Mosko S: Evolution and infant sleep: An experimental study of infant-parent co-sleeping and its implications for SIDS. Acta Paediatr Suppl 389:31, 1993.

60. Mitchell EA, Scragg R, Stewart AW, et al: Cot death supplement: Results from the first year of the New Zealand Cot Death Study. NZ Med J 104:71, 1991.

61. Montgomery DL, Splett PL: Economic benefit of breast-feeding infants enrolled in WIC. J Am Diet Assoc 97:379, 1997.

62. Mothers Survey: Updated Breast-feeding Trend through 1996. Ross Products Division, Abbott Laboratories, Columbus, Ohio, 1998.

63. Newton N: Psychologic differences between breast and bottle feeding. In Jelliffe DB, Jelliffe EFP (eds): Symposium: The Uniqueness of Human Milk. Am J Clin Nutr 24:993, 1971.

64. Pope John Paul II, Solemn Papal Audience: Breastfeeding: Science and society. Food Nutr Bull 17:289, 1996.

65. Popkin BM, Bilsborrow RE, Akin JS: Breastfeeding patterns in low-income countries. Science 218:1088, 1982.

66. Popkin BM, Canahauti J, Bailey PE, et al: An evaluation of a national breastfeeding promotion programme in Honduras. J Biosoc Sci 23:5, 1991.

67. Puffer RR, Serrano CV: Patterns of mortality in childhood. Scientific Pub. No. 262, Washington, DC, Pan American Health Organization, 1973.

68. Queenan JT: Breastfeeding: It's an important gift. Obstet Gynecol 102:3, 2003.

69. Ramos CV, Almeida JAG: Maternal allegations for weaning: Qualitative study. J Pediatr 79:385, 2003.

70. Raphael D: The Tender Gift: Breast Feeding. New York, Schocken, 1976.

71. Reamer SB, Sugarman M: Breastfeeding beyond six months: Mothers' perceptions of the positive and negative consequences. J Trop Pediatr 33:93, 1987.

72. Report of the Surgeon General's Workshop on Breastfeeding and Human Lactation. Pub. No. HRS-D-MC

84-2. Washington, DC, Department of Health and Human Services, 1984.

73. Report of the Second Surgeon General's Workshop on Breastfeeding and Human Lactation. Washington, DC, National Center for Education in Maternal and Child Health, 1991.

74. Romagnob D, DiAugustine RP: The mammary gland: Protein factory of the future. Environ Health Perspect 102:644, 1994.

75. Ruvalcaba RHA: Stress-induced cessation of lactation. West J Med 146:228, 1987.

76. Ryan AS: The resurgence of breastfeeding in the United States. Pediatrics 99:2, 1997 (electronic article).

77. Ryan AS, Martinez GA: Breastfeeding and the working mother: A profile. Pediatrics 83:524, 1989.

78. Ryan AS, Rush D, Krieger FW, et al: Recent declines in breastfeeding in the United States, 1984 through 1989. Pediatrics 88:719, 1991.

79. Sarett HP, Bain KR, O'Leary JC: Decisions on breastfeeding or formula feeding and trends in infant-feeding practices. Am J Dis Child 137:719, 1983.

80. Sauls HS: Potential effects of demographic and other variables in studies comparing morbidity of breast-fed and bottle fed infants. Pediatrics 64:523, 1979.

81. Schwartz K, D'Arcy HJS, Gillespie B, et al: Factors associated with weaning in the first 3 months postpartum. J Fam Practice 51:439, 2002.

82. Scrimshaw NS, Taylor CE, Gordon JE: Interaction of nutrition and infection. WHO Monograph, No 29. Geneva, World Health Organization, 1968.

83. Sloper K, McKean L, Baum JD: Patterns of infant feeding in Oxford. Arch Dis Child 49:749, 1974.

84. Taylor J: The duty of nursing children. In Ratner H: The nursing mother: Historical insights from art and theology. Child Fam 8(4):19, 1949.

85. Toubas PL: Forgotten lessons of the past. Pierre Budin Perinatal Section News 17:2, 1992.

86. United States Breastfeeding Committee: Benefits of breastfeeding [issue paper]. Raleigh, NC: United States Breastfeeding Committee, 2002.

87. U.S. Department of Health and Human Services: Healthy People 2010 (conference edition, in two volumes). Washington, DC, DHHS, Jan. 2000.

88. Victora CG: Infection and disease: The impact of early weaning. Food Nutr Bull 17:390, 1996.

89. Victora CG, Smith PG, Barros FC, et al: Risk factors for death due to respiratory infections among Brazilian infants. Int J Epidemiol 18:918, 1989.

90. Victora CG, Smith PG, Vaughan JP, et al: Evidence for protection by breastfeeding against infant deaths from infectious diseases in Brazil. Lancet 2:319, 1987.

91. Watkins CJ, Leeder SR, Corkhill RT: The relationship between breast and bottle feeding and respiratory illness in the first year of life. J Epidemiol Community Health 33:180, 1979.

92. West CP: Factors influencing the duration of breastfeeding. J Biosoc Sci 12:325, 1980.

93. WHO: Infant and young child nutrition and progress in implementing the International Code of Marketing of Breast-milk Substitutes. Report by the Secretariat. Geneva, World Health Organization, 2003.

94. WHO/UNICEF: Protecting, promoting and supporting breastfeeding: The special role of maternity services, a joint WHO/UNICEF statement. Geneva, World Health Organization, 1989.

95. WHO/FAO: Diet, nutrition and the prevention of chronic diseases, a joint WHO/FAO report. Geneva, World Health Organization, 2003.

96. Wickes IG: A history of infant feeding. I. Primitive peoples, ancient works, Renaissance writers. Arch Dis Child 28:151, 1953.

97. Wickes IG: A history of infant feeding. II. Seventeenth and eighteenth centuries. Arch Dis Child 28:232, 1953.

98. Wolf JH: Don't kill your baby: Public health and the decline of breastfeeding in the 19th and 20th centuries. Columbus, Ohio, Ohio State University Press, 2001.

99. Wolf JH: Low breastfeeding rates and public health in the United States. Am J Pub Health 93:2000, 2003.

100. Woodbury RM: The relation between breast and artificial feeding and infant mortality. Am J Hyg 2:668, 1922.

101. Woo-Iun M, Gussler J, Smith N (eds): The International Breast-Feeding Compendium, 3rd ed. Columbus, Ohio, Ross Laboratories, 1984.

102. World Health Organization: Contemporary patterns of breastfeeding. In Report on the WHO Collaborative Study on Breast-feeding. Geneva, World Health Organization, 1981.

103. Wright AL, Holberg C, Taussig LM, et al: Infant-feeding practices among middle-class Anglos and Hispanics. Pediatrics 82:496, 1988.

104. Yalom M: A history of the breast. New York, Knopf, 1997.

105. Young HB, Buckley AE, Hamza B, et al: Milk and lactation: Some social and developmental correlates among 1,000 infants. Pediatrics 69:169, 1982.

2

Anatomy of the human breast

GROSS ANATOMY

The *mammary gland,* as the breast is medically termed, received its name from *mamma,* the Latin word for breast. The human mammary gland is the only organ that is not fully developed at birth. It experiences dramatic changes in size, shape, and function from birth through pregnancy, lactation, and ultimately involution. The gland undergoes three major phases of growth and development before pregnancy and lactation: in utero, during the first 2 years of life, and at puberty.

Embryonic development

The milk streak appears in the fourth week, when the embryo is 2.5 mm long. It becomes the milk line, or ridge, during the fifth week (2.5 to 5.5 mm). Mammary glands begin to develop in the 6-week-old embryo, continuing their proliferation until milk ducts are developed by the time of birth[36] (Tables 2-1 and 2-2). Embryologically, the mammary glands develop as ingrowths of the ectoderm into the underlying mesodermal tissue.[16] In the human embryo a thickened, raised area of the ectoderm can be recognized in the region of the future gland at the end of the fourth week of pregnancy. The thickened ectoderm becomes depressed into the underlying mesoderm, and thus the surface of the mammary area soon becomes flat and finally sinks below the level of the surrounding epidermis. The mesoderm in contact with the ingrowth of the ectoderm is compressed, and its elements become arranged in concentric layers, which at a later stage give rise to the gland's stroma. The ingrowing mass of ectodermal cells soon becomes pouch or pear shaped and then grows out into the surrounding mesoderm as a number of solid processes that represent the gland's future ducts. These processes, by dividing and branching, give rise to the future lobes and lobules and, much later, to the alveoli.

By 16 weeks' gestation, the branching stage has produced 15 to 25 epithelial strips that represent future secretory alveoli. At this time the secondary mammary anlage (primordium) develops. The secondary mammary anlage then develops with elements of hair follicles, sebaceous glands, and sweat glands, as well as the Montgomery glands, around the alveoli. Mesenchymal cells differentiate into the smooth muscle of the nipple and areola between 12 and 16 weeks of gestation.[22] Thus far, development is independent of hormone stimulation. By 28 weeks' gestation, placental sex hormones enter the fetal circulation and induce canalization.[22]

The lumina develop in the outgrowths, forming the lactiferous ducts and their branches. The lactiferous ducts open into a shallow epithelial depression known as the *mammary pit.* The pit becomes elevated as a result of the mesenchymal proliferation

TABLE 2-1	**Embryonic timetable of breast development in the human**	
Age of embryo (wk)	**Crown-rump length of embryo (mean)**	**Developmental stage**
4	2.5 mm	Mammary streak
5	2.5–5.5 mm	Milk line, or milk ridge
6	5.5–11 mm	Parenchymal cells proliferate
7–8	11–25 mm	Mammary disk progresses to globular stage
9	25–30 mm	Cone stage: inward growth of parenchyma
10–12	30–68 mm	Epithelial buds sprout from invading parenchyma
12–13	68 mm–5 cm	Indentation buds become lobular with notching at epithelial-stromal border
15	10 cm	Buds branch into 15–25 epithelial strips
20–24	20 cm	Solid cords canalize by desquamation and lysis
24–32	30 cm	Further canalization
32–40	35–50 cm	Lobular-alveolar development

Data from Russo J, Russo IH: Development of the human mammary gland. In Neville MC, Daniel CW (eds): The Mammary Gland. New York, Plenum, 1987.

forming the nipple and areola. An inverted nipple is a result of the failure of the pit to elevate.[3] A lumen is formed in each part of the branching system of cellular processes after 32 weeks' gestation. Near term, about 15 to 25 mammary ducts form the fetal mammary gland (Fig. 2-1). Duct and sebaceous glands coalesce near the epidermis. Parenchymal differentiation occurs with the development of lobular-alveolar structures that contain colostrum. This change occurs at 32 to 40 weeks and is called the end-vesicle stage.

Fetal and prepubertal development

The mammary glands of male and female fetuses of 13 to 40 weeks' gestation were studied ultrastructurally by Tobon and Salazar.[32] This work confirms morphologic developments in the fetal breast tissue in response to hormonal stimuli that are similar to those in the maternal breast. The Golgi system and abundant reticula with dilated cisternae filled with finely granular material are present in the cellular structure. Abundant mitochondria and lipid droplets are observed. Proliferation and conditioning of the epithelial cells are evident, and in the last trimester there are microvilli along the ductal lumen accompanied by large cytoplasmic protrusions (see Table 2-2).

Study of the ultrastructure of the fetal breast may help in understanding the functional lactating breast. The secretion of a fluid resembling milk may take place at birth as a result of maternal hormones that have passed across the placenta into the fetal circulation. The lactiferous sinuses appear before birth as swellings of the developing ducts.

An extensive anatomic and histologic study of the human infant breast revealed an epithelial differentiation that followed a chronologic pattern, starting with secretory changes and apparently going through a period of apocrine metaplasia before the postsecretory changes and involution.[2] The embryonic fat probably plays a role in growth and morphogenesis of the ductal system. No distinguishing features were found between the breasts of female and male infants,[2] however.

The terminal end buds, lateral buds, and lobules of three to five alveolar buds predominate in prepubertal tissue. Lobules of alveolar buds and lobules of up to 60 ductules predominate in pubertal

TABLE 2-2 Stages of mammary development

Developmental stage	Hormonal regulation	Local factors	Description
Embryogenesis	???	Fat pad necessary for ductal extension	Epithelial bud develops in 18- to 19-week fetus, extending a short distance into mammary fat pad with blind ducts that become canalized; some milk secretion may be present at birth
Pubertal development	—	—	—
Prior to onset of menses	Estrogen, GH	IGF-1, HGF, TGF-β, ???	Ductal extension into the mammary fat pad; branching morphogenesis
After onset of menses	Estrogen, progesterone, PRL?		Lobular development with formation of terminal duct lobular unit
Development in pregnancy	Progesterone, PRL, placental lactogen	HER, ???	Alveolus formation; partial cellular differentiation
Transition: lactogenesis	Progesterone withdrawal, PRL, glucocorticoid	Unknown	Onset of milk secretion: stage I, midpregnancy; stage II, parturition
Lactation	PRL, oxytocin	FIL, stretch	Ongoing milk secretion, milk ejection
Involution	Withdrawal of prolactin	Milk stasis (FIL??)	Alveolar epithelium undergoes apoptosis and remodeling and gland reverts to pre-pregnant state

GH, growth hormone; IGF-1, insulin-like growth factor-1; HGF, human growth factor; TGF-β, transforming growth factor-β; PRL, prolactin; HER, herregulin; FIL, feedback inhibitor of lactation.
From Neville MC: Breastfeeding, part I: The evidence for breastfeeding. Anatomy and physiology of lactation. Pediatr Clin North Am. 48:13, 2001.

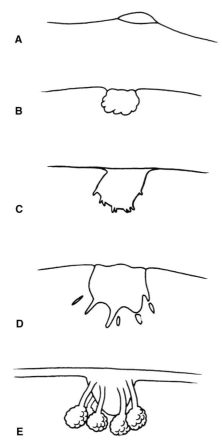

Figure 2-1. Evolution of nipple. **A,** Thickening of epidermis with formation of primary bud. **B,** Growth of bud into mesenchyma. **C,** Formation of solid secondary buds. **D,** Formation of mammary pit and vacuolation of buds to form epithelial-lined ducts. **E,** Lactiferous ducts proliferate. Areola is formed. Nipple is inverted initially. (Modified from Weatherly-White RCA: Plastic Surgery of the Female Breast. Hagerstown, Md., Harper & Row, 1980.)

females. In prepuberty, these epithelium-lined ducts will bud out to form alveoli when stimulated by hormones of menarche (Fig. 2-1).

The breast is made up of glandular tissue, supporting connective tissue, and protective fatty tissue. Immediately after birth, the newborn's breast may even be swollen and secreting a small amount of milk, often termed *witch's milk*. This phenomenon, common among both male and female infants,

is caused by the stimulation of the infant's mammary glands by the same hormones produced by the placenta to prepare the mother's breast for lactation. This secretory activity subsides within 3 to 4 weeks, and then the mammary glands are inactive until shortly before the onset of puberty, when hormones begin to stimulate growth again. During childhood (prepuberty), the gland merely keeps pace with physical growth (Figs. 2-2 and 2-3).

The molecular biology of mammary gland development depends on a combination of systemic mammotropic hormones plus local cell-to-cell interactions. A variety of growth factors mediate the local cell interactions. These factors include the epidermal growth factor (EGF), transforming growth factor-β (TGF-β), fibroblast growth factor (FGF), and the *Wnt* gene families. In the developing breast these factors are thought to act in concert with systemic hormones.[19]

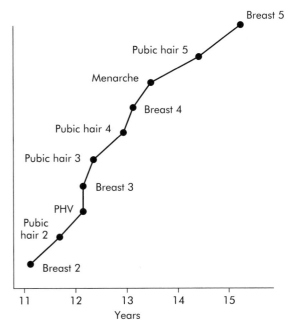

Figure 2-2. Pubertal development in the female. The sequence and mean ages of pubertal events in females, adapted from the data of Marshall and Tanner. PHV, peak height velocity. (From Root AW: Endocrinology of puberty. J Pediatr 83:1, 1973.)

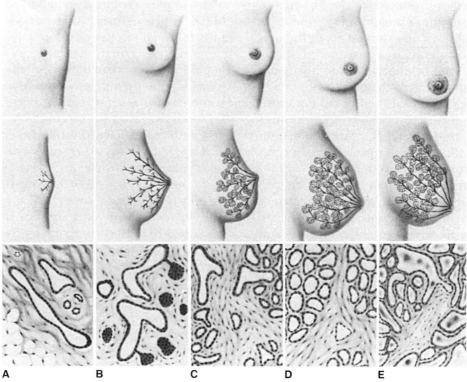

A   B   C   D   E

Figure 2-3.   Female breast from infancy to lactation with corresponding cross section and duct structure. **A, B,** and **C,** Gradual development of well-differentiated ductular and peripheral lobular-alveolar system. **D,** Ductular sprouting and intensified peripheral lobular-alveolar development in pregnancy. Glandular luminal cells begin actively synthesizing milk fat and proteins near term; only small amounts are released into lumen. **E,** With postpartum withdrawal of luteal and placental sex steroids and placental lactogen, prolactin is able to induce full secretory activity of alveolar cells and release of milk into alveoli and smaller ducts.

Pubertal development

The development of the human breast involves two distinct processes: organogenesis and milk production.[8] *Organogenesis* involves ductal and lobular growth and begins before and continues through puberty, resulting in growth of the breast parenchyma with its surrounding fat pad. When the female is between 10 and 12 years of age, just before puberty, the ductal tree extends and generates its branching pattern, lengthening the existing ducts, dichotomously branching the growing ductal tips, and monopodially branching with the growth of the lateral buds at the sides of the ducts (Tables 2-2 and 2-3). During this period of rapid growth, the ducts can develop bulbous terminal end buds. The formation of alveolar buds begins within a year or two of the onset of menses. The sprouting of new alveolar buds continues for several years, producing alveolar lobes.[26]

Anatomic location

The breast is located in the superficial fascia between the second rib and sixth intercostal cartilage and is superficial to the pectoralis major muscle.[18] It tends to overlap this muscle inferiorly

TABLE 2-3   Phases of breast development

Phase	Age (yr)	Developmental characteristics
I	Puberty	Preadolescent elevation of nipple with no palpable glandular tissue or areolar pigmentation
II	11.1 ± 1.1	Presence of glandular tissue in subareolar region; nipple and breast project as single mound from chest wall
III	12.2 ± 1.09	Increase in amount of readily palpable glandular tissue, with enlargement of breast and increased diameter and pigmentation of areola; contour of breast and nipple remains in single plane
IV	13.1 ± 1.15	Enlargement of areola and increased areolar pigmentation; nipple and areola form secondary mound above breast level
V	15.3 ± 1.7	Final adolescent development of smooth contour with no projection of areola and nipple

Modified from Tanner JM: Wachstun und Reifung des Menschen. Stuttgart, Thieme-Verlag, 1962.

to become superficial to the external oblique and serratus anterior muscles. It measures 10 to 12 cm in diameter. It is located horizontally from the parasternal to midaxillary line. The central thickness of the breast is 5 to 7 cm (Fig. 2-4).

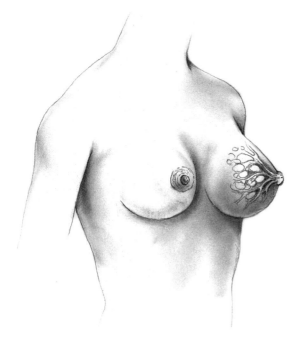

Figure 2-4. Mammary gland in longitudinal cross section showing mature, nonlactating duct system.

At puberty, the breasts in the female enlarge to their adult size, with the left frequently slightly larger than the right.[35] In a nonpregnant woman the mature breast weighs approximately 200 g. During pregnancy, breast size and weight increase; thus, when a pregnant woman is near term, the breast weighs 400 to 600 g. During lactation the breast weighs 600 to 800 g (see Fig. 2-3).

The shape of the breast varies from woman to woman, just as body build and facial characteristics do. Racial variations may be associated with discoidal, hemispheric, pear-shaped, or conical forms. Typically, the breast is dome-shaped or conic in adolescence, becoming more hemispheric and finally pendulous in the parous female. Mammary glandular tissue projects somewhat into the axillary region. This is known as the *tail of Spence* (see Fig. 2-6). Mammary tissue in the axilla, which is connected to the central duct system, becomes more obvious during pregnancy and produces milk during lactation, when it may cause various symptoms (see Chapter 8).[1] The tail of Spence is distinguished from a supernumerary gland because it connects to the normal duct system.

The three major structures of the breast are skin, subcutaneous tissue, and corpus mammae. The *corpus mammae* is the breast mass that remains after freeing the breast from the deep attachments and removing the skin, subcutaneous connective tissue, and adipose tissue.

The breasts of the adult female are always paired and develop from a line of glandular tissue found in the fetus and known as the *milk line*. This milk streak, or *galactic band*, develops from the axilla to the groin during the fifth week of embryonic life.[22] In the thoracic region, the band develops into a ridge, and the rest of the band regresses (Fig. 2-5).

Abnormalities

In some women, additional residual tissue of the galactic band remains as mammary tissue, which

can develop anywhere along this line. *Hypermastia* is the presence of accessory mammary glands, which are phylogenic remnants of the embryonic mammary ridge resulting from incomplete regression or dispersion of the primitive galactic band (see Fig. 2-5). Because of this origin, accessory nipples and glandular tissue may be found along these lines, which extend from the clavicular to the inguinal regions. Occasionally, supernumerary glands are found in the urogenital region, on the buttocks, or on the back as well.[36] The glands are derived from the ectoderm, whereas the connective tissue stroma is mesodermal in origin.

The accessory tissue may involve the corpus mammae, the areola, and the nipple.[23] From 2% to 6% of women have hypermastia. The response of hypermastia to pregnancy and lactation depends on the tissue present.

Box 2-1 defines other selected breast abnormalities. *Symmastia* is a webbing across the midline between the breasts, which are usually symmetric.[3] A more common variation is the presternal confluence representing blending of breast tissue associated with large breasts. These abnormalities are ectodermal in origin and have many variations, from an empty skin web to the presence of significant glandular tissue. Little is known about their function, but several procedures exist for their surgical amelioration.[3]

Congenital absence of the breast is called *amastia,* which is rare. When a nipple is present but there is no breast tissue, the condition is called

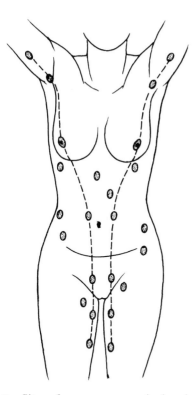

Figure 2-5. Sites of supernumerary nipples along milk line. Ectopic nipples, areolae, or breast tissue can develop from groin to axilla and upper inner arm. They can lactate or undergo malignant change. (Modified from Weatherly-White RCA: Plastic Surgery of the Female Breast. Hagerstown, Md., Harper & Row, 1980.)

BOX 2-1   Breast abnormalities

Accessory breast Any tissue outside the two major glands
Amastia Congenital absence of breast and nipple
Amazia Nipple without breast tissue
Hyperadenia Mammary tissue without nipple
Hypoplasia Underdevelopment of breast
Polythelia Supernumerary nipple(s) (also hyperthelia)
Symmastia Webbing between breasts

amazia. Another term for this condition when it occurs in addition to a normal breast is *hyperthelia.*

Some have suggested a relationship between *polythelia* (supernumerary nipple) and renal defect. Polythelia has also been associated with renal agenesis, renal cell carcinoma, obstructive disease, and supernumerary kidneys.[25] Others have described associations with congenital cardiac anomalies, pyloric stenosis, ear abnormalities, and arthrogryposis multiplex congenita.[3] After careful study of 65 patients with a supernumerary nipple, Hersh and associates[13] found 7 (11%) individuals who had significant renal lesions, somewhat less than the incidence reported originally. Apparently no association exists in blacks.

Poland syndrome, first described in 1841 (Box 2-2), includes absence of the pectoral muscle, chest wall deformity, and breast anomalies.[22] It is now known also to include symbrachydactyly, with hypoplasia of the middle phalanges and central skin webbing. *Breast hypoplasia* is underdevelopment of the breast. Although 90% of cases of breast hypoplasia are associated with hypoplasia of the pectoral muscles, 92% of women with pectoral muscle abnormalities have normal breasts. Box 2-2 lists

---

BOX 2-2   Types of breast hypoplasia, hyperplasia, and acquired abnormalities

Unilateral hypoplasia, contralateral breast normal
Bilateral hypoplasia with asymmetry
Unilateral hyperplasia, contralateral breast normal
Bilateral hyperplasia with asymmetry
Unilateral hypoplasia, contralateral breast hyperplasia
Unilateral hypoplasia of breast, thorax, and pectoral muscles (Poland syndrome)
Acquired abnormalities caused by trauma, burns, radiation treatment for hemangioma or intrathoracic disease, chest tube insertion in infancy, and preadolescent biopsy

Modified from Osbourne MP: Breast development and anatomy. In Harris JR, Lippman ME, Morrow M, Hellman S (eds): Diseases of the Breast. Philadelphia, Lippincott-Raven, 1996.

---

types of breast hypoplasia, *hyperplasia* (overdevelopment), and acquired breast abnormalities.

Hyperadenia is the presence of mammary tissue without nipples. The swelling and secretion of this tissue may produce pain during lactation. Occasionally, aberrant breast tissue can cause discomfort or embarrassment in adolescence and during menses, especially when located in the axilla.[15] Mammographic features of normal accessory axillary breast tissue were reviewed by Adler and coworkers[1] in 13 women who were diagnosed on routine mammography. Seven of these women had a mass or fullness on physical examination; one was seen post partum because of pain; nine were asymptomatic. They ranged in age from 31 to 67 years. Radiographically, the accessory tissue resembled the rest of the normal glandular tissue but was separate from it. It occurred on the right in 11 of the 13 women. The accessory tissue was recognized as a normal developmental variant, distinguishable from the frequent axillary tail of Spence, which represents a direct extension from the outer margin of the main mass of glandular tissue.

On mammography, accessory tissue is best visualized on oblique and exaggerated craniocaudal views. In rare cases, it may be appropriate to remove the tissue surgically, a treatment well known to experienced plastic surgeons. If treatment is not initiated before pregnancy and lactation in these women, pain and swelling will be intensified and may progress to mastitis or the necessity to terminate lactation.

Apart from physiologic variations, other conditions of abnormal anatomy include *hypomastia* (abnormally small breasts), hypertrophy, and inequality.

Acquired abnormalities

The most common cause of acquired breast abnormality is iatrogenic and most commonly caused by chest wall trauma in premature infants when chest tubes are inserted. Biopsy in prepubertal females may remove vital tissues. Cutaneous burns to the chest wall may result in scaring and breast deformity. Such findings do not automatically prevent breastfeeding. The lactation center at the University of Rochester has been consulted about several such women who have been able to breastfeed with assistance and encouragement in spite of scarring and seeming deformity.

Corpus mammae

The mammary gland is an orderly conglomeration of a variable number of independent glands. It undergoes a series of changes that can be divided into developmental and differentiation phases. Surgical dissection of many postoperative specimens has contributed more precise information about the anatomic structure of the breast.[6] The ramifications of the lactiferous ducts and stroma were carefully studied by Hicken,[14] who reported that in 95% of women the ducts ascend into the axilla, occasionally following the brachial plexus and axillary vessels into the apex of the axilla. Ducts are found in the epigastric region in 15% of women. In rare cases, ducts cross the midline (Fig. 2-6).

The morphology of the corpus mammae includes two major divisions, the parenchyma and the stroma.[1] The *parenchyma* includes the ductular-lobular-alveolar structures. It is composed of the alveolar gland with treelike ductular branching alveoli, which are approximately 0.12 mm in diameter. The ducts are approximately 2 mm in diameter. The lactiferous sinuses are 5 to 8 mm in diameter. The lobi, which are arranged like spokes converging on the central nipple, are 15 to 25 in number. Each lobus is divided again into 20 to 40 lobuli, and each lobulus is again subdivided into 10 to 100 alveoli, or tubulosaccular secretory units. The *stroma* includes the connective tissue, fat tissue, blood vessels, nerves, and lymphatics.[18]

The mass of tissue in the breast consists of the tubuloalveolar glands embedded in fat (the adipose tissue), giving the gland its smooth, rounded contour. The mammary fat pad is essential for the proliferation and differentiation of the mammary epithelium, providing the necessary space, support, and local control for duct elongation and, ultimately, lobuloalveolar proliferation. Each gland

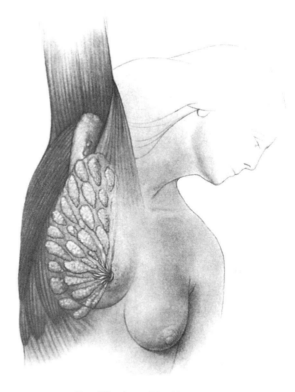

Figure 2-6. Ramification of lactiferous ducts and mammary tissue. Ducts extend onto upper medial aspect of arm, to midline, and into epigastrium. Composite drawing from mammographic studies. (Modified from Hicken NF: Mastectomy: Pathologic study demonstrating why most mastectomies result in incomplete removal of the mammary gland. Arch Surg 40:6, 1940.)

forms a lobe of the breast, and the lobes are separated by connective tissue septa. These septa attach to the skin. Each tubuloalveolar gland opens into a lactiferous duct, which leads into a more elastic area, the lactiferous sinus; there is a slight constriction before the sinus opens onto the surface of the nipple (Fig. 2-7). Extension of ducts within the fat pad is orderly. The fat pad is critical to the development of the arborization. An inhibitory zone into which other ducts cannot penetrate exists around each duct, and development does not normally proceed beyond the duct end-bud stage before puberty.[2]

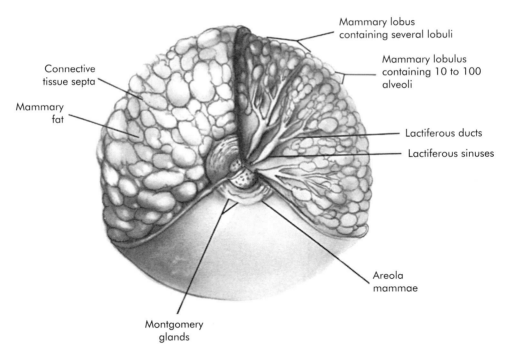

Figure 2-7.   Morphology of mature breast with dissection to reveal mammary fat and duct system.

Nipple and areola

The skin of the breast includes the nipple, areola, and general skin. The skin is the thin, flexible, elastic cover of the breast and is adherent to the fat-laden subcutaneous tissue. It contains hair, sebaceous glands, and apocrine sweat glands. The nipple, or *papilla mammae,* is a conic elevation located in the center of the areola at about the fourth intercostal space, slightly below the midpoint of the breast. Although very different in size, the nipples and areolae of women and men are qualitatively identical.[20] The nipple contains 15 to 25 milk ducts. Each of the tubuloalveolar glands that make up the breast opens onto the nipple by a separate opening. The nipple also contains smooth muscle fibers and is richly innervated with sensory nerve endings and Meissner corpuscles in the dermal papillae; it is well supplied with sebaceous and apocrine sweat glands but no hair.

The nipple is surrounded by the areola, or *areola mammae,* a circular pigmented area. It is usually faintly darker before pregnancy, turning reddish brown during pregnancy, and always maintaining some darker pigmentation thereafter. The average areola measures 15 to 16 mm in diameter, although the range is great, enlarging during pregnancy and lactation. The pigmentation results from many melanocytes distributed throughout the skin and glands. The understructure of the epidermis of the areola is not as elaborate as that of the nipple but is intermediate to that of the surrounding skin. The nipple and areola are extremely elastic.

Little or no true lobuloalveolar development occurs before the first pregnancy. A framework is laid down, within which the specialized secretory cells will proliferate (Fig. 2-8).[7] The framework forms a vital part of the gland's overall developmental course, and maldevelopment or trauma during fetal or juvenile life can seriously reduce the size and secretory potential of the mature gland.

Montgomery tubercles, containing the ductular openings of sebaceous and lactiferous glands, are

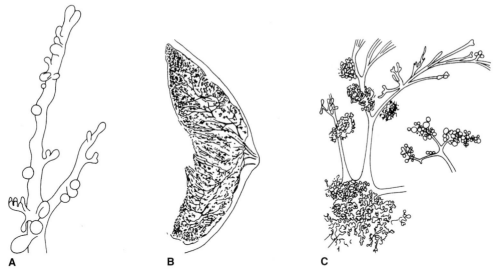

A   **B**   **C**

Figure 2-8. **A,** Duct end from a 15-year-old nulligravida on second day of menstruation showing typical form of puberty: a coarsely diversified system of thick, mostly well-filled ducts with round, often ball-shaped or half-ball-shaped ends. Note use of connective tissue as guiding tracts, circumvention of fat tissue, and paucity of secretory alveoli. **B,** Sagittal section through milk gland of a nulligravida 19-year-old between menses (died of skull fracture). Note massive body of connective tissue without preserved lobes of fatty tissue and richness of connective tissue with respective richness of parenchyma. Note also distribution of larger ducts in superficial parallel connective tissue septum of former subcutaneous fat tissue and smaller ducts in vertical septa. Thin section; drawing with Busch magnifying glasses. **C,** Gland of a nulligravida 19-year-old (part of a 4-mm-thick section). Bushy short sprout and duct build long sprout, with the latter in acute angled bifurcation, often lying very close to each other. This demonstrates development of ductal and secretory elements during menstrual cycle; however, connective tissue and fat are predominant. (From Dabelow A: Die Milchdrüse. In Handbuch der Mikroskopischen Anatomie des Menschen, Vol. III, Part 3. Berlin, Springer-Verlag, 1957.)

present in the areola,[30] as are sweat glands and smaller, free sebaceous glands. The Montgomery glands become enlarged and look like small pimples during pregnancy and lactation (Fig. 2-9). They secrete a substance that lubricates and protects the nipples and areolae during pregnancy and lactation. A small amount of milk is also secreted from these tubercles. After lactation, these glands recede again to their former unobtrusive state.

Light microscopy has shown that Morgagni was correct in 1719 when he first described the 12 to 20 areolar glands and noted them to be sebaceous and to include lactiferous structures as well. Building on the original work, in 1837 Montgomery pre-

pared a more detailed treatise on the tubercle itself and named it after himself. Serial sections of 35 tubercles also showed that there were lactiferous ducts from the deeper breast parenchyma ascending into the sebaceous glands of the tubercle (see Fig. 2-9). The sebaceous gland itself was no different from those of the skin or those associated with the terminal lactiferous ducts of the nipple. The mammary duct was lined with two layers of cuboidal to columnar cells. They arose from the underlying mammary lobules through the subcutaneous tissues and into the region of the sebaceous gland. The terminal portion of the mammary duct in some cases joined the duct to the sebaceous

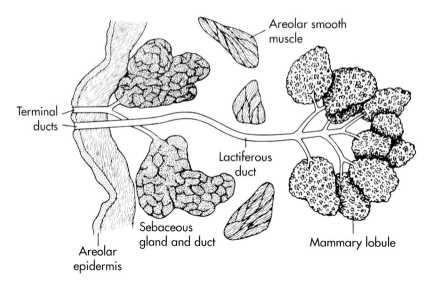

Figure 2-9. Tubercle of Montgomery and underlying structures. Lactiferous duct may join seba-ceous gland ducts and terminate at common opening in areolar epidermis as shown. (Modified from Smith DM, Peters TG, Donegan WL: Montgomery's areolar tubercle. A light microscopic study. Arch Pathol Lab Med 106:62, 1982.)

gland and in other cases opened separately but close to it. The ducts appear to be a miniature of the major mammary system. Sebaceous and mammary ductal components underlie the areolar tubercle.

The areola and nipple are darker than the rest of the breast, ranging from light pink in fair-skinned women to dark brown in others. The areola's darker color may be a visual signal to newborns so that they will close their mouth on the areola, not on the nip-ple alone, to obtain milk. Nipple erection is induced by tactile, sensory, and autonomic sympathetic stim-uli. The corium (dermis) of the areola lacks fat but contains smooth muscle and collagenous and elastic connective tissue fibers in radial and circular arrangements. The dermis of the nipple and the are-ola contains many multibranched, free nerve fiber endings. Local venostasis and hyperemia occur to enhance the process of erection of the nipple because the nipple and areola are rich in arteriove-nous anastomoses. The glabrous skin of the nipple is wrinkled, containing large papillae of the corium.

Each nipple contains 15 to 25 lactiferous ducts surrounded by fibromuscular tissue (Figs. 2-10,

2-11, 2-12, and 2-13). These ducts end as small ori-fices near the tip of the nipple. Within the nipple, the lactiferous ducts may merge. The ductular ori-fices therefore are sometimes fewer in number than the respective breast lobi. The milk ducts within the nipple dilate at the nipple base into the cone-shaped ampullae of milk sinuses. The ampullae function as temporary milk containers during a feeding but con-tain only epithelial debris in the nonlactating state. The use of ultrasound imagery of the contralateral

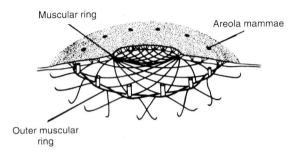

Figure 2-10. Nipple and areola with smooth muscula-ture structure.

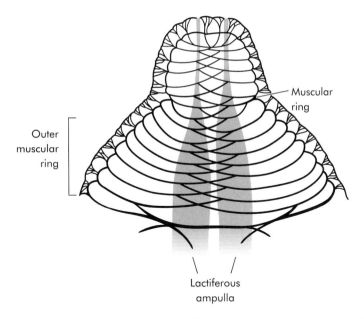

Figure 2-11. Smooth musculature of areola and nipple in cross section when contracted to make nipple erect.

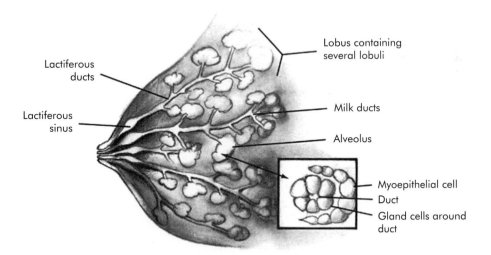

Figure 2-12. Simplified schematic drawing of duct system with cross section of myoepithelial cells around duct opening. Myoepithelial cells contract to eject milk.

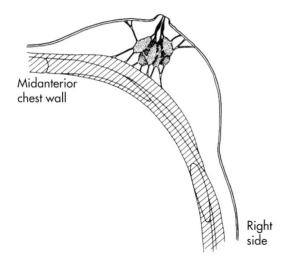

Midanterior
chest wall

Right
side

Figure 2-13. Horizontal cross section of breast ligaments, looking from head to foot. Ligaments of Cooper suspend 15 to 20 lobes of breast within matrix of fat. They are attached to lobes, skin, and deep fascia.

breast while the infant is nursing on the other breast or the other breast is being pumped has shown that the profound elasticity of the ductal system allows for an acute increase in milk duct diameter during let-down and milk production (see Fig. 2-12A). Contrary to the sketches of the breast in so many professional and lay journals, the ducts do not form sinuses just before the nipple.[12] The lining of the infundibular and ampullar parts of the lactiferous ducts consists of an 8- to 10-cell layered squamous epithelium. The bulk of the nipple is composed of smooth musculature, which represents a closing mechanism for the milk ducts and sinuses of the nipple (see Figs. 2-10 and 2-11). The milk ducts in the nipple are embedded in stretchable and mobile connective tissue. The inner longitudinal muscular arrangements and the outer, more circular and radial arrangements do not obstruct the milk ducts. Tangential fibers also branch off from the more circular muscular fibers of the nipple bases to the outer circular muscular range.

The functions of the muscular fibroelastic system of the areola and nipple include decreasing the surface area of the areola, producing nipple erec-

tion, and emptying the swollen ducts during nursing. When the nipple erects because of tactile, thermal, or sexual stimulation, the system causes the nipple to become smaller, firmer, everted, and more prominent (Fig. 2-11).

The mammary tissues are enveloped by the superficial pectoral fascia, and the breast is fixed by fibrous bands to the overlying skin and the underlying pectoral fascia, which are known as *ligaments of Cooper* (see Fig. 2-13). The glandular part of the breast is surrounded by a fat layer that seldom extends beyond the lower border of the pectoralis major muscle. The breast is attached to the muscles between the ribs, the clavicle, and the bones of the upper arm near the shoulder. The breast itself contains no supporting muscles and relies on ligaments to sustain its shape.

Blood supply

The blood supply to the breast is from branches of the intercostal arteries and the perforating branches of the internal thoracic artery; the third, fourth, and fifth are usually most prominent. The major blood supply to the breast is provided by the internal mammary artery and the lateral thoracic artery. A small supply is obtained from the intercostal arteries and the arterial branches of the axillary and subclavian arteries, but this contribution is minimal; 60% of the total breast tissue, especially the medial and central part, receives blood from the internal mammary artery. All the mammary branches of this artery lead transversely to the nipple and anastomoses, with branches coming from the lateral thoracic artery.[6] Anastomoses with intercostal arteries are less common, but the blood supply to the nipple is extensive and close to the surface, contributing to the richer color. Many areas of the breast are supplied by two or three arterial sources (Fig. 2-14).

The venous supply parallels the arterial supply and bears similar names. The veins drain the breast and enter the fascia, muscle layers, and intercostal spaces at the same point. The veins end in the internal thoracic and the axillary veins. Some veins may reach the external jugular vein. The veins create an

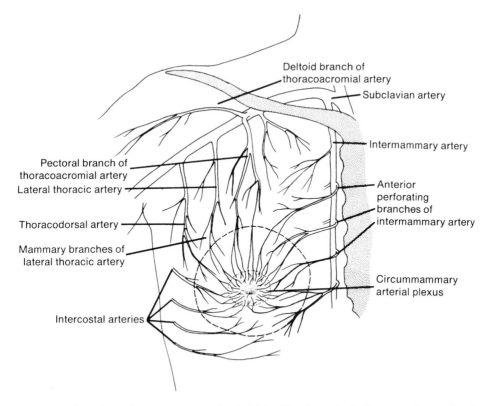

Figure 2-14. Blood supply to mammary gland. Major blood supply is from anterior perforating branches of internal mammary artery.

anastomotic circle around the base of the papilla, called the *circulus venosis*.[4]

Lymphatic drainage

The lymphatic drainage of the breast has been the subject of considerable study because of the frequency of breast cancer, but it has significance for the lactating breast as well. The lymphatic drainage can be quite extensive. The main drainage is to axillary nodes and to the parasternal nodes along the internal thoracic artery inside the thoracic cavity. The lymphatics of the breast originate in the lymph capillaries of the mammary connective tissue, which surrounds the mammary structures, and drain through the deep substance of the breast. The subepithelial or papillary plexus of the lympatics of the breast is confluent with the subepithelial lymphatics over the surface of the body. These valveless lymphatics communicate with subdermal lymphatic vessels and merge with the subareolar plexus.[22]

The lymph drainage of the breast consists of the superficial or cutaneous section, the areola, and the glandular or deep-tissue section. Other points of drainage are to pectoral nodes between the pectoralis major and minor muscles and to the subclavicular nodes in the neck deep to the clavicle. Flow from the deep subcutaneous and intramammary lymphatic vessels travels centrifugally toward the axilla and the internal mammary lymph nodes. The recent physiologic studies have disproved the former hypothesis of centripetal flow toward the subareolar plexus. About 97% of lymph flow is into the axillary nodes.[22] Some transmammary lymph drainage occurs to the opposite breast as well as to subdiaphragmatic lymphatics that lead ultimately to the liver and intraabdominal nodes (Fig. 2-15).

Innervation

The nerves of the breast are from branches of the fourth, fifth, and sixth intercostal nerves and consist of sensory fibers innervating the smooth muscles in the nipple and blood vessels. The sensory innervation of the nipple and areola is extensive and consists of both autonomic and sensory nerves. A detailed anatomic and clinical study of the nipple-areola complex showed that it is innervated from the lateral cutaneous branch of the fourth intercostal nerve, which penetrates the posterior aspect of the breast at the intersection of the fourth

intercostal space and the pectoralis major muscle (4 o'clock on the left breast and 8 o'clock on the right breast).[9] The nerve divides into five fasciculi, one central to the nipple, two upper, and two lower branches (always at 5 and 7 o'clock, left and right side, respectively) (Figs. 2-16 and 2-17).

The innervation of the corpus mammae is minimal by comparison and predominantly autonomic. No parasympathetic or cholinergic fibers supply any part of the breast. No ganglia are found in mammary tissue. Norepinephrine-containing nerve fibers are abundant among the smooth muscle cells of the nipple and at the interface between the media and adventitia of the breast arteries. Physiologic observations demonstrate that the efferent nerves to these structures are sympathetic adrenergic.

The majority of the mammary nerves follow the arteries and arterioles and supply these structures.

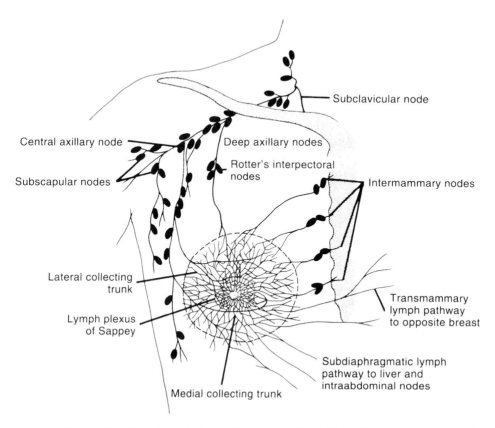

Figure 2-15.   Lymphatic drainage of mammary gland. Major drainage is toward axilla.

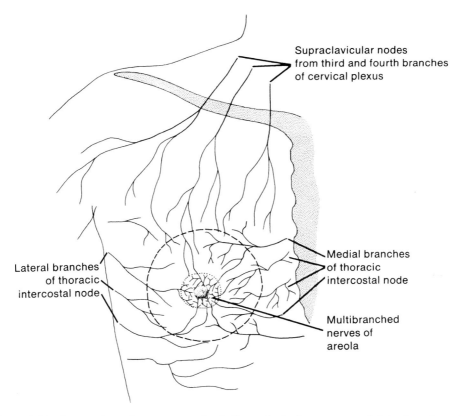

Supraclavicular nodes
from third and fourth branches
of cervical plexus

Lateral branches
of thoracic
intercostal node

Medial branches
of thoracic
intercostal node

Multibranched
nerves of
areola

Figure 2-16. Innervation of mammary gland. Supraclavicular nerves and lateral and medial branches of intercostal nerves provide sensory innervation. Sympathetic and motor nerves are provided by supracervical and intercostal nerves.

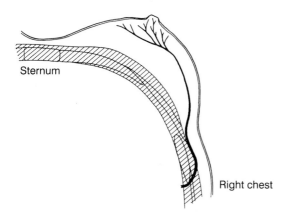

Sternum

Right chest

Figure 2-17. Cross section of nerve supply of breast and nipple. Cutaneous nerves run close to deep fascia before turning outward toward skin.

A few fibers from the perivascular networks course along the walls of the ducts. They may correspond to sensory fibers for sensing milk pressure. No innervation of mammary myoepithelial cells has been identified. It can therefore be concluded that secretory activities of the acinar epithelium depend on hormonal stimulation, such as that of oxytocin and other hormones, and are not stimulated via the nervous system directly.

Stimulation of the sensory nerve fibers or sensory receptors does induce the release of adenohypophyseal prolactin and neurohypophyseal oxytocin via an afferent sensory reflex pathway whereby stimuli reach the hypothalamus. Sympathetic mammary stimulation causes the contraction of the small myoepithelial cells of the areola and the nipple.

The locally released norepinephrine induces stimulation of the myoepithelial adrenergic receptors, causing muscular relaxation. In the absence of parasympathetic activity, a minor physiologic catamine inhibitory effect on the mammary myoepithelium may exist, which is overcome by oxytocin release during suckling, inducing myoepithelial contraction.

The supraclavicular nerves supply the sensory fibers for innervation of the upper cutaneous parts of the breast. Branches of the intercostal nerves provide the major sensory innervation of the mammary gland. The sympathetic sensory and motor fibers are derived from the supraclavicular and intercostal nerves, respectively. Sympathetic fibers run only along the mammary gland—supplying arteries to innervate the glandular body. There is relatively restricted innervation to the epidermal parts of the nipple and areola, leading to lack of superficial sensory acuity.

Courtiss and Goldwyn[5] measured breast sensation in a large number of women using a device that emitted a variable current producing a burning sensation when the threshold was exceeded. The areola was shown to be the most sensitive and the nipple the least sensitive, with the skin of the breast intermediate. Thus the skin in these areas responds only to major stimuli, such as sucking. The relatively large number of dermal nerve endings provides a high mammary responsiveness toward stimuli for elicitation of the sucking reflex. The neuroreflex induces adequate release of both prolactin and oxytocin. It appears that, in addition to the hormonal actions, breast nerves can also influence the mammary blood supply and milk secretion. Abnormalities of sensory or autonomic nerve distributions in the areola and nipple therefore could impair adequate lactation, especially in the functioning of the let-down reflex and the secretion of prolactin and oxytocin.

In summary, the somatic sensory cutaneous nerve supply of the breast includes the supraclavicular nerves and the thoracic intercostal nerves. The autonomic motor nerve supply of the breast is derived from the sympathetic fibers of the intercostal nerves, which supply the smooth muscula-ture of the areola and the nipple. The autonomic supply is also derived from sympathetic fibers of the accompanying arteries, which innervate the smooth musculature of the inner glandular blood vessel walls to produce constriction. The nerve supply to the area of the areola and the nipple includes free sensory nerve endings, tactile corpuscles to the papillae of the corium of the nipple and areola, and the fibers around the larger lactiferous duct and in the dermis of the areola and peripheral breast. All cutaneous nerves run radially to the glandular body toward the nipple. The nerve supply to the inner gland is sparse and contains only sympathetic nerves accompanying blood vessels (see Fig. 2-16).

MICROSCOPIC ANATOMY

After many decades of neglect since the phylogenic studies of the mammary gland in the 1800s and early 1900s, the mammary gland has become one of the most studied organs because of its usefulness as a tool in developmental biology, biochemistry, endocrinology and biology, histology, oncology, virology, and molecular biology.[29] No cell can exist independent of its surrounding cells. All cells have relations with neighboring cells and with cells at distant sites. The interactions of the epithelial parenchyma and mesenchymal stroma are most important in primary and secondary induction in organogenesis.

The mammary gland consists of a branching system of excretory ducts embedded in connective tissue.[11] The gland is composed of two layers of epithelial cells: luminal epithelium and basal layer epithelium, along with a few basal (stem) cells. The whole structure is surrounded by a basement membrane. In the ducts, elongated myoepithelial cells make up a continuous sheath. The luminal cell interaction with the extracellular matrix is mediated by the myoepithelium.

The integrity of the normal mammary gland is maintained by several adhesion systems.[11] The mammary gland is composed of epithelial parenchyma and two types of mesenchymal stroma: dense mammary mesenchyma and fatty stroma. The dense mammary mesenchyma is present in the embryonic stage, in end buds of puberty, and in cancers. It determines mammary epithelium and fixes the ability of the epithelium to interact with the fatty stroma. The fatty stroma is essential for typical mammary gland morphogenesis.[29]

The two types of mammary stroma synthesize different extracellular matrix proteins. Dense mesenchyma makes fibronectin and tenascin. Fatty stroma makes liminin, proteoglycans, and fibronectin.

In their structure and mode of development, the mammary glands somewhat resemble the sweat glands.[10] During embryonic life, their differentiation is similar in the two sexes. The male experiences little additional development postnatally. The female, in contrast, experiences extensive structural change paralleling her age and the functional state of the reproductive system.

Vogel and associates[34] studied histologic changes in the normal human mammary gland in association with the menstrual cycle. They describe five phases: proliferative (days 3 to 7), follicular phase of differentiation (days 8 to 14), luteal phase of differentiation (days 15 to 20), secretory (days 21 to 27), and menstrual (days 28 to 2). Table 2-4 outlines the morphologic criteria for these phases. These findings illustrate the correlation of morphologic response to hormonal stimulus of the mammary gland during normal cycling.

The greatest development in the female is reached by the 20th year. Gradual changes are correlated with the menstrual cycle, and major changes accompany pregnancy and lactation (see Fig. 2-8).

Russo and Russo[27] describe the development of the mammary gland as "an asynchronous process of progressive invasion of the mammary stroma by a parenchyma composed of ductal elements in which the advancing ends are the club-shaped terminal end buds (TEBs) that progressively differentiate into alveolar buds (ABs) or regress to terminal ducts (TDs)" (Fig. 2-18).

Mature mammary gland

The mammary gland is a compound tubuloalveolar gland containing 15 to 25 irregular lobes radiating from the nipple. Each lobe has a lactiferous duct (2 to 4 mm in diameter) lined by stratified squamous epithelium. The duct opens on the nipple and has an irregular angular outline. Beneath the areola, each duct finally emerges at the end of the nipple as a 0.4- to 0.7-mm opening. Each lobe is subdivided into lobules of various orders; the smallest are elongated tubules, the alveolar ducts, covered by small saccular evaginations, the alveoli. The interlobular connective tissue is dense; however, it is more cellular, has fewer collagenous fibers, and contains almost no fat. Greater distensibility is permitted by the looser connective tissue.

The ducts and ductules of mature women consist chiefly of two cell types: the inner lining of epithelial cells and the outer lining of myoepithelial cells. A basement membrane separates these structures from the stroma. Histochemical and immunocytochemical reagents can distinguish these elements, their positions, and their infrastructures. Rudland[26] has reported on the histochemical organization and cellular composition of ductal buds in the developing human breast. This work suggests that there are cytochemical intermediates between epithelial and myoepithelial cells. The undifferentiated peripheral cap cells may be transitional forms of the cortical epithelial cells that will line the lumina and of the myoepithelial cells of the subtending duct.

Transforming growth factors (TGF-β1, 2, and 3) are potent inhibitors of cell proliferation but play an important role in mammary gland development. They exhibit overlapping patterns of expression within the epithelium of the developing gland. TGF-β3 is detected in the myoepithelial progenitor cells of the growing end buds and the myoepithelial cells in the mature duct.[24]

The secretory portions of the gland, the alveolar ducts and the alveoli, have cuboidal or low-columnar secretory cells, resting on basal laminae and myoepithelial cells. These myoepithelial cells enclose the alveoli in a loosely meshed network

TABLE 2-4 Morphologic criteria for phase assignment in menstrual cycle

			Epithelium			
	Stroma	Lumen	Cell types	Orientation of epithelial cells	Mitoses	Active secretion
Phase I Days 3–7	Dense, cellular	Tight	Single predominant pale eosinophilic cell	No stratification apparent	Present, average 4/10 HPF	None
Phase II Days 8–14	Dense, cellular-collagenous	Defined	1. Luminal columnar basophilic cell 2. Intermediate pale cell 3. Basal clear cell with hyperchromatic nucleus (myoepithelial)	Radial around lumen	Rare	None
Phase III Days 15–20	Loose, broken	Open with some secretion	1. Luminal basophilic cell 2. Intermediate pale cell 3. Prominent vacuolization of basal clear cell (myoepithelial)	Radial around lumen	Absent	None
Phase IV Days 21–27	Loose, edematous	Open with secretion	1. Luminal basophilic cell 2. Intermediate pale cell 3. Prominent vacuolization of basal clear cell (myoepithelial)	Radial around lumen	Absent	Active apocrine secretion from luminal cell
Phase V Days 28–2	Dense, cellular	Distended with secretion	1. Luminal basophilic cell with scant cytoplasm 2. Extensive vacuolization of basal cells	Radial around lumen	Absent	Rare

HPF, high powered field.
Modified from Vogel PM, Georgiade NG, Fetter BF, et al:The correlation of histologic changes in the human breast with the menstrual cycle. Am J Pathol 104:23, 1981.

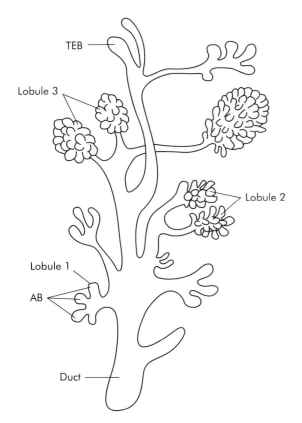

TEB

Lobule 3

Lobule 2

Lobule 1

AB

Duct

Figure 2-18. Schematic representation depicting various topographic compartments of human mammary gland: terminal end buds (TEB); alveolar buds (AB); lobules types 1, 2, and 3; and ducts. (Modified from Russo J, Russo IH: Development of human mammary gland. In Neville MC, Daniel CW [eds]: The Mammary Gland. New York, Plenum, 1987.)

with their many starlike branchings. The myoepithelial cells are stimulated by oxytocin and sex steroids. The presence of myoepithelial cells has been used as evidence that the mammary gland is related to the sweat gland.

In the resting phase, epithelial structures consist of the ducts and their branches. The presence of a few alveoli budding off from the ends of ducts is still under investigation. This variance may be caused by the effect of the menstrual cycle. The swelling and engorgement accompanying the menstrual cycle are associated with hyperemia and some edema of the connective tissue. Most significant is that the gland does not have a single duct but many. Each lobe is a separate compound alveolar gland whose primary ducts join into larger and larger ducts. These ducts drain into a lactiferous duct. Each lactiferous duct drains separately at the tip of the nipple.

The epidermis of the nipple and areola is invaded by unusually long dermal papillae whose capillaries richly vascularize the surface and impact the richer hue. Bundles of smooth muscle, placed longitudinally along the lactiferous ducts and circumferentially within the nipple and at its base, permit the erection of the nipple. In the areola are the areolar Montgomery glands, which are intermediate in their microscopic structure between sweat glands and true mammary glands. The periphery of the areola also has sweat glands and sebaceous glands (see Figs. 2-9 and 2-10).

Mammary gland in pregnancy

In the first 3 to 4 weeks of pregnancy, there is marked ductular sprouting with some branching and lobular formation, stimulated by estrogenic release. By 5 to 8 weeks, the breast changes are physically notable with dilation of the superficial veins, heaviness, and increased pigmentation of the nipple and areola. Changes in levels of circulating hormones result in profound changes in the ductular-lobular-alveolar growth during pregnancy (Fig. 2-19). During the first trimester there is rapid growth and branching from the terminal portion of the duct system into the adipose tissue. As the epithelial structures proliferate, the adipose tissue seems to diminish. During this time, increasing infiltration of the interstitial tissue occurs with lymphocytes, plasma cells, and eosinophils. The rate of hyperplasia levels off. In the last trimester, any enlargement is the result of parenchymal cell growth and distention of the alveoli with early colostrum, which is rich in protein and relatively low in lipid. Fat droplets gradually accumulate in the secretory alveolar cells. The interlobular connective tissue is noticeably decreased, and alveolar proliferation is extensive. In experimental studies,

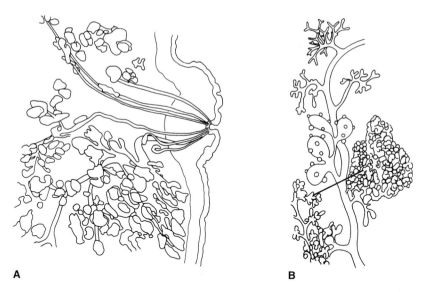

A   **B**

Figure 2-19. A, Milk gland of 21-year-old primigravida in second month of pregnancy. Development of small lobes has protruded almost to mammilla. Very regular development is shown over whole range of this thick section. Natural dimensions: 2.6 × 2.1 cm. **B,** Milk gland of same 21-year-old primigravida. Note very different forms of sprouting. Partly atypical sprouts above diagonal line are composed from same section; bifurcations below line are in natural position. Alveoli are beginning to resemble mature gland. (From Dabelow A: Die Milchdrüse. In Handbuch der Mikroskopischen Anatomie des Menschen, Vol. III, Part 3. Berlin, Springer-Verlag, 1957.)

these effects can be duplicated when estrogen and progesterone stimulate a release of prolactin-inhibiting factor (PIF). Prolactin is released in humans during pregnancy, thus stimulating epithelial growth and secretion. Prolactin levels increase over time during pregnancy.

The histologic appearance of the gland varies. The functional state appears to vary from dilated, thin-walled lumen to narrow-lumened, thick-walled glandular tissue. Epithelial cells vary, being flat to low columnar in shape with indistinct boundaries. Some cells protrude into the lumen of the alveoli; others are short and smooth. The lumen of the alveolus is crowded with fine granular material and lipid droplets similar to those protruding from the cells. The mammary alveoli but not the milk ducts lose the superficial layer of cells in the second trimester. The monolayer differentiates into a cell layer that accumulates eosinophilic cells, plasma cells, and leukocytes around the alveoli.

Lymphocytes, round cells, and desequamated phagocytic alveolar cells are also found in the lumen.

Lactating mammary gland

The lactating mammary gland is characterized by a large number of alveoli (Fig. 2-20). The alveoli of the lactating gland are made up of cuboidal epithelial and myoepithelial cells. Only a small amount of connective tissue separates the neighboring alveoli. Under special preparations, lipid can be seen as small droplets within the cells. These droplets become larger and are discharged into the lumen.

The functioning of the mammary gland depends on the interplay of multiple and complex nervous system and endocrine factors. Some factors are involved in the development of the mammary glands to a functional state *(mammogenesis),* others in the establishment of milk secretion *(lactoge-*

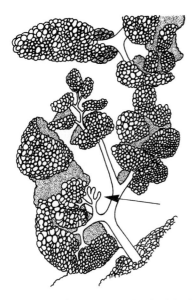

Figure 2-20. Part of mammary gland with significant milk obstruction in 26-year-old woman who died from food poisoning after ingesting spoiled fish 3 weeks post partum and who had not breastfed for 48 hours before death. In upper half, formed duct and lobes are located on alternating sides. This form results from different development of two parts of a dichotomized bifurcation: one takes over production of small lobes, while the other continues the stem. Thick section; *arrow*, very primitive, undeveloped sprouts. (From Dabelow A: Die Milchdrüse. In Handbuch der Mikroskopischen Anatomie des Menschen, Vol. III, part 3. Berlin, Springer-Verlag, 1957.)

nesis), and others in responsibility for the maintenance of lactation *(galactopoiesis).*

The division and differentiation of mammary epithelial cells and presecretory alveolar cells into secretory milk-releasing alveolar cells take place in the third trimester. Stimulation of ribonucleic acid (RNA) synthesis promotes galactopoiesis and apocrine milk secretion into the alveoli. The deoxyribonucleic acid (DNA) and RNA content of the cellular nuclei increases during pregnancy and is highest at lactation (see Fig. 2-3).

The former concepts of mammary gland secretion indicated that the mode of release was apocrine secretion. *Apocrine secretion* is the process by which the cell undergoes partial disintegration. A fat-filled portion projects into the lumen; the fat globule constricts at the base; and the cell replaces itself. Electron microscopy has shown that the cell has two distinct secretory products, formed and released by different mechanisms. The protein constituents of milk are formed and released identically to those of other protein-secreting glands, classified as *merocrine glands.* Secretory materials are passed out through the cell apex without appreciable loss of cytoplasm in merocrine glands.

The fatty components of milk arise as lipid droplets free in the cytoplasmic matrix. The droplets increase in size and move into the apex of the cell. They project into the lumen, covered by a thin layer of cytoplasm. The droplets are ultimately cast off, enveloped by a detached portion of the cell membrane and a thin rim of subjacent cytoplasm. (See Fig. 2-3 and Chapter 3 for further discussion.)

The ultrastructure of the human mammary gland during lactogenesis was studied by Tobon and Salazar,[33] who reviewed surgical specimens from seven lactating women 1 day to 5½ months post partum. They noted widespread hypertrophy and hyperplasia of the acini accompanied by dilatation and engorgement of the lumen by milk. The vascular channels were engorged. The lactogenic epithelial cells had rich cytoplasm, prominent layers of reticulum, and enlarged oval mitochondria. The Golgi apparatus was hypertrophied. The myoepithelium was stretched and thinned to contain the filled acini.

Postlactation regression of mammary gland

If milk is not removed from the breast, the glands become greatly distended and milk production gradually ceases. Part of the decrease results from the lack of stimulation of sucking, which initiates the neurohormonal reflex for maintenance of prolactin secretion. Perhaps a stronger effect is the engorgement of the breast with compression of blood vessels, causing diminished flow. The diminished blood flow results in decreased oxytocin to the myoepithelium. The alveoli are greatly distended and the epithelium flattened. The secretion remaining in the alveolar spaces and ducts is absorbed. The alveoli gradually collapse, with an increase in perialveolar connective tissue. The glandular elements gradually return to the resting state. Adipose tissue and macrophages increase. The gland does not return completely to the prepregnancy state in that the alveoli formed do not totally involute. Some appear as scattered, solid cords of epithelial cells.

Microscopically, increased autophagic and heterophagic processes occur in the first few days after weaning. Lysosomal enzymes increase, whereas nonlysosomal enzymes decrease. The gland undergoes alveolar epithelium apoptosis and remodeling reverting back to the prepregnant state with the loss of prolactin.

Although the process of regression has been studied carefully in animals, little study has been done in the human. Slow weaning, which usually takes 3 months, probably has a very different timetable from abrupt weaning, in which marked involution has been intense and rapid over days or weeks.

REFERENCES

1. Adler DD, Rebner M, Pennes DR: Accessory breast tissue in the axilla: Mammographic appearance. Radiology 163:709, 1987.
2. Anbazhagan R, Bartek P, Monaghan P, et al: Growth and development of the human infant breast. Am J Anat 192:407, 1991.
3. Bland KI, Romnell LJ: Congenital and acquired disturbances of breast development and growth. In Bland KI, Copeland EM III (eds): The Breast: Comprehensive Management of Benign and Malignant Diseases. Philadelphia, WB Saunders, 1991.
4. Clemente CD (ed): Gray's Anatomy of the Human Body. Philadelphia, Lea & Febiger, 1985.
5. Courtiss EH, Goldwyn RM: Breast sensation before and after plastic surgery. Plast Reconstr Surg 58:1, 1976.
6. Crafts RC: A Textbook of Human Anatomy. New York, Ronald Press, 1966.
7. Dabelow A: Die Milchdrüse. In Handbuch der Mikroskopischen Anatomie des Menschen, Vol. III, Part 3. Berlin, Springer-Verlag, 1957.
8. Egan RL: Breast embryology, anatomy, and physiology. In Breast Imaging: Diagnosis and Morphology of Breast Diseases. Philadelphia, WB Saunders, 1988.
9. Farina MA, Newby BG, Alani HM: Innervation of the nipple-areolar complex. Plast Reconstr Surg 66:497, 1980.
10. Fawcett DW: Bloom and Fawcett: A Textbook on Histology, 11th ed. Philadelphia, WB Saunders, 1986.
11. Glukhova M, Koteliansky V, Sastre X, et al: Adhesion systems in normal breast and in invasive breast carcinoma. Am J Pathol 146:706, 1995.
12. Hartmann PE, Cregan MD, Ramsay DT, et al: Physiology of lactation in preterm mothers: Initiation and maintenance. Pediatr Ann 32:351, 2003.
13. Hersh JH, Bloom AS, Cromer AO, et al: Does a supernumerary nipple/renal field defect exist? Am J Dis Child 141:989, 1987.
14. Hicken NF: Mastectomy: A clinical pathologic study demonstrating why most mastectomies result in incomplete removal of the mammary gland. Arch Surg 40:6, 1940.
15. Kaye BL: Axillary breasts: A significant esthetic deformity. Plast Reconstr Surg 53:61, 1974.
16. Knight CH, Peaker M: Development of the mammary gland: Symposium report no 19. Lactation. J Reprod Fertil 65:521, 1982.
17. Kreipe RE: Normal somatic adolescent growth and development. J Pediatr 83:1, 1973.
18. Larson BL (ed): Lactation. Ames, Iowa State University Press, 1985.
19. Liscia DS, Merlo G, Ciardiello F, et al: Transforming growth factor-alpha messenger RNA localization in the developing adult rat and human mammary gland by in situ hybridization. Dev Biol 140:123, 1990.
20. Montagna W, Macpherson EE: Some neglected aspects of the anatomy of human breasts. J Invest Dermatol 63:10, 1974.
21. Neville MC: Breastfeeding, part I: The evidence for breastfeeding. Anatomy and physiology of lactation. Pediatr Clin North Am 48:13, 2001.
22. Osbourne MP: Breast development and anatomy. In Harris JR, Lippman ME, Morrow M, Hellman S (eds): Diseases of the Breast. Philadelphia, Lippincott-Raven, 1996.
23. Pellegrin JR, Wagner RF Jr: Polythelia and associated conditions. Am Family Phys 28:129, 1983.
24. Pierce DF Jr, Johnson MD, Matsui Y, et al: Inhibition of mammary duct development but not alveolar outgrowth during pregnancy in transgenic mice expressing active TGF-β1. Genes Dev 7:2308, 1993.
25. Rahbar F: Clinical significance of supernumerary nipples in black neonates. Clin Pediatr 21:46, 1983.
26. Rudland PS: Histochemical organization and cellular composition of ductal buds in developing human breast: Evidence of cytochemical intermediates between epithelial and myoepithelial cells. J Histochem Cytochem 39:1471, 1991.

27. Russo IH, Russo J: Progestagens and mammary gland development: Differentiation versus carcinogenesis. Acta Endocrinol 125:7, 1991.

28. Russo J, Russo IH: Development of human mammary gland. In Neville MC, Daniel CW (eds): The Mammary Gland. New York, Plenum, 1987.

29. Sakakura T: New aspects of stroma-parenchyma relations in mammary gland differentiation. Int Rev Cytol 125:165, 1991.

30. Smith DM, Peters TG, Donegan WL: Montgomery's areolar tubercle. Arch Pathol Lab Med 106:60, 1982.

31. Tanner JM: Wachstun und Reifung des Menschen. Stuttgart, Thieme-Verlag, 1962.

32. Tobon H, Salazar H: Ultrastructure of the human mammary gland. I. Development of the fetal gland throughout gestation. J Clin Endocrinol Metab 39:443, 1974.

33. Tobon H, Salazar H: Ultrastructure of the human mammary gland. II. Postpartum lactogenesis. J Clin Endocrinol Metab 40:834, 1975.

34. Vogel PM, Georgiade NG, Fetter BF, et al: The correlation of histologic changes in the human breast with the menstrual cycle. Am J Pathol 104:23, 1981.

35. Vorherr H: The Breast: Morphology, Physiology, and Lactation. New York, Academic Press, 1974.

36. Weatherly-White RCA: Plastic Surgery of the Female Breast. Hagerstown, Md, Harper & Row, 1980.

$\mathscr{P}$hysiology of lactation

Lactation is the physiologic completion of the reproductive cycle. The human infant at birth is the most immature and dependent of all mammals except for marsupials. The marsupial joey is promptly attached to the teat of a mammary gland in an external pouch. The gland changes as the offspring develops, and the joey remains there until able to survive outside the pouch. In the human, throughout pregnancy the breast develops and prepares to take over the role of fully nourishing the infant when the placenta is expelled.

The breast is prepared for full lactation from 16 weeks' gestation without any active intervention from the mother. It is kept inactive by a balance of inhibiting hormones that suppress target cell response. In the first few hours and days post partum, the breast responds to changes in the hormonal milieu and the stimulus of the newborn infant's suckling to produce and release milk.[94]

The energy expenditure during lactation has suggested an efficiency of human milk synthesis greater than the 80% value previously hypothesized by investigators. Frigerio and associates[24] suggest, from work in Gambian women and extensive review of other studies, that the energy cost of human lactation is minimal and the process functions at 95% efficiency.

This chapter provides a review of the physiologic adaptation of the mammary gland to its role in infant survival. Several major reviews that include substantial bibliographies for readers who need the detailed reports of the original investigators are referenced.[19,49,56,60,63,64,94] Newer scientific techniques in the study of human lactation provide more precise, more detailed, and more integrated data on which the clinician can base a physiologic approach to lactation management.

Box 3-1 lists the abbreviations for the hormones that are involved in lactation and are discussed in this chapter.

HORMONAL CONTROL OF LACTATION

In contrast to most organs, which are fully developed at birth, the mammary gland undergoes most of its morphogenesis postnatally in adolescence and adulthood.[62] Lactation is an integral part of the reproductive cycle of all mammals, including humans. The hormonal control of lactation can be described in relation to the five major stages in the development of the mammary gland: (1) embryogenesis; (2) mammogenesis, or mammary growth; (3) lactogenesis, or initiation of milk secretion; (4) lactation (stage III lactogenesis), or full milk secretion; and (5) involution (Table 3-1).[62]

Current terminology divides lactogenesis into two stages.[32] Stage I takes place during pregnancy when the gland is sufficiently developed to actually produce milk. It begins about midpregnancy (approximately 16 weeks). It can be identified by measuring the levels of lactose and α (alpha)-lactalbumin.[2] Should the mother deliver at this point, milk would be produced. Some mothers can express colostrum during this time. As the

BOX 3-1	Hormone abbreviations
Adrenocorticotropic hormone	ACTH
Epidermal growth factor	EGF
Feedback inhibitor of lactation	FIL
Follicle-stimulating hormone	FSH
Growth hormone (human growth hormone)	GH (hGH), HGH
Heregulin	HER
Human growth factor	hGF, HGF
Human placental lactogen	hPL, HPL
Insulin-like growth factor 1	IGF-1
Prolactin	PRL
Prolactin-inhibiting factor	PIF
Thyroid-stimulating hormone	TSH
Thyrotropin-releasing hormone	TRH
Transforming growth factor beta	TGF-β

pregnancy proceeds, milk production is inhibited by high levels of circulating progesterone in most mammals and estrogen as well in humans.

Stage II of lactogenesis is the onset of copious milk production at delivery. In all mammals, it is associated with the drop in progesterone levels. This drop occurs to herald delivery in some species so that milk is copious when the young are born. In the human, these levels drop over the first 4 days post partum reflected by the milk "coming in" during this time. The drop in progesterone is accompanied by the transformation of the mammary epithelium over days to finally produce volumes of milk by the fifth day. This change includes a change in permeability of the paracellular pathway, changes in secretion of protective factors (i.e., lactoferrin, immunoglobulins), as well as increases

TABLE 3-1   Stages of mammary development*

Developmental stage	Hormonal regulation	Local factors	Description
Embryogenesis	?	Fat pad necessary for ductal extension	Epithelial bud develops in 18- to 19-week-old fetus, extending short distance into mammary fat pad with blind ducts that become canalized; some milk secretion may be present at birth
Mammogenesis			Anatomic development
Puberty			
Before onset of menses	Estrogen, GH	IGF-1, hGF, TGF-β, ? others	Ductal extension into mammary fat pad; branching morphogenesis
After onset of menses	Estrogen, progesterone, ? PRL		Lobular development with formation of terminal duct lobular unit (TDLU)
Pregnancy	Progesterone, PRL, hPL	HER, ? others	Alveolus formation; partial cellular differentiation
Lactogenesis	Progesterone withdrawal, PRL, glucocorticoid	Not known	Onset of milk secretion Stage I: midpregnancy Stage II: parturition
Lactation	PRL, oxytocin	FIL	Ongoing milk secretion
Involution	PRL withdrawal	Milk stasis, ? FIL	Alveolar epithelium undergoes apoptosis and remodeling; gland reverts to prepregnant state

*See Box 3-1 for abbreviations.

Modified from Neville MC: Mammary gland biology and lactation: A short course. Presented at biannual meeting of the International Society for Research on Human Milk and Lactation, Plymouth, Mass, October 1997.

in all milk components that parallel increased glucose production.

Over the next 10 days, the composition of the milk slowly changes to mature milk. Composition then changes slowly over the months of full exclusive breastfeeding.

Embryogenesis

Embryogenesis begins with the mammary band, which develops about the 35th embryonic day and progresses to a bud at the 49th day (see Chapter 2). Ducts continue to elongate to form a mammary sprout, which invades the fat pad, branches, and canalizes, forming the rudimentary mammary ductal system present at birth. After birth, growth of this set of small branching ducts parallels the child's linear growth but remains limited, probably controlled by growth hormone before onset of ovarian activity.

Under the influence of sex steroids, especially the estrogens, the mammary glandular epithelium proliferates, becoming multilayered. Buds and papillae then form. The growth of the mammary gland is a gradual process that starts during puberty. The process depends on pituitary hormones. Lobuloalveolar development and ductal proliferation also depend on an intact pituitary gland.

The following six well-documented factors help explain organization of mammary growth. Much of this work has resulted since the availability of "knockout" studies in mice and associated techniques.

1. Mammary ducts must grow into an adipose tissue pad if morphogenesis is to continue. Only adipose stroma supports ductal elongation.[16] The mammary epithelium is closely associated with the adipocyte-containing stroma in all phases of development. In midgestation during human fetal development, a fat pad is lain down as a separate condensation of mesenchyma. Rudimentary ducts expand into the fat pad but do not progress.[62] At puberty the ducts elongate to fill the entire fat pad, terminating growth as they reach the margins of the fat pad.

2. Estrogen is essential to mammary growth. Ductal growth does not occur in the absence of ovaries but can be stimulated when estrogen is provided. In the ovariectomized (oophorectomized) mouse, an estrogen pellet placed in the mammary tissue stimulates growth in that gland but not in the opposite gland. When the estrogen receptor is "knocked out" in the mouse, no mammary development occurs. The increase in estrogen at puberty results in mammary development. Although estrogen is essential, it is not adequate alone.[5]

3. The exact location of the estrogen receptors in the human breast is unclear. Estrogen receptors are not in the proliferating cells and have not been located in the stroma. Cells with estrogen receptors, however, secrete a *paracrine factor* that is responsible for the proliferation of ductal cells. This paracrine factor may hold the key to understanding both normal and abnormal breast development.

4. In addition to estrogen, the pituitary gland is necessary for breast development. Kleinberg[40] has identified growth hormone (GH) as important to pubertal development and development of the terminal end buds in the breast. Prolactin could not replace GH in these experiments, but insulin-like growth factor 1 (IGF-1) could. It is produced in the stromal compartment of the mammary gland under stimulation by GH, and together with estradiol from the ovaries, IGF-1 brings about ductal development at puberty.

5. Transforming growth factor beta (TGF-β) maintains the spacing of the mammary ducts as they branch and elongate.[62] These ducts exhibit unique behavior during growth, turning away to avoid other ducts and end buds. This avoidance behavior accounts for the orderly development of the duct system in the breast and the absence of ductal entanglements. This pattern provides ample space between ducts for later development of alveoli. TGF-β has been identified as the negative regulator and is found in many tissues, including breast tissue produced by an epithelial element. The pattern

formation in ductal development depends on the localized expression of TGF-β.[17]

6. Progesterone secretion brings about the side branching of the mammary ducts.[36] The presence of progesterone receptors in the epithelial cells has been confirmed by studies in knockout mice whose mammary glands develop to the ductal stage but not to alveolar morphogenesis. Ormandy and associates[68] established that prolactin is necessary for full alveolar development through prolactin receptor studies in knockout mice whose mammary glands do not develop beyond the ductal stage. This was further confirmed in murine mammary cultures when full development of the alveoli depends on prolactin. Further, when prolactin is withdrawn, apoptosis of the alveolar cells occurs.[99]

The coordination of epithelial and stromal activity in the mammary gland is complex. Hepatocyte growth and scatter factor has been associated with the process during puberty.[68] Another growth factor, heregulin, a member of the epidermal growth factor (EGF) family, has been identified in the stroma of mammary ducts during pregnancy.

Neville[62] has diagrammed the regulation of mammary development (Fig. 3-1). She notes that the concentrations of estrogen, progesterone, and lactogenic hormone in the form of prolactin or placental lactogen greatly increase, enhance alveolar development, and result in the differentiation of alveolar cells. Although many investigators have contributed pieces to the puzzle of mammogenesis, Neville has succeeded in creating the current visualization.

Mammogenesis: mammary growth

Prepubertal growth

Mammogenesis occurs in two phases as the gland responds to the hormones of puberty and later of pregnancy.[60] During the prepubertal phase the primary and secondary ducts that develop in the fetus in utero continue to grow in both the male and the female in proportion to growth in general. Shortly before puberty, a more rapid expansion of the duct system begins in the female. The growth of the duct system seems to depend predominantly on estrogen and does not occur in the absence of ovaries. The complete growth of the alveoli requires stimulation by progesterone as well.

Studies of hypophysectomized animals have shown failure of full mammary growth even with

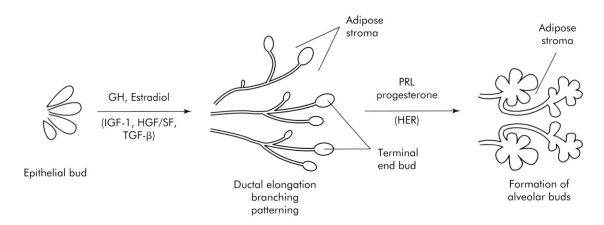

Figure 3-1. Scheme for regulation of mammary development in the mouse. (From Neville MC: Mammary gland biology and lactation: A short course. Presented at annual meeting of the International Society for Research on Human Milk and Lactation, Plymouth, Mass, October 1997.)

adequate estrogen and progesterone.[16] Secretion of prolactin and somatotropin by the pituitary gland results in mammary growth. Adrenocorticotropic hormone (ACTH) and thyroid-stimulating hormone (TSH) acting on the adrenal and thyroid glands also play a minor role in growth of the mammary gland.

Growth and development during organogenesis involve the interaction of cells with extracellular matrices and neighboring cells.[82] Necropsy breast specimens from six male and eight female infants ranging in age from 1 day to 9 months were studied to determine the process of organogenesis in the human.[1] Integrins were expressed in a pattern that correlates with morphologic and functional differentiation of the normal mammary gland. *Integrins* are transmembrane glycoproteins that form receptors for extracellular matrix proteins such as fibronectin, laminin, and collagen. Integrins are widely expressed in normal tissue and are considered critical to the control of cell growth and differentiation. This suggests integrin involvement in the functional characterization of the adhesion molecules in the breast.

Pubertal growth

When the hypophyseal-ovarian-uterine cycle is established, a new phase of mammary growth, which includes extensive branching of the system of ducts and proliferation and canalization of the lobuloalveolar units at the distal tips of the branches, begins. Organization of the stromal connective tissue forms the interlobular septa. The ducts, ductules (terminal intralobular ducts), and alveolar structures are all formed by double layers of cells. One layer, the epithelial cells, circumscribes the lumen. The second layer, the myoepithelial cells, surrounds the inner epithelial cells and is bordered by a basement lamina.

Menstrual cycle growth

The cyclic changes of the adult mammary gland can be associated with the menstrual cycle and the hormonal changes that control that cycle. Estrogens stimulate parenchymal proliferation, with formation of epithelial sprouts. This hyperplasia continues into the secretory phase of the cycle. Anatomically, when the corpus luteum provides increased amounts of estrogens and progesterone, there is lobular edema, thickening of the epithelial basal membrane, and secretory material in the alveolar lumen. Lymphoid and plasma cells infiltrate the stroma. Clinically, mammary blood flow increases in this luteal phase. This increased flow is experienced by women as fullness, heaviness, and turgescence. The breast may become nodular because of interlobular edema and ductular-acinar growth.

After onset of menstruation and reduction of sex steroid levels, milk-secretory prolactin action is limited. Postmenstrual changes occur rapidly, with degeneration of glandular cells and proliferation tissue, loss of edema, and decrease in breast size. The ovulatory cycle actually enhances mammary growth in the early years of menstruation (until about age 30) because the postmenstrual regression of the glandular-alveolar growth after each cycle is not complete. These changes of ductal and lobular proliferation, which occur during the follicular phase before ovulation, continue in the luteal phase and regress after the menstrual phase, exemplifying the sensitivity of this target organ to variations in the balance of hormones.

Fowler and associates[21] measured cyclic changes in composition and volume of the breast during the menstrual cycle using nuclear magnetic resonance T1 imaging. The T1 relaxation time (spin-lattice T1 relaxation) is a measure of the rate of energy loss from tissues after T1 excitation. This energy loss depends on the biophysical environment of the excited protons. A short T1, therefore, indicates the presence of lipids and organic structures that bind water tightly. A longer T1 occurs with greater hydration and with the greatest amount of cellular water. This study revealed the lowest total breast volume and parenchymal volume. T1 and water content occurred between days 6 and 15 of the cycle. Between days 16 and 28, T1 rose sharply and peaked on the 25th day. The rise in parenchymal volume in the second half of the cycle resulted from not only increased tissue water but also from growth and increased tissue fluid, according to Fowler and associates.[21]

Growth during pregnancy

Hormonal influences on the breast cause profound changes during pregnancy (Fig. 3-2). Early in

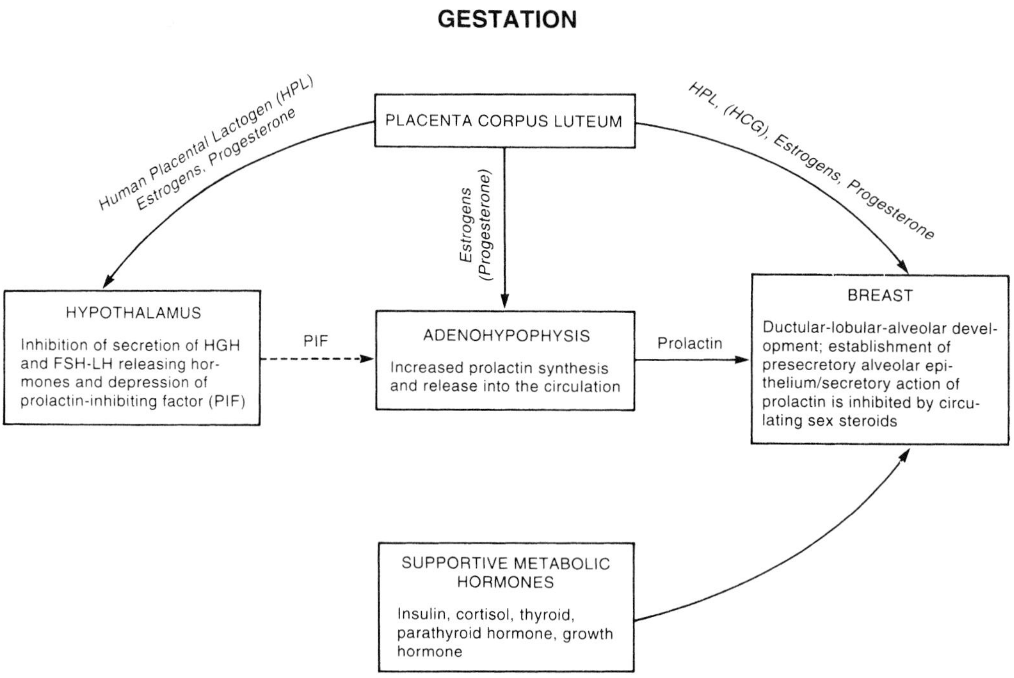

GESTATION

Figure 3-2.   Hormonal preparation of breast during pregnancy for lactation. (Modified from Vorherr H: The Breast: Morphology, Physiology and Lactation. New York, Academic Press, 1974.)

pregnancy, a marked increase in ductular sprouting, branching, and lobular formation is evoked by luteal and placental hormones.[102] Placental lactogen, prolactin, and chorionic gonadotropin have been identified as contributors to the accelerated growth (Fig. 3-3). The dichorionic ductular sprouting has been attributed to estrogen and lobular formation to progesterone.

Prolactin is essential for complete lobular-alveolar development of the gland. Almost complete growth of the mammary lobular-alveolar system can be obtained experimentally in the hypophysectomized-adrenalectomized rat if the animal receives estrogen, progesterone, and prolactin.[43] Prolactin, as with other protein hormones, exerts its effect through receptors for the initiation of milk secretion located on the alveolar cell surfaces. The induction of milk synthesis requires insulin-induced cell division and the presence of cortisol. Prolactin is secreted by the pituitary, which is neg-

atively controlled by prolactin-inhibiting factor (PIF) from the hypothalamus.[43]

From the third month of gestation, secretory material that resembles colostrum appears in the acini. Prolactin from the anterior pituitary gland stimulates the glandular production of colostrum. By the second trimester, placental lactogen begins to stimulate the secretion of colostrum. A mother who delivers after 16 weeks of gestation will secrete colostrum, even though she has had a nonviable infant. This demonstrates the effectiveness of hormonal stimulation on lactation.

An estrogen-mediated increase in prolactin secretion in pregnancy may produce as much as a 10-fold to 20-fold increase in plasma prolactin. This effect may be partially controlled by lactogen from the placenta, which inhibits the production of prolactin. Hormonal regulation of the growth and proliferation of the mammary gland cells has been carefully studied in many species.

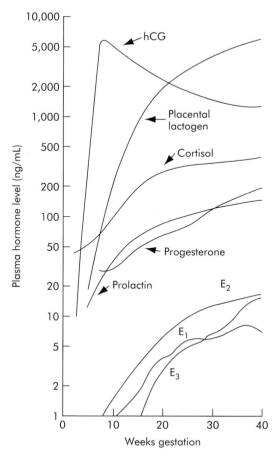

Figure 3-3. Plasma hormone levels during pregnancy. E₁, estrone; E₂, estradiol; E₃, estriol; hCG, human corticotropin. (From Neville MC, Morton J, Umemura S: The evidence for breastfeeding. Pediatr Clin North Am 48(1):42, 2001.)

Studies of mice in which receptors for each of the hormones have been ablated demonstrate that progesterone and prolactin (or possibly placenta lactogen) are key to alveolar development in pregnancy. The major inhibitor of milk production during pregnancy has been shown to be progesterone.[36]

A complex sequence of events, governed by hormonal action, prepares the breast for lactation (see Fig. 3-2). Estradiol-17β stimulates the ductal system of epithelial cells to elongate during pregnancy. In contrast to puberty, however, when estrogens appear to directly and indirectly stimulate breast development, estrogens have no indispensable role in mammary development during pregnancy except as a prolactin potentiator, according to Neville[59]; when estrogen levels are low in pregnancy, the breast still develops. Estrogen levels are normally high in pregnancy, but not for mammogenesis. Induced lactation in the cow is dependably reproduced with 7 days of estrogen and progesterone treatment. Progesterone, in turn, induces the specific epithelial cells of the tubular invaginations to produce distinct ducts, which branch from the main tubules. The end result of the combined actions of estrogen and progesterone is a richly branched arborization of the gland. Highly differentiated secretory alveolar cells develop at the ends of these ducts under the influence of prolactin (Fig. 3-4).

Serum growth factor, which is present in normal human serum, and insulin can stimulate the stem cells of the gland to proliferate. These dividing cells are further directed to the formation of alveoli by corticosteroid hormones. At least two types of cells are identified in the epithelial layer of the gland: stem cells and secretory alveolar cells. At this point in the pregnancy, prolactin influences the production of the constituents of milk.

TGF-β influences pattern formation in the developing mammary gland and may negatively regulate ductal growth as well.[17] The pattern of mammary ductal development varies widely among species and is a function of both genotype and hormonal status. Normal human breast cells secrete TGF-β and are themselves inhibited by it, suggesting an autoregulatory feedback circuit that may be modulated by estradiol. Growth and patterning of the ductal tree are regulated in part by TGF-β operating through an autocrine feedback mechanism and by paracrine circuits associated with epithelial-stromal interactions.[17]

The high circulating levels of prolactin in pregnancy are not associated with milk production partly because of the progesterone antagonism of the stimulatory action of prolactin on casein messenger ribonucleic acid (mRNA) synthesis. During late pregnancy the lactogenic receptors, which have similar affinities for both prolactin and human placental lactogen (HPL), are predominantly occupied

POSTPARTUM

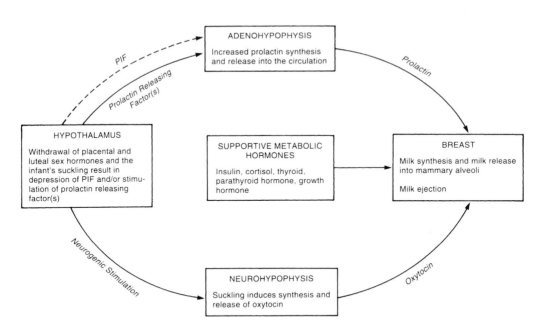

Figure 3-4. Hormonal preparation of breast post partum for lactation. PIF, prolactin-inhibitory factor. (Modified from Vorherr H: The Breast: Morphology, Physiology and Lactation. New York, Academic Press, 1974.)

by HPL. High doses of estradiol impair the incorporation of prolactin into milk secretory cells.

Prolactin is prevented from exerting its effect on milk excretion by the elevated levels of progesterone. Following the drop in progesterone and estrogen at delivery, copious milk secretion begins. The key hormone requirements for lactation to begin are prolactin, insulin, and hydrocortisone. A high level of plasma prolactin is essential to lactogenesis in humans as well. There is a question as to whether it is a surge in prolactin that is necessary for lactogenesis at parturition. Prolactin levels are now described as biphasic in humans for the initiation of lactogenesis at birth.[58] Prolactin stabilizes and promotes transcription of casein mRNA and stimulates synthesis of a lactalbumin that is the regulatory protein of the lactose-synthetase enzyme system.[69] Prolactin further increases the lipoprotein lipase activity in the mammary gland. Prolactin exists in three heterogenic forms of varying biologic activity. The monomer is in greatest quantity and is the most active form.

Lactogenesis: initiation of milk secretion

Stage I lactogenesis starts about 12 weeks before parturition and is heralded by significant increases in lactose, total proteins, and immunoglobulin and by decreases in sodium and chloride, and the gathering of substrate for milk production. The composition of prepartum secretion is fairly constant until delivery, as monitored by the milk protein α-lactalbumin.[31]

Lactogenesis is initiated in the postpartum period by a fall in plasma progesterone while prolactin levels remain high (see Fig. 3-4). The initiation of the process does not depend on suckling by the infant until the third or fourth day, when the secretion declines if milk is not removed from the breast.[100,101]

Stage II lactogenesis includes the increase in blood flow and oxygen and glucose uptake as well as the sharp increase in citrate concentration, considered a reliable marker for lactogenesis stage II. Stage II at 2 to 3 days post partum begins clinically when the secretion of milk is copious and biochemically when plasma α-lactalbumin levels peak (paralleling the period when "the milk comes in"). The major changes in milk composition continue for 10 days, when "mature milk" is established. The establishment of mature milk supply, once called *galactopoiesis,* is now referred to as *stage III of lactogenesis* (Figs. 19-2 to 19-4 and Fig. 3-5).[101,102]

The profound changes in milk composition have been established for the period of transitional to mature milk in relationship to increase in milk volume.[61] Detailed studies of successfully lactating women were performed by Neville and associates,[63] who report that a significant fall in sodium, chloride, and protein and a rise in lactose precede the major increase in milk volume during early lactogenesis. At 46 to 96 hours post partum, copious milk production is accompanied by an increase in citrate, glucose, free phosphate, and calcium concentrations and a decrease in pH (see Figs. 3-18 and 3-19).

The breast, one of the most complex endocrine target organs, has been prepared during pregnancy

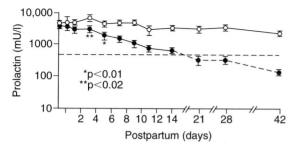

Figure 3-5. Prolactin levels in postpartum period in lactating (*open circles*) and nonlactating (*dots*) women. Levels in lactating women vary with intensity of suckling. (From Neville MC, Morton J, Umemora S: The evidence for breastfeeding. Pediatr Clin North Am 48(1):44, 2001.)

and responds to the release of prolactin by producing the constituents of milk (see Fig. 3-4). The lactogenic effects of prolactin are modulated by the complex interplay of pituitary, ovarian, thyroid, adrenal, and pancreatic hormones.

Prolactin

Human prolactin is a significant hormone in pregnancy and lactation.[22] Prolactin also has a range of actions in various species that is greater than any other known hormone. Prolactin has been identified in many animal species whether they nurse their young or not. Because of the original association with lactation, the term describes its action, "support or stimulation of lactation." Prolactin, however, has been shown to control nonlactating responses in other species and has been identified with more than 80 different physiologic processes. Study of prolactin was hampered until 1970, when it became possible to separate prolactin from human growth hormone (hGH) and to isolate and characterize prolactin from human pituitary glands.[91]

Before 1971, hGH and prolactin in humans were considered the same hormone. Until 1971, in fact, it was thought that prolactin did not exist in humans. hGH, however, is present in the human pituitary gland in an amount 100 times that of prolactin.[44]

Plasma prolactin varies in relation to psychosocial stress. Utilizing four different real-life stress studies in a longitudinal design, Theorell[92] found that change situations associated with passive coping are accompanied by increased plasma prolactin levels. Change situations associated with active coping are associated with unchanged or even lowered prolactin levels. The regulation of plasma prolactin is part of a dopaminergic system (see the list of pharmacologic suppressors in the next section).

In vitro, prolactin stimulates the synthesis of the mRNAs of specific milk proteins by binding to membrane receptors of the mammary epithelial cells. Prolactin has been demonstrated to penetrate the cytoplasm of these cells and even their nuclei. These specific actions in the gland require the presence of extracellular calcium ions. Some prolactin actually appears in the milk substrate itself, the functional significance of which is uncertain, although it is thought to influence fluid and ion absorption from the neonatal jejunum.

The effect of the stimulation of protein synthesis by allowing the expression of milk protein genes is not a direct effect of the hormone but rather the consequence of the activation of sodium/potassium adenosinetriphosphatase (Na/K ATPase) in the plasma membrane. The intracellular concentration of potassium is kept high and that of sodium low compared with the concentrations in extracellular fluid. As a result, the Na/K ratio is high both in the milk and in the intracellular fluid. Further action of prolactin has been identified in the development of the immune system in the mammary gland and, possibly more directly, in the lymphoid tissue. In conjunction with estrogen and progesterone, prolactin attracts and retains immunoglobulin A (IgA) immunoblasts from the gut-associated lymphoid tissue for the development of the immune system for the mammary gland. A very sensitive bioassay has been developed using the in vitro biologic effect of prolactin to stimulate the growth of cell cultures for malignant niobium (Nb) rat lymphomas.

The baseline levels of prolactin are essentially the same in the normal human male and female (Table 3-2). Moreover, both males and females experience a rise in prolactin levels during sleep.[87] There is also a normal diurnal variation in levels in both males and females. At puberty the increase in estrogens causes a slight but measurable increase in prolactin. Prolactin increases during the proliferative phase of the menstrual cycle but not during the secretory phase. A number of factors, including some that are significant for the nursing mother, such as psychogenic influence and stress, increase prolactin levels. Anesthesia, surgery, exercise, nipple stimulation, and sexual intercourse also produce increased amounts in both lactating and nonlactating females. Prolactin levels increase as serum osmolality increases.

Although prolactin levels in maternal serum are well established, less is known about prolactin levels in the milk and its role in the newborn. Prolactin in milk is known to be biologically potent and is absorbed by the newborn. In the intestine, prolactin influences fluid, sodium, potassium, and calcium transport. Prolactin content is highest in the early transitional milk just after the colostrum in the first postpartum week (levels of 43.1 ± 4 ng/mL).[107] Levels drop to 11.0 ± 1.4 ng/mL in mature milk over time until about 40 weeks post partum.

Prolactin-inhibiting factor

Prolactin-inhibiting factor (PIF) controls the secretion of prolactin from the hypothalamus. Prolactin thus is unusual among the pituitary hormones because it is inhibited by a hypothalamic substance. Catecholamine levels in the hypothalamus control the inhibiting factor, which is poured into the circulation as a result of dopaminergic impulses. Drugs and events that decrease catecholamines also decrease the inhibiting factor, causing a rise in prolactin. Dopamine itself can act directly on the pituitary gland to decrease prolactin secretion. Agents that increase prolactin by decreasing catecholamines and thus the PIF level include the phenothiazines and reserpine.

Thyrotropin-releasing hormone (TRH) is a strong stimulator of prolactin secretion, but its physiologic role is not clear, because thyrotropin levels do not rise during normal nursing. In the postpartum period, a dose of TRH will cause a marked increase in prolactin. Even the nonnursing postpartum mother will experience engorgement and milk release when stimulated with TRH. Ergot, which is frequently prescribed for the postpartum patient, inhibits prolactin secretion either by direct inhibition or by its effect on the hypothalamus.

Prolactin response to breast stimulation in lactating women is not mediated by endogenous opioids. Neither baseline nor stimulated prolactin values were affected by naloxone.[8]

The following factors affect prolactin release in normal humans:

Physiologic stimuli
   Nursing in postpartum women—breast stimulation
   Sleep
   Stress

TABLE 3-2   Prolactin levels*

	Range (ng/mL)	Average (ng/mL)
Males and prepubertal and postmenopausal females	2–8	
Females' menstrual life	8–14	10
Term pregnancy	200–500	200
Amniotic fluid	Up to 10,000	
Lactating women	Response to breastfeeding	
First 10 days	Baseline 200	Rise to 400
10–90 days	60–110	70–220
90–180 days	50	100
180 days to 1 year	30–40	45–80

*Collation of values from multiple studies and sources.

Sexual intercourse
Pregnancy
Pharmacologic stimuli
    Neuroleptic drugs
    Thyrotropin-releasing hormone (TRH)
    Metoclopramide (procainamide derivative)
    Estrogens
    Hypoglycemia
    Phenothiazines, butyrophenones
    Norepinephrine
    Histamine
    Acetylcholine
Pharmacologic suppressors
    L-Dopa
    Ergot preparations (2-Br-α-ergocryptine)
    Clomiphene citrate
    Large amounts of pyridoxine
    Monoamine oxidase inhibitors
    Prostaglandins E and $F_2\alpha$

In pregnancy, prolactin levels begin to rise in the first trimester and continue to rise throughout gestation. In the nonnursing mother, prolactin levels drop to normal in 2 weeks, independent of therapy to suppress lactation.

At delivery, with the expulsion of the placenta, levels of placental lactogen, estrogens, and progesterone abruptly decline.

Placental lactogen disappears within hours.[64] Progesterone drops over several days, and estrogens fall to baseline levels in 5 to 6 days (see Figs. 19-2 to 19-4 and Fig. 3-5). Prolactin in non-lactating women requires 14 days to reach baseline. Progesterone is considered the key inhibiting hormone, and decline in plasma progesterone levels is considered the lactogenic trigger for stage II lactogenesis.[59] However, progesterone does not inhibit established lactation because breast tissue does not contain progesterone-binding sites. Estrogens enhance the effect of prolactin on mammogenesis but antagonize prolactin by inhibiting secretion of milk. After delivery, there are low estrogen and high prolactin levels. Suckling provides a continued stimulus for prolactin release. If prolactin, essential for lactation, is diminished by hypophysectomy or medication, lactation ceases. Baseline prolactin levels do eventually diminish to more normal levels months after parturition, although lactation may continue.

The surge in prolactin over baseline levels, however, is critical to milk production, not the baseline levels (Figs. 3-5, 3-6, and 3-7). Although prolactin is necessary for milk secretion, the volume of milk secreted is not directly related to the concentration of prolactin in the plasma. Local mechanisms within the mammary gland that depend on the amount of milk removed by the infant are responsible for the day-to-day regulation of milk volume. Suckling stimulates the release of adenohypophyseal prolactin and neurohypophyseal oxytocin. These hormones

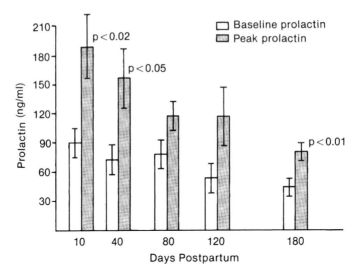

Figure 3-6. Prolactin levels after suckling. (From Battin DA, Marrs RP, Fleiss PM, et al: Effect of suckling on serum prolactin, luteinizing hormone, follicle-stimulating hormone, and estradiol during prolonged lactation. Obstet Gynecol 65:785, 1985.)

stimulate milk synthesis and production of milk-ejection metabolic hormones, which are also necessary in the process of milk synthesis.[59] Thus, suckling, emptying the breast, and receiving adequate precursor nutrients are essential to effective lactation (Fig. 3-8).

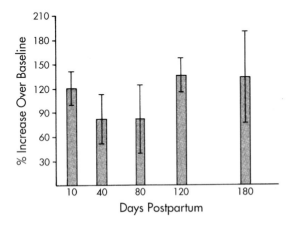

Figure 3-7. Percent increase in prolactin over baseline after suckling. (From Battin DA, Marrs RP, Fleiss PM, et al: Effect of suckling on serum prolactin, luteinizing hormone, follicle-stimulating hormone, and estradiol during prolonged lactation. Obstet Gynecol 65:785, 1985.)

When milk is not removed, secretion ceases in a few days, and the composition of the mammary secretion returns to a colostrum-like fluid. When the composition of the breast secretion of breastfeeding and nonbreastfeeding women was followed by Kulski and Hartmann,[42] it was the same for 3 to 4 days. Thereafter, the sodium and chloride concentrations in the nonbreastfeeding women increased rapidly.

The regulation of milk production in full lactation is based primarily on infant demand.[65] Maternal nutrition, age, body composition, and parity have only secondary impact. Suckling is a powerful stimulus to prolactin synthesis and secretion, and prolactin is necessary for milk secretion.[92] The pulsatile nature of prolactin secretion makes it difficult to measure over time. Milk yield is not directly correlated to prolactin levels. Evidence indicates that a proteinaceous factor in milk itself actually inhibits milk production and is associated with residual milk in the breast. This has been identified as a feedback inhibitor of lactation.

Prolactin circadian rhythm persists throughout lactation. Prolactin levels are notably higher at night than during the day, despite greater nursing times during the day. The highest levels in Stern

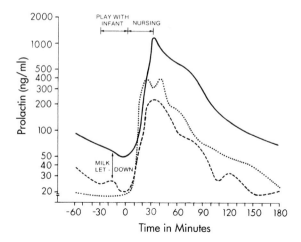

Figure 3-8. Plasma prolactin measured by radioimmunoassay before, during, and after period of nursing in three mothers, 22 to 26 days post partum. Prolactin levels rose with suckling and not with infant contact. (Modified from Josimovich JB, Reynolds M, Cobo E: Lactogenic hormones, fetal nutrition, and lactation. In Josimovich JB, Reynolds M, Cobo E (eds): Problems of Human Reproduction, Vol. 2. New York, John Wiley & Sons, 1974.)

and Reichlin's study were when the least nursing occurred.[87]

The most effective and specific stimulus to prolactin release is nursing. The stimulation is a result of nipple or breast manipulation, especially suckling, not a psychologic effect of the presence of the infant (see Fig. 3-8). The prolactin-release reflex during nipple stimulation is suppressed in some adult women, being evidenced only during pregnancy and lactation.[51]

During human pregnancy, when serum prolactin rises steadily to 150 to 200 ng/mL at term, there is a brief drop in levels hours before delivery and then a rise again as soon as the neonate is suckled.[47,56] The response to nipple stimulation can be abolished by applying local anesthetic.[57] On the other hand, trauma or surgery to the chest wall can initiate a prolactin rise and, in some reported cases, milk production.

Although it was initially reported that the high levels of prolactin measured in the first days and weeks of lactation dwindled to normal baseline by 6 months and showed no response to suckling stimulus, later studies clearly showed a different picture with more sensitive assays.[47] Prolactin does not drop to normal, but further stimulus causes a doubling of levels over baseline at all stages of lactation through the second year (see Table 3-2).

Acute prolactin and oxytocin responses were measured by Zinaman and associates,[108] who compared various mechanical pumping devices with manual expression and infant suckling. Prolactin response to mechanical expression in quantity and duration depended on the device used, with the full-size pulsatile electric pump (White River) eliciting the greatest response. This compared equally with infant suckling. There was no difference seen in oxytocin response with various devices. These data confirm that results in studies of milk production and release in humans also depend on the equipment used to stimulate the breast.[108]

Eight fully lactating women were followed through the first 6 months post partum at 10, 40, 80, 120, and 180 days, recording serum prolactin, luteinizing hormone (LH), follicle-stimulating hormone (FSH), and estradiol (zero time only) obtained just before the initiation of suckling and during the next 120 minutes.[3] Samples were obtained at 0, +15, +30, +60, and +120 minutes. Prolactin levels were high the first 10 days (90.1 ng/mL) but slowly declined over 180 days (44.3 ng/mL). The stimulus of suckling doubled the baseline values. Mean estradiol levels were low at 10 days (7.2 pg/mL), then gradually rose to a mean of 47.3 pg/mL at 180 days post partum in the subjects whose menses had resumed. In the amenorrheic subjects the estradiol levels remained low (4.25 pg/mL), whereas baseline prolactin remained high (63.6 ng/mL). The subjects were breastfeeding on demand, averaging 11 feedings (range 8 to 16) per day at 10 days and 8 feedings (range 5 to 12) at 120 and 180 days. All infants had stopped one night feeding, and two infants had started some solids between the third and fourth months.

The effort to relate the prolactin level to the volume of milk has not produced consistent findings.[10] Stimulating both breasts simultaneously, however, by either feeding two babies or "double pumping" (attachment to both breasts to pump via a Y tube) does produce a higher prolactin surge and a greater volume of milk totally as well as per unit of time. Howie and associates[35] reported the relationship between suckling-induced prolactin response and production of milk as being imprecise, finding no close temporal correlation between prolactin concentrations and milk yield. Milk yield was measured by electronic scale weighings before and after feedings. They calculated not only the peak prolactin level but also the area under the curve, and this latter value was consistent within the individual mother.

When specific binding sites for prolactin were looked for in the tammar wallaby, many sites were demonstrated in the lactating mammary gland but not the inactive gland.[49] Mammary prolactin receptors were also identified in the rabbit. Thus, the increased binding capacity would enhance tissue responsiveness, which may explain the maintenance of full lactation in the face of falling concentrations of prolactin. Prolactin also plays a critical role in increasing maternal bile secretory function post partum.[51]

Human placental lactogen and human growth hormone

Three main hormones are recognized in the lactogenic process: human placental lactogen (hPL), human growth hormone (hGH), and prolactin. The progressive rise in prolactin during pregnancy parallels the rise in hPL, becoming measurable at 6 weeks' gestation and increasing to 6000 ng/mL at term (see Fig. 3-3). This parallel action contributed to the belief that prolactin and hPL were the same. Although the principal function of hPL and prolactin in the human is a lactogenic one, no lactation ordinarily appears before delivery,[85] although some women report being able to express a few drops of colostrum.

First described in 1962, hPL has been studied more than lactogens from any other species.[57]

Extensive immunologic and structural homology exists between hGH and hPL, which probably explains their similar biologic activities. Concentrations of hPL increase steadily during gestation and decrease abruptly with the delivery of the placenta. A large-molecular-weight substance, hPL is derived from the chorion. Receptor sites that bind lactogen also bind protein and hGH.[98] hPL has been associated with mobilization of free fatty acid and inhibition of peripheral glucose utilization and lactogenic action.

hGH is secreted from the anterior pituitary eosinophilic cells. These cells have been identified by staining techniques that distinguish them from those that produce prolactin. Toward the end of pregnancy, the cells that produce prolactin are noticeably more numerous, whereas those that produce hGH are "crowded out." The role of hGH in the maintenance of lactation is poorly defined and may be synergistic with prolactin and glucocorticoids.

Prolactin, hGH, placental lactogen (PL), and chorionic somatotropin (CS) form a family of polypeptide hormones from the same ancestral gene, even though prolactin and hGH are produced by the pituitary and PL and CS by the placenta.[103] The suckling stimulus in postpartum lactation causes a rapid increase in serum hGH and prolactin. hGH and prolactin evolve from the same precursor, and although the hormones are distinct, the acute interruption of hGH secretion does not interfere with the milk secretion.

The possible role of TSH as a physiologic prolactin-releasing factor has been disproved by Gehlbach and associates,[26] who state that TSH is not responsible for the brisk release of prolactin with suckling. Normal lactation is possible in ateliotic dwarf women in the absence of detectable quantities of hGH.[79] For any hormone to exert its biologic effects, however, specific receptors for the hormone must be present in the target tissue. Changes in serum concentration have no effect if receptors are not present in the mammary gland to bind the hormone.

Oxytocin was the first hormone studied in relation to breastfeeding and to the let-down reflex. Studies first explored its role in the initiation and progression of labor. Because it was measurable and then isolated in the laboratory and finally manufactured synthetically, our knowledge of oxytocin was more extensive that it was for prolactin until the last 2 decades.

Oxytocin is not just a female hormone; it is produced by both males and females, and not just during reproduction in the female is it increased. It is now credited with producing increased responsiveness to receptivity, closeness, openness to relationships, and nurturing. The oxytocin circulating during breastfeeding has been credited with producing calm, lack of stress, and an enhanced ability to interact with the infant. The calm and connectedness system is part of a system of nerves and hormones that together trigger these effects.

Oxytocin is a polypeptide found in all mammalian species and works though a mechanisim whereby it activates receptors on the outer surface of the cell membrane. Oxytocin is produced in the supraoptic and paraventricular nuclei of the hypothalamus. Receptors have been identified for oxytocin in the uterus and the breast as well as the brain. It acts via the bloodstream and as a signaling substance in the nervous system. Substances that act to stimulate the release of oxytocin include serotonin, dopamine, noradrenaline, and glutamate. Others inhibit its release such as opiates, encephalin, and beta-endorphin. Spinal anesthesia has been associated with the inhibition of oxytocin release following childbirth. Estrogen can increase the number of receptors and stimulate the production of oxytocin. The release of oxytocin by repetitive soothing touches or when given via injection produces a calming reaction while lowering blood pressure and pulse rate. Uvnäs Moberg[95] has studied oxytocin extensively and calls it the hormone of calm, love, and healing.

Stage III lactogenesis (galactopoiesis): maintenance of established lactation

The maintenance of established milk secretion, originally called *galactopoiesis,* is now labeled *stage III lactogenesis,* or simply *lactation.* An intact hypothalamic-pituitary axis regulating prolactin and oxytocin levels is essential to the initiation and maintenance of lactation.[44] The process of lactation requires milk synthesis and milk release into the alveoli and the lactiferous sinuses. When the milk is not removed, the increased pressure lessens capillary blood flow and inhibits the lactation process. Lack of sucking stimulation means lack of prolactin release from the pituitary gland. Basal prolactin levels that are enhanced by the spurts that result from sucking are necessary to maintain lactation in the first weeks post partum. Without oxytocin, however, a pregnancy can be carried to term, but the female will fail to lactate because she will fail to let-down.

Sensory nerve endings, located mainly in the areola and nipple, are stimulated by suckling. The afferent neural reflex pathway, via the spinal cord to the mesencephalon and then to the hypothalamus, produces secretion and release of prolactin and oxytocin. Hypothalamic suppression of earlier PIF secretion causes adrenohypophyseal prolactin release. When prolactin is released into the circulation, it stimulates milk synthesis and secretion. A conditioned milk ejection can occur in lactating women without a concomitant release of prolactin, so that indeed the releases are independent, which may be significant in treating apparent lactation failure (Fig. 3-9).

Hormonal regulation of prolactin and oxytocin

The release of prolactin is inhibited by PIF.[45] The PIF has not been described but is closely associated with dopamine. There is also evidence of either serotonin release of prolactin or catecholamine-serotonin control of prolactin release. TSH has also been shown to simulate the release of prolactin. The amount of prolactin is proportional to the amount of nipple stimulation during early stages of lactation after the first 4 days. Milk synthesis proceeds for the first 4 days whether or not the breast is stimulated. At this time prolactin levels are the same for lactators and nonlactators.[58]

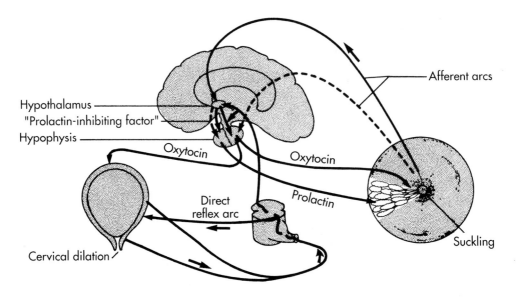

Figure 3-9. Neuroendocrine control of milk ejection. (Modified from Vorherr H: The Breast: Morphology, Physiology and Lactation. New York, Academic Press, 1974.)

Although both oxytocin and prolactin release are stimulated by nipple stimulation, some oxytocin is released by other sensory pathways, such as the visual, tactile, olfactory, and auditory.[66] Thus, a woman may release milk on seeing, touching, hearing, smelling, or thinking about her infant. Prolactin, however, is released only on nipple stimulation so that milk production is not initiated by other sensory pathways. Oxytocin is also released under physical stress, such as pain, exercise, cold, heat, changes in plasma osmolality, or hypovolemia, but these responses are blunted or reversed during lactation.[66]

When suckling occurs, oxytocin is released.[12] It enters the circulation and rapidly causes ejection of milk from alveoli and smaller milk ducts into larger lactiferous ducts and sinuses. This is the pathway of the let-down, or ejection, reflex. Oxytocin also causes contraction of the myometrium and involution of the uterus.

The polypeptide oxytocin is a messenger molecule with diverse physiologic actions as well as modes of delivery to its target sites. Oxytocin exerts effects as a hormone carried by the systemic circulation to distant targets in the uterus and the breast.[14] Oxytocin also serves as a hypophysiotropic factor, released from nerve terminals in the median eminence into the pituitary portal vasculature to affect anterior pituitary secretion. Its action here is as a peptidergic neurotransmitter or neuromodulator within the central nervous system, influencing a variety of neuroendocrine, behavioral, and autonomic functions. Its well-known role is related to reproduction and lactation, but it has other, less well explored physical and metabolic roles.[14]

After suckling is initiated, the oxytocin response is transient and intermittent rather than sustained. Plasma levels often return to basal between milk ejections, even though suckling continues. Ejection can be measured by placing a microcatheter in the mammary duct or can be noted subjectively by the mother as tingling or turgescence. The contractions last about 1 minute, with about 4 to 10 occurring in a 10-minute period. Corresponding pulses of oxytocin can be measured in the maternal bloodstream. The controls of oxytocin release are complex and are extensively described by Crowley and Armstrong.[14] That centrally released oxytocin is in control of the milk-ejection reflex was established in 1981 by Freund-Mercier and Richard.[23] They demonstrated in the rat that intracerebroventricular administration of oxytocin greatly increased the frequency and amplitude of pulsatile oxytocin release during suckling. Administration of oxytocin antagonists produced the opposite effect and suppressed responses.[23]

The human pituitary has an excessive storage capacity and contains 3000 to 9000 mU oxytocin, but the reflex milk ejection involves the release of only 50 to 100 mU.[104] Except in extreme cases (Sheenan syndrome), hormone depletion is rarely an issue, but hormone release and target-organ sensitivity are. Opiate and β-endorphin released during stress are known to block stimulus-secretion coupling by dissociating electrical activity at the terminal. This inhibition is naloxone reversible.

The mammary gland, from the platypus to the human, has an identical fine structure consisting of alveolar tissue that has increased its surface area 10,000-fold during gestation compared with the size of the gland.[53] It continuously produces milk throughout lactation, but the most complex issue is the release of milk. Because of the substantial surface tension forces opposing the movement of fluid in the small ducts, simple suction applied by suckling is relatively ineffective, especially in early lactation. Thus, the alveolus is enveloped in a basketlike network of myoepithelial cells that respond to oxytocin by contracting and expelling the milk into larger and larger ductules until it can be removed by the infant (Fig. 3-10). This is a classic example of a neuroendocrine reflex, a process that is remarkably uniform in all mammals.

Neuroendocrine control of milk ejection

Milk ejection involves both neural and endocrinologic stimulation and response. A neural afferent pathway and an endocrinologic efferent pathway are required.[57]

The ejection reflex depends on receptors located in the canalicular system of the breast. When the

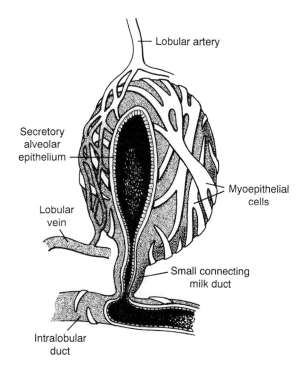

Figure 3-10. Fundamental mammary unit at lactation, with arrangement of secretory alveoli, myoepithelial cells, and vasculature. Secretory alveolar epithelium is monolayered, and epithelial lining of milk ducts consists of two layers. Between bases of glandular epithelial cells and tunica propria, starlike myoepithelial mammary cells surround alveolus in basketlike arrangement. (Modified from Vorherr H: The Breast: Morphology, Physiology and Lactation. New York, Academic Press, 1974.)

Labels in figure: Lobular artery; Secretory alveolar epithelium; Myoepithelial cells; Lobular vein; Small connecting milk duct; Intralobular duct

canaliculi are dilated or stretched, the reflex release of oxytocin is triggered. Tactile receptors for both oxytocin and reflex prolactin release are in the nipple. Neither the negative and positive pressures exerted by suckling nor the thermal changes trigger the milk-ejection reflex. Negative pressures have a minor effect, but tactile stimulation is the most important factor in milk ejection.

Studies in tactile stimulation show changes in sensitivity at puberty, during the menstrual cycle, and at parturition.[80] No difference exists in sensitivity between the sexes before puberty. In the female, tactile sensitivity increases after puberty and is increased at midcycle and during menstruation.

(Midcycle peak is absent in women taking oral contraceptives probably due to the suppression of ovulation.) Dramatic changes occur within 24 hours of delivery after several weeks of complete insensitivity. The nipple is the most sensitive area to both touch and pain, followed by the areola; the least sensitive area is the cutaneous breast tissue. The increased sensitivity of the breast continues several days post partum, even when the woman does not breastfeed. Estrogen treatment suppresses the induction of prolactin release on nipple stimulation, whereas on withdrawal of estrogen the prolactin response returns. Increased tactile sensitivity may be the key event activating the suckling-induced release of oxytocin and prolactin at delivery (Figs. 3-11 and 3-12).

The clinical study of oxytocin challenge tests for use in measuring the viability of the fetus has led to the study of breast stimulus on the uterus. Numerous studies have confirmed that oxytocin levels rise significantly during nipple stimulation, with short bursts of oxytocin during accompanying uterine contractions.[9] When the effect of breast stimulation on prostaglandin secretion was tested at 38 to 40 weeks' gestation, uterine contractions occurred and prostaglandin metabolite levels increased in all cases. Shalev and associates[83] suggest that the principal action of oxytocin is to stimulate prostaglandin synthesis in uterine tissues, which then becomes the primary cause of the uterine contractions.

The oxytocin-binding sites are located within the basement membrane of the mammary alveolus and along the interlobular ducts. A gradual 10-fold increase occurs in the concentration of oxytocin receptor sites in the mammary gland during pregnancy.[48] This contrasts sharply with the sudden 40-fold increase in oxytocin receptors in the uterus in the hours before delivery that then rap-

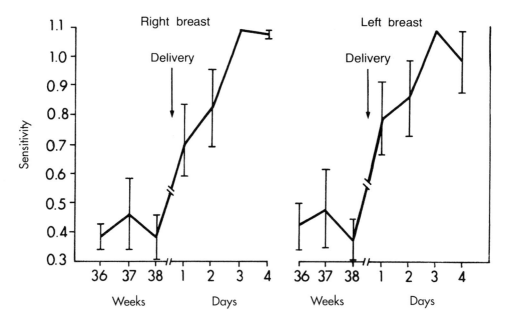

Figure 3-11. Changes in tactile sensitivity of cutaneous breast tissue in perinatal period. Sensitivity was calculated from two-point discrimination according to formula $K - \log^e$. K is an arbitrary figure employed to portray low two-point discrimination value as peaks of sensitivity. Dramatic increase in tactile sensitivity at delivery enhances response to suckling of newborn. (From Robinson JE, Short RV: Changes in breast sensitivity at puberty, during the menstrual cycle, and at parturition. Br Med J 1:1188, 1977.)

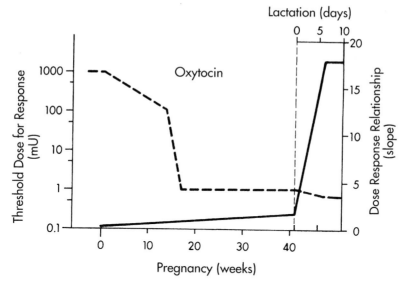

Figure 3-12.   Sensitivity of human mammary epithelium to oxytocin during pregnancy and lactation. Scale at left shows threshold dose necessary to evoke increase in intramammary pressure; scale at right shows maximum intramammary pressure obtained. (Modified from Caldeyro-Barcia R: Milk ejection in women. In Reynolds M, Folley SJ (eds): Lactogenesis: The Initiation of Milk Secretion at Parturition. Philadelphia, University of Pennsylvania Press, 1969.)

idly disappear. These changes in receptor availability may be why copious milk does not occur until shortly after delivery, because oxytocin first facilitates delivery and then promotes milk ejection sequentially. When the increase in intramammary pressure obtained with varying doses of oxytocin in nonpregnant, pregnant, and lactating women was recorded by Caldeyro-Barcia,[6] the amount of oxytocin required for a response dropped from 1000 mU in nonpregnancy to about 1 mU in late pregnancy and further to 0.5 mU in lactation (see Fig. 3-12).[59] The maximum intramammary pressure that could be evoked increased from 1 mm Hg early in pregnancy to a peak of 10 mm Hg 5 days post partum. Caldeyro-Barcia suggests that not only the sensitivity of the myoepithelial cells but the number of receptor sites increases as well during pregnancy.

Conflicting information exists regarding the exact nature of the release of oxytocin from the pituitary. The dose-response curve of the mammary gland has a very limited dynamic range, so that a bolus of 0.1 mU oxytocin (0.2 mg) given intravenously to a lactating rat fails to change intramammary pressure. An injection of 1.0 mU evokes an increase in pressure that begins after a delay of 10 seconds and peaks in 15 seconds at 8 to 10 mm Hg. A bolus has greater effect than a slow push, suggesting that a pulsatile pattern of hormone release would be the most effective way of utilizing oxytocin to produce milk ejection.[56]

Plasma oxytocin levels measured by Lucas and associates[53] with continuous sampling every 20 seconds revealed the hormone was released in surges and persisted in the circulation for less than 1 minute. The multiparas had a greater total response than primiparas, but with no difference between early (1 to 3 days post partum) and late (5 to 7 days). When a similar study was done by Dawood and associates[18] collecting samples only every 3 minutes, no pulsing was identified. Oxytocin was measurable within 2 minutes of suckling, peaked at 10 minutes, and had a bimodal curve dropping to a mean at 20 minutes comparable with that before suckling, which followed the burping and changing breasts at about 15 minutes.

A secondary peak occurred at 25 minutes. They found maximum response of intramammary pressures at the fifth to seventh day. McNeilly and associates[56] measured release of oxytocin in response to suckling in early and established lactation, drawing samples every 30 seconds. A catheter for blood sampling was placed in the forearm 40 minutes before lactation. Oxytocin levels increased 3 to 10 minutes before suckling in response to the baby crying or becoming restless or the mother preparing herself to feed. There was no prolactin response until suckling began.

Most results clearly showed response before tactile stimuli and then a second surge in response to suckling. The levels were pulsatile during suckling and not related to milk volume, prolactin response, or parity of the mother.

Significant elevations of the maternal oxytocin level occur at 15, 30, and 45 minutes after delivery when the infant is put skin to skin, compared with levels just before delivery during expulsion of the placenta.[67] Levels return to baseline after 60 minutes if the infant does not suckle. When oxytocin levels were measured after initiating breast stimulation with a mechanical breast pump in early lactation (10 to 90 days), midlactation (90 to 190 days), and late lactation (180 days to 12 months), baseline levels were similar in all three periods. The stimulated plasma oxytocin levels were greater in early than late lactation, but there was always a response. Thus, the oxytocin secretory reflex appears to continue for at least the first year of lactation.

The release of oxytocin by neurohypophyseal responses during lactation has been evoked both by infant's suckling and by mechanical dilatation of the mammary ducts. This release of oxytocin was demonstrated to be independent of vasopressin release. Conversely, further study[44,45] demonstrated that there could be stimulation of vasopressin release independent of oxytocin release.

When the levels of hGH, vasopressin, prolactin, calcitonin, gastrin, insulin, epinephrine, norepinephrine, and dopamine were measured in six lactating women during breastfeeding, Widstrom and associates[105] confirmed the rise in prolactin and demonstrated the progressive increase in insulin that may be secondary to prolactin rise and may participate in stimulating milk production. Gastrin level decreased, and there were no consistent findings for calcitonin, hGH, norepinephrine, or epinephrine and no change in dopamine and vasopressin. Vagally stimulated release of insulin and gastrin is antagonized when the tone of the sympathetic nervous system is increased, such as during stress, pain, or anxiety. Increased insulin also is known to stimulate the synthesis of casein and lactalbumin and thus secondarily milk production. It should be advantageous to breastfeed after a meal rather than before (practically, many mothers eat while feeding the infant).

Human myoepithelium, the effector tissue, is specifically stimulated by oxytocin, and this sensitivity and specificity increase throughout pregnancy. Suckling can induce milk secretion, which is under control of the adenohypophysis. In this case, oxytocin released by the neurohypophysis because of the suckling stimulus would cause both milk ejection and release of the anterior pituitary hormones responsible for milk secretion as well. This is probably the mechanism behind relactation and induced lactation in the woman who has never been pregnant. Mammary growth and lactogenesis may be induced by suckling, massage, and breast stimulation in many species.[20]

Alcohol has a dose-related effect on the central nervous system in inhibiting milk ejection. When intramammary pressure was measured in response to suckling by the infant while the mother received measured doses of alcohol, milk ejection was inhibited in a dose-dependent manner.[10] Doses up to 0.45 g/kg body weight (blood alcohol less than 0.1%), however, had no effect on intramammary pressure. Mechanical breast stimulation for 10 minutes and concomitant administration of intravenous fluid containing normal saline, naloxone, ethanol, or a combination of ethanol and naloxone were initiated in normal nonlactating women on day 22 of the regular menstrual cycle.[11] Plasma oxytocin levels rose twofold, with breast stimulation peaking at 10 minutes. Responses were unchanged by naloxone but were completely abolished by alcohol taken orally (approximately 110 mL of whiskey). Naloxone partially reversed the inhibiting effects of ethanol. The authors concluded that naloxone-sensitive endogenous opioids do not appear to be involved in the control of the oxytocin rise induced by breast stimulation and that opioid peptides are partly involved in the alcohol action.[11] Alcohol has been used in obstetrics to suppress premature labor in humans.

Normal alert newborns have been observed to "crawl" to the nipple and latch on unassisted when placed on the maternal abdomen following a normal delivery and the clamping and severing of the umbilical cord.[78]

Suckling brings about functional changes in the offspring. An infant who sucks on an artificial nipple quickly decreases the amount of body movement, increases mouth activity, and decreases crying. The suckling experience may affect infant behavior and mother-infant interaction. Nonnutritive sucking is observed in many species. In the human infant, nutritive sucking is shown to be a continuous stream of regular sucks with few, if any, pauses. Nonnutritive sucking has bursts of activity alternating with no sucking. Suckling can be altered by extraneous aural, visual, or olfactory stimuli. Response of breasts to different stimulation patterns of an electric breast pump was measured by Kent and associates. When cycles were 45 per minute, let-down occurred in 147 ± 13 seconds. In response to breastfeeding, let-down occurred after 56 ± 4 seconds. Volume was a reflection of negative pressure or vacuum applied but not the time for milk ejection.[39]

Maternal effects of suckling

Effects of suckling on the mother include the stimulation of afferent nerves for the removal of milk.[46] Reduction in sucking stimulus produces a reduction in prolactin and in milk synthesis. The lactating glands adjust the milk supply to demand, probably because of both a local and an endocrinologic mechanism. Variations in milk secretion are rapidly reflected in anatomic changes in the mammary gland. Mammary tissue shows regression after the first week or so, if unstimulated. Tissue regression proceeds at a rate

parallel to the demand for secretory tissue. Thus, when a suckling infant signals needs, the breast will respond.[81]

Effects on maternal behavior have been attributed to lactation. Maternal behavior is more easily defined in many other species, in which early nursing is initiated by the mother, who stimulates the neonate to suckle by grooming. She then presents her mammary gland to the offspring so that the nipple is located with minimal effort. All species of lactating females have a lessened response to stress. In the human, however, nursing behavior has a strong voluntary nature. When lactating women were stressed with graded treadmill exercise, significant decreases in plasma levels of ACTH, cortisol, and epinephrine were observed compared with a matched group of nonlactating women.[7] Plasma glucose levels did not increase in either group. Oxytocin pulse in the plasma in response to suckling was also accompanied by a decrease in plasma ACTH and cortisol in the lactating women.

Oxytocin administered intraventricularly to virgin rats induces maternal behavior. Local infusion of oxytocin antagonists to appropriate regions of the hypothalamus during parturition blocked the dams from pup retrieval, a measure of maternal behavior in rats.[74] Similar observations have been made in sheep.[75] The neurophysical mechanism is under study in the human. It is well established that oxytocin promotes the development of human maternal behavior and mother-infant bonding.[73] Some effects of oxytocin in the nipple and mammary gland appear to be caused by peptides released in the nipple from axon collaterals of somatosensory afferent nerves. Oxytocin is also present in neurons projecting to many areas in the brain and exerts many central actions. In addition to maternal behavior, oxytocin causes more nonspecific behavior changes, such as sedation or antistress effects, and optimizes transfer of energy to the mammary gland.[73]

Investigations of the agile wallaby, *Macropus agilis,* have revealed the let-down reflex as this species displays concurrent asynchronous lactation.[49] The young, weighing 35 g, attaches to the teat at birth. The lactating gland continues to grow for 200 days, increasing 10-fold in size. At 200 to 220 days, weighing 2500 g, the young first leaves the pouch. Twenty-six days later a second young is born, although the older one continues to suckle intermittently for another 160 days at the original teat. The second young attaches to an unused nipple, which begins to develop, displaying complete autonomy. Measurements of oxytocin during the initial lactation show an increase in intraductal pressure response with a decline in sensitivity over time. This permits milk ejection in response to a small release of oxytocin to be confined to the mammary gland to which the neonate is continuously attached. The release of large quantities of oxytocin in response to the suckling of the juvenile would cause release in both glands.[49]

Mammals have thus evolved diverse strategies for survival. Tandem nursing in the human has not been so carefully studied, but no known change occurs in let-down, although the milk reverts to colostrum at the birth of the new infant.

The spinothalamic tract is the most likely of the possible spinal and brainstem pathways by which the suckling stimulus reaches the forebrain. The areas of the forebrain influenced by the suckling stimulus include the hypothalamic structures that mediate oxytocin and prolactin release. The inhibition of milk ejection by visual and auditory stimuli, pinealectomy, and ventrolateral midbrain lesions in lactating rats has been studied to define further the neurohormonal pathways. In these experiments the pineal gland appeared to mediate an inhibitory visual reflex on both oxytocin release and milk ejection.[29,77]

A mechanism consisting of smooth muscle and elastic fibers acting as a sphincter at the end of the ducts in the nipple appears to prevent most unwanted loss of milk. Sympathetic control does not appear to be present in humans, although it is demonstrable in most other species.

As the end of pregnancy approaches, the breast is prepared to respond to the suckling offspring.[78] In the human this is evidenced by increased sensitivity of the breast to tactile stimulation; increased responsiveness of the ductiles to oxytocin, thus preparing to eject the milk; and increased response of the breast to signaling the release of prolactin to stimulate milk production. The signal for lactation occurs when the placenta is removed and the end organs in the breast can fully respond to the surge of prolactin resulting from suckling.[96]

Concentrations of oxytocin in milk

Human milk samples obtained by manual expression daily from the first to the fifth postpartum day were collected immediately before and after a feeding as well as 2 hours after nursing.[90] The baseline mean oxytocin concentrations were 3.3 to 4.7 mg/mL, increasing significantly with nursing. Oxytocin in milk is fairly stable compared with that in maternal serum, which is inactivated by oxytocinase in plasma, liver, and kidney. When oxytocin was administered to rat dams, it was also found in the suckling offspring's gastric contents, where it is stable in acid. Some is absorbed into the neonatal blood, where it is unstable. Levels of oxytocin in neonatal serum are produced predominantly by the neonate itself. Whether oxytocin has a physiologic role on the gut or other hormones is unknown.

Role of prostaglandins as milk ejectors

Because prostaglandins have many physiologic effects and are known to increase mammary duct pressure, Toppozada and associates[93] investigated their role as milk ejectors.[67] Comparison was made among three treatments: intravenous (IV) injections of oxytocin, PGE_2, and 16-phenoxy-PGE_2 given to one group of women on the third to sixth day post partum; IV oxytocin, 15-methyl-$PGF_2\alpha$, and $PGF_2\alpha$ tromethamine salt to a second group; and oxytocin and PGF intranasally to a third group. All combinations had some effect, with the IV route having a shorter latency period than the intranasal. $PGF_2\alpha$, the more potent of the prostaglandin preparations, was more potent via the nasal route than oxytocin nasally. The response lasted 25 minutes after intranasal instillation of 400 µg. PGE_2 and $PGF_2\alpha$

orally reduce prolactin levels and appear to be successful in suppressing lactation in the immediate postpartum period when given in large doses of 2 to 4 mg or in multiple doses up to 10 times greater. Although they are produced in larger quantities by the mammary gland in vitro and in vivo, the role of prostaglandins is still not clear, because these studies[93] are in conflict with previous results by Vorherr.[102] The practical application of this in lactation failure has not been reported.

Milk-borne prostaglandins clearly survive in the environment of the infant's gastrointestinal tract and are delivered in an active form to peripheral organs. The significance of this remains under investigation.[41]

Production of hormones by mammary gland

Hormones synthesized by the mammary gland may have endocrine, autocrine, or paracrine effects within the mother. The chemical mediators known to be synthesized by the mammary gland are epidermal growth factor (EGF), progesterone, prolactin, estrogens, and relaxin. Other hormones are transported to the gland.[71] These bioactive agents could have multiple roles in both mother and recipient infant. Insulin-like growth factors are found in high concentration in colostrum and at lower levels in mature milk. Milk factors other than nutrients are thought to control specific developmental processes in the infant. Because infants survive and grow on formula, this latter point is difficult to prove. Actions of milk regulatory substances are much more important in at-risk infants than in full-term infants.

Feedback inhibitor of lactation

The mammary gland is unique because, as an exocrine gland, it stores its secretion extracellularly. Storage within the gland's lumen suggests a local level of control on the rate of secretion.[62]

As stated earlier, milk is produced as long as it is removed from the mammary gland. Further, prolactin and oxytocin are responsible for the production and release of milk, allowing the infant to extract milk by suckling. The rate of milk secretion may differ between breasts if one breast is suckled more frequently or for a longer time. When lactating goats have an extra daily milking, the secretory rate is increased even if the milk is immediately replaced with an inert solution to maintain the gland's distention. The dilution of stored milk in the gland with an inert isotonic solution results in increased milk secretion, suggesting the dilution of a chemical inhibitor.

Identification of a factor that is produced and functions at the mammary level, called *feedback inhibitor of lactation* (FIL), has evolved from multiple studies.[76] Wilde and associates[106] described autocrine regulation of milk secretion by a previously unknown protein in the milk. When this active whey protein (FIL) was isolated and injected into the mammary gland of lactating goats, milk secretion was decreased temporarily. Similar work by Prentice and associates[76] has confirmed the presence of FIL in humans. FIL is able to exert reversible concentration-dependent autocrine inhibition on milk secretion in the lactating gland. It controls secretion of all milk constituents simultaneously; that is, it affects secretion, not composition.

The search for the mechanism that explains regulation of milk supply continues. When goats were studied, it was noted that when milk accumulated in the mammary gland, production decreased. When the milk was removed and replaced with isotonic sucrose solution to volume, the rate of milk produced increased. This finding supports the concept that it is a compound in the milk and not distention of the mammary gland that regulates synthesis. This factor, FIL, is an autocrine mechanism.

FIL cannot be the sole control of milk synthesis, or removal of milk would not stimulate milk production. Cregan and Hartmann speculate that the mechanism of local control of milk synthesis is related to the filling/emptying cycle of the alveoli.[13] Milk accumulation changes the morphology of the lactocytes lining the alveoli. When the luminal volume of mammospheres increased, according to St. Reuli and Edwards, it altered the interaction of the lactocytes with the basement membrane inhibiting prolactin receptors and further milk synthesis.[89]

Maternal adaptation to lactation

The hormonal trigger for lactogenesis is a decrease in progesterone while prolactin levels are maintained. Postpartum prolactin levels are comparable in breastfeeding and nonbreastfeeding women for a few days (see Figs. 19-2 to 19-4 and Fig. 3-5). Thus, the basic process occurs regardless of whether breastfeeding is initiated. The mammary epithelium must be adequately prepared by the hormones of pregnancy to respond by synthesizing milk.

Each mammalian species has evolved its own lactational strategies to meet the nutritional needs of its offspring, with influences from both genetic and environmental forces. The endocrine signals promote mammary development, inhibit milk production during gestation, and then promote development of enhanced metabolic and transport functions in adipose tissue, visceral organs, and reproductive organs.[70] Lactational adaptations of adipose tissue metabolism have been recognized in all species and may be most dramatic in seals, hibernating bears, and whales, who produce fat-rich milk from their fat stores while fasting. Lactation results in profound changes in adipose tissue metabolism to provide energy stores, modulate mammary development, affect appetite, and influence the immune system function.[97]

The substantial adaptation of the maternal intestine during lactation is the large increase in its size and complexity, which ensures adequate absorption of nutrients to meet the increased energy demand.[27] A corresponding increase occurs in liver and heart performance. In addition to extra fat demands, calcium concentration must be sufficient to maintain maternal stores while providing for the demands of milk synthesis, which are greater than those of pregnancy.[34] The estimated calcium requirement is 12 mg/kg/day in the human. The elevation in plasma dihydroxycholecalciferol, or $1,25\text{-}(OH)_2D_3$, during late gestation continues during early lactation. As lactation progresses beyond 3 months, plasma $1,25\text{-}(OH)_2D_3$ levels decline. This results in decreased calcium absorption, which is offset by greater maternal bone losses and reduced urinary calcium. Glucose requirements during lactation require major adjustments in glucose production and utilization in the maternal liver, adipose tissue, bone, muscle, and other tissues. Adaptation of folic acid metabolism is equally important, although less well studied.[70]

The mechanisms by which early pregnancy and lactation decrease the incidence of breast cancer are unclear. Close examination of the more differentiated mammary cell, which is less susceptible to the loss of growth regulation, is a next step, along with inspection of mucin, a glycoprotein and normal differentiation antigen expressed in both milk fat globules and mammary tumors.

Delay in the onset of lactogenesis

Clinically, it has been observed that delayed lactogenesis occurs in women who are diabetic, are stressed during delivery, and occasionally experience retained placenta. When signs of lactogenesis are absent in the first 72 hours, a cause should be sought. In diabetic women extra effort should be made that the process goes well with good hydration, adequate dietrary intake, insulin control, and attention to detail. After stressful deliveries, it may be necessary to initiate pumping if the infant is unable to adequately stimulate the breast. Again, close monitoring is essential prior to discharge. Retained placenta is discussed in Chapter 16. The treatment, dilatation and curettage, is definitive and dramatically therapeutic.

Anticipating problems and identifying early signals of faltering are key to ultimately improving lactogenesis.

LACTATION: SYNTHESIS OF HUMAN MILK

Computerized breast measurement (CBM) was developed by Hartmann and his colleagues[32] because of the inaccuracy of the established methods for measuring milk synthesis. The three other techniques utilized are (1) test weighing either the infant or the mother before and after every feeding for 24 hours; (2) isotope dilution used to estimate production over a 4- or 7-day period; and (3) breast expression in which the mother removes milk from breasts (this technique does not reflect the effect of the infant on milk production by suckling). CBM is designed to measure short-term rates of milk synthesis. This technique allows the appetite of the infant to dictate the amount of milk removed from the breast while also being able to measure the residual.

CBM measures changes in breast volume without interfering with the infant's pattern of breastfeeding. CBM allows not only measurement of change in breast volume and volume of milk removed during a feeding, but four additional parameters.

The first is the *short-term rate of milk synthesis* (S) between breastfeedings. The calculation takes the increase in breast volume from the end of one feeding (V_{B1}) to the beginning of the next (V_{B2}), divided by the time between these two measurements (T).

$$S = \frac{V_{B2} - V_{B1}}{T}$$

The second measures *storage capacity* (SC), which is defined by the authors as the maximum breast volume (V_{max}) minus the minimum breast volume (V_{min}) observed over a 24-hour period (Fig. 3-13).

$$SC = V_{max} - V_{min}$$

The third measurement is *the degree of fullness* (F), which is the ratio of any particular breast volume (V_B) divided by the storage capacity of the breast (SC).

$$F = \frac{V_B}{SC}$$

The range is from 1 when the breast is full to 0 when it is at minimum volume in a 24-hour period.

In addition, this technology (CBM) can be used to measure the increase in breast volume during pregnancy, thus measuring breast growth and breast involution after peak lactation.

The storage capacity was measured by Daly and associates[15] and varied from 80 to 600 mL. The rate of milk synthesis was minimal when the breast was full and maximum when the breast was emptied.

The function of the mammary gland is unique in that it produces a substance that makes tremendous demands on the maternal system without producing

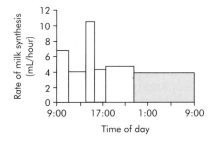
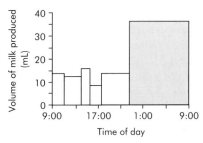

Figure 3-13. Rate of milk synthesis and volume of milk produced in one breast by an exclusively expressing mother over a 24-hour period. The shaded columns indicate the overnight period that had the lowest rate of milk synthesis but the highest volume expressed. (From Cregan MD, Hartmann PE: Computerized breast measurement from conception to weaning: Clinical implications. J Hum Lact 15:89, 1999.)

any physiologic advantage to the maternal organism. Because lactation is anticipated, the body prepares the breast anatomically and physiologically.[86] When lactation begins, the mother's metabolism changes greatly. The blood supply is redistributed, and the demand for nutrients increases, which requires an increased metabolic rate to accommodate their production. The mammary gland may need to produce milk at the metabolic expense of other organs. The supply of materials to the lactating breast for milk production and energy metabolism requires extensive cardiovascular changes in the mother. There is increased mammary blood flow, increased blood flow into the gastrointestinal tract and liver, and a high cardiac output. The mammary blood flow, cardiac output, and milk secretion are suckling dependent. Suckling induces the release of anterior pituitary hormones that act directly on breast tissue.

Milk is isosmotic with plasma in all species.[45] Human milk differs from many other milks in that the concentration of major monovalent ions is lower and that of lactose is higher; in other milks, the higher the ions, the lower the lactose, and vice versa. Many disparities in the intermediary metabolism among species of animals can be linked to evolutionary adaptations involving the digestive process.[44] Nonruminants rely on glucose, derived from carbohydrate in the diet. Ruminants, because of extensive fermentation in the rumen, absorb little glucose. The microbial fermentation products, which include acetate, propionate, and butyrate, play a significant part as energy and carbon sources for tissue metabolism. Amino acids are primary substitutes for glucose in ruminants.[45]

The biosynthesis of milk involves a cellular site where the metabolic processes occur. The epithelial cells of the gland contain stem cells and highly differentiated secretory alveolar cells at the terminal ducts. The stem cells are stimulated by hGH and insulin. Prolactin synergizes the insulin effect to stimulate the cells to secretory activity.

The cells of the acini and smaller milk ducts are active in milk synthesis and milk secretion into the alveoli and smaller milk ducts. Most milk is synthesized during the process of suckling; its production is stimulated by prolactin. Cortisol plasma levels are increased during suckling as well. The secretory cells are cuboidal, changing to a cylindric shape just before milk secretion, while cellular water uptake is increased. The cell's single nucleus is at the base in the dormant cell but migrates to the apex just before milk secretion.

The differentiated structure of the functional cell is acquired gradually during pregnancy, differing little from species to species. Very early in lactation, mammary cells show active synthesis and secretion of proteins and fat. The cells are polarized with abundant rough endoplasmic reticulum and Golgi dictyosomes above the nucleus, which is smooth and rounded with many mitochondria. The apical surface has microvilli, and the basal surface is extensively convoluted for the active transport of materials from the bloodstream into the cell. Fat droplets are in the cytoplasm and bulging at the membrane. Proteins, lactose, calcium, phosphate, and citrate are packaged into secretory vesicles and pass into the lumen of the alveolus by exocytosis.

The cytoplasm is finely granular in the resting phase but striated as milk secretion begins. As secretion commences, the enlarged cell with its thickened apical membrane becomes clublike in shape. The tip pinches off, leaving the cell intact. The protein is thus free in the secreted solution, retaining a cap of membrane (Fig. 3-14).

Function of cellular components of lactating breast

The schema of the mammary secretory cell is represented in Figures 3-15 and 3-16.

Nucleus

The nucleus is essential to the duplication of genetic material and the transcription of the genetic code.[100] The nucleus is also considered a regulatory organelle in cell metabolism, transmitting the design of the cell's enzymatic profile. The deoxyribonucleic acid (DNA) and RNA content of the cellular nuclei increases during pregnancy and is highest during lactation.

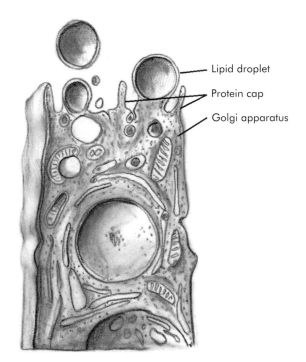

Lipid droplet

Protein cap

Golgi apparatus

Figure 3-14. Apocrine secretory mechanism for lipids, proteins, and lactose in milk.

Cytosol

The cytosol, which consists of the cytoplasm minus the mitochondrial and microsomal fractions, is also called the *particle-free supernatant.* The cytosol contains enzymes that involve key intermediates and cofactors essential to the process of milk synthesis.

Mitochondrial proliferation

The alveolar cell population of the mammary gland must have a greatly expanded oxidative capacity during lactation. It is supplied by an increase in size and function of the cell's mitochondrial population.[38] Mitochondria are increased in the epithelial cell at the onset of the lactation process. Mitochondrial proliferation has been observed in all cells with a high metabolic rate and high oxygen utilization.

During the presecretory differentiation phase in late pregnancy and early lactation, each mitochondrion undergoes a type of differentiation in which the inner membrane and matrix expand greatly. As with other cells, the mitochondria are key to the respiratory activity of the cell. Mitochondria control some cellular metabolism through differential permeability to certain anions. The citrate in the mitochondria is a major source of carbon for fatty acid biosynthesis. Mitochondria also supply the carbon for synthesis of nonessential amino acids.

Microsomal fraction

The microsomal fraction of the cell, which includes the Golgi apparatus, the endoplasmic reticulum, and the cell membranes, is involved in lipid synthesis. The role of the microsomal fraction is also to assemble the constituent parts (e.g., amino acids, glucose, fatty acids) into the final products of protein, carbohydrate, and fat for secretion.

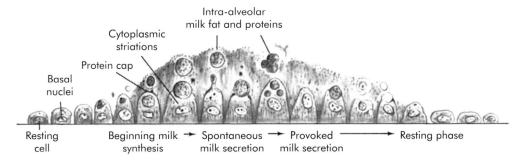

Intra-alveolar milk fat and proteins

Cytoplasmic striations

Protein cap

Basal nuclei

Resting cell — Beginning milk synthesis → Spontaneous milk secretion → Provoked milk secretion → Resting phase

Figure 3-15. Diagram of cycle of secretory cells from resting stage to secretion and return to resting stage. (Modified from Vorherr H: The Breast: Morphology, Physiology and Lactation. New York, Academic Press, 1974.)

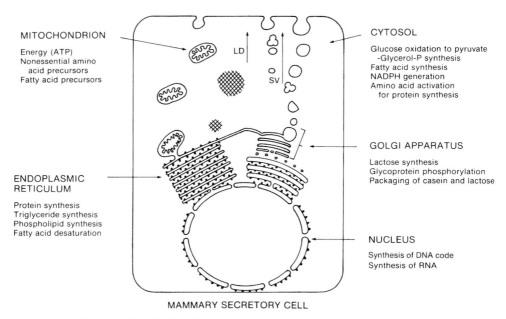

MAMMARY SECRETORY CELL

Figure 3-16. Schema of cytologic and biochemical interrelationships of secretory cell of mammary gland. LD, lipid droplet; SV, secretory vesicle.

Intermediary metabolism of mammary gland

The pathways identified for milk synthesis and secretion in the mammary alveolus, as described by Neville and associates,[60] include four major transcellular pathways and one paracellular pathway (Fig. 3-17):

1. Exocytosis of milk protein and lactose in Golgi-derived secretory vesicles
2. Milk fat secretion via the milk fat globule
3. Secretion of ions and water across the apical membrane
4. Pinocytosis-exocytosis of immunoglobulins
5. Paracellular pathway for plasma components and leukocytes

Carbohydrates

The major carbohydrate for most species is lactose, a disaccharide found only in milk. In addition to lactose, more than 50 oligosaccharides of different structures have been identified in human milk. One of the most important is glucose.

Glucose metabolism has a key function in milk production.[4] Glucose serves as the main source of energy for other reactions as well as a critical source of carbon. Glucose is critical to the volume of milk produced and is used in the production of lactose. The synthesis of lactose combines glucose and galactose, the latter originating from glucose-6-phosphate.[33]

Lactose synthesis is carried out by the following equations:

$$\text{UDP-galactose} + \textit{N}\text{-acetylglucosamine} \rightarrow$$
$$\textit{N}\text{-acetyllactosamine} + \text{UDP} \qquad \textbf{(1)}$$

$$\text{UDP-galactose} + \text{glucose} \rightarrow \text{lactose} + \text{UDP} \quad \textbf{(2)}$$

UDP is uridine diphosphogalactose. The catalyst in the first equation is a galactosyl transferase, *N*-acetyllactosamine synthetase. The reaction is activated by metal ions that bind to the galactosyl transferase.

Most of the intracellular glucose is derived from blood sugar. A specific whey protein, α-lactalbumin, catalyzes the lactose synthesis. It is

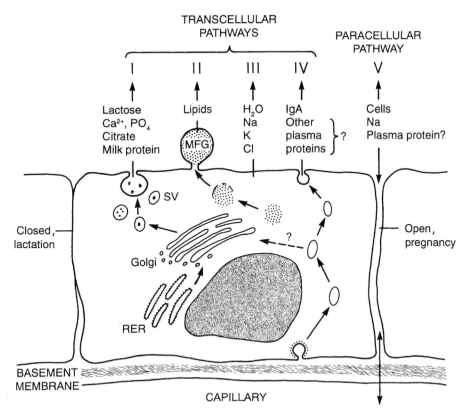

TRANSCELLULAR
PATHWAYS

PARACELLULAR
PATHWAY

I   II   III   IV   V

Lactose   Lipids   H₂O   IgA   Cells
Ca^{2+}, PO_4 Na   Other   Na
Citrate   K   plasma   Plasma protein?
Milk protein   Cl   proteins

MFG

SV

Closed,   Open,
lactation   pregnancy

Golgi

RER

BASEMENT
MEMBRANE

CAPILLARY

Figure 3-17. Pathways for milk synthesis and secretion into mammary alveolus. I, Exocytosis of milk protein and lactose in Golgi-derived secretory vesicles. II, Milk fat secretion via milk fat globule. III, Secretion of ions and water across apical membrane. IV, Pinocytosis-exocytosis of immunoglobulins.V, Paracellular pathway for plasma components and leukocytes. SV, secretory vesicle; RER, rough endoplasmic reticulum; MFG, milk fat globule. (Modified from Neville MC: The physiological basis of milk secretion. Part I. Basic physiology. Ann NY Acad Sci 586:1, 1990.)

a rate-limiting enzyme, which is inhibited by progesterone during pregnancy. In the absence of α-lactalbumin, little lactose is present. With the drop in progesterone and estrogen levels after the removal of the placenta at delivery, prolactin increases. The synthesis of α-lactalbumin becomes greater, and large amounts of lactose are produced from glucose. Progesterone regulates the onset of lactose synthesis, causing the initiation of production just as the infant is in need of nutrition.

Because lactose is synthesized only from glucose, maternal glucose utilization is increased by 30% in full lactation.[60]

Various aspects of lactose synthesis continue to be vigorously investigated.[33] The molecular mechanism of lactose synthesis is activated by metal ions, manganese (Mn), and calcium (Ca). Lactose synthesis takes place within the Golgi apparatus (see Fig. 3-17). The onset of copious milk secretion depends on rapid increase of lactose synthesis. Lactose synthetase performs the rate-limiting step in lactose synthesis, which is one of the few anabolic reactions involving glucose itself rather than a phosphorylated derivative.[4] Although progesterone, thyroxine, and lactogenic hormones are important in controlling synthesis, it is not known how they act in this system. The areas available for investigation about lactose synthesis remain vast.

Fat

Fat synthesis takes place in the endoplasmic reticulum. The alveolar cells are able to synthesize short-chain fatty acids, which are derived predominantly from acetate. Long-chain fatty acids, derived chiefly from blood plasma, are used in milk fat. Triglycerides are utilized from the plasma, as well as synthesized from intracellular glucose oxidized via the pentose pathway. Synthesis of fat from carbohydrate plays a predominant role in fat production in human milk.[37]

Two enzymes, lipoprotein lipase and palmitoyl-coenzyme A (CoA) l-glycerol-3-phosphate palmitoyl transferase, increase greatly after delivery. The lipase acts at the walls of the capillaries to catalyze the lipolysis and uptake of glycerol into the epithelial cells. The transferase catalyzes the process of synthesizing glycerides to triglycerides. It is believed that the marked increase of the lipase and transferase is stimulated by prolactin. Hormonal control of the glycerol precursors and the enzymatic release of fatty acids, leading to the formation of triglycerides, have been associated not only with prolactin but also with insulin, which stimulates the uptake of glucose into the mammary cells.

Esterification of fatty acids takes place in the endoplasmic reticulum. The triglycerides subsequently accumulate into fat droplets in several cisternae. The small droplets sit on the base of the cell and coalesce to large droplets that move toward the apex of the cell. The fat droplets are engulfed in the apical membrane and project into the alveolar lumen. The discharge of fat droplets involves the bulging of the cell apex to envelop the fat globules, protein, and a small amount of cytoplasm; with the pinching off, the globule becomes detached into the lumen. The membrane of the fat globule contains all the normal plasma enzymes. The fat droplets contain predominantly polar lipid and phosphatidyl choline.

Fatty acid synthesis involves a source of substrates and associated enzymes for their conversion to acetyl-CoA and reduced nicotinamide-adenine

dinucleotide phosphate (NADPH) in the cytoplasm of the cell and the conversion of acetyl-CoA to malonyl-CoA. The newly synthesized fatty acid is then released from the fatty acid-synthetase complex.

The milk-fat-globule membrane in human milk serves several roles. A layer of amphophilic (bipolar) substances at the globule/skim milk interface is required for the maintenance of emulsion stability of the fat globules.[37] This physiochemical fact applies to all emulsions and to the fat globules in the milk of all species. The globules and the milk-fat-globule membrane are compartments within the emulsion component of milk. Once in place, the components of the milk-fat-globule membrane, which is the oil-water interfacial compartment, are more or less firmly held in place by a variety of chemical and electrical forces. The stabilizing membrane acts as a reactive barrier on the interface between the globule and milk serum.[37] It is rate controlling for the binding of enzymes and trace elements, the controlled release of the products of lipolysis, the transfer of polar materials into milk serum, the maintenance of emulsion stability by the prevention of globule fission, and the availability of fatty acids and cholesterol for micellar absorption in the small intestine. All these interactions are dynamic. The envelopment mechanism involves rapid turnover of the plasma membrane lipids and proteins during milk production.

Protein

Most proteins in milk are formed from free amino acids in the secretory cells of the mammary gland. The definitive data confirming the origin of milk proteins were accumulated since 1980. The vast majority of proteins present in normal milk are specific to mammary secretions and are not identified in any quantity elsewhere in nature.[44]

The formation of milk protein and mammary enzymes is induced by prolactin and further stimulated by insulin and cortisol. De novo synthesis of protein uses both essential and nonessential plasma amino acids. Nuclear RNAs, induced by prolactin, stimulate synthesis of messenger RNA (mRNA) and transfer RNA (tRNA). The mRNA conveys the genetic information to the protein-synthesizing centers of the cells. The tRNA interprets the message to assemble the amino acids in the appropriate sequence of polypeptide chains of the specific milk proteins. The newly synthesized proteins are secreted into the milk during lactation. Casein, α-lactalbumin, and β-lactoglobulin from plasma amino acids are synthesized on the ribosomes of the endoplasmic reticulum, where they are condensed and appear as visible secretory granules moving toward the cellular apex.[55]

After some processing, the proteins pass to the Golgi complex, where they are further glycosylated and phosphorylated and then placed in secretory vesicles for export.[60] Alpha-lactalbumin, a protein necessary for lactose synthesis by the enzyme galactosyl transferase, is among the proteins synthesized in the mammary gland. Lactose is synthesized within the trans-Golgi complex and secreted together with the major milk proteins. The casein micelle is formed with calcium within the Golgi compartment, which presents a high concentration of calcium, phosphate, and protein via the milk. Most of the casein is bound in this manner. This pathway I (see Fig. 3-17) begins in the rough endoplasmic reticulum, where the proteins are inserted through the membrane into the lumen by exocytosis.[60]

The Golgi membrane is impermeable to lactose; thus the sugar is osmotically active. Water is drawn into the Golgi apparatus.[70] Casein micelle formation begins in the terminal Golgi vesicles, adding calcium in the secretory vesicle. These secretory vesicles move to the plasma membrane and through exocytosis extrude their contents into the alveolar lumen.[52]

Human casein micelles are smaller in size (30 to 75 nm in diameter) than bovine casein (600 nm). Human milk contains only β-casein and α-casein. Only 6% of calcium in human milk is bound to casein, compared with 65% in bovine milk. The gene for human β-casein has been cloned and sequenced.[70]

Some merocrine secretion also occurs, in which proteins and other cellular constituents are secreted, leaving the cell membrane intact. Protein caps, or signets, protruding into alveolar lumen, have been described on the outside of the apical membrane. Protein and lactose secreted into the lumen cannot be reabsorbed (Table 3-3).

The synthesis of proteins in the mammary gland follows the general pathway of all proteins under genetic control. Induction of synthesis is under hormonal control. This process involves synthesis from amino acids through the detailed system controlled by RNA and under genetic control of DNA. Glucocorticoid is required for the expression of the casein gene in the presence of prolactin. Cortisol is the limiting factor for casein gene expression.[25] Shennan[84] has reviewed the mechanisms of mammary gland ion transport.

Ions and water

Sodium, potassium, chloride, magnesium, calcium, phosphate, sulfate, and citrate pass through the membrane of the alveolar cell in both directions.[63] Water also passes in both directions, predominantly from the alveolar cells but also from the interstitial fluid. Plasma water passage depends on the amount of intracellular glucose available for lactose. The aqueous phase of milk is isosmotic to plasma. The major osmole of the aqueous phase of milk is lactose. The concentrations of sodium and chloride are less than those in plasma (Figs. 3-18 and 3-19).

Human milk differs from that of many other species in that the monovalent ions are in low concentration and lactose is in high concentration.[46] The osmolarity is the same, that is, isosmotic with plasma; thus the higher the lactose, the lower the

TABLE 3-3   **Alveolar epithelial membrane permeability**

Cell ↔ Alveolar lumen	Cell → Alveolar lumen
Glucose	Lactose
Water	Sucrose
Sodium	Citrate
Potassium	Proteins
Chloride	Fat
Iodine	Calcium
Sulfate	Phosphate

ions. It is presumed that the intracellular concentration of potassium is held high and that of sodium low by a pump on the basal membrane. The sodium and potassium ions are distributed according to the electrical potential gradient.[63] Milk is electrically positive compared with intracellular fluid. The sodium/potassium ratio is 1:3 in both milk and intracellular fluid. Vorherr[101,102] believes that lactose secretion is responsible for the potential difference across the apical membrane, thus keeping sodium and potassium ion concentration low.

The variation among species in the concentration of lactose and ions is caused by the rate of lactose synthesis, the permeability of the membrane, and the number of fixed negative charges on the membrane. The potential difference is higher in the human mammary gland than in any other species evaluated to date.

The relationship between intrastructure and function in the mammary gland changes from pregnancy to lactation. The junction between alveolar cells has attracted much interest. Cell junctions do not merely hold cells together but enable epithelia to function as permeable barriers, allowing communication between cells and coordination of activities. The three functions of cell junctions are adhesion, occlusion, and communication, which are carried out by desmosomes, tight junctions, and gap junctions, respectively. Changes in tight junctions may provide the basis for a reduction in permeability between cells. For instance, at the initiation of lactation, a tight junction changing from "leaky" to very tight blocks the paracellular movement of lactose and ions. This requires transport across cells of these materials and the maintenance of control of high intracellu-

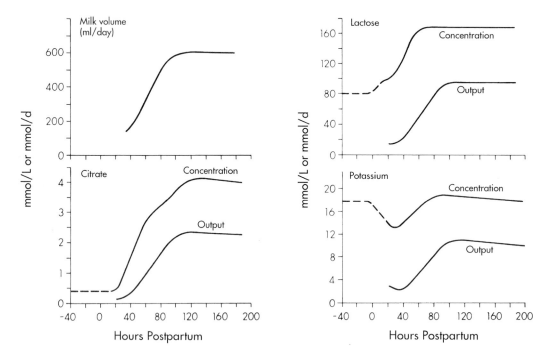

Figure 3-18. Concentrations and secretion rates of several milk components during lactogenesis. (Modified from Neville MC, Allen JC, Archer PC, et al: Studies in human lactation: Milk volume and nutrient composition during weaning and lactogenesis. Am J Clin Nutr 54:81, 1991.)

lar potassium and low intracellular sodium concentrations.[19]

Citrate is thought to be the harbinger of lactogenesis. Citrate plays a central role in the metabolism of all cells, but its significance and mode of secretion remain unknown.[72] In the final stages of lactogenesis in ruminants, the previously quiescent epithelial cells suddenly start to secrete large quantities of protein, fat, and carbohydrates. The exact lactogenic trigger is unknown, although significant hormonal changes occur. In women the onset of copious milk secretion does not begin until 3 to 4 days post partum. Significantly, citrate levels are low at delivery and rise quickly, reaching a peak on day 4 (see Fig. 3-19).[72] In the cow and the goat, copious production occurs at delivery, and the citrate levels begin to rise, increasing 10 to 100 times the baseline values.

Citrate is the main buffer system of milk.[63] It is formed within the secretory cell, but how it is secreted into the milk is not clear. Citrate and lactose may be secreted by a similar route. After dilution of milk in the gland with isosmotic lactose, the equilibrium is restored across the apical membrane in experimental models by the entrance of sodium, potassium, and chloride into the milk. No citrate, calcium, or protein enters in excess of the normal secretion rate. Inorganic phosphate is the

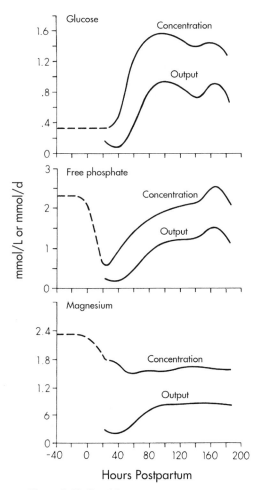
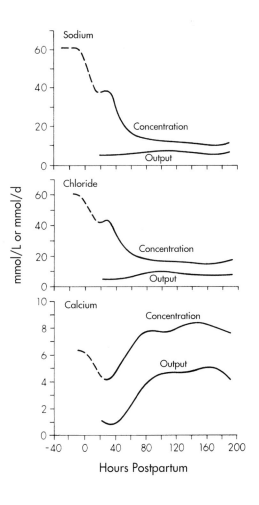

Figure 3-18. Cont'd.

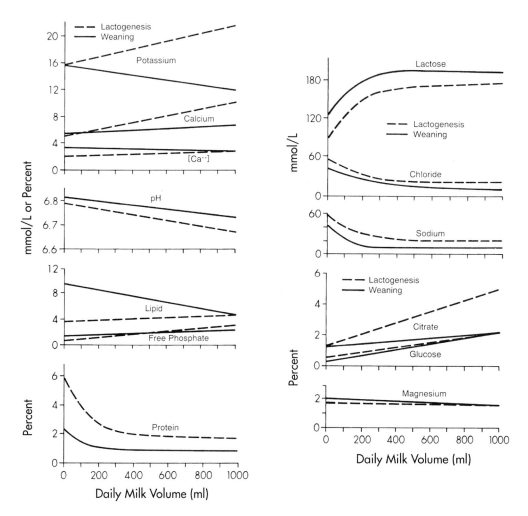

Figure 3-19. Comparison of relationship between milk volume and composition during lactogenesis (---) and weaning (—). (Modified from Neville MC, Allen JC, Archer PC, et al: Studies in human lactation: Milk volume and nutrient composition during weaning and lactogenesis. Am J Clin Nutr 54:81, 1991.)

other major buffer system, but how it is secreted is also unknown (see Fig. 3-18).

Calcium, much of which is bound to casein, enters the Golgi apparatus, where it is essentially trapped with casein in the micelle, and then enters the alveolar milk by unidirectional flow.

The mammary gland is unusual among exocrine glands because the rate of secretion slows and some secretion can be stored in its ducts.[84] Direct neural control of secretion is lacking. The

parenchyma of the gland also consists of ductal tissue in addition to secretory tissue. The ductal cells, however, are impermeable to the major milk ions during lactation, so they cannot modify the secretion, in contrast to the ductal cells of other exocrine glands (e.g., sweat, salivary) (see Fig. 3-19).[50]

A comparison of the levels of various constituents of the milk with corresponding plasma levels demonstrates the mechanism partly responsible for that mechanism (see Table 4-17).

Milk enzymes

Some milk enzymes enter the alveolar milk from the mammary blood capillaries via the intercellular fluid. Others come from the breakdown of the mammary secretory cells. The milk enzymes, xanthine oxidase, aldolase, and alkaline phosphatase, are contained in the fat globule, membrane, and milk serum. The most significant enzyme, lipase, splits triglycerides.

Human milk contains both proteolytic enzymes and protease inhibitors.[28] Amylase facilitates digestion of polysaccharides by the infant. Sulfhydryl (SH) oxidase catalyzes oxidation of SH groups. Glutathione peroxidase facilitates the delivery of selenium to the infant. Lysozyme and peroxidase are bactericidal.

Cellular components

Human milk has been called a "live fluid" by many and "white blood" in many ancient rites. Breast milk contains up to 4000 cells/mL, which have been identified with leukocytes and enter the milk via the paracellular pathway, pathway V.[100] The cell number is particularly high in colostrum. The cells in greatest number are the macrophages, which secrete lysozyme and lactoferrin. Lymphocytes, neutrophils, and epithelial cells are also present. Lymphocytes produce IgA and interferon.

Macrophages constitute a major cellular component in milk compared with levels in blood and can survive under conditions simulating the infant's gastrointestinal tract.[30] Because they release secretory IgA in association with phagocytosis, it is believed they play a role in host defense. Macrophage colony-stimulating factor in human milk and mammary gland epithelial cells are believed to be responsible for expansion of the macrophages in milk.

INVOLUTION: WEANING AND APOPTOSIS

During weaning, significant increases in milk protein, chloride, and sodium concentrations and a decrease in lactose occur when milk volumes fall below 400 mL/day. Glucose and magnesium levels are unchanged.[62] This suggests that volume is regulated differently during weaning than during lactogenesis. No sentinel substance is a reliable predictor of volume in all stages, but normal ranges of milk components during full lactation are sodium, 3 to 18 mmol/L; chloride, 8 to 24 mmol/L; protein, 8 to 23 g/L; and lactose, 140 to 230 mmol/L. Values outside these ranges suggest mastitis or weaning. During gradual weaning, between 6 and 15 months post partum, glucose, citrate, phosphate, and calcium levels decrease, whereas lipid, potassium, and magnesium increase[63] (see Fig. 3-19).

Postlactational involution of the mammary gland is characterized by two distinct physiologic processes.[54] First, secretory epithelial cells undergo apoptosis and programmed cell death. Second, the mammary gland's basement membrane undergoes proteolytic degradation. Apoptosis is almost absent during lactation but develops within 2 days of involution. In the initial phase of involution, apoptosis of fully differentiated mammary epithelial cells occurs without visible degradation of the extracellular matrix. The second phase consists of extracellular remodeling and altered mesenchymal-epithelial interactions followed by apoptosis of cells no longer differentiating.[88] During postlactational mammary gland involution, most mammary epithelium dies and is reabsorbed.

SUMMARY

In the human, lactogenesis occurs slowly over the first few days post partum as progesterone levels drop. Women experience "milk coming in" as a feeling of fullness between 40 and 72 hours, usually corresponding to the degree of parity, with multiparas sensing this more quickly than primiparas. Volume of milk increases over time for the first 2 weeks, starting at less than 100 mL/day and increasing to about 600 mL/day at 96 hours (Fig. 3-20). This parallels the rise in citrate production, reflecting the metabolic activity of the mammary gland. Lactose, sodium chloride, and protein rise promptly, stabilizing at 24 hours and reflecting the

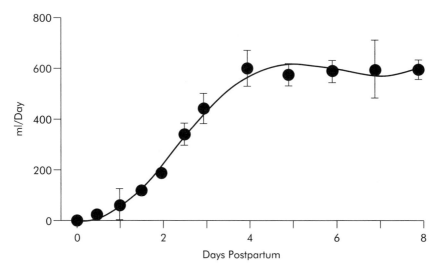

Figure 3-20. Milk volumes during first week postpartum. Mean values from 12 multiparous white women who test-weighed their infants before and after every feeding for first 7 days postpartum. (Redrawn from Neville MC: Determinants of milk volume and composition. In Jensen RG (ed): Handbook of Milk Composition. San Diego, Academic Press, 1995.)

closure of the pericellular pathway, which results in a decrease in direct flux into the milk. This suggests a two-step process of junctional closure followed by onset of secretory activity.

The changes in permeability of the tight junctions; rate of synthesis of lactose, lipids, and nutrient proteins; transport of glucose into the alveolar cells; transcytosis of secretory IgA; movement of immune cells into the alveolar lumen; and secretion of lactoferrin represent the distinct metabolic and cellular modifications. Neville[61] states, "The temporal sequence of these changes as they occur during lactogenesis suggests that they are either independently regulated or form part of an orderly cascade of temporally separate events." Figure 3-21 graphically illustrates these changes.

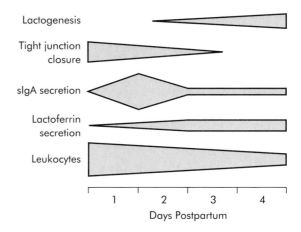

Figure 3-21. Summary model for temporal sequence of changes in mammary gland function during lactogenesis in women. (From Neville MC: Determinants of milk volume and composition. In Jensen RG (ed): Handbook of Milk Composition. San Diego, Academic Press, 1995.)

REFERENCES

1. Anbazhagan R, Bartek J, Stamp G, et al: Expression of integrin subunits in the human infant breast correlates with morphogenesis and differentiation. J Pathol 176:227, 1995.

2. Arthur PG, Hartmann PE, Smith M: Measurement of the milk intake of breastfed infants. J Pediatr Gastroenterol 6:419, 1989.

3. Battin DA, Marrs RP, Fleiss PM, et al: Effect of suckling on serum prolactin, luteinizing hormone, follicle-stimulating hormone, and estradiol during prolonged lactation. Obstet Gynecol 65:785, 1985.

4. Bell AW, Bauman DE: Adaptations of glucose metabolism during pregnancy and lactation. J Mammary Gland Biol Neoplasia 2:265, 1997.

5. Bochinfuso WP, Korach KS: Mammary gland development and tumorigenesis in estrogen receptor knockout mice. J Mammary Gland Biol Neoplasia 2:323, 1997.

6. Caldeyro-Barcia R: Milk ejection in women. In Reynolds M, Folley SJ (eds): Lactogenesis: The Initiation of Milk Secretion at Parturition. Philadelphia, University of Pennsylvania Press, 1969.

7. Chiodera P, Salvarani C, Bacchi-Modena A, et al: Relationship between plasma profiles of oxytocin and adrenocorticotropic hormone during suckling or breast stimulation in women. Horm Res 35:119, 1991.

8. Cholst IN, Wardlaw SL, Newman CB, et al: Prolactin response to breast stimulation in lactating women is not mediated by endogenous opioids. Am J Obstet Gynecol 150:558, 1984.

9. Christensson K, Nilsson BA, Stocks S, et al: Effect of nipple stimulation on uterine activity and on plasma levels of oxytocin in full term, healthy, pregnant women. Acta Obstet Gynecol Scand 68:205, 1989.

10. Cobo E: Effect of different doses of ethanol on the milk ejection reflex in lactating women. Am J Obstet Gynecol 115:817, 1973.

11. Coiro V, Alboni A, Gramellini D, et al: Inhibition by ethanol of the oxytocin response to breast stimulation in normal women and the role of endogenous opioids. Acta Endocrinol 126:213, 1992.

12. Cowie AT, Forsyth IA, Hart IC: Hormonal control of lactation. In Gross F, Grumbach MM, Labhart A, et al (eds): Monographs on Endocrinology, Vol. 15. New York, Springer-Verlag, 1980.

13. Cregan MD, Hartmann PE: Computerized breast measurement from conception to weaning: Clinical implications. J Hum Lact 15:89, 1999.

14. Crowley WR, Armstrong WE: Neurochemical regulation of oxytocin secretion in lactation. Endocr Rev 13:33, 1992.

15. Daly SEJ, Owens RA, Hartmann PE: The short-term synthesis and infant-regulated removal of milk in lactating women. Exper Physiol 78:209, 1993.

16. Daniel CW, Berger JJ, Strickland P, et al: Similar growth pattern of mouse mammary epithelium cultivated in collagen matrix in vivo and in vitro. Dev Biol 104:57, 1984.

17. Daniel CW, Robinson S, Silberstein GB: The role of TGF-α in faltering and growth of the mammary ductal tree. J Mammary Gland Biol Neoplasia 1:331, 1996.

18. Dawood MY, Khan-Dawood FS, Wahi RS, et al: Oxytocin release and plasma anterior pituitary and gonadal hormones in women during lactation. J Clin Endocrinol Metab 52:678, 1981.

19. Falconer IR, Rowe JM: Effect of prolactin on sodium and potassium concentration in the mammary alveolar tissue. Endocrinology 101:181, 1977.

20. Fournier PRJ, Desjardins PD, Friesen HG: Current understanding of human prolactin physiology and its diagnostic and therapeutic applications: A review. Am J Obstet Gynecol 118:337, 1974.

21. Fowler PA, Casey CE, Cameron GG, et al: Cyclic changes in composition and volume of the breast during the menstrual cycle, measured by magnetic resonance imaging. Br J Obstet Gynaecol 97:595, 1990.

22. Frantz AG: Prolactin. N Engl J Med 298:201, 1978.

23. Freund-Mercier MJ, Richard P: Excitatory effects of intra-ventricular injections of oxytocin on the milk ejection reflex in the rat. J Physiol 352:447, 1984.

24. Frigerio C, Schutz Y, Prentice A, et al: Is human lactation a particularly efficient process? Eur J Clin Nutr 45:459, 1991.

25. Ganguly R, Ganguly N, Mehta NM, et al: Absolute requirement of glucocorticoid for expression of the casein gene in the presence of prolactin. Proc Natl Acad Sci USA 77:6003, 1980.

26. Gehlbach DL, Bayliss P, Rosa C: Prolactin and thyrotropin responses to nursing during the early puerperium. J Reprod Med 34:295, 1989.

27. Hammond KA: Adaptation of the maternal intestine during lactation. J Mammary Gland Biol Neoplasia 2:243, 1997.

28. Hamosh M: Enzymes in milk: Their function in the mammary gland, in milk and in the infant. In Hanson LA (ed): Biology of Human Milk. Nestlé Nutrition Workshop Series, Vol 15. Philadelphia, Lippincott William & Wilkins, 1988, p. 45.

29. Hansen S, Gummesson BM: Participation of the lateral mid-brain tegmentum in the neuroendocrine control of sexual behavior and lactation in the rat. Brain Res 251:319, 1982.

30. Hara T, Irie K, Saito S, et al: Identification of macrophage colony-stimulating factor in human milk and mammary gland epithelial cells. Pediatr Res 37:437, 1995.

31. Hartmann PE: Changes in the composition and yield of the mammary secretion of cows during the initiation of lactation. J Endocrinol 59:231, 1973.

32. Hartmann PE, Saint L: Measurement of milk yield in women. J Pediatr Gastroenterol Nutr 3:270, 1984.

33. Healy DL, Rattigan S, Hartmann PE, et al: Prolactin in human milk: Correlation with lactose, total protein, and α-lactalbumin levels. Am J Physiol 238 (Endocrinol Metab 1):E83, 1980.

34. Horst RL, Goff JP, Reinhardt TA: Calcium and vitamin D metabolism during lactation. J Mammary Gland Biol Neoplasia 2:253, 1997.

35. Howie PW, McNeilly AS, McArdle T, et al: The relationship between suckling-induced prolactin response and lactogenesis. J Clin Endocrinol Metab 50:670, 1980.

36. Humphreys RC, Lydon J, O'Malley BW, et al: Mammary gland development is mediated by both stromal and epithelial progesterone receptors. Mol Endocrinol 11:801, 1997.

37. Jensen RG: The Lipids of Human Milk. Boca Raton, Fla, CRC Press, 1989.

38. Jones DH: The mitochondria of the mammary parenchymal cell in relation to the pregnancy-lactation cycle. In Larson BL (ed): Lactation, Vol 4. The Mammary Gland/Human Lactation/Milk Synthesis. New York, Academic Press, 1978.

39. Kent JC, Ramsay DT, Doherty D: Response of breasts to different stimulation patterns of an electric breast pump. J Hum Lact 19:179, 2003.

40. Kleinberg DL: Early mammary development: Growth hormone and IGF-1. Mammary Gland Biol Neoplasia 2:49, 1997.

41. Koldovsky O, Bedrick A, Rao R: Role of milk-borne prostaglandins and epidermal growth factor for the suckling mammal. J Am Coll Nutr 10:17, 1991.

42. Kulski JK, Hartmann PE: Changes in human milk composition during the initiation of lactation. Aust J Exp Biol Med 59:101, 1981.

43. Kwa HG, Bulbrook RD, Wang DY: An overall perspective on the role of prolactin in the breast. In Nagasawa H (ed): Prolactin and Lesions in Breast, Uterus and Prostate. Boca Raton, Fla, CRC Press, 1989.

44. Larson BL (ed): Lactation, Vol. 4. The Mammary Gland/Human Lactation/Milk Synthesis. New York, Academic Press, 1978.

45. Larson BL, Smith VR (eds): Lactation, Vol. 2. Biosynthesis and Secretion of Milk/Diseases. New York, Academic Press, 1974.

46. Larson BL, Smith VR (eds): Lactation, Vol. 3. Nutrition and Biochemistry of Milk/Maintenance. New York, Academic Press, 1974.

47. Leake RD, Waters CB, Rubin RT, et al: Oxytocin and prolactin responses in long-term breastfeeding. Obstet Gynecol 62:565, 1983.

48. Lincoln DW, Paisley AC: Neuroendocrine control of milk ejection. J Reprod Fertil 65:571, 1982.

49. Lincoln DW, Renfree MB: Mammary gland growth and milk ejection in the agile wallaby, Macropus agilis, displaying concurrent asynchronous lactation. J Reprod Fertil 63:193, 1981.

50. Linzell JL, Peaker M: The permeability of mammary ducts. J Physiol 216:710, 1971.

51. Liu Y, Hyde JF, Vore M: Prolactin regulates maternal bile secretory function postpartum. J Pharmacol Exp Ther 261:560, 1992.

52. Lönnerdal B, Atkinson S: Nitrogenous components of milk and human milk proteins. In Jensen RG (ed): Handbook of Milk Composition. San Diego, Academic Press, 1995.

53. Lucas A, Drewett RB, Mitchell MD: Breastfeeding and plasma oxytocin concentrations. Br Med J 281:834, 1980.

54. Lund LR, Rømer J, Thomasset N, et al: Two distinct phases of apoptosis in mammary gland involution: Proteinase-independent and -dependent pathways. Development 122:181, 1996.

55. Martin RH, Glass MR, Chapman C, et al: Human β-lactalbumin and hormonal factors in pregnancy and lactation. Clin Endocrinol 13:223, 1980.

56. McNeilly AS, Robinson ICA, Houston MJ, et al: Release of oxytocin and prolactin in response to suckling. Br Med J 286:257, 1983.

57. Meites J: Neuroendocrinology of lactation. J Invest Dermatol 63:119, 1974.

58. Neville MC: Anatomy and physiology of lactation. In Schanler RJ (ed): Breastfeeding Part I. Pediatr Clin North Am 48:35, 2001.

59. Neville MC: Regulation of mammary development and lactation. In Neville MC, Neifert MR (eds): Lactation: Physiology, Nutrition, and Breast-Feeding. New York, Plenum, 1983.

60. Neville MC: The physiological basis of milk secretion. Part I. Basic physiology. Ann NY Acad Sci 586:1, 1990.

61. Neville MC: Determinants of milk volume and composition. A. Lactogenesis in women: A cascade of events revealed by milk composition. In Jensen RG (ed): Handbook of Milk Composition. San Diego, Academic Press, 1995.

62. Neville MC: Mammary gland biology and lactation: A short course. Presented at biannual meeting of the International Society for Research on Human Milk and Lactation. Plymouth, Mass, October 1997.

63. Neville MC, Allen JC, Archer PC, et al: Studies in human lactation: Milk volume and nutrient composition during weaning and lactogenesis. Am J Clin Nutr 54:81, 1991.

64. Neville MC, Allen JC, Walters C: The mechanisms of milk secretion. In Neville MC, Neifert MR (eds): Lactation: Physiology, Nutrition, and Breast-Feeding. New York, Plenum, 1983.

65. Newton N: The relation of the milk-ejection reflex to the ability to breastfeed. Ann NY Acad Sci 652:484, 1992.

66. Newton N: The quantitative effect of oxytocin (Pitocin) on human milk yield. Ann NY Acad Sci 652:481, 1992.

67. Nissen E, Lilja G, Widström A-M, et al: Elevation of oxytocin levels early postpartum in women. Acta Obstet Gynecol Scand 74:530, 1995.

68. Ormandy CJ, Binart N, Kelly PA: Mammary gland development in prolactin receptor knockout mice. J Mammary Gland Biol Neoplasia 2:355, 1997.

69. Ostrom KM: A review of the hormone prolactin during lactation: Progress in food and nutrition. Science 14:1, 1990.

70. Patton S, Neville MC: Introduction: maternal adaptation to lactation. J Mammary Gland Biol Neoplasia 2:201, 1997.

71. Peaker M: Production of hormones by the mammary gland: Short review. Endocr Regul 25:10, 1991.

72. Peaker M, Linzell JL: Citrate in milk: a harbinger of lactogenesis. Nature 253:464, 1975.

73. Pederson CA: Oxytocin control of maternal behavior. Ann NY Acad Med 807:126, 1997.

74. Pederson CA, Prange AJ: Induction of maternal behavior in virgin rats after intracerebroventricular administration of oxytocin. Proc Natl Acad Sci 76:6661, 1979.

75. Pederson CA, Caldwell JD, Walker C, et al: Oxytocin activates the postpartum onset of rat maternal behavior in the ventral, tegmental and medial preoptic areas. Behav Neurosci 108:1163, 1994.

76. Prentice A, Addey CVP, Wilde CJ: Evidence for local feedback control of human milk secretion. Biochem Soc Trans 17:122, 1989.

77. Prilusky J, Deis RP: Inhibition of milk ejection by a visual stimulus in lactating rats: Implication of the pineal gland. Brain Res 251:313, 1982.

78. Richard L, Alade MO: Effect of delivery room routines on success of first breast-feed. Lancet 336:1105, 1990.

79. Rimoin DL, Holzman GB, Merimee TJ, et al: Lactation in the absence of human growth hormone. J Clin Endocrinol Metab 28:1183, 1968.

80. Robinson JE, Short RV: Changes in breast sensitivity at puberty, during the menstrual cycle, and at parturition. Br Med J 1:1188, 1977.

81. Robyn C, Meuris S: Pituitary prolactin, lactational performance and puerperal infertility. Semin Perinatol 6:254, 1982.

82. Rosen JM, Humphreys R, Krnacik S, et al: The regulation of mammary gland development by hormones, growth factors and oncogenes. Prog Clin Biol Res 387:95, 1994.

83. Shalev E, Weiner E, Tzabari A, et al: Breast stimulation in late pregnancy. Gynecol Obstet Invest 29:125, 1990.

84. Shennan DB: Mechanisms of mammary gland ion transport. Comp Biochem Physiol 97A:317, 1990.

85. Sherwood LM: Human prolactin. N Engl J Med 284:774, 1971.

86. Smith VR: Lactation, Vol. 1. The Mammary Gland/Development and Maintenance. New York, Academic Press, 1974.

87. Stern JM, Reichlin S: Prolactin circadian rhythm persists throughout lactation in women. Neuroendocrinology 51:31, 1990.

88. Strange R, Li F, Saurer S, et al: Apoptotic cell death and tissue remodeling during mouse mammary gland involution. Development 115:49, 1992.

89. St Reuli CH, Edwards GM: Control of normal mammary epithelial phenotype by integrins. J Mam Gland Biol Neoplasia 3:151, 1998.

90. Takeda S, Kuwabara Y, Mizuno M: Concentrations and origin of oxytocin in breast milk. Endocrinol Jpn 33:821, 1986.

91. Tanaka T, Shiu RPC, Gout PW, et al: A new sensitive and specific bioassay for lactogenic hormones: Measurement of prolactin and growth hormone in human serum. J Clin Endocrinol Metab 51:1058, 1980.

92. Theorell T: Prolactin: A hormone that mirrors passiveness in crisis situations. Integr Physiol Behav Sci 27:32, 1992.

93. Toppozada MK, El-Rahman HA, Soliman AY: Prostaglandins as milk ejectors: The nose as a new route of administration. In Samuelson B, Paoletti R, Rawell P (eds): Advances in Prostaglandin, Thromboxane, and Leukotrience Research, Vol. 12. New York, Raven, 1983.

94. Tyson JE: Mechanisms of puerperal lactation. Med Clin North Am 61:153, 1977.

95. Uvnäs-Moberg K: The oxytocin factor: Tapping the hormone of calm, love and healing. Cambridge, MA, Da Capo Press, 2003.

96. Uvnäs-Moberg K, Eriksson M: Breastfeeding: physiological, endocrine and behavioral adaptations caused by oxytocin and local neurogenic activity in the nipple and mammary gland. Acta Paediatr 85:525, 1996.

97. Vernon RG, Pond CM: Adaptations of maternal adipose tissue to lactation. J Mammary Gland Biol Neoplasia 2:231, 1997.

98. Vigneri R, Squatrito S, Pezzino V, et al: Spontaneous fluctuations of human placental lactogen during normal pregnancy. J Clin Endocrinol Metab 40:506, 1975.

99. Vonderhaar BK, Bremel RD: Prolactin, growth hormone, and placental lactogen. J Mammary Gland Biol Neoplasia 2:1, 1997.

100. Vorherr H: The Breast: Morphology, Physiology and Lactation. New York, Academic Press, 1974.

101. Vorherr H: Human lactation and breastfeeding. In Larson BL (ed): Lactation, Vol. 4. The Mammary Gland/Human Lactation/Milk Synthesis. New York, Academic Press, 1978.

102. Vorherr H: Hormonal and biochemical changes of pituitary and breast during pregnancy. In Vorherr H (ed): Human lactation. Semin Perinatol 3:193, 1979.

103. Wehrenberg WB, Gaillard RC: Neuroendocrine mechanisms regulating growth hormone and prolactin secretion during lactation. Endocrinology 124:464, 1989.

104. Weitzman RE, Leake RD, Rubin RT, et al: The effect of nursing on neurohypophyseal hormone and prolactin secretion in human subjects. J Clin Endocrinol Metab 51:836, 1980.

105. Widstrom AM, Winberg J, Werner S, et al: Suckling in lactating women stimulates the secretion of insulin and prolactin without concomitant effects on gastrin, growth hormone, calcitonin, vasopressin, or catecholamines. Early Hum Dev 10:115, 1984.

106. Wilde CJ, Addey CVP, Boddy LM, et al: Autocrine regulation of milk secretion by a protein in milk. Biochem J 305:51, 1995.

107. Yuen BH: Prolactin in human milk: the influence of nursing and the duration of postpartum lactation. Am J Obstet Gynecol 158:583, 1988.

108. Zinaman MJ, Hughes V, Queenan JT, et al: Acute prolactin and oxytocin responses and milk yield to infant suckling and artificial methods of expression in lactating women. Pediatrics 89:437, 1992.

$\mathscr{B}$iochemistry of human milk

The biochemistry of human milk encompasses a mammoth supply of scientific data and information, most of which has been generated since 1970. Each report or study adds a tiny piece to the complex puzzle of the nutrients that make up human milk. The answers to some questions still elude us. A question as simple as the volume of milk consumed at a feeding remains a scientific challenge. The methodology must be accurate, reproducible, noninvasive, and suitable for home use night or day and must not interrupt breastfeeding. The precision analysis available for measuring the concentration of the most minuscule of elements, however, is remarkably accurate and reproducible in the laboratory.

Advances in analytic methods bring greater sensitivity, resolving power, and speed to the analysis of milk composition. Previously unknown and unrecognized compounds have been detected. We now know milk brings both nutrients and nonnutritive signals to the neonate. With few exceptions, all milks contain the nutrients for physical growth and development. When the offspring develops rapidly, the milk is nutrient dense; when it develops slowly, the milk is more dilute. All milks contain fat, carbohydrate, and proteins, as well as minerals, vitamins, and other nutrients. The organization of milk composition includes lipids in emulsified globules coated with a membrane, colloidal dispersions of proteins as micelles, and the remainder as a true solution.[159] At no other time in life is a single food adequate as the sole source of nutrition.

The discussion in this chapter is limited to information perceived as immediately useful to the clinician. Considerable detail and species variability are overlooked to help focus attention on details directly influencing management. Extensive and exhaustive reviews are referenced to provide the reader with easy access to greater detail and validation of the general conclusions reported here.

Human milk is not a uniform body fluid but a secretion of the mammary gland of changing composition (Fig. 4-1). Foremilk differs from hindmilk. Colostrum differs from transitional and mature milks. Milk changes over time of day and as time goes by. As concentrations of protein, fat, carbohydrates, minerals, and cells differ, physical properties such as osmolarity and pH change. The impact of changing composition on the physiology of the infant gut is beginning to be appreciated. Many constituents have dual roles, not only nutrition but infection protection, immunity, or a host of other effects.

The more than 200 constituents of milk include a tremendous array of molecules whose descriptions continue to be refined as qualitative and quantitative laboratory techniques are perfected. Resolution of lipid chemicals has advanced dramatically in recent years, but new carbohydrates and proteins have been identified as well. Some of the compounds identified may well be intermediary products in the process

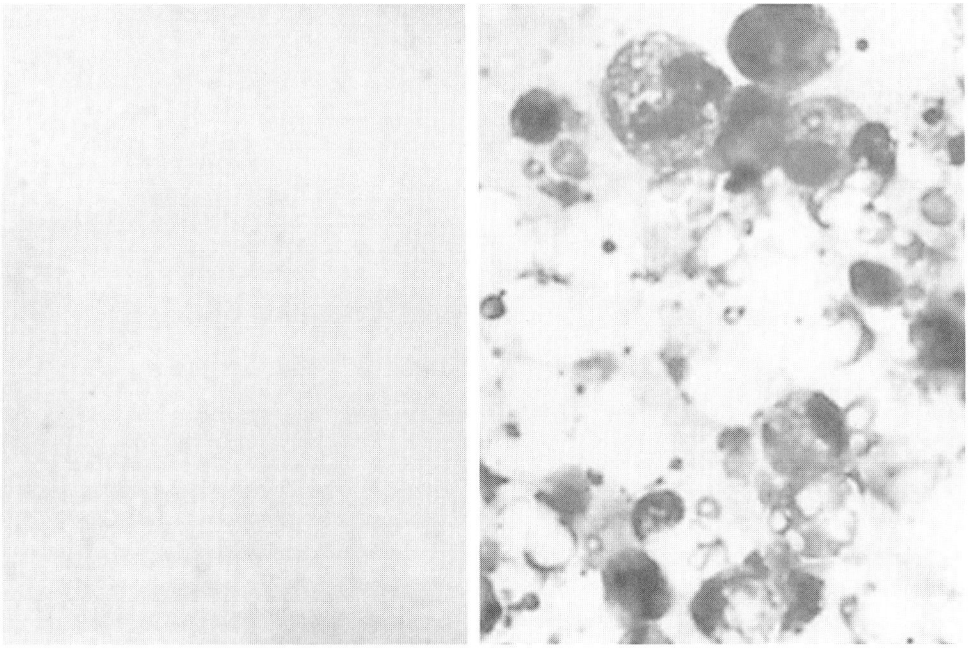

Formula vs Human Milk

Figure 4-1.   A comparison of formula (*left*) and human milk (*right*). Human milk is a dynamic colloidal solution of perfect nutrients and growth factors for infant. Formula is a totally homogenized solution of nutrient chemicals. (Courtesy of Nancy Wight, MD, San Diego, Calif.)

that occurs within the mammary cells and may be only incidental in the final product.[216] Milk includes true solutions, colloids, membranes, membrane-bound globules, and living cells.

Human and bovine milks are known in the greatest detail[83]; however, much information exists about the milk of the rat and the mouse, as well as five other species: the water buffalo, goat, sheep, horse, and pig. Several are listed in Table 4-1. Miscellaneous data are available on the milk of 150 more species but there are almost no data at all on another 4000 species. Jenness and Sloan[112] have compiled a summary of 140 species from which a sampling has been extracted (Table 4-2). The constituents of milk can be divided into the following groups, according to their specificity[112]:

1. Constituents specific to both organ and species (e.g., most proteins and lipids)

2. Constituents specific to organ but not to species (e.g., lactose)
3. Constituents specific to species but not to organ (e.g., albumin, some immunoglobulins)

NORMAL VARIATIONS IN HUMAN MILK

In defining the constituents of human milk, it is important to recognize that the composition varies with the stage of lactation, the time of day, the sampling time during a given feeding, maternal nutrition, and individual variation. Many early interpretations of the content of human milk were based on spot samples or even pooled samples from multiple donors at different times and stages of lactation. Samples obtained by pumping may

TABLE 4-1   **Composition of milks obtained from different mammals and growth rate of their offspring**

Species	Days required to double birth weight	Content of milk (%)			
		Fat	Protein	Lactose	Ash
Human	180	3.8	0.9	7.0	0.2
Horse	60	1.9	2.5	6.2	0.5
Cow	47	3.7	3.4	4.8	0.7
Reindeer	30	16.9	11.5	2.8	—
Goat	19	4.5	2.9	4.1	0.8
Sheep	10	7.4	5.5	4.8	1.0
Rat	6	15.0	12.0	3.0	2.0

From Hambraeus L: Proprietary milk versus human breast milk in infant feeding. A critical appraisal from the nutritional point of view. Pediatr Clin North Am 24:17, 1977.

vary from those obtained by the suckling infant, because some variation exists in content among the various methods of pumping.

Daytime consumption of milk in a given infant varies between 46% and 58% of the total 24-hour consumption, so that reliance on less than a 24-hour sampling may be misleading. Data from samples taken every 3 hours showed a variation in milk concentration of nitrogen, lactose, and fat, as well as in the volume of milk, by time of day (Fig. 4-2). Furthermore, there were statistically significant diurnal changes in the concentration of lactose and the volume within individual subjects, but the times of those changes were not consistent for each individual. Some individuals varied as much as twofold in volume production from day to day. These investigators also found a significant difference in the concentrations of fat and lactose and in the volume of milk produced by each breast. At the extreme, the less productive breast yielded only 65% of the volume of the other breast.

TABLE 4-2   **Constituents of milk (g/100 g) of specific mammals**

Mammalian species in taxonomic position	Total solids	Fat	Casein	Whey protein	Total protein	Lactose	Ash
Human	12.4	3.8	0.4	0.6	—	7.0	0.2
Baboon	14.4	5.0	—	—	1.6	7.3	0.3
Orangutan	11.5	3.5	1.1	0.4	—	6.0	0.2
Black bear	44.5	24.5	8.8	5.7	—	0.4	1.8
California sea lion	52.7	36.5	—	—	13.8	0.0	0.6
Black rhinoceros	8.1	0.0	1.1	0.3	—	6.1	0.3
Spotted dolphin	31.0	18.0	—	—	9.4	0.6	—
Domestic dog	23.5	12.9	5.8	2.1	—	3.1	1.2
Norway rat	21.0	10.3	6.4	2.0	—	2.6	1.3
Whitetail jackrabbit	40.8	13.9	19.7	4.0	—	1.7	1.5

Modified from Jenness R, Sloan RE: Composition of milk. In Larson BL, Smith VR (eds): Lactation, Vol. 3. Nutrition and Biochemistry of Milk/Maintenance. New York, Academic Press, 1974.

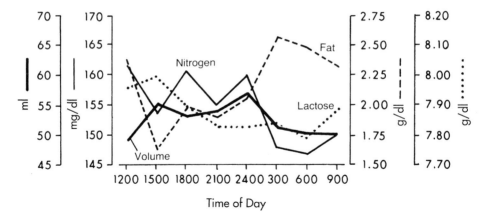

Figure 4-2. Mean concentrations of nitrogen, lactose, and fat in human milk by time of day. (Modified from Brown KH, Black RE, Robertson AD, et al: Clinical and field studies of human lactation: methodological considerations. Am J Clin Nutr 35:745, 1982.)

The variation in the fat content has received some attention. Fat content changes during a given feeding, increasing at the end of the feeding. Fat content rises from early morning to midday; the volume increased from two to five times, as reported in early studies when feedings were controlled. Multiple studies in different countries and different decades, summarized by Jackson and coworkers[108] reveal that some of the variation is related to other factors. Demand feeding (Thai mothers in 1988) has a different circadian variation than scheduled feeding (U.S. mothers in 1932) (Fig. 4-3). In the later part of the first year of lactation, the fat content diminishes. Work done by Atkinson and associates[13] and confirmed by other investigators has shown that the nitrogen content of the milk of mothers who deliver prematurely is higher than that of those whose pregnancies reach full term. For a given volume of milk, the premature infant would receive 20% more nitrogen than the full-term infant if each were fed his or her own mother's milk. Other constituents of milk produced by mothers who deliver prematurely have also been studied.

An additional consideration in reviewing information available on the levels of various constituents of milk is the technique used to derive the data. In 1975, Hambraeus[83] reported that there was less protein in human milk than originally calculated. The present techniques of immunoassay measure the absolute amounts, whereas earlier figures were derived from calculations based on measurements of the nitrogen content. About 25% of the nitrogen in human milk is nonprotein nitrogen. Cow milk has only 5% nonprotein nitrogen.

A major concern about variation in content of human milk is related to the mother's diet. Maternal diet is of particular concern when the mother is malnourished or eats an unusually restrictive diet. Malnourished mothers have approximately the same proportions of protein, fat, and carbohydrate as well-nourished mothers, but they produce less milk. Levels of water-soluble vitamins, such as ascorbic acid, thiamin, and vitamin B_{12}, are quickly affected by deficient diets. "From a nutritional perspective, infancy is a critical and vulnerable period. At no other stage in life is a single food adequate as a sole source of nutrition," writes Picciano.[177] This results from the immaturity of the tissues and organs involved in the metabolism of nutrients, which limits the ability to respond to nutrition excesses and deficiencies. The system is species-specific and depends on the presence of the self-contained enzymes and ligands to facilitate digestion at the proper stage while preserving function (such as sIgA). It continues to facilitate absorption and utilization.

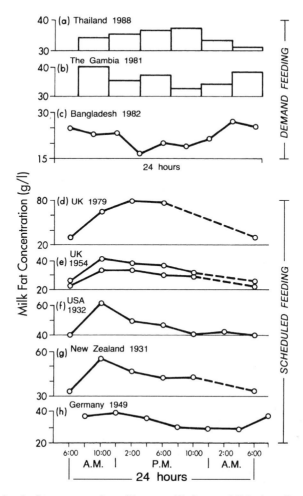

Figure 4-3. Circadian variation in fat concentration of breast milk from published studies. **A**, Thailand—Prefeed/post-feed expressed samples, 19 mothers studied for 24 hours each, infants aged 1 to 9 months. **B**, The Gambia (Prentice et al)—Demand feeding, pre/postexpressed samples, 16 mothers studied for 24 hours each, infants aged 1 to 18 months. **C**, Bangladesh (Brown et al)—Samples collected at scheduled intervals by total breast extraction (breast pump), seven mothers studied for 24 hours each, infants aged 1 to 9 months. **D**, United Kingdom (UK) (Hall)—Prefeed/postfeed expressed samples, one mother studied for 72 hours. **E**, UK: (Hytten)—Samples collected by total breast extraction (breast pump). Lower curve, 29 mothers studied for 24 hours each, infants aged 3 to 8 days. Upper curve, 20 mothers studied for 24 hours each, infants aged 21 days to 4 months. **F**, United States (USA) (Nims et al)—Samples collected by total breast extraction (manual), three mothers studied, but values given only for one mother, for 24 hours on six occasions and 72 hours on one occasion, infant aged 6 to 60 weeks. **G**, New Zealand (Deem)—Samples collected by total breast extraction (manual), 28 mothers studied for 24 hours each, infants aged 1 to 8 months. **H**, Germany (Gunther and Stainier)—Collection of samples by total breast extraction (manual), two mothers studied for 24 hours each, six mothers studied for 52 hours each, infants aged 8 to 11 days. (Modified from Jackson DA, Imong SM, Silprasert A, et al: Circadian variation in fat concentration of breast milk in a rural northern Thai population. Br J Nutr 59:349, 1988; see article for complete bibliography.)

Mother's milk is recommended for all infants under ordinary circumstances, even if the mother's diet is not perfect, according to the Committee on Nutrition during Pregnancy and Lactation of the Institute of Medicine.[158]

LACTOGENESIS STAGE I

Stage I lactogenesis is the onset of milk secretion and begins with the early changes in the mammary gland during pregnancy and continues until full lactation has occurred after delivery. Stage I begins when small quantities of milk components such as casein and lactose are secreted. This amount is held in check by high levels of circulating progesterone. The first milk obtained by the newborn at birth is called colostrum and the milk produced in the first 10 days is called transitional milk. Full volume is obtained in the next stage, lactogenesis II. Neville and associates[166] state that the terms "colostrum" and "transitional milk" do not describe the mammary secretion product during the first 4 days or from days 4 to 10 post partum. It has always been recognized that the content changes rapidly over the first 4 days and then more slowly over the next 6 or so days as a continuum. They suggest the abandonment of these terms. Colostrum and transitional milk are convenient clinical terms that are useful descriptive terms. The terms will be used in this text for clinical purposes.

Prepartum milk

Prepartum milk is the first stage of lactogenesis and is especially conspicuous in other species, such as the goat.[4] It provides evidence that the junctions between alveolar cells are "leaky" during pregnancy, allowing fluid and solutes to flow between the milk space and the interstitial fluid of the mammary gland. Figure 4-4 illustrates the composition of this milk. The lactose concentration is directly correlated with that of potassium, but sodium and chloride are inversely related to lactose (Tables 4-3 to 4-7).

Colostrum

The stages in the continuum of human milk are colostrum, transitional milk, and mature milk, and their relative contents are significant for newborns and their physiologic adaption to extrauterine life.

The mammary secretion during the first few days consists of a yellowish, thick fluid, colostrum. The residual mixture of materials present in the mammary glands and ducts at delivery and immediately after is progressively mixed with newly secreted milk, forming colostrum. Human colostrum is known to differ from mature milk in composition, both in the nature of its components and in the relative proportions of these components. The first changes are in sodium and chloride concentrations and an increase in lactose, probably due to the closure of the tight junctions. Colostrum's specific gravity is 1.040 to 1.060. The mean energy value is 67 kcal/dL compared with the 75 kcal/dL of mature milk. The volume varies between 2 and 20 mL per feeding in the first 3 days. The total volume per day also depends on the number of feedings and is reported to average, in the first 24 hours (which is different from the first day, depending on the time of delivery), 100 mL (Table 4-4). Tables 4-5 and 4-6 list the yield and composition of colostrum (1 to 5 days) and mature milk 14 days and beyond. The increased production of citrate is paralleled by the increase in volume (Figs. 4-5 and 4-6). The result is a decrease in sodium and chloride and an increase in lactose concentration due to water dilution.

The antepartum milk glucose level is 0.35 ± 0.16 mmol/L (see Table 4-3). Glucose levels vary among individuals. Glucose decreases during a feed as aqueous phase decreases and lipid increases. In early colostrum, glucose passes into the milk via the paracellular pathway and parallels lactose. When lactation is fully established, glucose levels are unrelated to lactose levels.[115] In mature milk, the level is 1.5 ± 0.4 mmol/L.

Dewey and associates[49] clearly demonstrate that in a well-established milk supply, volume depends on infant demand, and the residual milk available at each feeding is comparable in both low-intake and

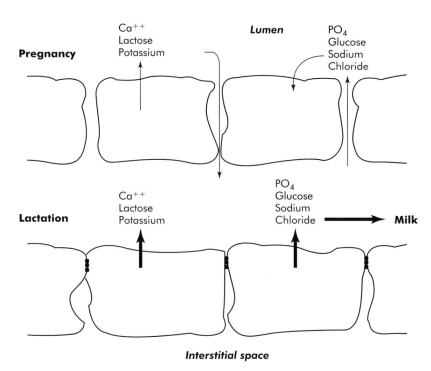

Figure 4-4. Model for directions of major fluxes of several macronutrients during pregnancy and lactation in women. (From Neville MC: Determinants of milk volume and composition. In Jensen RG (ed): Handbook of Milk Composition. San Diego, Academic Press, 1995.)

average-intake dyads. Infant birth weight, weight at 3 months, and total time nursing were positively associated with intake. The volume also varies with the mother's parity. Women who have had other pregnancies, particularly those who have nursed infants previously, have colostrum more readily available at delivery, and the volume increases more rapidly.

The yellow color of colostrum results from β-carotene. The ash content is high, and the concentrations of sodium, potassium, and chloride are

TABLE 4-3   Composition of prepartum human milk*

Milk component	Units	Mean ± SD (*n*)	Milk component	Units	Mean ± SD (*n*)
Mean days prepartum		20.21 ± 12.18 (11)	Calcium	mg/dL	25.35 ± 8.48 (10)
Lipid	%	2.07 ± 0.98 (11)	Magnesium	mg/dL	5.64 ± 1.44 (10)
Lactose	mM	79.78 ± 21.68 (9)	Citrate	mM	0.40 ± 0.17 (8)
Protein	g/dL	5.44 ± 1.71 (8)	Phosphate	mg/dL	2.32 ± 0.70 (9)
Glucose	mM	0.35 ± 0.16 (8)	Ionized calcium	mM	3.25 ± 0.84 (6)
Sodium	mM	61.26 ± 25.82 (10)	pH		6.83 ± 0.18 (6)
Potassium	mM	18.30 ± 5.67 (10)	Urea	mg/dL	14.87 ± 2.40 (9)
Chloride	mM	62.21 ± 17.44 (10)	Creatinine	mg/dL	1.47 ± 0.35 (9)

*Small samples of mammary secretion were obtained three times in prepartum period from each of 11 women. In some cases, volumes were insufficient for all analyses.
From Allen JC, Keller RP, Archer P, et al: Studies in human lactation: Milk composition and daily secretion rates of macronutrients in the first year of lactation. Am J Clin Nutr 54:69, 80, 1991.

TABLE 4–4 Average milk volume outputs (mL/24 hr) of well-nourished mothers who exclusively breastfed their infants

| | No. days | | Month of lactation | | | | | | | | | | | |
| Country | measured | Gender | <1 | | 1–2 | | 2–3 | | 3–4 | | 4–5 | | 5–6 | |
			n	mL/24 hr	n	mL/24 hr	n	mL/24 hr	n	mL/24 hr	n	mL/24 hr	n	mL/24 hr
U.S.	2	M, F	—	—	3	691	5	655	3	750	—	—	—	—
U.S.	1–2	M, F	46	681	—	—	—	—	—	—	—	—	—	—
Canada	?	M, F	—	—	—	—	—	—	33	793	31	856	28	925
Sweden	?	M, F	15	558	11	724	12	752	—	—	—	—	—	—
U.S.	3	M, F	—	—	11	600	—	—	2	833	—	—	3	682
U.S.	3	M, F	—	—	26	606	26	601	20	626	—	—	—	—
U.K.	4	M	—	—	27	791	23	820	18	829	5	790	1	922
		F	—	—	20	677	17	742	14	775	6	814	4	838
U.S.	1	M, F	16	673 ± 192 SD	19	756 ± 170	16	782 ± 172	13	810 ± 142	11	805 ± 117	11	896 ± 122

| | Month of lactation | | | | | |
Country	7	8	9	10	11	12
U.S.	875 ± 142 SD	834 ± 99	774 ± 180	691 ± 233	516 ± 215	759 ± 28

Modified from Ferris AM, Jensen RG: Lipids in human milk: A review. J Pediatr Gastroenterol Nutr 3:108, 1984.

TABLE 4-5   Yield and composition of human colostrum and milk from days 1 to 28

Component	Day post partum						
	1	2	3	4	5	14	28
Yield (g/24 hr)	50	190	400	625	700	1100	1250
Lactose (g/L)	20	25	31	32	33	35	35
Fat (g/L)	12	15	20	25	24	23	29
Protein (g/L)	32	17	12	11	11	8	9

Modified from Saint L, Smith M, Hartmann PE: The yield and nutrient content of colostrum and milk of women giving birth to 1 month post partum. Br J Nutr 52:87, 1984.

TABLE 4-6   Composition of human milk from days 1 through 36 post partum (mean ± SD), British and German donors

Day	Component (g/dL)		
	Total protein	Lactose	Triacylglycerols
1	2.95 ± 0.86	4.07 ± 0.98	2.14 ± 0.86
3	1.99 ± 0.22	4.98 ± 0.76	3.01 ± 0.77
5	1.82 ± 0.21	5.13 ± 0.54	3.06 ± 0.45
8	1.73 ± 0.27	5.38 ± 0.97	3.73 ± 0.70
15	1.56 ± 0.42	5.42 ± 0.76	3.59 ± 0.86
22	1.51 ± 0.27	5.34 ± 0.96	3.87 ± 0.68
29	1.5 ± 0.27	4.01 ± 1.13	4.01 ± 1.13
36	1.4 ± 0.26	5.34 ± 1.31	4.01 ± 1.20

Modified from Hibberd CM, Brooke DG, Carter ND, et al: Variation in the composition of breast milk during the first five weeks of lactation. Arch Dis Child 57:658, 1982.

greater than those of mature milk. Protein, fat-soluble vitamins, and minerals are present in greater percentages than in transitional or mature milk. Secretory immunoglobulin A (sIgA) and lactoferrin increase in concentration. The complex sugars, oligosaccharides, also increase, adding to the infection protection properties at this stage.

The higher protein, lower fat, and lactose solution is rich in immunoglobulins, especially sIgA. The number of immunologically competent mononuclear cells is at its highest level. Fat, contained mainly in the core of the fat globules, increases from 2% in colostrum, to 2.9% in transitional milk, and to 3.6% in mature milk. Concentration of fat in the prepartum secretion is only 1 g/dL, and the distribution among classes of lipids differs. Prepartum milk is 93% triglycerides, increasing to 97% in colostrum, with diglycerides, monoglycerides, and free fatty acids all increasing from prepartum to

TABLE 4-7   Fat distribution in milk

Measurement	Prepartum		Postpartum		
	Early	Late	Colostrum	Transitional	Mature
Fat (%)	—	2	2	2.9	3.6
Fat (g)	—	—	2.9	3.6	3.8
Lipid (g/dL)	1.15	1.28	3.16	3.49	4.14
Phospholipid (mg/dL)	37	40	35	31	27
Percent of total lipid	3.2	3.1	1.1	0.9	0.6
Cholesterol (mg/dL)	—	—	29	20	13.5

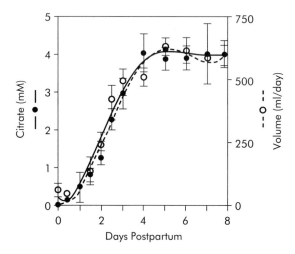

Figure 4-5. Changes in concentration of citrate in human milk in early postpartum period compared with increase in milk volume. (Data replotted from Neville et al, 1991.[163] Neville MC: Determinants of milk volume and composition. In Jensen RG (ed): Handbook of Milk Composition. San Diego, Academic Press, 1995.)

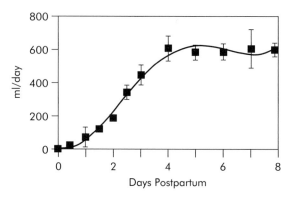

Figure 4-6. Milk volumes during first week post partum. Mean values from 12 multiparous white women who test-weighed their infants before and after every feeding for first 7 days post partum. (From Neville MC, Keller R, Seacat J, et al: Studies in human lactation: Milk volumes in lactating women during the onset of lactation and full lactation. Am J Clin Nutr 48:1375, 1988.)

postpartum secretions. Phospholipid levels decline during the same period. Prepartum secretions contain higher amounts of membrane components such as phospholipids, cholesterol, and cholesteryl esters, which decline from colostrum to mature milk.

Cholesterol appears to be synthesized in the mammary gland. The role of cholesterol in colostrum beyond its use in brain tissue development, the myelinization of nerves, and as the base of many enzymes remains elusive. Very little research has been done on cholesterol in colostrum.

Colostrum facilitates the establishment of *Lactobacillus bifidus* flora in the digestive tract. Colostrum also facilitates the passage of meconium. Meconium contains an essential growth factor for *Lactobacillus bifidus* and is the first culture medium in the sterile intestinal lumen of the newborn infant. Human colostrum is rich in antibodies, which may provide protection against the bacteria and viruses that are present in the birth canal and associated with other human contact. Colostrum also contains antioxidants, which may function as traps for neutrophil-generated reactive oxygen metabolites.[23]

The progressive changes in mammary secretion in both breastfeeding and nonbreastfeeding women between 28 and 110 days before delivery and up to 5 months after delivery were followed by Kulski and Hartmann[133] to study the initiation of lactation. During late pregnancy the secretion contained higher concentrations of proteins and lower concentrations of lactose, glucose, and urea than those contained in milk secreted when lactation was well established. The concentrations of sodium, chloride, and magnesium were higher and those of potassium and calcium lower in colostrum than in milk. The osmolarity was relatively constant throughout the study. The authors described a two-phase development of lactation, with an initial phase of limited secretion in late pregnancy and a true induction of lactation in the second phase, 32 to 40 hours post partum. Comparison with the nonlactating women revealed similar secretion during the first 3 days post partum. This, however, was abruptly reversed during the next 6 days as mammary involution progressed. Obtaining samples in these women, however, may have served to prolong the period of production. The authors[133] point out that although breastfeeding was not necessary for the initiation of lactation in this study, it was essential for the continuation of lactation.

The yield of milk has been calculated from absolute values to demonstrate the increase in output of milk constituents during lactogenesis (Fig. 4-7). Dramatic increases occurred in the production of all the milk constituents. The components synthesized by the mammary epithelium (lactose, lactalbumin, and lactoferrin) increased at a rate greater than those for IgA or proteins derived from the serum IgG and IgM. The greatest difference in yield between day 1 and day 7 post partum was for glucose.[162]

A survey of the fatty acid components shows the lauric acid and myristic acid contents to be low in concentration the first few days. When the lauric and myristic acids increased, C_{18} acids decreased. Palmitoleic acid increased at the same rate as the myristic acid. From this it was concluded that the early fatty acids are derived from extramammary sources, but the breast quickly begins to synthesize fatty acids for the production of transitional and mature milk (see Table 4-7). The total fat content may have a predictive value. It was shown that 90% of the women whose milk contained 20 g or more of fat per feeding on the seventh day were successfully breastfeeding 3 months later. Women who had only 5 to 10 g of fat on the seventh day had an 80% dropout rate by 3 months.

Colostrum's high protein and low fat are in keeping with the needs and reserves of the newborn at birth. Although the content of total nitrogen or any amino acid in breast milk in 24 hours is grossly related to the volume produced, the concentration in milligrams per deciliter (mg/dL) is not so related.[116] The relative distribution of the individual amino acids in each deciliter (100 mL) of milk differs in each mother. The colostrum may actually reflect a transitional maternal blood picture, which is associated with nitrogen metabolism of the postpartum period. The postpartum period is one of involution of body tissue and catabolism of protein in the mother (Fig. 4-8).

Colostrum contains at least two separate antioxidants, an ascorbate-like substance and uric acid.[23]

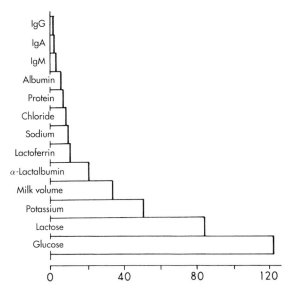

Figure 4-7. Relative increase in yield of milk components from day 1 to day 7 post partum. Values presented are for day 7 expressed as percentage increase over day 1. (Modified from Kulski JK, Hartmann PE: Changes in human milk composition during the initiation of lactation. Aust J Exp Biol Med Sci 59:101, 1981.)

These antioxidants may function in the colostrum as traps for neutrophil-generated, reactive oxygen metabolites. The aqueous human colostrum interferes with the oxygen metabolic and enzymatic activities of the polymorphonuclear leukocytes that are important in the reaction to acute inflammation.[23] This supports the belief that human milk is antiinflammatory.

The mineral and vitamin reserves of the newborn infant are related to the maternal diet. A fetal supply of vitamin C, iron, and amino acids is adequate because infant blood levels exceed those of the mother. Colostrum is rich in fat-soluble vitamin A, carotenoids, and vitamin E. The average vitamin A level on the third day can be three times that of mature milk. Similarly, carotenoids in colostrum may be 10 times the level in mature milk, and vitamin E may be two to three times greater than in mature milk.

Studies that looked at multiparas versus primiparas showed that the volume of milk was significantly

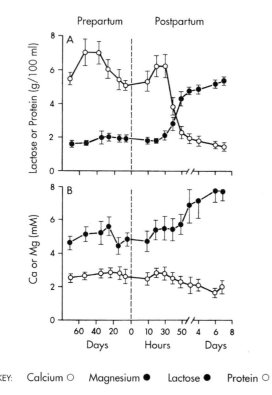

KEY: Calcium ○   Magnesium ●   Lactose ●   Protein ○

Figure 4-8. The levels of milk constituents pre partum and post partum change to reflect the maturation from colostrum to fully mature milk. Volume is driven by lactose production. (Modified from Dumas BR: Modifications of early milk composition during early states of lactation in nutritional adaptations of the gastrointestinal tract of the newborn. In Kretchmer N, Minkowski A (eds): Nutritional Adaptation of GI Tract of the Newborn, Vol. 3. New York, Nestlé Vevey/Raven, 1983.)

greater on day 5 with earlier appearance of the casein band in multiparas (Fig. 4-9).[34]

Sodium as a predictor of successful lactogenesis

Early in lactogenesis, the sodium levels are high but quickly drop from 60 mmol to 20 mmol by day 3 in women who have been fully feeding their infant. Observations by Morton[153] have shown that high breast milk sodium concentrations on day 3 are suggestive of impending lactation failure. Even women who remove only a small amount of milk daily for research purposes have the physiologic drop in sodium.

LACTOGENESIS STAGE II

Even though best practices recommend breastfeeding shortly after birth and frequently thereafter, Kulski and associates[133] showed that milk removal is not needed for the programmed physiologic changes in mammary epithelium to trigger lactogenesis II. Studies by Woolridge[221] confirmed this when there was no effect of breastfeeding in the first 24 hours on later milk transfer to the infants. However, time of first breastfeeding and frequency of breastfeeding on day 2 are correlated with milk volume by day 5.[34]

Transitional milk

The milk produced between the colostrum and mature milk stages is transitional milk; its content gradually changes. The transitional phase is approximately from 7 to 10 days post partum to 2 weeks post partum. The concentration of immunoglobulins and total protein decreases, whereas the lactose, fat, and total caloric content increases. The water-soluble vitamins increase, and the fat-soluble vitamins decrease to the levels of mature milk.

In a study of transitional milks, breast milk samples were obtained from healthy mothers of term infants on the 1st, 3rd, 5th, 8th, 15th, 22nd, 29th, and 36th days of lactation by Hibberd and associates,[97] who defined the first day of lactation to be the third day post partum. Twenty-four-hour samples were pooled for analysis and the remainder fed to the baby. The authors found a high degree of variability, not only among mothers but also within samples from the same mother. The maximum value in almost every case was more than twice the minimum. They were able to show, however, that the changes in composition were rapid before day 8, and then progressively less change took place until the composition was relatively stable before day 36 (see Tables 4-5 and 4-6).

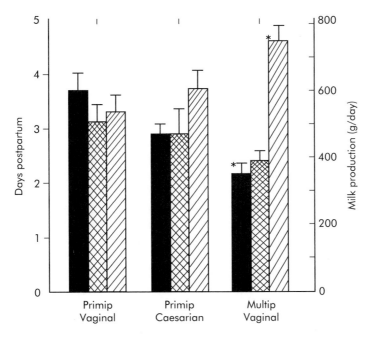

Figure 4-9. Effect of parity on measures of lactogenesis. Data show the mean time at which fullness of the breast was observed (solid bar), the day on which the casein band first appeared (cross-hatched bar) in an electrophoretic analysis of daily milk samples, and the volume of milk produced on day 5 (hatched bar) by primiparous women delivered vaginally ($n = 19$), primiparous (primip) women delivered by cesarian section ($n = 5$), and multiparous (multip) women delivered vaginally ($n = 16$). *Significant difference ($p < 0.05$) between multiparous and primiparous women delivered vaginally. The distance between the error bars represents two SEM. (Data from Chen DC, Nommsen-Rivers L, Dewey KG, et al: Stress during labor and delivery and early lactation performance. Am J Clin Nutr 68:335, 1998; Neville MC, Morton J, Umemura S: Breastfeeding 2001: The evidence for breastfeeding. Pediatr Clin North Am 48:35, 2001.)

Mature milk

Water

In almost all mammalian milks, water is the constituent in the largest quantity, with the exception of the milk of some arctic and aquatic species, who produce milks with high fat content (e.g., the northern fur seal produces milk with 54% fat and 65% total solids) (see Table 4-2). All other constituents are dissolved, dispersed, or suspended in water. Water contributes to the temperature-regulating mechanism of the newborn because 25% of heat loss is from evaporation of water from the lungs and skin. The lactating woman has a greatly increased obligatory water intake. If water intake is restricted during lactation, other water losses through urine and insensible loss are decreased before water for lactation is diminished. Because lactose is the regulating factor in the amount of milk produced, the secretion of water into milk is partially regulated by lactose synthesis. Investigations by Almroth[5] show that the water requirement of infants in a hot, humid climate can be provided entirely by the water in human milk.

Human milk is a complex fluid that scientists have studied by separating the several phases by physical forces.[114] These forces include settling; short-term, low-speed centrifugation; high-speed centrifugation; and precipitation by micelle-destroying treatments such as using the enzyme rennin (chymosin) or reducing the pH. On settling, the cream floats to the top, forming a layer of fat (about 4% by volume in human milk) (Table 4-8).[103] Lipid-soluble components such as cholesterol and phospholipid remain with the fat. With a slow-speed spin, cellular components form a pellet. The high-speed spin brings the casein micelles into a separate phase or forms a pellet. On top of the protein pellet is a loose pellet referred to as the "fluff," composed of membranes.[160,161] Casein precipitation (0.2% by weight) is caused by acid destruction of the micelles. The aqueous phase is whey, which also contains milk sugar, milk proteins, IgA, and the monovalent ions.

Lipids

Intense interest in the lipids in human milk has been sparked by the reports from long-range studies of breastfed infants that show more advanced development at 1 year,[147] 8 to 10 years,[148] and now 18 years of age[101] compared with formula-fed infants. This attention has resulted from the interest in supplementing formula with various missing factors, such as cholesterol and docosahexaenoic acid (DHA).[176] These compounds function in a milieu of arachidonic acid, lipases, and

TABLE 4-8   Estimates of the concentrations of nutrients in mature human milk

Nutrient	Amount in human milk*	Nutrient	Amount in human milk*
	g/liter ± SD		*μg/liter ± SD*
Lactose	72.0 ± 2.5	Vitamin A, RE	670 ± 200 (2230 IU)
Protein	10.5 ± 2.0	Vitamin D	0.55 ± 0.10
Fat	39.0 ± 4.0	Vitamin K	2.1 ± 0.1
	mg/liter ± SD	Folate	85 ± 37[‡]
Calcium	280 ± 26	Vitamin B$_{12}$	0.97[‖,§]
Phosphorus	140 ± 22	Biotin	4 ± 1
Magnesium	35 ± 2	Iodine	110 ± 40
Sodium	180 ± 40	Selenium	20 ± 5
Potassium	525 ± 35	Manganese	6 ± 2
Chloride	420 ± 60	Fluoride	16 ± 5
Iron	0.3 ± 0.1	Chromium	50 ± 5
Zinc	1.2 ± 0.2	Molybdenum	NR
Copper	0.25 ± 0.03		
Vitamin E	2.3 ± 1.0		
Vitamin C	40 ± 10		
Thiamin	0.210 ± 0.035		
Riboflavin	0.350 ± 0.025		
Niacin	1.500 ± 0.200		
Vitamin B$_6$	93 ± 8[†]		
Pantothenic acid	1.800 ± 0.200		

IU, international units; NR, not reported; RE, retinol equivalents; SD, standard deviation.

*Data from Pediatric Nutrition Handbook, 2nd ed. Elk Grove Village, Ill, AAP, 1985, p 363, unless otherwise indicated. Values are representative of amounts of nutrients present in human milk; some may differ slightly from those reported by investigators cited in text.

[†]From Styslinger L, Kirksey A: Effects of different levels of vitamin B-6 supplementation on vitamin B-6 concentrations in human milk and vitamin B-6 intakes of breastfed infants. Am J Clin Nutr 41:21, 1985.

[‡]From Brown CM, Smith CM, Picciano MF: Forms of human milk folacin and variation patterns. J Pediatr Gastroenterol Nutr 5:278, 1986.

[‖]From Sandberg DP, Begley JA, Hall CA: The content, binding, and forms of vitamin B$_{12}$ in milk. Am J Clin Nutr 34:1717, 1981.

[§]Standard deviation not reported; range 0.33 to 3.20.

From Report of Subcommittee, Institute of Medicine: Nutrition during Lactation. Washington, DC, National Academy Press, 1991.

other enzymes, and no evidence indicates that they are effective in isolation or that more is better. The value of supplementing the mother's diet in pregnancy and lactation is an equally important question, because dietary DHA levels have declined in the last half century as women have reduced eggs and animal organs in their diet (see Chapter 9).

Lipids are a chemically heterogeneous group of substances that are insoluble in water and soluble in nonpolar solvents. There are many classes and thousands of subclasses of lipids. The main constituents of human milk are triacylglycerols, phospholipids, and their component fatty acids, the sterols. Jensen, a renowned milk lipidologist, and his coauthors,[116] remind readers, in a comprehensive review of the lipids in human milk, of the nomenclature, such as palmitic acid (16:0), oleic acid (18:1), and linoleic acid (18:2). The figure to the left of the colon is the number of carbons and to the right is the number of double bonds. Polyunsaturated fatty acids (PUFAs) have a designation for the location of the double bond; in human milk, the designation is *cis* (*c*), which identifies the geometric isomer. Because milk is an exceptionally complex fluid, Jensen and associates[114,115] and other scientists have found it helpful to classify components according to their size and concentration, with solubility in milk or lack thereof as additional categories (Table 4-9). The lipids fulfill a host of essential functions in growth and development,[21,22] provide a well-tolerated energy source, serve as carriers of messages to the infant, and provide physiologic interactions, including the following[113]:

1. Allow maximum intestinal absorption of fatty acids.
2. Contribute about 50% of calories.
3. Provide essential fatty acids (EFAs) and PUFAs.
4. Provide cholesterol.

By percentage of concentration, the second greatest constituent in milk is the lipid fraction.

TABLE 4-9   Compartments and their constituents in mature human milk*

Compartment		Major constituents	
Description	Content (%)	Name	Content (%)
Aqueous phase	87.0	Compounds of Ca, Mg, PO_4, Na, K, Cl, CO_2, citrate, casein	0.2 as ash
True solution (1 nm)			
Whey proteins (3–9 nm)		Whey proteins: α-lactalbumin, lactoferrin, IgA, lysozyme, serum albumin	0.6
		Lactose and oligosaccharides; 7.0 and 1.0%	8.0
		Nonprotein nitrogen compounds: glucosamine, urea, amino acids; 20% of total N	35–50 mg N
		Miscellaneous: B vitamins, ascorbic acid	
Colloidal dispersion (11–55 nm, 10^{16}/mL)	0.3	Caseins: beta and kappa, Ca, PO_4	0.2–0.3
Emulsion			
Fat globules (4 μm, 1.1^{10}/mL)	4.0	Fat globules: triacylglycerols, sterol esters	4.0
Fat-globule membrane Interfacial layer	2.0	Milk-fat-globule membrane: proteins, phospholipids, cholesterol, enzymes, trace minerals, fat-soluble vitamins	2% of total lipid
Cells (8–40 μm, 10^4–10^5/mL)		Macrophages, neutrophils, lymphocytes, epithelial cells	

*All figures are approximate.
From Jensen RG: The Lipids of Human Milk. Boca Raton, Fla, CRC, 1989.

Milk lipids provide the major fraction of kilocalories in human milk.[113,116]

Lipids average 3% to 5% of human milk and occur as globules emulsified in the aqueous phase. The core or nonpolar lipids, such as triacylglycerols (TGs) and cholesterol esters, are coated with bipolar materials, phospholipids, proteins, cholesterol, and enzymes. This loose layer is called the *milk-lipid-globule membrane* (MLGM), which keeps the globules from coalescing and thus acts as an emulsion stabilizer.[116] Globules are 1 to 10 μm in diameter, with 1-μm globules predominating.[117]

Fats are also the most variable constituents in human milk, varying in concentration over a feeding, from breast to breast, over a day's time, over time itself, and among individuals (Table 4-10). This information is significant when testing milk samples for energy intake, fat-soluble constituents, and physiologic variation and when clinically managing lactation problems.[86] Much of the early work was based on lactation in women who "nursed by the clock" rather than tuned into infant needs. When circadian variation in fat content was studied in a rural Thai population who had practiced demand feeding for centuries, Jackson and associates[108] found fat concentrations in feeds in the afternoon and evening (1600 to 2000 hours) were higher than those during the night (400 to 800 hours). Fat concentrations at start and finish of feed

varied over 24 hours. The most important predictor of fat content was length of time since last feed; the longer the interval, the lower the fat concentration. Fat content at the end of a previous feed and milk intake at previous feed also influenced levels.

It is speculated that the altered posture at night, horizontal and relatively inactive, may redistribute fat. The larger the milk consumption at a feed, the greater is the increase in fat from beginning to end of the feed. Less fat change occurs during "sleep" feeds than in the daytime. Unless 24-hour samples are collected by standardized sampling techniques, results will vary. During the course of a feeding, the fluid phase within the gland is mixed with fat droplets in increasing concentration. The fat droplets are released when the smooth muscle contracts in response to the let-down reflex.

The lipid fraction of the milk is extractable by suitable solvents and may require more than one technique to extract all the lipids.[137] Complete extraction in human milk is difficult because the lipids are bound to protein. From 30% to 55% of the kilocalories are derived from fats; this represents a concentration of 3.5 to 4.5 g/dL. Milk fat is dispersed in the form of droplets or globules maintained in solution by an absorbed layer or membrane. The protective membrane of the fat globules is made up of phospholipid complexes. The rest of the phospholipids found in human

---

TABLE 4-10   Factors that influence human milk fat content and composition

Factor	Influence
Duration of gestation	Shortened gestation increases the long-chain polyunsaturated fatty acids secreted
Stage of lactation (↑)	Phospholipid and cholesterol contents are highest in early lactation
Parity (↓)	High parity is associated with reduced endogenous fatty acid synthesis
Volume (↓)	High volume is associated with low milk fat content
Feeding (↑)	Human milk fat content progressively increases during a single nursing
Maternal diet	A diet low in fat increases endogenous synthesis of medium-chain fatty acids (C6 to C10)
Maternal energy status (↑)	A high weight gain in pregnancy is associated with increased milk fat

(↑) increase; (↓) decrease.

Modified from Picciano MF: Nutrient composition of human milk. Breastfeeding 2001, Part I: The evidence for breastfeeding. Pediatr Clin North Am 48:53, 2001.

milk are dispersed in the skim milk fraction. Triglycerides, diglycerides, monoglycerides, free fatty acids, phospholipids, glycolipids, sterols, and sterol esters are found in human milk. Vitamin A esters, vitamin D, vitamin K, alkyl glyceryl ethers, and glyceryl ether diesters are also in the lipid fraction but do not fall into the classes listed.

Renewed interest in defining the constituents of human milk lipid has developed as investigators look for the causes of obesity, atherosclerosis, and other degenerative diseases and their relationship to infant nutrition. A number of reports of historic value are plagued with the technical problems of sampling. Because the fat content of a feeding varies with time, spot samples give spurious results. Ferris and Jensen[60] have reviewed the literature exhaustively and describe the fractionated lipid constituents in detail.

The average fat content of pooled 24-hour samples has been reported from multiple sources to vary in mature milk from 2.10% to 5.0% (Table 4-11). Maternal diet affects the constituents of the lipids but not the total amount of fat. A minimal increase in total lipid content was observed when an extra 1000 kcal of corn oil was fed to lactating mothers. A diet rich in polyunsaturated fats will cause an increased percentage of polyunsaturated fats in the milk without altering the total fat content. When the mother is calorie deficient, depot fats are mobilized, and milk resembles depot fat. When excessive nonfat kilocalories are fed, levels of saturated fatty acids increase as lipids are synthesized from tissue stores.

A 2-week crossover study of three nursing women was done by Harzer and associates,[88,89] alternating high fat/low carbohydrate and the reverse. The first diet was 50% fat, 15% protein, and 35% carbohydrate, for a total of 2500 calories. It resulted in a reduction of triglycerides (4.1% to 2.6%) and an increase in lactose (5.2% to 6.4%). See also Table 4-12.

The U.S. Department of Agriculture (USDA) has reported that the average American diet now includes 156 g of fat per day, up from 141 g in 1947. The significant change is from animal to vegetable

TABLE 4-11   Lipid class composition of human milk during lactation

Lipid class	Percentage of total lipids at lactation day:					Immediate extraction
	3	7	21	42	84	
Total lipid, % in milk[*]	2.04 ± 1.32	2.89 ± 0.31	3.45 ± 0.37	3.19 ± 0.43	4.87 ± 0.62	
Phospholipid	1.1	0.8	0.8	0.6	0.6	0.81
Monoacylglycerol	—	—	—	—	—	ND
Free fatty acids	—	—	—	—	—	0.08
Cholesterol (mg/dl)[†]	1.3 (34.5)	0.7 (20.2)	0.5 (17.3)	0.5 (17.3)	0.4 (19.5)	0.34
1,2-Diacylglycerol	—	—	—	—	—	0.01
1,3-Diacylglycerol	—	—	—	—	—	ND
Triacylglycerol	97.6	98.5	98.7	98.9	99.0	98.76
Cholesterol esters (mg)[‡]						
Number of women	39	41	25	18	8	6

ND, Not done.

*Mean ± SEM.

[†]Total cholesterol content ranges from 10 to 20 mg/dL after 21 days in most milks.

[‡]Not reported, but in Bitman et al (Bitman J, Wood DL, Mehta NR, et al: Comparison of the cholesteryl ester composition of human milk from preterm and term mothers. J Pediatr Gastroenterol Nutr 5:780, 1986) was 5 mg/dL at 3 days and 1 mg/dL at 21 days and thereafter.

From Jensen RG, Bitman J, Carlson SE: Milk lipids. In Jensen RG (ed): Handbook of Milk Composition. San Diego, Academic Press, 1995.

TABLE 4-12   **Effects of dietary cholesterol, phytosterol, and polyunsaturate (P)/saturate (S) ratio on human milk sterols**

Milk component	Maternal ad lib diet (P/S 0.53) (mg/100 g fat)	Low-cholesterol/high-phytosterol diet (P/S 1.8) (mg/100 g fat)	High-cholesterol/low-phytosterol diet (P/S 0.12) (mg/100 g fat)
Cholesterol	240 ± 40	250 ± 10	250 ± 20
Phytosterol	17 ± 3	220 ± 30	70 ± 10
Dietary cholesterol	450 ± 30	130 ± 5	460 ± 90
Dietary phytosterol	23 ± 8	790 ± 17	80 ± 1
Total fat (%)	3.58 ± 0.56	2.69 ± 0.17	2.66 ± 0.16

From Lammi-Keefe CJ, Jensen RG: Lipids in human milk: A review. J Pediatr Gastroenterol Nutr 3:172, 1984.

fat, which is now 39% of total dietary fats, especially resulting from the switch from butter and lard. A change in fatty acid content to more long-chain fatty acids and a twofold to threefold increase in linoleic acid have occurred. Except for 18:2 content in mature milk, the fatty acid composition is remarkably uniform unless the maternal diet is unusually bizarre.[137]

P/S ratio is the ratio of polyunsaturated to saturated fats; polyunsaturated fats include $C_{18:2}$ and $C_{18:3}$, or linoleic and linolenic acid. The bovine P/S ratio is 4. The P/S ratio has shifted as a result of recent dietary changes to 1.3 from 1.35 in human milk. The P/S ratio is significant in facilitating calcium and fat absorption. Calcium absorption is depressed by a 4:5 P/S ratio. The breast can dehydrogenate saturated and monounsaturated fatty acids in milk synthesis.

At least 167 fatty acids have been identified in human milk; possibly others are there in trace amounts. Bovine milk has 437 identified fatty acids. Major dietary changes would greatly change fatty acid composition.

Many investigators have studied essential fatty acid requirements for humans. Diets free from added fats or linoleic acid induce deficiency symptoms in infants, including skin lesions, insufficient weight gain, and poor wound healing. Low-fat diets in newborn rats have affected cerebral function. The American Academy of Pediatrics (AAP) has recommended that infant formulas contain a minimum of 3.3 g of fat per 100 kcal (30% of total kilocalories) and 300 mg of linoleic acid (18:2) per 100 kcal (about 1.7% of total kilocalories).[36,37] It did not set a limit on linoleic content of diet, because some human milks have 8% to 10% of the fat as linoleic acid. The AAP has no official policy on supplementation of either full term or premature formulas with LC-PUFA. There is no minimum or maximum of DHA or arachidonic acid (AA).

Milk from vegetarians (lacto-ovo) contained a lower proportion of fatty acids derived from animal fat and a higher proportion of polyunsaturated fatty acids derived from dietary vegetable fat. Women who consumed 35 g or more of animal fat per day had higher $C_{10:0}$, $C_{12:0}$, and $C_{18:3}$ but lower levels of $C_{16:0}$ and $C_{18:0}$. Finley and associates[62] suggest that a maximum amount of $C_{16:0}$ and $C_{18:0}$ can be taken up from the blood and subsequently secreted into milk (Table 4-13).

The milk of strict vegetarians has extremely high levels of linoleic acid, four times that of cow milk (see Table 4-13).[196] Some researchers include other long-chain fatty acids (e.g., $C_{20:2}$, $C_{20:3}$, $C_{24:4}$, $C_{22:3}$) as essential nutrients because they are structural lipids in the brain and nervous tissue. The effects of diet are also discussed in Chapter 9.

One important outcome of linoleic and linolenic acids is the conversion of these compounds into longer-chain polyunsaturates. These metabolites have been shown to be important for fluidity of membrane lipids and prostaglandin synthesis. They are

TABLE 4-13   Effects of maternal vegetarian diets on saturated and unsaturated fatty acids (wt%) in human milk lipids (mean ± SEM)

Lipid (%)/ fatty acid	Vegetarian[*]	Control[*]	Vegan[†]	Vegetarian[†]	Omnivore[†]
Number	12	7	19	5	21
Saturates					
6:0	—	—	—	—	—
8:0	0.16 ± 0.03	0.22 ± 0.01	—	—	—
10:0	1.56 ± 0.13	1.57 ± 0.09	1.8 ± 0.40	1.3 ± 0.51	0.4 ± 0.23
12:0	7.07 ± 0.78	5.47 ± 0.66	6.6 ± 0.54	3.2 ± 0.49	1.7 ± 0.35
14:0	8.16 ± 1.00	6.54 ± 0.73	6.9 ± 0.58	5.2 ± 0.50	4.5 ± 0.35
16:0	15.31 ± 0.73	20.48 ± 0.64	18.1 ± 1.34	21.2 ± 1.07	25.1 ± 0.78
18:0	4.48 ± 0.37	8.14 ± 0.55	4.9 ± 0.36	7.4 ± 0.35	9.7 ± 0.68
20:0	0.54 ± 0.02	0.57 ± 0.03	—	—	—
TOTAL	37.28	42.99			
Monounsaturates					
16:1	1.66 ± 0.14	3.35 ± 0.28	4.9 ± 0.24	2.9 ± 0.37	3.4 ± 0.35
18:1	26.89 ± 1.47	34.7 ± 0.86	32.2 ± 1.06	35.3 ± 1.94	38.7 ± 1.27
TOTAL	28.55	38.06	37.10	38.2	42.1
Polyunsaturates					
N-6 series					
18:2	28.82 ± 1.39	14.47 ± 1.98	23.8 ± 1.40	19.5 ± 3.62	10.9 ± 0.96
20:2	0.72 ± 0.03	0.50 ± 0.03	—	—	—
20:3	0.62 ± 0.03	0.56 ± 0.03	0.44 ± 0.03	0.42 ± 0.07	0.40 ± 0.08
20:4	0.68 ± 0.03	0.68 ± 0.03	0.32 ± 0.02	0.38 ± 0.05	0.35 ± 0.03
TOTAL	30.84	16.21	31.4	27.5	18.4
N-3 series					
18:3	2.76 ± 0.16	1.85 ± 0.16	1.36 ± 0.18	1.25 ± 0.22	0.49 ± 0.06
22:6	0.22 ± 0.08	0.27 ± 0.08	0.14 ± 0.06	0.30 ± 0.05	0.36 ± 0.07
TOTAL	3.05	2.12	1.50	1.55	0.86

Dietary information

Vegetarian (col. 2): whole cereal grains, 50%–60%; soup, 5%; vegetables, 20%–25%; beans and sea vegetables, 5%–10%; macrobiotic diet for a mean of 81 months; no meat or dairy products; occasional seafood, nuts, and fruit
Control: typical U.S. diet

Vegan: no foods of animal origin
Vegetarian (col. 5): exclude meat and fish
Omnivore: typical Western diet

[*]Modified from Specker BL, Wey HE, Miller D: Differences in fatty acid composition of human milk in vegetarian and nonvegetarian women: long-term effect of diet. J Pediatr Gastroenterol Nutr 6:764, 1987. New England donors: vegetarians, 3–13 months post partum; control subjects, 1–5 months; capillary gas-liquid chromatography (GLC) columns.

[†]Modified from Sanders TA, Reddy S: The influence of a vegetarian diet on the fatty acid composition of human milk and the essential fatty acid status of the infant. J Pediatr 120:S71, 1992. British donors: 6 weeks post partum; packed GLC columns.

From Jensen RG, Bitman J, Carlson SE: Milk lipids. In Jensen RG (ed): Handbook of Milk Composition. San Diego, Academic Press, 1995.

present in the brain and retinal cells. Long-chain polyunsaturates are needed for development of infant brain and nervous system.[62] When Gibson and Kneebore[70] studied fatty acid composition of colostrum and mature milk at 3 to 5 days and later at 6 weeks post partum, they reported that mature milk had a higher percentage of saturated fatty acids, including medium-chain acids, lower monounsaturates, and higher linoleic and linolenic acids and their long-chain polyunsaturated derivatives. The derivatives of these acids, often ignored by many investigators, have high biologic activity; thus, the reporting of only linoleic acid underestimates the essential fatty acid (EFA) levels in human milk.[137]

To address the issue of nutrition during brain development, it is important to consider the different periods of brain development that have been described biochemically. First, cell division occurs, with the formation of neurons and glial cells, and second, myelination. In the rat brain 50% of polyenoic acids of the gray matter lipids were laid down by the 15th day of life. The fatty acids characteristic of myelin lipids appeared later. Gray matter is largely composed of unmyelinated neurons, whereas white matter contains a very high proportion of myelinated conducting nerve fibers. Normal brain function depends on both. The synthesis and composition of myelin can be influenced by diet in the developing rat brain.

Myelin-specific messenger ribonucleic acid (mRNA) levels are developmentally regulated and influenced by dietary fat. The neonatal response to dietary fat is tissue specific at the mRNA level.[50]

The fatty acids characteristic of gray matter ($C_{20:4}$ and $C_{22:6}$) accumulate before the appearance of fatty acids characteristic of myelin ($C_{20:1}$ and $C_{24:1}$) in the developing brain. Arachidonic acid ($C_{20:4}$) and DHA ($C_{22:6}$) are synthesized from linoleic and linolenic acids, respectively, but the latter two must be obtained in the diet.

During the first year of life the human brain more than doubles in size, increasing from 350 to 1100 g in weight. Eighty-five percent of this growth is cerebrum; 50% to 60% of this solid matter is lipid.[223] Cortical total phospholipid fatty acid composition in both term and preterm infants is greatly influenced by dietary fat intake. Phospholipids make up about one quarter of the solid matter and are integral to the vascular system on which the brain depends.[58] Brain growth is associated with an increase in the incorporation of long-chain PUFAs into the phospholipid in the cerebral cortex.[109] Extreme dietary alterations in animal experiments have demonstrated an altered PUFA composition of the developing brain.

Such studies cannot be done in humans. Farquharson and associates[58] therefore examined the necropsy specimens of cerebrocortical gray matter obtained from 20 term and 2 premature infants, all of whom died within 43 weeks of birth. All were victims of sudden death and were genetically normal. The infants had either received exclusively breast milk or exclusively formula. The latter group was divided by formula type into three groups: mixture of formulas, SMA, or CGOST (cow milk or Osterfeed). (SMA and CGOST are formulas or mixtures of formulas sold in the UK.) Breastfed infants had greater concentrations of DHA in their cerebrocortical phospholipids than the formula-fed infants in all groups. A compensatory increase in n-6 series fatty acids (arachidonic, docosatetraenoic, and docosapentaenoic) occurred in the SMA group. No significant differences were seen between saturated and monounsaturated fatty acids. The two premature infants had the lowest levels of DHA.

Cerebrocortical neuronal membrane glycerophospholipids are composed predominantly (95%) of phosphatidylcholine (PC), phosphatidylethanolamine (PE), and phosphatidylserine (PS).[109] After birth, neuronal membranes and retinal photoreceptor cells derive most of their phospholipid DHA from diet and liver synthesis and not from fat reserves. Neither the liver nor the retinal and neuronal cells can synthesize DHA without reserves or a dietary supply. α-Linolenic acid, an essential fatty acid, is the precursor. If the enzymes are not activated or are inactivated by an excess of n-6 fatty acids, synthesis does not take place. Human milk provides the DHA and arachidonic acid (AA).[85]

Dietary supplementation with fish oil in the latter part of pregnancy resulted in increased DHA status at birth when measured in the umbilical blood.[150] When postpartum women were supplemented with DHA by capsule in a blind study, breast milk levels of DHA ranged from 0.2% to 1.7% of total fatty acids, increasing with dose. AA levels and antioxidant status of plasma AA and levels were unaffected.

Although DHA is essential to retinal development, levels peak in the retina at 36 to 38 weeks' gestation, suggesting that the most rapid rate of retinal accumulation occurs before term.[93] This further suggests that the premature infant is especially vulnerable to dietary deficiencies of DHA.

Dietary omega-3 (ω-3) fatty acids may not be essential to life, reproduction, or growth, but they are important for normal biochemical and functional development.[187] Long-chain ω-3 fatty acids, DHA in particular, form a major structural component of biologic membranes. When the ratio of omega-6 (ω-6) is high compared to ω-3, fatty acids aggravate the deficiency. Studies in monkeys have shown that DHA deficiency affects water intake and urine excretion, as well as ω-3 fatty acid levels in red blood cells.[187] Much remains to be learned about the effects of ω-3 fatty acids and DHA deficiency on the developing human infant.[215]

The EFAs, linoleic and linolenic acids, may have greater significance in the quality of the myelin laid down. Dick, observing the geographic distribution of multiple sclerosis worldwide, noted that the disease is rare in countries where breastfeeding is common.[51] He postulated that the development of myelin in infancy is critical to preventing degradation later. Dick investigated the difference between human milk and cow milk in relation to myelin production in multiple sclerosis.[51]

Experimental allergic encephalitis is a demyelinating condition and can be produced by shocking animals that have been sensitized to central nervous system (CNS) antigens. Newborn rats deficient in essential fatty acids are more susceptible to this disease, which has been described as resembling multiple sclerosis pathologically.

Widdowson and associates[220] analyzed the body fats of children from Britain and Holland. At birth, body fat was 1.3% linoleic acid for both groups of children. British infants received cow milk formulas that contained 1.8% linoleic acid. The Dutch infants received corn oil formulas that were 58.2% linoleic acid. The Dutch infants had body fat that was 25% linoleic acid at 1 month of age and 32% to 37% at 4 months of age. The British infants, receiving cow milk formulas, had 3% or less linoleic acid in their body fat. The Dutch infants had lower serum cholesterol levels. At approximately 10 years of age, the children appeared to be entirely normal.[220]

Other influences on fat content. Infections will alter milk composition. Mastitis does not alter fat content but does lower volume and lactose and increase sodium and chloride.

Parity has been cited as a major influence on fat content, with primiparous women having more fat than multiparous women. Prentice and associates[182] found a significant relationship between fat content and triceps skinfold thickness. The authors found seasonal changes in the Gambia, where volume and fat were lowest following the rainy season, when nutrient resources are scarce.

Hyperlipoproteinemias. Milk from women with type I hyperlipoproteinemia has been investigated.[117] Because the primary deficiency is serum-stimulated lipoprotein lipase in the plasma, resulting in reduced transfer of dietary long-chain fatty acids from blood to milk, levels of fat as fatty acids were abnormally low (about 1.5%) and the amounts of 10:0 and 14:0 higher than normal. (See Chapter 16.)

Cholesterol. Cholesterol is an essential component of all membranes and is required for growth, replication, and maintenance. Infants fed human milk have higher plasma cholesterol levels than formula-fed infants. Animal studies suggest that early postnatal ingestion of a diet high in cholesterol protects against high-cholesterol challenges later.[222]

The cholesterol content of milk is remarkably stable at 240 mg/100 g of fat when calculated by volume of fat. The range, depending on sampling techniques, is 9 to 41 mg/dL. The amount of cholesterol changed slightly over time, decreasing 1.7-fold over the first 36 days, as reported by Harzer and associates,[89] and stabilizing at about the 15th day postpartum at 20 mg/dL. This resulted in a change in the cholesterol/triglyceride ratio. The authors found no uniform pattern of circadian variations between mothers.

Neonatal plasma cholesterol levels range between 50 and 100 mg/dL at birth, with equal distribution of low-density lipoprotein (LDL) and high-density lipoprotein (HDL). Plasma cholesterol increases rapidly over the first few days of life, with LDL predominating regardless of mode of feeding.[106] In breastfed infants, however, there is a progressive increase in plasma cholesterol compared with that in infants fed low to no cholesterol and high-PUFA formulas. This may have a lasting effect on the individual's ability to metabolize cholesterol, a point yet to be confirmed.[107] Low-birth-weight (LBW) premature infants are at risk for stimulation of endogenous cholesterol biosynthesis, resulting in marked elevations in plasma cholesterol as a result of intravenous nutrition.

The effect of breastfeeding on plasma cholesterol, body weight, and body length was studied longitudinally in 512 infants by Jooste and associates.[120] Breastfed infants had higher plasma cholesterol than the formula-fed infants, created by a direct mechanism that persisted for as long as the infants were breastfed. Body length was similar in breastfed and formula-fed infants, but formula-fed infants weighed more.

Cholesterol has been a factor of great concern because of the apparent association with risk factors for atherosclerosis and coronary heart disease. At present, commercial formulas have high P/S ratios and little or no cholesterol compared with those of human milk. Dietary manipulation does not change the cholesterol level in the breast milk.[181] When the dietary cholesterol level is controlled, however, a fall in the infant's plasma cholesterol level is associated with an increase in the amount of linoleic acid present in the milk.[178]

Kallio and associates[124] followed 193 infants from birth, measuring concentrations of cholesterol, very low density lipoprotein (VLDL), LDL, HDL_2, and, on a limited group of 36, HDL_3 and apoprotein B. The largest differences between exclusively breastfed and weaned infants were at 2 months (0.8 mmol/L), 4 months (0.6 mmol/L), and 6 months (0.5 mmol/L). The LDL and apoprotein B concentrations were lower in weaned infants. VLDL and HDL_3 were independent of diet. The authors concluded that the low intake of cholesterol and high intake of unsaturated fatty acids greatly modify the blood lipid pattern in the first year of life.[124]

In a retrospective epidemiologic study of 5718 men in England born in the 1920s, 474 died of ischemic heart disease.[57] The infant-feeding groups were divided into those breastfed but weaned before 1 year, breastfed beyond a year, and bottle fed. The first group had the lowest death rate from ischemic heart disease and had lower total cholesterol, LDL cholesterol, and apolipoprotein B than those who were weaned after a year and especially those who were bottle fed. In all feeding groups, serum apolipoprotein B concentrations were lower in men with higher birth weights and weights at 1 year.

In a study of breastfed and formula-fed baboons that ate a high-fat carnivorous diet instead of their usual vegetarian fare, breastfeeding showed no protective effect.

No long-range effect of serum cholesterol level has been identified, although Osborn[175] described the pathologic changes in 1500 young people (newborns to age 20). He observed the spectrum of pathologic changes from mucopolysaccharide accumulations to fully developed atherosclerotic plaques. Lesions were more frequent and severe in children who had been bottle fed. Lesions were uncommon or mild in the breastfed children.

Animal investigations indicated that rats given high levels of cholesterol early in life were better able to cope with cholesterol in later life and maintained a lower cholesterol level.[50]

In a study of six breastfed and 12 formula-fed infants, ages 4 to 5 months, Wong and associates[222] measured the fractional synthesis rate (FSR). The breastfed infants had higher cholesterol intakes (18.4 ± 4.0 mg/kg/day) than formula-fed infants (only 3.4 ± 1.8 mg/kg/day). Plasma cholesterol levels were 183 ± 47 versus 112 ± 22 mg/dL; LDL cholesterol levels were 83 ± 26 versus 48 ± 16 mg/dL. An inverse relationship existed between the FSR of cholesterol and dietary intake of cholesterol. The authors concluded that the greater cholesterol intake of breastfed infants is associated with elevated plasma

LDL cholesterol concentrations. In addition, cholesterol synthesis in human infants may be efficiently regulated by coenzyme A (CoA) reductase when infants are challenged with dietary cholesterol.[222]

A carefully designed, well-controlled longitudinal study is needed to determine the long-range impact of cholesterol because it is a consistent constituent of human milk throughout lactation.

n-3 fatty acids. The n-3 fatty acids are important components of animal and plant cell membranes and are selectively distributed among the lipid classes. The role of DHA (22:n-3) in infantile nerve and brain tissue and retinal development has been discussed. It is also found in high levels in testis and sperm. Human milk contains DHA, and studies to evaluate the effects of "fish oil" supplements to the diet suggest an elevation of the dose-dependent levels.

Eicosapentaenoic acid (EPA, 20:5n-3) is part of another group of n-3 fatty acids, the eicosanoids, which comprise two families: the prostanoids (prostaglandins, prostacyclins, and thromboxanes) and the leukotrienes.[117] The *prostanoids* are mediators of inflammatory processes. *Leukotrienes* are key mediators of inflammation and delayed hypersensitivity. The eicosanoids are highly active lipid mediators in both physiologic and pathologic processes.[198] Eicosanoids provide cytoprotection and vasoactivity in the modulation of inflammatory and proliferative reactions. Long-chain polyunsaturated fatty acids (LCPUFA), their precursors, can affect the generation of eicosanoids. The role of eicosanoids in physiologic and pathophysiologic processes is beginning to be identified. It clearly goes beyond adding a little DHA to the brew. Sellmayer and Koletzko[198] reviewed this work.

In other species, restriction of n-3 fatty acids results in abnormal electroretinograms, impaired visual activity, and decreased learning ability. The influence of dietary n-3 fatty acids on visual activity development in very low birth weight (VLBW) infants was evaluated by Birch and associates,[20] using visual-evoked response (VER) and forced-choice preferential-looking (FPL) procedures at 36 and 57 weeks postconception. Feeding groups were randomized to one of three diets: corn oil (only linoleic), soy oil (linoleic and linolenic), and soy/marine oil (added n-3 fatty acids). The marine oil group matched the "gold standards" of VLBW infants fed human milk. Visual activity parameters in the other infants who did not receive n-3 oils were considerably lower.

The n-3 fatty acids appear to function in the membranes of photoreceptor cells and synapses. Jensen and Jensen[113] suggest a daily intake of 18:3n-3 (about 0.5% of calories) with the inclusion of n-3 long-chain PUFA, which is available in human milk. Many studies affirm the value of n-3 fatty acids in the diet and as protection against heart disease, chronic inflammatory disease, and possibly cancer.[203] When synthetic DHA and AA are added to infant formula, the measurements of visual acuity do not match that of human milk. The tolerance for these formulas is still undocumented and long-range outcomes unreported.

Proteins

All milks have been evaluated for their protein contents, which vary from species to species. Proteins constitute 0.9% of the contents in human milk and range up to 20% in some rabbit species. Proteins of milk include casein, serum albumin, α-lactalbumin, β-lactoglobulins, immunoglobulins, and other glycoproteins. Eight of 20 amino acids present in milk are essential and are derived from plasma. The mammary alveolar epithelium synthesizes some nonessential amino acids. Human milk amino acids occur in proteins and peptides, as well as a small percentage in the form of free amino acids and glucosamine (Table 4-14; Fig. 4-10).[2]

Tikanoja and associates[212] reported that postprandial changes in plasma amino acids in breastfed infants were proportional to dietary intake and were highest for the branched-chain amino acids. This was also found to be true for most semiessential and nonessential amino acids. The blood urea levels also reflect dietary intake, with values in breastfed infants being substantially lower than levels in bottle-fed infants.[45] The sum of plasma free amino acids rose and the glycine/valine ratio fell after a feed. When breastfed and formula-fed infants were compared by Järvenpää,[111] concentrations of citrulline, threonine, phenylalanine, and tyrosine

TABLE 4-14   Free amino acid concentrations in human milk

Amino acid	Colostral milk (μmol/dL)	Transitional milk (μmol/dL)	Mature milk (μmol/dL)
Glutamic acid	36–68	88–127	101–180
Glutamine	2–9	9–20	13–58
Taurine	41–45	34–50	27–67
Alanine	9–11	13–20	17–26
Threonine	5–12	7–8	6–13
Serine	12	6–11	6–14
Glycine	5–8	5–10	3–13
Aspartic acid	5–6	3–4	3–5
Leucine	3–5	2–6	2–4
Cystine	1–3	2–5	3–6
Valine	3–4	3–6	4–6
Lysine	5	1–11	2–5
Histidine	2	2–3	0.4–3
Phenylalanine	1–2	1	0.6–2
Tyrosine	2	1–2	1–2
Arginine	3–7	1–5	1–2
Isoleucine	2	1–2	1
Ornithine	1–4	1	0.5–0.9
Methionine	0.8	0.3–3	0.3–0.8
Phosphoserine	8	5	4
Phosphoethanolamine	4	8	10
α-Aminobutyrate	1	0.4–1.4	0.4–1
Tryptophan	5	1	1
Proline	—	6	2–3

From Carlson SE: Human milk nonprotein nitrogen: Occurrence and possible function. Adv Pediatr 32:43, 1985.

were higher in formula-fed than in breastfed infants. Concentrations of taurine were lower in the formula-fed infants. The peak time was different for formula-fed and breastfed infants, which points out the need to standardize sampling times.

The DARLING (Davis Area Research on Lactation, Infant Nutrition, and Growth) Study was the first longitudinal study to follow a large group of mother-infant dyads to 12 months.[49] The investigators report protein intake to be positively associated with milk lipid concentrations after 16 weeks. Milk protein concentration was negatively related to milk volume at 6 and 9 months and positively related to feeding frequency at these times. Milk composition is more sensitive to maternal factors such as body composition, diet, and parity during later lactation than during the first few months.[170]

Casein. Milk consists of casein, or curds, and whey proteins, or lactalbumins. The term *casein* includes a group of milk-specific proteins characterized by ester-bound phosphate, high-proline content, and low solubility at pH of 4.0 to 5.0.[114,143] Caseins form complex particles or *micelles,* which are usually complexes of calcium caseinate and calcium phosphate. When milk clots or curdles as a result of heat, pH changes, or enzymes, the casein is transformed into an insoluble caseinate–calcium phosphate complex. Physiochemical differences exist between human and cow caseins.[143] Casein has a species-specific amino acid composition.

When Lönnerdal and Forsum[143] originally measured the casein content of human milk by three different methods—isoelectric precipitation,

Distribution of the main protein fractions in human and bovine milks

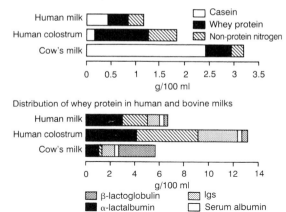

Figure 4-10. Distribution of main protein fractions (*top*) and whey protein (*bottom*) in human and bovine milk. (Modified from Dumas BR: Modifications of early human milk composition during early states of lactation in nutritional adaptation of the gastrointestinal tract of the newborn. In Kretchmer N, Minkowski A [eds]: Nutritional Adaptation of GI Tract of the Newborn, Vol. 3. New York, Nestlé Vevey/Raven, 1983.)

sedimentation by ultracentrifuge, and indirect analysis—they consistently had three separate results.

Utilizing two newer techniques, Kunz and Lönnerdal[135] report confirming results revealing that casein synthesis is low or absent in early lactation, then increases rapidly, and then decreases. The concentration of whey proteins decreases from early lactation. The whey protein/casein ratios change accordingly from 90:10 in early milk to 60:40 in mature milk and 50:50 in late lactation. The authors suggest whey and casein are regulated by different mechanisms.[135]

Methionine/cysteine ratio. The cysteine content is high in human milk, whereas it is very low in cow milk. Because the methionine content is high in bovine milk, the methionine/cysteine ratio is two to three times greater in cow milk than in the milk of most mammals and seven times that in human milk. Human milk is the only animal protein in which the methionine/cysteine ratio is close to 1. Otherwise, this ratio is seen only in plant proteins.

Two significant characteristics of amino acid composition of human milk are the ratio between the sulfur-containing amino acids methionine and cysteine and the low content of the aromatic amino acids phenylalanine and tyrosine. The newborn and especially the premature infant are poorly prepared to handle phenylalanine and tyrosine because of their low levels of the specific enzymes required to metabolize them.

Taurine. Taurine, 2-aminoethanesulfonic acid (so named because it was first isolated from the bile of the ox), is a third sulfur-containing amino acid that has been found in high concentrations in human milk and is virtually absent in cow milk. It is now being added to some prepared formulas. Free taurine and glutamic acid have been measured in breast milk in high concentration. Taurine has been associated in the body at all ages with bile acid conjugation; in the newborn, bile acids are almost exclusively conjugated with taurine.

Sturman and associates[209] suggest that taurine may also be a neurotransmitter or neuromodulator in the brain and retina. Taurine in the nutrition of the human infant was reviewed by Gaull[69] who reports that evidence is accumulating that taurine has a more general biologic role in development and membrane stability.

Taurine is found in very high concentrations in the milk of cats.[185] Kittens deprived of taurine by feeding with purified taurine-free casein diets after weaning develop retinal degeneration and blindness. The process can be reversed by feeding taurine, but not by feeding methionine, cysteine, or inorganic sulfate.[151] The structural integrity of the retina of the cat has been shown to be taurine dependent. The taurine levels were more severely depleted in the brain tissue, but the significance of this finding has not yet been determined.[209] Both humans and cats are unable to synthesize taurine to any degree as newborns and young infants and are therefore wholly dependent on a dietary supply. The process requires cystathionase and cysteine-sulfinic acid decarboxylase, which are enzymes that convert methionine, cysteine, or cystine to taurine.

In studies of amino acid levels, only the concentrations of taurine in plasma and urine of breastfed term infants were higher than those of preterm infants fed formula. Levels in term infants were higher than those of preterm infants fed pooled human milk at a fixed volume. The effects of feeding taurine-deficient formula to the human infant, which occurred before the addition of taurine to infant formula, are not as severe as seen in the kitten. The presence of taurine in human milk and predominance of taurine conjugates in the gut at birth suggest that bile acid conjugate status may be a controlling factor. When bile acid metabolism was measured in infants fed human milk, the infants consistently had higher intraluminal bile acid concentrations at all ages (1 week to 5 weeks) than did formula-fed infants with and without additional taurine. Human milk also facilitated intestinal lipid absorption.[217]

The human infant conjugates bile acids predominantly with taurine at birth but quickly develops the capacity to conjugate with glycine. Those infants fed human milk continue to conjugate with taurine, whereas those fed formulas soon conjugate with glycine predominantly. The cat, in contrast, uses only taurine throughout life.[217] In the human the various pools of taurine in the body cannot be predicted by measurement of plasma taurine alone.

Since 1968, when scientists' attention was drawn to taurine, more than a thousand reports, including reviews, have been published.[69] The physiologic actions of taurine have been reviewed exhaustively by Huxtable.[104] Nonmetabolic actions such as osmoregulation, calcium modulation, and interactions with phospholipid protein and zinc are reported. Taurine is also observed to be a product of metabolic action and a precursor of many other metabolic actions. All these actions demonstrate the careful balance in nature of a number of interdependent constituents. Taurine does not function in isolation. Because of the growing evidence for the role of taurine during development, the requirement for taurine for the neonate remains under investigation.[209]

Whey proteins. When clotted milk stands, the clot contracts, leaving a clear fluid called *whey,* which contains water, electrolytes, and proteins. The ratio of whey proteins to casein is 1.5 for breast

milk and 0.25 for cow milk; that is, 40% of human milk protein is casein and 60% lactalbumin, and cow milk is 80% casein and 20% lactalbumin.[143]

Human milk forms a flocculent suspension with zero curd tension. The curds are easily digested. The total amount of protein has been recently measured to be 0.9%, which is lower than the previously reported 1.2%. The discrepancy is caused by recalculation of the data, in which the total amount of protein was determined by measuring the nitrogen content and multiplying by 6.25. Of the nitrogen content, 25% is nonprotein nitrogen, whereas in bovine milk, 5% of the nitrogen is from nonprotein nitrogen. Hambraeus[83] has reported the composition of the nonprotein fraction to be urea, creatine, creatinine, uric acid, small peptides, and free amino acids (Table 4-15).

Closer examination of the whey proteins shows α-lactalbumin and lactoferrin to be the chief fractions, with no measurable β-lactoglobulin. Beta-lactoglobulin is the chief constituent of cow milk. The term *lactalbumin* includes a mixture of whey proteins found in bovine milk and should not be confused with α-lactalbumin, which is a specific protein that is part of the enzyme lactose synthetase. The α-lactalbumin content parallels lactose levels in different species. Human milk is high in both lactose and α-lactalbumin. Many investigators, however, have continued to measure nitrogen compounds in human milk (see Table 4-15).

Lactoferrin. Lactoferrin is an iron-binding protein that is part of the whey fraction of proteins in human milk. It appears in very low amounts in bovine milk. Lactoferrin has been observed to inhibit the growth of certain iron-dependent bacteria in the gastrointestinal tract. It has been suggested that lactoferrin protects against certain gastrointestinal infections in breastfed infants. Giving iron to newborn infants appears to inactivate the lactoferrin by saturating it with iron and promoting the growth of *Escherichia coli* in particular.

Immunoglobulins

The immunoglobulins in breast milk are distinct from those of the serum. The main immunoglobu-

TABLE 4-15   **Composition of protein nitrogen and nonprotein nitrogen in human milk and cow milk***

	Human milk			Cow milk		
Protein nitrogen			1.43	(8.9)		5.3	(31.4)
Casein nitrogen	0.40	(2.5)			4.37	(27.3)
Whey protein nitrogen	1.03	(6.4)			0.93	(5.8)
α-Lactalbumin	0.42	(2.6)			0.17	(1.1)
Lactoferrin	0.27	(1.7)			Traces	
β-Lactoglobulin	—				0.57	(3.6)
Lysozyme	0.08	(0.5)			Traces	
Serum albumin	0.08	(0.5)			0.07	(0.4)
IgA	0.16	(1.0)			0.005	(0.03)
IgG	0.005	(0.03)			0.096	(0.06)
IgM	0.003	(0.02)			0.005	(0.03)
Nonprotein nitrogen			0.50			0.28
Urea nitrogen	0.25				0.13
Creatine nitrogen	0.037				0.009
Creatinine nitrogen	0.035				0.003
Uric acid nitrogen	0.005				0.008
Glucosamine	0.047				?
α-Amino nitrogen	0.13				0.048
Ammonia nitrogen	0.002				0.006
Nitrogen from other components	?		——		0.074	——
Total nitrogen			1.93			5.31

*Values refer to grams of nitrogen per liter; values within parentheses, to grams of protein per liter.
From Forsum E, Lönnerdal B: Protein evaluation of breast milk and breast milk substitutes with special reference to the nonprotein nitrogen: Effect of protein intake on protein and nitrogen composition of breast milk. Am J Clin Nutr 33: 1809, 1980.

lin in serum is IgG, which is present in the amount of 1210 mg/dL. IgA is found in the serum at 250 mg/dL, one fifth the level of IgG. The reverse is true of human colostrum and milk. Colostrum IgA is 1740 mg/dL, and milk IgA level is 100 mg/dL. Colostrum has 43 mg/dL of IgG, and milk has 4 mg/dL. The IgA and IgG in human milk are derived from serum and from synthesis in the mammary gland.

The IgA is secretory IgA (sIgA), the principal immunoglobulin in colostrum and milk. Secretory IgA contains an antigenic determinant associated with a secretory component. It is synthesized in the gland from two molecules of serum IgA linked by disulfide bonds. The sIgA levels are very high in colostrum the first few days and then decline rapidly, disappearing almost completely by the 14th day. Secretory IgA is very stable at low pH and resistant to proteolytic enzymes. It is present in the intestine of breastfed infants and provides a protective defense against infection by keeping viruses and bacteria from invading the mucosa. The protective qualities are further described in Chapter 5.

Nonimmunoglobulins

Human milk contains numerous nonimmunoglobulins that are being identified and their actions isolated and quantified.[224] Mucins and sialic acid–containing glycoproteins have been isolated and demonstrated to inhibit rotavirus replication and prevent experimental gastroenteritis. The rotavirus has been observed to bind to the milk mucin complex, inhibiting its replication both in vitro and in vivo. (See later discussion under "Oligosaccharides and glycoconjugates.")

Lysozyme

Lysozyme is a specific protein and basic polypeptide with lytic properties[92] found in high concentration in egg whites and human milk but in low concentration in bovine milk. It has been identified as a nonspecific antimicrobial factor. This enzyme is bacteriolytic against Enterobacteriaceae and gram-positive bacteria. It has been found in concentrations up to 0.2 mg/mL. Lysozyme is stable at 100° C (212° F) and at an acid pH. Lysozyme contributes to the development and maintenance of specific intestinal flora of the breastfed infant. (See later discussion under "Enzymes" and Chapter 5.)

Polyamines

Polyamines are ubiquitous intracellular cationic amines recognized as participants in cell proliferation and differentiation in many tissues, especially those of intestinal tract development, absorption, and biologic activity, in both sucklings and adults of the species.[180] The synthesis of polyamines is an active process in the mammary gland throughout lactation.[14]

Putrescine, spermidine, and spermine have been identified and quantitated in human milk by Pollack and associates.[180] They reported mean values per liter of 0 to 615 nmol putrescine, 73 to 3512 nmol spermidine, and 722 to 4458 nmol spermine. In contrast, levels in formula are low and dependent on the protein source. Levels of spermine and spermidine increase greatly during the first few days of lactation, plateauing at levels 12 and 8 times, respectively, the levels immediately post partum.[12] These findings have been confirmed by Romain and associates,[191] who noted that levels in human milk remained stable throughout lactation. They demonstrated the effects of spermine or spermidine on maturation and "gut closure" and suggest a protective effect of spermine against alimentary allergies.

Nonprotein nitrogen

Nonprotein nitrogen (NPN) accounts for 18% to 30% of the total nitrogen in human milk,[30] compared with only 3% to 5% in cow milk. The NPN fraction of human milk is traditionally identified as the acid-soluble nitrogen remaining in the supernatant after protein precipitation or as the dialyzable nitrogen after dialysis of whole milk.[14] Because large-molecular-weight glycoproteins are also soluble in the acid, the fraction should be called *acid-soluble nitrogen* (ASN).[155]

Although there are large interindividual variations, ASN ranges from 350 to 530 mg/L. The total nitrogen ranges from 1700 to 3700 mg/L, depending on length of gestation, duration of lactation, and maternal diet. Some of the nitrogen contributes to the pool available for synthesis of nonessential amino acids in the neonate. Those compounds having more specialized roles are peptide hormone/growth factors, epidermal growth factor, amino sugars of oligosaccharides, free amino acids, amino alcohols of phospholipids, nucleic acids, nucleotides, and carnitine. Their importance is not based on percentage of concentration, because they may serve roles as catalysts. Many protein factors in human milk serve roles other than growth, such as the host resistance factors (lactoferrin, sIgA, and lysozyme).

Table 4-16 presents the significance of these compounds and their relative concentrations. The wide variety of nitrogenous compounds within the fraction of human milk is only beginning to be investigated and understood. This information clearly widens the chemical gap between human milk and proprietary formulas. Increasing evidence suggests that the premature infant reaps even more benefit than the term infant from mother's milk, based on the investigations of NPN alone.[30]

Maternal milk production and the protein nitrogen (but not NPN) fraction of human milk are well preserved when lactating women are subjected to marginal dietary protein intakes in the short term.[155] In nitrogen (N) balance studies on lactating poor Mexican women, equilibrium was attained at 178.9 ± 25.8 mg N (1.1 g protein/kg body weight/day), which is close to current dietary standards.[47]

Interest in urea levels has been stimulated because women with various stages of renal failure were concerned about the effect of high serum levels of urea on their milk urea levels. Urea is 30% to

TABLE 4-16   Levels and significance of nonprotein nitrogen (NPN) constituents of human milk

NPN	Concentration in milk		Significance
	Under 30 days	**Over 30 days**	
Amino sugars			
N-Acetylglucosamine	230 mg N/L	150 mg N/L	Low oral osmotic load; control gut colonization; constituents of ganglio-sides for brain development
N-Acetylneuraminic acid	63 mg N/L	3–27 mg N/L	Substrate for gut epithelium
Peptides	—	60 mg N/L	
Epidermal growth factor	88 ng/mL	—	Regulates intestinal mucosal development
Somatomedin-C/insulin-like growth factor	18 ng/mL	6–8 ng/mL	Stimulates DNA synthesis and cell division in gut
Delta sleep-inducing peptide	30 ng/mL	5 ng/mL	Diurnal pattern highest at 2 PM and 8 PM; ? influence sleep/awake patterns
Insulin	21 ng/mL	2 ng/mL	? Regulates development of gut
Free amino acids			
Taurine	41–45 μmol/dL	27–67 μmol/dL	See under "Taurine"
Glutamic acid/glutamine	2–9 μmol/dL	13–58 μmol/dL	Improves zinc absorption; precursor to brain glutamate
Carnitine	1.0 mg N/L	0.7 mg N/L	Brain lipid synthesis
Choline and ethanolamine	7–20 mg N/L	10–20 mg N/L	Possible growth requirement
Nucleic acid	—	19 mg N/L	Pool of DNA and RNA
Nucleotides	3 mg N/L	3 mg N/L	Growth and immune advantage
Polyamines	0.1 mg N/L	0.2 mg N/L	Increase rate of transcription, N/L nitrogen per liter; translation, and amino acid activation

DNA, deoxyribonucleic acid; N/L, nitrogen per liter; RNA, ribonucleic acid.

50% of the NPN in milk. Levels increase from colostrum to mature milk (3.2 g/dL N in colostrum to 1.7 g/dL in milk. If the original milk urea was provided solely by passive diffusion from the maternal blood, a constant level of urea nitrogen would be anticipated at all stages of lactation instead of increasing from colostrum to mature milk.[14]

Nucleotides

Increased attention has been paid to the presence and role of nucleotides in human milk, as their relative absence in bovine milk has led to experimental supplementation of some infant formulas. Nucleotides have been identified as playing key roles in biochemical processes within the cell, acting as metabolic regulators and altering enzyme activities. A dietary requirement has not been established because they can be synthesized de novo in the adult. Human milk provides 20% of NPN as nucleotides; furthermore, human milk provides a larger percentage (30%) of nitrogen as NPN, three times more than other species. The daily intake from human milk is 1.4 to 2.1 mg of nucleotide nitrogen.[184] Cytidine, adenine, and uridine compose the majority of soluble nucleotides.

Nucleotides are compounds derived from nucleic acid by hydrolysis and consist of phosphoric acid combined with a sugar and a purine or pyrimidine derivative. The level and components of acid-soluble nucleotides of several species, including humans, have been studied extensively. Work has shown a characteristic nucleotide composition in the milk that differs from that of the mammary gland. The large numbers of purine and pyrimidine nucleotides present in various tissues have a number of functions in the cell. They are part of nucleic acid synthesis and metabolism and are also part of milk synthesis. It is well known that adenosine triphosphate (ATP) supplies usable energy for biosynthetic reactions.

Free nucleotides in human milk have been recorded at 6.1 to 9.0 μmol/dL.[183,184] The levels in colostrum and mature milk are similar. The conspicuous difference in quality and quantity of nucleotides between the mammary gland and its secretion would indicate that nucleotides are secreted from the epithelial cells of the gland into the milk. There are distinct species differences in composition and content of nucleotides as well. Cytidine monophosphate (CMP) and uracil are the nucleotides in the highest concentration in human milk, which also contains uridine diphosphate-N-acetyllactosamine and other oligosaccharides. Human milk contains only a trace of orotic acid and no guanosine diphosphate fucose. Orotic acid is the chief nucleotide of bovine milk. Nucleotide levels fall rapidly in bovine milk to minimal levels in mature bovine milk. Synthetic nucleotides produced for formula have a very different profile.

When the nitrogen fraction of human milk was further identified over time at 2, 4, 8, and 12 weeks, a variance was noted in the pattern of nucleotides (Table 4-17).[184] Levels of cytidine-5'-monophosphate (CMP) and adenosine-5'-monophosphate (AMP) declined from 594 to 321 μg/dL and from 244 to 143 μg/dL, respectively, whereas levels of inosine-5'-monophosphate (IMP) increased from 158 to 290 μg/dL. The total nucleotide nitrogen remained constant, accounting for 0.10% to 0.15% of the total NPN. The average intake per day of a normal breastfed infant would be 1.4 to 2.1 mg of nucleotide nitrogen. Measurement of AMP and cyclic guanosine monophosphate (GMP) showed variation in concentration within 15 minutes, which fluctuated over 24 hours.[184] Milk concentration differed widely from maternal plasma levels collected at the same time.

TABLE 4-17 **Nucleotide content of human milk**	
Nucleotide	**Mean* (mg/dL)**
Cytidine monophosphate (CMP)	461 (17.9)
Uridine monophosphate (UMP)	179 (19.8)
Adenosine monophosphate (AMP)	175 (12.8)
Inosine monophosphate (IMP)	228 (14.5)
Guanosine monophosphate (GMP)	138 (8.5)
Uridine diphosphate (UDP)	174 (12.8)
Cytidine diphosphate (CDP)	474 (41.5)
Adenosine diphosphate (ADP)	69 (17.9)
Guanosine diphosphate (GDP)	96 (8.9)

*Mean nucleotide content of human milk at weeks 2, 4, 8, and 12 of lactation.
From Hendricks K: Semin Pediatr Gastroenterol Nutr 2:(1)14, 1991; Modified from Janas LM, Picciano MF: The nucleotide profile of human milk. Pediatr Res 16:659, 1982.

The biologic effects of dietary nucleotides involve the immune system, the intestinal microenvironment, and the absorption and metabolism of certain other nutrients (see Table 4-17). They are considered "semiessential" for newborns.[71] Whether IMP contributes to the superior iron absorption is still unanswered.

Metabolic disturbances in nucleotide metabolism can result in abnormal accumulation of specific intermediates in cells and tissues, causing a variety of diseases.[183] An example is Lesch-Nyhan syndrome, a genetic disease characterized by mental retardation, self-mutilation, and gout, which is caused by the absence of the purine salvage enzyme. On the other hand, disturbances from lack of nucleotides in the diet have not been identified.

Nucleotides are formed by de novo synthesis by capturing or scavenging partially degraded nucleotides or are obtained completely from diet. Dietary nucleotides are absorbed by action of the microvillus membrane as nucleosides. The developing neonate has a reduced capacity to synthesize or salvage nucleotides. Exogenous nucleotides are potential stimuli, modulating not only the gene control of their own metabolism but also that of a number of functions in cardiovascular, neurologic, and immune systems.[35] Nucleotides are important as coenzymes for the processes involved in the metabolism of lipids, carbohydrates, and proteins.

Nucleotides are recognized as an integral part of the immune system, acting as the host defense against bacteria, viruses, and parasites, as well as various malignancies.[17]

Nucleotides are important in the process of protein synthesis, which is enhanced in the newborn infant by a dietary supply of nucleotides. A statistically significant increase in weight was observed by György and his colleagues[79] in 1963 when weanling rats who had been fed a low-protein diet (10% casein) were given added nucleotides as compared with control rats without supplements of nucleotides. A high-protein diet (20%) did not produce significant growth increase when nucleotides were added. This result may explain the satisfactory growth pattern of breastfed infants on relatively low protein intake and the more efficient protein utilization of breastfed infants.

Study of the exact role of nucleotides continues in vivo, although some effort to supplement formula with synthetic nucleotides has already begun.

Carnitine

Carnitine is γ-trimethylamino-β-hydroxybutyrate and is essential for the catabolism of long-chain fatty acids. Only two conditions in life have been described when carnitine is indispensable: total parenteral nutrition lasting more than 3 weeks and early postnatal life. In older individuals it is synthesized in liver and kidney from essential amino acids lysine and methionine. Carnitine serves as an essential carrier of acyl groups across the mitochondrial membrane to sites of oxidation and therefore has a central role in the mitochondrial oxidation of fatty acids in the human.[174]

The newborn undergoes major metabolic changes during transition from fetal to extrauterine life, including the rapid development of the capacity to oxidize fatty acids and ketone bodies as fuel alternatives to glucose. The fatty acids derived from high-fat milk and endogenous fat stores become the preferred fuel of the heart, brain, and tissues with high-energy demands. In addition, a dramatic increase occurs in serum fatty acids in the first hours of life. After the interruption of the fetoplacental circulation and in the absence of an exogenous supply of carnitine, neonatal plasma levels of free carnitines and acylcarnitines decrease very rapidly. Carnitine administration seems to act by increasing ketogenesis and lipolysis.[171] When serum carnitine and ketone body concentrations were measured in breastfed and formula-fed newborn infants, lower carnitine levels were found in infants fed formulas than in those fed breast milk.[171]

The levels of carnitine range from 70 to 95 nmol/mL in breast milk (up to 115 nmol/mL in colostrum) and from 40 to 80 nmol/mL in commercial formula (Enfamil). The bioavailability of carnitine in human milk may be a significant factor in the higher carnitine and ketone body concentrations in breastfed babies. In omnivorous mothers, L-carnitine levels do not vary considerably over time.[18] Levels in the milk of lacto-ovovegetarian mothers were always consistently lower than those of omnivores. The lower serum level of lysine in these women is a possible cause of lower carnitine.

The carnitine levels in human milk were followed for 50 days post partum and the mean level was found to be 62.9 nmol/mL (56.0 to 69.8 nmol/mL range) during the first 21 days and 35.2 ± 1.26 nmol/mL until the 40th to 50th days. Levels were not related to volume of milk secreted.[171]

Carbohydrates

The predominant carbohydrate of milk is *lactose,* or milk sugar. It is present in high concentration (6.8 g/dL in human milk and 4.9 g/dL in bovine milk). Lactose is a disaccharide compound of two monosaccharides, galactose and glucose. Lactose is synthesized by the mammary gland.

A number of other carbohydrates are present in milk. They are classified as monosaccharides, neutral and acid oligosaccharides, and peptide-bound and protein-bound carbohydrates. Small amounts of glucose (1.4 g/dL) and galactose (1.2 g/dL) also are present in breast milk. Other complex carbohydrates are present in free form or bound to amino acids or protein, such as *N*-acetylglucosamine. The concentration of oligosaccharides is about 10 times greater than in cow milk. This difference arises from biosynthetic control mechanisms yet to be described. These carbohydrates and glycoproteins possess bifidus factor activity. Fucose, which is not present in bovine milk, may be important to the early establishment of *Lactobacillus bifidus* as gut flora. The nitrogen-containing carbohydrates are 0.7% of milk solids.

In a study of carbohydrate content over the first 4 months of lactation, Coppa and associates[39] observed that lactose concentrations increased from 56 ± 6 g/L on day 4 to 68.9 ± 8 g/L on day 120. Oligosaccharide levels decreased from 20.9 ± 5 g/L to 12.9 ± 3.30 g/L. Monosaccharides were only 1.2% of the total carbohydrates. The authors describe carbohydrate synthesis by the mammary gland as a dynamic process. Oligosaccharides represent a low osmolar source of calories, stimulate the growth of *L. bifidus* flora, and inhibit bacterial adhesion to epithelial surfaces, competing with cell receptors in the binding of pathogenic agents.

Lactose is hydrolyzed selectively by a brush border enzyme called *lactase* located predominantly in the tip of the intestinal villi. Digestion of lactose is the rate-limiting step in its absorption. Although lactase activity develops later in fetal life than that of other disaccharidases, it is present by 24 weeks of fetal life. Lactase concentration is greatest in the proximal jejunum. Levels continue to increase throughout the last trimester, reaching concentrations at term two to four times those levels at 2 to 11 months of age. Premature infants rapidly increase their lactase levels given a lactose challenge. A well-fed breastfed infant ingesting 150 mL of milk/kg/day receives 10 g of lactose/kg/day, which ensures the normal unstressed infant at least 4 mg/kg/min of glucose, which is considered the optimal rate.[139]

Lactose does appear to be specific, however, for newborn growth. It has been shown to enhance calcium absorption and has been suggested as being critical to the prevention of rickets, in view of the relatively low calcium levels in human milk. Lactose is a readily available source of galactose, which is essential to the production of the galactolipids, including cerebroside. These galactolipids are essential to CNS development.

Interesting correlations have been made between the amount of lactose in the milk of a species and the relative size of the brain (Fig. 4-11).[132] Because lactose is found only in milk and not in other animal and plant sources, its high level in human milk is even more significant. Lactose levels are quite constant throughout the day in a given mother's milk. Even in poorly nourished mothers, the levels of lactose do not vary. Because lactose is influential in controlling volume, the total output for the day may be diminished, but the concentration of lactose in human milk will be 6.2 to 7.2 g/dL.[162] An adequate source of carbohydrate is important for optimal lactation, which suggests that excessive amounts of sugar substitutes may have an effect on volume.[129]

Oligosaccharides and glycoconjugates

Oligosaccharides are the third largest solid component in milk after lactose and triglyceride. Most of the milk oligosaccharides contain lactose at the reducing end of the structure and may also contain fucose or sialic acid at the nonreducing end. More than 80 neutral and acidic oligosaccharides have been identified.[168]

Biochemically, oligosaccharides result from the sequential addition of monosaccharides to the lactose molecule in the mammary gland by glycoglytransferases. The presence and quantity of different types of oligosaccharides in human milk are genetically determined. Of the 21 oligosaccharides studied in depth, the highest amount is present by day 4 with gradual decreasing by 20% by day 30. The physiologic role of human milk and oligosaccharides had been limited to the enhancement of the growth of *L. bifidus* flora and indirectly to the protection against gastrointestinal infections. It is now known they have an important role in defenses against viruses, bacteria, and their toxins. It is their receptor-like mechanism that prevents the adhesion of the pathologic to the epithelial cells. Real efficacy has been demonstrated in core oligosaccharides against *Streptococcus pneumoniae, Helicobacter pylori, E. coli,* and influenza viruses.

Glycoproteins, glycosylated major milk proteins, include lactoferrin, immunoglobulins, and

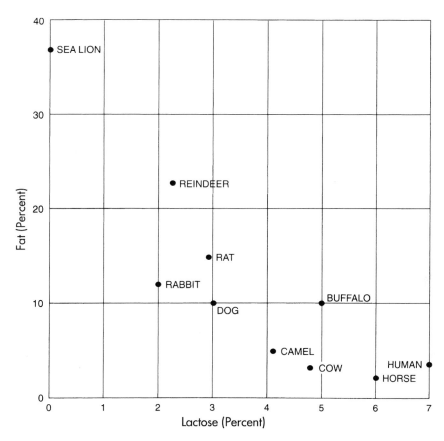

Figure 4-11. Concentration of lactose varies with source of milk. In general, less lactose, more fat, which can also be used by newborn animal as energy source. (From Kretchmer N: Lactose and lactase. Sci Am 227:73. Copyright ©1972 by Scientific American, Inc. All rights reserved.)

mucins. Their protective characteristics have been described to act as receptor homologs, inhibiting the binding of enteropathogens to their host receptors. Research continues to link specific carbohydrate structures with protection against specific pathogens. These nonimmunoglobulin agents are also active against whole classes of pathogens.[168] The protective glyconjugates and oligosaccharides are unique to human milk and to date have not been replicated synthetically.

Minerals

Minerals represent a special category of constituents whose pathways into milk vary from simple diffusion to both positive and negative pump mechanisms. Table 4-18 records the measurements of the constituents in human milk compared with maternal serum. By examining this relationship, it can be estimated how the particular constituent reaches the milk, that is, by passive diffusion or positive or negative pump.

The total ash content of milk is species specific and parallels the growth rate and body structure of the offspring. A number of metallic elements and organic and inorganic acids are present in milk as ions, un-ionized salts, and weakly ionized salts. Some are bound to other constituents. Sodium, potassium, calcium, and

TABLE 4-18   Difference in composition of human milk and blood plasma

	Specific gravity	Osmo-larity	pH	Calories	Water	Carbohy-drates	Fat	Protein		Iron	Na+	K+
								Albumin	Globulin			
Human mature milk	1031	295	7.3	65 kcal/dL	87.5 g%	7.0 g% (lactose)	3.7 g%	0.3 g%	0.2 g%	0.15 mg%	15 mg%	57 mg%
Blood plasma	1033	285	7.4	35 kcal/dL	92 g%	80 mg% (glucose)	200 mg%	4.5 g%	2.5 g%	125 µg%	320 mg%	18 mg%

	Ca^{2+}	Mg^{2+}	Cl$^-$	Phosphorus	Sulfur	Vitamins					
						A*	B$_1$	B$_2$	Niacin	C	D
Human mature milk	35 mg%	4 mg%	43 mg%	15 mg%	14 mg%	280 IU/dL	20 µg%	50 µg%	172 µg%	5 mg%	5 IU/dL
Blood plasma	10 mg%	2.5 mg%	365 mg%	4 mg%	2 mg%	50 µg%	10 µg%	0.5 µg%	500 µg%	1 mg%	188 IU/dL

*1 µg of vitamin A corresponds to the activity of 3 IU of vitamin A.
Modified from Vorheer H: The Breasts: Morphology, Physiology, and Lactation. New York, Academic Press, 1974.

magnesium are the major cations. Phosphate, chloride, and citrate are the major anions.[31]

The monovalent ions are sodium, potassium, and chloride. The divalent ions are calcium, magnesium, citrate, phosphate, and sulfate.[12] The monovalent ions are among the most prevalent and contribute 30 mosmol, or one tenth of the total osmolarity of human milk. The sum of the concentrations of the monovalent ions is inversely proportional to the lactose content across species. Monovalent ion concentration is regulated chiefly by the secretion mechanism in the alveolar cell, with the human having the highest lactose and lowest ion content.[167] This maintains osmolality close to that of serum.

Daily intakes of calcium, phosphorus, zinc, potassium, sodium, iron, and copper from breast milk were found to decrease significantly over the first 4 months of life, with only magnesium increasing. Despite seemingly low mineral intakes, growth during this time was found to be satisfactory by Butte and associates.[25] High mineral content is associated with a rapid growth rate of specific species.

Potassium and sodium. Potassium levels are much higher than those of sodium, which are similar to the proportions in intracellular fluids (Table 4-19). Although sodium, potassium, and chloride are pres-ent as free ions, the other constituents appear as complexes and compounds. Ions can pass through the secretory cell membrane in both directions and in and out of the lumen. Intracellular sodium, chloride, and potassium are in equilibrium with the ions of the plasma and alveolar milk. An apical pumping mechanism has been calculated for chloride release, whereas sodium, potassium, and intracellular chloride pass into milk because of their electrochemical gradients. The cellular pumping mechanism maintains the ionic concentrations in the extracellular fluid and alveolar milk.

The Committee on Nutrition of the American Academy of Pediatrics[38] has stated that the daily requirement of sodium for growth is 0.5 mEq/kg/day between birth and 3 months of age, decreasing to 0.1 mEq/kg/day after 6 months of age (Table 4-20). To cover dermal losses, an additional 0.4 to 0.7 mEq/kg/day is needed, with little for urine and stool losses. Infants fed human milk receive enough sodium to meet their needs for growth, dermal losses, and urinary losses. Studies by Keenan and associates[125] have demonstrated an apparent regulation in the levels of milk sodium and potassium concentrations by adrenocorticosteroids as well as a circadian rhythm.

Sodium levels in cow milk are 3.6 times those in human milk (human, 7 mEq/L or 16 mg/dL; bovine,

---

TABLE 4-19   Minerals in human milk and cow milk (per deciliter)

Minerals	Colostrum	Transitional	Mature	Cow milk
Calcium (mg)	39	46	35	130
Chlorine (mg)	85	46	40	108
Copper (μg)	40	50	40	14
Iron (μg)	70	70	100	70
Magnesium (mg)	4	4	4	12
Phosphorus (mg)	14	20	15	120
Potassium (mg)	74	64	57	145
Sodium (mg)	48	29	15	58
Sulfur (mg)	22	20	14	30
Total ash (mg)	—	—	200	700

From Food and Nutrition Board, National Research Council, National Academy of Sciences: Recommended Dietary Allowances, 10th ed. Washington, DC, U.S. Government Printing Office, 1989.

TABLE 4-20	Recommended dietary intake of electrolytes for infants		
Age	Sodium (mg)	Potassium (mg)	Chloride (mg)
To 6 mo	115–350 (11.5 mg/kg)	350–925	275–700
6 mo–1 yr	250–750 (23 mg/kg)	425–1500	400–1200

From Food and Nutrition Board, National Research Council. National Academy of Sciences: Recommended Dietary Allowances. 10th ed. Washington, DC. U.S. Government Printing Office, 1989.

22 mEq/L or 50 mg/dL). Hypernatremic dehydration has been associated with cow milk feedings. Experiments with newborn rats on high salt intakes have shown that hypertension can develop.

The diurnal variation in milk electrolytes was found to vary between 22% and 80%.[125] These changes varied as the lactation period progressed but were independent of mother's diet. Sodium restriction did not influence milk levels. In a longitudinal study, sodium levels fell from 20 mEq/L to 15 mEq/L in the first week. On day 8, levels were 8 mEq/L, and by the fifth week they were stabilized at 6 mEq/L.[165] Time-dependent changes in milk composition are also reported by Allen and associates[4] as a 25% or greater decrease in sodium, potassium, and citrate from 1 to 6 months. Calcium and glucose increase by 10% or more over this time. The authors suggest milk composition is always in transition.[4]

At a constant sodium intake, decreasing the sodium/potassium (Na/K) ratio in the diet by increasing potassium lowers blood pressure. The dietary Na/K ratio has an important role in determining the severity, if not the development, of salt-induced hypertension. The mechanism of potassium's antihypertensive effect is unclear, but the higher potassium and lower sodium levels of breast milk appear to be physiologically beneficial.

Chloride. Little attention has been paid to the adequacy of chloride in the diet, and it has always been assumed to be sufficient until recent events focused attention on this cation.

Chloride deficiency in infants has become associated with a syndrome of failure to thrive with hypochloremia and hypokalemic metabolic alkalosis. This was first described in infants fed formula that was deficient in chloride but has also been described in a breastfed infant whose mother's milk contained less than 2 mEq/L chloride (normal is greater than 8 mEq/L).[11] This is a rare phenomenon caused by unexplained maternal production. This mother had previously successfully nourished five other infants.

Total ash. Cow milk has three times the total salt content of human milk (Table 4-21). All the minerals that appear in cow milk also appear in human milk.[112] The phosphorus level is six times greater in cow milk; the calcium level is four times higher (Table 4-22).

The renal solute load of cow milk is considerably higher than that of breast milk. This is magnified by the metabolic breakdown products of the high protein content, which are in increased amounts as well.

TABLE 4-21	Principal salt constituents in bovine and human milks	
Constituent	Bovine (mg/dL)	Human (mg/dL)
Calcium	125	33
Magnesium	12	4
Sodium	58	15
Potassium	138	55
Chloride	103	43
Phosphorus	96	15
Citric acid	175	20–80
Sulfur (total)	30	14 (±2.6; 4.5 mmol/L)
Carbon dioxide	20	—

From Jenness R, Sloan RE: Composition of milk. In Larson BL, Smith VR (eds): Lactation. Vol. 3. Nutrition and Biochemistry of Milk/Maintenance. New York. Academic Press, 1974.

TABLE 4-22	**Recommended dietary intake of minerals for infants**[*]					
Age	Calcium (mg)	Phosphorus (mg)	Magnesium (mg)	Iron (mg)	Zinc (mg)	Iodine (mg)
To 6 mo	400	300	40	6	5	40
6 mo–1 yr	600	500	60	10	5	50

[*]Because there is little information on which to base allowances, these amounts are provided in the form of ranges of recommended intakes.
From Food and Nutrition Board, National Research Council, National Academy of Sciences: Recommended Dietary Allowances, 10th ed. Washington, DC. U.S. Government Printing Office, 1989.

This is shown in the high urea levels in formula-fed infants (Table 4-23). Although the mean urea levels in breast milk are 37 mg/dL and only 15 mg/dL in cow milk, the blood urea levels in breastfed infants are about 22 mg/dL, whereas those of infants fed formula are 47 mg/dL and those of infants fed formula plus solids are 52 mg/dL (see Table 4-23).[45] The plasma osmolarity of infants fed breast milk is lower and approximates the physiologic level of plasma.

Calcium/phosphorus ratio. The calcium/phosphorus (Ca/P) ratio is considerably lower in cow milk (1:4) than in human milk (2:2). Many investigators have studied calcium and phosphorus values in human milk and found some variation from mother to mother and from study to study. The Ca/P ratio varied from 1.8 to 2.4, with the absolute values for calcium varying from 20 to 34 mg/dL and those for phosphorus varying from 14 to 18 mg/dL. Fetal and newborn plasma concentrations for calcium decline sharply from 10.4 mg/dL at birth to 8.5 mg/dL by day 4. Unlike calcium, phosphorus concentrations rise in the postnatal period. The drop in serum calcium levels in the bottle-fed infants was more marked than in the breastfed infants. Infant serum phosphorus concentrations rise during the postnatal period. When gestation is prolonged or the mother has preeclampsia, the concentrations are even higher at birth.

Longitudinal studies by Greer and associates,[76] measuring calcium and phosphorus in human milk and maternal and infant sera, have shown progressive increases in infant serum calcium in association with decreasing phosphorus content of breast milk and infant serum. Maternal serum calcium also increased, although the mother's dietary intake was below recommended levels for lactating women. Calcium uptake in the maternal duodenum is enhanced during lactation.

TABLE 4-23	**Statistical analysis by Student's t-test of blood urea levels in 61 healthy infants age 1 to 3 months**			
			Individual values >40 mg/dL	
Infant group	Number	Blood urea, mean ± SE (mg/dL)	Number	Total observations (%)
A: breastfed	12	22.7 ± 1.6[*]	0	0[‡]
B: artificial milk alone	16	47.4 ± 2.0[†]	12	75[§]
C: artificial milk + solid foods	33	51.9 ± 1.8	29	88

[*]When compared with group B and group C: $p < 0.001$ ($t = 9.7$) and $p < 0.001$ ($t = 11.5$), respectively.
[†]When compared with group C: $p > 0.05$ ($t = 1.6$).
[‡]When compared with group B and group C: $p < 0.001$ ($t = 6.9$) and $p < 0.001$ ($t = 15.5$), respectively.
[§]When compared with group C: $p > 0.05$ ($t = 1.1$).
From Davies DP, Saunders R: Blood urea: Normal values in early infancy related to feeding practices. Arch Dis Child 48:563, 1973.

Although the Ca/P ratio has been stressed in the past, recent investigations have not found a statistical correlation between the calcium and phosphorus contents of plasma and corresponding breast milk Ca/P ratio. This suggested that Ca/P ratio is not critical in the low mineral loads present in breast milk. Calcium and phosphorus decrease over time during lactation.[9] When human milk was fractionated and analyzed for distribution of calcium, whole milk contained 241.2 ± 61.9 µg/mL, with most of the calcium in the skim fraction. Significant amounts were also found in the fat; less than 4% was found in the casein. A low-molecular-weight fraction contained 34% calcium, which may explain calcium's bioavailability. The total calcium requirements for maximum growth have been questioned by those who believe the total amount of calcium is too low in breast milk. The fact that rickets has not been seen in infants totally breastfed by well-nourished mothers is supportive circumstantial evidence. There is bone mobilization in the mother during lactation and recovery of bone mass during and after weaning.[207]

Lactating women contribute 210 mg of calcium per day in breast milk. A study of intestinal calcium absorption of women during lactation and after weaning revealed that serum calcium and phosphorus concentrations were greater in lactating compared with nonlactating postpartum women, but levels were the same after weaning.[121,122] Calcitrol, however, was greater in women after weaning compared with postpartum control subjects. Kalkwark and associates[123] concluded that lactation stimulates increases in fractional calcium absorption and serum calcitrol after the onset of menses or after weaning. Observations of these women using bone mineral content (BMC) and bone mineral density (BMD) technology showed that lactating women lost significantly more bone throughout the body and in the lumbar spine than nonlactating postpartum women in the first 6 months.[123] After weaning, the lactators regained significantly more bone in the lumbar spine than nonlactating women. Early resumption of menses was associated with a smaller loss and greater increase after weaning.[43] Parathyroid hormone

concentrations are reported to be higher only after weaning.

Calcium supplementation does not prevent bone loss during lactation and only slightly enhances the gain in bone density after weaning.[122] Supplementation did not affect levels in the milk. Krebs and associates[131] reported that excesses of protein have a negative effect on calcium absorption in lactating women. The calcium/protein ratio appears to be critical to efficient utilization. Estradiol stimulated the osteoblastic proliferation and enhanced the collagen gene expression. Calcium was shown to be well absorbed in 5- to 7-month-old breastfed infants who had begun to receive beikost (solids and semisolids).

Magnesium and other salts. Magnesium is present as a free ion and in complexes with casein and phosphate in caseinate micelles or citrate complexes. Cow milk has three times as much magnesium as human milk (12 mg/dL compared with 4 mg/dL) (Table 4-21). Magnesium was measured in human milk by Fransson and Lönnerdal,[67] who found 41.4 ± 15.4 µg/mL in whole milk samples, with most of the magnesium in the skim milk fraction but significant amounts in the fat fraction and less than 4% in the casein. The bound fraction was associated with low-molecular-weight proteins, thus enhancing bioavailability. Mineral intakes were shown to increase between 1 and 3 months post partum (1.15 to 1.36 mmol/L).[178]

Longitudinal magnesium concentrations were measured by Greer and associates[76] in milk and maternal sera and in the infants over a 6-month period. Progressive increases in serum magnesium level were seen in the breastfed infants in association with decreasing phosphorus content of the milk. Milk magnesium levels did not change significantly between 3 and 26 weeks. The authors suggested that the rising magnesium levels in infant serum may in part be caused by a decrease in dietary phosphorus in breastfed infants.

Citrate is found in the milks of many species and is three to four times higher in cow milk than in human milk (see Table 4-21). The distribution of ions and salts differs among various milks and depends on the relative concentrations of casein and citrate.[112]

Citrate is made in the mitochondria from pyruvate and transported into the cytoplasm, where it is available for lipid synthesis and for transport into the Golgi complex.[12] Citrate levels are not often measured in human milk, although citrate may be a marker of milk production potential (see Fig. 4-5). Levels are high the first few days and rise as calcium levels rise.

Most of the *sulfur* in milk is in the sulfur-containing amino acids, with only about 10% present as sulfate ion. Some organic acids are present, and they appear as anions in milk.

Trace elements. Tables 4-21 and 4-22 list the recommended daily intake of trace elements for infants.[63]

Iron. Because of the great emphasis on iron in the modern diet, and especially in the diet of the infant in the first year of life, the iron in human milk has been closely scrutinized. It has been determined that normal infants need 1500 mg of exogenous elemental iron in the first year of life, which can be translated into 8 to 10 mg/day (Table 4-23). Prepared infant formulas currently supply 10 to 12 mg/day. Human milk has 100 µg/dL, which does not meet the requirements just given. Historically, however, breastfed infants have not been anemic (Table 4-19).

In 350 samples of breast milk, there was a variation between less than 0.1 and 1.6 µg of iron/mL. Age, parity, and lactation history influenced the levels in some studies. The distribution of iron in various fractions of human milk of Swedish women was determined using multiple methods by Fransson and Lönnerdal,[66] who also found low levels, 0.26 and 0.73 ng/mL. The lipid fraction bound 15% to 46% of the iron; 18% to 56% of the iron was in the low-molecular-weight protein fraction, with only a small amount bound to lactoferrin. Feeley and associates[59] studied 102 American women by stage of lactation; 96% of the women took prenatal iron supplements. A diurnal variation was observed, and a significant decrease occurred from 4 to 45 days post partum. The authors estimated that fully breastfed infants would receive 0.10 mg/kg/day of iron.[59]

Iron absorption from human milk is more efficient and has been noted to be 49% of iron available, whereas only 10% of cow milk iron and 4% of iron in iron-fortified formulas are absorbed. Hematologic values of bottle-fed infants were abnormal, whereas those of breastfed infants were not. The breastfed infants had high ferritin levels, indicating a long-term adequacy of iron assimilation.

The infant who is exclusively breastfed for the first 6 months of life is not at risk for iron deficiency anemia or the depletion of iron stores during that time, according to iron depletion studies of Duncan and associates.[53] Studies in adults given tagged iron in human milk and in cow milk show better absorption from the human milk solution.

Other factors that influence iron absorption include higher amounts of vitamin C. Lactose, which promotes iron absorption, is in higher concentration in breast milk, especially compared with prepared formulas, which may not contain lactose. Calcium and phosphorus may interfere with iron absorption, as may high protein levels. Considerable doubt still exists as to whether it is physiologically sound to increase the hemoglobin of an infant with exogenous iron. All species of mammals have low iron content in their milks. All mammals investigated so far have a drop in their hemoglobin levels after birth and a gradual rise to adult levels for the species.

A study of 40 normal, full-term infants followed in an Argentinian clinic found that the exclusively breastfed infants had a 27% incidence of anemia compared with a 7% rate in those who received iron-supplemented formula.[27] There was no storage iron in the anemic breastfed infants. The average incidence of anemia in children in Argentina is 46%. The mothers had been instructed to start beef, liver, and orange juice at 6 months. Most of the iron was present in hemoglobin, the body storage iron being a small fraction of total body iron (2.05% for breastfed and 2.79% for formula-fed infants).[27]

Pisacane and associates[179] studied the iron status of 30 infants breastfed until their first birthday who never received cow milk, supplemental iron, or iron-enriched formula. Examination of their iron stores and hematocrits revealed that those exclusively breastfed for 6½ months versus 5½ months were less likely to be anemic.[179] None of the infants exclusively breastfed for 7 months was anemic and all of these infants continued to have good iron status at 12 and 24 months.

The relationship between plasma concentration of ferritin and body iron stores has not been clearly established; the explanation of iron absorption and use in breastfed infants is still under study.

Absorption of iron from breast milk by 5- to 7-month-old infants receiving solid foods was studied using stable isotope Fe.[1] Iron was well absorbed from human milk in older infants after the introduction of solid foods to the diet.[1]

After extensive studies in Sweden and in Honduras, it was concluded that iron stores in human milk provide sufficient iron for full term, normal birth weight infants with good prenatal iron stores. Infants who are at risk for iron deficiency at 6 months are low birth weight or preterm or with inadequate prenatal iron stores. At 9 months, infants with iron deficiency absorb more iron than infants with normal iron stores. There was no effect on weight gain in infants with normal hemoglobins who received iron supplements from 4 to 9 months. There was, however, slower gain in linear growth and in head circumference in the infants supplemented with iron. When the hemoglobin was normal, the incidence of diarrheal disease was also greater in the supplemented group.

Zinc. Zinc has been identified as essential to the human.[90] Its chief roles described to date are as part of the enzyme structure and as an enzyme activator. Zinc has been identified as a first limiting nutrient in breast milk when anthropometric indicators of growth were correlated with zinc levels in healthy breastfed infants.[52] Zinc deficiency has been described as well, most dramatically in newborns and premature infants on hyperalimentation regimens. The chief clinical symptoms are failure to thrive and typical skin lesions. Human milk has been identified as a food with bioavailable zinc.[118]

Zinc absorption from human milk, cow milk, and infant formula was tested in healthy adults with labeled zinc chloride, using ^{65}Z. The absorption was 41% from human milk, 28% from cow milk, 31% from standard infant formula, and 14% from soy

formula. The dietary zinc intake of both lactating and nonlactating postpartum women was found by Moser and Reynolds[154] to be 42% of recommended allowances. No correlation was found between zinc concentrations in breast milk and maternal dietary zinc and maternal plasma and erythrocyte zinc.

Changes in hair zinc concentrations of breastfed and bottle-fed infants during the first 6 months of life were measured by MacDonald and associates.[149] Only the bottle-fed males had a significant decline in hair zinc concentration. There was no decline of zinc in any breastfed infant, which supports the concept of the superior bioavailability of zinc in breast milk.

Picciano and Guthrie[178] studied milk from 50 mothers in 350 samples. They found zinc levels to average 3.95 µg/mL and to be consistent regardless of time of day, duration of lactation, or other variables. They estimated that breastfed infants receive 0.35 mg of zinc/kg/day. They found zinc levels to decline slightly from the first to the third month post partum (33.8 to 29.5 µmol/L). At 6 months, zinc levels are 1.1 mg/L, and they are 0.5 mg/L at 1 year. Longitudinal changes in dietary zinc requirements for infants acquiring new lean body mass through growth were studied by Krebs and Hambidge.[130] As growth velocity declines, zinc requirements decline in the male infant from a high of 780 µg/day at 1 month to 480 µg/day in the 5th through 12th months. Meanwhile, the percentage of absorption increased over time.

Human milk was fractionated and analyzed by Fransson and Lönnerdal[67] for the distribution of zinc. Most of the zinc was found in the skim milk fraction, but significant amounts were found in the fat associated with the fat globule membrane; less than 4% was found in the casein.

Longitudinal zinc balances in breastfed and formula-fed infants revealed that the median daily zinc intake in breastfed infants decreased from 0.59 mg/kg to 0.15 mg/kg in the first 17 weeks of life.[202] Comparable values for the formula-fed infants were 0.58 mg/kg and 0.67 mg/kg. The median retention of zinc was 27% in breastfed versus 21% in bottle-fed infants. Considering the minimal urinary and fecal losses in the breastfed infants, a daily intake of zinc of 0.3 to 0.5 mg/kg is sufficient. Zinc intake in breastfed infants from 6 to 12 months may be low in some populations. There is little evidence it is a problem in the normal population.[48]

Khoshoo and associates[126] reported zinc deficiency in a full-term, breastfed infant, previously reported in a breastfed premature infant. This case was diagnosed at 7 months of age by the characteristic perineal and perioral rash in an otherwise healthy, well-grown infant. The presumed cause was defective zinc uptake by the mammary gland, because the milk level was only 0.13 mg/L. The infant responded promptly to oral zinc supplements.

In a 9-week-old infant with an intractable diaper rash, the mother's milk was noted to have low zinc levels after the rash responded to zinc therapy.[10] She had nursed two other children without difficulty. Analyzing a small series of cases, Atkinson and associates[15] concluded that lowered zinc levels in milk were caused by decreased zinc uptake by the mammary gland, because the maternal plasma levels were normal. Maternal diet does not influence zinc concentrations in the milk.

Cow milk zinc is associated with high-molecular-weight fractions, and zinc in human milk is associated with low-molecular-weight fractions. The association of zinc with low-molecular-weight components of milk is related in part to protein content and composition and to the relative zinc concentration.[102] When adult females were given oral doses of zinc with human milk, cow milk, casein hydrolysate formula, and soy-based formula, the plasma response with human milk was significantly (three times) greater than with any of the other milks.[32]

The low-molecular-weight ligand has been proved to be readily absorbed. Breast milk has been therapeutic in the treatment of acrodermatitis enteropathica, an inherited zinc metabolism disorder, whereas cow milk formulas are ineffective.

Copper, selenium, chromium, manganese, molybdenum, and nickel. Trace elements constitute less than 0.01% of body weight; however, their atoms are present in large numbers and play a critical role in growth and development. The technical ability to measure these elements is expanding.[200] The effects of trace element deficiencies in fetal and neonatal development are yet to be understood.

Picciano and Guthrie[178] studied *copper* levels in human milk and noted that the content varied considerably among women and within each woman. The range was 0.09 to 0.63 µg/mL. Copper levels were higher in the morning. Dietary supplements did not alter results. Age, parity, and lactation history showed that older mothers and multiparas had higher levels. The fully breastfed infant would receive 0.05 mg of copper/kg/day (Table 4-24).

Fractionated analysis by Fransson and Lönnerdal[67] revealed whole milk concentration of copper to be 0.27 ± 0.13 µg/mL, with most of the copper in the skim milk fraction, significant amounts in the fat, and little in the casein. The predominant binding was with low-molecular-weight proteins, which would enhance bioavailability.[67]

MacDonald and associates[149] studied changes in hair copper concentrations among breastfed and bottle-fed infants. Hair copper levels rose in the first 3 months in all infants and then declined, regardless of feeding or gender of infant. The

TABLE 4-24	**Recommended dietary intake of trace elements for infants**[*]					
Age	Copper (mg)	Manganese (mg)	Fluorine (mg)	Chromium (mg)	Selenium (mg)	Molybdenum (mg)
To 6 mo	0.4–0.6	0.3–0.6	0.1–0.5	0.01–0.04	0.01–0.04	0.015–0.03
6 mo–1 yr	0.6–0.7	0.6–1.0	0.2–1.0	0.02–0.06	0.015–0.06	0.02–0.04

*Because the toxic levels for many trace elements may be only several times the usual intakes, the upper levels for the trace elements given in this table should not be habitually exceeded.
From Food and Nutrition Board, National Research Council, National Academy of Sciences: Recommended Dietary Allowances, 10th ed. Washington, DC. U.S. Government Printing Office, 1989.

authors associated this with the redistribution of copper in early infancy (see Table 4-19). Copper is a component of a number of metalloenzymes.

The bioavailability of *selenium* depends on the sources and chemical form, and the quantitative significance is under investigation. Except for Keshan disease, a potentially fatal cardiomyopathy seen in infants in China, no convincingly associated clinical deficiency syndrome has been reported. Dietary recommendations have been based on those for adults. Dietary intakes less than the lower limits, however, should not be considered deficient, especially in breastfed infants.[225]

Selenium concentrations in human milk are consistent in samples collected from many parts of the world, according to work by Hadjimarkos and Shearer.[80] The mean value was 0.020 ppm, which was similar to the value from many parts of the United States, where the range was 0.007 to 0.033 ppm.

Increased selenium requirements have been observed in pregnant and lactating women. Supplementation with different compounds, such as selenium-enriched yeast and selenomethionine, significantly influenced selected indices of selenium status, including milk concentrations.[3]

Selenium is considered an essential nutrient in humans. It is an integral component of glutathione peroxidase, an enzyme known to metabolize lipid peroxides, and deficiency states have been described. Questions have been raised about the detrimental effects of high selenium intake on dentition. Smith and associates[204] assessed selenium status in infants exclusively fed human milk or infant formula for 3 months. Foremilk samples had a mean concentration of 15.7 ng/mL, hindmilk mean concentration was 16.3 ng/mL, and mean formula concentration was 8.6 ng/mL. Breastfed infants have greater intakes and higher serum levels of selenium than formula-fed infants in the first 3 months (see Table 4-24).

The concentration of *chromium* is highest in the organs of the newborn and declines rapidly during the first years of life. A longitudinal study of chromium in human milk was undertaken by Kumpulainen and Vuori.[134] Mothers collected samples at 8 to 18 days, 47 to 54 days, and 128 to 159 days post partum, representing every feed during a 24-hour period with equal portions of foremilk and hindmilk. The mean concentration was 0.39 (SD = 0.15) ng/mL and the intake 0.27 (SD = 0.11) μg/day. The values did not change over time. These values are the same as those in human serum and urine. The mothers' dietary intake averaged about 30 μg/day, which is lower than the 50 to 200 μg recommended daily allowance.

When chromium metabolism was studied in 17 lactating postpartum subjects, breast milk chromium content was independent of dietary chromium intake and serum and urinary values.[8] Chromium intake did not correlate with serum or urinary chromium.

An HDL cholesterol level can be increased with chromium supplementation. Chromium also is reported to have a favorable effect on serum lipid profiles. Deficiency of chromium in infancy may be an issue with LBW infants or those with inadequate fetal stores.[134] It is present in all tissues of the body and is in high levels in nucleic acids.[200]

Mainly because of a lack of information, little is known about *manganese* in infant nutrition.[144] Manganese is a component of comparatively few metalloenzymes, including pyruvate carboxylase and mitochondrial superoxide dismutase. It does, however, activate others. Deficiencies cause impaired growth and skeletal abnormalities in all species studied. In human milk the major fraction of manganese is the 71% found in the whey, with 11% in the casein and 18% in the lipid. Levels in human milk in the first month of lactation decreased from a mean of 5.4 ± 1.6 μg/dL on day 1 to 2.7 ± 1.6 ng/mL from day 5 through day 28. The average intake of the infant in the first month was 2.0 mg/day.

The main biochemical role of *molybdenum* in mammals is as a cofactor for several enzymes.[31] Deficiencies are rare, usually occurring in those receiving total parenteral nutrition. Molybdenum levels in human milk were measured from day 1 through day 38. Levels began at 15.0 ± 6.1 μg/dL and leveled off at 1 to 2 μg/dL at 1 month.[31]

Nickel is generally accepted as an essential trace element for animals, but its role in humans is undefined. Levels in human milk are stable over time at 1.2 µg/dL. The average daily intake of nickel at 1 month was 0.8 µg.

Fluorine. Fluorine has been widely accepted as a significant dietary factor in decreasing dental caries (see Table 4-24). The effect has been associated with the conversion of the enamel hydroxyapatite to fluorapatite with a reduction in acid solubility. The presence of fluorine during the formation of hydroxyapatite may create less soluble, more resistant crystals.

Conflicting reports of the fluorine levels in human milk have led to the belief that breastfed infants needed supplementation.[142] More accurate studies in communities where fluoride has been in the public drinking water supply show 7 µg of fluorine per liter (range 4 to 14 µg/L).[56] The American Academy of Pediatrics no longer recommends routinely supplementing breastfed infants with fluorine (see Chapter 9).

The significant development of deciduous and permanent teeth occurs after birth and depends on fetal stores of fluorine as well as on fluorine available in the diet. Studies comparing breastfed and bottle-fed infants show a distinct difference, with fewer dental caries and better dental health in breastfed infants. The role of fluorine and other factors, such as selenium, that predispose the breastfed infant to healthier teeth has yet to be defined completely. Nursing-bottle caries add to the total dental caries of the bottle fed infant.

Iodide

Iodide levels have rarely been studied, although it was recognized that levels in the milk could be raised above those in the serum (in which radioactive iodine compounds have been examined). Mean breast milk iodide levels were 178 µg/L (range 29 to 490 µg/L), which is about four times the recommended daily allowance for infants.[78] Levels in milk were unrelated to the infant's age but directly related to maternal intake calculated in the diet.

pH and osmolarity

The pH range in human milk is 6.7 to 7.4, with a mean of 7.1. The mean pH of cow milk is 6.8. The caloric content of both human and cow milk is 65 kcal/dL or 20 kcal/oz. The specific gravities are 1.031 and 1.032, respectively.

The osmolarity of human milk approximates that of human serum, or 286 mosmol/kg of water, whereas that for cow milk is higher, 350 mosmol.[44] The renal solute load of human milk is considerably lower than that of cow milk. Renal solute load is roughly calculated by totaling the solutes that must be excreted by the kidney. It consists primarily of nonmetabolizable dietary components, especially electrolytes, ingested in excess of body needs, and metabolic end products, mainly from the metabolism of protein. Renal solute load can be estimated by adding the dietary intake of nitrogen and three minerals—sodium, potassium, and chloride. Each gram of protein is considered to yield 4 mosmol (as urea), and each milliequivalent of sodium, potassium, and chloride is 1 mosmol. The renal solute load of cow milk is 221 mosmol, compared with 79 mosmol for human milk.

Dearlove and Dearlove[46] investigated osmoregulation in human lactation in an effort to determine whether fluid loading was a valid clinical maneuver. It is known that an oral hypotonic fluid load results in suppression of prolactin in adults. After an intravenous hypotonic saline infusion, a significant correlation was seen between serum osmolarity and prolactin. No changes in serum prolactin, milk yield, serum, or breast milk osmolarity were noted, however, when normal lactating women were given a hypotonic fluid load in a controlled study.

Vitamins

Vitamin A. Vitamin A content is 75 µg/dL or 280 international units (IU) in mature human milk and 41 µg/dL or 180 IU in cow milk (Table 4-25). Thus, the supply of vitamin A and its precursors, carotenoids (e.g., β-carotene), is considered adequate to meet the estimated daily requirement, which varies from 500 to 1500 IU/day if the infant consumes at least 200 mL of breast milk per day (Table 4-26). There is twice as much vitamin A in colostrum as in mature milk. During the first 6 months, retinol equivalent (RE) content of term milk in developing countries is only 330 µg RE/L compared to 660 µg in developed

TABLE 4-25 **Vitamins and other constituents of human milk and cow milk (per deciliter)**

Milk elements	Colostrum	Transitional	Mature	Cow milk
Vitamin A (μg)	151.0	88.0	75.0	41.0
Vitamin B$_1$ (μg)	1.9	5.9	14.0	43.0
Vitamin B$_2$ (μg)	30.0	37.0	40.0	145.0
Nicotinic acid (μg)	75.0	175.0	160.0	82.0
Vitamin B$_6$ (μg)	—	—	12.0–15.0	64.0
Pantothenic acid (μg)	183.0	288.0	246.0	340.0
Biotin (μg)	0.06	0.35	0.6	2.8
Folic acid (μg)	0.05	0.02	0.14	0.13
Vitamin B$_{12}$ (μg)	0.05	0.04	0.1	0.6
Vitamin C (mg)	5.9	7.1	5.0	1.1
Vitamin D (μg)	—	—	0.04	0.02
Vitamin E (mg)	1.5	0.9	0.25	0.07
Vitamin K (μg)	—	—	1.5	6.0
Ash (g)	0.3	0.3	0.2	0.7
Calories (kcal)	57.0	63.0	65.0	65.0
Specific gravity	1050.0	1035.0	1031.0	1032.0
Milk (pH)	—	—	7.0	6.8

From Food and Nutrition Board, National Research Council, National Academy of Sciences: Recommended Dietary Allowances, 10th ed. Washington, DC, U.S. Government Printing Office, 1989.

countries.[169] Retinol content of milk of mothers who deliver prematurely is even higher. A single 60-mg supplement of β-carotene sustained elevated β-carotene concentrations in serum and milk longer than 1 week in normal mothers but did not affect concentrations of other major carotenoids, retinol, or tocopherol.[28] Vitamin A intake and serum vitamin A concentrations during pregnancy influence the com-

position of breast milk. Human milk is a vital source of vitamin A in developing countries, even beyond the first year of life.[173]

Vitamin D. Vitamin D has always been included in the fat-soluble vitamin group because that is the form in which it had been identified in nature. The levels in human milk were 0.05 μg/dL, previously reported in the fat fraction. Human milk was shown

TABLE 4-26 **Recommended daily dietary allowances of fat-soluble vitamins for infants***

Age	Weight		Height		Protein (g)	Vitamin A (μg RE)[†]	Vitamin D (μg)[‡]	Vitamin E (mg αTE)[§]
	(kg)	(lb)	(cm)	(in)				
To 6 mo	6	13	60	24	kg × 2.2	395	7.5	3
6 mo–1 yr	9	20	71	28	kg × 1.6	375	10	4

*The allowances are intended to provide for individual variations among most normal persons as they live in the United States under usual environmental stresses. Diets should be based on a variety of common foods in order to provide other nutrients for which human requirements have been less well defined.
[†]Retinol equivalents. 1 RE = 1 μg retinol or 6 μg carotene.
[‡]As cholecalciferol, 10 μg cholecalciferol = 400 IU vitamin D.
[§]α-Tocopherol equivalents. 1 mg d-α-tocopherol = 1 αTE.
From Food and Nutrition Board, National Research Council, National Academy of Sciences: Recommended Dietary Allowances, 10th ed. Washington, DC, U.S. Government Printing Office, 1989.

to have vitamin D in both the fat and the aqueous fractions. Investigators measured the water-soluble sulfate conjugate of vitamin D and evaluated the biologic activity of the water-soluble metabolites. The water-soluble fraction is considered to be inactive metabolites. When activity is calculated by an assay that measures stimulation of intestinal calcium transport, human milk is found to contain 40 to 50 IU/L of vitamin D activity. The metabolite 25-hydroxyvitamin D_3 accounts for 75% of the activity; vitamins D_2 and D_3 account for 15%. Vitamin D sulfate, or any other as yet unidentified water-soluble metabolite of vitamin D, has not been proved to have significant biologic activity.

The impact of the maternal diet content of vitamin D was measured in a double-blind study of white mothers in a temperate climate in the winter.[192] A direct relationship was seen between maternal and infant levels of 25-OH-vitamin D_3 and maternal diet. An additional group of infants, whose mothers' diets were unsupplemented, received 400 IU vitamin D per day and had even higher serum concentrations of 25-OH-vitamin D_3. When mothers have been given large doses of vitamin D, the content of vitamin D and D_3 in their milk increases as it does with exposure to sunshine. The level of 25-OH-vitamin D does not change. The majority of the activity in human milk is in the form of 25-OH-vitamin D. This may be an advantage for the breastfed infant, who utilizes this form most readily. Clearly the levels vary and may be inadequate in human milk in some situations, especially in cold climates in the winter with little sunshine and for dark-skinned individuals.

In a review of vitamin D in adults, especially pregnant women, Hollis[100] demonstrated clearly that traditional levels of vitamin D of 400 IU/day or less are grossly inadequate today when few women get adequate sun exposure or wear sunscreen or clothing that obstructs the exposure. Most recommendations were done before it was possible to measure circulating 25-(OH)-vitamin D, the true indicator of nutritional vitamin D status. The dose of 10 μg or 400 IU daily had little effect on adult 25-(OH)-vitamin D levels. When submariners were given 600 IU/day for several months, they failed to maintain adequate 25-

(OH)-vitamin D levels.[98] The dose that is adequate during pregnancy is unknown, although it is greater than 400 IU.[100] Doses of 10,000 IU daily in adults did not elevate circulating 25-(OH)-D above the normal range, and doses of 1000 IU may not maintain normal levels. The resurgence of rickets in infants may well begin with inadequate levels in pregnancy.

Cases of vitamin D-deficiency hypocalcemia and rickets in nonwhite infants have been reported in increasing numbers in exclusively breastfed infants.[33] The epidemic is aggravated by the use of sunscreen, ethnic traditions of covering the body, and lack of sunshine. Serum 1,25-dihydroxyvitamin D concentrations are significantly higher in lactating compared with nonlactating women and among vegetarian compared with nonvegetarian women, reports Specker and associates.[208] All lactating women in a study by Chang[33] had elevated serum parathyroid hormone levels (see Table 4-26). Levels of vitamin D are higher in colostrum than in mature milk.[136] Studies are under way providing high levels of vitamin D (4000 IU/day) to mothers to increase their milk levels.[217] It has been recommended that all breastfed infants receive 200 IU vitamin D beginning at 2 months of age.[7] Until pregnant and lactating women who are at risk for inadequate intake are supplemented, it will be necessary to supplement normal breastfeeding infants.

The concern for toxicity of excessive vitamin D was based on the reported relationship with cardiac disease and supravalvular aortic stenosis syndrome (SAS) and William syndrome, which has been proved to be genetic. Hypervitaminosis from high levels of vitamin D has resulted from therapeutic misadventures resulting in hypercalcium when the circulating 25-(OH)-D concentrations were over 100 ng/mL (normal levels of 25-(OH)-D are over 15 ng/mL serum). No case of hypervitaminosis D has been reported from sun exposure even though one half hour in the summer sun between 10 AM and 2 PM in a bathing suit (about 3 minimal erythermal dose exposure) will release about 50,000 IU or 1.25 μg/day vitamin D within 24 hours in most whites.[100]

Vitamin E. Vitamin E has been a subject of much interest. Levels in colostrum are 1.5 mg/dL, whereas transitional milk has 0.9 mg/dL and mature milk has 0.25 mg/dL. The difference at different stages has been found to be caused by α-tocopherol, because the contents of β- and γ-tocopherol are similar. Total tocopherol in mature milk correlates with total lipid and linoleic acid contents. Significantly higher tocopherol/linoleic acid ratios are found in both colostrum and transitional milk than in mature milk.[110]

Cow milk has 0.07 mg/dL of vitamin E (see Table 4-25). Correspondingly, serum levels in breastfed infants rise quickly at birth and maintain a normal level, whereas cow milk–fed infants have depressed levels. Vitamin E includes a group of fat-soluble compounds (α-, β-, γ-, and δ-tocopherol), and their unsaturated derivatives (α-, β-, γ-, and δ-tocotrienol). An international unit of vitamin E is equal to 1 mg of synthetic α-tocopherol or 0.74 mg of natural α-tocopherol acetate.

Vitamin E is required for muscle integrity, resistance of erythrocytes to hemolysis, and other biochemical and physiologic functions. The requirement for vitamin E is related to the polyunsaturated fatty acid (PUFA) content of the cellular structures and of the diet (see Table 4-26). Satisfactory plasma levels are 1 mg/dL, and these levels can be maintained by feedings with a vitamin E/PUFA ratio of 0.4 mg/g. The requirement for infants up to age 6 months is 3 mg/day and after 6 months 4 mg/day. The requirement during lactation is 14 mg during the first 6 months and 17 mg/day after 6 months post partum.

An estimate of the tocopherol/linoleic acid ratio in mature milk is 0.79 mg α-tocopherol equivalents per gram, which is comparable to a daily requirement of 0.5 mg for term infants but may be low for premature infants, especially those receiving iron supplements.[137] Ordinarily, this would be supplied by 4 IU of vitamin E per day. Because human milk contains 1.8 mg/L or 40 µg of vitamin E per gram of lipid, it supplies more than adequate levels of vitamin E.[136]

Vitamin K. Vitamin K is essential for the synthesis of blood-clotting factors, which are normal in the serum at birth. The previous levels of vitamin K reported in human milk (15 µg/dL) have been replaced with those calculated by more accurate techniques and are lower, 2.1 µg/L for mature milk and 2.3 µg/L for colostrum,[137] which are less than the recommended daily intake of 12 µg/day (Table 4-27).

The measurement of the homologs of vitamin K have been equivocal. When mothers are given a single dose of 20 mg phylloquinone (K_1), the milk level increases from 1 to 140 µg/L in 12 hours, dropping to 5 µg/L in 48 hours.[75] When infants are given 1 mg vitamin K_1 at birth, as is the practice in many countries, the concentration of K_1 in both breastfed and formula-fed infants in the first week of life remains elevated. When no neonatal prophylaxis is given, Büller and associates[24] reported no difference in coagulating factors among a sample of 113 breastfed, formula-fed, or combination-fed infants. They reported a case of low vitamin K levels in the milk of a mother whose infant died at 6 weeks from intracranial bleeding without neonatal prophylaxis.

Vitamin K is produced by the intestinal flora but takes several days in the previously sterile neonatal gut to be effective. Vitamin K–dependent clotting factors in normal breastfed infants were normal. The prothrombin time and partial thromboplastin time were similar in breastfed and bottle-fed infants. The normotest and thrombotest were significantly prolonged in the breastfed group. The authors concluded that 5% of breastfed children have possible vitamin K deficiency. In several case

TABLE 4-27   Recommended daily dietary allowances of vitamins for infants*

Age	Vitamin K (µg)	Biotin (µg)	Pantothenic acid (mg)
To 6 mo	5 (1 µg/kg)	10	2
6 mo–1 yr	10	15	3

*The allowances are intended to provide for individual variations among most normal persons as they live in the United States under usual environmental stresses. Diets should be based on a variety of common foods in order to provide other nutrients for which human requirements have been less well defined.

From Food and Nutrition Board, National Research Council, National Academy of Sciences: Recommended Dietary Allowances, 10th ed. Washington, DC, U.S. Government Printing Office, 1989.

reports,[172] infants exclusively breastfed with no vitamin K given at birth developed late-onset hemorrhagic disease that responded to vitamin K administration. O'Connor and associates[172] note the association of vitamin K deficiency with home birth and suggest that the physician give vitamin K immediately as recommended by the American Academy of Pediatrics if it has been omitted.

At 3 months of age, 165 breastfed infants who had received 1 mg vitamin K_1 at birth had reduced serum levels of vitamin K_1. Their clotting factors were unchanged. For complete protection, Cornelissen and associates[42] recommend a second oral dose of vitamin K_1 at 3 months. In a similar study, Greer and associates[73] found that despite low plasma phylloquinone concentrations in the breastfed infant (less than 0.25 ng/mL) for the first 6 months, continued vitamin K_1 supplementation was not recommended. Canfield and associates[29] confirm the low levels of vitamin K_1 in breastfed infants compared with those in infants fed formula containing many times the recommended daily dose (0.5 ng/day). No requirements have been set for breastfed infants. No data are available regarding the potential toxicity of excessive vitamin K.

It is recommended that all infants receive vitamin K at birth, regardless of feeding plans, to prevent hemorrhagic disease of the newborn caused by vitamin K deficiency in the first few days of life.[36]

The vitamin content of common foods has been recalculated downward so that diets of average women are probably deficient in vitamin K. Furthermore, vitamin K levels in serum of lactating women are not good markers of deficiency. Carboxylated prothrombin (des-γ-carboxyprothrombin [PIVKA]) is produced in the absence of vitamin K and is a marker of vitamin K deficiency. Greer and associates[74] followed breastfed infants and found normal PIVKA at birth and 4 weeks but elevations by 8 weeks. The authors recommend maternal supplementation during lactation.

Vitamin C. Vitamin C is part of several enzyme and hormone systems, as well as of intracellular chemical reactions. It is essential to collagen synthesis (Tables 4-28 and 4-29).

Human milk is an outstanding source of water-soluble vitamins and reflects maternal dietary intake (see Table 4-26). Increased vitamin C has been measured in the milk within 30 minutes of a bolus of vitamin C being given to the mother. Human milk contains 43 mg/dL (fresh cow milk contains up to 21 mg). Levels obtained in normal lactating women 6 months post partum were 35 mg/L in those on normal diets and 38 mg/L in those supplemented with multivitamins containing 90 mg vitamin C.[211] Levels obtained in 16 lactating women of low socioeconomic level were 53 mg/L for unsupplemented and 65 mg/L for supplemented mothers at 1 week post partum and 61 mg/L and 72 mg/L, respectively, at 6 weeks post partum. Several subjects in the unsupplemented low socioeconomic group had levels too low to provide 35 mg vitamin C per day to their infants.

TABLE 4-28	Recommended daily dietary allowances of water-soluble vitamins for infants*						
Age	Vitamin C (mg)	Thiamin (mg)	Riboflavin (mg)	Niacin (mg NE)†	Vitamin B_6 (mg)	Folacin‡ (μg)	Vitamin B_{12} (μg)
To 6 mo	30	0.3	0.4	5	0.3	25	0.3
6 mo–1 yr	35	0.4	0.5	6	0.6	35	0.5

*The allowances are intended to provide for individual variations among most normal persons as they live in the United States under usual environmental stresses. Diets should be based on a variety of common foods in order to provide other nutrients for which human requirements have been less well defined.
†1 NE (niacin equivalent) is equal to 1 mg of niacin or 60 mg of dietary tryptophan.
‡The folacin allowances refer to dietary sources as determined by *Lactobacillus casei* assay after treatment with enzymes ("conjugases") to make polyglutamyl forms of the vitamin.
From Food and Nutrition Board, National Research Council, National Academy of Sciences: Recommended Dietary Allowances, 10th ed. Washington, DC, U.S. Government Printing Office, 1989.

TABLE 4-29 Estimated secretion of nutrients in mature human milk compared with increments in recommended dietary allowances (RDAs) for lactating women

A. Energy, protein, and fat-soluble vitamins

Measure	Energy (kcal)	Protein (g)	Vitamin A (µg RE)	Vitamin D (µg)	Vitamin E (mg of α-TE)	Vitamin K (µg)
Estimated secretion in milk*	420–700	6.3–10.5	400–670	0.3–0.6	1.4–2.3	1.3–2.1
Increment in RDAs†,‡ for following lactation periods:						
0–6 mo	500	15	500	5	4	0
6–12 mo	500	12	400	5	3	0
Comments	Estimated 80% efficiency in conversion to milk energy	Estimated 70% efficiency in conversion to milk protein	None	Increment advised in part to maintain calcium balance	Estimated 75% absorption	No increment listed because intakes usually exceed RDA

B. Water-soluble vitamins

Measure	Vitamin C (mg)	Thiamin (mg)	Riboflavin (mg)	Niacin (mg of NE)	Vitamin B₆ (mg)	Folate (µg)	Vitamin B₁₂ (µg)
Estimated secretion in milk*	24–40	0.13–0.21	0.21–0.35	0.9–1.5	0.06–0.09	50–83	0.6–1.0
Increment in RDAs†,‡ for following lactation periods							
0–6 mo	35	0.5	0.5	5	0.5	100	0.6
6–12 mo	30	0.5	0.4	5	0.5	80	0.6
Comments	Estimated 85% absorption	Increment higher than secretion because of increased energy needs	Estimated 70% utilization for milk production	Increment higher than secretion because of increased energy needs	Milk concentration used is for unsupplemented women	Estimated 50% absorption; RDA based on 50 rather than 83 µg/L	RDA based on 0.6 rather than 1.0 µg/L

c. Minerals

Measure	Calcium (mg)	Phosphorus (mg)	Magnesium (mg)	Iron (mg)	Zinc (mg)	Iodine (µg)	Selenium (µg)
Estimated secretion in milk*	168–280	84–140	21–35	0.18–0.30	0.9–1.5[||] 0.3–0.5[¶]	66–110	12–20
Increment in RDAs[†,‡] for following lactation periods:							
0–6 mo	400	400	75	0	7	50	20
6–12 mo	400	400	60	0	4	50	20
Comments	None	Based on desired 1:1 ratio for calcium/phosphorus intake	Estimated 50% absorption	Secretion during lactation is less than menstrual loss	Estimated 20% absorption	Based on need of infant, not maternal loss in milk	Estimated 80% absorption

α-TE, α-tocopherol equivalents; NE, niacin equivalents; RE, retinol equivalents
*At volumes of 600–1000 mL/day, based on milk composition shown in Table 4–13.
[†]From National Research Council (NRC) (1989).
[‡]Women aged 25 to 50.
[||]0 to 6 months.
[¶]6 to 12 months.
From Report of Nutriton during Lactation Subcommittee, Institute of Medicine: Nutrition during Lactation. Washington, DC, National Academy Press, 1991.

When lactating women were given 250, 500, or 1000 mg/day vitamin C for 2 days, milk levels remained within the range of 44 to 158 mg/L and did not differ significantly between dosages, even at 10 times the recommended dietary allowance (RDA).[26] Total intake of the infant through the milk ranged from 49 to 86 mg/day. These findings suggest a regulatory mechanism for vitamin C levels in milk. When women received high doses of vitamin C, levels of the vitamin excreted in the urine also increased proportionately.[177]

Vitamin B complex

Vitamin B1. Vitamin B_1, or *thiamin,* levels increase with the duration of lactation but are lower in human milk (160 μg/dL) than in cow milk (440 μg/dL) (see Tables 4-28 and 4-29). In a study by Nail and associates,[157] levels obtained by normal lactating women showed significant increases between 1 and 6 weeks post partum, but there was no difference in levels between supplemented (1.7 mg daily) and unsupplemented women. Cases of beriberi in infants have been associated with a deficiency in the mother.

Because urinary excretion of thiamin is significantly higher in supplemented than in unsupplemented women, the amount of vitamin transferred into milk appears to be limited.[177] Malnourished women, however, do show significant increases in their milk when supplemented.[142] Thiamin is essential for the use of carbohydrates in the pyruvate metabolism (cofactor in pyruvic acid decarboxylation) and for fat synthesis. Insufficient thiamin produces insufficient carbohydrate oxidation with accumulation of intermediary metabolites such as lactic acid.

Vitamin B2. Vitamin B_2, or *riboflavin,* is significant for the newborn in whom intestinal tract bacterial synthesis is minimal (see Tables 4-28 and 4-29). Riboflavin is involved in oxidative intracellular systems and is essential for protoplasmic growth. Levels are 36 μg/dL in human milk and 175 μg/dL in cow milk.

Levels obtained in normal lactating women showed significantly lower levels of riboflavin in the milk of the unsupplemented women (36.7 μg/dL) at 1 week compared with the milk of the supplemented women, who received 2 mg/day in a multivitamin (80.0 μg/dL). No significant difference was seen between 1 and 6 weeks in either group.[157]

Niacin. Niacin *(nicotinamide)* is an essential part of the pyridine nucleotide coenzymes and is part of the intracellular respiratory mechanisms. There are 147 μg/dL in human milk and 94 μg/dL in cow milk (see Tables 4-28 and 4-29). Levels respond to dietary supplementation.

Vitamin B6. Vitamin B_6 *(pyridoxine)* forms the enzyme group of certain decarboxylases and transaminases involved in metabolism of nerve tissue. The supply of vitamin B_6 is vital to deoxyribonucleic acid (DNA) synthesis, which is needed to form the cerebrosides in the myelination of the CNS. There are 12 to 15 μg/dL of vitamin B_6 in human milk and 64 μg/dL in cow milk (see Tables 4-28 and 4-29). The principal form of vitamin B_6 in human milk is *pyridoxal* (PL), whereas pyridoxine (PN) is the principal form of vitamin B_6 fortification in infant formulas.[214] Levels of vitamin B_6 in the milk of mothers consuming more than 2.5 mg of the vitamin daily (RDA for lactating women is 2.5 mg/day) were significantly higher in the first week than were levels in the unsupplemented mothers' milk. Average maternal diets in several studies were consistently below the recommended levels of vitamin B_6.[189]

The accumulated stores of vitamin B_6 during pregnancy are significant for the maintenance of adequate vitamin B_6 status of infants during the early months of breastfeeding. For some infants, human milk alone without supplementary foods may be insufficient to meet vitamin B_6 needs after 6 months of age.[94] The recommended daily intake for infants under 6 months of age is 0.30 mg. Vitamin B_6 deficiency has been associated with CNS disorders in three breastfed infants.[127]

Long-term use of oral contraceptives has been shown to result in low levels of vitamin B_6 in maternal serum in pregnancy and at delivery and low levels in the milk of these mothers.[190] The relationship of vitamin B_6 supplements to suppression of prolactin and the treatment of galactorrhea is discussed under lactation failure (see Chapter 16). The doses used to suppress lactation (600 mg/day) far exceed the levels in multiple vitamins (1 to 10 mg) (see Table 4-29).

Pantothenic acid. Pantothenic acid is part of coenzyme A, a catalyst of acetylation reactions. The reaction of coenzyme A with acetic acid to form acetyl-CoA is prime to intermediary metabolism. The levels of pantothenic acid in human milk were restudied by Johnston and associates[119] because of the range of values in the literature. They found the mean to be 670 μg/dL in foremilk and hindmilk samples. No change occurred in concentrations from 1 to 6 months post partum. They did find a positive correlation with dietary intake.

Folacin. Folacin (*folic acid*) is part of the conversion of glycine to serine. It is also involved in the methylation of nicotinamide and homocysteine to methionine. It is essential for erythropoiesis (see Table 4-28).

The folate (anionic form of folic acid) content of human milk produced by well-nourished women averages 80 to 130 μg/L (see Table 4-29).[172] These values are substantially greater than those reported in the literature previously because of difficulty in the analysis. Folate in human milk is quantitatively bound to folate-binding proteins and presents in multiple labile forms. Folate values typically increase as lactation progresses and are even maintained as maternal stores begin to be depleted.

Supplementation with folic acid in deficient mothers caused prompt increase in levels in the milk. When mothers and their infants were evaluated, folate levels were two to three times higher in the breastfed infants than in their mothers, and there was a correlation between levels in the milk and in the infants' plasma.[193] Folic acid has also been identified as a critical element in deficiency states during pregnancy, being associated with abruptio placentae, toxemia, and intrauterine growth failure as well as megaloblastic anemia.

Vitamin B$_{12}$. Early studies reported that vitamin B$_{12}$ is found in human milk in low concentration, 0.3 μg/L, whereas cow milk has 4.0 μg/mL. Well-nourished mothers on balanced diets appear to have adequate amounts for their infants. Microbiologic assay has demonstrated that very high concentrations of vitamin B$_{12}$ appear in early colostrum but level off in a few days to those of serum. Samples of colostrum reported by Samson and McClelland[194] have a mean binding capacity of 72 ng/mL; in mature milk the capacity is one third of this value. Vitamin B$_{12}$ levels were compared by Sandberg and associates[195] in supplemented and unsupplemented mothers and were not significantly different. Levels were 33 to 320 ng/dL, with a mean of 97 ng/dL. When nutritionally deficient, low-socioeconomic lactating women were studied by Sneed and associates,[205] supplementation with a multivitamin did result in elevated vitamin B$_{12}$ levels. This was true for folate as well.

Although cow milk has five to ten times more vitamin B$_{12}$ than mature human milk, cow milk has little vitamin B$_{12}$–binding capacity, which is substantial in human milk. Vitamin B$_{12}$ functions in transmethylations such as synthesis of choline from methionine, serine from glycine, and methionine from homocysteine. It is involved in pyrimidine and purine metabolism. Vitamin B$_{12}$ also affects the metabolism of folic acid. Megaloblastic anemia is a common symptom of vitamin B$_{12}$ deficiency. Vitamin B$_{12}$ occurs exclusively in animal tissue, is bound to protein, and is minimal or absent in vegetable protein.

The 1989 recommendation for the minimum daily requirement for infants is 0.3 μg/day in the first year of life, when growth is rapid (see Table 4-28). Based on their data on omnivorous and vegetarian women, Specker and associates[206] conclude that the current RDA for infants provides little margin for safety (see Table 4-29).

Enzymes

Considerable data have been collected on the enzymatic activities of many milks. Jenness and Sloan[112] report 44 enzymes detected in bovine, human, and other milks. Xanthine oxidase, lactoperoxidase, uridine diphosphogalactose, galactosyl transferase, ribonuclease, lipase, alkaline phosphatase, acid phosphatase, and lysozyme have been isolated in crystalline form.

The role and significance of enzymes in human milk were reviewed by Hamosh,[84] who confirmed that more than 20 active human milk enzymes exist (Table 4-30). They can be categorized into three general groups by their activity: *mammary gland function,* which reflects physiologic changes occurring in the mammary gland itself during lactation; *compensatory digestive enzymes* in human milk, which have digestive functions in the neonate; and *milk enzymes,* important in stimulating neonatal development.[84] Some enzyme levels are significantly higher in colostrum than in mature milk. Most are whey proteins and contribute minimally to milk proteins. Some enzymes, like other proteins in milk, are probably produced elsewhere and transported to the breast via the bloodstream. The evidence to support the concept of local synthesis includes the demonstration of secretory tissue in the mammary gland. Amylase levels are twice as high in milk as in serum.[95,140] Casein proteins have been synthesized in vitro in cell-free mammary-derived messenger ribonucleic acid (mRNA)-enriched systems. Mammary explants from mice, monkeys, and humans have accumulated lactose synthetase B. The enzymes of possible importance in infant digestion are those with pancreatic analogs: amylase, lipases, protease(s), and ribonuclease.[199]

Amylase. Amylase, the chief polysaccharide-digesting enzyme, is not developed at birth even in full-term infants, who have only 0.2% to 0.5% of adult values. Mammary amylase is present, however, throughout lactation, with levels higher in colostrum than in mature milk. Human milk levels are 0.5 to 1.0 g/dL oligosaccharides of varying chain length. Milk levels of preterm mothers are comparable to term milk levels.

Milk levels are twice those of serum in the first 90 days and remain higher than serum over 6 months. When exposed to a pH of 5.3, this salivary-type amylase remains active; at a pH of 3.5, one half the original activity is present at 2 hours and one third at 6 hours. Amylase is stable at −20° C to −70° C (−4° F to −94° F) for storage and at least for 24 hours at 15° C to 38° C (59° F to 100° F). Much milk amylase activity remains in the duodenum after a meal of human milk. This is significant for the digestion of starch because pancreatic amylase is still low in infants. Mammary amylase may be an alternate pathway of digestion of glucose polymers, as well as of starch (Table 4-31).

Milk amylase is part of the isozyme group as salivary amylase and is thought to inhibit the growth of certain microorganisms.

Lipases. Milk fat is almost completely digestible. The emulsion of fat in breast milk is greater than in cow milk, resulting in smaller globules. Milk lipases play an active role in creating the emulsion, which yields a finer curd and facilitates the digestion of triacylglycerols (TGs). The newborn easily digests and completely uses the well-emulsified small fat globules of human milk. Free fatty acids are important sources of energy for the infant.

Lipase in human milk was first described in 1901. At least two different lipases (glycerol ester hydrolases) were described then. The lipases in human milk make the free fatty acids available in a large proportion even before the digestive phase of the intestine. The lipolytic milk-enzyme activity is similar to the activity of pancreatic lipase, breaking down triglycerides to free fatty acids and glycerol. One enzyme is present in the fat fraction and is inhibited by bile salts.[84]

Milk from undernourished mothers may lose some of its ability to hydrolyze milk lipid esters over the course of lactation; this ability remains constant in well-nourished mothers.[54] This would have an effect on the utilization of the esters of lipid-soluble vitamins A, D, and E.

It appears that the function of this enzyme, inhibited by bile salts, is to facilitate the uptake by the mammary gland of fatty acids from circulating triglycerides for incorporation with milk lipids, because lipase in vivo depends on added serum for activity. Its presence in milk probably represents "leakage" from the mammary gland, and it is unlikely to play a major physiologic role in the lipolysis of milk triglycerides.[96]

Additional lipases in the skim milk fraction are stimulated by *bile salts.* Bile salt–stimulated lipase (BSSL) has greater activity and splits all three ester bonds of the triglyceride. This lipase is also stable in

TABLE 4-30	**Component functions in human milk**	
Function	**Component**	**Process**
Biosynthesis of milk components in mammary gland	Phosphoglucomutase	Synthesis of lactose
	Lactose synthetase	Synthesis of lactose
	Fatty acid synthetase	Synthesis of medium-chain fatty acids
	Thioesterase	Uptake of circulating triglyceride fatty acids
	Lipoprotein lipase	Uptake of circulating triglyceride fatty acids
Digestive function in infant	Amylase	Hydrolysis of polysaccharides
	Lipase (bile salt dependent)	Hydrolysis of triglycerides
	Proteases	Proteolysis (not verified)
	Xanthine oxidase	Carrier of iron, molybdenum
	Glutathione peroxidase	Carrier of selenium
	Alkaline phosphatase	Carrier of zinc, magnesium
Preservation of milk components	Antiprotease	Protection of bioactive proteins, i.e., enzymes and immunoglobulins
	Sulfhydryl oxidase	Maintenance of structure and function of proteins containing disulfide bonds
Antiinfective agents	Lysozyme	Bactericidal
	Peroxidase	Bactericidal
	Lipases (lipoprotein lipase, bile salt-dependent lipase)	Release of free fatty acids that have antibacterial, antiviral, and antiprotozoan actions
Antiinflammatory agents	Vitamins A, C, and E	Scavenges oxygen radicals
	Catalase	Degrades hydrogen peroxide
	Glutathione peroxidase	Prevents lipid peroxidation
	Platelet-activating factor acetylhydrolase	Degrades platelet-activating factor
	α_1-antitrypsin	Inhibits inflammatory proteases
	α_1-antichymotrypsin	Inhibits inflammatory proteases
	Prostaglandin 1	Cytoprotective
	Prostaglandin 2	Cytoprotective
	Epidermal growth factor	Promotes gut growth and function
	Transforming growth factor-α	Promotes epithelial cell growth
	Transforming growth factor-β	Suppresses lymphocyte function
	Interleukin 10	Suppresses function of macrophages and natural killer and T cells
	Transforming growth factor-α receptors I and II	Binds to and inhibits transforming growth factor-α

From Hamosh M: Enzymes in human milk: Their role in nutrient digestion, gastrointestinal function and nutrient delivery to the newborn infant. In Lebenthal E (ed): Textbook of Gastroenterology and Nutrition in Infancy, 2nd ed. New York, Raven, 1989; Hamosh M: Bioactive factors in human milk. Breastfeeding 2001, Part I: The evidence for breastfeeding. Pediatr Clin North Am 48: 69, 2001.

TABLE 4-31   Characteristics of milk enzymes active in infant digestion

Characteristic	Amylase	BSSL*
High parity (≥10)	Low activity	?
Malnutrition	?	Decrease in activity
Diurnal and within feed activity	Constant	Constant
Prepartum	?	Present
Presence in preterm (PT) and term (T) milk	Equal activity PT and T	Equal activity PT and T
Pattern through lactation	Colostrum greater than milk	Colostrum lower than milk
Weaning	?	Activity constant independent of milk volume
Distribution in milk	Skim milk	Skim milk
Effect of milk storage		
−20° to −70° C	Stable years	Stable years
15 to 38° C	Stable (≤24 hours)	Stable (≤24 hours)
Stability to low pH (passage through stomach)	pH > 3.0	pH > 3.0
Optimum pH	6.5–7.5	7.4–8.5
Enzyme characteristics	Salivary amylase isozyme	Identical with pancreatic carboxyl ester hydrolase
Evidence of activity in infant's intestine	Yes	Yes
Presence in milk of other species	?	Primates, carnivores, and rodents

*BSSL, Bile salt-stimulated lipase

From Hamosh M: Enzymes in human milk. In Jensen RG (ed): Handbook of Milk Composition. San Diego, Academic Press, 1995; Hamosh M: Bioactive factors in human milk. Breastfeeding 2001, Part I: The evidence for breastfeeding. Pediatr Clin North Am 48: 69, 2001.

the duodenum and contributes to the hydrolysis of the TGs in the presence of the bile salts.[96] BSSL is identical to carboxyl ester hydrolase (carboxylesterase), a pancreatic enzyme. BSSL activity is lower in colostrum than in mature milk. No correlation appears to exist between the volume of milk at various stages and the volume of enzyme secreted.[64] BSSL is present in early prepartum secretions less than 2 months before delivery and in the milk expressed during weaning. For a given well-nourished woman, levels remain stable even after prolonged lactation. BSSL activity is protective against infection by virtue of the production of free fatty acids and monoglycerides, products of fat digestion that have antiinfective properties (see Table 4-31).[64]

The enzyme activity of BSSL is remarkably stable during prolonged storage up to 2 years at either −20° C or −70° C (−4° F or −94° F). It has

also been noted to be stable at 15°, 25°, and 38° C (59°, 77°, and 100° F).[86]

Contrary to earlier suggestions, no association exists between jaundice and increased levels of free fatty acids produced as a result of high activity of milk lipase.[64]

Investigators have continued to study the action of these lipases in the presence of bile salts.[81,82,96] The BSSL remains active during passage through the stomach because it is stable above pH 3.5 and only slowly inactivated by pepsin. The optimal bile salt concentration for activity is about 2 mmol/L, which is within the physiologic range in the newborn. Bile salts protect the enzyme from tryptic activity.[96]

Glucose-6-phosphate dehydrogenase. Glucose-6-phosphate dehydrogenase (G-6-PD) is rich in the milk of mothers with normal red blood cell dehydrogenase and absent in mothers with G-6-PD deficiency. Its levels depend on the increased rate of carbohydrate metabolism in the mammary gland.[199]

Lactic and malic acid dehydrogenases. Lactic and malic acid dehydrogenase levels are high in colostrum, are lower in mature milk, and increased at the end of a feeding. The levels are higher in species with small body size; thus, mice and humans have more than cows.[16] Because no correlation exists with serum levels, these enzymes are thought to be synthesized in the mammary gland. A change occurs in these enzymes during lactation.

Lactose synthetase. Lactose synthetase catalyzes the synthesis of lactose from UDP-galactose and glucose. This enzyme has two components: A-protein, a glycoprotein, and B-protein, an α-lactalbumin. The control mechanism for lactose biosynthesis by the A-protein and α-lactalbumin ensures that lactose is synthesized in the mammary gland only in response to specific hormones.

Lysozyme. Lysozyme is a thermostable, nonspecific antimicrobial factor that catalyzes the hydrolysis of β-linkage between *N*-acetylglucosamine and *N*-acetylmuramic acid in the bacterial cell wall. It is bacteriolytic toward Enterobacteriaceae and gram-positive bacteria and is considered to play a role in the antibacterial activity of milk as well as a significant role in the development of intestinal flora. It also hydrolyzes mucopolysaccharides. Human lysozyme is antigenically and serologically different from the bovine enzyme. The content in human milk is 3000 times that in bovine milk and the activity 100 times that of bovine milk. Lysozyme is considered to be a spillover product from breast epithelial cells.

Phosphatases. *Acid phosphatase* is similar in human and bovine milk, but *alkaline phosphatase* is much less active in human milk by a factor of 40. Its level increases with the increase in fat concentration and increases as the feeding progresses. In 199 samples from 20 donors, no relationship to age, nationality, or other characteristics of the donor was found, except for a tendency for alkaline phosphatase to increase over time. Alkaline phosphatase concentrations appeared to be related to the fat concentration in human milk. Levels increased

as lactation progressed.[2] Alkaline phosphatase is a metal-carrying enzyme with four zinc molecules and two magnesium atoms. It differs from the placental alkaline phosphatase.

Serum alkaline phosphatase is increased in pregnancy. The placenta produces alkaline phosphatase, which may contribute to this increase. The liver does not enlarge. The histologic appearance is normal. The spider angiomata and palmar erythema that are observed are attributed to the increase in estrogen.[68]

Proteases and antiproteases. Several enzymes have caseinolytic activity and elastase-like activity. Beta casein and V-casein and galactothermin are probably the by-products of endogenous human milk proteolytic activity.[87] There are also small peptides of only three to eight amino acids derived from a casein group called β-casomorphins with specific physiologic activity. These peptides may be associated with the sleeping patterns of neonates and even have relevance to postpartum psychosis.[141]

Proteases catalyze the hydrolysis of proteins. High levels of protease are found in human milk, suggesting that enzymes may provide the breastfed infant with significant digestive assistance immediately after birth.

Antiproteases' physiologic role is not entirely clear. The main protease inhibitors in human milk are α_1-*antichymotrypsin* and α_1-*antitrypsin*.[84] Trace amounts of others have been identified. One function may be to protect the mammary gland from local proteolytic activity by leukocytic and lysosomal proteases during different stages of lactogenesis. They may prevent the breakdown of proteins in stored milk.[87] The protection of immunoglobulins that are transferred intact to the neonate and the protection of growth hormones are probably other roles of the antiproteases. The presence of such inhibitors may restrain the invading bacterial enzymes in the host tissue (breast) or secretion (milk). Thus, the presence of these inhibitors may protect the mammary gland and the recipient infant from infection.

Xanthine oxidase. Xanthine oxidase catalyzes the oxidation of purines, pyrimidines, and aldehydes. Although bovine milk contains high levels, it was only after much effort that investigators were able to identify it in human milk.[226] The activity in human milk peaks on the third day after birth and decreases with the progression of lactation. It differs from that in bovine milk in that it is not of bacterial origin and its activity is correlated with protein concentration.

Many enzymes are being studied in the human and other species. See Table 4-30 for a summary of the most significant enzymes. For an extensive discussion, see Hamosh.[84]

Hormones

Protein hormones, especially prolactin, and steroid hormones, such as gestagens, estrogens, corticoids, androgens, and opiate-like peptides, can be detected in human milk and in the milk of other mammals.[197] Animal studies have shown that at least some of these hormones retain physiologic activity when ingested but not when pasteurized. Although their presence was recognized in the 1930s, advances in hormone assay techniques have brought more information to light.[128] Hormones with simple structures, such as steroids and *thyroxine* (T_4), can pass easily by diffusion into the milk from circulating blood. Peptide hormones such as hypothalamic-releasing hormones, because of their small size, also would be expected to appear in milk. Of the larger-molecular-weight pituitary hormones, only prolactin has been found so far. The hormones identified in human milk include gonadotropin-releasing hormone, thyroid-releasing hormone (TRH), thyroid-stimulating hormone (thyrotropin, TSH), prolactin, gonadotropins, ovarian hormones, corticosteroids, erythropoietin, cyclic adenosine monophosphate (cAMP), and cyclic guanosine monophosphate (cGMP) (Tables 4-32 and 4-33).

The concentration of hormones changes during lactation, with prolactin decreasing over time and *triiodothyronine* (T_3) and T_4 increasing. Evidence indicates that the gastrointestinal tract of suckling mammals possesses the ability to absorb various proteins with substantial preservation of their immunologic properties. The absorption of large-molecular-weight hormones has been demonstrated

TABLE 4-32   Nonpeptide hormone in human milk

Hormone	Concentration (ng/mL)
Thyroid	
Thyroxine (T_4)	1–4
	0.3–2.0
	12.0
	1.16–2.4
	0.8–2.3
Triiodothyronine (T_3)	0.02–0.40
	0.05–0.10
Reverse T_3	0.008–0.15
Adrenal gland: Cortisol	0.2–32.0 (5:10)*
	3.7
Sexual	
Progesterone	10–40
Pregnanediol	0–450
Estrogens	15–840 (15:60)*
Contraceptives	Biologically significant quantities

*Ratio of values in colostrum/values in mature milk.
Modified from Koldovsky O, Strbak V: Hormones and growth factors in human milk. In Jensen RG (ed): Handbook of Milk Composition, San Diego, Academic Press, 1995.

in suckling rats and mice, with measurable amounts appearing in serum and other tissues.

The thyroid hormones have received considerable attention because of the apparent protection of hypothyroid infants who are breastfed. TSH content was investigated by both direct [118]I-TSH radioimmunoassay and indirect radioimmunoassay.[210] TSH was present in human milk in low concentrations comparable to those normally found in the serum of euthyroid adults. Experimentally, thyroidectomy of the lactating rat led to the disappearance of measurable T_4 and an increase in the level of TSH in the milk. In contrast, administration of T_3 decreased the TSH in the rat model.

Prolactin has been identified as a normal constituent of human milk. Levels are high in the first few days post partum but subsequently decline rapidly. "Prolactin-like" biologic activity is measurable in human colostrum, with the highest levels on day 1. Concentrations in the milk tend to parallel concen-

TABLE 4-33   Hormonally active peptides in human milk

Peptide	Concentration	Ratio (colostrum/mature milk)
Erythropoietin	Bioassay	?
Growth factors		
Epidermal growth factor (EGF)	3–107 ng/mL	2:10
Insulin	0–80 µU/mL	3:10
Insulin-like growth factor 1 (IGF-1)	1.3–7 ng/mL	2:3
Nerve growth factor (NGF)	Present	
Transforming growth factor alpha (TGF-α)	0–8.4 ng/mL	1
Other growth factors	Present	?
Gastrointestinal regulatory peptides		
Gastrin	10–30 pg/mL	2:3
Gastric inhibitory peptide (GIP)	33–59 ng/mL	1
Gastric regulatory peptide (GRP)	31–55 pg/mL 60–430 pg/mL	2:3
Neurotensin	7–15 pg/mL	2:3
Peptide histidine methionine (PHM)	3–32 pg/mL	5:10
Peptide YY (PYY)	15–30 pg/mL	2:3

Modified from Koldovsky O, Strbak V: Hormones and growth factors in human milk. In Jensen RG (ed): Handbook of Milk Composition, San Diego, Academic Press, 1995.

trations in the blood plasma among different species. Three stages of neuroendocrine development are theorized: placental, milk, and autonomous, in which the milk phase is the adaptation to extrauterine life.[84]

The exact mechanism by which prolactin enters the milk is unclear. Prolactin-binding sites have been identified within the alveolar cells.[91] The functional significance of prolactin also remains unclear. In rodents, milk prolactin influences fluid and ion absorption from the jejunum. It also may influence gonadal and adrenal function, as demonstrated in other species.

Endocrine responses in the neonate differ between breastfed and formula-fed infants.[145] In a study of 34 healthy, 6-day-old full-term infants who were formula fed, plasma concentrations of insulin, motilin, enteroglucagon, neurotensin, and pancreatic polypeptide changed significantly after a feeding. Similar levels were measured in 43 normal breastfed infants, and little or no change was noted. Further, the basal levels of gastric inhibitory polypeptide, motilin, neurotensin, and vasoactive intestinal peptide were also higher in the bottle-fed than in the breastfed infants. Whether pancreatic and gut hormone-release changes affect postnatal development is yet to be determined.

Erythropoietin (EPO) is synthesized in the maternal kidney and targets bone marrow where it stimulates erythropoiesis. The bioavailablity of EPO enterally is thought to be insufficient; however, when present in human milk, it may be different for newborns. In the rat model it has been shown to stimulate erythropoiesis in the suckling rat. It may have a physiologic effect on human breastfed newborns.[19]

Prostaglandins

In the investigation of the factors in human milk that may modify or supplement physiologic functions in the neonate, the role of prostaglandins comes under review. Prostaglandins include any of a class of physiologically active substances present in many tissues and originally described in genital fluid and accessory glands. Among the many effects are those of vasodepression, stimulation of intestinal smooth muscle, uterine stimulation, aggregation of blood platelets, and antagonism to hormones influencing lipid metabolism. Prostaglandins are a group of prostanoic acids often abbreviated PGE, PGF, PGA, and PGB with numeric subscripts according to structure.

The synthesis of prostaglandins occurs when dietary linoleic acid is converted in the body by a series of steps involving chain lengthening and dehydration to arachidonic acid, the principal (but not the only) precursor of prostaglandins. Although the prostaglandins are similar in structure, the biologic effects of various prostaglandins produced from a single unsaturated fatty acid can be profoundly different and, in some cases, antagonistic.

Because of the possible beneficial effects of prostaglandins on the gastrointestinal (GI) tract of infants, several investigators[6,146,186] have measured levels in human milk. The measurements were made in colostrum, transitional milk, and mature milk with collections of both foremilk and hindmilk. PGE and PGF have been shown to be present in breast milk in more than 100 times the concentration in adult plasma (Fig. 4-12). The ratio of the principal metabolite of PGFM to PGF itself suggests a relatively long half-life. Although prostaglandins occur in cow milk, none was measurable in cow milk–based formulas. Two inactive metabolites were found in milk in levels similar to those in the control adult plasma.

It is thought that prostaglandins play a role in gastrointestinal motility, possibly assisting peristalsis physiologically. Infantile diarrhea may occasionally be caused by excessive prostaglandin secretion into the mother's milk during menstruation, when maternal plasma levels of PGF may be raised. The difference in stool patterns between infants who are breastfed versus formula fed may be partially attributable to the presence of prostaglandins in human milk and not in formulas. The role of prostaglandins in the pathogenesis of food intolerance is also under study, because prostaglandins have a cytoprotective effect on the upper bowel and reportedly are increased in patients with abnormal peristalsis and irritable bowel syndrome.[138]

Prostaglandins E_1, E_2, and $F_2\alpha$ (PGE_1, PGE_2, $PGF_2\alpha$) were determined in milk and plasma from mothers of term and preterm infants by Shimizu and associates.[201] They found the concentration of PGE_1 in milk to be similar to that in plasma and the concentrations of PGE_2 and $PGF_2\alpha$ to be about 1.2 to 2 times higher in milk than in plasma. Foremilk and hindmilk levels, however, were similar, as were term and preterm levels. Levels appeared to be constant throughout lactation. PGE_1 is credited with a variety of physiologic effects on the GI tract, including cytoprotection and a diarrhea-producing action. Other actions are expected and yet to be identified because of prostaglandins' stability throughout lactation and lack of degradation in milk and in the lumen of the gut.

In addition, the human infant may require PGE_2 for maintenance of gastric mucosal integrity, as do adults. Therefore, it is not surprising that the use of prostaglandin synthesis inhibitors, such as indomethacin for closure of a patent ductus, is associated with necrotizing enterocolitis. PGE_2 in human milk may also promote the accumulation of phospholipids in the neonatal stomach, enhancing the gastric mucosal barrier.

Relaxin. Relaxin is a hormone with a polypeptide structure similar to that of insulin. It is produced by the corpus luteum during pregnancy as well as by the decidua and the placenta. Relaxin induces cervical softening, loosens the pelvic girdle, and decreases myometrial activity during pregnancy in many species.[55] Its role in humans remains under study.

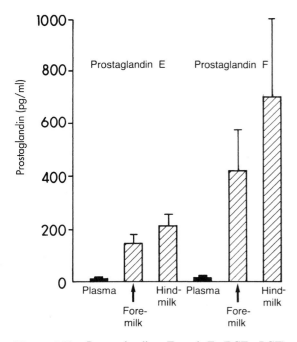

Figure 4-12. Prostaglandins E and F (PGE, PGF) (pg/mL ± SEM) in human milk and adult plasma. (From Lucas A, Mitchell MD: Prostaglandins in human milk. Arch Dis Child 55:950, 1980.)

It has been postulated that human mammary tissue is a target and a source of relaxin synthesis. Relaxin was measured by specific human relaxin radioimmunoassay in milk and sera of women delivering at term, prematurely at 3 days, and at 6 weeks post partum.[55] Sera and milk levels were similar in term and preterm mothers; however, at 6 weeks, relaxin concentrations in milk were higher in the preterm group. The presence in milk at 6 weeks suggests a nonluteal site of synthesis. The authors suggest that before lactation, relaxin may aid the growth and differentiation of mammary tissue, and then in the neonate, it may act directly on the GI tract.

Bile salts

Another limiting factor in digestion in the newborn is the decreased bile salt pool and the low concentration of bile salts in the duodenum. The presence of some biologically active substances in human milk contributes to digestion in the newborn. For this reason, the role of bile salts was investigated, and cholate and chenodeoxycholate were found in all samples of milk obtained from 28 lactating women in the first postpartum week.[65] In both colostrum and milk, cholate predominated. Samples were randomly collected, and the range of concentration was wide. The ratio of maternal serum to milk levels was 1:1 for cholate and 4:1 for chenodeoxycholate. The significance of these findings is under study.

Epidermal growth factor

Epidermal growth factor (EGF) is a small polypeptide mitogen that has been identified in many species and isolated and characterized in human milk. Of the growth factors that have been purified to date, EGF is one of the most biologically potent and best characterized as to its physical, chemical, and biologic properties. EGF has been associated with neonatal maturation, mechanisms of milk collection, and various protective effects. It is well established that EGF stimulates the proliferation of epidermal and epithelial tissues and has significant biologic effects in the intact mammal, particularly in the fetus and the newborn.[152] Effects verified in humans also include increased growth and maturation of the fetal

pulmonary epithelium, stimulation of ornithine decarboxylase activity and DNA synthesis in the digestive tract, and acceleration of the healing of wounds of the corneal epithelium. Quite unrelated is the observation that EGF inhibits histamine- or pentagastrin-induced secretion of gastric acid. It has a maturational effect on duodenal mucosal cells and increased lactase activity and net calcium transport in suckling rats. EGF has been identified in plasma, saliva, urine, amniotic fluid, and milk. Human milk is known to be mitogenic for cultured cells. EGF is active when administered orally, stable in acid, and resistant to trypsin digestion.

Newborn puppies, fed their mother's milk, were found to have hyperplasia of the enteric mucosa as compared with formula-fed littermates. Furthermore, the intestinal weight, length, and DNA and RNA content were greater in the puppies fed their mother's milk.

Previous studies specified the presence of EGF in the aqueous portion of human milk only; however, Gullett and associates[77] have established that EGF and its receptor are found in all human milk compartments: aqueous, liposomal, and membranes (MFGM).

Studies of EGF in human milk first reported that human milk stimulates DNA synthesis in cell cultures in which growth had been arrested.[152] The mitogenic activity of the milk was neutralized by the addition of antibody to human EGF. These findings support the concept that EGF is a major growth-promoting agent in breast milk. Actual measurements of EGF in the milk of 11 mothers who delivered at term and 20 who delivered prematurely were also done. EGF concentrations were 68 ± 19 ng/mL (mean $\pm$ SEM) in those who delivered at term and 70 ± 5 ng/mL (mean $\pm$ SEM) in the milk of those who delivered prematurely. There was no significant change over 7 weeks and no diurnal variation. The total EGF content was closely correlated with the volume of milk expressed, suggesting to the authors that EGF has a passive transport from the circulation as a function of plasma concentration.[152]

Using various techniques for assay, Iacopetta and associates[105] found 30 to 40 ng/mL in human milk, less than 2 ng/mL in bovine milk, and none in several bovine milk-based formulas. Little change occurred with refrigeration or freezing. The

role of EGF in promoting normal growth and functional maturation of the intestinal tract continues to be under study.

REFERENCES

1. Abrams SA, Wen J, Stuff JE: Absorption of calcium, zinc and iron from breast milk by five- to seven-month-old infants. Pediatr Res 41:384, 1996.
2. Adcock EW, Brewer ED, Caprioli RM, et al: Macronutrients, electrolytes and minerals in human milk: Differences over time and between population groups. In Howell RR, Morriss FH, Pickering LK (eds): Human Milk in Infant Nutrition and Health. Springfield, Ill, Charles C Thomas, 1986.
3. Alaejos MS, Romero CD: Selenium in human lactation. Nutr Rev 53:159, 1995.
4. Allen JC, Keller RP, Archer P, et al: Studies in human lactation: Milk composition and daily secretion rates of macronutrients in the first year of lactation. Am J Clin Nutr 54:69, 1991.
5. Almroth SG: Water requirements of breastfed infants in a hot climate. Am J Clin Nutr 31:1154, 1978.
6. Alzina V, Puig M, de Echániz L, et al: Prostaglandins in human milk. Biol Neonate 50:200, 1986.
7. American Academy of Pediatrics: Pediatric Nutrition Handbook, 5th ed. Elk Grove, Ill, American Academy of Pediatrics, 2003.
8. Anderson RA, Bryden NA, Patterson KY, et al: Breast milk chromium and its association with chromium intake, chromium excretion and serum chromium. Am J Clin Nutr 57:519, 1993.
9. Anderson RR: Variations in major minerals of human milk during the first 5 months of lactation. Nutr Res 12:701, 1992.
10. Ando K, Goto Y, Matsumoto Y, et al: Acquired zinc deficiency in a breast-fed mature infant: A possible cause of acquired maternal decreased zinc uptake by the mammary gland. J Am Acad Dermatol 29:111, 1993.
11. Asnes RS, Wisotsky DH, Migel PF, et al: The dietary chloride deficiency syndrome occurring in a breast-fed infant. J Pediatr 100:923, 1982.
12. Atkinson S, Alston-Mills B, Lönnerdal B, et al: Major minerals and ionic constituents of human and bovine milks. In Jensen RG (ed): Handbook of Milk Composition. San Diego, Academic Press, 1995.
13. Atkinson SA, Bryan MH, Anderson GH: Human milk: Differences in nitrogen concentration in milk from mothers of term and premature infants. J Pediatr 93:67, 1978.
14. Atkinson SA, Lönnerdal B: Nonprotein nitrogen fractions of human milk. In Jensen RG (ed): Handbook of Milk Composition. San Diego, Academic Press, 1995.
15. Atkinson SA, Whelan D, Whyte RK, et al: Abnormal zinc content in human milk. Am J Dis Child 143:608, 1989.
16. Auricchio S, Rubino A, Mürset E: Intestinal glycosidase activities in the human embryo, fetus, and newborn. Pediatrics 35:944, 1965.
17. Barness LA, Carver J: Nucleotides and immune function, Semin Gastroenterol Nutr 2:11, 1991.
18. Barth CA, Roos N, Nottbohm B, et al: L-Carnitine concentrations in milk from mothers on different diets. In Schaub J (ed): Composition and Physiological Properties of Human Milk. Amsterdam, Elsevier, 1985.
19. Bernt KM, Walker WA: Human milk as a carrier of biochemical messages. Acta Paediatr Suppl 430:27, 1999.
20. Birch EE, Birch DG, Hoffman DR, et al: Dietary essential fatty acid supply and visual activity development. Invest Ophthalmol Vis Sci 33:3242, 1992.
21. Bitman J, Wood DL, Mehta NR, et al: Comparison of the phospholipid composition of breast milk from mothers of term and preterm infants during lactation. Am J Clin Nutr 40:1103, 1984.
22. Bitman J, Wood DL, Neville MC, et al: Lipid composition of prepartum, preterm and term milk. In Hamosh M, Goldman AS (eds): Human Lactation, Vol. 2. Maternal and Environmental Factors. New York, Plenum, 1986.
23. Buescher ES, McIlheran SM: Colostral antioxidants: Separation and characterization of two activities in human colostrum. J Pediatr Gastroenterol Nutr 14:47, 1992.
24. Büller H, Peters M, Burger B, et al: Vitamin K status beyond the neonatal period. Eur J Pediatr 145:496, 1986.
25. Butte NF, Garza C, Smith EO: Macro- and trace mineral intakes of exclusively breastfed infants. Am J Clin Nutr 45:42, 1987.
26. Byerley LO, Kirksey A: Effects of different levels of vitamin C intake on the vitamin C concentration in human milk and the vitamin C intakes of breastfed infants. Am J Clin Nutr 41:665, 1985.
27. Calvo EB, Galindo AC, Aspres ND: Iron status in exclusively breastfed infants. Pediatrics 90:375, 1992.
28. Canfield LM, Giuliano AR, Neilson EM, et al: Beta carotene in breast milk and serum is increased after a single beta carotene dose. Am J Clin Nutr 66:52, 1997.
29. Canfield LM, Hopkinson JM, Lima AF, et al: Vitamin K in colostrum and mature human milk over the lactational period: A cross-sectional study. Am J Clin Nutr 53:730, 1991.
30. Carlson SE: Human milk nonprotein nitrogen: Occurrence and possible function. Adv Pediatr 32:43, 1985.

31. Casey CE, Smith A, Zhang PC: Microminerals in human and animal milks. In Jensen RG (ed): Handbook of Milk Composition. San Diego, Academic Press, 1995.

32. Casey CE, Walravens PA, Hambidge KM: Availability of zinc: Loading tests with human milk, cow's milk, and infant formulas. Pediatrics 68:394, 1981.

33. Chang YT, Germain-Lee EL, Doran TF, et al: Hypocalcemia in non-white breastfed infants. Clin Pediatr 31:695, 1992.

34. Chen DC, Nommsen-Rivers L, Dewey KG, et al: Stress during labor and delivery and early lactation performance. Am J Clin Nutr 68:335, 1998.

35. Chu SW: Nucleotides: Biochemistry and metabolism. Semin Gastroenterol Nutr 2:11, 1991.

36. Committee on Nutrition, American Academy of Pediatrics: Vitamin K supplementation for infants. Pediatrics 48:483, 1971.

37. Committee on Nutrition, American Academy of Pediatrics: Nutrition and lactation. Pediatrics 68:435, 1981.

38. Committee on Nutrition, American Academy of Pediatrics: Sodium intake of infants in the United States. Pediatrics 68:445, 1981.

39. Coppa GV, Gabrielli O, Pierani P, et al: Changes in carbohydrate composition in human milk over 4 months of lactation. Pediatrics 91:637, 1993.

40. Coppa GV, Pierani P, Zampini L, et al: Oligosaccharides in human milk during different phases of lactation. Acta Paediatr Suppl 430:89, 1999.

41. Coppa GV, Pierani P, Zampini L, et al: Oligosaccharides in human milk during different phases of lactation. Acta Paediatr Suppl 430:89, 1999.

42. Cornelissen EAM, Kollee LAA, DeAbreu RA, et al: Effects of oral and intramuscular vitamin K prophylaxis on vitamin K1, PIVKA-II and clotting factors in breastfed infants. Arch Dis Child 67:1250, 1992.

43. Cross NA, Hillman LS, Allen SH, et al: Calcium homeostasis and bone metabolism during pregnancy, lactation, and post weaning: A longitudinal study. Am J Clin Nutr 61:514, 1995.

44. Dale G, Goldfinch ME, Sibert JR, et al: Plasma osmolality, sodium, and urea in healthy breastfed and bottle-fed infants in Newcastle upon Tyne. Arch Dis Child 50:731, 1975.

45. Davies DP, Saunders R: Blood urea: Normal values in early infancy related to feeding practices. Arch Dis Child 48:563, 1973.

46. Dearlove JC, Dearlove BM: Prolactin, fluid balance, and lactation. Br J Obstet Gynaecol 88:652, 1981.

47. DeSantiago S, Villalpando S, Ortiz N, et al: Protein requirements of marginally nourished lactating women. Am J Clin Nutr 62:364, 1995.

48. Dewey KG, Cohen RJ, Landa Rivera I, et al: Effects of age of introduction of complementary foods on iron status of breastfed infants in Honduras. Am J Clin Nutr 67:878, 1998.

49. Dewey KG, Heinig MJ, Nommsen LA, et al: Maternal versus infant factors related to breast milk intake and residual milk volume: The DARLING Study. Pediatrics 87:829, 1991.

50. DeWille JW, Farmer SJ: Postnatal dietary fat influences mRNAs involved in myelination. Dev Neurosci 14:61, 1992.

51. Dick G: The etiology of multiple sclerosis. Proc R Soc Med 69:611, 1976.

52. Dorea JG: Is zinc a first limiting nutrient in human milk? Nutr Res 13:659, 1993.

53. Duncan B, Schifman RB, Corrigan JJ, et al: Iron and the exclusively breastfed infant from birth to six months. J Pediatr Gastroenterol 4:421, 1985.

54. Dupuy P, Sauniere JF, Vis HL, et al: Change in bile salt dependent lipase in human breast milk during extended lactation. Lipids 26:134, 1991.

55. Eddie LW, Sutton B, Fitzgerald S, et al: Relaxin in paired samples of serum and milk from women after term and preterm delivery. Am J Obstet Gynecol 161:970, 1989.

56. Ekstrand J, Spak CJ, Falch J, et al: Distribution of fluoride to human breast milk following intake of high doses of fluoride. Caries Res 18:93, 1984.

57. Fall CHD, Barker DJP, Osmond C, et al: Relation of infant feeding to adult serum cholesterol concentration and death from ischaemic heart disease. Br Med J 304:801, 1992.

58. Farquharson J, Cockburn F, Patrick WA, et al: Infant cerebral cortex phospholipid fatty-acid composition and diet. Lancet 340:810, 1992.

59. Feeley RM, Eitenmiller RR, Jones JB, et al: Copper, iron, and zinc contents of human milk at early stages of lactation. Am J Clin Nutr 37:443, 1983.

60. Ferris AM, Jensen RG: Lipids in human milk: A review. I. Sampling, determination and content. J Pediatr Gastroenterol Nutr 3:108, 1984.

61. Filteau SM: Milk components with immunomodulatory potential. In Woodward B, Draper HH (eds): Advances in Nutritional Research, Vol. 10. New York, Kluwer Academic/Plenum Publishers, 2001, p 327.

62. Finley DA, Lönnerdal B, Dewey KG, et al: Breast milk composition: Fat and fatty acid composition in vegetarians and non-vegetarians. Am J Clin Nutr 41:787, 1985.

63. Food and Nutrition Board, National Research Council, National Academy of Sciences: Recommended Dietary Allowances, 10th ed. Washington, DC, U.S. Government Printing Office, 1989.

64. Forsyth JS, Donnet L, Ross PE: A study of the relationship between bile salts, bile salt stimulated lipase, and free fatty acids in breast milk: Normal infants and those with breast milk jaundice. J Pediatr Gastroenterol Nutr 11:205, 1990.

65. Forsyth JS, Ross PE, Bouchier IAD: Bile salts in breast milk. Eur J Pediatr 140:126, 1983.

66. Fransson GB, Lönnerdal B: Iron in human milk. J Pediatr 96:380, 1980.

67. Fransson GB, Lönnerdal B: Zinc, copper, calcium and magnesium in human milk. J Pediatr 101:504, 1982.

68. Gabbe SG, Niebyl JR, Simpson JL, et al: Obstetrics: Normal and Problem Pregnancies, 4th ed. Philadelphia, Churchill Livingstone, 2002, pp 92–93.

69. Gaull GE: Taurine in the nutrition of the human infant. Acta Paediatr Scand Suppl 269:38, 1982.

70. Gibson RA, Kneebore GM: Fatty acid composition of human colostrum and mature breast milk. Am J Clin Nutr 34:252, 1981.

71. Gil A, Uauy R: Nucleotides and related compounds in human and bovine milk. In Jensen RG (ed): Handbook of Milk Composition. San Diego, 1995, Academic Press.

72. Greer F, Gartner L: Prevention of rickets and vitamin D deficiency: New guidelines for vitamin D intake. Pediatrics 111: 908, 2003.

73. Greer FR, Marshall S, Cherry J, et al: Vitamin K status of lactating mothers, human milk, and breastfeeding infants. Pediatrics 88:751, 1991.

74. Greer FR, Marshal SP, Foley AL, et al: Improving vitamin K status of breastfeeding infants with maternal vitamin K supplements. Pediatrics 99:88, 1997.

75. Greer FR, Mummah-Schendel LL, Marshall S, et al: Vitamin K1 (phylloquinone) and vitamin K2 (menaquinone) status in newborns during the first week of life. Pediatrics 81:137, 1988.

76. Greer FR, Tsang RC, Levin RS, et al: Increasing serum calcium and magnesium concentrations in breastfed infants: Longitudinal studies of minerals in human milk and in sera of nursing mothers and their infants, J Pediatr 100:59, 1982.

77. Gullett SL, Baatz JE, Forsythe DW, et al: Establishing the presence of epidermal growth factor (EGF) and the EGFR in human milk's compartments. ABM News & Views 9(4):26, 2003.

78. Gushurst CA, Mueller JA, Green JA, et al: Breast milk iodide: Reassessment in the 1980's. Pediatrics 73:354, 1984.

79. György P: Biochemical aspects. In Jelliffe DB, Jelliffe EFP (eds): The uniqueness of human milk. Am J Clin Nutr 24:970, 1971.

80. Hadjimarkos DM, Shearer TR: Selenium in mature human milk. Am J Clin Nutr 26:583, 1973.

81. Hall B: Changing composition of human milk and early development of an appetite control. Lancet 1:779, 1975.

82. Hall B, Muller DPR: Studies on bile-salt-stimulated lipolytic activity in human milk. II. Demonstration of two groups of milk with different activities. Pediatr Res 17:716, 1983.

83. Hambraeus L, Forsum E, Lönnerdal B: Nutritional aspects of breast milk and cow's milk formulas. In Hambraeus L, Hanson L, MacFarlane H (eds): Symposium on Food and Immunology. Stockholm, Almqvist and Wiksell, 1975.

84. Hamosh M: Enzymes in human milk. In Howell RR, Morriss FH, Pickering LK (eds): Human Milk in Infant Nutrition and Health. Springfield, Ill, Charles C Thomas, 1986.

85. Hamosh M: Breast milk jaundice. J Pediatr Gastroenterol Nutr 11:145, 1990.

86. Hamosh M: Lipid metabolism in pediatric nutrition. Pediatr Clin North Am 42:839, 1995.

87. Hamosh M, Hong MH, Hamosh P: β-Casomorphins: Milk β-casein derived opioid peptides. In Lebenthal E (ed): Textbook of Gastroenterology and Nutrition in Infancy, 2nd ed. New York, Raven, 1989.

88. Harzer G, Dieterich I, Haug M: Effects of the diet on composition of human milk. Ann Nutr Metab 28:231, 1984.

89. Harzer G, Haug M, Dieterich I, et al: Changing patterns of human milk lipids in the course of the lactation and during the day. Am J Clin Nutr 37:612, 1983.

90. Harzer G, Kauer H: Binding of zinc to casein. Am J Clin Nutr 35:981, 1982.

91. Healy DL, Rattigan S, Hartmann PE, et al: Prolactin in human milk: Correlation with lactose, total protein, and β-lactalbumin levels. Am J Physiol 238 (Endocrinol Metab 1):E83, 1980.

92. Heine W, Braun OH, Mohr C, et al: Enhancement of lysozyme trypsin-mediated decay of intestinal bifidobacteria and lactobacilli. J Pediatr Gastroenterol Nutr 21:54, 1995.

93. Heird WC, Prager TC, Anderson RE: Docosahexaenoic acid and development and function of the infant retina. Curr Opin Lipidol 8:12, 1997.

94. Heiskanen K, Siimes MA, Perheentupa J, et al: Risk of low vitamin B6 status in infants breast-fed exclusively beyond six months. J Pediatr Gastroenterol Nutr 23:38, 1996.

95. Heitlinger LA, Lee PA, Dillon WP, et al: Mammary amylase: A possible alternate pathway of carbohydrate digestion in infancy. Pediatr Res 17:15, 1983.

96. Hernell O, Bläckberg L: Digestion of human milk lipids: Physiologic significance of sn-2 monoacylglyceral hydrolysis by bile salt-stimulated lipase. Pediatr Res 16:882, 1982.

97. Hibberd CM, Brooke OG, Carter ND, et al: Variation in the composition of breast milk during the first five weeks of lactation: Implications for the feeding of preterm infants. Arch Dis Child 57:658, 1982.

98. Holick MF: Evolution, functions, and RDA. In Holick MF (ed): Vitamin D: Physiology, Molecular Biology, and Clinical Applications. Totowa, NJ, Humana Press, 1999, p 1.

99. Hollis BW: Comparison of equilibrium and disequilibrium assay conditions for ergocalciferol, cholecaliferol and their major metabolites. J Steroid Biochem 21:81, 1984.

100. Hollis BW: Daily reference intake and lowest observed adverse effect level for vitamin D in the adult human subject with special emphasis on the pregnant women: A comparison of new and past data. Am J Clin Nutr. 79:17, 2004.

101. Horwood LJ, Fergusson DM: Breastfeeding and later cognitive and academic outcomes. Pediatrics 101:e9, 1998.

102. Howell RR, Palma PA, West MS, et al: Trace elements in human milk: Differences over time and between population groups. In Howell RR, Morriss FH, Pickering LK (eds): Human Milk in Infant Nutrition and Health. Springfield, Ill, Charles C Thomas, 1986.

103. Huston GE, Patton S: Membrane distribution in human milks throughout lactation as revealed by phospholipid

and cholesterol analyses. J Pediatr Gastroenterol Nutr 5:602, 1986.

104. Huxtable RJ: Physiological actions of taurine. Physiol Rev 72:101, 1992.

105. Iacopetta BJ, Grieu F, Horlsberger M, et al: Epidermal growth factor in human and bovine milk. Acta Paediatr Scand 81:287, 1992.

106. Innis SM: Human milk and formula fatty acids. J Pediatr Suppl 120:556, 1992.

107. Innis SM, Hamilton JJ: Effects of developmental changes and early nutrition on cholesterol metabolism in infancy: A review. J Am Coll Nutr 11:635, 1992.

108. Jackson DA, Imong SM, Silprasert A, et al: Circadian variation in fat concentration of breast milk in a rural northern Thai population. Br J Nutr 59:349, 1988.

109. Jamieson EC, Abbasi KA, Cockburn F, et al: Effect of diet on term infant cerebral cortex fatty acid composition. In Galli C, Simopoulis AP, Tremoli E (eds): Fatty Acids and Lipids: Biological Aspects. World Rev Nutr Diet (Basel Karger) 75:139, 1994.

110. Jansson L, Akesson B, Holmberg L: Vitamin E and fatty acid composition of human milk. Am J Clin Nutr 34:8, 1981.

111. Järvenpää AL, Rassin DK, Raiha NCR, et al: Milk protein quantity and quality in the term infant. II. Effects on acidic and neutral amino acids. Pediatrics 70:221, 1982.

112. Jenness R, Sloan RE: Composition of milk. In Larson BL, Smith VR (eds): Lactation, Vol. 3. Nutrition and Biochemistry of Milk/Maintenance. New York, Academic Press, 1974.

113. Jensen GL, Jensen RG: Specialty lipids for infant nutrition. II. Concerns, new developments and future applications. J Pediatr Gastroenterol Nutr 15:382, 1992.

114. Jensen RG: Introduction. In Jensen RG (ed): Handbook of Milk Composition. San Diego, Academic Press, 1995.

115. Jensen RG: Lipids in human milk: A review. Lipids 34:243, 1999.

116. Jensen RG, Bitman J, Carlson SE: Milk lipids. A. Human milk lipids. In Jensen RG (ed): Handbook of Milk Composition. San Diego, Academic Press, 1995.

117. Jensen RG, Ferris AM, Lammi-Keefe CJ: Lipids in human milk and infant formulas. Ann Rev Nutr 12:417, 1992.

118. Johnson PE, Evans GW: Relative zinc availability in human breast milk, infant formulas, and cow's milk. Am J Clin Nutr 31:416, 1978.

119. Johnston L, Vaughn L, Fox HM: Pantothenic acid content of human milk. Am J Clin Nutr 34:2205, 1981.

120. Jooste PL, Roosouw LJ, Steenkamp HJ, et al: Effect of breastfeeding on the plasma cholesterol and growth of infants. J Pediatr Gastroenterol Nutr 13:139, 1991.

121. Kalkwarf HJ, Specker BL: Bone mineral loss during lactation and recovery after weaning. Obstet Gynecol 86:26, 1995.

122. Kalkwarf HJ, Specker BL, Bianchi DC, et al: The effect of calcium supplementation on bone density during lactation and after weaning. N Engl J Med 337:523, 1997.

123. Kalkwarf HJ, Specker BL, Heubi JE, et al: Intestinal calcium absorption of women during lactation and after weaning. Am J Clin Nutr 63:526, 1996.

124. Kallio MJT, Salmenperä L, Siimes MA, et al: Exclusive breastfeeding and weaning: Effect on serum cholesterol and lipoprotein concentrations in infants during the first year of life. Pediatrics 89:663, 1992.

125. Keenan BS, Buzek SW, Garza C: Cortisol and its possible role in regulation of sodium and potassium in human milk. Am J Physiol (Endocrinol Metab 7) 244:E253, 1983.

126. Khoshoo V, Kjarsgaar DJ, Krafchick B, et al: Zinc deficiency in a full term breastfed infant: Unusual presentation. Pediatrics 89:1094, 1992.

127. Kirksey A, Roepke JLB: Vitamin B6 nutriture of mothers of three breastfed neonates with central nervous system disorders. Fed Proc 40:864, 1981.

128. Koldovsky O, Strbak V: Hormones and growth factors in human milk. In Jensen RG (ed): Handbook of Milk Composition. San Diego, Academic Press, 1995.

129. Koski KG, Hill FW, Lönnerdal B: Altered lactational performance in rats fed low carbohydrate diets and its effect on growth of neonatal rat pups. J Nutr 120:1028, 1990.

130. Krebs NF, Hambidge KM: Zinc requirements and zinc intakes in breastfed infants. Am J Clin Nutr 43:288, 1986.

131. Krebs NF, Reidinger CJ, Robertson AD, et al: Bone mineral density changes during lactation: Maternal, dietary, and biochemical correlates. Am J Clin Nutr 65:1738, 1997.

132. Kretchmer N: Lactose and lactase. Sci Am 227:73, 1972.

133. Kulski JK, Hartmann PE: Changes in human milk composition during the initiation of lactation. Aust J Exp Biol Med Sci 59:101, 1981.

134. Kumpulainen J, Vuori E: Longitudinal study of chromium in human milk. Am J Clin Nutr 33:2299, 1980.

135. Kunz C, Lönnerdal B: Re-evaluation of whey protein/casein ratio of human milk. Acta Paediatr Scand 81:107, 1992.

136. Lammi-Keefe CJ: Vitamin D and E in human milk. In Jensen RG (ed): Handbook of Milk Composition. San Diego, Academic Press, 1995.

137. Lammi-Keefe CJ, Jensen RG: Lipids in human milk: A review. 2. Composition and fat-soluble vitamins. J Pediatr Gastroenterol Nutr 3:172, 1984.

138. Lessof MH, Anderson JA, Youlten LJ: Prostaglandins in the pathogenesis of food intolerance. Ann Allergy 51:249, 1983.

139. Lifschitz CH: Carbohydrate needs in preterm and term newborn infants. In Tsang RC, Nichols BL (eds): Nutrition during Infancy. St Louis, Mosby, 1988.

140. Lindberg T, Skude G: Amylase in human milk. Pediatrics 70:235, 1982.

141. Lindstrom LH, Nyberg F, Terenius L, et al: CSF and plasma-casomorphine-like opioid peptides in postpartum psychosis. Am J Psychiatry 141:1059, 1984.

142. Lönnerdal B: Effects of maternal dietary intake on human milk composition. J Nutr 116:499, 1986.

143. Lönnerdal B, Forsum E: Casein content of human milk. Am J Clin Nutr 41:113, 1985.

144. Lönnerdal B, Keen CL, Hurley LS: Manganese binding proteins in human and cow's milk. Am J Clin Nutr 4:550, 1985.

145. Lucas A, Blackburn AM, Aynsley-Green A, et al: Breast vs bottle: Endocrine responses are different with formula feeding. Lancet 1:1267, 1980.

146. Lucas A, Mitchell MD: Prostaglandins in human milk. Arch Dis Child 55:950, 1980.

147. Lucas A, Morley R, Cole TJ, et al: Breast milk and subsequent intelligence quotient in children born preterm. Lancet 339:261, 1992.

148. Lucas A, Morley R, Cole TJ, et al: A randomised multicentre study of human milk versus formula and later development in preterm infants. Arch Dis Child 70:F141, 1994.

149. MacDonald LD, Gibson RS, Miles JE: Changes in hair zinc and copper concentrations of breastfed and bottle-fed infants during the first six months. Acta Paediatr Scand 71:785, 1982.

150. Makrides M, Neumann MA, Gibson RA: Effect of maternal docosahexaenoic acid (DHA) supplementation on breast milk composition. Eur J Clin Nutr 50:352, 1996.

151. Malloy MH, Rassin DK, Gaull GE, et al: Development of taurine metabolism in beagle pups: Effects of taurine-free total parenteral nutrition. Biol Neonate 40:1, 1981.

152. Moran JR, Courtney ME, Orth DN, et al: Epidermal growth factor in human milk: Daily production and diurnal variation during early lactation in mothers delivering at term and at premature gestation. J Pediatr 103:402, 1983.

153. Morton JA: The clinical usefulness of breast milk sodium in the assessment of lactogenesis. Pediatrics 93:802, 1994.

154. Moser PB, Reynolds RD: Dietary zinc intake and zinc concentrations of plasma, erythrocytes, and breast milk in antepartum and postpartum lactating and nonlactating women: A longitudinal study. Am J Clin Nutr 38:101, 1983.

155. Motil KJ, Thotathuchery M, Bahar A, et al: Marginal dietary protein restriction, reduced nonprotein nitrogen, but not protein nitrogen, components of human milk. J Am Coll Nutr 14:184, 1995.

156. Mott GE, Lewis DS, McGill HC Jr: Programming of cholesterol metabolism by breast or formula feeding. The childhood environment and adult disease. Ciba Found Symp 156:56, 1991.

157. Nail PA, Thomas MR, Eakin R: The effect of thiamin and riboflavin supplementation on the level of those vitamins in human milk and urine. Am J Clin Nutr 33:198, 1980.

158. National Academy of Science: Nutrition during Lactation. Institute of Medicine, Washington, DC, National Academy Press, 1991.

159. Neville MC: Mammary gland biology and lactation: A short course. Presented at biannual meeting of the International Society for Research on Human Milk and Lactation. Plymouth, Mass, October 1997.

160. Neville MC: Sampling and storage of human milk. In Jensen RG (ed): Handbook of Milk Composition. San Diego, Academic Press, 1995.

161. Neville MC: Determinants of milk volume and composition. In Jensen RG (ed): Handbook of Milk Composition. San Diego, Academic Press, 1995.

162. Neville MC: Volume and caloric density of human milk. In Jensen RG (ed): Handbook of Milk Composition. San Diego, Academic Press, 1995.

163. Neville MC, Allen JC, Archer PC, et al: Studies in human lactation: Milk volume and nutrient composition during weaning and lactogenesis. Am J Clin Nutr 54:81, 1991.

164. Neville MC, Casey C, Hay WW: Endocrine regulation of nutrient flux in the lactating woman. In Allen L, King J, Lonnerdal B (eds): Nutrient Regulation during Pregnancy, Lactation, and Infant Growth. New York, Plenum Press, 1994, p 85.

165. Neville MC, Keller R, Seacat J, et al: Studies in human lactation: Milk volumes in lactating women during the onset of lactation and full lactation. Am J Clin Nutr 48:1375, 1988.

166. Neville MC, Morton J, Umenura S: Lactogenesis: The transition from pregnancy to lactogenesis. Pediatr Clin North Am 48:35, 2001.

167. Neville MC, Zhang P, Allen JC: Minerals, ions, and trace elements in milk. A. Ionic interactions in milk. In Jensen RG (ed): Handbook of Milk Composition. San Diego, Academic Press, 1995.

168. Newburg DS: Oligosaccharides and glycoconjugates in human milk: Their role in host defense. J Mammary Gland Biol Neoplasia 1:271, 1996.

169. Newman V: Vitamin A and breastfeeding: A comparison of data from developed and developing countries. San Diego, Wellstart International, 1993.

170. Nommsen LA, Lovelady CA, Heinig MJ, et al: Determinants of energy, protein, lipid, and lactose concentrations in human milk during the first 12 months of lactation: The DARLING study. Am J Clin Nutr 53:457, 1991.

171. Novak M, Monkus EF, Chang D, et al: Carnitine in the perinatal metabolism of lipids. I. Relationship between maternal and fetal plasma levels of carnitine and acylcarnitines. Pediatrics 67:95, 1981.

172. O'Connor DL, Tamura T, Picciano MF: Pteroylpolyglutamates in human milk. Am J Clin Nutr 53:930, 1991.

173. Ortega RM, Andres P, Martinez RM, et al: Vitamin status during the third trimester of pregnancy in Spanish women: Influence on concentrations of vitamin A in breast milk. Am J Clin Nutr 66:564, 1997.

174. Orzali A, Donzelli F, Enzi G, et al: Effect of carnitine on lipid metabolism in the newborn. Biol Neonate 43:186, 1983.

175. Osborn GR: Relationship of hypotension and infant feeding to aetiology of coronary disease. Coll Int Cont Natl Res Sci 169:193, 1968.

176. Oski FA: What we eat may determine who we can be. Nutrition 13:220, 1997.

177. Picciano MF: Vitamins in milk. A. Water-soluble vitamins in human milk composition. In Jensen RG (ed): Handbook of Milk Composition. San Diego, Academic Press, 1995.

178. Picciano MF, Guthrie HA: Copper, iron, and zinc contents of mature human milk. Am J Clin Nutr 29:242, 1976.

179. Pisacane A, DeVizia B, Valiante A, et al: Iron status in breast-fed infants. J Pediatr 127:429, 1995.

180. Pollack PF, Koldovsky O, Nishioka K: Polyamines in human and rat milk and in infant formulas. Am J Clin Nutr 56:371, 1992.

181. Potter JM, Nestel PJ: The effects of dietary fatty acids and cholesterol on the milk lipids of lactating women and the plasma cholesterol of breastfed infants. Am J Clin Nutr 29:54, 1976.

182. Prentice A, Roberts SB, Prentice AM, et al: Dietary supplementation of lactating Gambian women. I. Effect on breastmilk volume and quality. Hum Nutr Clin Nutr 37C:53, 1983.

183. Quan R, Barness LA, Uauy R: Do infants need nucleotide supplemented formula for optimal nutrition? J Pediatr Gastroenterol Nutr 11:429, 1990.

184. Quan R, Uauy R: Nucleotides and gastrointestinal development. Semin Gastroenterol Nutr 2:3, 1991.

185. Rassin DK, Sturman JA, Gaull GE: Taurine in milk: Species variation. Pediatr Res 11:449, 1977.

186. Reid B, Smith H, Friedman Z: Prostaglandins in human milk. Pediatrics 66:870, 1980.

187. Reisbick S, Neuringer M, Connor WE, et al: Postnatal deficiency of omega-3 fatty acids in monkeys: Fluid intake and urine concentration. Physiol Behav 51:473, 1992.

188. Report of the Subcommittee on Nutrition during Lactation, The Institute of Medicine, National Academy of Sciences, Washington, DC, National Academy Press, 1991.

189. Roepke JLB, Kirksey A: Vitamin B6 nutriture during pregnancy and lactation. I. Vitamin B6 intake, levels of the vitamin in biological fluids, and condition of the infant at birth. Am J Clin Nutr 32:2249, 1979.

190. Roepke JLB, Kirksey A: Vitamin B6 nutriture during pregnancy and lactation. II. The effect of long-term use of oral contraceptives. Am J Clin Nutr 32:2257, 1979.

191. Romain N, Dandrifosse G, Jeusette F, et al: Polyamine concentration in rat milk and food, human milk and infant formulas. Pediatr Res 32:58, 1992.

192. Rothberg AD, Pettifor JM, Cohen DF, et al: Maternal-infant vitamin D relationships during breastfeeding. J Pediatr 101:500, 1982.

193. Salmenperä L, Perheetupa J, Siimes MA: Folate nutrition is optimal in exclusively breastfed infants but inadequate in some of their mothers and in formula-fed infants. J Pediatr Gastroenterol Nutr 5:283, 1986.

194. Samson RR, McClelland DBL: Vitamin B12 in human colostrum and milk. Acta Paediatr Scand 69:93, 1980.

195. Sandberg DP, Begley JA, Hall CA: The content, binding, and forms of vitamin B12 in milk. Am J Clin Nutr 34:1717, 1981.

196. Sanders TAB, Ellis FR, Dickerson JWT: Studies of vegans: The fatty acid composition of plasma choline phosphoglycerides, erythrocytes, adipose tissue, and breast milk, and some indicators of susceptibility to ischemic heart disease in vegans and omnivore controls. Am J Clin Nutr 31:805, 1978.

197. Schams D, Karg H: Hormones in milk. Ann NY Acad Sci 464:75, 1986.

198. Sellmayer A, Koletzko B: Long chain polyunsaturated fatty acids and eicosanoids in infants: Physiological and pathophysiological aspects and open questions. Lipids 34:199, 1999.

199. Shahani KM, Kwan AJ, Friend BA: Role and significance of enzymes in human milk. Am J Clin Nutr 33:1861, 1980.

200. Shaw JCL: Trace elements in the fetus and young infant. Am J Dis Child 134:74, 1980.

201. Shimizu T, Yamashiro Y, Yabuta K: Prostaglandin E1, E2, and F2a in human milk and plasma. Biol Neonate 61:222, 1992.

202. Sievers E, Oldigs H-D, Dörner K, et al: Longitudinal zinc balances in breastfed and formula-fed infants. Acta Paediatr Scand 81:1, 1992.

203. Simopoulas AP: Omega-3 fatty acids in health and disease in growth and development. Am J Clin Nutr 54:438, 1991.

204. Smith AM, Picciano MF, Milner JA: Selenium intakes and status of human milk and formula-fed infants. Am J Clin Nutr 35:521, 1982.

205. Sneed SM, Zane C, Thomas MR: The effects of ascorbic acid, vitamin B6, vitamin B12 and folic acid supplementation on the breast milk and maternal nutritional status of low socioeconomic lactating women. Am J Clin Nutr 34:1338, 1981.

206. Specker BL, Black A, Allen L, et al: Vitamin B12: Low milk concentrations are reported to correspond to low serum concentrations in vegetarian women and to methylmalonic aciduria in their infants. Am J Clin Nutr 52:1073, 1990.

207. Specker BL, Tsang RC, Ho ML: Changes in calcium homeostasis over the first year postpartum: Effect of lactation and weaning. Obstet Gynecol 78:56, 1991.

208. Specker BL, Tsang RC, Ho ML, et al: Effect of vegetarian diet on serum 1,25-dihydroxyvitamin D concentrations during lactation. Obstet Gynecol 70:870, 1987.

209. Sturman JA, Rassin DK, Gaull GE: Taurine in the developing kitten: Nutritional importance. Pediatr Res 11:450, 1977.

210. Tenore A, Oberkotter LV, Koldovsky O, et al: Thyrotropin in human breast milk. Horm Res 14:193, 1981.

211. Thomas MR, Sneed SM, Wei C, et al: The effects of vitamin C, vitamin B6, and vitamin B12, folic acid, riboflavin, and thiamin on the breast milk and maternal status of well-nourished women at 6 months postpartum. Am J Clin Nutr 33:2151, 1980.

212. Tikanoja T, Simell O, Viikari M, et al: Plasma amino acids in term neonates after a feed of human milk or formula. II. Characteristic changes in individual amino acids. Acta Paediatr Scand 71:391, 1982.

213. Tomashek K, Nesby-O'Dell S, Scanlon KS, et al: Nutritional rickets in Georgia. Pediatrics 107, 2001.

214. Vanderslice JT, Brownlee SG, Maire CE, et al: Form of vitamin B6 in human milk. Am J Clin Nutr 37:867, 1983.

215. Van Houwelingen AC, Sorensen JD, Hornstra G, et al: Essential fatty acid status in neonates after fish-oil supplementation during late pregnancy. Br J Nutr 74:723, 1995.

216. Vorherr H: The Breast: Morphology, Physiology, and Lactation. New York, Academic Press, 1974.

217. Wagner CL, Howard C, Lawrence RA, et al: Maternal vitamin D supplementation during lactation: A viable alternative to infant supplementation. Pediatr Res 53: 255A, 2003.

218. Watkins JB: Bile acid metabolism in the human infant: Role of taurine supplementation and human milk. In Filer LJ, Fomon SJ (eds): The Breastfed Infant: A Model for Performance. Columbus, Ohio, Ross Laboratories, 1986.

219. Welch T, Bergstrom W, Tsang R: Vitamin D-deficient rickets: The reemergence of a once-conquered disease. J Pediatr 137:143, 2000.

220. Widdowson EM, Dauncey MJ, Gardner DM, et al: Body fat of British and Dutch infants. Br Med J 1:653, 1975.

221. Woolridge MW, Greasley V, Silpisornkosol S: The initiation of lactation: The effect of early versus delayed contact for suckling on milk intake in the first week post-partum. A study in Chiang Mai, Northern Thailand. Early Hum Dev 12:269, 1985.

222. Wong WW, Hachey DL, Insull W, et al: Effect of dietary cholesterol on cholesterol synthesis in breast-fed and formula-fed infants. J Lipid Res 34:1403, 1993.

223. Work Group on Breastfeeding, American Academy of Pediatrics: Breastfeeding and the use of human milk. Pediatrics 100:6, 1997.

224. Yolken RH, Peterson JA, Vonderfecht SL, et al: Human milk mucin inhibits rotavirus replication and prevents experimental gastroenteritis. J Clin Invest 90:1984, 1992.

225. Young VR, Nahapetian A, Janghorbani M: Selenium bioavailability with reference to human nutrition. Am J Clin Nutr 35:1076, 1982.

226. Zikakis JP, Dougherty TM, Biasotto HO: The presence and some properties of xanthine oxidase in human milk and colostrum. J Food Sci 41:1408, 1976.

$\mathcal{H}$ost-resistance factors and immunologic significance of human milk

ROBERT M. LAWRENCE

Some of the most dramatic and far-reaching advances in the understanding of the immunologic benefits of human milk have been made using newer techniques to demonstrate the specific contribution of the numerous "bioactive factors" contained in human milk. The multifunctional capabilities of the individual factors, the interactive coordinated functioning of these factors, and the longitudinal changes in the relative concentrations of them over the duration of lactation make human milk unique. The immunologically active components of breast milk make up an important aspect of the host defenses of the mammary gland in the mother; at the same time, they complement, supplement, and stimulate the ongoing development of the infant's immune system.

The explosion of research on all the immunologic properties and actions of breast milk over the last 15 years makes it impossible to summarize all the important aspects of what we now know about the immunologic benefits of breast milk. This chapter emphasizes the important concepts of these immunologic benefits and refers the interested reader to the most recent literature for more extensive information on the many specific components.

OVERVIEW

The immunologic benefits of human milk can be analyzed from a variety of perspectives:
1. Reviewing the published information on the protection of infants from specific infections comparing breastfed and formula fed infants.
2. Comparing the documented deficiencies in the infant's developing immune system and the actions of bioactive factors provided in breast milk.
3. Examining the proposed function of the active components contained in human milk: antimicrobial, antiinflammatory, and immunomodulating.
4. Considering the nature of the different factors: soluble, cellular, and hormone-like.

5. Determining the site of the postulated action of the specific factors (e.g., in the breast or in the infant) at the mucosal level (respiratory tract or gastrointestinal tract) or at the systemic level.

6. Classifying the factors relative to their contribution to the constitutive defenses versus the inducible defenses of the infant's immune system.

7. Clarifying the mechanism of action of the proposed immunologic benefit (the mucosal-associated lymphoid tissue formation of bioactive factors at the level of the mucosa and their subsequent action at the breast or in the infant).

8. Examining the contribution of breast milk to immune function of the mammary gland and the infant as an evolutionary process.

Breast milk's protective effect against infection was documented as early as 1892 in the medical literature by data proving that milk from various species, including humans, was protective for the offspring, containing antibodies against a vast number of antigens.[1] Veterinarians have long known the urgency of offspring receiving the early milk of the mother. Death rates among newborns not suckled at the breast in the Third World are at least five times higher than among those who receive colostrum and mother's milk. The evidence that a lack of breastfeeding and poor environmental sanitation have a pernicious synergistic effect on infant mortality rate has been presented by Habicht[2] after studying 1262 women in Malaysia.

The evidence that breastfeeding protects against infections in the digestive and respiratory tracts has been reported for several decades.[3] However, many of the older studies were criticized for flawed methodology and because they were performed in "developing countries" where the risk of infection due to poor sanitation was expected to be higher.[2,4,5] Various researchers have proposed specific criteria for assessing the methodology of studies reporting on the protective effects of breast milk, clearly identifying measurable outcomes and the definition of breastfeeding along with other methods to limit bias and to control for confounding variables.[4,6,7,8] More recent studies, which have incorporated many of the proposed methodologic criteria, continue to document that breastfeeding protects infants against diarrhea, respiratory infections, and otitis media.[9-15] A recent paper on the benefits of breastfeeding by M. Jane Henig, PhD, nicely reviews studies that utilized the criteria described by Bauchner and associates[4] and focused the research in industrialized countries.[5]

One of the important considerations relative to measuring the immunologic benefits of breast milk is the exclusivity and duration of breastfeeding. The basic idea is identifying a dose-response relationship between the amount of breast milk received by the infant over the period of observation and the immunologic benefit gained with greater exclusivity and duration. There is also the issue of the potential effect of other foods and fluids in an infant's diet influencing the immunologic benefits of breast milk. Dr. Labbok and others have carefully defined breastfeeding in terms of the patterns of breastfeeding relative to the amount of supplementation with formula (full/nearly full, medium or equal, low partial, or token) in order to standardize the use of equatable terms in different studies.[6] Raisler and associates[184] referred to a dose-response relationship when they studied the effect of "dose" of breast milk on preventing illness in over 7000 infants. "Full breastfeeding" was associated with the lowest rates of illness (diarrhea, cough, or wheeze) and even children with "most" or "equal" breastfeeding had evidence of lower odds ratios of ear infections and certain other illnesses. A number of other long-term studies have demonstrated greater protection from infection with increased exclusivity of breastfeeding and durations of at least 3 months.[9-11,14-21] The current recommendations from the American Academy of Pediatrics reinforce the importance of the dose-response relationship between breastfeeding and the benefits of breastfeeding when they recommend exclusive breastfeeding for the first 6 months of life and at least partial breastfeeding after the introduction of solid foods, for an additional 12 months or longer.[22]

The newborn infant's immune system is immature and inadequate at birth. There are rapid adaptations to the immune system in the early postnatal period related to the natural maturation of the skin and mucosal barriers as well as to the exposure of the infant to various infectious agents in the extrauterine environment. The infant's immune system continues to develop over at least the first 2 years of life. Overall, the infant has a limited ability to respond effectively and quickly to infectious challenges, which explains the infant's ongoing susceptibility to infection.[23-26] The activation and responsiveness of the mucosa-associated lymphoid tissue (MALT) develops during infancy.[27,28] The systemic cell-mediated immune response and neutrophil activity of the infant are also developmentally delayed during the first months of life. There are numerous immune components that are produced in limited amounts in infancy including complement, interferon-gamma, secretory IgA, interleukins (IL-3, IL-6, IL-10), tumor necrosis factor-alpha (TNF-α), lactoferrin, and lysozyme[23,24] The development of effector and memory T cells and the production of IgG in response to certain T-cell–dependent antigens are also poor. Relative to these various immune deficits in the infant, one can find various bioactive and immunomodulating factors in breast milk that are potentially capable of complementing and enhancing the development of the infant's mucosal and systemic immune system.[24,29]

This concept of bioactive and immunomodulating factors in breast milk is an important area of evolving research that has been extensively reviewed in the literature.[24,29-31] The most intense focus of this research centers on the effects of human milk on the infant's gastrointestinal tract.[32,33] The bioactive factors being studied are as diverse as proteins (lactoferrin, lysozyme, etc.), hormones (erythropoietin, prolactin, insulin, etc.), growth factors (epithelial growth factor, insulin-like growth factor, etc.), neuropeptides (neurotensin, somatostatin, etc.), cytokines (TNF-α, IL-6, etc.), antiinflammatory agents (enzymes, antioxidants, etc.), and nucleotides. This concept encompasses most of what one might consider the immunologic benefits of breast milk to be.

From an evolutionary perspective, maternal antibody is transmitted to the fetus by different pathways in different species.[24,34,35] An association has been recognized between the number of placental membranes and the relative importance of the placenta and the colostrum as sources of antibodies. By this analysis, the horse, with six placental membranes, passes little or no antibodies transplacentally and relies totally on colostrum for protection of the foal. Humans and monkeys, having three placental membranes, receive more of the antibodies via the placenta and less from the colostrum. The transfer of immunoglobulin G (IgG) in the human is accomplished by active transport mechanism of the immunoglobulin across the placenta. Secretory IgA (sIgA) immunoglobulins are found in human milk and provide local protection to the mucous membranes of the gastrointestinal (GI) tract. Other investigations have established that the mammary glands and their secretion of milk are important in protecting the infant not only through the colostrum but also through mature milk from birth through the early months of life.

Although the predominance of IgA in human colostrum and milk had long been described, the importance of this phenomenon was not fully appreciated until the discovery that IgA is a predominant immunoglobulin present in mucosal secretions of other glands in addition to the breast. Mucosal immunity has become the subject of extensive research.[25,27,28] It is clear that considerable traffic of cells occurs between mucosal epithelia and secretory or lymphoid tissue sites. The data support the concept of a general system of MALT, which includes the gut, lung, mammary gland, salivary and lacrimal glands, and the genital tract (see Fig. 5-3). Through the immune response of MALT, a reaction to an immunogen at a mucosal site may be an effective means of producing immunity at distant sites. Antibodies against specific antigens found in the milk have also been found in the saliva, evidence for transfer of protection to two different distant sites simultaneously. Evidence suggests that the mammary glands may act as extensions of the gut-associated lymphoid tissue

(GALT) and possibly the bronchiole-associated lymphoid tissue (BALT). The ability of epithelial surfaces exposed to the external environment to defend against infectious agents has been well documented for the GI, genitourinary, and respiratory tracts.[36] Secretory IgA and secretory IgM produced through the adaptive response of the mucosal-lymphoid immune system act by blocking colonization with pathogens and limiting the passage of harmful antigens across the mucosal barrier. Activated B cells and cytokines pass to the mammary gland where they contribute to the production of secretory IgA in breast milk. Direct contact between the antigen and the lymphoid cells of the breast is unlikely.[37] Peyer's patches, tonsils, and other MALT structures appear to be well developed at birth.[38] Nevertheless, the actual effective production of sIgA to various antigens presented to the infant's mucosal surfaces (respiratory and gastrointestinal tracts) is still inadequate to protect against infection. The breastfeeding infant, as part of the maternal-infant dyad exposed to the same antigens via their mucosal services, can receive protective sIgA and sIgM in the mother's breast milk produced by the mother's MALT (see Fig. 5-3).

The protective properties of human milk can be divided into cellular factors and humoral factors for facility of discussion, although they are closely related in vivo. A wide variety of soluble and cellular components and hormone-like agents have been identified in human milk and colostrum (Table 5-1). Although the following discussion separates these elements, it is important to emphasize that the constituents of human milk are multifunctional and their functioning in vivo is interactive and probably coordinated and complementary.

CELLULAR COMPONENTS OF HUMAN COLOSTRUM AND MILK

Cells are an important postpartum component of maternal immunologic endowment. Over 100 years ago, cell bodies were described in the colostrum of animals. As with much lactation research, further study of colostral corpuscles was undertaken by the dairy industry for commercial reasons in the early 1900s. This research afforded an opportunity to make major progress in the understanding of cells in milk. Initially, it was believed that these cells represented a reaction to infection in the mammary gland and were even described as "pus cells."

It has become clear that the cells of milk are normal constituents of colostrums in all species. Cells include macrophages, lymphocytes, neutrophils, and epithelial cells, and they total approximately 4000/mm^3. Cell fragments and epithelial cells were examined by electron microscope in fresh samples from 30 women by Brooker.[39] He found that the membrane-bound cytoplasmic fragments in the sedimentation pellet outnumbered intact cells. The fragments were mostly from secretory cells that contained numerous cisternae of rough endoplasmic reticulum, lipid droplets, and Golgi vesicles containing casein micelles. Secretory epithelial cells were found in all samples and, after the second month post partum, began to outnumber macrophages. Ductal epithelial cells were about 1% of the population of cells for the first week or so and then disappeared. All samples contained squamous epithelial cells originating from galactophores and the skin of the nipple.

Living leukocytes are normally present in human milk.[36] The overall concentration of these leukocytes is of the same order of magnitude as that seen in peripheral blood, although the predominant cell in milk is the macrophage rather than the neutrophil. Macrophages compose about 90% of the leukocytes, and 2000 to 3000/mm^3 are present. Lymphocytes make up about 5% to 10% of the cells (200 to 300/mm^3), which is a much lower concentration than in human blood.[40] The number of cells found in human milk increases with mastitis. There are large and small lymphocytes. By indirect immunofluorescence with anti-T-cell antibody to identify thymus-derived lymphocytes, it has been shown that 50% of human colostral lymphocytes are T cells, and in human milk up to 80% of the lymphocytes are T cells.[41] Immunofluorescence procedures to detect surface immunoglobulins characteristic of B lymphocytes identified 34% as B lymphocytes.

TABLE 5-1   Immunologically and pharmacologically active components and hormones observed in human colostrum and milk

Soluble	Cellular	Hormones and hormonelike substances
Immunologically specific	*Immunologically specific*	Epidermal growth factor (EGF)
Immunoglobulin	T-lymphocytes	Prostaglandins
sIgA (11S), 7S IgA, IgG, IgM	B-lymphocytes	Relaxin
IgE, IgD, secretory component		Neurotensin
	Accessory cells	Somatostatin
T-cell products	Neutrophils	Bombesin
	Macrophages	Gonadotropins
Histocompatibility antigens	Epithelial cells	Ovarian steroids
		Thyroid-releasing hormone (TRH)
Nonspecific factors		Thyroid-stimulating hormone (TSH)
Complement		Thyroxine and triiodothyronine
Chemotactic factors		Adrenocorticotropin
Properdin (factor P)		Corticosteroids
Interferon		Prolactin
α-Fetoprotein		Erythropoietin
Bifidus factor		Insulin
Antistaphylococcal factor(s)		Cytokines
Antiadherence substances		Interleukins
Epidermal growth factor (EGF)		
Folate uptake enhancer		
Antiviral factor(s)		
Migration inhibition factor (MIF)		
Gangliosides		
Nucleotides		
Carrier proteins		
Lactoferrin		
Transferrin		
Vitamin B_{12}-binding protein		
Corticoid-binding protein		
Enzymes		
Lysozyme		
Lipoprotein lipase		
Leukocyte enzymes		

Modified from Ogra PL, Fishaut M: Human breast milk. In Remington JS, Klein JO, editors: Infectious diseases of the fetus and newborn infant, 4th ed. Philadelphia, Saunders, 1995.

The number of leukocytes and the degree of mitogenic stimulation of lymphocytes sharply decline during the first 2 or 3 months of lactation to essentially undetectable levels, according to Goldman and associates (Fig. 5-1).[42] Enumeration of the total cell numbers in milk has been difficult, but when various techniques are compared (Coulter electronic particle counter, visual cell counting with special stains, filter trapping with fluorescent detection, and automated fluorescent cell counting)

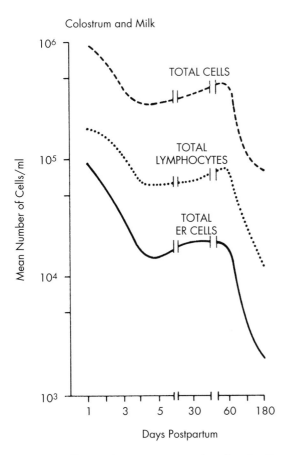

Colostrum and Milk

Figure 5-1. Geometric mean concentration of total cells, lymphocytes, and E (erythrocyte) rosette-forming cells (ER) in colostrum and milk of 200 lactating women. (Modified from Ogra SS, Ogra PL: Immunologic aspects of human colostrum and milk. I. Distribution characteristics and concentrations of immunoglobulins at different times after the onset of lactation. J Pediatr 92:546, 1978.)

stains for deoxyribonucleic acid (DNA) were superior to the other techniques.

Macrophages

Macrophages are large-complex phagocytes that contain lysosomes, mitochondria, pinosomes, ribosomes, and a Golgi apparatus. The monocytic phagocytes are lipid laden and were previously called the *colostral bodies of Donne*. They have the same functional and morphologic features as those of other human tissue sources. These features include ameboid movement, phagocytosis of microorganisms (fungi and bacteria), killing of bacteria, and production of complement components C3 and C4, lysosome, and lactoferrin. Other milk macrophage activities include the following[43]:

  Phagocytosis of latex, adherence to glass
  Secretion of lysozyme, complement components
  C3b-mediated erythrocyte adherence
  IgG-mediated erythrocyte adherence and phagocytosis
  Bacterial killing
  Inhibition of lymphocyte mitogenic response
  Release of intracellular IgA in tissue culture
  Giant cell formation
  Interaction with lymphocytes

Data suggest these macrophages also amplify T-cell reactivity by direct cellular cooperation or by antigen processing. The colostral macrophage has been suggested as a potential vehicle for the storage and transport of immunoglobin. A significant increase in IgA and IgG synthesis by colostral lymphocytes, when incubated with supernatants of cultured macrophages, has been reported.[44]

The macrophage may also participate in the biosynthesis and excretion of lactoperoxidase and cellular growth factors that enhance growth of intestinal epithelium and maturation of intestinal brush-border enzymes.

The mobility of macrophages is inhibited by the lymphokine migration inhibitor factor (MIF), which is produced by antigen-stimulated sensitized lymphocytes. The activities of macrophages have been demonstrated in both fresh colostrum and colostral cell culture, and certain functions are altered compared with their counterpart in human peripheral blood.

Polymorphonuclear leukocytes

The highest concentration of cells occurs in the first few days of lactation and reaches more than a million per milliliter of milk.

Colostrum (1 to 4 days post partum) contains 10^5 to 5×10^6 leukocytes/mL, and 40% to 60% are polymorphonuclear cells (PMNs). Mature milk (i.e., beyond 4 days) has fewer cells (Fig. 5-2), about 10^5/mL with 20% to 30% PMNs. Beyond 6 weeks, there are few PMNs. The functions of the PMNs normally include microbial killing, phagocytosis, chemotactic responsiveness, stimulated hexose monophosphate shunt activity, stimulated nitroblue tetrazolium dye reduction, and stimulated oxygen consumption.[45] When milk PMNs are compared with those in the serum, their activity is often less than that of serum PMN cells. Whether milk PMNs actually perform a role in protection of the infant has been studied by many investigators using many techniques. Animal studies, in summary, have shown that (1) the mammary gland is susceptible to infection in early lactation, (2) a dramatic increase in PMNs occurs with mammary inflammation, and (3) in the presence of peripheral neutropenia during chronic mastitis, severe infection of the gland occurs. This implies, according to Buescher and

Pickering,[45] that the primary function of milk PMNs is as defense of the mammary tissue per se and not to impart immunocompetence to the newborn. This may explain the presence of large numbers of PMNs that are relatively hypofunctional early and then disappear over time. There is evidence that neutrophils found in human milk demonstrate signs of activation including increased expression of CD11b (an adherence glycoprotein), decreased expression of L-selectin, production of granulocyte-macrophage colony-stimulating factor (GM-CSF) spontaneously, and the ability to transform into CD1+ dendritic cells (DCs).[46] Human milk macrophages have the morphology and motility of activated cells. The movement of these cells in a three-dimensional system is greater than that of monocytes, their counterparts in peripheral blood. Such activated neutrophils may play a role in phagocytosis at the level of the mucosa of the gastrointestinal tract, supplementing the infant's poor ability to recruit phagocytes to that site.[47]

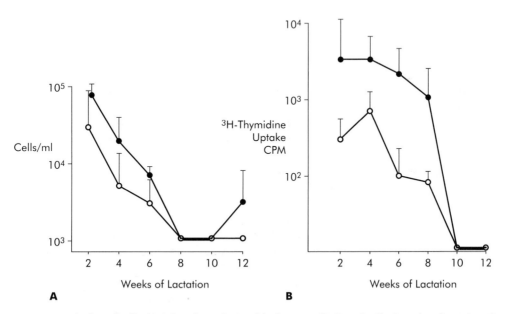

Figure 5-2. A, Longitudinal study of numbers of leukocytes. **B,** Longitudinal study of uptake of ^{3}H-thymidine in lymphocytes. Same subjects were examined during second through twelfth week of lactation. Data are presented as means ± SD of macrophages-neutrophils (•) and lymphocytes (○) in **A** and of stimulated (•) and unstimulated (○) lymphocytes in **B**. (From Goldman AS, Garza C, Nichols BL, et al: Immunologic factors in human milk during the first year of lactation. J Pediatr 100:563, 1982.)

Lymphocytes

Both T and B lymphocytes are present in human milk and colostrum and are part of the immunologic system in human milk. T cells make up about 80% of the lymphocytes in breast milk. Human milk lymphocytes respond to mitogens by proliferation, with increased macrophage-lymphocyte interaction and the release of soluble mediators, including MIF. Cells destined to become lymphopoietic cells are derived from two separate influences, the thymus (T) and the bursa (B) or bursal equivalent tissues. The population of the *B cells* makes up the smaller part of the total. They synthesize IgA antibody. The term *B cell* is derived from its origination in a different anatomic site from the thymus; in birds, it has been identified as the bursa of Fabricius. The B cells can be identified by the presence of surface immunoglobulin markers. The B cells in human milk include cells with IgA, IgM, and IgG surface immunoglobulins. B cells transform into plasma cells and remain sessile in the tissues of the mammary gland.

T-cell system

More rapid mitotic activity occurs in the thymus gland than in any other lymphatic organ, yet 70% of the cells die within the cell substance. The thymus is the location for much of the T-cell differentiation and selection and plays a major role in the development of the infant's immune system. Thymosin has been identified as a hormone produced by thymic epithelial cells to expand the peripheral lymphocyte population. After emergence from the thymus gland, T cells acquire new surface antigen markers. The T cells circulate through the lymphatic and vascular systems as long-lived lymphocytes, which are called the "recirculating pool." They then populate restricted regions of lymph nodes, forming thymic-dependent areas.[41] It is interesting to note that exclusively breastfed infants have a significantly larger thymus than formula fed infants at 4 and 10 months.[48] The significance of the lymphocytes in human milk in affording immunologic benefits to the breastfed infant continues to be investigated. It is suggested

that lymphocytes can sensitize, induce immunologic tolerance, or incite graft-versus-host reactions. According to Head and Beer,[49] lymphocytes may be incorporated into the suckling's tissues, achieving short-term adoptive immunization of the neonate.

Studies of the activities of lymphocytes have been carried out by a number of investigators who collected samples of milk from lactating women at various times post partum, examined the number of cell types present, and then studied the activities of these cells in vitro.[36,50] Ogra and Ogra collected samples from 200 women and measured the cell content from 1 through 180 days (see Fig. 5-1).[51] They then compared the response of T lymphocytes in colostrum and milk with that of the T cells in the peripheral blood (see Fig. 5-2). T-cell subpopulations have also been shown by surface epitopes to be similar to those in the peripheral blood.

The greatest number of cells appeared on the first day, with the counts ranging from 10,000 to 100,000/mm^3 for total cells. By the fifth day, the count had dropped to 20% of the first day's count. In addition, the number of E (erythrocyte) rosette-forming cells was determined by using sheep erythrocyte-rosetting technique. The E rosette formation (ERF) lymphocytes constituted a mean 100/mm^3 on the first day and a tenth of that by the fifth day.

At 180 days, total cells were 100,000/mm^3, lymphocytes were 10,000/mm^3, and ERF lymphocytes were 2000/mm^3. The investigators compared the values with those in the peripheral blood of each mother; the levels remained essentially constant.[51] In a similar study, Bhaskaram and Reddy[52] sampled milk over time from 74 women and found comparable cell concentrations. They examined the bactericidal activity of the milk leukocytes and found it to be comparable with that of the circulating leukocytes in the blood, irrespective of the stage of lactation or state of nutrition of the mother.

Ogra and Ogra[37] also studied the lymphocyte proliferation responses of colostrum and milk to antigens. Their data show response to stimulation from the viral antigens of rubella, cytomegalovirus, and mumps. Analysis of cell-mediated immunity to microbial antigens shows milk lymphocytes are limited in their potential for recognizing or responding to certain infectious agents as compared with cells from the peripheral circulation. This is believed to be an intercellular action and not caused by lack of external factors. In contrast, the T cells and B cells have been shown to have unique reactivities not seen in peripheral blood.

Colostral lymphocytes are derived from mature rather than immature T-cell subsets. The distribution of T-cell subsets in colostrum includes both CD4+ and CD8+ cells.[53] The distribution of CD4 cells in colostrum and human milk is lower than in the serum, and fewer CD4 cells exist than CD8 cells.[41] The percentage of CD4 cells is higher than in the serum of either postpartum donors or normal control subjects. No correlation exists with length of gestation and number of cells (in normal blood there are usually twice as many CD4+ as CD8+ lymphocytes).[54]

Parmely and associates[55] partially purified and propagated milk lymphocytes in vitro to study their immunologic function. Milk lymphocytes responded in a unique manner to stimuli known to activate T lymphocytes from the serum. The authors found milk lymphocytes to be hyporesponsive to nonspecific mitogens and histocompatibility antigens on allogenic cells in their laboratory. They found them unresponsive to *Candida albicans*. Significant proliferation of lymphocytes occurred in response to K_1 capsular antigen of *Escherichia coli*.[56] Lymphocytes from blood failed to respond to the same antigen. This supports the concept of local mammary tissue immunity at the T-lymphocyte level.

More recent experiments in rodents have provided evidence that T lymphocytes reactive to transplantation alloantigens can adoptively immunize the suckling newborn. Foster nursing experiments performed in rodents have shown that newborn rats exposed to allogenic milk manifested alterations in their reactivity to skin allografts of the foster mother's strain. In animals, mothers may give their suckling newborn immunoreactive lymphocytes. The influence of maternal milk cells on the development of neonatal immunocompetence

has been demonstrated in several different immunologic contexts. Congenitally, athymic nude mice nursed by their phenotypically normal mothers or normal foster mothers had increased survival. The mothers contributed their T-cell-helper activity to the suckling newborn.

Colostral lymphocytes proliferate in response to various mitogens, alloantigens, and conventional antigens. Colostral cells survive in the neonatal stomach and in the gut of experimental animals, some remaining viable in the upper GI tract for a week. No evidence, however, indicates that transepithelial migration takes place when neonatal mice are foster-nursed by newly delivered animals whose colostral cells were tagged with ^{3}H-thymidine.[45]

Cells in human milk have been studied using the same markers employed with cells in the peripheral blood. About 80% of the lymphocytes are T cells that are equally distributed between CD4+ and CD8+ subpopulations, and their T-cell receptors (TCRs) are principally of the α/β type. CD4+ cells are common leukocyte cells of the helper and suppressor-inducer subsets, and CD8+ cells are leukocytes of the cytotoxic and noncytotoxic subsets. T cells in human milk are presumed activated because they display increased phenotypic markers of activation including HLA-DR and CD25 (IL-2 receptor). The majority of T cells in human milk are CD45RO+ consistent with effector and memory T cells.[41] These cells are effective producers of interferon-γ, in keeping with their phenotypic features. Here again, human milk may supplement the infant with a functioning immune cell to compensate for an identified deficiency in the infant, a paucity of memory T cells.

B-cell system

Juto[54] studied the effect of human milk on B-cell function. Cell-free, defatted, filtered colostrum as well as mature breast milk showed an enhancing effect on B-cell proliferation and generation of antibody secretion. This was not seen with formula. Juto suggested that this could represent an important immunologic mechanism. Goldblum and associates[57] were able to show a B-cell response in human colostrum to *Escherichia coli* given to the mother orally, which was not accompanied by a systemic response in the mother. This suggests that the breast and breast milk reflect sites of local humoral or cell-mediated immunity, which were initially induced at a distant site such as the gut and transferred via reactive lymphoid cells migrating to the breast. Head and Beer[49] provided a scheme to describe this mechanism (Fig. 5-3). The diagram depicts the progeny of specifically sensitized lymphocytes that originated in GALT, specifically Peyer's patches, as they migrate to the mammary gland. As they infiltrate the mammary gland and its secretion, they supply the breast with immune cells capable of selected immune responses. Ogra and Ogra[37, 51] suggest that the cells may selectively accumulate in the breast during pregnancy. The responses of milk cells and their antibodies are not representative of the individual's total immunity.[55] Most of these immunocompetent cells, initially stimulated in GALT, recirculate to the external mucosal surface and populate the lamina propria as antibody-producing plasma cells. A substantial number of these antigen-sensitized cells selectively home in to the stroma of the mammary glands and initiate local IgA antibody synthesis against the antigens initially encountered in the respiratory or intestinal mucosa.[52]

The accumulated research data support the concept that lymphocytes from colostrum and milk provide the human infant with immunologic benefits. Both T and B lymphocytes are reactive against organisms invading the intestinal tract. Investigations on allergy, necrotizing enterocolitis, tuberculosis, and neonatal meningitis support the concept that human milk fulfills a protective function.

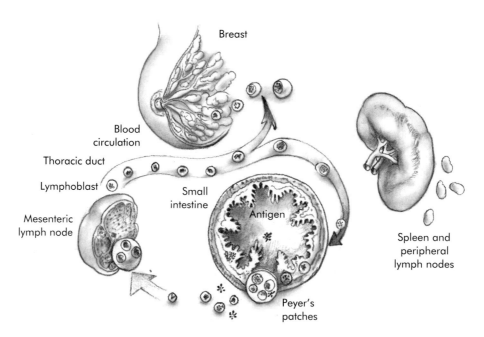

Figure 5-3. Schema of mechanism by which progeny of specifically sensitized lymphocytes originating from gut-associated lymphoid tissue may migrate to and infiltrate mammary gland and its secretions, supplying breast with immune cells. (Modified from Head JR, Beer AE: The immunologic role of viable leukocytic cells in mammary exosecretions. In Larson BL (ed): Lactation, Vol. IV. Mammary Gland/Human Lactation/Milk Synthesis. New York, Academic Press, 1978.)

SURVIVAL OF MATERNAL MILK CELLS

Although it is clear that cells are provided in the colostrum and milk, the effectiveness and impact of these cells on the neonate depend on their ability to survive in the GI tract. It has been demonstrated in several species, including humans, that the pH of the stomach can be as low as 0.5, but the output of hydrochloric acid (HCl) is minimal for the first few months, as is the peptic activity. Immediately after a feeding begins, the pH rises to 6.0 and returns to normal in 3 hours. The cells from milk tolerate this. Studies have also shown that intact nucleated lymphoid cells are found in the stomach and intestines.[58] These cells, when removed from rat stomachs, are capable of phagocytosis. Lymphoid cells in milk have been shown to traverse the mucosal wall.

When human milk is stored, however, the cellular components do not tolerate heating to 63° C (145.4° F), cooling to −23° C (−9.4° F), or lyophilization. Although a few cells may be identified, they are not viable.[59]

HUMORAL FACTORS
Immunoglobulins

All classes of immunoglobulins are found in human milk. The study of immunoglobulins has been enhanced through the techniques of electrophoresis, chromatographics, and radioimmunoassay. More than 30 components have been identified; of these, 18 are associated with proteins in the maternal serum, and the others are found exclusively in milk. The concentrations are highest in the colostrum of all species, and the concentrations change as lactation proceeds.[60] IgA, principally sIgA, is highest in colostrum. Although postpartum levels fall over the next 4 weeks, substantial levels are maintained throughout the first year, during gradual weaning between 6 and 9 months, and even during partial breastfeeding (when infant receives solid foods) in the second year of life (Figs. 5-4 and 5-5 and Table 5-2). Specific sIgA antibodies to *E. coli* persist through lactation and may even rise (see Fig. 5-4).

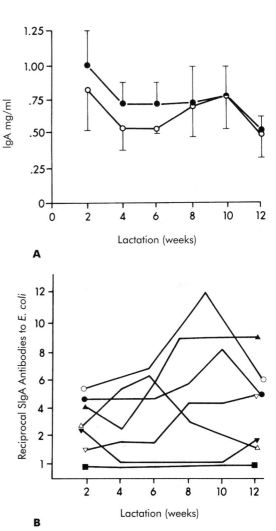

Figure 5-4. Same subjects in Figure 5-2 were examined during second through twelfth week of lactation. Total (•) and secretory IgA (○) data are presented as mean ± SD. The sIgA antibody titers to *E. coli* somatic antigens from each subject are represented by different symbols. **A,** Longitudinal study of total IgA and sIgA. **B,** Longitudinal study of reciprocal of sIgA antibody titers to *E. coli* somatic antigens in human milk. (From Goldman AS, Garza C, Nichols BL, et al: Immunologic factors in human milk during the first year of lactation. J Pediatr 100:563, 1982.)

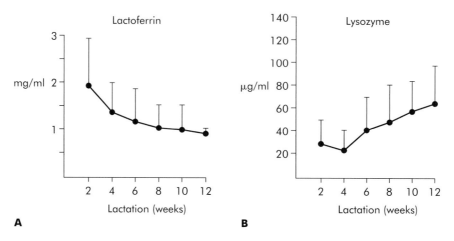

Figure 5-5. Same subjects in Figure 5-2 were examined during second through twelfth week of lactation. Data in longitudinal studies are presented as mean ± SD. **A,** Concentration of lactoferrin progressively decreased through first 8 weeks ($r = 0.69$) (2 vs. 8 weeks; $p < 0.02$), but not thereafter. **B,** In contrast, lysozyme levels steadily increased from fourth through twelfth week ($r = 0.76$) (4 vs. 12 weeks; $p < 0.01$). (From Goldman AS, Garza C, Nichols BL, et al: Immunologic factors in human milk during the first year of lactation. J Pediatr 100:563, 1982.)

The main immunoglobulin in human serum is IgG; IgA content is only one fifth the level of IgG. In milk, however, the reverse is true. IgA is the most important immunoglobulin in milk, not only in concentration but also in biologic activity. Secretory IgA is likely synthesized in the mammary alveolar cells[61] or by lymphocytes that have migrated from Peyer's patches in the gastrointestinal tract or from lymphoid tissue in the respiratory tract via the lymphatics to the breast. Cytokines cause isotype switching of local IgM+ B cells to become IgA+ B lymphocytes.[62-64] These isotype switched cells travel to the breast where they are transformed into plasma cells producing secretory, dimeric IgA. It is through this "enteromammary" pathway that the mother provides increased amounts of sIgA to the

TABLE 5-2   Concentrations of immunologic components in human milk collected during second year of lactation

Component	Duration of lactation (months)		
	12	13–15	16–24
IgA (mg/ml)			
Total	0.8 ± 0.3	1.1 ± 0.4	1.1 ± 0.3
Secretory (sIgA)	0.8 ± 0.3	1.1 ± 0.3	1.1 ± 0.2
Lactoferrin (mg/mL)	1.0 ± 0.2	1.1 ± 0.1	1.2 ± 0.1
Lysozyme (µg/mL)	196 ± 41	244 ± 34	187 ± 33
sIgA antibodies (reciprocal titers to *E. coli* somatic antigens)	5 ± 6	9 ± 10	6 ± 3

Data are presented as the mean ± SD.
From Goldman AS, Goldblum RM, Garza C: Immunologic components in human milk during the second year of lactation. Acta Paediatr Scand 72:461, 1983.

infant against the microorganisms present in the mother's and infant's environment.[35]

Brandtzaeg and associates have proposed a model for the transport of IgA (polymeric) and IgM (pentameric), produced by plasma cells, across the secretory epithelium with the formation of secretory IgA and IgM through binding with the secretory component (SC) attached to the epithelial membrane.[28] This occurs in the membrane of mammary epithelial cells during lactation.[65,66]

Quantitative determinations of immunoglobulins in human milk were made from milk collected at birth up to as long as 27 months post partum by Peitersen and associates[67] and by Goldman and associates.[42] The IgA content was high immediately after birth, dropping in 2 to 3 weeks, and then remaining constant. Similar observations were made on IgG levels and IgM levels. Ogra and Ogra[37,51] have compared serum and milk levels at various times post partum. Samples obtained separately from the left and right breasts showed similar values. The levels remained constant during a given feeding and throughout a 24-hour period. In all quantitative determinations, IgA is the predominant immunoglobulin in breast milk, constituting 90% of all the immunoglobulins in colostrum and milk.

Ogra and Ogra[37,51,68] studied the serum of postpartum lactating mothers and nonpregnant matched control subjects and noted that the individual and mean concentrations of all Ig classes were lower in the postpartum subjects. The levels were statistically significant for IgG; they were 50 to 70 mg higher in the nonpregnant women.

Immunoglobulin levels, particularly IgA and IgM, are very high in colostrum and drop precipitously in the first 4 to 6 days, but IgG does not show this decline. The volume of mammary secretion, however, increases dramatically in this same period; thus, the absolute amounts of immunoglobulins remain more nearly constant than it would first appear. Local production and concentration of IgA and probably IgM may take place in the mammary gland at delivery.

IgE and IgD have also been measured in colostrum and milk. Using radioimmunoassay techniques, colostrum was found to contain concentrations of 0.5 to 0.6 IU/mL IgE in 41% of samples and less in the remainder.[69] IgD was found in all samples in concentrations of 2 to 2000 µg/dL. Plasma levels were poorly correlated. The findings suggest possible local mammary production rather than positive transfer. The question of whether IgE or IgD antibodies in breast milk have similar specificities for antigens as the IgA antibodies in milk remains unanswered.[70] Keller and associates[71] examined the question of local mammary IgD production and its possible participation in a mucosal immune system by comparing colostrum and plasma levels of total IgD with specific IgD antibodies. From their work comparing colostrum/plasma ratios for IgG, IgD, and albumin and measuring IgD against specific antigens, the authors reported evidence for IgD participation in the response of the mucosal immune system, with increases in total IgD and IgD against specific antigens found in colostrum.

To address the question of total quantities of immunologic components secreted into human milk per day and available to the infant, Butte and associates[72] measured the amounts of sIgA, sIgA antibodies to *E. coli,* lactoferrin, and lysozyme ingested per day and per kilogram per day in the first 4 months of life (Figs. 5-6 to 5-10). Lactoferrin, sIgA, and sIgA antibodies gradually declined in amount ingested per day and per kilogram per day. Lysozyme, in contrast, rose during the same period in total amount available and amount per kilogram per day. The authors[72] suggest that production and secretion of these immunologic factors by the mammary gland may be linked to the catabolism of the components at the infant's mucosal tissues. When the concentrations of sIgA, IgG, IgM, α_1-antitrypsin, lactoferrin, lysozyme, and globulins C3 and C4 were compared in relationship to parity and age of the mother, there was no consistent trend. When maturity of the pregnancy was considered, however, mean concentrations of all these proteins were higher, except for IgA, when the delivery was premature. Because several proteins in human milk have physiologic function in the infant, Davidson and Lönnerdal[73] examined the survival of human milk proteins through the GI tract. Crossed immunoelectrophoresis

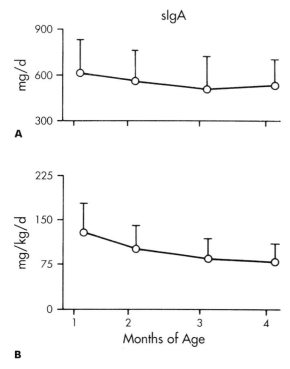

A

B

Figure 5-6. Amounts of sIgA and sIgA antibodies to *E. coli* somatic antigens in human milk ingested per day, **A**, and per kilogram per day, **B**. Data are presented as mean ± SD. (From Butte NF, Goldman RM, Fehl LM, et al: Daily ingestion of immunologic components in human milk during the first four months of life. Acta Paediatr Scand 73:296, 1984.)

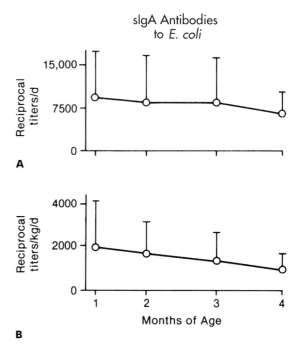

A

B

Figure 5-7. Amounts of sIgA antibodies to *E. coli* somatic antigens in human milk ingested as reciprocal titers per day, **A**, and per kilogram per day, **B**. Data are presented as mean ± SD. (From Butte NF, Goldman RM, Fehl LM, et al: Daily ingestion of immunologic components in human milk during the first four months of life. Acta Paediatr Scand 73:296, 1984.)

showed that three human milk proteins transversed the entire intestine and were present in the feces: lactoferrin, sIgA, and α_1-antitrypsin.

Miranda and associates[74] reported on the effect of maternal nutritional status on immunologic substances in human colostrum and milk. Maternal malnutrition was characterized as lower weight-to-height ratio, creatine/height index, total serum proteins, and IgG and IgA. In malnourished mothers, the colostrum contained one third the normal concentration of IgG, less than half the normal level of albumin, and lower IgA and complement C4. Lysozyme, complement C3, and IgM levels were normal. Levels improved with development of mature milk and improvement in maternal nutrition.

According to one 2003 report, moderate exercise during lactation does not affect the levels of IgA, lactoferrin, or lysozyme in breast milk.[75] Immunologic components contained in human milk during the second year of lactation become a significant point as more infants are nursed longer. For a longitudinal study of lactation into the second year, women were included who had fully breastfed their infants for 6 months to a year, and were continuing to partially breastfeed.[76] Samples were collected by fully emptying the breast by electric pump. Table 5-2 summarizes the concentrations of the measured factors. No leukocytes were detected. Concentrations of total IgA and sIgA, lactoferrin, and lysozyme were similar to those 7 to 12 months post partum and during gradual weaning. sIgA antibodies

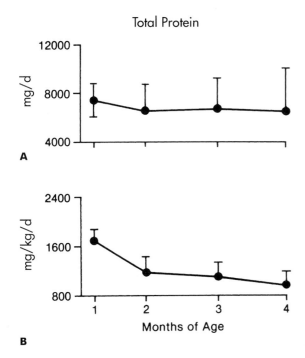

Figure 5-8. Amount of total protein in human milk ingested per day, **A**, and per kilogram per day, **B**. Data are presented as mean ± SD. (From Butte NF, Goldblum RM, Fehl LM, et al: Daily ingestion of immunologic components in human milk during the first four months of life. Acta Paediatr Scand 73:296, 1984.)

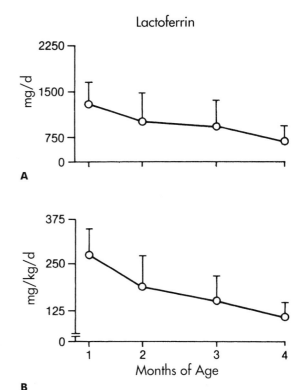

Figure 5-9. Amount of lactoferrin in human milk ingested per day, **A**, and per kilogram per day, **B**. Data are presented as mean ± SD. (From Butte NF, Goldblum RM, Fehl LM, et al: Daily ingestion of immunologic components in human milk during the first four months of life. Acta Paediatr Scand 73:296, 1984.)

to *E. coli* were produced in the second year, demonstrating significant immunologic benefit to the infant with continued breastfeeding.[76] IgA, IgM, and IgG were measured in nursing women from the beginning of lactation and simultaneously in the feces of their children by Jatsyk and associates[77] at the Academy of Medicine in Moscow. They reported IgA to be very high in the milk and rapidly increasing in the feces. IgG and IgM levels, however, were low in both milk and feces. In normal full-term bottle-fed infants, IgA appeared in the feces at 3 to 4 weeks of age but at much lower levels than in breastfed infants. Koutras reported that in the first 8 weeks of life, there are increased amounts of sIgA in the stools of breastfed infants compared with formula fed infants. The authors ascribed this phenomenom to the presence of sIgA

in human milk and a stimulation of the local gastrointestinal production of immunoglobulin.[78]

Savilahti and associates[79] measured serum levels of IgG, IgA, and IgM in 198 infants at 2, 4, 6, 9, and 12 months of age. By 9 months, the infants exclusively breastfed had IgG and IgM levels significantly lower than those who had been weaned early (before 3.5 months) to formula. Six infants were still exclusively breastfed at 12 months, and their IgA levels had also lowered to levels found at 2 months with bottle feeders. Infection rates were similar. Two months after the children were weaned to formula, the IgG and IgM levels were comparable. Iron and zinc levels were the same in all children.

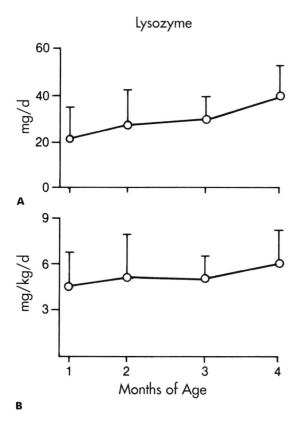

A

B

Figure 5-10. Amount of lysozyme in human milk ingested per day, **A**, and per kilogram per day, **B**. Data are presented as mean ± SD. (From Butte NF, Goldblum RM, Fehl LM, et al: Daily ingestion of immunologic components in human milk during the first four months of life. Acta Paediatr Scand 73:296, 1984.)

Specificity of immunoglobulins

Secretory IgA antibodies have been identified in human milk that recognize a large variety of microorganisms. The sIgA antibodies that recognize viruses are listed in Table 5-3. Goldman has reported that there are sIgA antibodies that recognize a long list of bacteria, including *E. coli*, *Shigella*, *Salmonella*, *Campylobacter*, *V. cholerae*, *Hae-mophilus influenzae*, *Streptococcus pneumoniae*, *Clostridium difficile*, *Clostridium botulinum*, *Klebsiella pneumoniae* as well as *Giardia* and *Candida albicans*.[63] Noguera-Obenza and Cleary reviewed the role of breast milk sIgA in provid-

ing protection for infants against various agents causing bacterial enteritis.[80]

Stability of immunoglobulins

Preservation of human milk at −20° C alters the levels of IgA, IgM, C3, C4, α_1-antitrypsin, and sIgA antibodies to *E. coli* and lactoperoxidase.[81] Heat treatments include low-temperature, short-time (LTST), 56° C for 15 minutes; Holder pasteurization (HP), 62.5° C for 30 minutes; and high-temperature, short-time (HTST), 70° C for 15 seconds. Boiling essentially destroys 100% of immunologic activity. Secretory IgA and lysozyme activities drop by 20% with HP and by 50% at 65° C. Neither LTST nor HTST reduces the sIgA or lysozyme content. IgG and IgM are greatly reduced by HP (see Table 5-3).

Secretory IgA differs antigenically from serum IgA. IgA can be synthesized in the nonlactating as well as in the lactating breast. It is a compact molecule and resistant to proteolytic enzymes of the intestinal tract and the low pH of the stomach. sIgA present in human milk is primarily manufactured by plasma cells in the mammary gland, modified in its translocation across the mammary epithelia and only minimally produced by the cellular lymphocytes in milk. Levels in milk are 10 to 100 times higher than in serum. Levels in cow milk are very low, that is, a tenth of the level in mature human milk (0.03 mg/dL). Later in life, the human intestinal tract's subepithelial plasma cells secrete IgA, but this does not occur in the neonatal period.

Discussion continues as to whether any antibodies are absorbed from the intestinal tract, although probably 10% are absorbed. Almost 75% of ingested IgA from milk survives passage through the intestinal tract and is excreted in the feces. All immunoglobulin classes have been identified in the feces.[82] A large body of evidence demonstrates the activity of the immunoglobulins, especially IgA, at the mucosal level of the gastrointestinal and respiratory tracts. These antibodies provide local intestinal protection against microorganisms, which may infect the mucosa or enter the body through the gut or respiratory tract.

TABLE 5-3   Antiviral antibody in human milk

Factor	Shown, in vitro, to be active against:	Assay	Effect of heat
Secretory IgA	Enteroviruses		
	Poliovirus types 1, 2, 3	ELISA, NA, Precipitan	Stable at 56° C for 30 min;
	Coxsackievirus types A_9, B_3, B_5	NA	some loss (0%–30%)
	Echovirus types 6 and 9	NA	Stable at 62.5° C for 30 min; destroyed by boiling
	Herpesvirus		
	Cytomegalovirus	ELISA, IFA, NA	
	Herpes simplex virus	NA	
	Semliki Forest virus	IFA	
	Respiratory syncytial virus	IFA	
	Rubella	IFA, HAI	
	Reovirus type 3	ELISA, NA	
	Rotavirus		
IgM, IgG	Cytomegalovirus		Stable at 56° C for 30 min;
	Respiratory syncytial virus		IgG decreased by a third at
	Rubella		62.5° C for 30 min

ELISA, enzyme-linked immunosorbent assay; HAI, hemagglutination inhibition; IFA, immunofluorescent assay; NA, neutralizing assay.

Bifidus factor

It has been established since the work of Tissier in 1908 on the newborn's intestinal flora that the predominant bacteria of the breastfed infant are bifid bacteria. *Bifid bacteria* are gram-positive, nonmotile anaerobic bacilli. Many observers have shown the striking difference between the flora of the guts of breastfed and bottle-fed infants. György[83] demonstrated the presence of a specific factor in colostrum and milk that supported the growth of *Lactobacillus bifidus.* Bifidus factor has been characterized as a dialyzable, nitrogen-containing carbohydrate that contains no amino acid.

In vitro studies by Beerens and associates[84] showed the presence of a specific growth factor for *Bifidobacterium bifidum* in human milk, which they called BB. Other milks, including cow milk, sheep milk, pig milk, and infant formulas, did not promote the growth of this species but did show some activity supporting *B. infantis*

and *B. longum*. This growth factor was found to be stable when the milk was frozen, heated, freeze-dried, and stored for 3 months. Growth-promoting factors were present for the six strains studied, which varied in their resistance to physical change. Because all these factors were active in vitro, they did not require the presence of intestinal enzymes for activation. It has not been possible to show the presence of this growth factor in other mammalian milks; thus it may contribute to the implantation and persistence of *B. bifidum* in the breastfed infant's intestine.

Lactobacillus has been described as one of a number of probiotic bacteria, which provide an immune protective benefit to their host. Lactobacillus reportedly stimulates antibody production and improves phagocytosis by blood leukocytes.[85,86] The use of probiotic bacteria has reportedly produced benefits in a variety of situations associated with infections. The addition of such bacteria to formula is another example of trying to make formula better by making it more like breast milk. Hatakka and associates examined the possible effect of adding probiotic bacteria to formula on the occurrence of infection in children attending day care. They reported modest reductions in the number of children with complicated respiratory infections or lower respiratory tract infections as well as the number of children receiving antibiotics for a respiratory infection in the group of children receiving formula supplemented with *Lactobacillus rhamnosus* GG compared with children receiving unsupplemented formula.[87]

Resistance factor

It was well known in the preantibiotic era that human milk protects the human infant throughout lactation against staphylococcal infection. György[83] identified the presence of an "antistaphylococcal factor" in experiments with young mice that had been stressed with staphylococci. This factor, with no demonstrable direct antibiotic properties, was termed *resistance factor* and described as nondialyzable, thermostable, and part of the free fatty acid part of the phosphide fraction, probably $C_{18:2}$, but distinct from linoleic acid.

Lysozyme

Human milk contains a nonspecific antimicrobial factor, lysozyme, which is a thermostable, acid-stable enzyme. This enzyme is a 130-amino-acid-containing glycoprotein which can hydrolyze the 1-4 linkage between *N*-acetylglucosamine and *N*-acetylmuramic acid in bacterial cell walls. It is found in large concentrations in the stools of breastfed infants and not in stools of formula fed infants; it thus is thought to influence the flora of the intestinal tract.

Goldman and associates[42] describe an initial fall in lysozyme levels from 85 to 90 mg/mL to 25 mg/mL at 2 to 4 weeks and then a rise over 6 months to 250 mg/mL (see Fig. 5-5). Lysozyme levels show an increase over time during lactation; this finding is more apparent in Indian women than in those of the Western world. Reddy and associates[88] studied the levels of lysozyme in well-nourished and poorly nourished women in India and

found no difference between them (Table 5-4). As shown in this study, lysozyme levels increase during lactation. Levels in human milk are 300 times the level in cow milk. Lysozyme is bacteriostatic against Enterobacteriaceae and gram-positive bacteria.[43] It is secreted by neutrophils and some macrophages and is present in many body secretions in the adult.

In a study of immunologic components in human milk in the second year of lactation, Goldman and associates[76] reported that concentrations of lysozyme, lactoferrin, and total and secretory IgA were similar to those in uninterrupted lactation and in gradual weaning at 6 to 9 months. sIgA antibodies to *E. coli* were also produced during the second year. The authors state that "this supports the idea that the enteromammary lymphocyte traffic pathway, which leads to the development of lymphoid cells in the mammary gland that produce IgA antibodies to enteric organisms, operates throughout lactation."[76] When cow milk formula is added to human milk, it reduces the effect of lysozyme; however, powdered human milk fortifier (Enfamil) did not inhibit the antiinfective properties.[89]

Lactoferrin

Lactoferrin is an iron-binding protein closely related to the serum iron transport protein, transferrin. A bacteriostatic effect of lactoferrin is well established for a wide range of microorganisms, including gram-positive and gram-negative aerobes, anaerobes, and yeasts. The original proposed mechanism of action for its bacteriostatic effect was depriving the microorganism of iron. Now it is considered a multifunctional, immunoregulatory protein.

The biologic role of lactoferrin has been reviewed in several studies.[90-92] They point out that lactoferrin reversibly binds two ferric ions and that its affinity for iron is 300 times greater than that of transferrin, retaining iron down to a pH of 3. Human lactoferrin is strongly basic. Lactoferrin is normally unsaturated with iron,[93] and it is usually less than 10% saturated with iron in human milk.[92,94] Oral iron therapy for the infant can interfere with the bacteriostatic action of lactoferrin, which

TABLE 5-4 Antibacterial factors in colostrum and mature milk in well-nourished and undernourished Indian women

Group	Hemoglobin (g/dL)	Serum albumin (g/dL)	Immunoglobulins (mg/dL)			Lysozyme (mg/dL)	Lactoferrin (mg/dL)
			IgA	IgG	IgM		
Colostrum (1 to 5 days)							
Well-nourished women	11.5 ± 0.37	2.49 ± 0.065	335.9 ± 37.39 (17)*	5.9 ± 1.58 (17)	17.1 ± 4.29 (17)	14.2 ± 2.11 (15)	420 ± 49.0 (28)
Undernourished women	11.3 ± 0.60	2.10 ± 0.081	374.3 ± 42.13 (10)	5.3 ± 2.30 (10)	15.3 ± 2.50 (10)	16.4 ± 2.39 (21)	520 ± 69.0 (19)
Mature milk (1 to 6 months)							
Well-nourished women	12.8 ± 0.43	3.39 ± 0.120	119.6 ± 7.85 (12)	2.9 ± 0.92 (12)	2.9 ± 0.92 (12)	24.8 ± 3.41 (10)	250 ± 65.0 (17)
Undernourished women	12.6 ± 0.56	3.47 ± 0.130	118.1 ± 16.2 (10)	5.8 ± 3.41 (10)	5.8 ± 3.41 (10)	23.3 ± 3.53 (23)	270 ± 92.0 (13)

*Figures in parentheses indicate number of samples analyzed.
From Reddy V, Bhaskaram C, Raghuramula N, et al: Antimicrobial factors in human milk. Acta Paediatr Scand 66:229, 1977.

depends on its unsaturated state for some portion of its bacteriostatic function. Reddy and associates[88] showed that giving iron to the mother did not interfere with the saturation of lactoferrin in the milk or thus its potential bacteriostatic effect. Protein energy malnutrition, rather than iron supplies, influences lactoferrin synthesis in the mammary gland. Malnourished but non-iron-deficient mothers are lactoferrin deficient.

The concentration of lactoferrin is high in colostrum—600 mg/dL—then progressively declines over the next 5 months of lactation, leveling off at about 180 mg/dL. Breast milk also contains small amounts of transferrin (10 to 15 μg/mL). Lactoferrin makes up about 10% to 15% of the total protein content of human milk.[90] Lactoferrin is resistant to proteolysis, especially in its iron-saturated form. Intact lactoferrin is detectable in the stool of infants, with higher proportions of lactoferrin measurable in the stool of premature infants.[95] Both intact lactoferrin and fragments have been detected in the urine of premature infants, although absorption is less likely in full-term infants.[96]

Many bacteria require iron for normal growth, and the bacteriostatic effect of lactoferrin has been ascribed to its iron-binding action. In neutrophils, lactoferrin within neutrophilic granules tightly binds iron, but neutrophils with excessive iron are inefficient at destroying bacteria. Lactoferrin does not limit the growth of all microorganisms; *Helicobacter pylori* and *Neisseria, Treponema,* and *Shigella* species all have receptors for lactoferrin, directly binding iron and allowing adequate growth.

Some evidence supports various other proposed mechanisms of action for lactoferrin's antimicrobial effect. Pepsin hydrolysate products of lactoferrin (B or H) may exert a direct bactericidal effect by binding to lipopolysaccharide of gram-negative organisms and disrupting bacterial membranes.[97] Lactoferrin may cause an increased release of cytokines by cells.[98] Others have shown that lactoferrin suppresses the release of interleukin 1 and 2 (IL-1, IL-2) and tumor necrosis factor-alpha (TNF-α), which would be more of an immune-modulating effect.[90]

Several other effects have been proposed for lactoferrin, including inhibition of hydroxyl radical formation, decreasing local cell damage; lipopolysaccharide binding, also leading to a diminished inflammatory response; and DNA binding, affecting transcription and possibly regulation of the production of cell products.[91] Activation of natural killer (NK) cells, modulation of complement activity, and blocking of adhesion of enterotoxigenic *E. coli* and *Shigella flexneri*[99] are other proposed actions of lactoferrin.

A specific region of lactoferrin, near the N terminus of the molecule, is strongly basic and is reported to mediate some of lactoferrin's antimicrobial activity. "Lactoferricins," small peptides containing this basic region, produced by proteolytic cleavage reportedly bind to lipopolysaccharide (LPS), leading to disruption of the cell wall and cytoplasmic membrane.[97]

The exact roles and possible mechanisms of action of lactoferrin in the breastfed infant must be more specifically clarified.

Interferon

Colostral cells in culture have been shown to be stimulated to secrete an interferon-like substance with strong antiviral activity up to 150 National Institutes of Health (NIH) units/mL.[43] This property has not yet been identified in the supernatant of colostrum or milk. Interferon-γ has been produced by T cells from human milk when stimulated in vitro.[43] The T cells isolated from human milk were the CD45RO phenotype and have been identified as a source of interferon. Srivastava and associates[100] have measured low levels of interferon-γ in not only colostrum but also transitional and mature milk. They postulated that the low level of interferon-γ (0.7 to 2 pg/mL) might be adequate to protect against infection without hyperactivation of T cells. Interferon is produced by natural killer cells and by T cells, phenotypically Thy0 and Thy1. It can cause increased expression of major histocompatibility complex (MHC) molecules, increase macrophage function, inhibit IgE and IL-10 production, and produce antitumor and antiviral activity.

The exact role of interferon-γ in breast milk has not been delineated.

Complement

The C3 and C4 components of complement, known for their ability to fuse bacteria bound to a specific antibody, are present in colostrum in low concentrations as compared with their levels in serum. IgG and IgM activate complement. C3 proactivator has been described, and IgA and IgE have been identified as stimulating the system. Activated C3 has opsonic, anaphylactic, and chemotactic properties and is important for the lysis of bacteria bound to a specific antibody. No functional role for complement in breast milk has been identified.

Vitamin B$_{12}$–binding protein

Unsaturated vitamin B$_{12}$–binding protein of high molecular weight has been found in very high levels in human milk and in the meconium and stools of breastfed infants as compared with its levels in infant formulas and the infants who are formula fed. The protein binding renders the vitamin B$_{12}$ unavailable for bacterial growth of *E. coli* and *Bacteroides*.[101]

Glycoconjugates, gangliosides, and oligosaccharides

Glycoconjugates are complex carbohydrates that are present in large amounts in human milk. They include glycoproteins, glycolipids (gangliosides), glycosaminoglycans, mucins, and oligosaccharides. Oligosaccharides compose the major portion of glycoconjugates in milk and are present in the milk-fat globule membrane and in skim milk.[102,103] Gangliosides are glycolipids found in the plasma membrane of cells, especially in cells in the gray matter of the brain. More specifically, gangliosides are glycosphingolipids that contain sialic acid, hexoses, or hexose amines as the carbohydrate component and ceramide as the lipid component of the molecule. The predominant gangliosides in human milk are GM$_1$, GM$_2$, GM$_3$, and GD$_3$, as reported by

Newburg.[104] There is a diverse abundance of these complex carbohydrates, synthesized by the many glycosyltransferases contained in the mammary gland. Mucin and lactadherin are two glycoproteins included in this group of antimicrobial factors. Some of these carbohydrate molecules are structurally similar to glycans on the surface of small intestine epithelial cells that act as receptors for microorganisms. One proposed mechanism for the antimicrobial effect of these soluble substances is direct binding with the potential pathogenic organisms. Schroten and associates proposed that mucins contained in the human milk fat-globule membrane can block bacterial adhesion throughout the intestine after studying the adhesion of S-fimbriated *E. coli* to buccal epithelial cells.[105]

Gangliosides appear to be responsible for blocking the activity of heat-labile enterotoxin from *E. coli* and the toxin from *Vibrio cholerae* in rat intestinal loop preparations.[106] Another toxin from *Campylobacter jejuni,* with similar binding specificity, also seems to be inhibited by GM$_1$.[107,108] Globotriaosylceramide (Gb3), another glycolipid in human milk, is the natural cell surface receptor for the toxin from *Shigella dysenteriae* and verotoxin released by enterohemorrhagic *E. coli*.[109] The proposed mechanism of action of these glycolipids is that by binding to the toxin, they form a stable complex that prevents the toxin from binding to the appropriate receptors on intestinal cells; however, Crane and associates proposed from their studies that the oligosaccharide binds to the toxin receptor to block the action of the heat-stable enterotoxin of *E. coli*.[110] Human milk gangliosides may be important in protecting infants against toxin-induced diarrhea, but this has not been specifically demonstrated in vivo (Table 5-5).[106,109]

Chaturvedi and associates have recently examined the survival of oligosaccharides from human milk in infants' intestines.[111] They demonstrated that the concentrations of oligosaccharides were higher in the infants' feces than in mothers' milk and higher in feces than urine. The profile of oligosaccharides found in the infants was similar to that found in their mothers' milk. The formula fed infants had lower concentrations of oligosaccharides and the profiles

TABLE 5-5   Nonimmunoglobulin antipathogens from human milk

Antipathogen	Pathogen
Ganglioside GM$_1$	Cholera toxin
	Labile toxin of *Escherichia coli*
	Toxin of *Campylobacter jejuni*
Globotriaosylceramide (Gb3)	*Shigella* toxin I
	Shigalike toxin of *E. coli*
Fatty acids	Enveloped viruses
	Giardia lamblia
Glycoprotein (mucin)	Inhibition: rotavirus in vitro and in vivo
Glycoprotein (mucin, glycosaminoglycan)	Human immunodeficiency virus (HIV)
Mucin	Adherence: S-fimbriated *E. coli*
Glycoprotein (mannosylated)	*E. coli* intestinal adherence
Large macromolecule	Respiratory syncytial virus
Oligosaccharides	Adherence: *Streptococcus pneumoniae* and *Haemophilus influenzae* adherence of enteropathogenic *E. coli*
Fucosylated oligosaccharide	Adherence: invasion, *C. jejuni* toxicity of stabile toxin of *E. coli* (ST) in vivo

From Newburg DS: Mammary Gland Biol Lactation Newslett 11:10, 1992.

of the oligosaccharides were different from those found in the breastfed infants. The oligosaccharides remained intact passing through the intestine and were absorbed and excreted intact in the urine. Therefore, the oligosaccharides were available at these sites to block intestinal and urinary pathogens.

Interleukins

Interleukins (ILs) are now considered a "subgroup" of cytokines.[112] Originally, when cytokines were first hypothesized, it was believed that they were primarily produced by leukocytes and acted on other leukocytes, and therefore, they could be called interleukins. Although much of their effect is on lymphocyte activation and differentiation, it is now known that interleukins act on and are produced by a variety of cells.[40]

Goldman and associates[40] identified IL-1β, IL-6, IL-8, and IL-10 in breast milk (Table 5-6). Srivastava and associates[100] reported measuring moderate amounts of IL-6, IL-8, and IL-10 in the different stages of breast milk. Very low amounts of IL-1β were detected, especially in comparison with the amount of IL-1 receptor antagonist (RA), which presumably could block the activity of the small amount of IL-1. Hawkes and associates reported on the amount of cytokines in breast milk over the first 12 weeks of lactation.[113] The proposed "proinflammatory" cytokines, IL-1β, IL-6, and TNF-α, were present in only 7 of 36 mothers who donated samples at each point throughout the study. There was a broad range of concentrations of each of these cytokines over the course of the study. The "antiinflammatory" cytokines, TGF-β$_1$ and TGF-β$_2$, were present in significant amounts in all samples.

IL-6 has been identified in breast milk by other investigators, especially in the first 2 days of life.[114,115] The authors suggest that IL-6 in human milk may augment the newborn's immune functions before the body can begin full production of cytokines. Specifically, this is accomplished by increasing antibody production, especially IgA;

TABLE 5-6   **Bioactivity and concentrations of cytokines in human milk**

Agents	Bioactivity in milk	Concentrations*
IL-1β	±	1130 ± 478
IL-6	+	151 ± 89
IL-8	?	3684 ± 2910
IL-10	+	3400 ± 3800
TNF-α	+	620 ± 183
G-CSF	?	~358
M-CSF	+	17,120
Interferon-γ	?	?
EGF	+	~200,000
TGF-α	+	~2200–7200
TGF-β₂	+	130 ± 108

From Goldman AS, Chheda S, Garofalo R, Schmalstieg FC: Cytokines in human milk properties and potential effects upon the mammary gland and the neonate. J Mammary Gland Biol Neoplasia 1(3):251, 1996.

IL, Interleukin; *TNF*, tumor necrosis factor; *CSF*, colony-stimulating factor; *M*, macrophage; *G*, granulocyte; *EGF*, epidermal growth factor; *TGF*, transforming growth factor.

*The concentrations of these agents were determined by enzyme-linked immunosorbent assay (ELISA) except for IL-1β and EGF by radioimmunoassay. Concentrations are expressed as pg/mL except for M-CSF (U/mL).

enhancing phagocytosis; activating T cells; and increasing α_1-antitrypsin production by mononuclear phagocytes.

IL-8 is a chemokine capable of attracting and activating neutrophils and attracting CD45RA+ T cells. IL-8 is produced by mammary epithelial cells.[114] Srivastava and associates[100] also detected messenger ribonucleic acid (mRNA) for IL-8, suggesting that cells in breast milk were capable of producing IL-8. The exact function of IL-8 in breast milk remains to be elucidated.

IL-10 is believed to have antiinflammatory effects, including decreasing the production of interferon-γ, IL-12, and other proinflammatory cytokines. It has been reported to enhance IgA, IgG, and IgM synthesis.

IL-18 has been identified in colostrum, early milk, and mature milk with the highest levels occurring in colostrum and in association with preterm deliveries and complications of pregnancy in the mothers.[116] The levels of IL-18 were correlated with soluble Fas ligand in colostrum. IL-18 was detected by immunohistochemical staining in actively secreting epithelial cells in the lactating breast. IL-18 has been shown to be produced by intestinal epithelial cells and activated macrophages. It leads to the production of other chemokines (GM-CSF, IL-2, TNF-α). It induces the expression of Fas ligand on lymphocytes. The authors suggested that IL-18 present in colostrum may play a role in stimulating a systemic T_H1 response and causing NK cell and macrophage activation in neonates.

The interaction and the direct effect of these interleukins in breast milk must be clarified. The amount of T cells bearing markers of recent activation is increased in human milk compared with the results in peripheral blood of adults. Wirt and associates[41] have described a marked shift from virginal to antigen-primed (memory) T cells in human milk, which suggests certain functional capacities for these cells. The phenotypic pattern of T cells may result from T-cell-activating substances or selective homing of T cells to the breast. These activated T-cell populations are transferred to the infant through breast milk along with a variety of interleukins at a time when infants are capable of only limited production of interleukins. A complex interaction of interleukins and cells in human milk and at the mucosal level may provide antimicrobial and antiinflammatory benefits to the infant.

Cytokines

Of the many bioactive substances that have been identified in human milk, cytokines are some of the most recently identified and investigated agents, although their existence has long been suspected in attempts to explain certain immunologic and protective effects of breast milk on infants. More than 40 cytokines have been described,[117] and more than 10 of these have been identified in human milk.[40,100] Cytokines are small proteins or glycoproteins that, through binding to receptors on immune and nonimmune cells, produce a broad range of effects (many still unidentified) through autocrine, paracrine, and endocrine actions. Cytokines are produced predominantly by immune cells and function in complex associations with other cytokines to stimulate and control the development and normal functioning of the immune system. The nomenclature and abbreviations used are complicated and confusing. Newer systems of classification have been established according to which cells produce them or what their general functions are[112] or based on the relative position of their cysteine residues or their receptor types (CCR, CXCR, CX3CR).[117] Box 5-1 provides a simplified list with abbreviations.

Little evidence demonstrates specific in vivo activity of the different cytokines. Based on general information on the function and interaction of the particular cytokines, as well as consideration of as yet unexplained effects of breast milk, proposed

functions of the cytokines include initiation of development of host defense, stimulation of host defenses, prevention of autoimmunity, antiinflammatory effects in the upper respiratory tract and GI tract, and stimulation of the development of the digestive system, especially the mucosal immune system of the alimentary tract and the proximal respiratory tract. The maternal breast may respond to feedback stimulation or suppression by secreted cytokines, influencing the growth, differentiation, and secretory function of the breast. As shown in other situations, cytokines may enhance receptor expression on cells in the respiratory and GI tracts for MHC molecules or immunoglobulins. Various cell types in the mucosal immune system may be activated or attracted to specific sites in the GI tract.

The actual measurement of cytokines in breast milk has been complicated by a number of factors, including different assays used (bioassays, ELISA, radioimmunoassay), binding to proteins, their existence in monomeric or polymeric forms,[118] the presence of antagonists, and their varying presence in colostrum, early milk, or mature milk. Goldman and associates[40] reported on the bioactivity and concentration of cytokines in breast milk from their own work and that of others (see Table 5-6). Srivastava and associates[100] obtained some conflicting results using different assays in colostrum, early milk, and mature milk. They confirmed the presence of M-CSF throughout lactation, as well as TGF-β_1 and -β_2, IL-1RA, GRO-α, MCP-1, RANTES, and IL-8, but reported insignificant amounts of GM-CSF, SCF, LIF, MIP-1α, IL-2, IL-4, IL-11, IL-12, IL-13, IL-15, sIL-2R, and IFN-α (see Box 5-1 for nomenclature). Srivastava and associates[100] also used reverse transcriptase polymerase chain reaction (PCR) to measure the production of cytokine mRNA by cells in breast milk. They reported the presence of mRNA for MCP-1, IL-8, TGF-β_1, TGF-β_2, M-CSF, IL-6, and IL-1β, which may be another source of these cytokines in breast milk. Hawkes and associates demonstrated that human milk cells (HMC) from lactating women at 5 weeks post partum are capable of active cytokine production in vitro (IL-1β, IL-6, TNF-α) with and without exposure to lipopolysaccharide.[113]

BOX 5-1   Nomenclature and abbreviations for various cytokines

Interferon alpha, beta, gamma	IFN-α, -β, -γ
Granulocyte colony-stimulating factor	G-CSF
Macrophage colony-stimulating factor	M-CSF
Stem cell factor	SCF
Interleukin 1, 2, 4, 6, 8, 10	IL-1, -2, -4, -6, -8, -10
Interleukin 1 beta	IL-1β
Interleukin 1 receptor antagonist	IL-1RA
Soluble interleukin 2 receptor	sIL-2R
Transforming growth factor beta$_2$	TGF-β_2
Tumor necrosis factor alpha	TNF-α
Transforming growth factor alpha	TGF-α
Macrophage inflammatory protein	MIP
Regulated on activation, normal T cell expressed and secreted	RANTES
Epidermal growth factor	EGF
Growth-regulated oncogene	GRO
Monocyte chemoattractant protein 1	MCP-1
Leukocyte inhibitory factor	LIF

Continued cytokine production by human milk cells is another explanation for the variable amounts of cytokines identified in breast milk and is further evidence that the cells are capable of responding to an infectious stimulus.

In their investigations of the possible antiinflammatory effects of breast milk, Buescher and Malinowska[119] examined milk for the presence of soluble receptors and cytokine antagonists. They demonstrated sICAM-1 (soluble intercellular adhesion molecule 1), sVCAM-1 (soluble vascular cell adhesion molecule 1), and sE-selectin (soluble E-selectin) in colostrum and at lower levels in mature milk, as well as high levels of sTNF-αRI (soluble TNF-α receptor I), sTNF-αRII, and IL-1RA. Also, they identified that most TNF-α did not exist "free" in breast milk but was associated with TNF receptors. The in vivo significance of these findings remains to be assessed.

Given the complex interaction and regulation of cytokine production and cytokines' relation to co-ordinated inflammatory and antiinflammatory responses in tissues, one should assume that the interaction of cytokines in breast milk and the effect of cytokines, cytokine receptors (soluble and expressed on various cell types), and cytokine antagonists on the infant will be equally complex. Continued investigation is essential to understanding the significance and specific effects of these substances in breast milk.

Nucleotides

Nucleotides, nucleosides, nucleic acids, and related metabolic products are essential to many biologic processes. Although they are not essential nutrients because they can be synthesized endogenously, their presence in the diet may carry significant benefits in various situations. In situations of disease, stress, rapid growth, or limited dietary intake, supplementation of the diet with nucleotides may decrease energy expenditure to synthesize or salvage nucleotides, which optimizes the host response to these adverse situations.

Nucleotides exist in relatively large amounts in human milk, about 15% to 20% of the nonprotein nitrogen (NPN), suggesting that they have some nutritional significance, although no clinical syndromes have been associated with nucleotide deficiency to date. Nucleotides are present in the natural milk of different species in varying amounts and composition. The nucleotide content and composition of bovine milk are particularly less and different from that of human milk, and subsequently the same has been true of infant formulas (see Chapter 4). Considerable debate surrounds the logic, the need, and the practical issues of adding nucleotides to formula.[120-122] Mammalian cells contain a large variety of nucleotides and related products, which have many metabolic functions, including the following[123]:

1. Energy metabolism: adenosine triphosphate (ATP) is a major form of available cellular energy.
2. Nucleic acid precursors: the monomeric units for RNA and DNA are present.
3. Physiologic mediators: cyclic adenosine monophosphate (cAMP) and cyclic guanosine monophosphate (cGMP) serve as "messengers" for cellular processes; adenosine diphosphate (ADP) is necessary for platelet aggregation; and adenosine has been shown to affect vasodilatation.
4. Related products function as coenzymes in metabolic pathways: nicotinamide-adenine dinucleotide (NAD), flavin adenine dinucleotide (FAD), and coenzyme A (CoA).
5. Related products function as intermediate carrying molecules in synthetic reactions: uridine diphosphate (UDP) glucose in glycogen synthesis and guanosine diphosphate (GDP) mannose, GDP-fucose, UDP-galactose, and cytidine monophosphate (CMP) sialic acid in glycoprotein synthesis.
6. Allosteric effectors: the intracellular concentrations of nucleotides influence the progression of certain steps of metabolic pathways.
7. Cellular agonists: extracellular nucleotides influence intracellular signal transduction (e.g., cAMP and inositol-calcium pathway).

Nucleotide concentrations in cells and tissues are maintained by de novo synthesis and salvage from

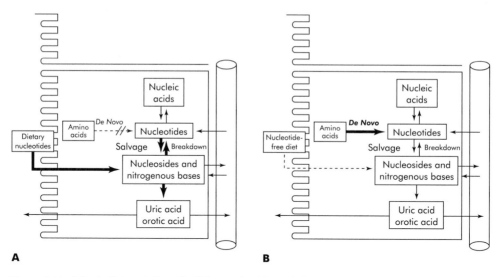

Figure 5-11. Metabolic regulation of cellular nucleotide pools in presence and absence of nucleotide in diet. **A,** Effect of dietary nucleotide activating salvage pathway. **B,** De novo nucleotide synthesis is enhanced with nucleotide-free diet. (From Quan R, Barness LA: Do infants need nucleotide supplemented formula for optimal nutrition? J Pediatr 11(4):429, 1990.)

intermediary metabolism and diet (Fig. 5-11).[121] Nucleosides are the predominant product absorbed in the small intestine. Nucleosides are probably transported by passive diffusion and a carrier-mediated process; purines and pyrimidines are transported by passive diffusion at high concentrations and by a sodium-dependent active mechanism at low concentrations (Fig. 5-12).[121] The digestion and absorption of nucleotides, nucleosides, and pyrimidines and purines also involve polymeric and monomeric nucleotides and other adducts (nucleosides in a biologically active moiety).

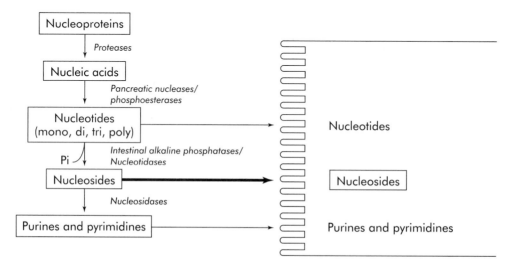

Figure 5-12. Digestion and absorption of nucleic acids and their related products. (From Quan R, Barness LA: Do infants need nucleotide supplemented formula for optimal nutrition? J Pediatr 11(4):429, 1990.)

In early reports on the nucleotide and nucleoside content of milk, various methods of measurement were used, and the amounts were described as either the monomeric fraction of nucleotides or the total RNA. Leach and associates,[124] recognizing the complex nature of digestion and absorption of nucleotides and related products, attempted to measure the total potentially available nucleosides (TPANs) in human milk using solid-phase extraction, high-performance liquid chromatography (HPLC) analysis, and enzymatic hydrolysis of the various fractions. They analyzed breast milk samples at various stages throughout lactation (colostrum; transitional, early, and late mature milk) from 100 European women and 11 American women. They used an aqueous TPAN-fortified solution containing ribonucleosides, 5′-mononucleotides, polymeric RNA, and nucleoside-containing adducts to estimate the accuracy of their process.

The mean ranges of TPAN values were similar for European women from different countries and American women, although broad ranges were seen and the composition of individual nucleotides varied.[124] The mean TPAN value was lowest in colostrum but did not show a consistent upward or downward trend in transitional, early, or late mature milk. The mean ranges of TPAN values were 82 to 164 µmol/L for colostrum, 144 to 210 µmol/L for transitional milk, 172 to 402 µmol/L for early mature milk, and 156 to 259 µmol/L for late mature milk (Table 5-7). Monomeric and polymeric nucleotides were the predominant forms of TPAN in pooled samples. Cytidine, guanosine, and adenosine were found mainly in these fractions, whereas uridine was found primarily as free nucleotide and adduct (Table 5-8). The methods used recovered 90% to 95% of the true TPAN values compared with the TPAN-fortified solution, although the uridine and guanosine content was underestimated. Tressler and associates measured the TPAN in pooled breast milk samples from Asian women demonstrating average levels in colostrum, transitional milk, and mature milk and found it to be similar to the levels in European and American women.[125]

Leach and associates[124] concluded that their process of estimating TPANs, including sequential enzymatic hydrolyses, and measuring the entire nucleotide fraction provides a reasonable estimate of the in vivo process and the nucleotides available to the infant from human milk.

Proposed effects of dietary nucleotides include effects on the immune system, iron absorption, intestinal flora, plasma lipoproteins, and growth of intestinal and hepatic cells. Effects on the immune system, related to nucleotide supplementation to the diet, have mainly been reported from animal studies and include increased mortality rate from graft-versus-host disease, improved delayed-type cutaneous hypersensitivity and alloantigen-induced lymphoproliferation, reversal of malnutrition and starvation-induced immunosuppression, increased resistance to challenge with *Staphylococcus aureus* and *Candida albicans,* and enhanced T-cell maturation and function.[120] Spleen cells of mice fed a nucleotide-free diet produce lower levels of IL-2, express lower levels of IL-2 receptors, and have decreased natural killer (NK) cell activity and macrophage activity.[126,127] Presumably these nucleotide-associated changes are related to T-helper/inducer cells and the initial phases of antigen processing and lymphocyte proliferation.[123,127,128]

In vitro and in vivo experiments have documented that ingested nucleotides increased iron absorption, perhaps affecting xanthine oxidase.[121] Although in vitro studies showed that added nucleotides enhanced the growth of bifidobacteria, conflicting results have been obtained on the influence of dietary nucleotides on the fecal flora of infants receiving breast milk or nucleotide-supplemented formula.[121,129] Clinical studies in infants receiving nucleotide-supplemented formula demonstrated increased high-density lipoprotein (HDL) cholesterol, lower very low density lipoprotein (VLDL) cholesterol, increased long-chain polyunsaturated fatty acids (PUFAs), and changes in red blood cell (RBC) membrane phospholipid composition.[121] Supplementation studies in animals have shown enhanced GI tract growth and maturation, improved intestinal repair

TABLE 5-7 **Nucleotide and total potentially available nucleoside (TPAN) in pooled human milk by stage of lactation (μmol/L)***

	Uridine	Cytidine	Guanosine	Adenosine	TPAN
Colostrum					
Site 1	27	84	22	20	153
Site 2	21	33	15	13	82
Site 3	30	82	26	26	164
Site 4	24	84	20	22	150
Mean	26	71	21	21	137
Transitional milk					
Site 1	23	82	22	19	146
Site 2	33	76	19	17	144
Site 3	37	84	43	42	206
Site 4	36	100	36	38	210
Mean	32	86	30	29	177
Early mature milk					
Site 1	30	86	28	28	172
Site 2	50	79	23	21	173
Site 3	44	96	36	37	214
Site 4	67	146	91	97	402
Mean	48	102	45	46	240
Late mature milk					
Site 1	36	73	22	25	156
Site 2	58	106	29	27	219
Site 3	49	81	20	24	173
Site 4	45	124	40	49	259
Mean	47	96	28	31	202
Grand mean	38	88	31	32	189
SD	13	24	18	20	70
Range	21–67	33–146	19–92	13–97	84–402
American pool[†]	37	70	30	24	161

*Data from 100 individual samples collected at four sites and combined into 16 pooled samples (5 to 7 individual samples per site per stage of lactation). *Site 1*, Rouen and Mount Saint Aignau, France; *Site 2*, Mainz, Germany; *Site 3*, Bolzano, Italy; *Site 4*, Treviso, Italy.
†Pooled sample of milk collected from 11 American women between 2 and 4 months post partum.
From Leach JL, Baxter JH, Molitor BE, et al: Total potentially available nucleosides of human milk by stage of lactation. Am J Clin Nutr 61:1224, 1995.

after diarrhea, stimulation of hepatic growth, and augmented recovery from hepatectomy.[120]

Studies in human infants of the effect of dietary nucleotides on the immune system and protection against infection are limited. Carver and associates[127] compared infants receiving breast milk to those receiving commercially available infant formula and formula supplemented with nucleotides at a level of 32 mg/L. At 2 and 4 months, NK cell activity and IL-2 production were higher in the breastfed and nucleotide-supplemented groups compared with those receiving formula without

TABLE 5-8   Percentage of total potentially available nucleoside (TPAN) in pooled human milk as adducts, polymeric nucleotides, monomeric nucleotides, and nucleosides[*]

	Uridine	Cytidine	Guanosine	Adenosine	TPAN
Polymeric nucleotides	19 ± 7	57 ± 12	59 ± 21	47 ± 11	48 ± 8
Monomeric nucleotides	36 ± 12	37 ± 13	34 ± 14	35 ± 10	36 ± 10
Nucleosides	18 ± 14	5 ± 5	1 ± 2	5 ± 4	8 ± 6
Adducts[†]	27 ± 12	1 ± 1	7 ± 15	13 ± 9	9 ± 4

[*]$\bar{x} \pm$ SD. Based on the mean of entire pool of human milk collected from 100 individuals at four stages of lactation at four sites.
[†]Adducts are of the form nucleoside-phosphate-phosphate-X, where X is a biologically relevant moiety (e.g., uridine diphosphate–galactose or NAD).
From Leach JL, Baxter JH, Molitor BE, et al: Total potentially available nucleosides of human milk by stage of lactation. Am J Clin Nutr 61:1224, 1995.

nucleotide supplements. Infections occurred infrequently in all groups, but slightly less in the breastfed group. No differences were noted in hematologic profiles and plasma chemistry values, and no toxicity or intolerance was associated with nucleotide supplementation. The sample size was small, marked variability was seen in the IL-2 measurements, and the differences noted at 4 months were less than at 2 months. Therefore, the authors concluded that dietary nucleotides may contribute to improved immunity in breastfed infants.

Brunser and associates[130] examined the effect of a nucleotide-supplemented formula on the incidence of diarrhea in 392 Chilean infants, studied through 6 months of age. Although the infants receiving the supplemented formula (20 mg/L) experienced less diarrhea, the difference in the duration of diarrhea was small. The numbers were too small to comment on the causative agents of diarrhea, although there was no apparent protection against any one agent. The beneficial effect of nucleotides against diarrhea was proposed to be secondary to enhanced immune response to intestinal pathogens or improved intestinal integrity or a combination of both. In a larger study of 3243 infants younger than 6 months of age, the severity of the diarrhea (duration and number of bowel movements) as well as the incidence of diarrhea was lower in the nucleotide supplemented group.[131]

Two groups of premature infants fed either nucleotide supplemented (20 mg/L) or unsupplemented formula were followed, measuring the concentration of plasma immunoglobulins over the first 3 months of life.[132] IgG plasma concentrations were not different in the two groups over the study period. IgM plasma levels were higher in the nucleotide supplemented group at 20 to 30 days and 3 months of life, while IgA plasma levels were significantly higher at 3 months of age in the supplemented group.

Pickering and associates[120] published a 12-month, controlled, randomized study of 311 infants to examine the effect of added nucleotides at levels comparable to human milk on the infant's immune response to various vaccine antigens. Nonrandomized, 103 infants received breast milk for at least 2 months and then either human milk or a standard infant formula. Another 208 infants were randomized to receive either a standard infant formula or one supplemented with nucleotides. The amount and actual nucleotide content added were based on TPANs, as measured by Leach and associates[124] equaling 72 mg/L. Overall growth and nutrition tolerance were similar in each group. The nucleotide group had significantly higher geometric mean titers of Hib (*Haemophilus influenzae* type b) antibody and diphtheria antibody than the control group or the breastfed infants. No significant difference was seen between the nucleotide and control groups for the IgG response to oral poliovirus vaccine (OPV) or tetanus. Infants breastfed for longer than 6 months had significantly higher antibody responses to OPV than children breastfed for less than 6 months or either of the two formula fed groups. No significant differences were found between the different groups with respect to total IgG, IgA, or IgE. Differences were seen in the number of children who experienced at least one episode of diarrhea: the nucleotide group (4/27, 15%) versus the control group (13/32, 41%, $p < 0.05$) and the breastfed group (6/27, 22%). Notably, the breastfed group was very heterogeneous relative to the amount of breast milk received and the duration of feeding, whereas the nucleotide group received supplementation for the entire 12 months.

Questions that remain concerning nucleotides and their proposed beneficial effects in an infant's diet include the following:

- What are the mechanisms of action of these proposed benefits?
- What form and concentration of nucleotides are necessary to effect these benefits?
- Is adequate information available to justify using nucleotides in infant formula in higher amounts and different compositions than are currently used?

Debate and research to answer these and other questions concerning nucleotides will continue.

BACTERIAL FLORA OF THE INTESTINAL TRACT

As noted earlier, the normal flora of the intestinal tract of the breastfed infant is *Lactobacillus bifidus*. The gram-negative population in the gut is kept small.[133]

In a prospective study of breastfed Mayan Indian infants from birth to 3 years of age, bifid bacteria predominated and constituted 95% to 99% of the flora. Other culturable microorganisms were *Streptococcus, Bacteroides, Clostridium, Micrococcus, Enterococcus*, and *E. coli*. A change occurred when large amounts of solid foods were added at about 1 year of life. The solids were notably protein poor. *E. coli* progressively increased in numbers. *Lactobacillus bifidus* metabolizes milk saccharides, producing large amounts of acetic acid, lactic acid, and some formic and succinic acids, which create the low pH of the stool of breastfed infants. *L. bifidus* also produces short-chain fatty acids in the course of colonization. Large numbers of bifidobacteria can lower the pH of the intestine, which limits the growth of some pathogens such as *E. coli, Bacteroides*, and staphylococci. The intestinal flora of bottle fed infants is made up of predominantly gram-negative bacteria, especially coliform organisms and *Bacteroides*.

The flora of bifid bacteria is inhibitory to certain pathogenic bacteria. Substantial clinical evidence is available to demonstrate protection against intestinal infections from *Staphylococcus aureus, Shigella, Salmonella, Vibrio cholerae, E. coli*, rotavirus, *Campylobacter,* and protozoa.[134]

Two actions are apparent. The first encourages the growth of *L. bifidus* and thus crowds out the growth of other bacteria. In the second, the number of pathogens is also kept low by the direct action of lysozyme and lactoferrin. When the number of pathogenic bacteria is kept low; immune antibodies can keep the growth under control and prevent the absorption of bacteria through the gut wall into the bloodstream.

EFFECTIVENESS OF HUMAN MILK IN CONTROLLING INFECTION

The properties of human milk do appear to control infection. Specific disease entities have shown a clear differential in the incidence between infants fed cow milk and those fed human milk.[135,136]

Protection against bacterial infection

Breast milk IgA has antitoxin activity against enterotoxins of *E. coli* and *V. cholerae* that may be significant in preventing infantile diarrhea. Antibodies against O antigen of some of the most common serotypes of *E. coli* were found in high titer in breast milk samples collected from healthy mothers in Sweden. The infants who had consumed reasonable amounts of breast milk with high titers of *E. coli* antibodies had antibodies in their stool.[1] Protection against cholera in breastfed children by antibodies in breast milk was studied by Glass and associates.[134] A prospective study in Bangladesh showed cholera antibody levels to vary in the colostrum and milk. The correlation among colonization, disease, and milk antibodies led the authors to conclude that breast milk antibodies against cholera do not protect children from colonization with *V. cholerae,* but they do protect against disease.

Salmonella infection was simila[r]
France and associates[137] to evalua[te]
logic mechanisms in host colostrum[,]
cific for salmonellae. Vigorous
colostral and milk cells against th[e]
and nonspecific opsonizing capacity [of the]
phase of colostrum and milk were de[?]

Gothefors and associates[138] show[ed that]
isolated from stools of breastfed infants differed from strains found in formula fed infants in two respects. First, *E. coli* strains were more sensitive to the bactericidal effect of human serum. Second, and more often, spontaneously agglutinated bacteria from other sites, such as the prepuce or periurethral area, were less sensitive in breastfed infants. These findings support the theory that breast milk favors proliferation of mutant strains, which have decreased virulence. This mutation of bacterial strains is another way breastfeeding may protect against infection.

It has been suggested that milk immunization is a dynamic process because a mother's milk has been found to contain antibody to virtually all her infant's strains of intestinal bacteria. The mother exposed to the infant's microorganisms through either the breast or the gut responds immunologically to those microorganisms and thus automatically protects her immunologically immature infant.

The orderly review of data on the presence of antibodies in human milk has produced a substantial list of affected organisms. In addition to *E. coli,* antibodies to *Bacteroides fragilis, Clostridium tetani, Haemophilus pertussis, Diplococcus pneumoniae, Corynebacterium diphtheriae, Salmonella, Shigella, Chlamydia trachomatis, V. cholerae, S.*

aureus, and several strains of *Streptococcus* (Table 5-9) have been identified. Noguera-Obenza and Cleary have summarized the contribution of secretory IgA in breast milk in protecting infants from bacterial enterititis.[80]

A study in Oslo by Hanson[1] of an outbreak of severe diarrhea caused by *E. coli* strain 0111 showed that six severely ill children were formula fed. Two infants who were breastfed had *E. coli* strain 0111 in their stools but showed few symptoms. Their mothers had no detectable antibodies for strain 0111 in their milk, which would suggest that other factors in human milk protect the infant from serious illness when there are no antibodies in the milk. Hanson[1] also showed in another study that after colonization with a specific strain of *E. coli,* mothers had large numbers of lymphoid cells in their milk with antibodies to that *E. coli.* Their serum produced no such response. This supports the concept that antigen-triggered lymphoid cells from Peyer's patches seek out lymphoid-rich tissue, producing IgA in the mammary gland. The mother is immunized in the gut at the same time as her milk. It has also been shown that *E. coli* enteritis can be cured by feeding human milk.

Schlesinger and Covelli[139] studied possible cell-mediated immunity in breastfed infants. They showed that tuberculin-positive nursing mothers had reactive T cells in their colostrum and early milk. Furthermore, 8 of 13 infants nursed by tuberculin-positive mothers had tuberculin-reactive [periphera]l blood T cells after 4 weeks. Cord blood [had no su]ch activity. There are no clinical or [other d]ata available suggesting a protective [effect of thi]s apparently induced tuberculin reactiv[ity in infan]ts.

[Protecti]on against viral infection

[Protection a]gainst viruses has been the subject of similar studies. Breast milk contains antibodies against poliovirus, coxsackievirus, echovirus, influenzavirus, reovirus, respiratory syncytial virus, rotavirus, and rhinovirus.[140] It has been confirmed that human milk inhibits the growth of these viruses in tissue culture. Nonspecific

TABLE 5-9 Nonantibody, antibacterial protective factors in human milk

Factors	Proposed mechanisms of action	Organisms affected	Effect of heat
Bifidus factor	Inhibits replication of certain bacteria in gastrointestinal tract by causing proliferation of lactobacilli	Enterobacteriaceae, including shigellae, salmonellae, and some *E. coli*	Stable to boiling
Complement components	Opsonic, chemitactic, and bacteriolytic activity	*E. coli*	Destroyed by heating at 56° C for 30 min
Lysozyme	With IgA, peroxide, or ascorbate, causes lysis of bacteria	*E. coli* Salmonellae	Some loss (0%–23%) at 62.5° C for 30 min; essentially destroyed by boiling for 15 min
Lactoferrin (nutrient binders)	Binds ferric iron	*E. coli* *Candida albicans*	Two-thirds destroyed at 62.5° C for 30 min
Lactoperoxidase	Oxidizes bacteria	*E. coli* *Salmonella typhimurium*	Presumably destroyed by boiling
Nonantibody proteins: receptor-like glycolipid or glycoprotein	Inhibit bacterial adherence	*Vibrio cholerae*	Stable to boiling for 15 min
Gangliosides (GM1-like)	Interfere with attachment of enterotoxin to GM1 cell membrane ganglioside receptors	*E. coli* and *V. cholerae* enterotoxins	Stable to boiling
Nonlactose carbohydrate factors	Prevent action of stable toxin (ST)	*E. coli* ST	Stable at 85° C for 30 min
Milk cells (macrophages, polymorphonuclear leukocytes, B- and T-lymphocytes)	By phagocytosis and killing: *E. coli*, *S. aureus*, *S. enteritidis* By sensitized lymphocytes: *E. coli* By phagocytosis: *C. albicans* lymphocyte stimulation by *E. coli* K antigen		Destroyed at 62.5° C for 30 min

Modified from May JT: Antimicrobial properties and microbial contaminants of breast milk—An update. Aust Paediatr J 20:265, 1984; and Pickering LK, Kohl S: Human milk humoral immunity and infant defense mechanisms. In Howell RR, Morriss RH Jr, Pickering LK, editors: Human Milk and Infant Nutrition and Health, Springfield, Ill, Thomas, 1986.

substances in human milk are active against arbovirus and murine leukemia virus, according to work by Fieldsteel.[141]

A high degree of antiviral activity against Japanese B encephalitis virus as well as the two leukemia viruses has been found in human milk. The factor was found in the fat fraction and was not destroyed by extended heating, which distinguishes it from antibodies. May[135] believes the nonimmunoglobulin macromolecule antiviral activity in human milk is caused by specific fatty acids and monoglycerides (Table 5-10).

Specimens of human colostrum have been found to contain neutralizing activity against *respiratory syncytial virus* (RSV). RSV has become a major threat in infancy and is the most common reason for hospitalization in infancy in some developed countries. It has a high mortality rate. Epidemics have occurred in special care nurseries. Statistically significant data collected by Downham and associates[142] showed that few breastfed babies (8 of 115) were among the infants hospitalized for RSV infection, compared with uninfected control subjects who were breastfed (46 of 167).

Fishaut and associates[143] studied the immune response to RSV prospectively in 26 nursing mothers over several months. Antiviral IgM and IgG were rarely found in colostrum or milk. RSV-specific IgA, however, was identified in 40% to 75% of specimens. Two mothers with the disease had specific IgG, IgM, and IgA antibody in serum and nasopharyngeal secretions, but only IgA was found in their milk. This confirms that IgA antibody to specific respiratory tract pathogens is present in the products of lactation. Because RSV appears to replicate only in the respiratory tract, the authors suggest that viral-specific antibody activity in the mammary gland may be derived from the bronchus-associated lymphoid tissue (BALT).

Necrotizing enterocolitis has been a serious threat to premature infants in acute care nurseries. Animal studies have demonstrated a protective quality to breast milk. Efforts to confirm a similar relationship in human infants have been encouraging but not conclusive. Leukocytes in milk fulfill a protective function in premature infants, possibly

as a consequence of their natural transplantation, according to Beer and Billingham.[58]

In a controlled prospective study of high-risk, low-birth-weight infants in India using donor human milk, there were significantly fewer infections and no major infections in the group receiving human milk, although the control infants experienced diarrhea, pneumonia, septicemia, and meningitis.[136]

The relationship of *sudden infant death syndrome* (SIDS) to formula feeding is supported by circumstantial evidence and retrospective studies. The fact remains that in all series reported, SIDS is rare in breastfed infants. Whether this is related to protection against infection is not clear.

The apparent predisposition of bottle fed infants to purulent otitis media as compared with the predisposition of breastfed infants may result from IgA-conferred immunity in human milk. It may also be caused by the mechanics of bottle feeding. Of a group of infants with otitis media, 85% had their bottles propped up, whereas only 8% of a matched bottle feeding control group who did not have otitis media had their bottles propped up. When an infant swallows fluid lying flat on the back, it is possible to regurgitate it into the eustachian tube.[144]

Antiprotozoan factors

In human milk, bile salt-stimulated lipase (BSSL) has been found to be the major factor inactivating protozoans (Table 5-11).[135] The mechanism by which lipase acts is not known, although it may generate fatty acids and monoglycerides, which inactivate enveloped bacteria, viruses, or protozoa. A nonimmunoglobulin, nonlipase, heat-stable factor has been identified in human milk that can inactivate *Giardia lamblia*.

ANTIINFLAMMATORY PROPERTIES

Human milk protects against many intestinal and respiratory pathogens with minimal evidence of inflammation. Goldman and associates[145] hypothesize that human milk is poor in initiators and

TABLE 5-10 **Nonantibody, antiviral, and antiprotozoan factors in human milk**

Factors	Proposed mechanisms of action	Organisms affected	Effect of heat
Lipids (unsaturated fatty acids and monoglycerides)	Inactivate lipid-enveloped virus	Herpes simplex Semliki Forest Influenza Ross River	Stable to boiling for 30 min
Macromolecules	Inhibit attachment and penetration	Herpes simplex Coxsackievirus B$_4$ Cytomegalovirus Rotavirus	Most stable at 56° C for 30 min Destroyed by boiling for 30 min
α_2-Macroglobulin protein	Inhibits hemagglutinin activity	Influenza Parainfluenza	Stable to boiling for 15 min
α_1-Antitrypsin Bile salt-stimulated lipase	Trypsin-dependent inhibition May generate fatty acids and monoglycerides that inactivate organisms	Rotavirus Giardia lamblia Entamoeba histolytica	Stable to boiling for 10 min
Nonlipase macromolecule	Unknown	G. lamblia	
Milk cells	Induced interferon by virus or phytohemagglutinin (PHA); induced lymphokine (LDCF) by PHA; induced cytokine by herpes simplex virus; lymphocyte stimulation by rubella, cytomegalovirus, herpes, measles, mumps		Destroyed at 62.5° C for 30 min

Modified from May JT: Antimicrobial properties and microbial contaminants of breast milk—An update. Aust Paediatr J 20:265, 1984; and Pickering LK, Kohl S: Human milk humoral immunity and infant defense mechanisms. In Howell RR, Morriss RH Jr, Pickering LK, editors: Human Milk and Infant Nutrition and Health, Springfield, III, Thomas, 1986.

TABLE 5-11   Antiprotozoan factors in human milk

Factor	Organisms affected (in vitro)	Effect of heat
Bile salt-stimulated lipase	*Giardia lamblia* *Entamoeba histolytica* *Trichomonas vaginalis*	Destroyed at 62.5° C for 1 min
Nonimmunoglobulin, nonlipase macromolecule	*G. lamblia*	Stable to boiling for 20 min

Modified from May JT: Antimicrobial properties and microbial contaminants of breast milk—An update. Aust Paediatr J 20:265, 1984.

mediators of inflammation but rich in antiinflammatory agents. Several major biochemical pathways of inflammation, including the coagulation system, the fibrinolytic system, and complement, are poorly represented in human milk. Box 5-2 outlines the antiinflammatory properties of various constituents and the paucity of certain proinflammatory mediators in breast milk.

The interaction of factors in the milk with one another or with host defenses cannot be entirely predicted by examining each factor separately. When the decreased response of human milk leukocytes to chemoattractant peptides was demonstrated by Thorpe and associates,[146] the failure of the response of human milk leukocytes was not caused by alterations in maternal peripheral blood leukocytes. This suggests that inhibitors are in the milk and that the human milk leukocytes may be modified in the mammary gland to protect through noninflammatory mechanisms.[146] Many other studies have documented the decreased function of milk polymorphonuclear leukocytes and macrophages in both colostrum and mature milk.[147]

The antioxidant properties of human colostrum were demonstrated by Buescher and McIlheran[148] using aqueous human colostrum on human PMNs. The colostrum significantly interfered with PMN oxygen metabolic and enzymatic activities that are important in the mediation of acute inflammation. Other antioxidants include an ascorbate-like compound, uric acid, α-tocopherol, and β-carotene. Blood levels of α-tocopherol and β-carotene are higher in breastfed than unsupplemented formula fed infants.

Additionally, specific cytokines that can exhibit antiinflammatory effects have also been identified in human colostrum and milk: TGF-β_1 and -β_2[149,150,151] and IL-10.[152] A cytokine antagonist, IL-1RA, and soluble receptors for TNF-α are also found in colostrum and milk.[100,119] Palkowetz and associates have reported that IL-1RA can decrease the action of IL-1β.[114]

Both human colostrum and milk cause a diminished influx of polymorphonuclear cells to a local site of inflammation in two different in vivo models of inflammation in rats.[153,154]

The inflammatory response can be protective for the host at the same time as it can produce the symptoms of clinical illness. Breast milk contains a large variety of antimicrobial factors that exert their protective effect without causing significant inflammation (e.g., secretory IgA, oligosaccharides, lactoferrin, nucleotides, etc.). Many other cells and factors in breast milk participate in a complex interaction to both protect the infant and limit the potential damaging effects of an uncontrolled inflammatory response. Further study into the dynamic interplay of the many factors in breast milk with the developing infant's mucosal barriers and immune system is needed to fully understand the protective immune response and the antiinflammatory benefits of human milk.

MUCOSAL BARRIER SYSTEM

Significant differences exist between the biophysical and biochemical organization and function of the mucosal barrier system.[155] The microvillous membrane of the neonate's intestinal tract

---

BOX 5-2 Antiinflammatory features of human milk

Paucity of initiators and mediators

Foreign antigens
IgG antibodies
Complement system
Fibrinolytic system
Coagulation system
Kallikrein system

Antiinflammatory agents

Lactoferrin	Inhibits complement
Secretory IgA	Prevents bacterial adherence
	Inhibits neutrophil chemotaxis
	Limits antigen penetration
Lysozyme	Inhibits neutrophil chemotaxis, generation of toxic oxygen radicals
Catalase	Destroys hydrogen peroxide
α-Tocopherol	Scavengers of oxygen radicals
Cysteine	
Ascorbic acid	
Histaminase	Degrades histamine
Arylsulfatase	Degrades leukotrienes
α_1-Antichymotrypsin	Neutralizes enzymes that act in inflammation
α_1-Antitrypsin	
Prostaglandins (E_2, $F_2\alpha$)	Cytoprotective: inhibits neutrophil degranulation, lymphocyte activation
Pregnancy-associated α_2-glycoprotein	Inhibits lymphocyte blastogenesis
Oligosaccharides	Inhibits microbial attachment
Epidermal growth factors	Strengthens mucosal barriers

Special features of leukocytes

No basophils, mast cells, eosinophils, or platelets
T lymphocytes respond poorly to allogeneic cells
Low natural killer cell activity or antibody-dependent cytotoxicity
Poor response of neutrophils and macrophages to chemoattractants

Modified from Goldman AS, Thorpe LW, Goldblum RM, et al: Anti-inflammatory properties of human milk. Acta Paediatr Scand 75:689, 1986.

---

permits increased attachment of certain pathogenic enterobacteria and their toxins to epithelial cells. Growth factors in human milk, such as epidermal growth factor, lactoferrin, cortisol, and several hormones, have a stimulating effect on the neonatal gut development and increase the effectiveness of the epithelial barrier. Platelet activating factor (PAF) has been associated with the pathogenesis of necrotizing enterocolitis in sick newborns.[156] A substance in the leukocytes in the aqueous phase of human milk, an acetylhydrolase that breaks down PAF, is known to exist in low levels in premature infants. These are important observations toward understanding the role of the antiinflammatory function of human milk and how human milk contributes to a more effective barrier.[140] Many of the contributions of breast milk to an effective mucosal barrier have been discussed relative to secretory IgA and other humoral factors that function at the mucosal level.

ALLERGIC PROTECTIVE PROPERTIES

In discussing the allergic protective properties of human milk, it is difficult to identify specific protective factors that are proved to protect against allergy. It is equally difficult to discuss the proposed mechanisms of protection because the exact mechanism of "oral tolerance" remains theoretical and the relative importance of contributing factors to hypersensitivity must still be adequately defined. Some of the important variables concerning tolerance and sensitization are genetic background of the host, nature and dose of the antigen, frequency of exposure, timing (age) at first and subsequent exposures, immunologic status of the host, and route of exposure.

During the neonatal period the small intestine has increased permeability to macromolecules. Infants have more serum and secretory antibodies against dietary proteins than children or adults. Production of IgA in the intestinal tract is delayed until 6 weeks to 3 months of age. IgA in colostrum and breast milk prevents the absorption of foreign macromolecules when the infant's immune system is immature. Mucin, oligosaccharides, and other factors within breast milk may affect antigen presentation. Protein of breast milk is species specific and therefore nonallergic for the human infant. No antibody response has been demonstrated to occur with human milk in infants. It has also been shown that macromolecules in breast milk are not absorbed.

Indirect evidence can be inferred from a demonstration of an infant's response to cow milk protein. Within 18 days of taking cow milk, the infant will begin to develop antibodies. Since the advent of prepared formulas, in which the protein has been denatured by heating and drying, the incidence of cow milk allergy has been considered to be 1%. The most reliable means of diagnosing cow milk allergy is by challenging with isolated cow milk protein. Although circulating antibodies and coproantibodies have been identified, these are not reliable techniques for the clinician involved in patient care.

The allergic syndromes that have been associated with cow milk allergy include gastroenteropathy, atopic dermatitis, allergic rhinitis, chronic pulmonary disease, asthma, eosinophilia, failure to thrive, and SIDS, or cot death, which has in some cases been attributed to anaphylaxis to cow milk.[157,158] The GI symptoms have received the greatest attention and include spitting, colic, diarrhea, blood in the stools, frank vomiting, weight loss, malabsorption, colitis, and failure to thrive. Cow milk has been associated with the GI protein and blood loss. The diagnosis is best made by elimination of cow milk from diet and, when appropriate, challenge tests. Cutaneous testing is of little help. Cow milk allergy has been described in breastfed infants, and exclusive breastfeeding alone is not sufficient to protect an infant at high risk to become sensitized to cow milk proteins.[159] The incidence of cow milk allergy in exclusively breastfed infants has been estimated as 0.4% to 0.5% compared with the overall incidence ranging from 1.9% to 7.5% in population-based studies.[159]

Murray[160] showed the association of nasal secretion eosinophilia with infants freely fed cow milk or solid foods as compared with eosinophilia in strictly breastfed infants. In infants receiving cow milk, 32% had high eosinophilic secretions, and only 11% of breastfed infants had eosinophils present in nasal secretions.

Not surprisingly, many different antigenic specificities are recognized when the colostrum or milk of one species is fed to or injected into another species. Cow milk is high on the list of food allergens, particularly in children; sensitivity to cow milk is responsible for at least 20% of all pediatric allergic conditions, according to Gerrard.[161] Evidence indicates that IgA antibodies play an important role in confining food antigens to the gut. Food antigens given to bottle fed infants before they can make their own IgA, and when they are deprived of that in human milk and the plasma cells, may be expected to be more readily absorbed.

Glaser[162] first made the association between the drop in breastfeeding and the rise in allergy. He pioneered the theory of prophylactic management of allergy. Allergy in infancy is associated with a familial history of atopic disease and elevated cord blood IgE levels. The introduction of "foreign" proteins to the infant's diet and even to the mother's diet in the breastfeeding dyad can lead to allergic symptoms in the infant. Exclusive breastfeeding does not protect high-risk children from allergic symptoms unless the mother also adheres closely to a restrictive diet that excludes common allergens.[163,164]

There is a large body of literature examining whether breastfeeding protects against atopic disease. In 1988, Kramer defined 12 standards for methodology and the study of allergy and breastfeeding. The standards clarified the definitions of breastfeeding, measurable outcomes, and the diagnostic criteria for specific allergic syndromes, defined children at high risk for atopic disease, and addressed methods to decrease bias and control for confounding variables.[8] Several recent large meta-analyses have been performed assessing the protective effect of breastfeeding against allergic rhinitis, atopic dermatitis, and asthma.[165-167] Exclusive breastfeeding during the first 3 months of life protected against allergic rhinitis (summary odds ratio 0.74 (95% confidence interval 0.54 to 1.01) with or without a family history of atopy.[165] Exclusive breastfeeding for at least 3 months was associated with lower rates of atopic dermatitis in children with a family history of atopy.[167] Exclusive breastfeeding in the first months of life was protective against asthma during childhood [odds ratio 0.70 (95% confidence interval 0.60 to 0.81)].[166]

Chapter 18 discusses the prophylactic management of the potentially allergic infant. Chapters 8 and 15 outline the management of specific syndromes such as colic and colitis.

PROTECTION AGAINST INFECTION OUTSIDE THE GASTROINTESTINAL TRACT

Although protection against GI disease while exclusively being breastfed is well recognized, protection against infections in other organ systems is less well documented.[168] More than 1000 healthy infants followed in a health maintenance organization by Wright and associates[15] were found to have significantly fewer lower respiratory tract infections in the first 4 months of life if they were breastfed. A study of 128 infants with urinary tract infection (UTI) and 128 matched control subjects confirmed protection against UTI in the ever-breastfed infant. Infants breastfed at time of study had a very low risk of UTI, but ever-breastfeeding provided some protection.[169] Several authors have reported a decreased likelihood of neonatal sepsis in breastfed infants, in both developing and developed countries.[170-172]

PROTECTION AGAINST CHRONIC DISEASE IN CHILDHOOD

The major elements of the immune system in human milk are direct-acting antimicrobial factors, antiinflammatory factors, and immunomodulating bioactive compounds.[168] Epidemiologic studies have produced compelling information suggesting that breastfeeding for 4 months or longer can provide some immunologic protection against some childhood-onset diseases.[40,63,173]

An increase in childhood-onset diabetes was correlated with a decrease in breastfeeding in Scandinavia, retrospectively. In 1991, Viitanen and associates[174] reported a prospective long-term study among children in Finland that showed a significantly lower incidence of childhood-onset diabetes in those at-risk children who had been breastfed for 4 months or longer. Other epidemiologic studies have demonstrated a decreased incidence of insulin-dependent diabetes mellitus in breastfed children.[173,175,176] These clinical observations have been supported in the laboratory by studies of diet control in diabetic mice. The isolation of a bovine albumin peptide as a possible trigger of insulin-dependent diabetes mellitus makes further study imperative.[177]

The review of the national perinatal collaborative study by Davis and associates[178] showed a protective effect against development of childhood cancer by being breastfed for 4 months or longer for children followed for 10 years. The effect was greater for acute leukemia and lymphoma. The role of infant feeding practices showed a similar effect of breastfeeding as protective in postponing or decreasing the occurrence of inflammatory bowel disease in childhood.[179,180] Greco and associates reported a decreased risk of celiac disease in breastfed infants.[181]

Maternal renal allografts have a better survival rate in individuals who were breastfed in infancy when compared with those who were not breastfed.[182,183] The mechanism of these apparent long-term immunologic benefits remains unclear, although theories abound.[63] Confirmation of these proposed benefits by additional carefully controlled trials is required, given the potential for confounding factors and bias in large long-term studies.

SUMMARY

An increasing amount of accumulated epidemiologic literature, utilizing improved methodology and statistics, demonstrates the protective benefits of human milk for infants. A large number of bioactive factors have been identified and measured in breast milk over the period of lactation. Additional research is needed to clarify the interactions and the mechanisms of action of the many bioactive factors in human milk and then correlate these immunomodulatory actions with specific protective benefits for the infant.

REFERENCES

1. Hanson LA: The mammary gland as an immunological organ. Immunol Today 3:168, 1982.
2. Habicht JP, DaVanzo J, Butz WP: Mother's milk and sewage: Their interactive effects on infant mortality. Pediatrics 81(3):456, 1988.
3. Villalpando S, Hamosh M: Early and late effects of breast-feeding: Does breast-feeding really matter? Biol Neonate 74(2):177, 1998.
4. Bauchner H, Leventhal JM, Shapiro ED: Studies of breast-feeding and infections. How good is the evidence? JAMA 256(7):887, 1986.
5. Heinig MJ: Host defense benefits of breastfeeding for the infant. Pediatr Clin North Am 48(1):105, 2001.
6. Labbok M, Krasovec K: Toward consistency in breastfeeding definitions. Stud Fam Plan 21(4):226, 1990.
7. Coffin CJ, Labbok MH, Belsey M: Breastfeeding definitions. Contraception 55(6):323, 1997.
8. Kramer MS: Infant feeding, infection, and public health. Pediatrics 81(1):164, 1988.
9. Cushing AH, Samet JM, Lambert WE, et al: Breastfeeding reduces risk of respiratory illness in infants. Am J Epidemiol 147(9):863, 1988.
10. Dewey KG, Heinig MJ, Nommsen-Rivers LA: Differences in morbidity between breast-fed and formula-fed infants. J Pediatr 126(5, pt 1):696, 1995.
11. Howie PW, Forsyth JS, Ogston SA, et al: Protective effect of breast feeding against infection. BMJ 300(6716):11, 1990.
12. Margolis PA, Greenberg RA, Keyes LL, et al: Lower respiratory illness in infants and low socioeconomic status. Am J Publ Health 82(8):1119, 1992.
13. Popkin BM, Adair L, Akin JS, et al: Breast-feeding and diarrheal morbidity. Pediatrics 86(6):874, 1990.
14. Scariati PD, Grummer-Strawn LM, Fein SB: A longitudinal analysis of infant morbidity and the extent of breastfeeding in the United States. Pediatrics 99(6):E5, 1997.
15. Wright AL, Holberg CJ, Martinez FD, et al: Breast feeding and lower respiratory tract illness in the first year of life. Group Health Medical Associates. BMJ 299(6705):946, 1989.
16. Aniansson G, Alm B, Andersson B, et al: A prospective cohort study on breast-feeding and otitis media in Swedish infants. Pediatr Infect Dis J 13(3):183, 1994.
17. Beaudry M, Dufour R, Marcoux S: Relation between infant feeding and infections during the first six months of life. J Pediatr 126(2):191, 1995.
18. Duncan B, Ey J, Holberg CJ, et al: Exclusive breast-feeding for at least 4 months protects against otitis media. Pediatrics 91(5):867, 1993.
19. Owen MJ, Baldwin CD, Swank PR, et al: Relation of infant feeding practices, cigarette smoke exposure, and group child care to the onset and duration of otitis media with effusion in the first two years of life. J Pediatr 123(5):702, 1993.
20. Duffy LC, Faden H, Wasielewski R, et al: Exclusive breast-feeding protects against bacterial colonization and day care exposure to otitis media. Pediatrics 100(4):E7, 1997.
21. Duffy LC, Byers TE, Riepenhoff-Talty M, et al: The effects of infant feeding on rotavirus-induced gastroenteritis: A prospective study. Am J Publ Health 76(3):259, 1986.
22. AAP Working Group on Breastfeeding: Breastfeeding and the use of human milk. Pediatrics 106:1035, 1997.

23. Chheda S, Palkowetz KH, Garofalo R, et al: Decreased interleukin-10 production by neonatal monocytes and T cells: Relationship to decreased production and expression of tumor necrosis factor-alpha and its receptors. Pediatr Res 40(3):475, 1996.

24. Goldman AS, Chheda S, Garofalo R: Evolution of immunologic functions of the mammary gland and the postnatal development of immunity. Pediatr Res 43:155, 1998.

25. Holt PG: Postnatal maturation of immune competence during infancy and childhood. Pediatr Allergy Immunol 6(2):59, 1995.

26. Xanthou M: The development of the immune system. In Xanthou M, Bracci R, Prindull G (eds): Neonatal Haematology and Immunology. II. Amsterdam, Elsevier, 1993, pp 113–122.

27. Brandtzaeg P: Development and basic mechanisms of human gut immunity. Nutr Rev 56(1, pt 2):S5, 1998.

28. Brandtzaeg P: Mucosal immunity: Integration between mother and the breast-fed infant. Vaccine 21(24):3382, 2003.

29. Hanson LA, Silfverdal SA, Korotkova M, et al: Immune system modulation by human milk. Adv Exp Med Biol 503:99, 2002.

30. Goldman AS, Chheda S, Garofalo R: Spectrum of immunomodulating agents in human milk. Int J Pediatr Hematol Oncol 4:491, 1997.

31. Koldovsky O, Goldman AB: Growth Factors and Cytokines in Milk, 2nd ed. San Diego, Academic Press, 1999.

32. Goldman AS: Modulation of the gastrointestinal tract of infants by human milk. Interfaces and interactions. An evolutionary perspective. J Nutr 130(2S suppl):426S, 2000.

33. Ogra PL, Mestecky J, Lamm ME, et al: Mucosal Immunology, 2nd ed. New York, Academic, 1999.

34. Lewis-Jones DI, Lewis-Jones MS, Connolly RC, et al: The influence of parity, age and maturity of pregnancy on antimicrobial proteins in human milk. Acta Paediatr Scand 74(5):655, 1985.

35. Telemo E, Hanson LA: Antibodies in milk. J Mammary Gland Biol Neoplasia 1(3):243, 1996.

36. Kleinman RE, Walker WA: The enteromammary immune system: An important new concept in breast milk host defense. Dig Dis Sci 24(11):876, 1979.

37. Ogra SS, Ogra PL: Immunologic aspects of human colostrum and milk. II. Characteristics of lymphocyte reactivity and distribution of E-rosette forming cells at different times after the onset of lactation. J Pediatr 92(4):550, 1978.

38. Brandtzaeg P, Nilssen DE, Rognum TO, Thrane PS: Ontogeny of the mucosal immune system and IgA deficiency. Gastroenterol Clin North Am 20(3):397, 1991.

39. Brooker BE: The epithelial cells and cell fragments in human milk. Cell Tissue Res 210(2):321, 1980.

40. Goldman AS, Chheda S, Garofalo R, Schmalstieg FC: Cytokines in human milk: Properties and potential effects upon the mammary gland and the neonate. J Mammary Gland Biol Neoplasia 1(3):251, 1996.

41. Wirt DP, Adkins LT, Palkowetz KH, et al: Activated and memory T lymphocytes in human milk. Cytometry 13(3):282, 1992.

42. Goldman AS, Garza C, Nichols BL, Goldblum RM: Immunologic factors in human milk during the first year of lactation. J Pediatr 100(4):563, 1982.

43. Pickering LK, Kohl S: Human milk humoral immunity and infant defense mechanisms. In Howell RR, Morriss RH, Pickering LK (eds): Human Milk in Infant Nutrition and Health. Springfield, Ill, Thomas, 1986.

44. Pitt J: The milk mononuclear phagocyte. Pediatrics 64(5, pt 2 suppl):745, 1979.

45. Buescher ES, Pickering LK: Polymorphonuclear leukocytes in human colostrum and milk. In Howell RR, Morriss RH, Pickering LK (eds): Human Milk in Infant Nutrition and Health. Springfield, Ill, Thomas, 1986.

46. Ichikawa M, Sugita M, Takahashi M, et al: Breast milk macrophages spontaneously produce granulocyte-macrophage colony-stimulating factor and differentiate into dendritic cells in the presence of exogenous interleukin-4 alone. Immunology 108(2):189, 2003.

47. Keeney SE, Schmalstieg FC, Palkowetz KH, et al: Activated neutrophils and neutrophil activators in human milk: Increased expression of CD11b and decreased expression of L-selectin. J Leukoc Biol 54(2):97, 1993.

48. Hasselbalch H, Engelmann MD, Ersboll AK, et al: Breast-feeding influences thymic size in late infancy. Eur J Pediatr 158(12):964, 1999.

49. Head JR, Beer AE: The Immunologic Role of Viable Leukocytic Cells in Mammary Gland/Human Lactation/Milk Synthesis, Vol. 4. New York, Academic Press, 1978.

50. Keller MA, Faust J, Rolewic LJ, Stewart DD: T cell subsets in human colostrum. J Pediatr Gastroenterol Nutr 5(3):439, 1986.

51. Ogra SS, Ogra PL: Immunologic aspects of human colostrum and milk. I. Distribution characteristics and concentrations of immunoglobulins at different times after the onset of lactation. J Pediatr 92(4):546, 1978.

52. Bhaskaram P, Reddy V: Bactericidal activity of human milk leukocytes. Acta Paediatr Scand 70(1):87, 1981.

53. Richie ER: Lymphocyte subsets in colostrum. In Howell RR, Morriss RH, Pickering LK (eds): Human Milk in Infant Nutrition and Health. Springfield, Ill, Thomas, 1986.

54. Juto P: Human milk stimulates B cell function. Arch Dis Child 60(7):610, 1985.

55. Parmely MJ, Beer AE, Billingham RE: In vitro studies on the T-lymphocyte population of human milk. J Exp Med 144(2):358, 1976.

56. Ho PC, Lawton JW: Human colostral cells: Phagocytosis and killing of E. coli and C. albicans. J Pediatr 93(6):910, 1978.

57. Goldblum RM, Ahlstedt S, Carlsson B, et al: Antibody-forming cells in human colostrum after oral immunisation. Nature 257(5529):797, 1975.

58. Beer AE, Billingham RE: Immunologic benefits and hazards of milk in maternal-perinatal relationship. Ann Intern Med 83(6):865, 1975.

59. Goldman AS: Immunologic system in human milk. J Pediatr Gastroenterol Nutr 5(3):343, 1986.

60. Michael JG, Ringenback R, Hottenstein S: The antimicrobial activity of human colostral antibody in the newborn. J Infect Dis 124(5):445, 1971.

61. Stoliar OA, Pelley RP, Kaniecki-Green E, et al: Secretory IgA against enterotoxins in breast-milk. Lancet 1(7972):1258, 1976.

62. Schultz CL, Coffman RL: Control of isotype switching by T cells and cytokines. Curr Opin Immunol 3:350, 1991.

63. Goldman AS: The immune system of human milk: Antimicrobial, antiinflammatory and immunomodulating properties. Pediatr Infect Dis J 12(8):664, 1993.

64. Whitmore AC, Prowse DM, Haughton G, Arnold LW: Ig isotype switching in B lymphocytes. The effect of T cell-derived interleukins, cytokines, cholera toxin, and antigen on isotype switch frequency of a cloned B cell lymphoma. Int Immunol 3(1):95, 1991.

65. Brandtzaeg P: Mucosal and glandular distribution of immunoglobulin components: Differential localization of free and bound SC in secretory epithelial cells. J Immunol 112:1553, 1974.

66. Goldman AS, Chheda S, Keeney SE, et al: Immunologic protection of the premature newborn by human milk. Sem Perinatol 18:495, 1994.

67. Peitersen B, Bohn L, Andersen H: Quantitative determination of immunoglobulins, lysozyme, and certain electrolytes in breast milk during the entire period of lactation, during a 24-hour period, and in milk from the individual mammary gland. Acta Paediatr Scand 64(5):709, 1975.

68. Ogra SS, Weintraub DI, Ogra PL: Immunologic aspects of human colostrum and milk: Interaction with the intestinal immunity of the neonate. Adv Exp Med Biol 107:95, 1978.

69. Bahna SL, Keller MA, Heiner DC: IgE and IgD in human colostrum and plasma. Pediatr Res 16(8):604, 1982.

70. McClelland DB: Antibodies in milk. J Reprod Fertil 65(2):537, 1982.

71. Keller MA, Heiner DC, Myers AS, Reisinger DM: IgD in human colostrum. Pediatr Res 19(1):122, 1985.

72. Butte NF, Goldblum RM, Fehl LM, et al: Daily ingestion of immunologic components in human milk during the first four months of life. Acta Paediatr Scand 73(3):296, 1984.

73. Davidson LA, Lonnerdal B: Persistence of human milk proteins in the breast-fed infant. Acta Paediatr Scand 76(5):733, 1987.

74. Miranda R, Saravia NG, Ackerman R, et al: Effect of maternal nutritional status on immunological substances in human colostrum and milk. Am J Clin Nutr 37(4):632, 1983.

75. Lovelady CA, Hunter CP, Geigerman C: Effect of exercise on immunologic factors in breast milk. Pediatrics 111(2):48, 2003.

76. Goldman AS, Goldblum RM, Garza C: Immunologic components in human milk during the second year of lactation. Acta Paediatr Scand 72(3):461, 1983.

77. Jatsyk GV, Kuvaeva IB, Gribakin SG: Immunological protection of the neonatal gastrointestinal tract: The importance of breast feeding. Acta Paediatr Scand 74(2):246, 1985.

78. Koutras AK, Vigorita VJ: Fecal secretory immunoglobulin A in breast milk versus formula feeding in early infancy. J Pediatr Gastroenterol Nutr 9(1):58, 1989.

79. Savilahti E, Salmenpera L, Tainio VM, et al: Prolonged exclusive breast-feeding results in low serum concentrations of immunoglobulin G, A and M. Acta Paediatr Scand 76(1):1, 1987.

80. Noguera-Obenza M, Cleary T: The role of human milk secretory IgA in protecting. Adv Nutr Res 10:213, 2001.

81. Ford JE, Law BA, Marshall VM, Reiter B: Influence of the heat treatment of human milk on some of its protective constituents. J Pediatr 90(1):29, 1977.

82. Remington JS, Klein JO: Current concepts of infections of the fetus and newborn infant. In Remington JS, Klein JO (eds): Infectious Diseases of the Fetus and Newborn Infant, 5th ed. Philadelphia, WB Saunders, 2001, pp 1–69.

83. Gyorgy P: A hitherto unrecognized biochemical difference between human milk and cow's milk. Pediatrics 11(2):98, 1953.

84. Beerens H, Romond C, Neut C: Influence of breast-feeding on the bifid flora of the newborn intestine. Am J Clin Nutr 33(11 suppl):2434, 1980.

85. Kaila M, Isolauri E, Soppi E, et al: Enhancement of the circulating antibody secreting cell response in human diarrhea by a human lactobaccillus strain. Pediatr Res 32:141, 1992.

86. Pelto L, Isolauri E, Lilius E-M, et al: Probiotic bacteria down-regulate the milk-induced inflammatory response in milk-hypersensitive subjects but have an immunostimulatory effect in healthy subjects. Clin Exp Allergy 28:1474, 1998.

87. Hatakka K, Savilahti E, Ponka A, et al: Effect of long term consumption of probiotic milk on infections in children attending day care centres: Double blind, randomised trial. BMJ 322(7298):1327, 2001.

88. Reddy V, Bhaskaram C, Raghuramulu N, Jagadeesan V: Antimicrobial factors in human milk. Acta Paediatr Scand 66(2):229, 1977.

89. Kerner JA, Yang CC, Stevenson DK: Effects of nutritional supplements on anti-infective factors in human milk. Gastroenterology 94:118, 1988.

90. Lonnerdal B: Lactoferrin in milk. Ann Nestlé 54(3):79, 1996.

91. Nuijens JH, van Berkel PH, Schanbacher FL: Structure and biological actions of lactoferrin. J Mammary Gland Biol Neoplasia 1(3):285, 1996.

92. Sanchez L, Calvo M, Brock JH: Biological role of lactoferrin. Arch Dis Child 67(5):657, 1992.

93. Bullen JJ: Iron-binding proteins and other factors in milk responsible for resistance to Escherichia coli. Ciba Found Symp 42:149, 1976.

94. Fransson GB, Lonnerdal B: Iron in human milk. J Pediatr 96(3, pt 1):380, 1980.

95. Donovan SM, Atkinson SA, Whyte RK, Lonnerdal B: Partition of nitrogen intake and excretion in low-birth-weight infants. Am J Dis Child 143(12):1485, 1989.

96. Hanson LA, Adlerberth I, Carlsson B, et al: Host defense of the neonate and the intestinal flora. Acta Paediatr Scand Suppl 351:122, 1989.

97. Tomita M, Takase M, Wakabayshi H, et al: Antimicrobial peptides of lactoferrin. Adv Exp Med Biol 357:107, 1995.

98. Crouch SP, Slater KJ, Fletcher J: Regulation of cytokine release from mononuclear cells by the iron-binding protein lactoferrin. Blood 80(1):235, 1992.

99. Guigliano L, Ribeiro STG, Vaninstein MH, et al: Free secretory components and lactoferrin of human milk inhibit the adhesion of enterotoxigenic Escherichia coli. J Med Microbiol 42:3, 1995.

100. Srivastava MD, Srivastava A, Brouhard B, et al: Cytokines in human milk. Res Commun Mol Pathol Pharmacol 93(3):263, 1996.

101. Gullberg R: Possible influence of vitamin B 12-binding protein in milk on the intestinal flora in breast-fed infants. II. Contents of unsaturated B 12-binding protein in meconium and faeces from breast-fed and bottle-fed infants. Scand J Gastroenterol 9(3):287, 1974.

102. Newburg DS, Neubauer SH: Carbohydrates in Milks: Analysis, Quantities and Significance. New York, Academic Press, 1995.

103. Newburg DS: Human glycoconjugates that inhibit pathogens. Curr Med Chem 6(2):117, 1999.

104. Newburg DS: Oligosaccharides and glycoconjugates in human milk: Their role in host defense. J Mammary Gland Biol Neoplasia 1(3):271, 1996.

105. Schroten H, Hanisch FG, Plogmann R, et al: Inhibition of adhesion of S-fimbriated Escherichia coli to buccal epithelial cells by human milk fat globule membrane components: A novel aspect of the protective function of mucins in the nonimmunoglobulin fraction. Infect Immun 60(7):2893, 1992.

106. Otnaess AB, Laegreid A, Ertresvag K: Inhibition of enterotoxin from Escherichia coli and Vibrio cholerae by gangliosides from human milk. Infect Immun 40(2):563, 1983.

107. Laegreid A, Kolsto Otnaess AB: Trace amounts of ganglioside GM1 in human milk inhibit enterotoxins from Vibrio cholerae and Escherichia coli. Life Sci 40(1):55, 1987.

108. Ruiz-Palacios G, Torres J, Torres NI, et al: Cholera-like enterotoxin produced by Campylobacter jejuni. Infect Immun 43:314, 1984.

109. Newburg DS, Chaturvedi P: Neutral glycolipids of human and bovine milk. Lipids 27(11):923, 1992.

110. Crane JK, Azar SS, Stam A, Newburg DS: Oligosaccharides from human milk block binding and activity of the Escherichia coli heat-stable enterotoxin (Sta) in T84 intestinal cells. J Nutr 124:2358, 1994.

111. Chaturvedi P, Warren CD, Buescher CR, et al: Bioactive Components of Human Milk. New York, Plenum Publishers, 2001.

112. Liles WC, Van Voorhis WC: Review: Nomenclature and biologic significance of cytokines involved in inflammation and the host immune response. J Infect Dis 172(6):1573, 1995.

113. Hawkes J, Bryan D-L, James M, Gibson R: Cytokines (IL-1[beta], IL-6, TNF-[alpha], TGF-[beta]1, and TGF-[beta]2) and prostaglandin E2 in human milk during the first three months postpartum. Pediatr Res 46(2):194, 1999.

114. Palkowetz KH, Royer CL, Garofalo R, et al: Production of interleukin-6 and interleukin-8 by human mammary gland epithelial cells. J Reprod Immunol 26(1):57, 1994.

115. Rudloff HE, Schmalstieg FC Jr, Palkowetz KH, Goldman AS: Interleukin-6 in human milk. J Reprod Immunol 23(1):13, 1993.

116. Takahata Y, Takada H, Nomura A, et al: Interleukin-18 in human milk. Pediatr Res 50(2):268, 2001.

117. Luster AD: Chemokines—Chemotactic cytokines that mediate inflammation. N Engl J Med 338(7):436, 1998.

118. Baggiolini M, Dewald B, Moser B: Human chemokines: An update. Annu Rev Immunol 15:675, 1997.

119. Buescher ES, Malinowska I: Soluble receptors and cytokine antagonists in human milk. Pediatr Res 40(6):839, 1996.

120. Pickering LK, Granoff DM, Erickson JR, et al: Modulation of the immune system by human milk and infant formula containing nucleotides. Pediatrics 101(2):242, 1998.

121. Quan R, Barness LA: Do infants need nucleotide supplemented formula for optimal nutrition? J Pediatr Gastroenterol Nutr 11(4):429, 1990.

122. Yu VY: Scientific rationale and benefits of nucleotide supplementation of infant formula. J Paediatr Child Health 38(6):543, 2002.

123. Carver JD, Walker WA: The role of nucleotides in human nutrition. J Nutr Biochem 6:58, 1995.

124. Leach JL, Baxter JH, Molitor BE, et al: Total potentially available nucleosides of human milk by stage of lactation. Am J Clin Nutr 61(6):1224, 1995.

125. Tressler RL, Ramstack MB, White NR, et al: Determination of total potentially available nucleosides in human milk from Asian women. Nutrition 19(1):16, 2003.

126. Carver JD. Dietary nucleotides: Cellular immune, intestinal and hepatic system effects. J Nutr 124(1 suppl):144S, 1994.

127. Carver JD, Pimentel B, Cox WI, Barness LA: Dietary nucleotide effects upon immune function in infants. Pediatrics 88(2):359, 1991.

128. Van Buren CT, Kulkarni AD, Fanslow WC, Rudolph FB: Dietary nucleotides, a requirement for helper/inducer T lymphocytes. Transplantation 40(6):694, 1985.

129. Balmer SE, Hanvey LS, Wharton BA: Diet and faecal flora in the newborn: Nucleotides. Arch Dis Child Fetal Neonatal Ed 70(2):F137, 1994.

130. Brunser O, Espinoza J, Araya M, et al: Effect of dietary nucleotide supplementation on diarrhoeal disease in infants. Acta Paediatr 83(2):188, 1994.

131. Lama RA, Gil-Alberdi B: Efecto de la suplementacion dietetica con nucleotidos sobre la diarrea en el lactante sano. An Esp Pediatr 48:371, 1998.

132. Navarro J, Maldonado J, Narbona E, et al: Influence of dietary nucleotides on plasma immunoglobulin levels and lymphocyte subsets of preterm infants. BioFactors 10:67, 1999.

133. Yoshioka H, Iseki K, Fujita K: Development and differences of intestinal flora in the neonatal period in breast-fed and bottle-fed infants. Pediatrics 72(3):317, 1983.

134. Glass RI, Svennerholm AM, Stoll BJ, et al: Protection against cholera in breast-fed children by antibodies in breast milk. N Engl J Med 308(23):1389, 1983.

135. May JT: Antimicrobial properties and microbial contaminants of breast milk—An update. Aust Paediatr J 20(4):265, 1984.

136. Narayanan I, Prakash K, Gujral VV: The value of human milk in the prevention of infection in the high-risk low-birth-weight infant. J Pediatr 99(3):496, 1981.

137. France GL, Marmer DJ, Steele RW: Breast-feeding and Salmonella infection. Am J Dis Child 134(2):147, 1980.

138. Gothefors L, Olling S, Winberg J. Breast feeding and biological properties of faecal E. coli strains. Acta Paediatr Scand 64(6):807, 1975.

139. Schlesinger JJ, Covelli HD: Evidence for transmission of lymphocyte responses to tuberculin by breast-feeding. Lancet 2(8037):529, 1977.

140. Newburg DS: Antiviral components of human milk. Mammary Gland Biol Lactation Newsletter 11:10, 1992.

141. Fieldsteel AH: Nonspecific antiviral substances in human milk active against arbovirus and murine leukemia virus. Cancer Res 34(4):712, 1974.

142. Downham MA, Scott R, Sims DG, et al: Breast-feeding protects against respiratory syncytial virus infections. Br Med J 2(6030):274, 1976.

143. Fishaut M, Murphy D, Neifert M, et al: Bronchomammary axis in the immune response to respiratory syncytial virus. J Pediatr 99(2):186, 1981.

144. Beauregard WG: Positional otitis media. J Pediatr 79(2):294, 1971.

145. Goldman AS, Thorpe LW, Goldblum RM, Hanson LA: Anti-inflammatory properties of human milk. Acta Paediatr Scand 75(5):689, 1986.

146. Thorpe LW, Rudloff HE, Powell LC, Goldman AS: Decreased response of human milk leukocytes to chemoattractant peptides. Pediatr Res 20(4):373, 1986.

147. Buescher ES: Bioactive Components of Human Milk. New York, Kluwer Academic/Plenum Publishers, 2001.

148. Buescher ES, McIlheran SM: Antioxidant properties of human colostrum. Pediatr Res 24(1):14, 1988.

149. Noda K, Umeda M, Ono T: Transforming growth factor activity in human colostrum. Gann 75(2):109, 1984.

150. Saito S, Yoshida M, Ichijo M, et al: Transforming growth factor-beta (TGF-beta) in human milk. Clin Exp Immunol 94(1):220, 1993.

151. Strober W, Kelsall B, Fuss I, et al: Reciprocal IFN-gamma and TGF-beta responses regulate the occurrence of mucosal inflammation. Immunol Today 18:61, 1997.

152. Garofalo RP, Goldman AS: Expression of functional immunomodulatory and anti-inflammatory factors in human milk. Clin Perinatol 26(2):361, 1999.

153. Murphey DK, Buescher ES: Human colostrum has anti-inflammatory activity in a rat subcutaneous air pouch model of inflammation. Pediatr Res 34(2):208, 1993.

154. Grazioso CF, Werner AL, Alling DW, et al: Anti-inflammatory effects of human milk on chemically induced colitis in rats. Pediatr Res 42(5):639, 1997.

155. Pang KY, Bresson JL, Walker WA: Development of the gastrointestinal mucosal barrier. Evidence for structural differences in microvillus membranes from newborn and adult rabbits. Biochim Biophys Acta 727(1):201, 1983.

156. Caplan MS, Kelly A, Hsueh W: Endotoxin and hypoxia-induced intestinal necrosis in rats: The role of platelet activating factor. Pediatr Res 31(5):428, 1992.

157. Johnstone DE, Dutton AM: Dietary prophylaxis of allergic disease in children. N Engl J Med 274(13):715, 1966.

158. Lebenthal E: Cow's milk protein allergy. Pediatr Clin North Am 22(4):827, 1975.

159. Jarvinen KM, Suomalainen H: Development of cow's milk allergy in breast-fed infants. Clin Exp Allergy 31(7):978, 2001.

160. Murray AB: Infant feeding and respiratory allergy. Lancet 1(7697):497, 1971.

161. Gerrard JW: Allergy in infancy. Allerg Pediatr Ann 3:9, 1974.

162. Glaser J: The dietary prophylaxis of allergic disease in infancy. J Asthma Res 3(3):199, 1966.

163. Bardare M, Vaccari A, Allievi E, et al: Influence of dietary manipulation on incidence of atopic disease in infants at risk. Ann Allergy 71(4):366, 1993.

164. Arshad SH, Tariq SM, Matthews S, Hakim E: Sensitization to common allergens and its association with allergic disorders at age 4 years: A whole population birth cohort study. Pediatrics 108(2):E33, 2001.

165. Mimouni Bloch A, Mimouni D, Mimouni M, Gdalevich M: Does breastfeeding protect against allergic rhinitis during childhood? A meta-analysis of prospective studies. Acta Paediatr 91(3):275, 2002.

166. Gdalevich M, Mimouni D, Mimouni M: Breast-feeding and the risk of bronchial asthma in childhood: A systematic review with meta-analysis of prospective studies. J Pediatr 139(2):261, 2001.

167. Gdalevich M, Mimouni D, David M, Mimouni M: Breast-feeding and the onset of atopic dermatitis in childhood: A systematic review and meta-analysis of prospective studies. J Am Acad Dermatol 45(4):520, 2001.

168. Hanson LA, Karlberg J, Ashraf R, et al: Health and Human Potential. Diseases. The State of Health of Children in the

Developing World. Rome, Pontifical Academy of Sciences, The Vatican, 1992.

169. Pisacane A, Graziano L, Mazzarella G, et al: Breast-feeding and urinary tract infection. J Pediatr 120(1):87, 1992.

170. Ashraf RN, Jalil F, Zaman S, et al: Breast feeding and protection against neonatal sepsis in a high risk population. Arch Dis Child 66(4):488, 1991.

171. Winberg J, Wessner G: Does breast milk protect against septicaemia in the newborn? Lancet 1(7709):1091, 1971.

172. Hanson LA: The role of breastfeeding in prevention of neonatal infection. Semin Neonatol 7:275, 2002.

173. Mayer EJ, Hamman RF, Gay EC, et al: Reduced risk of IDDM among breast-fed children. The Colorado IDDM Registry. Diabetes 37(12):1625, 1988.

174. Viirtanen SM, Rasanen L, Aro A, et al: Infant feeding in Finnish children less than 7 yr of age with newly diagnosed IDDM. Childhood Diabetes in Finland Study Group. Diabetes Care 14(5):415, 1991.

175. Borch-Johnsen K, Joner G, Mandrup-Poulsen T, et al: Relation between breast-feeding and incidence rates of insulin-dependent diabetes mellitus. A hypothesis. Lancet 2(8411):1083, 1984.

176. Norris JM, Scott FW: A meta-analysis of infant diet and insulin-dependent diabetes mellitus: Do biases play a role? Epidemiology 7(1):87, 1996.

177. Karjalainen J, Martin JM, Knip M, et al: A bovine albumin peptide as a possible trigger of insulin-dependent diabetes mellitus. N Engl J Med 327(5):302, 1992.

178. Davis MK, Savitz DA, Graubard BI: Infant feeding and childhood cancer. Lancet 2(8607):365, 1988.

179. Koletzko S, Sherman P, Corey M, et al: Role of infant feeding practices in development of Crohn's disease in childhood. BMJ 298(6688):1617, 1989.

180. Rigas A, Rigas B, Glassman M, et al: Breast-feeding and maternal smoking in the etiology of Crohn's disease and ulcerative colitis in childhood. Ann Epidemiol 3(4):387, 1993.

181. Greco L, Auricchio S, Mayer M, Grimaldi M: Case control study on nutritional risks in celiac disease. J Pediatr Gastroenterol Nutr 7:395, 1998.

182. Campbell DA Jr, Lorber MI, Sweeton JC, et al: Breast feeding and maternal-donor renal allografts. Possibly the original donor-specific transfusion. Transplantation 37(4):340, 1984.

183. Kois WE, Campbell DA Jr, Lorber MI, et al: Influence of breast feeding on subsequent reactivity to a related renal allograft. J Surg Res 37(2):89, 1984.

184. Raisler J, Alexander C, O'Campo P: Breast-feeding and infant illness: A dose-response relationship? Am J Public Health 89:25, 1999.

6

$\mathcal{P}$sychological impact
of breastfeeding

Although the previous chapters provide more than adequate information to support the preference for breastfeeding in almost every case, the critical impact in the return to breastfeeding in modern cultures rests with the issue of the mother's role and her perception of breastfeeding as a biologic act. The maternal influences include psychophysiologic reactions during nursing, long-term psychophysiologic effects, maternal behavior, sexual behavior, and attitudes toward men. All professionals providing support care in the perinatal period need to have a clear view not only of the biologic benefits of breastfeeding but also of their own psychological attitudes about the breast itself.

"For men, breasts are sexual ornaments—the crown jewels of femininity."[92] This is not true worldwide, however, and other body parts (e.g., small feet, nape of neck, buttocks) are sexually charged, with much of the fascination resulting from full or partial concealment. Until the 14th century, the nursing Madonna was the prevailing image, but in truth, the availability of a mother's milk meant life or death for every newborn.

The breast has assumed many roles throughout history, moving from sacred to domestic to political, to erotic. The definition of the breast has been provided by moralists, historians, poets, pornographers, lovers, and women themselves. Much of the rhetoric today is about the breast in crisis: "The breast is torn between nurturance, eroticism, and the fear of cancer."[92] In the eyes of the beholder, babies see food, men see sex, physicians see disease, business sees dollar signs, and religion sees spiritual symbols. Psychoanalysis places breasts in the center of the unconscious. The breast has a privileged place in human thought. Perhaps the love affair with science has turned women from being comfortable with their breasts as a source of infant nurturance to being uncomfortable and ashamed of breastfeeding, and yet has them searching through science and medicine for the perfect size or shape.[92]

The breast has been regarded as a sex object in the Western world for more than a century, and its biologic benefits have been downplayed. This is clearly demonstrated by the conflicting mores that permit pornographic pictures in newspapers, movies, and nude theaters but insist on the arrest of a mother for indecent exposure who is discreetly nursing her baby in public.

Proponents of breastfeeding have generally accepted, even before the upsurge of interest and research in attachment, that the major reason to breastfeed is to provide the special relationship and closeness that accompany nursing. Conversely, the major contraindication to breastfeeding was lack of desire to do so. This was evidenced by it being considered more appropriate to present breastfeeding as a matter of personal choice with no compelling reasons to urge a mother to consider nursing. The concern over creating guilt in the mother who chooses not to nurse has been significant and often resulted in a passive attitude on the part of the clinician so that the mother received no prenatal counseling about infant feeding.[46] As efforts to educate the public in general and women in particular about the benefits of breastfeeding have been increased, guilt is being used as a defense for doing nothing. Far more disturbing have been the aggressive attacks on breastfeeding promotion justified by the fear of producing guilt in the mother who chooses not to breastfeed. Other public health campaigns have not been muted or halted for fear of producing guilt in the obese, the smoker, or the drug abuser.

MOTHER-INFANT INTERACTION

The studies performed to understand bonding have largely been done without reference to breastfeeding. A supposedly comprehensive book, *Attachment and Loss,* by Bowlby,[10] which reviews early mother-infant interactions extensively, never mentions breastfeeding. In addition, sucking is given extensive treatment without making a distinction between bottle and breast or implying that an alternative to the bottle exists. The emphasis in the 1940s was on the effects of disrupting already-formed attachments. Separation in the neonatal period was ignored, and infant socialization was studied from 6 months of age.

Work by Spitz[80] and others has identified the devastating effects on the infant deprived of long-term maternal contact. These investigators demonstrated major deficits in both mental and motor development, as well as general failure to thrive. The impact on the mother had not yet been described. Klaus and Kennell[42] provided those data in their many writings on mother-infant interaction, which are summarized in their book, *Parent-Infant Bonding.* Evidence indicates that the maternal-infant bond is the strongest human bond when two major facts are considered: the infant's early growth is within the mother's body, and survival after birth depends on her care. Although the process had not been meticulously described yet,

Budin[13] noted in 1907 that when a mother was separated from her infant and was unable to provide the early care of her sick child, she lost interest and even abandoned the infant.

The immediate emotional reactions of mothers to their newborns were studied by Robson and Kumar[75] in 193 women (two groups of primiparas, $n = 112$ and $n = 41$, and one group of multiparas, $n = 40$). About 40% of the primiparas and 25% of the multiparas recalled that their predominant emotional reaction when holding their babies for the very first time had been indifference. Maternal affection was more likely to be lacking if the mother had had an amniotomy or painful labor or had received more than one dose of meperidine (Pethidine) unrelated to cesarean birth or forceps delivery. The authors found no difference between breastfeeding and bottle feeding mothers. The feelings of indifference persisted for a week or longer. This study points out that normal women may be indifferent toward their babies initially, whereas others experience great elation.

The development of positive feelings in primiparous women toward their normal newborns occurred before delivery in a third of women, immediately at birth or on the first day for 42%, and by the second or third day for an additional 19% in a study by Pascoe and French.[66] Breastfeeding mothers were more likely to express positive feelings. Labors of less than 9 hours were associated with positive feelings, but there was no association with social class, infant gender, type of delivery, or duration of initial mother-infant contact.

Klaus and Kennell[42] noted that mothers in the United States showed different attachment behavior when permitted early contact with their premature infants compared with mothers who had first contact at 3 weeks of age. Mothers of full-term infants who were allowed contact within the first 2 hours and subsequent extra contact behaved differently at 1 month and 1 year with their babies, compared with control subjects. Jackson and associates[38] made similar observations in the Yale Rooming-In Unit from 1945 to 1955 but failed to provide control observations.

In part because of the thought-provoking work of Klaus and Kennell[42] in the 1970s, remarkable changes have taken place in labor, delivery, and postpartum services in hospitals in the United States and around the world. Mothers have been "allowed" to have their infants to hold and cuddle as soon as possible after delivery, and fathers have been "allowed" to participate in the birth experience. The take-charge attitude of health care professionals has relaxed, and gradually hospital perinatal care has been humanized. In the meantime, a number of investigators have challenged the power of bonding. In a critical review of early and extended maternal-infant contact research, Siegel[77] suggests that although many longitudinal experiences affect parenting behavior in complex ways, reasonable judgment supports early and extended contact whenever possible.

When a normal, healthy infant born to an unmedicated mother is placed on the mother's abdomen immediately after the cord is cut, the infant crawls to the breast, finds the nipple, and latches on, beginning to suckle.[74] This event takes place unassisted by the mother or an attendant. The warmth of the mother maintains the infant's body temperature. This is described as a series of events beginning with the infant resting and occasionally looking at the mother, then moving toward the breast with some lip smacking and mouthing. Approaching the breast, the infant turns from one to the other breast before finally moving toward one nipple, bobbing over it, and grasping the areola and suckling. Experiments that involve washing one breast demonstrate the infant chooses the unwashed breast. When the mother has been medicated during labor, the "medicated" infant struggles to find the breast and often fails. Infants who are left with their mothers seldom cry during this awake, alert period.[74] If unimpeded, this process takes 40 to 45 minutes, which suggests the original baby-friendly mandate of initiating breastfeeding within a half hour may have been hasty. Physiologically, the stimulus to the mother's nipple and the stimulus to the infant's mouth trigger the release of vital hormones in both mother and infant, beginning the maturation of the intestinal mucosa and enhancing nutrient absorption for both mother and infant (Fig. 6-1).

This awake, alert period immediately after delivery provides an opportunity for receiving the first measure of colostrum, which is not only nourishing but also protective from an immunologic and infectious standpoint.

When the newborn is separated from the mother in the first hours post partum, crying occurs and stops on reunion.[40] The cry has been studied by sound spectrographic analysis in a group of infants in contact with their mothers for the first 90 minutes compared to those kept in a crib. The separated infants cried 10 times more than the contact infants. On analysis, the cry was characterized as a discomfort cry as compared with patterns seen in cries of hunger or pain.[56]

The impact of early mother-infant interaction and breastfeeding on the duration of breastfeeding has been reported; no data appear to be available as to whether mothering is different between breastfeeding and bottle feeding mothers in this early period.[37] Sosa and associates[79] reported the effect of early mother-infant contact on breastfeeding, infection, and growth. Breastfeeding mothers who were permitted early contact but not early breastfeeding were compared with mothers without early contact who also breastfed. The mothers with early contact were observed to nurse 50% longer than the control subjects. The early-contact infants were heavier and had fewer infections. Sosa and associates[79] conducted a similar study in Brazil, in which each mother nursed immediately on delivery and the infant was kept beside the mother's bed until they went home. At home, they had a special nurse make continual contacts to help in the breastfeeding. The control subject had traditional therapy, that is, contact at feeding times after an early glimpse. Infants were housed in a separate nursery. At 2 months, 77% of the early-contact mothers and only 27% of the control mothers were successfully nursing. The early and continued contact may have been accompanied by increased support and assistance from the nursery staff. This added support could facilitate breastfeeding and thus be the cause of the improved outcome.

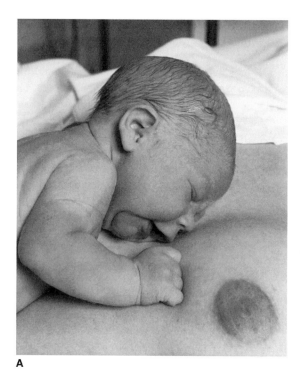

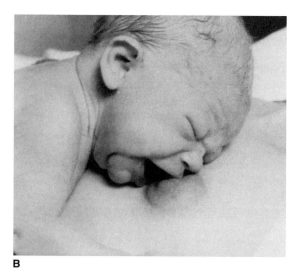

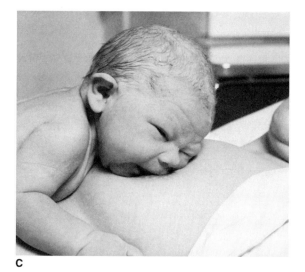

Figure 6-1. Infant crawling to breast (**A**), making mouthing and sucking movements (**B**), then taking breast (**C**). (From Righard L, Alade MO: Effect of delivery room routines on success of first breast-feed. Lancet 336:1105, 1990.)

An additional study of early contact by deChâteau and associates[20] in Sweden investigated a group of 21 mothers with early contact and 19 control mothers, all of whom were breastfeeding in the hospital. The only difference in management was the first 30 minutes of early contact, because 24-hour rooming-in was provided for all mothers after 2 hours post partum. The length of breastfeeding differed: for the early-contact group, 175 days, and for the control subjects, 105 days. Follow-up observations at 3 months showed different mothering behavior. The study group displayed more attachment behavior, fondling, caressing, and kissing than the control group.

Unless heavy medication or difficult delivery intervenes, an infant experiences a period when the eyes are wide open and the infant can see, has visual preferences, turns to the spoken word, and responds to the environment.[43] Similar periods in the state of consciousness of the infant may last only a few seconds or minutes over the next 1 to 2 days.

Although some mothers begin the attachment process when the decision to have an infant is made, after conception the physiologic changes in the maternal body strengthen the developing bond.[29] During pregnancy, listening to the fetal heart and watching echocardiographic images of fetal movements are confirming factors created by modern medicine. The first picture in the infant's scrapbook may be of the infant as a 12-week fetus. The moment of delivery, the first glimpse, and the first hours are intense opportunities for further "bonding" to occur. For some, however, the process will take a day or a week before the mother feels true love for this infant. Unfortunately, studies investigating this time line do not distinguish breastfeeding from bottle feeding women.

As in every area of medicine, new ideas and new theories invite criticism. The best type is neither partisan nor polemical and serves to repeat dispassionately the studies and confirm or disprove.[15,28] Many investigators have affirmed the "bonding" theory. Other critics,[4,15,17,27-29,44] however, have been hostile yet unable to disprove that biologic factors might play a significant role in a mother's response to her infant. A new group has called the theories "a bogus notion," reflecting medicine's need to control women and to enhance market demands and the status of medicine itself.[23] Further, it is argued that bonding is demeaning to women because it rests on the idea of instinct. These critics agree that increased contact between mother and infant in the first few days increases maternal emotional response, that early contact enhances breastfeeding, and that early extended contact decreases the incidence of child abuse, with effects solely on the parents, not the child.

Further study is needed, although randomly assigning a mother to a restricted contact control group would be difficult, if not unethical, today. Skin-to-skin versus clothed contact and hormonal components in relationship to behaviors remain to be explored. The father's and siblings' roles also deserve additional attention. Lamb,[44] however, has been supportive of the trend toward humanizing childbirth to provide a rich emotional experience for parents, in spite of his criticism of bonding research.

Sensitive periods in biologic phenomena are times when events alter later behavior. The existence of a sensitive period in human behavior is disputed, although it has been shown to exist in other species. There is a longer period of time during which human bonding occurs.[44] The power of attachment enables mother and father to make the many sacrifices necessary for their infant.[41] More than 30 years of investigation have confirmed the observations that the human maternal-infant bond can be facilitated, supported, and encouraged by more caring sensitive processes beginning in labor and throughout the perinatal period.

Human relationships are complex. A newborn brings joy, fear, anxiety, frustration, and triumph, reminds Richards.[73] Adaptability and compensation in the developmental processes are part of human existence. The concept of bonding has drawn attention to this period of life and begun the process of understanding the mother-infant relationship.[43]

BODY CONTACT AND CULTURAL TRADITION

If we look at other mammals, lactation behavior, including the duration and frequency of feedings, is species specific and predictable because it is a genetically controlled behavioral characteristic of the species. Only those animals kept in zoos or laboratories reject their young. Among higher primates, learning plays a significant role; monkeys reared without role models have to be taught how to groom and feed their young. In the human, breastfeeding behavior is highly variable from one culture to the next. Different cultures of the world have different sets of "rules" about lactation as they do about many other aspects of life and even death. Cultural tradition dictates the initiation, frequency, and termination of breastfeeding. Learning plays a key role in the lactation process, but the learning is focused on the beliefs, attitudes, and values of the culture.

The degree of body contact permitted by the culture is a fundamental difference among these cultures. Simpson-Herbert[78] describes the degree of mother-infant body contact as the physical and social distance that mothers keep from their babies. The physical distance is viewed as a reflection of the social distance sanctioned by the culture.

Cultures prescribe how often infants will be held or carried and how they will be carried (e.g., in the arms, a pouch, or a sling, or on a cradleboard). How infants are clothed, where they are placed when not held, and where they spend the night are all culturally determined and also affect breastfeeding. The cultural constraints that control maternal behavior include those on the kinds and amounts of maternal clothing, acceptability of breast exposure, and beliefs on frequency and length of feedings.

The effect of increased carrying of infants was studied by Hunziker and Barr[36] in a group of primiparous breastfeeding women in Montreal. The crying pattern of normal infants in industrialized societies has been reported to increase until 6 weeks of age, followed by a decline to 4 months, with most crying occurring in the evening. The investigators had the study families increase carrying the infants either in the arms or in a carrier to a minimum of 3 hours a day, whereas control infants were placed in a crib or a seat with a mobile in view. At 6 weeks, there was significantly less (43%) crying in the "carried" infants, especially in the evening. Similar but smaller differences were noted at 4, 8, and 12 weeks.

When Cunningham and associates[18] randomly provided either soft baby carriers or plastic infant seats to a group of low-income women in a clinic in New York City, they found the infants carried in a soft carrier were more securely attached than those placed in a seat when tested with the Ainsworth Strange-Situation Study. The study and control infant groups had an equal number of breastfeeders, and thus, the authors found no effect of breastfeeding on study results. They concluded that in low-income groups, mother-infant relationships benefited from early use of soft carriers and "contact comfort."[18]

Although the mean length of breastfeeding was similar in both groups, the breastfeeding was not defined, that is, as exclusive, partial, or minimal. Also, time spent holding to breastfeed versus time spent holding to bottle feed was not noted. There were 21 breastfeeders and 28 bottle feeders.[18] Although it is helpful to use carriers with bottle fed infants, it should not be done to the abandonment of breastfeeding support programs.

Anthropologic studies of 60 societies by Whiting[90] considered mother-infant body contact. He classified these cultures as high or low in contact as follows:

Culture classification	Minimum distance between mother and child
High contact: ↓ Symbiotic identification ↓ Long breastfeeding	1. Infant almost continuously carried by mother in the early months. 2. Little or no clothing separates the mother and infant so that they are in skin-to-skin contact. 3. Infant sleeps with mother.
Low contact: ↓ Ambivalent dependency ↓ Early weaning	1. Infant is separated from mother at birth. 2. Infant is often swaddled or elaborately clothed. 3. Infant is kept in a crib or cradle-board. 4. Infant does not sleep with mother at night.

Other factors influence the development of cultural mores, including climate and means of food gathering. Simpson-Herbert[78] points out that when infants are heavily clothed and swaddled, as in cold climates, they are neat packages that can be put down easily. The Eskimo is an exception, however, keeping the infant inside her parka for warmth and frequent feeding. Breastfeeding is almost axiomatic in warm climates where clothing is loose or absent; there is frequent holding and carrying, and the breast is readily accessible.

The diet of the hunter-gatherer society is not conducive to early weaning because meat, roots, nuts, and berries are difficult for infants to chew and digest, whereas the softer foods of the agricultural societies can be prepared for early infant feeding.

Study of specific world societies reveals that North American and European women are concerned with the beliefs that it is indecent to expose the breast, it is possible to spoil an infant with too much handling, and early weaning is a sign of infant development. Western mothers keep their distance from their babies. Mothers in high-body contact societies spend at least 75% of the time in contact with their babies, whereas low-contact societies spend less than 25%.

Since the 1990s, infant care in Western societies has included carrying infants in carriers close to the parent's body. Co-sleeping with the infant for easy access to the breast through the night and the concept of the family bed have emerged as more conducive to good parent-infant attachment. Their role in sudden infant death syndrome (SIDS) is being evaluated. Data on bottle feeding and co-sleeping are not available.

The practice of co-sleeping and bed sharing, although customary in many cultures, is rare in industrialized societies. Careful scientific study of co-sleeping has revealed a number of benefits, but present custom is based on the bottle feeding philosophy that embraces separation of parent and child. Where the infant sleeps is not just a family issue but a medical one according to McKenna,[54] who has performed the seminal studies on co-sleeping and pointed out the benefits of bed sharing. As a result of extensive study on the subject, the Academy of Breastfeeding Medicine has developed "A Guideline on Co-Sleeping and Breastfeeding" (Box 6-1).[1]

Box 6-1   Safe sleeping environments for infants

Families should be given all the information that is known about safe sleep environments for their infants, including the following:
- Place babies in a supine position for sleep.
- Use a firm, flat surface and avoid waterbeds, couches, sofas, pillows, soft materials, and loose bedding.
- Use only a thin blanket to cover the infant. Assure the head will not be covered. In a cold room the infant could be kept in an infant sleeper to maintain warmth.
- Avoid the use of quilts, duvets, comforters, pillows, and stuffed animals in the infant's sleep environment.
- Never put an infant down to sleep on a pillow or adjacent to a pillow.
- Never leave an infant alone on an adult bed.
- Inform families that adult beds have potential risks and are not designed to meet federal safety standards for infants.
- Ensure that there are no spaces between the mattress and headboard, walls, and other surfaces that may entrap the infant and lead to suffocation.

From Academy of Breastfeeding Medicine: A guideline on co-sleeping and breastfeeding. ABM News Views 9:10, 2003.

Breastfeeding is often enhanced by bed sharing, and provided the precautions are noted, bed sharing is safe and healthy.

PSYCHOLOGICAL DIFFERENCE BETWEEN BREASTFEEDING AND BOTTLE FEEDING

Professionals have spent decades reassuring mothers that they can capture the same emotional and behavioral experience by feeding an infant from a bottle as they can feeding at the breast, with the same warmth and love. Technically speaking, the same warmth is not there, because the lactating breast has been shown to be warmer than the nonlactating breast. This warmth can be demonstrated by infrared pictures and thermograms. Responses to stress appear to be muted in lactating women. Using graded treadmill exercises, lactating women had significantly decreased plasma levels of ACTH (adrenocorticotropic hormone, or corticotropin), cortisol, and epinephrine compared to match-control nonlactating women. Plasma glucose did not rise as it did in nonlactating women.

Mezzacappa and Katkin[55] examined subjective stress as well as individual differences in both breastfeeding and bottle feeding mothers at 1 to 12 months post partum. They administered the Perceived Stress Scale (PSS) and the trait component of the State-Trait Personality Inventory (STPI). The 10-item PSS is widely used to index subjective stress, and the STPI is a 30-item questionnaire assessing anxiety, anger, and curiosity. Breastfeeding mothers had significantly less perceived stress in the month preceding the test than did the bottle feeders. There were no significant differences among groups in anxiety, anger, or curiosity. Maternal age, time post partum, parity, and work status were controlled for. In a second experiment, the authors examined the acute psychological effects of breastfeeding and bottle feeding. Positive and negative mood were assessed in the same mother before and after a feeding. They recruited mothers who were both breastfeeding and bottle feeding, studying them in two sessions a week apart, randomly sequenced. The mothers completed the Positive and Negative Affect Scale (PANAS), rested 10 minutes, fed the infant, rested 10 minutes, and retook the PANAS. The mood became significantly less positive after bottle feeding than after breastfeeding. Mood became significantly less negative after breastfeeding than after bottle feeding. A possible explanation is the surge of oxytocin during let-down. Uvnäs-Moberg[85,86] has reported mood effects of breastfeeding mediated by oxytocin. She describes oxytocin levels as inversely related to negative moods and emotions. The higher the levels of oxytocin, the more calm the mother.

Mezzacappa and Katkin conclude that the results confirm that breastfeeding buffers mood. They attributed this to psychological effects of breastfeeding itself and not to the differences between breastfeeders and bottle feeders, because the participants did both and were their own controls.

Newton and Newton[63] suggest that special caution should be used in evaluating statistical associative studies that purport to investigate the hypothesis that breastfeeding and bottle feeding are psychological equivalents. "Because breastfeeding involves a large measure of personal choice and because it is related to attitudinal and personality factors, no groups of breastfeeders and bottle feeders are likely to be equal in other respects. Therefore the relation of breastfeeding to any particular psychosocial measure may not be cause and effect, but simply the differences due to other uncontrolled covariables."[63] A human mother's care of her infant is derived from a complex mixture of her genetic endowment, the response of the infant, a long history of interpersonal relationships, her family constellation, this and previous pregnancies, and the community and culture.

The method chosen to feed a baby is but one item in a whole style of maternal-child interaction. It is unlikely that this style is determined by the method of feeding, according to Richards.[72] Breastfeeding is a very different activity when it is carried out by a small minority compared with breastfeeding that is commonplace in the community.

In a study of patterns of variation in breastfeeding behaviors, Quandt[70] offers three explanations: cultural, biologic, and biocultural. Predictions of exclusive breastfeeding duration were most accurate for women with a breastfeeding style of infrequent feedings and therefore early weaning, whereas predictions for women with a style of frequent feeding were confounded by cultural factors that independently affected supplementation.

Before reviewing specific psychological attributes relating to breastfeeding, the distinction between styles of nursing in Western societies should be considered. The Interagency Group for Action on Breastfeeding developed a schema for breastfeeding definitions. Newton and Newton,[63] however, have described two distinct styles, unrestricted breastfeeding and token breastfeeding, which are important to understanding maternal choices.

Unrestricted breastfeeding

Unrestricted breastfeeding means the infant is put to the breast whenever he or she cries or fusses. Feeding is ad lib and not by the clock, usually leading to 10 or more feedings a day. The infant receives no bottles, and solids are not introduced until the second half of the first year. Breast milk continues to be a major source of nourishment beyond the first year of life. It is interesting that this was routine practice in the United States in the beginning of the 20th century, as attested by writings on the subject of child rearing.

Token breastfeeding

Token breastfeeding means feeding characterized by rules and regulations. Both frequency and duration of feeding are determined by the clock. It is deemed unnecessary to permit unlimited suckling. Weaning usually occurs by the third month, if not before. Supplementary bottles and solids are not uncommon. As a result, the let-down reflex is never well established. Engorgement may occur. The infant is frequently too frantic from crying or too sleepy to feed well at the appointed times.

New definitions of breastfeeding (i.e., exclusive, partial) have been published to standardize statistical comparisons (see Chapter 1) but do not reflect the psychosocial differences between unrestricted and token breastfeeding. The American Academy of Pediatrics Section on Breastfeeding recommends exclusive breastfeeding for 6 months and the gradual inclusion of solids (never before 4 months), preferably at 6 months or later.

A University of Rochester study[45] of urban physicians revealed that those pediatricians who prescribed solids by 3 months or earlier also suggested supplementary bottles and had been in practice 20 years or longer. Most of the physicians in the family medicine program in the same community, however, provided no supplements and no solids until 6 months and had been in practice less than 20 years. More than 50% of mothers in that community who planned to breastfeed had made contact with some childbirth or breastfeeding program and chose their physician according to practice style.

Definition of breastfeeding in the United States has been undertaken by the Breastfeeding Promotion Consortium (BPC) convened by the U.S. Department of Agriculture semiannually since 1990. The report points out that there are many definitions (legal, programmatic [for WIC food allotments], surveillance, and monitoring) for policies and guidelines and for research. Descriptively, it includes initiation, duration, and intensity. The BPC is concerned about monitoring for surveillance purposes. The clinician needs to know frequency per day, length of a feeding, and the provision of any other liquids or foods.[46]

Imprinting, pacifiers, and dummies

Scores of infants are being introduced to pacifiers or dummies shortly after birth, all too often by an impatient perinatal staff member who knows a breastfed infant should not be bottle fed. Free pacifiers are being provided as gifts by some formula companies eager to beat the competition. The UNICEF/WHO 10 steps to becoming a Baby Friendly Hospital (see Chapter 1) includes the exclusion of pacifiers from the hospital's provisions. Do pacifiers have a long-range impact on infants? For bottle fed infants, probably not, if possible dental problems are excluded; a pacifier will provide the sucking a bottle fed infant may not receive during a feeding. For a breastfed infant, the answer may be different.

Human imprinting is little discussed in pediatric textbooks and rarely noted when discussing infant feeding, yet the human infant, as does any other mammalian newborn, recognizes the mother by the oral, tactile, and olfactory modes. "The most sensitive organ and the one over which a newborn mammal has the most control, its mouth, is the organ central to mammalian and human imprinting," states Mobbs.[57] It is believed that the imprinting process, or "stamping," as it was termed in the 1930s and 1940s, takes place for a brief period early in postnatal development when an animal seeks a particular class of stimuli (i.e., objects of a particular shape).[57] Having found such an object or one resembling it, the animal responds with an unlearned pattern of attachment behavior. The process is innate. Comfort sucking and formation of nipple preference are genetically determined behaviors for imprinting to the mother's nipple. The recognition of the mother is at first through the distinctive features of the nipple. Although imprinting is multisensory and varies from species to species, it is oral/tactile for the human and other higher mammals.

Mistakes and mishaps can occur in the process when the newborn fixes on a rubber nipple (bottle), thumb, or pacifier (Table 6-1). Geese have imprinted to a man's boot. In birds, innate responses are preferentially selective to supernormal-size stimuli. Nonnutritive sucking on thumbs or pacifiers is displacement activity that would normally be directed at imprinting to mother's nipple and reflects a tendency toward supernormal size. In other species with multiple births or litters, the offspring imprints to one teat throughout the lactation period. The one nipple preference sometimes reflects emotional attachment to the object rather than a preoccupation with a need for sucking. According to Passman and Halonen,[67] who found 42% of the interaction with the dummy to be nonsucking attachment, the preference for one nipple was maintained.

Mothers of thumb-sucking infants are less likely to breastfeed successfully, as was demonstrated in a study of 93 mother-infant pairs. Those who used a dummy or pacifier breastfed a shorter period (mean of 5.5 months compared with 7.5 months). Nonnutritive sucking on objects was added to the list of causes of lactation failure by Lilburne and associates[50] following this study. Margaret Mead stated that in those societies where access to the breast is unlimited and frequent suckling is accepted, there is no thumb sucking.[71]

A randomized prospective study of 750 mother-infant pairs performed by Howard and associates.[34] The pairs were randomly assigned to early pacifier at 2 weeks or no pacifier. There was a significant negative impact on duration of breastfeeding in the group given early pacifier.

Although the term "nipple confusion" has not yet been accepted in the medical literature, strong psychosomatic evidence suggests that human imprinting can be altered by introducing a foreign object during the process of imprinting.

PERSONALITY DIFFERENCES BETWEEN BREASTFEEDING AND BOTTLE FEEDING MOTHERS

Clear differences exist between mothers who practice unrestricted breastfeeding and those who bottle feed. There are even some distinctions between token breastfeeders and bottle feeders. It has been said that maternal personality is more important than either breastfeeding or bottle feeding per se to the development of the infant's personality.

TABLE 6-1   **Instinctive fixation on sucking objects in the process of oral, tactile, mother recognition**

	Objects of fixation			
	Human breast	**Filled nursing bottle**	**Thumb/finger/ knuckles**	**Empty bottle/pacifier (dummy)/cloth**
Nutritive	Yes	Yes	No	No
Animate	Yes	No	Yes	No
Non-self	Yes	Yes	No	Yes
Infant control	No	No	Yes	No

From Mobbs EJG: Human imprinting and breastfeeding: Are the textbooks deficient? In Llewellyn-Jones D, Abraham S (eds): Proceedings 16th Annual Congress, Australian Society for Psychosomatic Aspects of Reproductive Medicine, Pokolbin, South Wales, March 1989.

Experimenters looking at these factors have provided a wealth of somewhat conflicting information. Chamberlain[16] studied the differences between mothers who bottle fed and those who practiced unrestricted breastfeeding with their second child. The groups were similar in age, education, parity, intelligence, and socioeconomic status. The breastfeeding mothers were less defensive about their method of feeding, were more oriented toward home life, and had higher radicalism scores. The bottle feeding mothers confirmed the hypothesis that they had problems in trying to breastfeed their first child because of inadequate lactation, possibly a psychosomatic reaction. They also had a greater incidence of sexual performance problems, as indicated by a higher surgency score.* The breastfeeding mothers wanted their children to do things typical of children; the bottle feeding mothers preferred their children to be conservative and other-person oriented and urged them to be more adult.

Call[14] studied the emotional factors favoring successful breastfeeding and noted that of 104 consecutive mothers delivering at an Air Force hospital, 42.6% of the multiparas and 50% of the primiparas chose bottle feeding. Of the breastfeeding mothers, 48% of those multiparas and 40% of the primiparas were successful beyond 3 weeks. Failure was associated with engorgement, lack of let-down reflex, and psychological conflict. The two conflicts seen in those who did not nurse and those who failed were as follows:

1. They had a conflict in accepting the biologic maternal role in relation to the infant versus other roles society holds for women. The maternal role is considered a general class attitude in middle-class American society.
2. They had a conflict regarding the functioning of the breast itself, that is, as an organ for nourishment of the young versus a sexual organ, affording the breast the same psychological value as the penis in the male. Nursing thus became a "castration" threat.

PSYCHOPHYSIOLOGIC REACTIONS DURING NURSING

Newton and Newton[63] have equated psychophysiologic reactions during nursing to the degree of successful lactation. During unrestricted suckling, the gentle stroking of the nipple by undulating motion of the infant tongue occurs 3000 to 4000 times in a single feeding. This should result in an increase in temperature of the mammary skin and rhythmic contraction of the uterus. Failure to experience these signs in early lactation is related to failure to produce adequate milk.

Let-down reflex

The unrestricted breastfed infant cries, and the mother has the urge to suckle the infant because the cry has triggered her let-down reflex. The breast is turgescent and ready for the infant. Unrestricted crying is rarely seen in these infants. With token breastfeeding, such a response does not occur on schedule, and from feeding to feeding the milk supply may be little or, conversely, gushing. The infant is unable to cope with the unpredictability. Insufficient milk is rarely a problem when infants are carried and fed frequently.

The role of various hormones in inducing maternal behaviors in animals has been extensively studied. Rosenblatt[76] showed that both male and female rats, including virgin females, manifest maternal behavior after 5 to 7 days of contact with foster pups. Manipulation of estrogen, progesterone, and prolactin has demonstrated that estrogen is the most potent inducer of maternal behavior, progesterone usually is inhibitory, and prolactin strangely ineffective.

More recently, evidence indicates that prolactin does have a role in stimulating maternal behaviors in the rat, but only when it is primed by placental lactogens that affect the maternal brain (medial preoptic area) in regard to maternal responses at

---

*A higher surgency score indicates increased gaiety, enthusiasm, effervescence, and impulsiveness and an increase in conversion reaction symptoms (hysteria) and sexual anomalies.

birth.[12] The brain of the maternally behaving rat is altered as a result of the dam's behavior toward her pups. Morphologic changes are seen in the supraoptic nucleus, which contains oxytocinergic neurons important for lactation. The supraoptic nuclei of lactating animals have a higher incidence of dendritic bundling compared with those of non-maternal virgin rats.[59] These experiments support the concept that maternal behavior in lactating animals can have a profound effect on the morphology and physiologic functioning of oxytocinergic neurons in the hypothalamus.

When levels were measured in 22 puerperal women, the suckling-induced oxytocin during nursing was pulsatile, with discrete, short pulses.[84] When the women were subjected to the stress of loud noise (70 dB) by earphones or to the stress of performing mathematical problems, the frequency of pulsatile release of oxytocin was significantly lower. No difference was seen in prolactin levels or milk yield. These data suggest that psychological relaxation is necessary for a successful let-down response, confirming what Newton and Newton[63] had observed more than 30 years ago.

The induction of maternal behavior after administration of oxytocin experimentally in rats by Pedersen and Prange[68] demonstrated that estrogen priming is necessary for the effect, but oxytocin may be the triggering hormone for maternal behaviors. A strong relationship between the peptide hormones native to the central nervous system and the reproductive hormones results not only in endocrine effects but also in behavioral effects.[33]

The long-term psychophysiologic response to unrestricted nursing is a more even mood cycle than the mood swings associated with ovulation and menstruation. Unrestricted nursing is associated with secondary amenorrhea for as long as 16 months.

From studies in animals, Thoman and associates[82] have noted:

> The present experiments do indicate that there is a unique buffering system which appears to protect the lactating female from large variations in responsiveness during the process of lactating. Inasmuch as there exists considerable information that indicates that maternal factors have profound and long-lasting effects on the psychophysiologic function of offspring in adulthood, the existence of such buffering systems in the lactating females would appear to be of importance in the mother-young interaction.

In relating the rate of success in breastfeeding to experiences at birth, Jackson and associates[38] reported that the more difficult the labor, the less successful the breastfeeding. A direct correlation has also been made with the amount of medication and anesthetic given during labor and delivery and subsequently the sleepiness of the infant and, ultimately, the inadequacy of the suckling. Newton and Newton[63] observed that mothers who talked to their babies on the second day nursed their babies longer, that is, beyond the second month.

Modahl and Newton[58] measured mood state differences between breastfeeding and bottle feeding mothers when feeding and not feeding. They used the Curran and Cattep questionnaire, which measures transient mood states rather than personality traits. Bottle feeders showed significantly more anxiety, stress, depression, regression, fatigue, and guilt than breastfeeders. Mothers measured while bottle feeding reported higher levels of these states and more extroversion than the control group of bottle feeders tested in a nonfeeding situation. Another control group who were lactating but also gave bottles were measured while not feeding and showed less anxiety, stress, depression, regression, fatigue, and guilt than the average population. Measurements were taken at home with no examiner present.

The psychophysiologic responses of breastfeeding and bottle feeding mothers to their infants' signals were measured by Wiesenfeld and associates,[91] using physiologic monitoring, while mothers observed previously prepared videotapes of their own infants while they smiled, were quiescent, and cried. Strikingly different response patterns characterized breastfeeding and bottle feeding mothers across all response measures. Breastfeeding mothers were physiologically more relaxed but were more apt to want to interact with their child and expressed greater satisfaction with the feeding experience. The authors interpreted these patterns as suggesting a physiologic influence of breastfeeding rather than maternal personality factors influencing the choice of feeding mode.

When 60 primiparous mothers' maternal role adjustments were analyzed by measuring mother-infant mutuality and maternal anxiety scores, the infant-feeding method (breast, bottle, or both) was found to account for considerable variation by Virden.[88] Women who breastfed had scores indicating less anxiety and more mutuality, a central factor in maternal adjustment, than women who bottle fed. The Maternal Attitude Scale (MAS) was used. The findings are compatible with other studies showing breastfeeding to be emotionally gratifying and as stimulating a sense of emotional union between mother and infant.[48]

IMPACT OF SOCIETY, MEDICAL PROFESSION, AND FAMILY

Society

Newton[62] has pointed out that a woman's joy in and acceptance of the female biologic role in life may be an important factor in her psychosexual behavior, which includes lactation. She found that women who wished to bottle feed also often believed that the male role was the more satisfying role. Nulliparous women who planned to breastfeed their children more often stated their satisfaction with the female role, according to Adams.[2] Breastfeeding behavior has been related to a woman's role in life as influenced by her cultural locale, education, social class, and work. Breastfeeding rates and weaning times vary in the United States by geographic area. The smaller the community, the longer is the duration of breastfeeding. Cross-cultural studies in large cities show variation in rates of nursing. These rates are influenced by education, and in the current generation, the higher the education, the higher the incidence of breastfeeding.

Medical profession

The enthusiastic physician can influence the number of breastfeeding mothers in the practice;

this has been demonstrated. If the physician provides knowledgeable medical and psychological support, the success rate of the patients who intended to breastfeed will increase. Some patients who had not formed an opinion or given it any thought in their preparation for motherhood will be persuaded to try. In addition, this physician will attract patients to the practice who are already successfully breastfeeding but find their own physician unable or unwilling to support their efforts.

A study was done at the University of Rochester in a small community where more than 50 pediatricians practiced.[47] The pediatricians described their own practices according to the number of breastfeeding mothers (high, 75%; moderate, 50%; low, 25%). They were also asked when they started solid foods, general practice "regulations," and finally, how their own children were fed. The physicians with a high incidence of breastfeeding in their practices started solids after 4 months and had few rules and regulations about the practice, and usually their own children had been breastfed. The physicians with a high number of bottle feeders started solids by 6 weeks and had many rules and regulations about the practice, and their own children had been bottle fed. When asked about using lay groups to help their patients breastfeed, the female physicians were more apt than the male physicians to discredit what these lay mothers could do to help other mothers.

A national survey conducted among a representative sample of obstetricians, pediatricians, and family physicians by mailed questionnaire reinforced the observation that the physician's attitude and personal beliefs about breastfeeding influence the advice given.[45] It further confirmed that not all physicians were informed about current knowledge on human lactation, not all physicians discussed lactation with their pregnant patients, and not all believed it was worth counseling time when problems arose. Results in 1993 were similar to those of the previous decade, despite national efforts to increase the physician's knowledge base regarding breastfeeding.[46]

The family

Impact on the infant

For the infant, differences exist between breast-feeding and bottle feeding in the alleviation of hunger, the mother-infant interaction, oral gratification, activity, development, personality, and adaptation to the environment. Often mother and baby are alone together during breastfeeding, and the mother gives her full attention to the baby with stroking and fondling. Social interaction with the baby is less frequent during bottle feeding, and the mother is often in a distracting social situation or someone else feeds the infant. The breastfed infant has control of what is happening, or at least shares control, whereas the mother controls the bottle and the bouts of sucking.

In a study of newborns at 6 to 7 days of age, the effects of breastfeeding, giving breast milk by bottle, and just holding the infant were measured.[52] Results suggest that the total mother-infant interaction during breastfeeding has a positive influence on neonatal behavior. It induces a more stable state for an infant compared with that generated by giving the same human milk in a bottle and increases some sucking and holding times.

The attitudes of the husband, close family, and friends influence the mother's attitude toward breastfeeding. More important, these attitudes influence the rate of success and the age at weaning more negatively than positively. One study showed that a grandmother's interest did not influence the mother's decision to nurse as frequently as did a friend's (peer's) decision to bottle feed. A woman whose husband is not supportive of breastfeeding weans early, or does not start at all.[39]

Development. Early assessment of newborns in the first and second weeks of life shows more body activity with breastfed than bottle fed infants. They are more alert and have stronger arousal reaction. Statistics reported by Douglas[22] on age of learning to walk in Great Britain showed a distinct difference, with breastfed infants starting 2 months earlier than bottle fed infants. The longer the infant was nursed, the more striking the differences. Thus, prolonged breastfeeding does not impede development, as has been implied by advocates of early weaning. A study in Illinois in 1929 compared children exclusively breastfed for 4 months, 9 months, and over a year with bottle fed infants.[32] The children who were exclusively breastfed for 4 and 9 months scored significantly higher on achievement tests, but the difference was reversed beyond a year. Exclusively breastfeeding beyond a year increased morbidity as well, which is in keeping with the concept that solids should be added in the second half of the first year.

A cross-cultural study of 50 3-year-old children in Hawaii, reflecting the cultural diversity of the islands, provided periodic behavioral assessments as part of the Heptaclor study. The study, which used the McCarthy scales, showed that the duration of breastfeeding was correlated with general cognition, verbal and quantitative scores, and memory, regardless of socioeconomic status, gender, or pesticide exposure. There were no associations in this study to motor skills at 3 years of age.[7]

An extensive study by Morrow-Tlucak and associates[61] investigated differences between breastfed and bottle fed infants. Batteries of infant assessment measures and maternal interviews were conducted by trained examiners blind to the risk factors during home visits when the infant was 6, 12, and 24 months of age. The 350 children were born to women at the Cleveland Metropolitan General Hospital who were part of a study of child development and psychosocial risk factors. The Bayley scales and the Home Observation Measurement of Environment (HOME) were done. A significant difference among bottle fed children, children breastfed 4 months or less, and those breastfed 4 months or more was found at all points, with extended breastfeeding having a positive effect.[61]

Animal research has also shown a relationship of weaning time to learning skills. Since it has become evident that species-specific proteins and amino acids exist, it is possible that the brain develops more physiologically with the precise basic nutrients. Comparisons with animal species show that the more intelligent and skillful groups within a species are nursed longer.

Personality. The personality and adjustment of infants as related to their early feeding experiences have been the subject of much discussion. The personality of the mother and the temperament of the child need to be considered. Some conflicting information is reported in studies retrospectively analyzing the effects of breastfeeding on outcome in terms of security and behavior. The emphasis has been on the duration of the breastfeeding rather than on the quality of the relationship.

In a prospective study of a birth cohort of New Zealand children followed up to the age of 8 years, both maternal and teacher assessments of conduct disorder showed a statistically significant tendency for conduct disorder scores to decline with increasing duration of breastfeeding.[25] Overall, however, the authors suggest no real evidence indicates that breastfeeding is protective against conduct disorders.

When abrupt weaning takes place, it may be psychologically very traumatic for the infant and the mother. In animals, when the mother is stressed while lactating, the nursling's plasma cortisone levels are elevated. The psychologically depressed mother may not experience postpartum depression until the infant is weaned from the breast. It has been accepted that early experience, including feeding experience, does influence later behavior in the long run. The performance in young college women on an anxiety scale questionnaire (IPAT) and a personality inventory (EPI) showed that those women who had been bottle fed had higher anxiety scores and greater neuroticism than the women who had been breastfed, irrespective of duration of breastfeeding.[35] Much more study must be done before the impact of nursing at the breast is truly understood in the complexity of life's events.

Impact on the father

Since the birthing process moved into the hospital setting, fathers have been moved farther from the nucleus of the new family. In recent years, this trend has been reversed. Research on interaction with the infant focused on the mother until Parke and associates[64] observed all three together. In the triadic situation, the father tends to hold the baby twice as much and touches the baby slightly more but smiles significantly less than the mother. The father plays the more active role when both are present. The study was conducted with middle-class participants who had been to childbirth classes, but the same results were obtained among low-income families without preparation or the presence of the father in the labor and delivery room. The infant had to be relatively active and responsive to capture the father's attention. The investigators believed that fathers were far more involved in and responsive toward their infants than our culture had acknowledged. Other studies have shown that when fathers were asked to undress their babies and establish eye contact with them in the first few days of life, they showed more caregiving behavior 3 months later than did control subjects.

Newton and Newton[63] describe the early attachments of the new family as follows:

Father interacts with baby: engrossment
Mother interacts with baby: bonding
Baby interacts with mother: attachment

The father has been brought back into the childbirth scene as a coach. The coach role has been described as the father's role in shared childbirth. The idea of coaching has negative connotations, because a coach is one who presses the players to work and try harder but always to win. Ideally, the father should be a partner and supporter in labor, delivery, and breastfeeding. Raphael[71] has suggested that the father may well play the role of the doula. The *doula* is one who provides psychological encouragement and physical assistance to the newly delivered mother. Raphael further indicates that the lack of a doula to support the mother predisposes her to failure with breastfeeding.[71]

The stress placed on sharing responsibilities of parenthood implies an across-the-board division of labor. This implies that parenting is equal for women and men. There are complementary activities for fathers and mothers. Parents are not equally able to do all things. There is more to nurturing the infant than to feeding. The father therefore should play a very significant role with the infant. For instance, when the infant is fussy and does not need to be fed, comforting is often best done by the father. Nonnutritive cuddling is best done by the father.

According to Waletzky,[89] the father's most common negative reaction to breastfeeding is jealousy of the physical and emotional closeness of the nursing mother and child. The degree of jealousy may reflect how much and how happily the mother breastfeeds. Actually, fathers may express distress because they have no similar way to bring food and contentment to their baby. Male envy of female sex characteristics and reproductive capacity has been identified by Lerner[49] as "a widespread and conspicuously ignored dynamic." Improving the birth experience for husbands is a significant means of helping them feel closer to their baby and better about themselves as fathers, according to Waletzky.[89]

Fathers who object to their wives' breastfeeding may do so because they do not want to share this part of their lover with an infant. Some fathers express concern that the breast will leak and destroy any sexual mystique. On the other hand, many men take great pride in the knowledge that their infants will be breastfed and support their wives in this effort. The decision to breastfeed should be made with the full involvement of the father.

Impact on siblings

Although there is some information about siblings and breastfeeding with regard to behavior patterns, no known studies compare siblings of bottle fed and breastfed infants. Just as siblings frequently want to try the infant's bottle, they may want to nurse at the breast. The child will reflect the mother's attitude toward the breast and nursing. If the mother nurses secretly or in private and isolates herself from the family, it may cause concern in the sibling and produce feelings of shame or guilt toward the breasts.

Breastfeeding and feminism

"Breastfeeding empowers women and contributes to gender equality [and therefore] is an important feminist, human rights and women's issue," states Van Esterik.[87] Despite Eyer's statement that the results of mother-infant research "will be shaped to address social and political agendas . . . and women inspired by feminism helped to precipitate a reform movement that actively embraces bonding,"[23] Van Esterik points out that writers on feminist theory almost always ignore the breast and ignore motherhood as well. Breastfeeding advocates have been criticized as wanting to tie women down. Van Esterik[87] makes the following suggestions for women's groups:

- Request that policy makers consult with women's groups before breastfeeding legislation is drafted.
- Recognize that breastfeeding is an emotional issue for many women, and develop strategies for framing the issue in nonjudgmental ways.
- Plan how to counter possible negative effects, such as employers threatening to fire women rather than provide maternity entitlements.
- Ensure that breastfeeding campaigns stress the welfare of both mother and child.

Intimacy and breastfeeding

Breastfeeding is an intimate activity for some women, but most health professionals tend to present it in the context of the biopsychosocial model.[21] The closeness of the mother-infant dyad is a feminine image.

According to McAdams,[53] the definition of intimacy includes 10 characteristics in the exchange between people: joy and mutual delight, reciprocal dialogue, openness, contact, union, receptivity, perceived harmony, concern for the other's well-being, surrender of manipulative control and the desire to master, and being in an encounter.

The theoretical definition for intimacy, states Timmerman,[83] is "a quality of a relationship in which the individuals must have reciprocal feelings of trust and emotional closeness toward each other and are able to openly communicate thoughts and feelings with each other. The conditions that must be met for intimacy to occur include reciprocity of trust, emotional closeness and self-disclosure."

Breastfeeding provides body contact with another and is the source of comfort, security, warmth, and nourishment for the infant and reciprocity for the mother. The mother's perception of breastfeeding as intimate describes her concept of the mother-infant relationship. The spouse's perception, however, may have the greatest effect on the success and duration of breastfeeding. Jordan and Wall[39] suggest that "supporting the father during breastfeeding may help improve the mother's satisfaction with breastfeeding, the duration of breastfeeding and adaptation of both parents to parenting."

WHY SOME WOMEN DO NOT BREASTFEED

Before the trend toward bottle feeding can be reversed, one has to understand why some women do not breastfeed. It cannot be blamed on society or the medical profession when a woman cannot accept this as part of the biologic role of a mother. A physician who does not understand the complexities of rejecting breastfeeding cannot hope to assist a mother to succeed in breastfeeding.

Exploring the question of whether body satisfaction and maternal attachment affect breastfeeding, 38 women at about 35 weeks' gestation were given the Maternal Foetal Attachment Scale, the Eating Disorders Examination, and the Body Satisfaction Scale.[27] Women who intended to breastfeed were more satisfied with their gravid shape and had higher levels of maternal-fetal attachment. The mother's age and body mass index did not differ between breastfeeders and bottle feeders. Mothers with high body dissatisfaction did not breastfeed. Not surprisingly, five mothers with a history of bulimia had difficulty breastfeeding, and three thought it was distasteful and adversely affected their appearance.[80] In a report of six women with bulimia nervosa who had bilateral reduction mammaplasty, the surgeons report that postoperatively the women were relieved of their physical symptoms and had improvement in their psychological well-being. Previously women with

eating disorders had been disqualified for plastic surgery. Macromastia can cause a distortion of the body image and in such cases can be the root cause of the bulimia.[51]

Our society has assumed that no valid intellectual stimulation can occur in the company of young children. Mothers are made to feel intellectually stagnant and uncreative while breastfeeding. Indeed, they are also made to feel asexual at the peak of their sexual cycle. In response, new mothers struggle in panic to maintain their social and professional ties. They feel they must produce tangible works to be productive. Bloom[9] points out poignantly that one of the greatest intellectual voyages of our time was undertaken when Jean Piaget sat at his son's crib and observed the child's successive attempts to grasp a rattle. A nursing mother learns about her child through many internal, subjective, and kinesthetic modes that were not open to Piaget. When a mother wrote of her observations in this setting, her writing was ignored as unscientific and trivial.

Bentovim[8] has taken a systems approach to successful breastfeeding, pointing out that a range of physical, psychological, and sociologic factors are involved. "Breastfeeding is a systemic product of many interacting factors rather than a product of individual behavior only,"[8] according to Bentovim. A good experience with breastfeeding can ensure an intense interaction and synchronous response of giving and taking. According to Brazelton,[11] this is the essence of the infant's beginning to create a secure world for the self.

Beliefs and attitudes toward breastfeeding influence the choice and the success of breastfeeding. Bentovim points out that it may be possible to restore breastfeeding as the natural choice.[8] This would depend on society finding a system in which the breast can be accepted not only as good for the infant and development, but also as the object of less ambivalent and secret pleasure. Bentovim[8] suggests, "The role of the health professionals in this area is important in that only through the right relationship with the mother will a new source of mothering be found that can act as a form of extended family for the woman to identify with and to counteract personal, family, and cultural influences." Hendrickse[31] confirms this view and states that the biggest block in the minds of women relates to feelings of shame associated with breastfeeding. More than half the women in the Newcastle survey were prevented from breastfeeding because of a sense of shame.[5] The shame is a result of relating the breast to concepts of sexuality.

Failure at breastfeeding: grief, shame, guilt, or anger

When a mother who had planned to breastfeed is unable to because of illness in herself or her baby, or when a mother begins to breastfeed and must stop, there is a grief reaction. The mother experiences a great loss. Prolonged mourning and depression may occur. Some women report feeling more distant from this child than from her other children if the others had been successfully breastfed. The stronger the commitment had been to breastfeed, the stronger is the grief reaction. Few mothers found help, according to Richards[72] in this study, from either professionals or lay support groups. Professionals failed to understand the feeling of failure or loss. The support groups tended to magnify the guilt and sense of failure.

The emotions are complex surrounding this intimate activity. Physicians who must recommend discontinuing breastfeeding for medical reasons should be aware of the impact and provide for appropriate support for the mother. A woman's choice of feeding method does not make her a good or bad mother, and her inability to produce adequate milk for her infant does not make her a bad mother. Lactation failure is often a reflection on the system and the culture rather than the person.

A random sampling of educated middle-class women in a university neighborhood revealed a number of women who had had difficulty breastfeeding. The study did not describe methodology or how it was randomized, but the report reflected much shame, guilt, and finally anger.[26] Failure of breastfeeding by a woman or her friends can be a powerful influence against deciding to breastfeed a future child.

Fear, shame, and guilt were regarded by Freud as different forms of anxiety. Objective anxiety is fear (fear of failure) and arises from external dangers; social anxiety is shame resulting from the criticisms of others; and conscience anxiety is guilt.[19] Real external dangers produce normal anxiety, but when one overreacts, this is neurotic anxiety. Defenses against guilt feelings include repression, rationalization, and projection. Any guilt can be borne more easily if someone else has had a similar experience.[24] Thus, knowing other women have failed to breastfeed successfully helps relieve the guilt.

Lasting anger following lactation failure has become more visible. The woman who writes an angry tirade against breastfeeding in a letter to the editor after a news story supporting breastfeeding deserves understanding and support. She is likely a victim of poor medical management and inadequate social support to breastfeed. Letter writing can be therapeutic, but it is never a cure for the underlying hurt.

In our clinical experience, well-educated women who have difficulty producing enough milk or who have an infant who fails to thrive are driven to find out why. The Lactation Study Center has received many calls from women who may even have had trouble feeding one or more other infants and want to be "tested" to find the cause. Testing resources are limited and reveal little more than can be identified with a good history of breast response in pregnancy and post partum. The mother's need usually involves a desire to know that the situation is out of her control. The best management beyond ruling out simple remediable causes (positioning, timing, or reduction of fatigue) may be the therapy of a good listener and the reassurance that one is still a good mother. Confirming that the prolactin levels are low can be a great source of comfort for the mother that it was not her fault.

Avoiding guilt as a reason not to promote breastfeeding

In many interactions physicians, especially obstetricians, are encouraged to provide enough information about breastfeeding to a woman prenatally to allow her to make an informed choice. The response often is, "No, I don't want to make a mother feel guilty, so I say nothing."

No studies in the literature support this position. In the dozens of reports on efforts to increase breastfeeding among many cultures, there is no report of producing guilt feelings. Women interviewed with open-ended questionnaires have not mentioned guilt feelings in response to the questioning. The only individuals who ever mention guilt are the older generation whose daughters are now choosing breastfeeding. The grandmother feels guilty because no one ever told her; no one ever encouraged her to breastfeed. "If only she had known . . . if only her doctor had told her. . . ." In the interest of good health, physicians counsel their patients about good nutrition, weight gain, smoking, drinking, and a number of detrimental personal behaviors without any concern for the guilt they might produce because of the importance of the issue. The feeding choice has an equally important impact for both mother and infant.

In a study at the University of Rochester prenatal clinic, women were randomly assigned to the group attending the Best Start program to encourage breastfeeding or to the control group spending the same time in "counseling" about pregnancy and delivery but nothing about breastfeeding.[47] After delivery, interviewed mothers in both groups were comfortable about their own infant-feeding decision. Those who received breastfeeding encouragement and chose to bottle feed said it was right for them and denied any guilt feelings.

SUMMARY

Decades of research have shown that the breast plays an important role in the growth, development, identity, and psychological well-being of women. Not all women have the same level of comfort with their breasts or see them in the same light with respect to their primary purpose, the nourishment of the newborn offspring. The infant, on the other hand, when given the opportunity, will find the breast, seek out and latch on, and suckle. Infants at birth are programmed to breastfeed. Their innate reflexes of rooting and suckling are designed for breastfeeding. Infants also can be taught other mechanisms for feeding. The intricacies of how women choose infant-feeding methods remain to be identified. This choice is influenced by culture, community, personal experiences, education, and the opinions of those close to the mother.

The physician can make a difference. Women indicate that they rely heavily on the messages they hear from their physicians. The issue of guilt regarding choices is no more important in choosing to breastfeed than it is in choosing to smoke, drink, abuse drugs, or give in to problems of overeating. The physician's role in the latter situations has always been clear: take a firm stand and provide guidelines for the patient. In addition to providing information and support regarding infant-feeding choices, the physician is also in a very critical position to facilitate breastfeeding in its early hours and to be supportive and constructive in ensuring its success with appropriate monitoring of progress, not only in the hospital but in the first weeks and months of the infant's life.

The impact of breastfeeding on the mother herself is more difficult to identify. Mothers who breastfeed are not different at the onset but do change in their relationship with their infant. Breastfeeding does have an impact psychologically on both mother and infant.

REFERENCES

1. Academy of Breastfeeding Medicine: A guideline on co-sleeping and breastfeeding. ABM News Views 9:10, 2003.
2. Adams AB: Choice of infant feeding technique as a function of maternal personality. J Consult Clin Psychol 23:143, 1959.
3. Alder EM, Cox JL: Breastfeeding and post-natal depression. J Psychosom Res 27:139, 1983.
4. Anisfeld E, Lipper E: Early contact, social support, and mother-infant bonding. Pediatrics 72:79, 1983.

5. Bacon CJ, Wylie JM: Mother's attitudes to infant feeding at Newcastle General Hospital in summer 1975. Br Med J 1:308, 1976.

6. Barr RG, Elias MF: Nursing interval and maternal responsivity: Effect of early infant crying. Pediatrics 81:529, 1988.

7. Bauer G, Ewald S, Hoffman J, et al: Breastfeeding and cognitive development of three year old children. Psychol Rep 68:1218, 1991.

8. Bentovim A: Shame and other anxieties associated with breast feeding: A systems theory and psychodynamic approach. In Ciba Foundation Symposium, No. 45. Breast Feeding and the Mother. Amsterdam, Elsevier Scientific, 1976.

9. Bloom M: The romance and power of breast feeding. Birth Fam J 8:259, 1981.

10. Bowlby J: Attachment and Loss. London, Hogarth, 1969.

11. Brazelton TB: The early mother-infant adjustment. Pediatrics 32:931, 1963.

12. Bridges RS: The role of lactogenic hormones in maternal behavior in female rats. Acta Paediatr Suppl 397:33, 1994.

13. Budin P: The Nursling. London, Caxton, 1907.

14. Call JD: Emotional factors favoring successful breast-feeding of infants. J Pediatr 55:485, 1959.

15. Campbell SBG, Taylor PM: Bonding and attachment: Theoretical issues. Semin Perinatol 3:3, 1979.

16. Chamberlain RE: Some personality differences between breast and bottle feeding mothers. Birth Fam J 3:31, 1976.

17. Chess S, Thomas A: Infant bonding: mystique and reality. Am J Orthopsychiatry 52:213, 1982.

18. Cunningham N, Anisfeld E, Casper V, et al: Infant carrying, breastfeeding and mother-infant relations. Lancet 1:379, 1987 (letter).

19. Davids A, Engrew T: Introductory Psychology. New York, Random House, 1975.

20. deChâteau P, Holmberg H, Jakobsson K, et al: A study of factors promoting and inhibiting lactation. Dev Med Child Neurol 19:575, 1977.

21. Dignam DM: Understanding intimacy as experienced by breastfeeding women. Health Care Women Int 16:477, 1995.

22. Douglas JWB: The extent of breast feeding in Great Britain in 1946, with special reference to health and survival of children. J Obstet Gynaecol Br Empire 57:335, 1950.

23. Eyer D: Mother-Infant Bonding: A Scientific Fiction. New Haven, Yale University Press, 1992.

24. Fenichel O: Psychoanalytic Therapy for Neurosis. New York, Norton, 1975.

25. Fergusson DM, Horwood LJ, Shannon FT: Breastfeeding and subsequent social adjustment in six- to eight-year-old children. J Child Psychol Psychiatr 28:378, 1987.

26. Fisher PJ: Breast or bottle: A personal choice. Pediatrics 72:434, 1983 (letter).

27. Foster SF, Slade P, Wilson K: Body image, maternal fetal attachment and breast feeding. J Psychosom Res 41:181, 1996.

28. Goldberg S: Parent-infant bonding: Another look. Child Dev 54:1355, 1983.

29. Grossman ER: The parent-infant bonding controversy: A critique of the critics. Dev Behav Pediatr 15:379, 1994.

30. Grummer-Strawn L: Defining Breastfeeding in the United States. United States Breastfeeding Committee, 2003.

31. Hendrickse RG: Discussion from Ciba Foundation Symposium, No. 45. Breast Feeding and the Mother. Amsterdam, Elsevier Scientific, 1976.

32. Hoefer C, Hardy MC: Later development of breast fed and artificially fed infants. JAMA 92:615, 1929.

33. Hollander E, Liebowitz MR, Cohen B, et al: Prolactin and sodium lactate-induced panic. Psychiatr Res 28:181, 1989.

34. Howard CR, Howard FM, Lanphear B, et al: A randomized clinical trial of pacifier use and bottle or cupfeeding and their effect on breastfeeding. Pediatrics 111:511, 2003.

35. Hughes RN, Hawkins AB: EPI and IPAT anxiety scale performance in young women as related to breastfeeding during infancy. J Clin Psychol 31:663, 1975.

36. Hunziker UA, Barr RG: Increased carrying reduces infant crying: A randomized controlled trial. Pediatrics 77:64, 1986.

37. Hwang C-P: Aspects of the mother-infant relationship during nursing, 1 and 6 weeks after extended post-partum contact. Early Hum Dev 5:279, 1981.

38. Jackson EB, Wilkin LC, Auerbach H: Statistical report on incidence and duration of breast feeding in relation to personal-social and hospital maternity factors. Pediatrics 17:700, 1956.

39. Jordan PL, Wall VR: Supporting the father when an infant is breastfed. J Hum Lact 9:31, 1993.

40. Kennell JH, Klaus MH: Bonding: Recent observations that alter perinatal care. Pediatr Rev 19:4, 1998.

41. Kennell JH, Trause MA, Klaus MH: Evidence for a sensitive period in the human mother. In Ciba Symposium, No. 33. Parent-Infant Interaction. Princeton, NJ, Excerpta Medica, Associated Scientific Publishers, 1975.

42. Klaus M, Kennell J: Parent-Infant Bonding. St Louis, Mosby, 1982.

43. Klaus M, Kennell J: Parent to infant bonding: Setting the record straight. J Pediatr 102:575, 1983.

44. Lamb M: Early contact and maternal-infant bonding: One decade later. Pediatrics 70:763, 1982.

45. Lawrence RA: Practices and attitudes toward breast-feeding among medical professionals. Pediatrics 70:912, 1982.

46. Lawrence RA: Review of the Surgeon General's Workshop in Breastfeeding and Human Lactation for the American Public Health Association Meetings, San Diego, CA, November 1984.

47. Lawrence RA: Unpublished data, 1996.

48. Leifer M: Psychological changes accompanying pregnancy and motherhood. Genet Psychol Monogr 95:57, 1977.

49. Lerner H: Early origins of envy and devaluation of women: Implications for sex role stereotypes. Bull Menninger Clin 38:538, 1974.

50. Lilburne AM, Oates RK, Thompson S, et al: Infant feeding in Sydney: A survey of mothers who bottlefeed. Aust Paediatr J 24:49, 1988.

51. Losee JE, Serletti JM, Kreipe RE, Caldwell EH: Reduction mammaplasty in patients with bulimia nervosa. Ann Plast Surg 39(5):443, 1997.

52. Maekawa K, Nara T, Hoash E: Influence of breastfeeding on neonatal behavior. Acta Paediatr Jpn 27:608, 1985.

53. McAdams D: Power, Intimacy, and the Life Story: Personological Inquiries into Identity. New York, Guilford, 1988.

54. McKenna JJ, Thoman EB, Anders TF, et al: Infant-parent co-sleeping in an evolutionary perspective: Implications for understanding infant sleep development and the sudden infant death syndrome. Sleep 16:263, 1993.

55. Mezzacappa ES, Katkin ES: Breast-feeding is associated with reduced perceived stress and negative mood in mothers. Health Psychol 21:187, 2002.

56. Michelsson K, Christensson K, Rothgänger H, et al: Crying in separated and non-separated newborns: Sound spectrographic analysis. Acta Paediatr 85:471, 1996.

57. Mobbs EJG: Human imprinting and breastfeeding: Are the textbooks deficient? In Llewellyn-Jones D, Abraham S (eds): Proceedings 16th Annual Congress, Australian Society for Psychosomatic Aspects of Reproductive Medicine, Pokolbin, South Wales, March 1989.

58. Modahl C, Newton N: Mood state differences between breast and bottle feeding mothers. In Carenza L, Zinchella L (eds): Emotion and reproduction. Proc Serano Symp 20B:819, 1979.

59. Modrey BK, Hatton GI: Maternal behaviors: Evidence that they feed back to alter brain morphology and function. Acta Paediatr Suppl 397:29, 1994.

60. Montague A: Touching. New York, Harper & Row, 1986.

61. Morrow-Tlucak M, Haude RH, Ernhart CB: Breastfeeding and cognitive development in the first two years of life. Soc Sci Med 26:635, 1988.

62. Newton N: Psychologic differences between breast and bottle feeding. In Jelliffe DB, Jelliffe EFR (eds): Symposium: The uniqueness of human milk. Am J Clin Nutr 24:993, 1971.

63. Newton N, Newton M: Psychologic aspects of lactation. N Engl J Med 277:1179, 1967.

64. Nordstrom UL, Dallas JH, Morton HG, et al: Mothering problems and child morbidity amongst "mothers with emotional disturbances." Acta Obstet Gynecol Scand 67:155, 1988.

65. Parke RD, O'Leary S, West S: Mother-father-newborn interaction: Effects of maternal medication, labor and sex of infants. J Perspect Soc Psychol 23:243, 1972.

66. Pascoe JM, French J: The development of positive feelings in primiparous mothers toward their normal newborns: A descriptive study. Am J Dis Child 142:382, 1988 (abstract).

67. Passman RH, Halonen JS: A developmental survey of young children's attachments to inanimate objects. J Genet Psychol 134:165, 1979.

68. Pedersen CA, Prange AJ: Induction of maternal behavior in virgin rats after intracerebroventricular administration of oxytocin. Proc Natl Acad Sci USA 76:6661, 1979.

69. Petersen M: Breastfeeding ads delayed by a dispute over content. The New York Times C1, C4, December 4, 2003.

70. Quandt SA: Patterns of variation in breastfeeding behaviors. Soc Sci Med 23:445, 1986.

71. Raphael D: The Tender Gift: Breastfeeding. New York, Schocken, 1976.

72. Richards MPM: Breast feeding and the mother-infant relationship. Acta Paediatr Scand Suppl 299:33, 1982.

73. Richards MPM: Bonding babies. Arch Dis Child 60:293, 1985.

74. Righard L, Alade MO: Effect of delivery room routines on success of first breast-feed. Lancet 336:1105, 1990.

75. Robson KM, Kumar R: Delayed onset of maternal affection after childbirth. Br J Psychiatry 136:347, 1980.

76. Rosenblatt JS: Nonhormonal basis of maternal behavior in the rat. Science 156:1512, 1967.

77. Siegel E: Early and extended maternal-infant contact. Am J Dis Child 136:251, 1982.

78. Simpson-Herbert M: Breast feeding and body contact. Populi 7:17, 1980.

79. Sosa R, Kennell JH, Klaus M: The effect of early mother-infant contact on breast feeding: Infection and growth. In Ciba Foundation Symposium, No. 45. Breast Feeding and the Mother. Amsterdam, Elsevier Scientific, 1976.

80. Spitz RA: An inquiry into the psychiatric conditions in early childhood. Psychoanal Study Child 1:53, 1945.

81. Stein A, Fairburn C: Children of mothers with bulimia nervosa. Br Med J 299:777, 1989.

82. Thoman EB, Wetzel A, Levine S: Lactation prevents disruption of temperature regulation and suppresses adrenocortical activity in rats. Part A. Community Behav Biol 2:165, 1968.

83. Timmerman G: A concept analysis of intimacy. Issues Ment Health Nurs 12:19, 1991.

84. Ueda T, Yokoyama Y, Irahara M, et al: Influence of psychological stress on suckling-induced pulsatile oxytocin release. Obstet Gynecol 84:259, 1994.

85. Uvnäs-Moberg K, Widstrom AM, Nissen E, Bjorvell H: Personality traits in women 4 days postpartum and their correlation with plasma levels of oxytocin and prolactin. J Psychosom Obstet Gynaecol 11:261, 1990.

86. Uvnäs-Moberg K: The Oxytocin Factor. Cambridge, MA, DaCapo Press, Perseus Books Group, 2003.

87. Van Esterik P: Breastfeeding and feminism. Int J Gynaecol Obstet 47(suppl):S41, 1994.

88. Virden SF: The relationship between infant feeding method and maternal role adjustment. J Nurse Midwifery 33:31, 1988.

89. Waletzky LR: Husband's problems with breast feeding. Am J Orthopsychiatry 49:349, 1979.

90. Whiting JWM: Causes and consequences of the amount of body contact between mother and infant. In Munroe RL, Munroe RD, Whiting BB (eds): Handbook of Cross-Culture Human Development. New York, Garland, 1980.

91. Wiesenfeld AR, Malatesta CZ, Whitman PB, et al: Psychophysiological response of breast and bottle feeding mothers to their infant's signals. Psychophysiology 22:79, 1985.

92. Yalom M: A History of the Breast. New York, Knopf, 1997.

$\mathcal{M}$aking an informed decision about infant feeding

BENEFITS OF BREASTFEEDING FOR INFANT

In any statement about breastfeeding and breast milk (human milk), it is important first to establish breast milk's distinct and irreplaceable value to the human infant.

Species specificity

Species specificity encompasses all the benefits of being breastfed for the human infant, as breast milk is more than just good nutrition. Human breast milk is specific for the needs of the human infant, just as the milk of thousands of other mammalian species is specifically designed for their offspring. For optimal growth of brain and body, as well as protection against infection and development of immunity, human milk is specifically designed for the human infant.

Nutritional benefits

The unique composition of breast milk provides the ideal nutrients for human brain growth, especially in the first year of life. Cholesterol, docosahexaenoic acid (DHA), and taurine are particularly

important. Cholesterol is part of the fat globule membrane and is present in about equal amounts in both cow milk and breast milk. Maternal dietary intake of cholesterol has no impact on breast milk's cholesterol content. Formula naturally lacks human DHA and taurine. The cholesterol in cow milk, however, has been removed in infant formulas, which are cholesterol-free. These elements, cholesterol, DHA, and taurine, are readily available from breast milk, and are the essential nutrients for the human infant.

The maximum bioavailability of essential nutrients, including the microminerals, means that digestion and absorption are highly efficient. Comparison of the biochemical percentages of constituents of breast milk and infant formula fails to reflect the highly efficient bioavailability and utilization of constituents in breast milk compared with modified cow milk, from which only a small fraction of some nutrients is absorbed.

Nourishment with breast milk is a combination event, in which nutrient-to-nutrient interaction is significant. The process of mixing isolated single nutrients in formula does not guarantee the nutrient or nonnutrient benefits that result from breastfeeding. The composition of human milk is a delicate balance of macronutrients and micronutrients, each in the proper proportion to enhance absorption. Ligands bind to some micronutrients to enhance their absorption. Enzymes also contribute to the digestion and absorption of all nutrients.

An excellent example of balance is the action of lactoferrin, which binds iron to make it unavailable for *Escherichia coli*, which depends on iron for growth. When the iron is bound, *E. coli* cannot flourish and the normal flora of the newborn gut, *Lactobacillus bifidus (Bifidobacterium bifidum)*, can thrive. In addition, the small amount of iron in human milk is almost totally absorbed, whereas only about 10% of the iron in formula is absorbed by the infant.[111] Nutrients such as proteins are examples of constituents in human milk with multiple functions, which include preventing infection and inflammation, promoting growth, transporting microminerals, catalyzing reactions, and synthesizing nutrients.[128]

For decades, growth in infancy had been measured according to data collected on infants who were exclusively formula fed, until the publication of data in the 1990s on the growth curves of infants who were exclusively breastfed.[14] The physiologic growth curves of breastfed infants show a pattern similar to that of formula fed infants at the 50th percentile, with significantly fewer breastfed infants in the 90th percentile. This is most evident in the examination of the Z-scores, which indicate that formula fed infants are heavier compared with breastfed infants, meaning that more are obese.[17,33,34]

Infection protection

Leukocytes, specific antibodies, and other antimicrobial factors protect the breastfed infant against many common infections. Protection against gastrointestinal infections is well documented.[27] Protection against infections of the upper and lower respiratory system and the urinary tract is less recognized but equally well documented. These infections lead to more emergency room visits, hospitalizations, treatments with antibiotics, and health care costs for the infant who is not breastfed.[5]

The incidence of acute lower respiratory infections in infants has been evaluated in a number of studies examining the relationship between respiratory infections and breastfeeding or formula feeding in these infants.[10,106] These studies confirm that breastfed infants are less likely to be hospitalized for respiratory infection and, if hospitalized, are less seriously ill. In a study of infant deaths from infectious disease in Brazil, the risk of death from diarrhea was 14 times more frequent in the formula fed infant, and the risk of death from respiratory illness was four times more frequent.[141] The association of wheezing and allergy with infant feeding patterns has also shown a significant advantage to breastfeeding. In a report from a 7-year prospective study in South Wales, the advantage of breastfeeding persisted to age 7 years in nonatopic infants, and in at-risk infants who were breastfed the risk of wheezing was 50% lower (after accounting for employment status, passive smoking, and overcrowding).[16] Breastfeeding is thought to confer long-term protection against respiratory infection as well.

Upper and lower respiratory tract infections have been evaluated in case-control studies, cohort-based studies, and mortality studies in both clinic and hospitalized children in many countries of the developed world.[22,27,31,47,76] The results all show clearly that breastfeeding has a protective effect, especially in the first 6 months of life. A randomized controlled trial indicated that withholding cow milk and giving soy milk provided no such protective effect.[16] The incidence of acute otitis media in formula fed infants is dramatically higher than in breastfed infants,[1,7] not only because of the protective constituents of human milk but also because of the process of suckling at the breast, which protects the inner ear.[76] When an infant feeds by bottle, the eustachian tube does not close, and formula and secretions are regurgitated up the tubes. Child care exposure increases the risk of otitis media, and bottle feeding amplifies this risk.[22,76]

Immunologic protection

In addition to the protection provided by breastfeeding against acute infections, epidemiologic studies have revealed a reduced incidence of childhood lymphoma,[31] childhood-onset insulin-dependent diabetes,[142] as well as diabetes type 2 and Crohn's disease[71] in infants who have been exclusively breastfed for at least 4 months, compared with formula fed infants.

Allergy prophylaxis

Breastfed infants at high risk for developing allergic symptoms such as eczema and asthma by 2 years of age show a reduced incidence and severity of symptoms in early life.[16] Some studies suggest the protective effect continues through childhood.[16,44,68] A significant reduction in risk of childhood asthma at age 6 years was reported by Oddy and associates[101] if exclusive breastfeeding is continued for at least 4 months.

Psychological and cognitive benefits

Newton[98] noted that children who had been breastfed were more mature, secure, and assertive, and they progressed further on the developmental scale than nonbreastfed children. More recently, studies by Lucas and associates[83] and other investigators[60] have found that premature infants who received breast milk provided by tube feeding were more advanced developmentally at 18 months and at 7 to 8 years of age than those of comparable gestational age and birth weight who had received formula by tube. Such observations suggest that breast milk has a significant impact on the growth of the central nervous system. This suggestion is further supported by studies of visual activity in premature infants who were fed breast milk compared with those who were fed infant formula.[95] When similar studies were performed in term infants, visual acuity developed more rapidly in the breastfed infants.[62] Even when docosahexanoic acid (DHA) was added to formula, the performance by the breastfed infants was still better.[61]

An 18-year longitudinal study reported by Horwood and Fergusson[55] demonstrates a small but detectable increase in childhood cognitive and educational achievement in infants who were breastfed. The effects were confirmed in a range of measures, including standardized tests, teacher ratings, and academic outcomes in high school and young adulthood. More than 1000 children in New Zealand participated. Children who were breastfed for 8 months or longer had a mean test score at age 18 that was 0.11 to 0.30 standard deviation (SD) units higher than those not breastfed.

In order to examine the association between duration of infant breastfeeding and intelligence in young adult life, Mortensen and associates[92] conducted a prospective longitudinal cohort study of over 3000 individuals in Denmark born between 1959 and 1961. They concluded that, independent of a wide range of possible confounding factors, a significant positive association between duration of breastfeeding and intelligence test results existed, using two separate intelligence tests.

In an effort to examine the minimum duration of exclusive breastfeeding for optimal neurologic outcome, Bouwstra and associates[12] assessed the quality of general movements (GMs) at 3 months of 147 breastfeeding healthy term infants. General movement quality is considered a sensitive marker of neurologic status according to the authors. They demonstrated a positive effect between breastfeeding duration and GM quality with a saturation effect at about 6 weeks. They concluded that exclusive breastfeeding for at least 6 weeks might improve neurologic outcome.

BENEFITS OF BREASTFEEDING FOR MOTHER

Breastfeeding may provide the mother with a number of benefits, which should be included during a discussion about making an informed decision regarding how to feed one's infant.

Empowerment

In addition to clinically proven medical benefits, breastfeeding empowers a woman to do something special for her infant.[126] The relationship of a mother with her suckling infant is considered the strongest of human bonds. Holding the infant to the mother's breast to provide total nutrition and nurturing creates an even more profound and psychological experience than carrying the fetus in utero. These observations have been tested in animal experiments in which oxytocin and prolactin have triggered parenting behavior with nonpregnant subjects.

In studies of young women enrolled in the Women, Infants, and Children (WIC) program in Kentucky who were randomly assigned to breastfeed or not to breastfeed and who were provided with a counselor/support person throughout the first year post partum, the women who breastfed changed their behavior.[15,46] They developed self-esteem and assertiveness, became more outgoing, and interacted more maturely with their infants than did the women assigned to artificial feeding. The women who breastfed turned their lives around by completing school, obtaining employment, and providing for their infants.

Postpartum recovery

Women who breastfeed return to prepregnancy state more promptly than women who do not, and they have a lower incidence of obesity in later life (Box 7-1).[104,128] The presence of oxytocin stimulates the uterus to contract and involute with each feeding so that the uterus returns to the prepregnant

---

BOX 7-1   Benefits of breastfeeding

Infant
- Species specificity
- Nutritional advantages
- Infection protection
- Immunologic protection
- Allergy prophylaxis
- Psychological benefits

Mother
- Postpartum recovery
- Psychological benefits, empowerment
- Improved health risks

---

state within 6 weeks. The extra pregnancy tissue storage is utilized in the production of milk, and the return to prepregnancy weight is thus facilitated.

Decreased risk of osteoporosis

The risk of osteoporosis in later life is greatest for women who have never borne an infant, somewhat less for those who have borne infants, and measurably less for those who have borne and breastfed infants.[64,65] The bone mineral loss experienced during pregnancy and lactation is temporary. Bone mineral density returns to normal following pregnancy and even following extended lactation when mineral density may exceed the original baseline.[64] Serum calcium and phosphorus concentrations are greater in lactating than in nonlactating women. Lactation stimulates the greatest increases in fractional calcium absorption and serum calcitriol after weaning.[65] Postweaning concentrations of parathyroid hormone are significantly higher than in other stages, and urinary calcium loss is significantly lower.[26]

Protection against ovarian cancer

There is general agreement that a woman's increasing number of pregnancies, increasing length of oral contraceptive use, and increasing duration of lactation are protective against ovarian cancer.[146] When the relationship between lactation and epithelial ovarian cancer was studied from a multinational database, short-term lactation was as effective as long-term lactation in decreasing the incidence of ovarian cancer in developed countries where ovulation suppression may be less prolonged in relation to lactation.[113] In a study of black women, who are known to have a lower incidence of ovarian cancer, breastfeeding for 6 months or longer, as well as four or more pregnancies and oral contraceptive use, further reduced the incidence of ovarian cancer.[59]

Siskind and associates[122] studied the modifying effect of menopausal status on the association between lactation and risk of ovarian cancer in 824 cancer patients and 855 community control subjects. No association was noted in women whose cancer occurred postmenopausally; however, breastfeeding was somewhat protective against ovarian cancer before menopause in this study.

Reduced incidence of breast cancer

A mother with a new diagnosis of breast cancer should not nurse her infant in the interest of having definitive treatment immediately, because prolactin levels remain very high during lactation, and the role of prolactin in the advancement of mammary cancer is still in dispute.[54] Although endogenous prolactin by itself may not be a risk factor, it could, along with sex steroids, contribute to the acceleration of malignant growth.[133] All lumps in the lactating breast are not cancer and are not even benign tumors. The lactating breast is lumpy, and the "lumps" shift day by day. If a mass is located and the physician thinks it should be biopsied, this can be done under local anesthesia without weaning the infant.

University of Rochester (New York) surgeons have performed many such procedures following referrals in the past 35 years without postoperative complications. The diagnosis of a benign mass was made in almost all cases. Immediate surgery relieved tremendous anxiety without unnecessarily sacrificing breastfeeding. With noninvasive mammary imaging techniques such as ultrasound, computed tomography (CT) scanning, and magnetic resonance imaging (MRI), careful diagnosis can be carried out without interfering with lactation and without delaying diagnosis.

Relationship to breastfeeding

Is cancer more or less common in women who breastfeed? The answer is not easy to find, but in countries where breastfeeding is common, breast cancer is uncommon. In the United States the incidence of breast cancer has steadily risen while the frequency of breastfeeding has declined. It has been suggested that nursing protects a woman against breast cancer. This concept has been investigated in many international studies. Breastfeeding

does not predispose a woman to cancer and may protect her.[40]

A case-controlled study of 453 white females with breast cancer and 1365 white females without breast cancer from upstate New York showed an inverse relationship between length of breastfeeding and incidence of breast cancer in premenopausal women that has not been seen in postmenopausal women.[17] The authors found this apparent protective effect persisted throughout the childbearing years, with statistical control for age, parity, age at first pregnancy, age of menarche, and education. The women with cancer had had a higher incidence of lactation failure caused by "insufficient milk." The authors[17] suggest that the significance of this study may be that women who are unsuccessful at lactation are at increased risk for cancer rather than that breastfeeding is protective.

Kalache and associates[63] studied 707 married women ages 16 to 50 years with breast cancer in eight teaching hospitals in Oxford and London. Data were collected on duration of breastfeeding of each child and on detailed medical information on study patients and 707 control subjects. They found no correlation between breastfeeding and cancer.[63] The combination of low parity and late age at first birth was associated with a sevenfold increase in risk of breast cancer at ages 66 to 80 in a study by Lubin and associates[82] of more than 1400 women in Canada. At all ages, the authors found an increased cancer risk associated with relative infertility, benign breast disease, and not breastfeeding.

Marriage has been established as a negative risk factor for breast cancer. Mortality rates for most causes of death are higher among single women than among ever-married women.[58]

The statistics associating pregnancy and breast cancer influence the picture. In an epidemiologic study, the risk of breast cancer had a linear relationship to the time interval between puberty and childbirth.[90,97] The risk was reduced by one third for women who bore their first child before 18 years of age compared with those women who have their first infant when they are older. The risk of breast cancer for women who become pregnant before age 20 was about half that of those who first become pregnant after 25 years of age. Births after the first full-term pregnancy did not influence the statistics. Women whose first pregnancy appeared after 30 to 35 years of age had a risk of breast cancer four times that of nulliparous women in the same age group.[90,97]

The incidence of breast cancer is low among groups who had nursed their infants, including lower economic groups, foreign-born groups, and those in sparsely populated areas.[90,97] The frequency of breast cancer in mothers and sisters of a woman with breast cancer is two to three times that expected by chance. This influence could be genetic or environmental. Since the isolation of the "breast cancer gene," women are being identified who are at risk. Cancer actually is equally common on both sides of the family of an affected woman. If breast milk were the cause, it should be transmitted from mother to daughter. When mother-daughter incidence of cancer was studied, no relationship was found to breastfeeding. The association between breastfeeding and the incidence of breast cancer among 89,887 women in the U.S. Nurses Healthy Study was sought through an additional questionnaire. The authors[87] suggest that there was no important association between breastfeeding and the occurrence of breast cancer.

Unilateral breastfeeding (limited to the right breast) is a custom of Tanka women of the fishing villages of Hong Kong. Ing and associates[56] investigated the question, "Does the unsuckled breast have an altered risk of cancer?" They studied breast cancer data from 1958 to 1975. Breast cancer occurred equally in the left and the right breast. Comparison of patients who had nursed unilaterally with nulliparous patients and patients who had borne children but had not breastfed indicated a highly significantly increased risk of cancer in the unsuckled breast. The authors conclude that in postmenopausal women who have breastfed unilaterally, the risk of cancer is significantly higher in the unsuckled breast. They believe that breastfeeding may help protect the suckled breast against cancer.[56]

Other authors[72] have suggested that Tanka women are ethnically a separate people and that it is possible that left-sided breast cancer is related

to their genetic pool and not to their breastfeeding habits. No mention has been made of other possible influences, for instance, the impact of their role as "fishermen" or any inherent trauma to the left breast.[104]

As early as 1926, Lane-Claypon[75] stated that the breast that had never lactated was more liable to become cancerous. Nulliparity and absence of breastfeeding had been considered important risk factors for breast cancer.

In a collective review of the etiologic factors in cancer of the breast in humans, Papaioannou concludes, "Genetic factors, viruses, hormones, psychogenic stress, diet and other possible factors, probably in that order of importance, contribute to some extent to the development of cancer of the breast."[104]

Gradually, studies have appeared challenging the dogma. Brinton and associates,[14] McTiernan and Thomas,[86] and Layde and associates[78] all showed the clearly protective effects of breastfeeding. Another example is a study conducted to clarify whether lactation has a protective role against breast cancer in an Asian people, regardless of confounding effects of age at first pregnancy, parity, and closely related factors.[151] Similar results were reported by Zheng and colleagues[153] in a study in Shandong Province, China, in both pre- and postmenopausal women who had a reduced risk of breast cancer. The longer the total months of breastfeeding, the lower the risk. In a hospital-based case-control study of 521 women with breast cancer and 521 women without breast cancer, statistical adjustment for potential confounders and a likelihood ratio test for linear trend were done by unconditional logistic regression. Total months of lactation regardless of parity was the discriminator. Regardless of age at first pregnancy and parity, lactation had an independent protective effect against breast cancer in Japanese women.[151] Although breast cancer incidence is influenced by genetics, stress, hormones, and pregnancy, clearly breastfeeding has a protective effect. "There is a reduction in the risk of breast cancer among premenopausal women who have lactated. No reduction in the risk of breast cancer occurred among postmenopausal women with a history of lactation," according to Newcombe and coworkers,[96] reporting a multicentered study in 1993.

Two large prospective studies[72,87] did not report a protective effect of breastfeeding. Populations of 50,274 and 89,887 identified 2130 and 459 breast cancer patients. The odds ratios indicate 1.01 (0.98 to 1.05) and 0.95 (0.86 to 1.06), respectively. As with most studies of this nature, the cancers are well defined but not the breastfeeding. No attempt was made to note exclusivity and associated amenorrhea. The studies obtained breastfeeding histories when the women were over 45 years old and included those who ever breastfed.

The concern for exposure to estrogen early in life has been part of breast cancer assessment. In utero exposure to estrogen is greater in twin pregnancies and when the mother is older. Estrogen levels in smokers, however, are lower. Weiss and associates[145] analyzed cancer risk in a population-based case-control study in the United States (2202 with breast cancer and 2009 control subjects under 55 years of age). Twins were at greater risk than singletons, but no association with maternal age at delivery was found. A reduced breast cancer risk was seen among women who had themselves been breastfed as infants. Nielsen and O'Hara[99] followed Cochrane guidelines in performing a MEDLINE search of papers from 1990 to 2002 and reported a reduction of women's relative risk of breast cancer and a protective effect against ovarian cancer in women who breastfed their children.

In an effort to understand the relationship between breastfeeding and breast cancer, Newton[97] points out that over the past two centuries, women have changed from being pregnant or lactating 60% of the time between menarche and menopause to fewer pregnancies and shorter lactation periods. Thus, the amount of time a woman lives with unopposed estrogen (the proliferative phase of the menstrual cycle) was 15% in 1800 and 45% in 1996. Case-control epidemiologic studies consistently show a protective effect (Table 7-1). The most important predictors may be duration of the amenorrheal/hypoestrogenic state and the exposure to breast milk as an infant, according to Newton.[97]

Radiation therapy to breast

Ionizing radiation is carcinogenic to female mammary tissue. Women in Hiroshima and Nagasaki and those subjected to therapeutic radiation for mastitis were followed for many years.[121] The risk of cancer is 3.2 times greater in irradiated breasts, increasing over time after the irradiation. A linear relationship to radiation dose also exists.

TABLE 7-1   Breast cancer and lactation

| Study | Population | Likelihood of breast cancer | |
		Odds ratio	(95th confidence interval)
Michels et al[87]	All	0.93	(0.83–1.03)
	BF > 2 yr	1.11	(0.90–1.38)
Katsouyanni et al[67]	Premenopausal, BF > 2 yr	0.53	(0.23–1.41)
Romieu et al[112]	All	0.39	(0.25–0.62)
Brinton et al[14]	BF > 2 wk	0.87	(0.7–1.0)
Yang et al[150]	Premenopausal, failed to BF	3.0	(1.6–5.4)
Yoo et al[151]	All	0.62	(0.37–1.04)
	Premenopausal, BF > 7 mo	0.39	(0.15–0.97)

BF, breastfeed
From Newton ER Jr: Does breastfeeding protect women from breast cancer? ABM News Views 2(2):1, 1996.

In the late 1940s and early 1950s, radiation of the breast was performed as a treatment for mastitis. Although this approach seems irrational today, no antibiotics were readily available at that time, and women were hospitalized for mastitis. Sulfa drugs were not identified until the 1940s and penicillin shortly thereafter. The compounds were used only for life-threatening diseases. The effect of radiation on the infected breast was to clear the mastitis dramatically, stop lactation overnight, and seemingly solve the problem. The mother would continue to nurse on the other breast. The long-term follow-up of these women reveals a high incidence of cancer in the radiated breast.[121]

Radiation usually causes destruction to lobules, condensation of the cytoplasm in cells lining the ducts, and fibrosis. Successful lactation following radiation for carcinoma, however, has been reported in a 36-year-old woman with one previous pregnancy and lactation experience 6 years previously.[29]

Protective effect of being breastfed

Davis[31] first reported the reduction of childhood-onset cancers in children who have been exclusively breastfed for at least 4 months. The fear of cancer in the breastfed female offspring of a woman with breast cancer does not justify avoiding breastfeeding. Breastfed women have the same breast cancer experience as nonbreastfed women, and no increase occurs in benign tumors. Daughters of breast cancer patients have an increased risk of developing benign and malignant tumors by merit of their heredity, not their breastfeeding history.[88,90] This is confirmed with the identification of a breast cancer gene.

The critical question remains: does being breastfed increase any child's risk of developing breast cancer, especially in female offspring? This haunting question, first posed by an experimental scientist, created tremendous publicity and genuine concern among physicians queried by patients. One needs to explore the available data.[117]

No documented evidence indicates that women with breast cancer have ribonucleic acid (RNA) of tumor virus in their milk. No correlation between RNA-directed deoxyribonucleic acid (DNA) polymerase activity has been found in women with a family history of breast cancer. RNA-directed DNA polymerase activity, a reverse transcriptase, is a normal feature of the lactating breast.[21,38,114–116]

CONTRAINDICATIONS TO BREASTFEEDING

In reviewing the contraindications to breastfeeding, it is important to look at the entities that put the mother or infant at significant risk and are not remedial. Contraindications are medical; the disadvantages tend to be social. The physician needs to have a clear understanding of the benefits of breastfeeding to measure the risks for a particular mother-infant dyad. The risk/benefit ratio can be determined only by the clinician in a position to weigh all the data, usually the pediatrician for the infant or the obstetrician for the mother or the family physician.

Infectious diseases

In general, acute infectious diseases in the mother are not a contraindication to breastfeeding, if such diseases can be readily controlled and treated.[22] In most cases the mother develops the infection during breastfeeding. By the time the diagnosis has been made, the infant has already been exposed, and the best management is to continue breastfeeding so that the infant will receive the mother's antibodies and other host resistance factors in breast milk.[119] This is true for respiratory infections such as the common cold. Infections of the urinary tract or other specific closed systems such as the reproductive tract or gastrointestinal tract do not pose a risk for excreting the virus or bacteria in the breast milk unless there is generalized septicemia. In certain situations, given the relative virulence and infectivity of the organism, such as with β-hemolytic streptococcus group A, both mother and infant should be treated, but breastfeeding is not contraindicated (Table 7-2).[22,76] When the offending organism is especially virulent or infection

TABLE 7-2   **Summary of medical contraindications to breastfeeding***

Problem	Breastfeeding	Conditions
Infectious diseases		
Acute infectious disease	Yes	Respiratory, reproductive, gastrointestinal infections
HIV	No	HIV positive in developed countries
Active tuberculosis	Yes	After mother has received 2 or more weeks of treatment
Hepatitis		
A	Yes	As soon as mother receives gamma globulin
B	Yes	After infant receives HBIG, first dose of hepatitis B vaccine should be given before hospital discharge
C	Yes	If no coinfections (e.g., HIV)
Venereal warts	Yes	
Herpesviruses		
Cytomegalovirus	Yes	
Herpes simplex	Yes	Except if lesion on breast
Varicella-zoster (chickenpox)	Yes	As soon as mother becomes noninfectious
Epstein-Barr	Yes	
Toxoplasmosis	Yes	
Mastitis	Yes	
Lyme disease	Yes	As soon as mother initiates treatment
HTLV-I	No	
Over-the-counter/prescription drugs and street drugs (see Chapter 11)		
Antimetabolites	No	
Radiopharmaceuticals		
Diagnostic dose	Yes	After radioactive compound has cleared mother's plasma
Therapeutic dose	No	
Drugs of abuse	No	Exceptions: cigarettes, alcohol
Other medications	Yes	Drug-by-drug assessment
Environmental contaminants		
Herbicides	Usually	Exposure unlikely (except workers heavily exposed to dioxins)
Pesticides		
DDT, DDE	Usually	Exposure unlikely
PCBs, PBBs	Usually	Levels in milk very low
Cyclodiene pesticides	Usually	Exposure unlikely
Heavy metals		
Lead	Yes	Unless maternal level ≥ 40 µg/dL
Mercury	Yes	Unless mother symptomatic and levels measurable in breast milk
Cadmium	Usually	Exposure unlikely
Radionuclides	Yes	Risk greater to bottle fed infants

*This table provides a brief summary. Each situation must be decided individually. Contraindications are rare.
DDE, dichlorodiphenyldichloroethane; DDT, dichlorodiphenyltrichloroethane; HBIG, hepatitis B immune globulin; HIV, human immunodeficiency virus; HTLV-1, human T-cell leukemia virus type 1; PBBs, polybrominated biphenyls; PCBs, polychlorinated biphenyls
Modified from Lawrence RA: A review of the medical benefits and contraindications to breastfeeding in the United States. In Maternal and Child Health Technical Information Bulletin, Arlington, VA, National Center for Education in Maternal and Child Health, 1997.

occurs through direct contact or respiratory droplets, separation of the infant and mother is indicated regardless of the mode of feeding (formula or breast milk). Examples of such infections include smallpox and tuberculosis. In these situations giving the infant expressed breast milk without maternal contact is appropriate. See Chapter 16 for discussion of management of infectious diseases during lactation.

Many agents in breast milk protect against infection, and their presence is not affected by nutritional status. Protection against infection is important in the United States, especially among infants exposed to multiple caregivers, child care outside the home, compromised environments, and less attention to the spread of organisms.[46] One of the most important and thoroughly studied agents in breast milk is secretory immunoglobulin (sIg, specifically, sIgA), which is present in high concentrations in colostrum and early breast milk and in lower concentrations throughout lactation, when the volume of milk is increased.[46] Secretory IgA antibodies may neutralize viruses, bacteria, or their toxins and are capable of activating the alternate complement pathway.[22] The normal flora of the intestinal tract of the breastfed infant, as well as the offspring of all other mammalian species studied until weaning, is bifidobacteria or lactobacilli.[46] These bacteria further inhibit the growth of bacterial pathogens by producing organic acids. This is in striking contrast to the formula fed infant, who has comparatively few bifidobacteria and many coliform bacteria and enterococci. In addition, although the attack rates of certain infections are similar in breastfed and formula fed infants in the same community, the manifestations of the infections are much less evident in the infants who are breastfed. This appears to result from antiinflammatory agents in breast milk.[76]

For a few specific infectious diseases, the possible infectious risk of breastfeeding outweighs the benefits.[22,76] See the following sections on HIV-1, HIV-2, and HTLV-I and -II, or refer to Chapter 16.

Human immunodeficiency virus type 1

Human immunodeficiency virus type 1 (HIV-1) is transmitted through human milk. Refraining from breastfeeding is a crucial aspect of preventing perinatal HIV infection in the United States and many other countries. The dilemma is the use of replacement feeding in countries where breastfeeding provides infants with significant protection from illness and death due to other infections.

The question of the contribution of breastfeeding in mother-to-child HIV-1 transmission is not a trivial one when one considers the following:

1. The World Health Oganization (WHO) has estimated that 40 million people were living with HIV-1 in 2003.
2. More than 90% of the children younger than 13 years old have been infected by mother-to-child transmission.
3. WHO estimates that 5 million people were newly infected with HIV-1 in 2003, with children younger than 15 years old accounting for 700,000 of that 5 million.
4. Breastfeeding contributes an estimated 10% to 20% increase in the overall mother-to-child transmission rates, over and above intrauterine and intrapartum transmission of HIV from mother to child.

The evidence of HIV transmission via breastfeeding is irrefutable. Two recent summaries document nicely the current proof in the literature.[108,135]

In summary, breastfeeding of infants by HIV-positive mothers does lead to an increased risk of HIV infection in the infant. There is much still to be understood about the mechanisms of HIV transmission via breast milk and the action and efficacy of interventions to prevent such transmission. The complete avoidance of breastfeeding remains a crucial component for the prevention of perinatal HIV infection in the United States and in many other developed countries. In resource-poor settings, where breastfeeding is the norm and where it provides vital nutritional and infection protective benefits, the WHO, UNICEF, and UNAIDS recommend education, counseling, and support for HIV-infected mothers so they can make an informed choice concerning infant feeding.[149] Mothers choosing to breastfeed should receive additional education, support, and medical care to minimize the risk of HIV transmission and to optimize their own health status during and after breastfeeding. Mothers choosing to use replacement feedings should receive parallel education, support, and medical care for themselves and their infants to minimize the effect of the lack of breastfeeding. The decision about infant feeding for the HIV-positive mother remains a true dilemma, a choice between two equally unsatisfactory alternatives. Only through continued research and education concerning the potential interventions to prevent HIV transmission via breast milk can we minimize transmission and optimize infant nutrition and health.

It is probable that HIV-2 transmission via breast milk is less common than that of HIV-1, but there are insufficient data to say the risk of transmission is zero. HIV-2–positive women should be tested for HIV-1, and guidelines for breastfeeding should follow those for HIV-1 until additional information is available.

Human T-cell leukemia virus type I

The occurrence of human T-cell leukemia virus type I (HTLV-I) is endemic in parts of southwestern Japan,[148,43] the Caribbean, South America,[43] and sub-Saharan Africa. HTLV-I is associated with adult T-cell leukemia/lymphoma (ATL) and a chronic progressive neuropathy. The progressive neuropathy is called HTLV-I-associated myelopathy or tropical spastic paraparesis (HAM/TSP). Other illnesses, including dermatitis, uveitis, arthritis, Sjögren syndrome in adults, and infective dermatitis and persistent lymphadenitis in children, have been reported in association with HTLV-I infection. Transmission of HTLV-I occurs most often through sexual contact, via blood or blood products, and via breast milk. Infrequent transmission does occur in utero or at delivery and with casual or household contact. HTLV-I is not a major disease in the United States.[128]

HTLV-I antigen has been identified in breast milk of HTLV-I-positive mothers.[69] Another report shows that basal mammary epithelial cells can be infected with HTLV-I and can transfer infection to peripheral blood monocytes.[80] HTLV-I-infected lymphocytes have been found in the milk of infected mothers, 10% of whose milk cells are T lymphocytes, of which 1% are infected. It is estimated that 1 mL of milk harbors 1000 infected T cells (Table 7-3).

If the risk of lack of breast milk is not too great, and formula is readily available and culturally acceptable, then the proscription of breastfeeding or at least a recommendation to limit the duration of breastfeeding to 6 months or less is appropriate to limit the risk of HTLV-I transmission to the infant. Freezing and thawing breast milk before giving it to the infant might be

TABLE 7-3   HTLV-I transmission related to the duration of breastfeeding

Author (reference)	Duration (months)	Seroconversion rate	Number of children*
Takahashi et al[130]	≤ 6 months	4.4%	4/90
	≥ 7 months	14.4%	20/139
	(bottle fed)	5.7%	9/158
Takezaki et al[131]	≤ 6 months	3.9%	2/51
	> 6 months	20.3%	13/64
Wiktor et al[147]	< 12 months	9%	8/86
	≥ 12 months	32%	19/60

*Number of children positive for HTLV-I over the number of children examined.
HTLV-I, human T-cell leukemia virus type I.

another reasonable intervention to decrease the risk of transmission. Neither immune globulin nor antiviral agents against HTLV-I are available at this time.

Human T-cell leukemia virus type II

Human T-cell leukemia virus type II (HTLV-II) is endemic in specific geographic locations, including Africa, the Americas, the Caribbean, and Japan. Transmission is primarily through intravenous drug use (IVDU), contaminated blood products, and breastfeeding. Sexual transmission occurs, but its overall contribution to the prevalence of HTLV-II in different populations remains uncertain. Many studies have examined the presence of HTLV-I and -II in blood products. Polymerase chain reaction (PCR) testing and selective antibody tests suggest that about one half of the HTLV seropositivity in blood donors is caused by HTLV-II.

HTLV-II has been recently associated with two chronic neurologic disorders similar to those caused by HTLV-I: tropical and spastic ataxia.[81] A connection between HTLV-II and glomerulonephritis, myelopathy, arthritis, T-hairy cell leukemia, and large granulocytic leukemia has been reported.

Mother-to-child transmission has been demonstrated in both breastfed and formula fed infants. It appears that the rate of transmission is greater in breastfed infants.[41,48,57,73,74,100,140,143] HTLV-II has been detected in breast milk.[48] Nyambi and associates reported that HTLV-II transmission did correlate with the duration of breastfeeding. The estimated rate of transmission was 20%. The time to serconversion (after the initial loss of passively acquired maternal antibodies) for infected infants seemed to range between 1 and 3 years of age.[100] Avoidance of breastfeeding and limiting the duration of breastfeeding are the only two possible interventions with evidence of effectiveness for preventing HTLV-II mother-to-child transmission.

Life-threatening illnesses

Life-threatening or debilitating illness in the mother may necessitate avoiding lactation. This clinical judgment should be made with the mother and father, with all facts presented. Although one woman may be able to overcome all obstacles and prove she can nurse her baby, it does not necessarily mean that another patient with the same diagnosis can.[13] If the mother wants some lay reading on the subject, the clinician should be familiar with available material so any apparent inconsistencies of opinion can be discussed. (See management of specific maternal illnesses in Chapter 15.)

Over-the-counter/prescription drugs and street drugs
Medications

Much concern and anxiety have been expressed regarding the question of medications taken by lactating women and the risk to the suckling infant. In reality, very few drugs are contraindicated during breastfeeding.[77] Each situation should be evaluated on a case-by-case basis by the physician. The important factors include the pharmacokinetics of the drug in the maternal system and the absorption, metabolism, distribution, storage, and excretion in the recipient infant. Variables to consider in the decision include gestational age, chronologic age, body weight, breastfeeding pattern, and other dietary practices. Ultimately, the decision is made by assessing the risk/benefit ratio (i.e., the risk of a small amount of the drug compared with the tremendous benefit of being breastfed).

See Chapter 11 for a full discussion of drugs, medications, and environmental toxins. The contraindications are few but include radioactive medications, antimetabolites, and street drugs (see Table 7-2 and Appendix D).

Drug abuse

Breastfeeding is contraindicated in women who are intravenous (IV) drug abusers.[128] The possibility of the infant receiving substantial amounts of drug through the milk is real; deaths have been reported in the recipient neonate. IV drug abusers have high incidences of hepatitis, HTLV-I/II, or HIV, which may be transmitted to the breastfed infant from the infected mother (see Chapter 11 and Appendix D for specific drugs of abuse).

DISADVANTAGES OF BREASTFEEDING

Disadvantages to breastfeeding are those factors perceived by the mother as an inconvenience to her, because no known disadvantages exist for the normal infant. (In the rare circumstance of galactosemia in the neonate, which involves an inability to tolerate lactose, breastfeeding is contraindicated; see Chapter 15). In cultures in which nursing in public is commonplace, nursing is not considered inconvenient because the infant and the feeding are always available.

The mother's commitment to the infant for 6 to 12 feedings a day for months may be overwhelming to a woman who has been free and independent. Motherhood itself changes a woman's lifestyle.

Guilt from failure, shame, and other anxieties are of considerable concern. Surveys evaluating the decline of breastfeeding have revealed that mothers describe feelings of shame, modesty, embarrassment, and distaste. These feelings are more common in lower social groups. Research on wider sociologic and psychological factors regarding the feelings and attitudes toward breastfeeding can have considerable influence on the choice to breastfeed and will be helpful in dealing with these issues.

Professionals and lay persons, under the banner of "supporting breastfeeding," occasionally get caught up in a rush to "convert" all mothers and parents to breastfeeding. Sometimes the push is to change many hospital routines and regulations to facilitate without assessing the full impact of those changes on all the mothers and infants. A sense of balance should be maintained. It is important to appreciate that some normal women cannot or will not nurse their babies. Their babies will survive and grow normally. Each woman, infant, and family should be supported in their choice of infant feeding; it is their choice to make. The education and support should be specific for the particular needs of each mother-infant dyad.

The sharp letter by Fisher[39] brings this to focus when she describes the frustrations and disappointments of others and dispels what she calls the myths about breastfeeding. She expresses anger over her failure to successfully breastfeed her child. Her anger is an outward sign of inner guilt about this perceived failure.

The popular press has drawn attention to parenting trends that divide responsibility for the infant equally between mother and father after the birth.[126] This, of course, necessitates some bottle feeding. The justification is division of labor and equal opportunity for both parents to do good things for the baby. This is probably another way of expressing breast envy and jealousy. Some husbands are jealous because they have no similar way to bring food and contentment to their infant, according to Waletzky.[144] "A certain manliness was required to foster breastfeeding in one's family when society as a whole was hostile to it," according to Pittenger and Pittenger.[107] They point out that the perinatal period is a breeding ground for marital and parental maladjustment.

Many writers, however, have described participation in childbirth as a potentially beneficial experience for men. The father's feelings are useful during labor and delivery. These experiences contribute to heightened self-concepts and better adjustments to roles as husband and father. The quality of the birth experience has been cited as the major determinant of paternal attachment. Paternal attachment has led to a greater pride in breastfeeding and a more secure, self-confident support person for the mother who is breastfeeding.

Perinatal counseling of prospective new parents may anticipate these reactions, and in turn the professional will have an opportunity to facilitate the best experience possible.

REFERENCES

1. Alho OP, Koivu M, Sorri M, et al: Risk factors for recurrent acute otitis media and respiratory infection in infancy. Int J Pediatr Otorhinolaryngol 19:151, 1990.
2. Ando Y, Kakimoto K, Tanigawa T, et al: Effect of freeze-thawing breast milk on vertical HTLV-I transmission from seropositive mothers to children. Jpn J Cancer Res 80:405, 1989.
3. Ando Y, Matsumoto Y, Nakano S, et al: Long-term follow-up study of HTLV-I infection in bottle-fed children born to seropositive mothers. J Infect 46:9, 2003.
4. Ando Y, Matsumoto Y, Nakano S, et al: Long-term follow up study of vertical HTLV-I infection in children breast-fed by seropositive mothers. J Infect 46:177, 2003.
5. Ando Y, Saito K, Nakano S, et al: Bottle feeding can prevent transmission of HTLV-I from mothers to their babies. J Infect 19:25, 1989.
6. Ando Y, Nakano S, Saito K, et al: Transmission of adult T-cell leukemia retrovirus (HTLV-I) from mother to child: Comparison of bottle- with breast-fed babies. Jpn J Cancer Res 78:322, 1987.
7. Aniansson G, Alm B, Andersson B, et al: A prospective cohort study on breastfeeding and otitis media in Swedish infants. Pediatr Infect Dis J 13:183, 1994.
8. Bener A, Denic S, Galadari S: Longer breast-feeding and protection against childhood leukaemia and lymphomas. Eur J Cancer 37:234, 2001.
9. Bertolli J, St Louis ME, Simonds RJ, et al: Estimating the timing of mother-to-child transmission of human immunodeficiency virus in a breast-feeding population in Kinshasa, Zaire. J Infect Dis 174(4):722, 1996.
10. Beudry M, Dufour R, Marcoux S: Relation between infant feeding and infections during the first six months of life. J Pediatr 126:191, 1995.
11. Blanche S, Rouzioux C, Moscato ML, et al. A prospective study of infants born to women seropositive for human immunodeficiency virus type 1. HIV Infection in Newborns French Collaborative Study Group. N Engl J Med 320:1643, 1989.
12. Bouwstra H, Boersma ER, Boehm G, et al: Exclusive breastfeeding of healthy term infants for at least 6 weeks improves neurological condition. Nutritional Neurosciences Research Communication. J Nutr 133:4243, 2003.
13. Brewster DP: You Can Breast Feed Your Baby . . . Even in Special Situations. Emmaus, PA, Rodale Press, 1979.
14. Brinton LA, Potischman NA, Swanson CA, et al: Breastfeeding and breast cancer risk. Cancer Causes Control 6:199, 1995.
15. Bryant CA: Overcoming breastfeeding barriers. Presented at U.S. Department of Health and Human Services Region IV Nutrition Conference, Building Support Networks for Breastfeeding, Atlanta, 1986.
16. Burr ML, Limb ES, Maguire MJ, et al: Infant feeding, wheezing, and allergy: A prospective study. Arch Dis Child 68:724, 1993.
17. Byers T, Graham S, Rzepka T, et al: Lactation and breast cancer. Am J Epidemiol 121:664, 1985.
18. Centers for Disease Control and Prevention, U.S. Public Health Service Working Group: Recommendations for counseling persons infected with human T-lymphotropic virus, types I and II. MMWR 42(RR-9):1, 1993.
19. Centers for Disease Control and Prevention: Testing for antibodies to HIV-2 in the United States. MMWR 41:1, 1992.
20. Chantry CJ, Howard CR, Auinger P: Breastfeeding fully for 6 months vs. 4 months decreases risk of respiratory tract infection. ABM News Views 9:29, 2003.
21. Chopra H, Ebert P, Woodside N, et al: Electron microscopic detection of simian-type virus particles in human milk. Nature N Biol 243:159, 1973.
22. Committee on Infectious Diseases, American Academy of Pediatrics: Report of the Committee on Infectious Diseases, 6th ed. Elk Grove Village, IL, American Academy of Pediatrics, 2003.
23. Coutsoudis A, Coovadia H, Pillay K, Kuhn L: Are HIV-infected women who breastfeed at increased risk of mortality? AIDS 15:653, 2001.
24. Coutsoudis A, Pillay K, Kuhn L, et al: Method of feeding and transmission of HIV-1 from mothers to children by 15 months of age: prospective cohort study from Durban, South Africa. South African Vitamin A Study Group. AIDS 15:379, 2001.
25. Coutsoudis A, Pillay K, Spooner E, et al: Influence of infant-feeding patterns on early mother-to-child transmission of HIV-1 in Durban, South Africa: A prospective cohort study. South African Vitamin A Study Group. Lancet 354:471, 1999.
26. Cross NA, Hillman LS, Allen SH, et al: Calcium homeostasis and bone postweaning: A longitudinal study. Am J Clin Nutr 61:514, 1995.
27. Cunningham AS, Jelliffe DB, Jelliffe EFP: Breast-feeding and health in the 1980s: A global epidemiologic review. J Pediatr 118:659, 1991.
28. Datta P, Embree JE, Kreiss JK, et al: Mother-to-child transmission of human immunodeficiency virus type 1: Report from the Nairobi Study. J Infect Dis 170:1134, 1994.
29. David FC: Lactation following primary radiation therapy for carcinoma of the breast. Int J Radiat Oncol Biol Phys 11:1425, 1985.
30. Davis MK: Human milk and HIV infection: Epidemiologic and laboratory data. In Mestecky J, Blair C, Ogra PL (eds): Immunology of Milk and the Neonate. New York, Plenum, 1991.
31. Davis MK: Review of the evidence for an association between infant feeding and childhood cancer. In

International Union Against Cancer (UICC, WHO) Workshop: Nutritional morbidity in children with cancer: Mechanisms, measures and management. Int J Cancer 11 (suppl):29, 1998.

32. De Martino M, Tovo PA, Tozzi, et al: HIV-1 transmission through breast-milk: Appraisal of risk according to duration of feeding. AIDS 6:991, 1992.

33. Dewey KG, Heinig MJ, Nommsen LA, et al: Growth of breast-fed and formula-fed infants from 0 to 18 months: The DARLING study. Pediatrics 89(6, pt 1):1035, 1992.

34. Dewey KG, Peerson JM, Brown KH, et al: Growth of breastfed infants deviates from current reference data: A pooled analysis of US, Canadian, and European data sets, World Health Organization Working Group on Infant Growth. Pediatrics 96(3, pt 1):495, 1995.

35. Ekpini ER, Wiktor SZ, Satten GA, et al: Late postnatal mother-to-child transmission of HIV-1 in Abidjan, Cote d'Ivoire. Lancet 349:1054, 1997.

36. Enger JM, Ross RK, Henderson B, et al: Breastfeeding history, pregnancy experience and risk of breast cancer. Br J Cancer 76:118, 1997.

37. European Collaborative Study: Children born to women with HIV-1 infection: Natural history and risk of transmission. Lancet 337:253, 1991.

38. Fieldsteel AH: Nonspecific antiviral substances in human milk active against arbovirus and murine leukemia virus. Cancer Res 34:712, 1974.

39. Fisher PJ: Breast or bottle: A personal choice. Pediatrics 72:435, 1983 (letter).

40. Fraumeni JF, Miller RW: Breast cancer from breast feeding. Lancet 2:1196, 1971.

41. Fujino T, Nagata Y: HTLV-I transmission from mother to child. J Reprod Immunol 47(2):197, 2000.

42. Fujiyama C, Fujiyoshi T, Miura T, et al: A new endemic focus of human T-lymphotropic virus type II carriers among Orinoco natives in Colombia. J Infect Dis 168:1075, 1993.

43. Gotuzzo E: HTLV-1: A new problem for Latin America. ASM News 67(3):144, 2001.

44. Gruskay FL: Comparison of breast, cow and soy feedings in the prevention of onset of allergic disease: A 15-year prospective study. Clin Pediatr 21:486, 1982.

45. Guay LA, Hom DL, Mmiro F, et al: Detection of human immunodeficiency virus type 1 (HIV-1) DNA and p24 antigen in breast milk of HIV-1-infected Ugandan women and vertical transmission. Pediatrics 98(3, pt 1):438, 1996.

46. Gussler JD, Bryant CA (eds): Helping mothers to breastfeed: Program strategies for minority communities. Lexington, KY, Nutrition and Health Education Division, Lexington-Fayette County Health Department, 1984.

47. Hanson LA, Adlerberth I, Carlsson B, et al: Host defense of the neonate and the intestinal flora. Acta Paediatr Scand 351(suppl):122, 1989.

48. Heneine W, Woods T, Green D, et al: Detection of HTLV-II in breastmilk of HTLV-II infected mothers. Lancet 340:1157, 1992.

49. Hino S, Katamine S, Kawase K, et al: Intervention of maternal transmission of HTLV-I in Nagasaki, Japan. Leukemia 94:S68, 1993.

50. Hino S, Katamine S, Miyata H, et al: Primary prevention of HTLV-I in Japan. J Acquir Immune Defic Syn Hum Retrovirol 13S: S15, 1996.

51. Hino S: Milk-borne transmission of HTLV-I as a major route in the endemic cycle. Acta Paediatr Jpn 31:428, 1989.

52. Hino S, Sugiyama H, Doi H, et al: Breaking the cycle of HTLV-I transmission via carrier mothers' milk. Lancet 2:158, 1987.

53. Hisada M, Maloney EM, Sawada T, et al: Virus markers associated with vertical transmission of human lymphotropic virus type 1 in Jamaica. Clin Infect Dis 34:1551, 2002.

54. Hornstein E, Skornick Y, Rozin R: The management of breast carcinoma in pregnancy and lactation. J Surg Oncol 21:179, 1982.

55. Horwood LJ, Fergusson DM: Breastfeeding and later cognitive and academic outcomes. Pediatrics 101:e9, 1998 (electronic article).

56. Ing R, Ho JHC, Petrakis NL: Unilateral breast feeding and breast cancer. Lancet 2:124, 1977.

57. Ishak R, Harrington WJ, Azeuedo VN, et al. Identification of human T-cell lymphotropic virus type IIa infection in the Kayapo, an indigenous population of Brazil. AIDS Res Hum Retrovirol 11(7):813, 1995.

58. Janerich DT, Hoff MB: Evidence for a crossover in breast cancer risk factors. Am J Epidemiol 116:737, 1982.

59. John EM, Whittemore AS, Harris R, et al: Characteristics relating to ovarian cancer risk: Collaborative analysis of seven US case-control studies—Epithelial ovarian cancer in black women. Collaborative Ovarian Cancer Group. J Natl Cancer Inst 85:142, 1993.

60. Johnson DL, Swank PR, Howie VM, et al: Breastfeeding and children's intelligence. Psychol Rep 79:1179, 1996.

61. Jonsbo F, Jorgensen MH, Michaelsen KF: The importance of n-3 and n-6 fatty acids for visual function and development in newborn infants. Ugeskrift Laeger 157:1987, 1995.

62. Jorgensen MH, Hernell O, Lund P, et al: Visual acuity and erythrocyte docosahexaenoic acid status in breast-fed and formula-fed term infants during the first four months of life. Lipids 31:99, 1996.

63. Kalache A, Vessey MP, McPherson K: Lactation and breast cancer. Br Med J 1:223, 1980.

64. Kalkwarf HJ, Specker BL, Heubi JE, et al: Intestinal calcium absorption of women during lactation and after weaning. Am J Clin Nutr 63:526, 1996.

65. Kalkwarf HJ, Specker BL: Bone mineral loss during lactation and recovery after weaning. Obstet Gynecol 86:26, 1995.

66. Kaplan JE, Abrams E, Shaffer N, et al: Low risk of mother-to-child transmission of human T lymphotropic virus type II in non-breastfed infants. J Infect Dis 166:892, 1992.

67. Katsouyanni K, Lipworth L, Trichopoulou A, et al: A case-control study of lactation and cancer of the breast. Br J Cancer 73:814, 1996.

68. Kern RA: Prophylaxis in allergy. Ann Intern Med 12:1175, 1939.

69. Kinoshita K, Hino S, Amagasaki T, et al: Demonstration of adult T-cell leukemia virus antigen in milk from three seropositive mothers. Gann 75:103, 1984.

70. Kinoshita K, Yamanouchi K, Ikeda S, et al: Oral infection of a common marmoset with human T-cell leukemia virus type I (HTLV-I) by fresh human milk of HTLV-I carrier mothers. Jpn J Cancer Res 76:1147, 1985.

71. Koletzko S, Sherman P, Corey M, et al: Role of infant feeding practices in development of Crohn's disease in childhood. Br Med J 298:1617, 1989.

72. Kvale G, Heuch I: Lactation and cancer risk: Is there a relation specific to breast cancer? J Epidemiol Community Health 42:30, 1987.

73. Lal RB, Owen SM, Segurado AAC, Gongora-Biachi RA: Mother-to-child transmission of human T-lymphotropic virus type II (HTLV-II). Ann Intern Med 120:300, 1994.

74. Lal RB, Renan A, Gongora-Biachi A, et al: Evidence for mother-to-child transmission of human T-lymphotropic virus type II. J Infect Dis 168:586, 1993.

75. Lane-Claypon JE: A further report on cancer of the breast, with special reference to its associated antecedent conditions. Report No. 32. London, England, Reports of the Ministry of Health, 1926.

76. Lawrence R: The clinician's role in teaching proper infant feeding techniques. J Pediatr 126:S112, 1995.

77. Lawrence RA: A review of the medical benefits and contraindications to breastfeeding in the United States. In Maternal and Child Health Technical Information Bulletin. Arlington, VA, National Center for Education in Maternal and Child Health, 1997.

78. Layde PM, Webster LA, Baughman AL, et al: The independent associations of parity, age at first full term pregnancy, and duration of breastfeeding with risk of breast cancer. J Clin Epidemiol 42:963, 1989.

79. Leroy V, Newell ML, Dabis F, et al: International multicentre pooled analysis of late postnatal mother-to-child transmission of HIV-1 infection. Ghent International Working Group on Mother-to-Child Transmission of HIV. Lancet 352(9128):597, 1998.

80. LeVasseur RJ, Southern SO, Southern PJ: Mammary epithelial cells support and transfer productive human T cell lymphotropic virus infections. J Hum Virol 1:214, 1998.

81. Lowis GW, Sheremata WA, Minagar A: Epidemiologic features of HTLV-II: Serologic and molecular evidence. Ann Epidemiol 12:46, 2002.

82. Lubin JH, Burns PE, Blot WJ, et al: Risk factors for breast cancer in women in northern Alberta, Canada, as related to age at diagnosis. J Natl Cancer Inst 68:211, 1982.

83. Lucas A, Morley R, Cole TJ, et al: Breast milk and subsequent intelligence quotient in children born preterm. Lancet 339:261, 1992.

84. Mbori-Ngacha D, Nduati R, John G, et al: Morbidity and mortality in breastfed women: A randomized clinical trial. JAMA 286(19):2413, 2001.

85. McManus IC: Predominance of left-sided breast tumours. Lancet 2:297, 1977.

86. McTiernan A, Thomas DB: Evidence for a protective effect of lactation on risk of breast cancer in young women: Results from a case-control study. Am J Epidemiol 124:353, 1986.

87. Michels KB, Willet WC, Rosner BA: Prospective assessment of breastfeeding and breast cancer incidences among 89,887 women. Lancet 347:431, 1996.

88. Miller RW, Fraumeni JF: Does breast feeding increase the child's risk of breast cancer? Pediatrics 49:645, 1972.

89. Miotti PG, Taha TE, Kumwenda NI, et al: HIV transmission through breastfeeding: A study in Malawi. JAMA 282(8):781, 1999.

90. Morgan RW, Vakil DV, Chipman ML: Breast feeding, family history, and breast disease. Am J Epidemiol 99:117, 1974.

91. Mortensen EL, Michaelsen KF, Sanders SA, et al: The association between duration of breastfeeding and adult intelligence. JAMA 287:2365, 2002.

92. Nakano S, Ando Y, Ichijo M, et al: Search for possible routes of vertical and horizontal transmission of adult T-cell leukemia virus. Gann 75:1044, 1984.

93. Nduati RW, John GC, Richardson BA, et al: Human immunodeficiency virus type 1-infected cells in breast milk: Association with immunosuppression and vitamin A deficiency. J Infect Dis 172:1461, 1995.

94. Nduati R, Richardson BA, John G, et al: Effect of breastfeeding on mortality among HIV-1 infected women: A randomised trial. Lancet 357:1651, 2001.

95. Neuringer M, Reisbick S, Janowsky J: The role of n-3 fatty acids in visual and cognitive development: Current evidence and methods of assessment. J Pediatr 125:S39, 1994.

96. Newcombe PA, Storer BE, Longnecker MP: Lactation and a reduced risk of premenopausal breast cancer. N Engl J Med 330:81, 1994.

97. Newton ER Jr: Does breastfeeding protect women from breast cancer? ABM News Views 2(2):1, 1996.

98. Newton N: Psychological differences between breast and bottle feeding. Am J Clin Nutr 24:993, 1971.

99. Nielsen M, O'Hara M: The effects of breastfeeding on maternal health. ABM News Views 9:28, 2004.

100. Nyambi PN, Ville Y, Louwagie J, et al: Mother-to-child transmission of human T-cell lymphotropic virus types I and II (HTLV-I/II) in Gabon: A prospective follow-up of 4 years. J Acquir Immune Defic Syn Hum Retroviral 12:187, 1996.

101. Oddy WH, Holt PG, Sly PD, et al: Association between breast feeding and asthma in 6 year old children: Findings of a prospective birth cohort study. BMJ 319:815, 1999.

102. Ory H, Cole P, MacMahon B, et al: Oral contraceptives and reduced risk of benign breast diseases. N Engl J Med 294:419, 1976.

103. Palasanthiran P, Ziegler JB, Stewart GJ, et al: Breast-feeding during primary maternal human immunodeficiency virus infection and risk of transmission from mother to infant. J Infect Dis 167:441, 1993.

104. Papaioannou AN: Etiologic factors in cancer of the breast in humans: Collective review. Surg Gynecol Obstet 138:257, 1974.

105. Pillay K, Coutsoudis A, York D, et al: Cell-free virus in breast milk of HIV-1 seropositive women. J Acquir Immune Defic Syn 24(4):330, 2000.

106. Pisacane A, Graziano L, Zona G, et al: Breast feeding and acute lower respiratory infection. Acta Paediatr 83:714, 1994.

107. Pittenger JE, Pittenger JG: The perinatal period: Breeding ground for marital and parental maladjustment. Keeping Abreast J 2:18, 1977.

108. Read JS, Committee on Pediatric AIDS: Human milk, breastfeeding, and transmission of human immunodeficiency virus type 1 in the United States. Pediatrics 112:5, 2003.

109. Rebuffe-Scrive M, Enk L, Crona N, et al: Fat cell metabolism in different regions in women: Effect of menstrual cycle, pregnancy, and lactation. J Clin Invest 75:1973, 1985.

110. Richardson BA, John-Steward GC, Hughes JP, et al: Breast-milk infectivity in human immunodeficiency virus type 1-infected mothers. J Infect Dis 187:736, 2003.

111. Rios E, Hunter RE, Cook J: The absorption of iron as supplements in infant cereal and infant formulas. Pediatrics 55:686, 1975.

112. Romieu I, Hernandez-Avila M, Lazcano E, et al: Breast cancer and lactation history in Mexican women. Am J Epidemiol 143:543, 1996.

113. Rousseau CM, Nduati RW, Richardson BA, et al: Longitudinal analysis of human immunodeficiency virus type 1 RNA in breast milk and of its relationship to infant infection and maternal disease. J Infect Dis 187(5):741, 2003.

114. Roy-Burman P, Rongey RW, Henderson BE, et al: Attempts to detect RNA tumour virus in human milk. Nature N Biol 244:146, 1973.

115. Ruff AJ, Coberly J, Halsey NA, et al: Prevalence of HIV-1 DNA and p24 antigen in breastmilk and correlation with maternal factors. J AIDS 7:68, 1994.

116. Sanner T: Removal of inhibitors against RNA-directed DNA polymerase activity in human milk. Cancer Res 36:405, 1976.

117. Sarkar NH, Charney J, Doion AS, et al: Effect of human milk on mouse mammary tumor virus. Cancer Res 33:626, 1973.

118. Sawada T, Iwahara Y, Ishii K, et al: Immunoglobulin prophylaxis against milkborne transmission of human T cell leukemia virus type 1 in rabbits. J Infect Dis 164:1193, 1991.

119. Schreiner RL, Coates T, Shackelford PG: Possible breast milk transmission of group B streptococcal infection. J Pediatr 91:159, 1977 (letter).

120. Semba RD, Kumwenda N, Hoover DR, et al: Human immunodeficiency virus load in breast milk, mastitis and mother-to-child transmission of human immunodeficiency virus type 1. J Infect Dis 180:93, 1999.

121. Shore RE, Hildreth N, Woodard E, et al: Breast cancer among women given x-ray therapy for acute postpartum mastitis. J Natl Cancer Inst 77:689, 1986.

122. Siskind V, Green A, Cain C, et al: Breastfeeding, menopause, and epithelial ovarian cancer in young women. Epidemiology 8:188, 1997.

123. Slusher T, Slusher I, Biomdo M, et al: Electric breast pump use increases maternal milk volume in African nurseries. Poster/oral presentation. ILCA annual conference Sydney, Australia, 2003.

124. Sowers MF, Corton G, Shapiro B, et al: Changes in bone density with lactation. JAMA 269:3130, 1993.

125. Stiehm ER, Vink P: Transmission of human immunodeficiency virus infection by breastfeeding. J Pediatr 118:410, 1991.

126. Stone E: A feminist fad? Ms 11(8):68, 1983.

127. Stuver SO, Hsieh C-C, Bertone E, et al: The association between lactation and breast cancer in an international case-control study: A re-analysis by menopausal status. Int J Cancer 71:166, 1997.

128. Subcommittee on Nutrition During Lactation, Food and Nutrition Board, Institute of Medicine, National Academy of Sciences. Washington, DC, National Academy Press, 1991.

129. Sugiyama H, Doi H, Yamaguchi K, et al: Significance of postnatal mother-to-child transmission of HTLV-I on the development of adult T-cell leukemia/lymphoma. J Med Virol 20:253, 1986.

130. Takahashi K, Takezaki T, Oki T, et al: Inhibitory effect of maternal antibody on mother-to-child transmission of human T-lymphotropic virus type I. The Mother-to-Child Transmission Study Group. Int J Cancer 49:673, 1991.

131. Takezaki T, Tajima K, Ito M, et al: Short-term breast-feeding may reduce the risk of vertical transmission of HTLV-I. The Tsushima ATL Study Group. Leukemia 11(suppl 3):60, 1997.

132. Tess BH, Rodrigues LC, Newell ML, et al: Infant feeding and risk of mother-to-child transmission of HIV-1 in Sao Paulo State, Brazil. Sao Paulo Collaborative Study for Vertical Transmission of HIV-1. J Acquir Immune Defic Syn Hum Retrovirol 19:189, 1998.

133. Thomas MR, Kawamoto J: Dietary evaluation of lactating women with or without vitamin and mineral supplementation. J Am Diet Assoc 74:669, 1979.

134. U.S. Public Health Service recommendations for human immunodeficiency virus counseling and voluntary testing for pregnant women. MMWR 44(RR-7):1, 1995.

135. UNAIDS/UNICEF/WHO: HIV and infant feeding. A review of HIV transmission through breastfeeding. Geneva, Switzerland, WHO/UNAIDS, 1998. Available at http://www.unaids.org/publications/documents/mtct/hivmod3.doc (accessed Jan. 21, 2004).

136. United States Breastfeeding Committee: Benefits of Breastfeeding [issue paper]. Raleigh, NC, United States Breastfeeding Committee, 2002.

137. Ureta-Vidal A, Angelin-Duclos C, Tortevoye P, et al: Mother-to-child transmission of human T-cell leukemia/lymphoma virus type I: Implication of high antiviral antibody titer and high proviral load in carrier mothers. Int J Cancer 82(6):832, 1999.

138. Van de Perre P, Simonon A, Msellati P, et al: Postnatal transmission of the human immunodeficiency virus type 1 from mother to infant: A prospective cohort study in Kigali, Rwanda. N Engl J Med 3325:593, 1991.

139. Van de Perre P, Simonon A, Hitimana D, et al: Infective and antiinfective properties of breastmilk from HIV-1 infected women. Lancet 341:914, 1993.

140. Van Dyke RB, Heneine W, Perrin ME, et al: Mother-to-child transmission of human T-lymphotropic virus type II. J Pediatr 127:927, 1995.

141. Victora CG, Smith PG, Vaughan JP, et al: Evidence for protection by breastfeeding against infant deaths from infectious diseases in Brazil. Lancet 2(8554):319, 1987.

142. Virtanen SM, Räsänen L, Aro A, et al: Infant feeding in Finnish children less than 7 years of age with newly diagnosed IDDM. Childhood Diabetes in Finland Study Group. Diabetes Care 14:415, 1991.

143. Vitek CR, Gracia FI, Giusti RA, et al: Evidence for sexual and mother-to-child transmission of human T lym-photrophic virus type II among Guaymi Indians, Panama. J Infect Dis 171:1022, 1995.

144. Waletzky LR: Husbands' problems with breastfeeding. Am J Orthopsychiatry 49:349, 1979.

145. Weiss HA, Potischman NA, Brinton LA, et al: Prenatal and perinatal risk factors for breast cancer in young women. Epidemiology 8:181, 1997.

146. Whittemore AS: Characteristics relating to ovarian cancer risk: implications for prevention and detection. Gynecol Oncol 55(3, pt 2):S15, 1994.

147. Wiktor SD, Pate EJ, Rosenberg PS, et al: Mother-to-child transmission of human T-cell lymphotropic virus type I associated with prolonged breast-feeding. J Hum Virol 1:37, 1997.

148. Wong-Staal F, Gallo RC: Human T-lymphocyte retroviruses. Nature 312:395, 1985.

149. World Health Organization/United National Children's Fund: HIV and breastfeeding consensus statement. Geneva, Switzerland, May 1992.

150. Yang CP, Weiss NS, Band PR, et al: History of lactation and breast cancer risk. Am J Epidemiol 138:1050, 1993.

151. Yoo K-Y, Tajima K, Kuroishi T, et al: Independent protective effect of lactation against breast cancer: A case-control study in Japan. Am J Epidemiol 135:726, 1992.

152. Yoshinaga M, Yashiki S, Fujiyoshi T, et al: A maternal factor for mother-to-child transmission: Viral antigen-producing capacities in culture of peripheral blood and breast milk cells. Jpn J Cancer Res 86:649, 1995.

153. Zheng T, Duan L, Liu Y, et al: Lactation reduces breast cancer risk in Shandong Province, China. Am J Epidemiol 152:1129, 2000.

154. Ziegler JB, Cooper DA, Johnson RO, et al: Postnatal transmission of AIDS-associated retrovirus from mother to infant. Lancet 1:896, 1985.

8

$\mathscr{M}$anagement of the mother-infant nursing couple

Successful nursing depends on the successful interaction of mother and infant, with appropriate support from the father, the family, and available health care resources. Because both mothers and infants vary, no simple set of rules in hospitals can be outlined to guarantee success. In fact, one of the difficulties has been that a rigid system was established for initiating lactation in the hospital that did not fit all mother-infant couples. Furthermore, physicians have not received formal education about breastfeeding; thus, they resort to gaining information from a variety of sources, including personal experiences, and may assume that this is the correct way to approach the situation.

Nowhere in medicine do one's personal interests or prejudices become more evident than in the area of counseling about childbirth and breastfeeding. Having a child does not make one an expert on the subject. Conversely, not having a child does not preclude the development of exceptional skills. Some of the world's most revered experts in human lactation have neither had a child nor nursed an infant, but they have brought to the situation the eye of a skilled observer and the experience of a broadly trained clinician unencumbered by emotional bias and personal prejudices.

Historically, rigid dogmas have directed management of lactation. In the effort to replace these

with what was perceived as more rational management, new dogmas have arisen. Once there was a paucity of literature, now there is a deluge from all sources, some very valid, others questionable. The very careful art and science of breastfeeding are being lost in the rage of righteousness. The clinician must be careful in choosing to employ the guidelines used in any other phase of medical and health care. No rules exist for breastfeeding. As in all phases of medicines, the clinician adapts the recommendations to the individual patients and their circumstances.[182]

It is not ordinarily the physician's role to teach the mother how to breastfeed. Instead, all the nursing staff who interact in the perinatal period, including obstetric office nursing, labor/delivery, nursery, postpartum, birth center, and pediatric office personnel, as well as midwives, have job descriptions that include hands-on assistance for the mother in the process of breastfeeding. The physician does, however, need to understand the anatomy and physiology and the basics of breastfeeding to recognize problems and determine their solutions. This chapter addresses the basic breastfeeding process. It is not a "how-to" manual for mothers, but the physician should be familiar with one or two good sources of information to suggest for patients, such as K. Huggins' *The Nursing Mother's Companion*,

255

or *The Womanly Art of Breastfeeding* from La Leche League International (see Appendix K for organizations providing materials).

The references for this chapter are not an exhaustive list of all material written on the topic; rather, they are intended to assist the reader in locating research that supports the evidence-based concepts described here.

The key to the management of the mother-infant nursing couple is establishing a sense of confidence in the mother and supporting her with simple answers to her questions when they arise. Good counseling also depends on understanding the science of lactation. Then, when a problem arises, a mechanism already is in place for the mother to receive help from her physician's office before the problem creates a serious medical complication.

THE SCIENCE OF SUCKLING

The ability to lactate is characteristic of all mammals, from the most primitive to the most advanced. The divergence of suckling patterns, however, makes it urgent that human patterns be studied specifically.[19] Some aquatic mammals such as whales nurse under water; others such as the seal and sea lion nurse on land. A variety of erect or recumbent postures are assumed by different terrestrial mammals.[34] Nursing may be continuous, as in the joey attached to a marsupial teat, or at widely different intervals characteristic of the species and parallel to the nutrient concentrations of the milk. The interval may be a half hour in the dolphin, an hour in the pig, a day in the rabbit, 2 days in the tree shrew, or a week in the northern fur seal.

Although many anatomic distinctions exist as well, the principal mechanism of milk removal common to all mammals is the contractile response of the mammary myoepithelium under the hormonal influence of oxytocin released from the neurohypophysis.[172]

The key function in all species is effective control of milk delivery to the young in the right amount and at the appropriate intervals, which requires a production system, exit channels, a pre-

hensile appendage, an expulsion mechanism, and a retention mechanism. The primary, secondary, and tertiary ducts form an uninterrupted channel for the passage of milk from the milk-producing alveoli to the mammary sinuses. A process of erection of the areolar region facilitates prehension by the young during suckling. The principal object of the suction produced by the facial musculature of the young is to draw the nipple into the mouth and retain it there. Positive pressure is used to expel milk from the gland by the contractile changes in the mammary gland provided by the myoepithelial cells (see Fig. 3-9). The sympathetic nervous stimuli can oppose milk ejection by increasing vasoconstrictor tone, thereby reducing access of circulating oxytocin to the mammary myoepithelium. Sympathetic activity also can occur during conditions of apprehension or muscular exertion. The milk-ejection reflex can be blocked by emotional disturbance or reflex excitation of the neurohypophysis. The central nervous system control of milk ejection indeed suggests that restraining mechanisms exist to ensure that milk ejection can only occur under circumstances wholly conducive to the effective removal of milk by the suckling young.

In all species that have been studied, a rise in intramammary pressure and flow of milk occur as a reflex event in suckling. The excitation of the neurohypophysis results in the release of oxytocin, which is conveyed via the bloodstream to mammary capillaries, where it evokes contraction of the myoepithelium.[32] The successive ejection pressure peaks, demonstrated in lactating women, can be duplicated more accurately by a series of separate oxytocin injections than by the same total dose as a single injection or by a continuous infusion of the hormone. This strongly suggests that oxytocin is released from the neurohypophysis in spurts. The study of suckling patterns in all species shows a high degree of ritualization, which in turn suggests a close neural connection between cognitive or behavioral and hormonal responses.

Attention has focused on the mechanisms that control suckling behavior, on its incidence, on events that precipitate and terminate it, on the effects of stress, and on how development modifies it. Suckling is characteristic of each species and is vital for survival. *Suckling* means to take nourishment at the breast and specifically refers to "breastfeeding" in all species. *Sucking,* however, means to draw into the mouth by means of a partial vacuum, which is the process employed when bottle feeding. Sucking also means to consume by licking.

Although suckling has been studied in the young and the mother in other species, a large portion of the human data has been collected using a rubber nipple and bottle. Other mammals suck only in the nutritive mode, whether receiving milk from the nipple or not. Human infants were noted to have two distinct patterns with rubber nipples: a nutritive mode, and a nonnutritive mode.[173,174] When this work was repeated using the breastfeeding model, there was no difference between nutritive and nonnutritive suckling rates but rather a continuous variation of suckling rate in response to milk-flow rate.[20] Suckling rates in other species correlate with milk composition and species-specific feeding schedules (one suck per second in great apes and four to five sucks per second in sheep and goats).

In further experiments, an inverse linear relationship was found between milk flow and suckling rate. Thus, the higher the milk flow, the lower is the suckling rate. In human infants younger than 12 weeks of age, suckling will terminate with sleep and be reinstated on awakening, a pattern that is well described in other species.[19] In infants older than 12 weeks, suckling is not terminated by sleep.[3] At 12 to 24 weeks, infants will play with the nipple and explore the mother and not always elicit nipple attachment. Continuous measurement of milk intake during a given feeding from one breast showed a progressive reduction in intake volume per suck and an increase in the proportion of time spent pausing between bursts of sucking.

Using the miniature Doppler ultrasound flow transducer, Woolridge and associates[177,178] have studied 32 normal mother-baby pairs from 5 to 9 days post partum. Intakes during trials averaged 34.2 g (±3.7 g) on the first breast and 26.2 g (±3.5 g) on the second breast. At the start of feeds the average suck volume was about 0.14 mL/suck,

which decreased to about 0.10 mL/suck or less. The mean latency for release of milk was 2.2 minutes after the infant began to suckle. The researchers also noted that on the first breast the flow increased and stabilized after 2 minutes, with concomitant slowing and stabilizing of sucking pattern over the remainder of the feed. On the second breast the suck volume fell off dramatically toward the end of the feed (50% reduction from peak to end of feed) (see Fig. 8-22).

These observations support the theory that infants become satiated at the breast and milk remains unconsumed in the breast. Over the first month of life, infants consume a given amount of fluid with decreasing investment of time.[177] The amount of fluid per suck increases over time. The control of intake appears to come under intrinsic control of the infant during the first month of life.[123]

When sucking was studied using a multisensor nipple for recording oral variables, such as lip and tongue movements and fluid flow, it was observed that fluid flow begins as the intranipple pressure decreases and tapers off as the intranipple pressure increases.[23] One flow pattern is seen in each sucking movement.

The development of the sucking response in the normal newborn with a rubber nipple transducer in a nonnutritive mode has been reported immediately after birth.[7] Pressure exerted immediately was 5 mm Hg at birth, peaking at 103 mm Hg at 90 minutes. Infants less than 24 hours old demonstrate a significantly different sucking pattern than a 3-day-old infant. The younger infants' duration of burst was longer (3.7 versus 2.8 seconds), frequency was lower in amplitude (1.7 versus 2.0 hertz), and the variability was greater. These evaluations were carried out in breastfeeding infants with a pacifier with a transducer and no nutrient reward.[55] No data are available on optimal pressures or on pressures developed with immediate breastfeeding.

The movement of the lips and tongue have been more difficult to study. A cineradiographic study of breastfeeding was done by Ardran and associates[10] in 1957 and compared with a similar study of bottle feeding.[11] The nipples and areolae of 41 breastfeeding mothers were coated with a paste of barium sulfate in lanolin, and cineradiographic films were taken with the infant at breast. These were then reviewed meticulously. Box 8-1 lists the authors' conclusions in their original description. These observations are of historic interest, but newer techniques in imagery have more accurately described the understanding of human suckling.

In a similar study of bottle feeding by Ardran and associates,[10] cineradiographic films were taken of infants, lambs, and kid goats, taking a mixture of milk and barium from a bottle. In the 1950s, when Ardran and associates[10,11] made their landmark studies of bottle feeding, the rubber nipples used were different in size, shape, and consistency, so some of their observations may not pertain to present equipment. They concluded that gravity was key to the operation and that infants are not able to suck and swallow with a bottle while taking a breath.

The development of real-time ultrasound improved the definition of images. Several studies have been published using this noninvasive technique to observe the action of the infant's tongue and buccal mucosa and the maternal nipple areola. Using a videorecorder that allowed frame-by-frame analysis and recorded simultaneous respiration, the pattern of suck, swallow, and breathing was documented over a period of active suckling at the breast. A *suck* was defined by Weber and associates[165] as the beginning of one indentation of the nipple by the tongue to the beginning of the next. Weber and associates had examined six breastfed and six bottle fed infants between 1 and 6 days of life. Not all sucks were associated with a swallow. Box 8-2 summarizes the process.

Observations of suckling using newer techniques over time from 2 to 26 weeks showed that suckling starts with a series of fast sucking movements and then stabilizes. In a 2-week-old breastfeeding infant, sucking and breathing pattern proportions alternated smoothly at about two sucks to one breath, with swallowing occurring with every suckle. Bottle feeding patterns were variable and sometimes asynchronous with sucking and breathing.

BOX 8-1   Radiographic interpretation of suckling at the breast

---

1. The nipple is sucked to the back of the baby's mouth and a teat is formed from the mother's breast.
2. When the jaw is raised, this teat is compressed between the upper gum and the tip of the tongue resting on the lower gum. The tongue is applied to the lower surface of the teat from the front backward, pressing it against the hard palate: the teat is reduced to approximately half its former width. As the tongue moves toward the posterior edge of the hard palate, the teat shortens and becomes thicker.
3. When the jaw is lowered, the teat is again sucked to the back of the mouth and restored to its previous size.
4. Each cycle of jaw and tongue movement takes place in approximately 1.5 seconds. The pharyngeal cavity becomes airless and the larynx closes every time the upward movement of the tongue against the teat and hard palate is completed.
5. The teat is formed from the nipple and the adjacent areola and underlying tissues.

From Ardran GM, Kemp FH, Lind J: A cineradiographic study of breast feeding. Br J Radiol 31:156, 1958.

BOX 8-2   Ultrasound interpretation of suckling at the breast

---

1. The lateral margins of the tongue cup around the nipple, creating a central trough.
2. The suck is initiated by the tip of the tongue against the nipple followed by pressure from the lower gum.
3. There is peristaltic action of the tongue toward the back of the mouth.
4. The tongue elevation continues to move the bolus of milk into the pharynx.

Modified from Weber F, Woolridge MW, Baum JD: An ultrasonographic study of the organization of sucking and swallowing by newborn infants. Dev Med Child Neurol 28:19, 1986.

The process of suckling has been described as a pulsating process similar to peristalsis along the rest of the gastrointestinal tract. This undulating motion, as described by cineradiography, did not involve stroking or friction, as was clearly pointed out by Woolridge.[175,180] The nipple should not move in and out of the infant's mouth if the breast is positioned correctly. The tip of the tongue does not move along the nipple. The positive pressure of the tongue against the teat (areola and nipple), coupled with ejection of the milk from increased intraductal pressure, evacuates the milk, not suction. The negative pressure created in the mouth holds the nipple and breast in place and reduces the "work" to refill the ampullae and ducts. Visual observations and videotapes made in our laboratory to study suckling show the undulating motion of the external buccal surfaces even in newborns. Ultrasound confirms the molding of buccal mucosa and tongue around the teat, leaving no space.

In breastfeeding the tongue action is a "rolling," or peristaltic, action from the tip of the tongue to the base, not side to side. In the bottle feeder the tongue action is more pistonlike or squeezing. When the infant rests between sucks, the human nipple is indented by the tongue, and the latex teat is expanded in bottle feeding (Figs. 8-1 and 8-12).

The change in nipple dimensions during suckling is detailed by Smith and associates,[147,148] who also used ultrasound and examined 16 term infants ages 60 to 120 days and their mothers. They demonstrated that the human nipple is highly elastic and elongates during active feeding, including about 2 cm of areola, to form a teat approximately twice its resting length. They also showed that the infant's cheeks (buccal membranes) with their thick layer of fatty tissue, known as *sucking fat pads,* act to make a passive seal to create a vacuum (as opposed to the concept that the cheeks are sucked in by the negative pressure). Milk ejection was noted to occur after maximal compression of the nipple.

Although the firm texture of the latex teat was more difficult for the infant to compress, Weber and associates[165] did not observe any practical differences between breast and bottle sucking. Softer latex nipples do not readily reexpand and so do not

solve the suckling problem. Ultrasound as a study tool will continue to clarify sucking patterns in neonates and can also be useful as a diagnostic tool in presumed sucking disorders before "suck training or retraining" is considered.

Coordination of suck and swallow

The ability to swallow is developed in utero during the second trimester and has been well demonstrated by fetal ultrasound. Fetal swallowing of amniotic fluid is an important part of the complex regulation of amniotic fluid. The suck is actually part of the oral phase of the swallow. Little was done to examine the role of swallowing on the suckling rate until Burke[25] studied the role of swallowing in the organization of suckling behavior, although with a bottle and solutions of 5% and 10% sucrose solution. The author reported two major observations: "First, the frequency of swallowing in newborns increased significantly as a function of increasing concentration and amount of sucrose solution given per criterion suck. Second, there was a significant difference in the duration of the sucking interresponse times which immediately followed the onset of swallowing and the duration of interresponse times not associated with swallowing." These observations explain those of previous investigators regarding nutritive and nonnutritive sucking.

The coordination of sucking and swallowing was observed by ultrasound by Weber and associates[165] as a movement of the larynx. By 4 days of age, both breastfed and bottle fed infants were swallowing with every suck. Later in the feeding the ratio of sucks to swallows changed to 2:1 or more until sucking stopped. Swallowing occurred in the end-expiratory pause between expiration and inspiration (see Fig. 8-1). The change in suck/swallow ratio seemed to be a function of the availability of milk.

Factors that influence sucking

As one manages infants with difficulty feeding, a number of rituals are often initiated to enhance

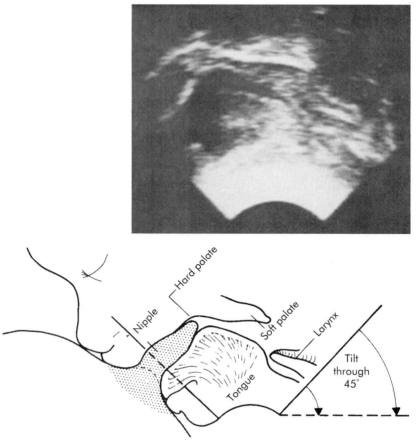

Figure 8-1. Ultrasound of infant at breast. Still picture of ultrasound scan frame from videorecording. Scanner head is at bottom, with a sector view of 90 degrees. Below is artist's impression of image showing key features. Image is seen best when tilted through 45 degrees, so that infant's head is vertical. Picture corresponds to point in sucking cycle when maximum point of compression of nipple by tongue has almost reached tip of nipple. Once nipple has become fully expanded, fresh cycle of compression will be initiated at base of nipple and will then move back. (From Weber F, Woolridge MW, Baum JD: An ultrasonographic study of the organization of sucking and swallowing by newborn infants. Dev Med Child Neurol 28:19, 1986.)

infant behavior. Only a few of these have been evaluated for their effect.[120] The effect of the infant's position, that is, supine or supported upright to a 90-degree angle, was found to have no influence on the sucking pattern or pressure. The effect of temperature, however, was found to be significant. Sucking pressure decreased as environmental temperature increased from 80° to 90° F (26.6° to 32.2° C), which may have application in

encouraging an infant to nurse. This effect was shown to increase from the third to the fifth day of life. Higher sucking pressures have been recorded in the morning than in the afternoon.[7]

When the size of latex nipples was studied, the large nipple elicited fewer sucks and a slower sucking rate than smaller nipples, although the volume of milk delivered was the same in this study with all nipple sizes.[31] Although human nipple size cannot be altered, this knowledge may help in assessing the response of a newborn in specific situations. Increasing nipple size and decreasing sucking rate may be significant in considering using an adult finger for finger feeding.

The volume of each swallow was calculated during breastfeeding in 1905 by Süsswein,[152] who counted swallows and made test weighings. His observations have now been confirmed with elaborate electronic equipment.[176] The average swallow of a newborn is 0.6 mL, which is also the exact amount drawn from a bottle equipped with an electromagnetic flowmeter transducer and a valve that responds to negative pressure at each suck in modern studies, even though the sucking mechanism between breast and bottle is different.[141] When a conventional bottle without a valve is used, the volume is reduced to one third, to 0.19 mL/suck. The valve removes the need for the infant to suck against the negative pressure created in the bottle. This supports the fact that a bottle fed infant with a poor suck does better with a boat-shaped bottle, in which the distal end is kept open, or with a collapsible bag as a source of milk, such as in the Playtex nurser. The size of the hole in the nipple influences the volume of the suck only in the valved bottle. When breastfed infants were compared with a group fed by cup from birth and a group fed by bottle, the breastfed infants had a stronger suck than either of the other two groups, who did not differ from each other in sucking skill.[34,37]

Lucas and associates[96] studied patterns of milk intake using electronic weighings in interrupted feeds. They reported that 50% of a feed from each breast was consumed in 2 minutes and 80% to 90% by 4 minutes, with minimal feeding from each breast in the last 5 minutes. Bottle fed infants, evaluated with the same technique of test weighings, took 84% of the feeding in the first 4 minutes. Bottle feeding patterns were linear, whereas the breastfed infant had a biphasic pattern when nursed on both breasts. The total intake of the two types of feeds was similar in volume in the same 25 minutes of total time.

Fat content and suckling

The high concentration of fat in breast milk toward the end of a feed was hypothesized as a satiety signal to terminate the feeding.[56] When this was studied using high- and low-fat formulas, it was found that high-fat milk did not act to cue babies to slow or stop feeding.[41,117,118] In fact, babies appeared to feed more actively on high-fat milk, sucking in longer bursts with less resting. When human milk of low- and high-fat content was fed from bottles, switching the baby from low-fat breast milk to high-fat breast milk, the babies did not alter either milk intake rate or sucking patterns.

To test the hypothesis fully, a study carefully observed infants switching from the first to the second breast and back to the first breast.[41] Infants were 2 months old and well established at exclusive breastfeeding. No significant difference was seen in the time taken to attach to the new breast and the time taken to reattach to the previously suckled breast. Mean milk intake from the first breast was 91.7 g (range 58 to 208 g), higher than that from the second breast (mean 52.5 g, range 8 to 75 g). The mean fat contents before and after nursing on the first breast were 23 g/L and 52 g/L, whereas on the second breast they were 24 g/L and 48 g/L. This shows that infants will nurse when fat content is higher, contrary to the theory that increasing fat causes satiation.[118]

Studies of 3-day-old bottle fed infants fed sucrose and glucose solutions show that they manifest tongue movements of greater amplitude when fed stronger concentrations of carbohydrate even though they do not respond to fat content in formula.[117] Sensory apparatus responsible for assessing sweetness is apparently competent in the newborn.

Breathing and sucking while feeding

Breathing and sucking during feeding were addressed by Johnson and Salisbury,[78] who studied normal full-term infants from 1 to 10 days of age, measuring breathing, sucking, and flow of fluid from a feeding bottle with a flowmeter. No infant aspirated water, but 8 of 18 infants inhaled saline. Even from a bottle, breast milk was associated with more regular breathing than was formula feeding. It has been demonstrated in other species that newborns will become apneic when fed milk from species other than their own. The coordination of breathing and swallowing improves with increase in milk availability and with the maturity of the infant, according to Weber and associates.[165]

Suckling patterns as indicators of problems or pathology

The behavior of the infant at birth is the first opportunity to observe the infant's adeptness at suckling. In a careful analysis of videotapes of newborns in the first 90 minutes of life, Widström and Thingström-Paulsson[169] observed a consistent pattern. Licking movements preceded and followed the rooting reflex in alert infants. The tongue was placed in the bottom of the mouth cavity during distinct rooting. The authors suggest that forcing the infant to the breast might disturb reflex and tongue position. They further observe that a healthy infant should be given the opportunity to show hunger and optimal reflexes and attach to mother's nipple by itself.

Righard and Alade[134] observed that an infant placed on the mother's abdomen will self-attach to the breast and suckle correctly in less than 50 minutes. They further reported that when the infants were separated from their mothers for delivery room procedures, the initial suckling attempts were disturbed, and many infants were too drowsy to suckle at all.[134]

Righard and Alade also investigated the prognostic value of suckling technique (faulty versus correct) during the first week after birth in relation to the long-term success of breastfeeding.[135] Eighty-two healthy mother-infant pairs were observed before discharge for assessment of breastfeeding technique. The authors defined correct sucking as the infant's mouth being wide open, the tongue under the areola, and the milk expressed in slow, deep sucks. Incorrect sucking is defined as infant positioned as if bottle feeding, using the nipple as a teat. The *oral searching reflex* is defined as the infant opening the mouth wide in response to proximity of the nipple to the lips and thrusting the tongue forward in preparation to taking the breast. This reflex is a part of the normal response to circumoral stimulus resulting in rooting by the infant, who comes forward, opens the mouth wide, and extends the tongue when stimulated centrally on the lower lip and even the upper lip. Stimulus on the side of the mouth elicits turning to that side.

In the study,[135] all the infants were assessed by the same observer before discharge from the hospital. If there was an incorrect suck, the mother-infant pairs were randomly assigned to a no-intervention group or to a group in which mothers received brief instruction on proper positioning. Telephone follow-up occurred at 2 weeks and monthly for 4 months. Switching to bottle was 10 times more common in the nipple-sucking group (9/25 or 36%) than in both the correct and the corrected group (2/57 or 3.5%). Table 8-1 lists the duration of breastfeeding in the various groups. Eighty-eight percent of the nipple-sucking group had further breastfeeding problems, with a high incidence of insufficient milk and sore nipples.[135]

It was first noted by Barnes and associates[15] that mothers with difficult labors and deliveries had more problems breastfeeding. The influence of mode of delivery on the initiation of breastfeeding was reported by Vestermark and associates.[161] For infants delivered by vacuum extraction or cesarean section, suckling was delayed and they received more supplements. Parity increases chances of success in lactation according to Dewey and associates.[39] They confirmed the influence of mode of delivery, duration of labor, labor medications, and the use of artificial feedings and pacifiers as well. When these factors are present, extra care should be made to support the mother's efforts to breastfeed (Fig. 8-2).[40]

Medications during labor

Newborn infants whose mothers received a single dose of 200 mg secobarbital as obstetric sedation during labor sucked at significantly lower rates and pressures and consumed less nutrient than did

	Exclusively breastfeeding 5 days	Exclusively and partly breastfeeding			
Sucking technique		1 mo	2 mo	3 mo	4 mo
No. (%) incorrect at discharge	25 (100)	16 (64)	12 (48)	11 (44)	10 (40)
No. (%) correct at discharge	57 (100)	55 (96)	48 (84)	45 (79)	42 (74)
p		<0.001	<0.01	<0.01	<0.01

TABLE 8-1   Duration of breastfeeding with different sucking techniques

From Righard L, Alade MO: Sucking technique and its effect on the success of breastfeeding. Birth 19:185, 1992.

infants whose mothers received no medication.[84] The effect persisted for 4 days. Similar effects have been seen in Brazelton's examination.[21] A single dose of 50 mg meperidine also altered suckling. The clinician must be aware of the perinatal history of medication during labor so that early identification of any effect on suckling can be made. The mother of an infant with a poor suck may need some additional stimulus by electric pump to facilitate milk production. The infant may require extra assistance in latching on and obtaining sufficient nourishment the first few days.

Epidural anesthesia

Because of repeated concerns about the possible effect of intrapartum epidural anesthesia on the newborn infant's ability to suckle and the rising incidence of epidurals in some hospitals (more than 50% of vaginal deliveries), Rosen and Lawrence[139] investigated 83 mother-infant dyads who either exclusively breastfed or bottle fed. The infant's ability to nurse at the breast or take the bottle was scored from multiple observations. Weight loss in the first few days was also evaluated. Epidural anesthesia had no apparent effect (although analgesics showed a relationship) on ability to feed or initial weight loss, although prolonged epidural use (beyond 4 hours or repeated dosing) may well have an effect because the drug has time to be absorbed into the systemic circulation.

The question of duration of epidural anesthesia was investigated by Bader and associates,[14] who found that maternal venous and umbilical venous levels of fentanyl and bupivacaine were relatively constant whether the epidural lasted 1 hour or up to 15 hours. Total doses varied between 27 and 200 mg for bupivacaine and 22 to 300 μg for fentanyl. Significantly, however, bupivacaine was measurable

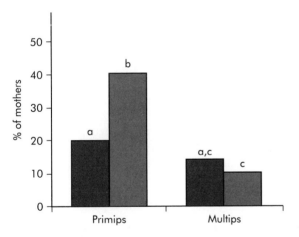

Figure 8-2. Percentage of mothers with delayed onset of milk production, by parity and infant birth weight, adjusted for mode of delivery, duration of stage II labor, maternal body mass index, and flat or inverted nipples (bars with different letters are significantly different, $p <$ 0.05). Vertical bars, birth weight ≤3600 g; horizontal bars, birth weight >3600 g. N = 69 primiparas with infants ≤3600 g, 61 primiparas with infants >3600 g, 40 multiparas with infants ≤3600 g, and 71 multiparas with infants >3600 g. (From Dewey KG, Nommsen-Rivers LA, Heinig MJ, Cohen RJ: Risk factors for suboptimal infant breastfeeding behavior, delayed onset lactation, and excess neonatal weight loss. Pediatrics 112:607, 2003.)

in the umbilical venous sample of the infants (0.15 ± 0.06 µg/mL). The significance of fetal tissue uptake is unclear. Umbilical artery blood gases (ABGs) and neurobehavioral scores were normal. Neonatal urine in another study had small but measurable bupivacaine metabolites 36 hours after delivery when spinal anesthesia was used for cesarean birth. It is noteworthy that usually the infant is delivered within 15 minutes of medication administration for cesearean birth.[85]

The effect on infants of different doses of meperidine given to mothers in labor was clearly demonstrated by Hodgkinson and associates[66] in a double-blind comparison of neurobehaviors of 920 neonates. They used the Early Neonatal Neurobehavior Scale (ENNS), which consists of 13 assessments, including general levels of alertness, rooting, and sucking. Meperidine was associated with broad depression of most items on ENNS on both the first and the second days of life, increasing with increasing dosages of 50, 75, and 150 mg. The best scores were achieved by infants whose mothers received chloroprocaine epidural anesthesia without meperidine (280 infants whose mothers received mean dose of 510 ± 255 mg chloroprocaine over 2.3 ± 1.1 hours; 177 mothers did not receive meperidine, and 81 did). Chloroprocaine is rapidly metabolized, whereas bupivacaine is bound to maternal plasma proteins.

The sucking rhythms of infants with a normal perinatal course were compared with those of infants with perinatal distress. The analysis showed that rhythms of nonnutritive sucking were significantly different from rhythms of normal control subjects even when there were no gross neurologic signs.[21,88] Subtle difficulties with feeding are sometimes the only perinatal evidence of the impact of hypoxia, as noted by low Apgar scores.

Infants whose mothers received bupivacaine epidural anesthesia were described to be less alert and have less ability to orient over the first month of life. Belfrage and associates[16] have reported bupivacaine and its metabolites in the circulation of infants for the first 3 days of life whose mothers had epidural anesthesia. Murray and associates[106] reported similar results using the Brazelton scale

and mother-infant interaction during feeding and mothers' perception of their infants. Levels of bupivacaine were measurable in the cord blood of all these infants as well, about 100 ng/mL. More recent studies report the use of lower doses of bupivacaine and either fentanyl or sufentanil.[92] Less sufentanil appeared in the cord blood. Measurable effects on the neonate's neurobehavior were seen in the Murray and associates study,[106] but not in the study by Bader and associates,[14] who observed epidurals of fentanyl and bupivacaine from 1 to 15 hours of infusion and saw no signs of accumulation in the cord blood and no adverse neonatal effects, as measured by umbilical ABGs and neurobehavioral scores. These studies did not note sucking ability. Only the Rosen and Lawrence study[139] reported the effects of epidural anesthesia on feeding ability of the neonates.

Perioral stimulation

Perioral stimulation facilitated nutritive sucking abilities in high-risk newborns (29 to 30 weeks' gestation), with each subject serving as his or her own control.[88] The stimulation was applied manually with quick touch-pressure stimulus for 1 second over the buccal fat pad. Similar stimulation has been used in children with central nervous system dysfunction in an effort to facilitate better sucking and swallowing. Such studies have not been reported during breastfeeding.[47]

Sucking stimulus and prolactin

When lactating postpartum women nurse their infants, the prolactin level increases from a high baseline level to levels several times over the mean baseline.[5] When nursing women played with but did not feed their infants, prolactin did not rise despite the initiation of milk dripping. Substitution of a breast pump at regular intervals caused prolactin elevations similar in timing and magnitude to those induced by sucking. When normal, menstruating, nonlactating adult women were stimulated with the breast pump for 30 minutes, significant prolactin increases occurred in 7 of the 18 women. No response was obtained in normal men.

When the prolactin response was used as a measure of "success" in establishing lactation in the first week post partum, no difference in prolactin levels was seen between women who had been considered good producers and those who were considered poor producers.[70] Mothers whose infants were in the special care unit and who were using a breast pump to establish lactation had minimal prolactin response to pumping but produced a mean of 86 g of milk per pumping. A similar study had been carried out previously, in which different responses in prolactin levels to suckling were found in good, fair, and poor producers.[68] When prolactin levels were measured after use of the breast pump at uniform settings, all three groups were similar.[9] This and the work of others[27,108] suggest that infant suckling plays a significant role in adequate milk production.

Conclusions

Knowledge about infant suckling has been accumulating rapidly, but little of it involves study of suckling at the breast. It has been established that the patterns are different mechanically. At the breast, nutritive and nonnutritive suckling vary only in rate, not in pattern. Infants can suckle immediately at birth and tolerate mother's milk (colostrum) best as the pattern of respirations remains physiologic. Inadequate suckling can influence maternal production, but inadequate suckling can be improved.

· · ·

Management of breastfeeding is best discussed in terms of the three stages: (1) prenatal period, (2) immediate postpartum, or hospital, period, and (3) postnatal, or posthospital, period.

PRENATAL PERIOD

It is most effective to prepare for breastfeeding well in advance of delivery. Prospective parents should consider feeding plans for the infant during the prenatal period, after the pregnancy is well established. Once quickening has occurred, the infant becomes more of a reality for the mother and she can relate to planning. Except in sophisticated cultures, the parents generally will not initiate this decision-making discussion, and it is appropriately introduced by the obstetrician, family physician, or midwife in the second trimester. Since the ready use of ultrasound and the presentation of an ultrasound picture of the fetus to the parents, the reality of a baby comes more quickly. Particularly with first children, it is appropriate to suggest to the parents that they select a pediatrician early. They should request a prenatal conference with the pediatrician to discuss not only feeding but also points of management and child rearing about which they might have questions. If the mother is receiving prenatal care from a family practice physician, this step is automatic.

Many studies of infant feeding choices have been reported in the literature reviewing the reasons women breastfeed. Universally, mothers breastfeed because it is best for the infant. Many decide long before the pregnancy, but those who choose bottle feeding admit they could have been persuaded if only someone had cared enough to tell them how important breastfeeding is to the infant. All women know mother's milk is best. Clearly, health care providers have made breastfeeding too complicated and burdened mothers with so many rules and regulations that they cannot cope and default to bottle feeding. When health care workers try to persuade a woman to breastfeed, they perpetuate the image of an impossible feat by saying, "Why not give it a try? It's not that bad," or "You'll be surprised. It isn't that hard," instead of conveying opportunity and good experience with, "It is a marvelous opportunity for you and your baby," or "It will be a special joy." Employment is often cited as the cause of early weaning, but it is actually unemployed women who are at home bottle feeding (see Chapter 13). Any time spent breastfeeding is worthwhile for the working mother and her infant.

The medical profession has been hesitant to take anything but a neutral position in discussions of breastfeeding for fear of pressuring the mother.[17] The evidence is stronger than ever that breastfeeding has distinct advantages for the infant and mother. Parents have the right to hear the data.

They can make their own choice. Fear of instilling guilt is a poor reason to deprive a mother of an informed choice, especially because women generally do not feel guilty about their own informed decision. After interviews with hundreds of mothers, half of whom chose to bottle feed, not one felt guilty, but some were disappointed that their physician did not discuss infant feeding.[139]

The prenatal discussion should also include any questions the parents may have about the lactation process and mother's ability to provide adequately for the infant. An examination of the breasts is part of good prenatal care and an excellent opportunity to discuss breastfeeding. If any anatomic abnormalities exist, they should be discussed. The breast tissue should be checked for lumps and cysts that might need treatment. The amount of mammary tissue is not correlated with the ability to produce milk. The more generous gland usually results from a more generous fat pad. During pregnancy the fat is replaced by proliferating acini. A woman with small breasts should not be discouraged from nursing; she may be the mother who most needs to prove herself.

Breast texture should be assessed by palpation. The inelastic breast gives the impression it is firmly knit together and the overlying skin is taut and firm so it cannot be picked up. The elastic breast is looser and the overlying skin is free, and the tissue is more easily picked up. Inelastic breasts are more prone to engorgement and seem improved by prepartum massaging and close attention to prevention of engorgement (Fig. 8-3).

Examination of the areola and nipple is equally important to identify any anatomic problems that may need attention before delivery. Gross malformations and inversion of the nipple can be easily detected, but lesser problems may go unnoticed. One must test for freedom of protrusion. When the areola is compressed and the nipple retracts, it indicates a "tied nipple" or inverted nipple caused by the persistence of fibers from the original invagination of the mammary dimple (Fig. 8-4).

The physician may provide literature on breastfeeding or suggest reading sources for the patient. One should avoid dismissing the parents' questions by merely suggesting appropriate readings because their decision making will be enhanced by open discussion with a knowledgeable professional. Although parents may have access to childbirth preparation programs in the community, they should not be put off to seek all their information from such sources. When parents have no opportunity to discuss with their care provider such issues

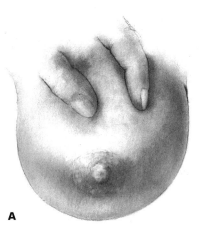
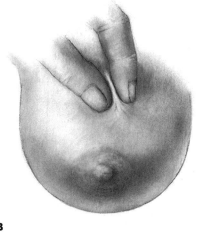

A   **B**

Figure 8-3. Texture of breast tissue can be assessed by picking up skin of breast. **A,** Inelastic breast tissue. **B,** Elastic breast tissue.

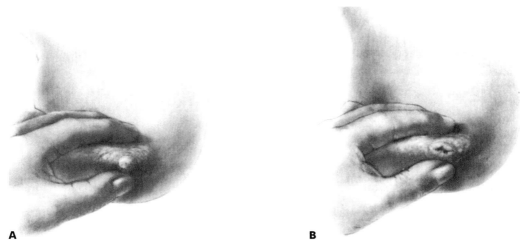

Figure 8-4. **A,** Normal nipple everts with gentle pressure. **B,** Inverted or tied nipple inverts with gentle pressure.

as early infant contact, nursing the infant in the delivery room, and family-centered maternity care, they often experience tremendous disappointment and misunderstanding.

The concerns most frequently expressed by mothers considering breastfeeding are related to themselves, not the infant. Mothers who are more concerned about their own well-being have more trouble adjusting to motherhood and should be provided with more support in adapting to the role. They may be helped by selecting a doula to support them, because our modern culture tends to isolate the young couple. Raphael describes a doula as one of "those individuals who surround, interact with, and aid the mother at any time within the perinatal period, which includes pregnancy, birth and lactation."[127] "The doula" has been further studied by Klaus and Klaus, who found a clear relationship between the presence of a doula in labor and the outcome of the delivery and the mother's personal experience and her recovery period (including breastfeeding).[82]

Concerns most frequently expressed prenatally by mothers include the following:

1. What is the effect on the mother's figure? Data indicate that the breast is affected by heredity, age, and pregnancy in that order and only minimally by lactation. Women who have never borne children may "lose their figures" long before a multipara who nurses her infants. Pregnancy enlarges breasts temporarily, as does early lactation, but the effect is temporary. Poor diet and lack of exercise will destroy a figure in both the male and the female long before any other influence.

2. What is the effect on the mother's freedom? Obviously, only a mother can breastfeed the infant; however, ample data support that it is possible to maintain a career, keep a job, or just get away from the house and still nurse in today's world. Actually, mothers in primitive cultures have returned to the fields or some form of productivity outside the home out of sheer necessity for generations. Mothers concerned about this often are best reassured by their peers, that is, mothers who are nursing. In communities with nursing mother groups, it is a simple referral. Employment statistics have revealed that women do successfully return to the work force and continue breastfeeding. Employment is rarely a reason for not breastfeeding, but it may influence duration (Chapter 13).

3. Many women are concerned with exposing the breasts. Despite the constant barrage of publicity about the breast in the modern press, many women are embarrassed to consider baring their breasts. As pointed out in Chapter 6, shame is an important consideration when helping a mother accept breastfeeding. Bentovim[17] suggests that shame and anxieties arise from the influence of one's life history and current events; thus, intervention is necessary at many levels. Clothes that make discreet breastfeeding possible are readily available and fashionable. Considerable body exposure is not necessary for breastfeeding. In a public survey performed in the Midwest for Surgeon General Koop in 1985, few people, male or female, in any age group considered breastfeeding embarrassing, and 82% would want their child breastfed. Universal publicity about breastfeeding in public places has created a more accepting attitude in most people, so that a nursing mother no longer needs to go and hide to feed her infant.[143]

Preparation of the breasts

The prenatal period is a time for the couple to prepare for their new role as parents and to learn as much as possible about breastfeeding. Most mothers do no special preparation and are very successful. Carefully controlled studies do not support the contention that fair-skinned women, especially redheads, are more prone to developing cracked, sore nipples than are others. Mothers who have had trouble with tender, cracked nipples when nursing a previous infant will need extra assistance in putting the infant to breast properly in the first few days, but elaborate rituals prenatally may actually cause problems. Nipple preparation has a negative effect on some women who are not ready to handle their breasts during pregnancy.

Bathing should be as usual, with minimal or no soap directly on the nipples and thorough rinsing. Some recommend patting the nipple dry with a soft towel, but this should not be done except after a shower or bath. Persistent removal of natural oils of the nipple and areola actually predisposes the skin to irritation. Montgomery glands in the areola secrete a sebaceous material for the cleansing and lubrication of the areola and nipple. This should not be removed by soaps or chemicals. Tincture of benzoin, alcohol, and other drying agents are contraindicated because they predispose the nipples to cracking during early lactation. Wearing protective brassieres, modern women do not experience the friction to the nipples that looser clothing provides, which may be why cracked nipples are a common problem in modern society but almost unheard of in developing countries and among other mammals. In Scandinavia, it is suggested that the pregnant woman get as much air and sunshine as possible directly on the breasts before delivery. Wearing a nursing brassiere with the flaps down to expose the nipples under loose clothing will serve the same purpose. However, aggressive and abrasive treatment of the nipples does not prevent nipple pain post partum and may aggravate it. Gentle love making involving the breasts is usually safe and is the most effective preparation.[62]

The use of lanolin, which is miscible with water and thus allows normal evaporation from the skin, does no apparent harm but in controlled studies also made no difference prenatally. Women allergic to wool will also be allergic to lanolin. Lanolin has been confirmed to contain insecticide residuals such as DDT and dioxins because sheep are routinely dipped in insecticides before shearing. The preparation Lansinoh is derived from natural lanolin with the contaminants and allergens removed and can be safely used if an ointment is indicated. Use of A and D ointment prophylactically also makes no difference, having an effect only in the treatment of fissures later. As with Lansinoh, mothers disliked the odor of this ointment. Petrolatum and other ointments made the skin more macerated and susceptible to irritation. Ointment should not be applied over the end of the nipple and the ducts.[137] It may also clog the Montgomery glands. In climates with average to high humidity, ointments are not routinely recommended for the breasts and may interfere with Montgomery gland secretion. In extremely dry climates, using ointments sparingly may be necessary.

Soap, alcohol, and tincture of benzoin have been shown to cause damage to tissue of the areola and nipple.[108]

Some believe gentle traction to the point of discomfort, but not pain, reduces perception of pain in the first week of lactation. A study carefully controlled to eliminate subjective discrepancies of interpretation revealed no significant difference in nipple sensitivity or trauma in those who practiced prenatal nipple rolling, application of breast cream, or expression of colostrum, as compared with those who had untreated breasts.[62] No increased pain or trauma was reported among the fair-skinned participants in this study, treated or untreated. Because many women are not inclined to manipulate their breasts before delivery and might be discouraged from breastfeeding if it is implied that this must be done, physicians should prescribe treatment only when an indication exists.[174]

Preparation of the nipples

Flat nipples or inverted nipples do not preclude breastfeeding. Flat nipples respond to the same passive treatment with a breast shell that works for inverted nipples. The shells can be worn during the last trimester by women who choose to do so (Figs. 8-5 and 8-6). They should be recommended only after careful examination and discussion about advantages and disadvantages by the physician. Follow-up at subsequent prenatal visits is also appropriate.

Alexander and associates[2] estimated that about 10% of pregnant women have inverted or nonprotractile nipples, which are thought to contribute to breastfeeding problems.[2] Breast shells (plastic disks with holes in the center and a domed cover) (see Fig. 8-5) and Hoffman exercises (stretching and pulling of the nipple and areola) are the most common treatments suggested. Alexander and associates[2] compared use of shells with no treatment and found more sustained improvement in the untreated group. The difference in use of shells/no shells was 52% and 60%, which is not significant.

A large multicenter trial of shells, Hoffman exercises, and no prenatal treatment showed "no treatment" to be most effective.[131] Exercises have had no significant impact and are contraindicated because of their tendency to initiate uterine contractions. The most significant finding was that more women who were instructed to wear shells or do nipple exercises than control subjects who had no prenatal preparation never initiated breastfeeding at delivery. More women also discontinued breastfeeding by 6 weeks compared with control subjects. The women complained that shells caused discomfort, embarrassment, sweating, rash, or milk leakage, or were conspicuous.

Such studies illustrate some of the risks of using untried methods to solve problems, although some women probably benefit by using shells. The question deserves further study. The process of assessing anatomic problems and initiating management should not be a deterrent to breastfeeding. Although discussion is appropriate prenatally, such assessment may best be delayed until the first few days of lactation when the mother is focused on feeding and the baby.

Inverted nipples (see Fig. 8-4) can be diagnosed by pressing the areola between the thumb and the forefinger. A flat or normal nipple will protrude: a

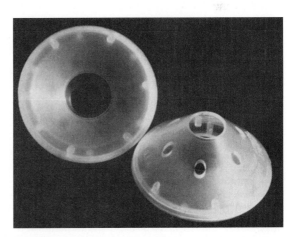

Figure 8-5. Breast shells: Vented domes worn over ring that allows nipple to evert. Shell is slipped into cup of well-fitting brassiere. Available in several styles and designs.

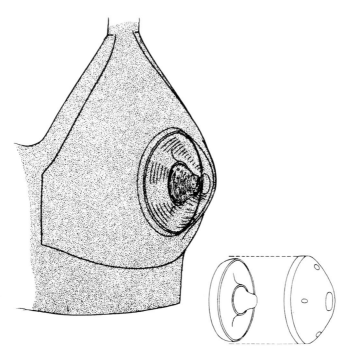

Figure 8-6.   Breast shell in place inside brassiere to evert nipple.

truly inverted nipple will retract. True inverted nipples are actually rare.

Treatments for inverted nipples

Exercises to evert inverted nipples are rarely successful and may be dangerous. The obstetric literature abounds with articles about the use of nipple stimulation in place of the traditional oxytocin challenge test to induce uterine contraction; only a few are cited here.[8,9,30,101] Using the breast pump or manual expression to produce colostrum is reported to induce labor or increase the strength of contractions in desultory labor.

Taylor and Green[154] reported a case of severe abruptio placentae after nipple stimulation. A series of patients induced labor with self-manipulation of the breasts with a 45% success rate. All patients in the series showed some ripening of the cervix with dilatation and effacement over 3 days of breast stimulation. Lipitz and associates[91] and others[4,154]

reported a relatively high incidence (45.5%) of exaggerated uterine activity in response to a breast-stimulation stress test, usually within 7 minutes of initiation of stimulation. Although all the cases and series cannot be reported here, it is clear that nipple stimulation in the third trimester can initiate uterine contractions and, in some, labor. Under the direction of an obstetrician, breast stimulation can be effective therapeutically, but it should not be recommended without obstetric evaluation.

Suggesting stretching (Hoffman) exercises is not advised, especially in women with a tendency to early labor. No study since Hoffman's initial report of two cases[67] has shown the process to be effective. Stretching the areola forcefully can damage the delicate Montgomery glands. Prepartum mastitis has also occurred with prenatal expression of colostrum. Whether manipulating the breast prenatally provides the mother with greater comfort in breastfeeding has not been demonstrated. Mothers who choose to bottle feed have told us that having to "exercise" their breasts is one of the "rules" that kept them from breastfeeding.

The Hoffman exercises[67] involve placing the thumbs or forefingers opposite each other close to the base of the nipple and slowly pushing away from the areola. Done in a vertical line and then a horizontal line in the form of an imaginary cross, this is intended to stretch and break the fibers that "tie" the inverted nipple.

Pumping with a pulsatile electric pump with a soft silastin flange (White River personal or institutional model) has been shown to facilitate latch-on with flat or inverted nipples after delivery. The breast is gently pumped on low settings until the teat is drawn out and the infant offered the breast. Similar pumping is done on the second breast, when that nipple is also inverted, before placing the infant on that breast. Usually the pumping can be discontinued after a few days, or a hand pump is adequate if prefeed pumping needs to be continued at home.

A readily available, inexpensive device can be prepared in the hospital from a standard syringe, selecting the size (10 or 20 mL) that best fits the nipple's diameter. The end of the barrel of a syringe with the piston removed is cut off with a sharp blade. The piston is then replaced from the cut end. This provides a smooth surface to place over the nipple, with the piston gradually withdrawn to create gentle suction for about a minute, then repeating. Mother can comfortably do this herself, repeating the procedure before each feeding as necessary.[80]

These approaches avoid the risk of never initiating breastfeeding identified in the Alexander and associates study.[2] They also provide one-on-one support from the nursing staff, which is very different from sending the mother home to use a strange plastic device.

The infant breastfeeds. The infant does not nipple-feed. If the nipples are flat or inverted, extra care is needed to provide enough areolar tissue in the infant's mouth to allow latch-on.

Surgical correction

Inverted nipples have been known to medicine for centuries, and treatment has included various exercises or use of older vigorous infants to suckle and use of adults who hired out for this purpose in difficult cases. The first surgical procedure was described in 1873. Other techniques have since been advanced.[58,126,146] A primary indication for surgical repair of the inverted nipple has been the chronic occurrence of central pockets of inflammation of the nipple, leading to spread of infection and suppurative mastitis. A simple method for correction without division of the lactiferous ducts involves using a purse-string suture and traction of holding sutures. The procedure can be done in the office under local anesthesia, according to Hauben and Mahler.[58] A truly inverted nipple may have fewer ducts. The microscopic pathologic examination of severely inverted nipples indicates the ducts are abnormal.

Hand expression prenatally

Some breastfeeding instructions suggest hand-expressing the breast to produce a few drops of colostrum every day for the last few weeks of pregnancy. Fortunately, the instructions usually suggest the patient consult her physician first. Manual or any kind of pumping of the breasts may stimulate the uterus to contract. Hand expression has no particular benefit and means that the early sequestered cells are expressed away in the drops of colostrum before delivery and are lost to the infant. Occasionally, prepartum mastitis has developed from this treatment. The risks far outweigh any seeming benefit.

Summary

1. During the first trimester, make the initial breast examination. Open the discussion about how the infant is to be fed and the benefits of breastfeeding. If anatomic variations may interfere with lactation, mention them and discuss possible remedies.
2. At each prenatal visit, offer information about breastfeeding.
3. Investigate the mother's knowledge of breastfeeding and document her information base to fill in the gaps and correct misinformation.

Also inquire about any treatments or routines she has initiated on her own so that the total management is appropriate.

4. Once quickening has been experienced, the parents are ready to plan more concretely about the baby. Suggest a visit with the pediatrician.

5. As delivery approaches, initiate discussion about feeding the infant immediately after birth, feeding protocols, and the mother's special needs or requests.

6. Be familiar with community resources so that patients can be wisely referred for peer support or assistance unavailable from one's office staff.

IMMEDIATE POSTPARTUM PERIOD

Immediately after the placenta has separated, the establishment of lactation begins. This is a critical period because many mothers who do not receive the proper support in the hospital are driven to failure at breastfeeding by inept management.

Nursing at delivery

The mother will probably want to nurse her infant immediately after birth if she has read the popular childbirth literature. Even if she does not ask, the obstetrician and delivery room staff should suggest and facilitate it.[90,134,170] Data confirm the view that delivery room or birthing center protocols that intercept interaction and suckling between mother and infant also have a negative impact on long-term lactation success.

Oxytocin levels at 15, 30, and 45 minutes after delivery are significantly elevated, coinciding with the expulsion of the placenta. Oxytocin has been associated with positive maternal feelings and with maternal bonding; thus, it is appropriate to optimize mother-infant interaction at this point of high oxytocin levels by facilitating suckling.

Disease-oriented physicians who have been trained to give trials of water first, hours after delivery, are always concerned that the infant may aspirate. Clinical signs of potential for aspiration include low Apgar score, increased secretions, and polyhydramnios. Actually, most infants in the world go straight to the breast on delivery, which has a physiologic effect on the uterus, causing it to contract. Because sugar water and cow milk formulas are very irritating if aspirated, delay in feeding has been the rule in the United States, where most infants are bottle fed. Colostrum is not irritating, however, and is readily absorbed by the respiratory tree if aspirated. Putting the infant to the breast within the first hour is optimal and compatible with Baby Friendly hospital guidelines.

A few possible obstacles exist to immediate nursing: (1) a heavily medicated mother, (2) an infant with a 5-minute Apgar score under 6, and (3) a premature infant under 35 weeks of gestation. The concern for the infant with a *tracheoesophageal* (TE) *fistula* is important, but a few precautions should suffice. If there is hydramnios or excess secretions at birth, a tube should be passed to the stomach to make sure the esophagus is patent. If all is well, the infant may nurse. If a TE fistula is found, it is a surgical emergency. *Choanal atresia* is another anomaly that would be of concern, but infants cannot suck on the breast or on anything if they cannot breathe through the nose. Usually an infant with choanal atresia has a low Apgar score or needs some assistance in establishing respirations.

As noted earlier, healthy newborns placed on the mother's abdomen will find their way to the breast and latch on if unimpeded.[134] For this first breastfeeding, it may be best to have the mother on a bed wide enough to have the infant lie beside her. Newer delivery tables are wide enough. The infant should not be dangled in midair over the breast. The mother should be assisted to turn onto her side and the infant presented to the breast, with the ventral surface to the ventral surface of the mother. The infant should not have to turn the head toward the breast. The mother may need assistance in holding her breast so as to present the nipple squarely into the infant's mouth, which is stimulated to open by stroking the center of the lower lip with the nipple.

When the lower lip is touched by the nipple, the infant will open widely, extending the tongue under the nipple. The breast will be drawn into the mouth, the nipple and areola elongated into a teat, and the suckling reflex initiated.[135]

Both mother and infant will do better if there is an atmosphere of tranquility in the room.[129] The only other risk to the infant is thermal stress. If the room is air-conditioned, it may be necessary to provide a radiant warmer over the infant and mother, especially if the infant is naked for skin-to-skin contact. Some mothers have shaking chills following the strenuous event of labor and cannot provide adequate warmth for the infant without some external source of heat or a blanket.

Chilling an infant may set off a chain of events from hypothermia to hypoglycemia to tachypnea to mild acidosis to the extent of requiring a septic workup. Hypothermia is therefore more easily prevented than treated.

If possible, mother, father, and infant should remain together for the next hour or so. The first hour for the infant is usually one of quiet alertness, a state that will usually recur only briefly again in the next few days. It is important to delay the instillation of prophylactic eye drops until after this time spent with the mother. If the drops are put into the eyes, blepharospasm will prevent the infant from opening the eyes and will mar the eye-to-eye contact. Only if there is a known risk of gonorrhea should the drops be put in immediately. If the mother has delivered in a birthing center, early contact and nursing should be part of the routine; however, it is equally important for all deliveries.

Two natural hand positions for the mother to introduce the breast are used most often. With attention to a few details, either position works (one is not right and the other wrong). The *scissor grasp* is the placement of the thumb and index finger above the areola and the other three fingers below the breast for support, thus allowing some compression of the areola. Care should be taken that the hand is not in the way of the infant's getting sufficient areola into the mouth (Fig. 8-7). This grip has been used for centuries and was shown in sketches and paintings even before the Christian

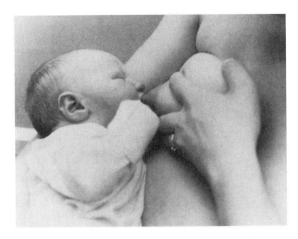

Figure 8-7. Scissor grasp, presenting breast while supporting infant.

era. If the hand is large or the breast small, it may work better than the palmar grasp.

The *palmar grasp* is the placement of all the fingers under the breast and only the thumb above (Fig. 8-8). This has been called the C-hold but is actually a V-hold, depending on the size of the breast and the size of the hand. This gives firm

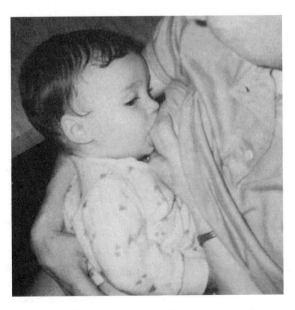

Figure 8-8. Palmar grasp for initiating breastfeeding.

support to the breast. It permits directing the breast squarely into the infant's mouth and avoids the need to press the breast away from the infant's nose. The palmar grasp is similar to the prehensile grasp of the apes when they nurse their young.

The apes, however, are unable to assume another hand posture neurologically or anatomically. If too much pressure is exerted by the human thumb, the nipple will be tipped upward (Fig. 8-9B), causing abrasion of the underside of the nipple. It is prefer-

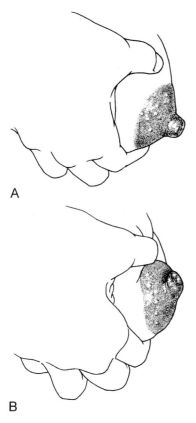

Figure 8-9. Palmar grasp (C-hold). **A,** When palm and fingers cup breast with support and thumb rests lightly above areola, nipple projects straight ahead or slightly downward (correct). **B,** When fingers come forward and thumb presses firmly above, nipple tips up and causes improper positioning. Improper positioning is a common cause of nipple abrasion (lower half) and pain with suckling. (Modified from Higgins K: The Nursing Mother's Companion, 2nd ed. Boston, Harvard Common Press, 1990.)

able that the nipple be directed horizontally as it is placed in the mouth (Fig. 8-9A) or tipped down slightly. The palmar grasp can be used when there is nipple pain, soreness, or trauma. It is also useful when the mother's hand is too small for a large breast. The mother should be encouraged to use the most natural and comfortable hand position.

Days in the hospital

The physician should see that patients are permitted to have their infants with them as much as they wish, within the guidelines of reasonable medical care. Only the few patients with difficult deliveries, cesarean birth with medication, postpartum complications, or eclampsia need to be excluded, but the mother's physician should make that judgment.

The influence of mode of delivery on initiation of breastfeeding was examined in 370 primiparas. Cesarean birth and other surgical delivery procedures (e.g., vacuum extraction) were associated with a sleepy infant, late start to feeding after delivery, increased incidence of bottle supplementation, less frequent night feedings, and delayed milk production in the hospital.[161] However, only 2.2% were not breastfeeding at discharge, and 52% were still breastfeeding at 6 months. Thus, despite many interventions, breastfeeding can succeed with sufficient support. An experienced nursing staff is critical to the management of the nursing mother in the first few days post partum.[93] Advice should be reasonable and consistent, and nurses should be cautioned against interjecting their own personal opinion or experience. When too many individuals may be involved in postpartum care, mothers are easily overwhelmed with information, especially if each person says something different.

Key points in management should include the following:

1. Feed when showing signs of hunger (Box 8-3).
2. Help the mother find a comfortable position. No rules should exist about sitting up or lying down.
3. Help the infant to the breast. The infant should be held so that the ventral surface of the infant faces the ventral surface of the mother.

BOX 8-3   **Signs of hunger in the infant**

1. Begins to stir
2. Brings hand(s) to mouth
3. Shows increasing efforts to root
4. Increasing activity, arms and legs flexed, hands in fist
5. If not picked up, progresses to frantic movements, wimpering
6. Crying is a late sign of hunger

4. Help the mother hold her breast for her baby, choosing the better grasp for the situation, and draw the baby to the breast by moving her arm toward her chest. Note: Never push the infant's head toward the breast because the infant will push back, often arching away from the breast. Holding or pushing the infant's head has been associated with persistent arching by the infant (arching reflex).

5. Help the mother reposition the infant on the second breast if the infant is still interested after releasing the first side. Moving may be difficult for the mother immediately post partum.

6. If the infant falls asleep after the first breast, the mother should be shown how to break the suction with her finger. Nonnutritive suckling while asleep is especially irritating to the nipple in the first few days. The mother should wait a little, wake the baby, and then move the infant to the second side.

7. When waking an infant to initiate feeding, unwrapping the blanket and using gentle stimulus are appropriate. Jackknifing is never appropriate and may cause regurgitation, aspiration, or trauma to vital organs. Usually infants are fed when they are ready.

8. The infant will nurse on the first breast until satisfied. After gentle burping, if the infant is still awake, the second side can be offered. The next feeding should be initiated on the other side. This will balance the stimulus to the breasts in the critical early days when milk production is just beginning.

9. Signs of satiety: sounds of swallowing dwindle and stop, nonnutritive suckling occurs in brief bursts, arms and legs relax, infant falls asleep and usually releases the nipple.

Stopwatch timing is not appropriate. It takes 2 to 3 minutes for the let-down reflex to produce milk in the early days, so the feeding must allow for the letdown. It is helpful for some mothers to have guidelines or estimates from which to work. Usually, infants nurse about 10 to 15 minutes per feeding in the first days. Nursing continually hour after hour may be counterproductive. Frequent small feedings will provide good stimulation to the breast without stressing the mother. The milk supply, however, is best stimulated by suckling.[123] The policy of the nursery should be to have all breastfed infants taken to their mothers when they awaken during the night,[89] if they are not rooming-in.

In keeping with the Baby Friendly Hospital Initiative (see Chapter 1), infants should be nursed on demand around the clock and receive no other food or drink. A mother and infant should be housed together unless there is a medical contraindication. Modern hospitals are a hubbub of activity, though, and with liberal visiting hours, the mother has no time to rest unless naps are scheduled. In the early days of the Rooming-In Unit at the Yale–New Haven Hospital, Jackson[15] insisted that all postpartum mothers have a nap after lunch. Every day the shades were drawn and traffic decreased on the unit for an hour. This is part of mothering the mother. In primitive cultures, mothers are groomed, fed, and protected after delivery, often for weeks. Furthermore, adequate rest is essential to successful lactation. In 1953, Jackson, along with Barnes and her colleagues,[15] prepared a classic description of the management of breastfeeding that remains the single most valuable source of information on the subject.

Diagnosing breastfeeding problems

To solve the problem of unsuccessful nursing, one should observe the mother feeding the infant. Often the problem is a simple one, such as a mother so uncomfortable and tense that the let-down reflex will not trigger, or perhaps an infant with a poor suck or poor latch. In these cases and others the diagnosis can be made most easily by direct observation.

In addition to mother's hand position, the manner in which the infant is held or placed to breastfeed is important. There is no one right position. Shortly after birth, lying down may be preferable for the mother. She lays on her side and the infant is placed on his or her side facing the breast, which the mother supports with her upper hand. She can use her lower hand to cradle the infant and bring him close. Pillows help sustain mother's position with one against her back and one between her knees. The latter is essential to keep her from rolling over should she drift asleep. When mother

is sitting up, the cradle position with mother bringing infant to the breast while cradling the infant in her bent elbow is the most common and natural position. Cross-cradle means the infant is held to one breast with the opposite arm so the body extends beyond the mother's lap. The football hold is a misnomer as the infant is not tucked under the arm like a football but rather forward so that mother supports the infant's head with her hand and the infant is supported by the mother's arm. The infant must be squarely facing the breast.

Introducing all the possible positions is overwhelming at first. With a little practice, mother will find what works best.

Understanding the mechanism of suckling in the neonate (Fig. 8-10), however, is essential to recog-

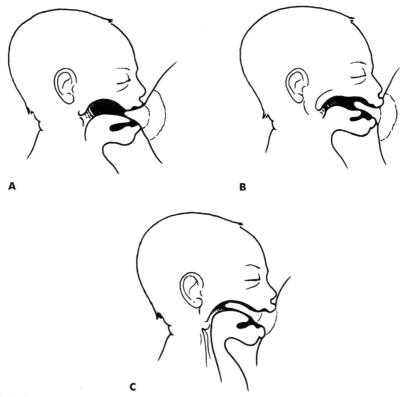

Figure 8-10. **A,** As infant grasps breast, tongue moves forward to draw in nipple. **B,** Nipple and areola move toward palate as glottis still permits breathing. **C,** Tongue moves along nipple, pressing it against hard palate and creating pressure. Ductules under areola are milked, and flow begins as a result of peristaltic movement of tongue. Glottis closes. Swallow follows.

nizing ineffective sucking. As the breast is offered to the infant, the mouth opens wide and the tongue is extended as the nipple is drawn into the mouth (Fig. 8-11). In a rhythmic motion, the tongue moves up against the hard palate, as it draws the nipple and areola into the mouth, creating an elongated teat. The cheeks fill the mouth because of the sucking fat pads and provide further negative pressure because they do not collapse. The tongue undulates along the teat, while remaining in place, compressing the collecting ductules in the areola and "milking" them toward the nipple. Milk flows from the nipple and is swallowed as the swallowing reflex is triggered and the peristaltic wave continues to the posterior tongue and pharynx and down the esophagus.

If the infant has a fluttering tongue that is discoordinate, it may not be as productive in stimulating ejection. If the infant cannot coordinate suck and swallow, choking occurs. Sometimes if let-down is strong, the first rush of milk will cause choking. Stopping and starting again should solve the prob-

lem. If the mother's milk flows abundantly with first let-down, she may need to express manually (and save) the first few milliliters to avoid choking the infant. Usually the flow moderates in the next few days. This problem is only temporary or is limited to times when the infant has not been nursed for an unusually long interval.

If the infant's jaw is slightly receding, the nipple may not stay in place. Gentle support from the mother's index finger at the angle of the jaw bringing it forward will help. She may always have to support the breast with her hand.

An infant who is given a bottle or rubber nipple to suck can become confused because the milking action is different (Fig. 8-12). The relatively inflexible rubber nipple may keep the tongue from its usual rhythmic action. In addition, the flow from the bottle may be so rapid, even without sucking, that the infant learns to put the tongue against holes in the rubber nipple to slow down the flow. Some infants who have been breastfed gag when the

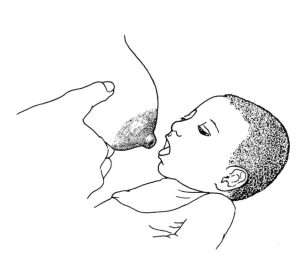

Figure 8-11. Latch-on response. In response to stimulating infant's lower lip with nipple, mouth opens wide. This response has been called oral searching reflex. It is part of circumoral rooting reflex. (From Righard L, Alade MO: Sucking technique and its effect on success of breastfeeding. Birth 19:185, 1992.)

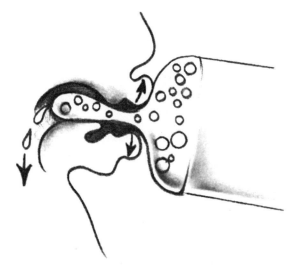

Figure 8-12. Infant sucking on rubber nipple, which fills mouth and thus prevents tongue action and provides flow without tongue movement. Flow occurs even if lips not tight around rubber hub.

relatively large rubber nipple is put in their mouths. When infants use the same tongue action needed for a rubber nipple while at the breast, they may even push the human nipple out of the mouth. When infants cannot grasp an engorged areola properly, they will clamp down on the nipple with the jaws, causing pain in the nipple and disrupting the ejection reflex. Manual expression of a little milk will soften the areola, permitting compression by mother's hand and an easier grasp by the infant.

When observing an infant being breastfed, take note of the following:

1. Position of mother, body language, and tension. Pillows may provide support for the arms or the infant.
2. Position of infant. Ventral surface should be to mother's ventral surface, with lower arm, if not swaddled, around mother's thorax. Infant cannot swallow if head has to turn to breast, and grasp of areola will be poor. Infant's head should be in crook of arm and moved toward breast by the mother's arm movement if cradle hold is used.
3. Position of mother's hand on breast not in way of proper grasp by infant.
4. Position of infant's lips on areola about 1 to 1½ inches (2.5 to 3.7 cm) from base of nipple.
5. Lips flanged and lower lip not folded in so that infant does not suck it.
6. Actual events around presenting breast and assisting infant to latch on.
7. Response of infant to lower lip stimulus by opening mouth wide (see Fig. 8-11).
8. Motion of masseter muscle during suckling and sounds of swallowing.
9. Ratio of sucks to swallows should move to 1:1 as feeding progresses.
10. Mother is comfortable with no breast pain.

Engorgement

The best management of engorgement is prevention. The degree of engorgement lessens for a woman with each infant because the time during which the milk "comes in" seems to shorten in multiparas. The primipara suffers most from engorgement.

Breast engorgement was carefully documented by Humenick and associates[71] for 14 days post partum in 114 breastfeeding women. Four distinct patterns emerged, varying from minimal engorgement to intense engorgement and including a bell-shaped pattern and a multimodal pattern. Characteristics of mothers, infants, and feeding frequency were similar across all patterns. Engorgement in these women was increased in second-time breastfeeders, with first-time feeders peaking at about 108 hours and second-time feeders at 100 hours. Engorgement cleared more quickly the second time. Clearly, mothers' experiences differ under seemingly similar circumstances. With early discharge, mothers are already home when it occurs.

A number of often conflicting theories and explanations regarding engorgement have been proposed in the professional and lay literature. The dictionary defines engorgement as "swollen with blood," and pathologists define it as "congestion." Engorgement of the breast involves three elements: (1) congestion and increased vascularity, which is the physiologic response that follows removal of the placenta and does not depend on suckling; (2) accumulation of milk, also a physiologic response to placental removal; and (3) edema secondary to the swelling and obstruction of drainage of the lymphatic system by vascular increases and fullness of the alveoli. No parallel exists in nature because the underlying process is physiologic. Engorgement is not injury, hemorrhage, or trauma. When the physiologic process proceeds smoothly, no pain, discomfort, or excessive swelling occurs. When edema is identifiable, the surface of the breast pits with pressure; the process is out of control, and intervention is necessary.[65]

Engorgement may involve only the areola, only the body of the breast (so-called peripheral engorgement), or both. Some engorgement is normal. When the breast does not respond with "fullness," this is abnormal and requires attention.

Areolar engorgement. When the areola is engorged, it obliterates the nipple and makes properly grasping the areola impossible for the infant. If the infant sucks only the nipple, it is exquisitely painful, because this is the only area of the breast with pain fibers. In addition, the collecting ductules are not "milked" and therefore do not empty, and the infant is frustrated by lack of milk.

The treatment is directed toward reducing the engorgement so that the infant can nurse effectively, which will further reduce the overdistended ducts. Gentle manual expression by the mother usually produces a small amount of flow and softens the areola. The presence of milk on the nipple will further encourage the infant's sucking. Warm soaks just before a feeding may facilitate manual expression. A mother should be taught how to express milk manually (Fig. 8-13). Placing the thumb and forefinger at the margins of the areola and pressing back in toward the chest and then bringing the fingers together, rhythmically simulating the action of the infant's jaw, will start the flow and soften the tense tissue (see Appendix G). When the infant is put to the breast, the mother should compress the areola between two fingers to make it easier for the infant to grasp. Offering the breast this way makes it easier for any infant to grasp, especially when the infant needs encouragement to nurse (Fig. 8-14).

Peripheral engorgement. Initially the breasts increase in vascularity and begin to swell. This usually starts in the second 24-hour period after delivery. Engorgement at this stage is vascular; thus, pumping mechanically briefly to stimulate the breast when the infant is not nursing adequately is appropriate. Pumping "to relieve engorgement" will yield little milk and may traumatize the hypervascular breast.

The mother should be advised to wear a well-fitting but adjustable nursing brassiere that does not have thin straps or permanent plastic lining. She should wear it 24 hours a day. With moderately severe engorgement, the breasts become full, hard, and tender. The swelling starts at the clavicle and goes to the lower rib cage and from the midaxillary line to the midsternum. The breasts may even become hard, tense, and warm. The mother complains of throbbing and aching pain and can find no comfortable position except to lie flat on her back and very still (Fig. 8-15).

Management centers on making the mother comfortable so that she can continue to nurse and stimulate milk production as well as nourish the infant. Proper support to elevate the breasts is important. The axillae are particularly painful, probably as a result of the tension on Cooper's ligament. Cold packs reduce vascularity. Warm packs

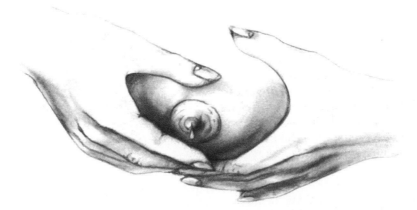

Figure 8-13. Position for manual expression of breast. Thumbs are brought toward areola, compressing areola between thumb and supporting fingers. With areola grasped, pressure is applied toward chest wall, and then pressure is released. This compression and pressure stimulate milking action (see also Appendix H).

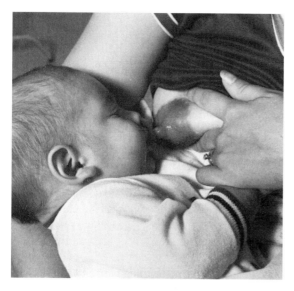

Figure 8-14. When breast is offered to infant, areola is gently compressed between two fingers and breast is supported to ensure that infant is able to grasp areola adequately.

aggravate the swelling. Having the mother stand in a warm shower and manually express some milk at the same time may be the best preparation to feed the infant. Some find comfort in alternating hot and cold water. Other mothers find leaning over a large

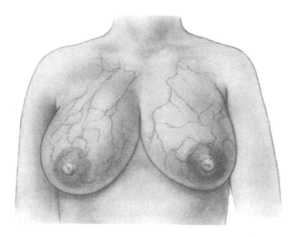

Figure 8-15. Marked mammary engorgement, predominantly vascular in nature.

mixing bowl of warm water just before feeding facilitates let-down and milk flow and is less disruptive than a shower.

After a feeding, cold packs reduce the swelling, edema, warmth, and pain. Acetaminophen or ibuprofen may give the mother some relief and are safe for the nursing infant. A codeine preparation can be recommended if there is no response to the simple medications. Codeine is cleared well by the mother, peaking in her serum at 30 to 60 minutes. The mother may need some sleep medication. Medications should be timed so that the least amount possible reaches the mother's milk and the baby. If medication is taken immediately before nursing, the pain will be relieved, but the drug will not reach the milk for more than ½ hour in the case of ibuprofen, acetaminophen, codeine, or short-acting barbiturates.

It is important to maintain drainage during this period of engorgement to prevent back pressure in the ducts from developing and eventually depressing milk production. Intraductal pressure can lead eventually to atrophy of both the secreting and the myoepithelial cells and a diminishing milk supply. The best treatment is breastfeeding frequently around the clock because suckling by the infant is the most effective mechanism for removal of milk. Relief is based on establishment of flow. The infant may have trouble grasping or may not be interested in nursing frequently in the first few days, so manual expression may also be necessary. Every mother should be taught manual expression by the perinatal nursing staff before discharge.[108]

The mother should support the breast with her fingers and place her thumbs distally and massage gently toward the areola, rotating gradually around the breast to include all quadrants. Then, once the peripheral lobules have been softened, areolar expression as previously described should be used to encourage complete emptying of the collecting ducts in the areola. This is a procedure best done by the mother, but it takes a skilled and experienced nurse to teach this technique (Appendix G). In women with significant engorgement, it may be helpful to use an electric pump, which is very effective because of its gentle milking action

(Chapter 21). The breast should be massaged distally before and during pumping.

Hand pumps can be used but exert only negative pressure on the areola. Unless accompanied by manual expression of the distal segments, they are only temporizing.

Treatment with cabbage leaves

A favorite treatment for severe engorgement is cabbage leaves. Cabbage leaves have been used in Europe for generations to relieve edema in other body parts, including the ankles. Chopped fresh leaves are applied to ankles overnight as a poultice and wrapped with a towel. When chilled whole cabbage leaves and chilled gel packs were compared as breast treatments for engorgement, no difference was found. Pain was relieved within 1 to 2 hours with both treatments in 68% of women. The mothers preferred the cabbage treatment.[138]

Severe engorgement occurs between the third and seventh day post partum, and the breasts are described as full, red, hard, and warm. The literature on this therapy is sparse, but two reports have been published. An Australian study involved a series of cases in which the treatment was applied.[140] There were no failures, but in several women the treatment was interrupted by other staff who applied ice and medications for pain without success. When cabbage leaves were reapplied, symptoms were relieved in 2 to 24 hours. Relief was often within 2 hours. Clinicians treated 30 patients and reported on nine in detail. Rosier[140] tried the treatment first with women who were engorged but were not nursing. No side effects have been reported.

A second randomized, controlled trial was undertaken in South Africa by Nikodem and associates,[114] who studied 120 breastfeeding women. At 72 hours post partum they were randomized to control or treatment group. Treatment was application of cool (from refrigerator) cabbage leaves to breasts, leaving just the nipple exposed. The leaves were applied after four feedings for 20 minutes or so until the leaves wilted. The cabbage used was *Brassica oleracea L var. capitata.* All mothers were also taught routine breast exercises,

which consisted of bending the arms at the elbow, moving the arms across the chest, with hands facing the same shoulder, so elbows touched, and swiping across the breast a total of 10 times. This exercise, known by various names, including the Johannesburg salute, is used as a preventive treatment for engorgement. Although the experimental group reported less engorgement, it was not statistically significant. Exclusive breastfeeding at 6 weeks was 76% compared with 58% among controls ($p = 0.09$). Mean duration of breastfeeding was 36 versus 30 days in control subjects ($p = 0.04$). However, this study had more multiparas in the control group, and engorgement is rarely a serious problem in multiparas.

Whether cabbage leaves have prophylactic value may be challenged, but their value in the therapy of severe engorgement is worth noting. Whether it is the coolness of the leaves or an innate property of cabbage itself that is therapeutic has not been proved. In Duke's *Handbook of Medicinal Herbs,** cabbage *(Brassica oleracea)* is referred to as a *galactogogue.* The most common variety, *B. capitata,* is the one used in engorgement therapy. This handbook also lists cabbage with other angiosperms as capable of causing hypoglycemia. Cabbage is noted to contain sinigrin (allyl isothiocyanate) and rapine. Herbalists consider rapine to be an antifungal antibiotic. The text lists galactogogues and lactation suppressants found in other plants but does not mention any mammary effects of cabbage.

A new product is available on the market called Cabbage Gel (Pure Necessities, 15036 Beltway, Addison, TX 75244). This pale green gel has a gentle odor of peppermint, is made of aloe vera, and contains peppermint oil and "herbal infusions" and apparently no cabbage. It is intended for use alone or with fresh cabbage leaves to help keep them in place and cool the engorged breast. Care must be taken to remove the gel before feeding the infant because aloe vera can be a powerful purgative.

---

*Duke J: Handbook of Medicinal Herbs. Boca Raton, FL, CRC Press, 1985.

Going home from the hospital

Currently, maternity patients are going home from the hospital in 2 to 3 days or sooner, which is certainly before lactation is well established but possibly before engorgement is full blown. When maternity floors were run so rigidly that ad lib breastfeeding was an impossible feat, it was often suggested that a mother go home and get away from the negative hospital atmosphere to a place where she could relax and concentrate on feeding the infant and resting. This is the point at which the doula, so well described by Raphael,[127] could make the difference between success and failure. It may be appropriate for the obstetrician to order the mother to have some assistance at home, whether from her husband, her mother, or a friend. "The common denominator for success in breastfeeding is the assurance of some degree of help from some specific person for a definite period of time after childbirth."[127]

Raphael studied mothers in the cycle of anxiety while she became the doula for them at about 6 to 10 days post partum. The calm that can be experienced in the presence of a confident, caring person will relax the mother. The infant senses the calm and confidence and sleeps. When feeding again, the infant nurses well. Breaking the cycle of panic that seizes a new mother when she finds herself home alone with a new infant who needs frequent feeding requires someone to instill confidence. This individual does not need to be a health professional, but should be a calm, reassuring, nonthreatening person who is supportive of breastfeeding.

Although physicians cannot be the doula, they can be sure that the family understands the need and can suggest community resources if no personal ones are available. Successful breastfeeding is not automatic, as demonstrated by the failure rate. Some problems have been generated by the disturbance of the synchronized interaction between mother and infant by rigid hospital protocol. This is continued at home when feeding is by the clock rather than by instinct. The office practice should be available by telephone. Ideally, the office nurse practitioner makes a home visit in the first week. An office visit should be scheduled within a week of birth, or sooner if a problem exists, especially for a weight check.

Most communities have a licensed, certified lactation consultant available for new mothers or any mother with a problem. The physician should be familiar with the available lactation consultants if the practice does not provide one on its staff.

Nipples

Painful nipples. Presumably the nipples will adapt to the nursing experience naturally; however, discomforts often arise. The initial grasp of the nipple and first suckles typically cause discomfort in the first few days of lactation because it is a new experience for the mother. This is not cause for alarm but requires maternal reassurance. The sensation is created by the negative pressure on the ductules, which are not yet filled with milk. Later, when lactation is well established and the let-down reflex has matured, mothers describe a *turgescence,* which is the increased fluid pressure being relieved by suckling. If the pain persists throughout the feeding, the situation demands immediate attention. It should not hurt to breastfeed.

Nipple pain was studied in 102 women in the first 96 hours post partum.[89] Engorgement was most closely associated with nipple discomfort, which may be enhanced by the general discomfort of the breast. Prenatal breast preparation was unrelated to soreness. Length of time spent suckling was also unrelated. No record was kept on nonnutritive suckling, although others have found suckling without swallowing to be more stressful early in lactation. How the breast is presented to the infant is the most critical factor (maternal hand position and infant squarely facing breast).[49] This is the time to observe the feeding, to check the latch, and to look for malpositioning or other abnormalities.

The most common cause of painful nipples in the first few days is positioning. This should be reviewed in detail, being certain the areola is softened sufficiently to have the infant grasp adequately.[113] The infant's lower lip is checked to ensure it is flanged around the breast and not drawn into the mouth, which can abrade the nipple. The tongue should be under the teat and cupped around it.

Specific areas of pain may have specific causes. Soreness on the top of the nipple or on the tip usually results from poor latch-on or tongue thrusting in an infant who is also bottle fed. Soreness can also be caused by tipping the nipple upward so that it grazes the hard palate from overzealous use of the palmar grasp or C-hold. Pain on the underside of the nipple is caused by presenting the breast with the nipple tipped up, usually because of more pressure by the mother's thumb on top than the fingers below the breast, so the infant "strokes" the underside of the nipple. The tip of the nipple may also graze the hard palate. The nipple may be bruised, scabbed, or blistered, depending how long the problem has continued (Fig. 8-16). Normally, the peristaltic motion of the tongue below the nipple is not uncomfortable.

If no abnormality is found, the pain may be caused by a "barracuda baby" with a vigorous suck. Occasionally, an infant will have a discordant suck, clamping down on the nipple. This may have a neurologic cause. Suck training may help.* The breast will gradually adapt, and this pain will not last indefinitely. Sometimes the maternal tissues are unusually tender and delicate. Brief dry heat may help between feedings in humid climates. The mother should remove the waterproofing from her brassiere and expose her breasts to air briefly after each feeding. A and D ointment may help in dry climates.

Even more effective, especially in humid climates, is the use of an electric hair dryer, set on warm and fanned across the breast about 6 to 8 in. (15 to 20 cm) away only for 2 to 3 minutes to avoid overdrying. This brings remarkable comfort and

---

*Suck training is a special technique developed to help an infant who cannot coordinate the undulating (peristaltic) motion of the tongue. It involves using the gloved finger of the lactation consultant and stimulating the infant's tongue with the finger pad to the tongue. The infant will gradually learn to suck. Using a feeding tube attached to a syringe of milk along the finger will provide the infant with milk when sucking is correct. This is called finger feeding.

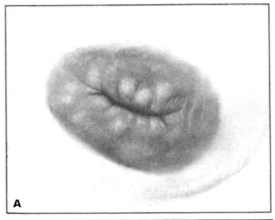

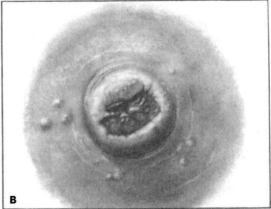

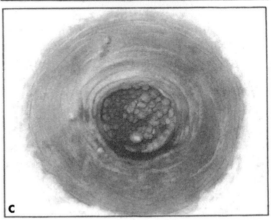

Figure 8-16. Various types of cracks in abraded lactating nipples. **A**, Crack across nipple. **B**, Multiple cracks (stellate). **C**, Crack at lower base.

can be done sitting, standing, or lying down. In dry climates, however, wetting the tissues is the preferred treatment. The breast will be moist with milk right after a feeding. This should not be wiped away but allowed to dry on the skin. Many primitive cultures treat irritation of the skin with human milk.[123] The surface-drying effect of the treatment helps counteract the increase in moisture experienced in the first days of lactation. This is neither necessary nor appropriate in arid climates.

Stabbing pain that radiates through the breast so that mother feels like the ducts are liquid fire may be associated with *Candida* infection of the breasts, often seen after antibiotic treatment. The infant may or may not have visible thrush. This deserves special attention.[42] Not all burning pain is due to thrush. Sore nipples that occur beyond the first weeks of breastfeeding may be caused by infections due to *Candida albicans* or *Staphylococcus* or even vasospasm. These causes are discussed in Chapters 16 and 17.

Ointments. The appropriate treatment of sore nipples is based on removing the cause and facilitating healing. Positioning is the most common cause, but repositioning will not heal a seriously damaged nipple without some medical intervention. The most appropriate application depends not only on cause but also on environmental conditions. With high humidity, greasy moisture-sealing ointments aggravate the skin. If the atmosphere is very dry (e.g., at the high altitudes of Denver or in the desert climate of the Southwest), creams may be appropriate.

All treatments are not appropriate to all lesions. Cool, wet tea bags, for instance, serve as an astringent because of the tannic acid, causing drying and cracking, and are not usually recommended. One study compared tea bag therapy with water compresses and no treatment. Both tea bags and water compresses were more effective than no treatment. Given the taste, smell, and astringent effect of the tannic acid in the tea bag, this study would further confirm that the same effect can be obtained with plain water.[87] Pugh and associates[125] examined three treatments for nipple soreness: USP modified lanolin, warm water compresses (a warm wet washcloth), and expressed breast milk with air drying. The use of warm compresses appeared to be the most effective of the three treatments.

The routine application of ointments to the nipple, areola, or breast should be discouraged except in cases of extremely dry skin where the tissue needs to be lubricated.

Lanolin is most hazardous to anyone with a wool allergy. Lansinoh is a purified, alcohol-free, and "allergen-free" ointment, however, and should be safe if an ointment is indicated. Some ointments and creams have irritants.[60] The sebaceous and Montgomery glands of the areola and nipple are easily plugged by repeated applications of oily substances during pregnancy and lactation. Preparations with vitamins A and D are innocuous, but those with vitamin E or hormones are unsafe unless prescribed for a specific problem by the physician.

Moist wound healing for sore or cracked nipples has been proposed by some dermatologists and is comparable to treatment for other areas of the body.[145] Early soreness may be caused by insufficient moisture present in the skin coupled with the friction of malpositioning.[131] Wetness on the surface caused by the milk and occlusive plastic-lined nursing pads does cause irritation. The moisture within the tissue, however, should be preserved by the application of a nonirritating ointment after a feeding when the nipple has been gently dried, according to Sharp.[145]

Local anesthetic creams should not be used because they can lead to allergic reactions, but more important, they can interrupt the let-down reflex and affect the infant by numbing the mouth and throat. The use of ice to numb the pain before feeding does not correct the cause and may interfere with the let-down reflex, which is easily intercepted by cold as well as by pain. If ice numbs the areola, it may numb the nervous response. Irritation or rash should first be treated by discontinuing any ointments or other self-medicating material. This is usually the first step in the treatment of any dermatologic problem.

Nipple shields. A nipple shield is a device made of rubber or synthetic materials that is worn over the nipple and areola while the infant is suckling.

A makeshift shield of a nursing-bottle nipple should never be used. Shields differ from the shells designed to evert nipples (Fig. 8-17). Shells should never be worn while breastfeeding, and any milk that drips into them should not be saved to feed the infant because it is heavily contaminated and of lower fat content. A study of the effect of a thin latex nipple shield on suckling showed no difference in length of suckling time and no difference in cortisol levels or prolactin levels, which were correlated with length of time suckling.[178] Wearing the shield without suckling had no effect on prolactin levels. The amount of milk received by the infant, however, was significantly reduced.

Nipple shields should not be used unless prescribed because it often becomes hard to wean the infant back to the bare breast. The infant becomes confused in learning the sucking routine, although there is the advantage that the mother can see the milk being transferred. Glass or plastic shields with a rubber nursing nipple never work well and should be abandoned. The effect of a traditional red rubber nipple shield (see Fig. 8-17) was compared to a new thin latex nipple shield referred to as a "Mexican hat." Normal mothers with no problems lactating nursed their infants using the shields.[178] The red rubber shield reduced the milk transfer by 58% and increased the infants' sucking rate and time spent resting. The thin latex shield reduced

milk by 22% but had no effect on sucking patterns. Many lactation experts consider the use of a breast shield a sign of failure of proper lactation guidance and a preventable situation. In the case of a large maternal nipple, however, the shield tapers the nipple so the infant can grasp it as an elongated teat.

Small or flat nipples. When the nipples are small or flat, special attention to compress the breast and areola between two fingers to provide as much nipple as possible to the infant will assist the infant in getting a hold. Using the breast shell between feedings will help draw the nipple to greater prominence. Softening the areola before a feed to make it more compressible also helps.

Drawing the nipple out with a hospital electric pump before each feeding should help facilitate latch-on and train the infant to a proper grasp. A day or two of such preparation with the pump is usually sufficient if the infant is full term with a good suck. Once engorgement is diminished and nursing is well established, small or flat nipples are usually no longer a problem.

Large nipples. Large nipples are occasionally a problem with a small infant or an infant with an indecisive suck. The shells do not help the infant cope at first, and it is best just to work patiently with the infant. Manual expression, which softens the areola to make it more pliable before putting the infant to the breast, often helps. Preparation

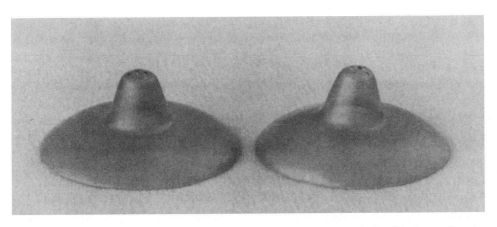

Figure 8-17.   Nipple shield made of tasteless, odorless silicone in very thin flexible form referred to as "Mexican hat."

with an electric pump may also facilitate the infant's latch-on by drawing the nipple into a teat. A thin silastin nipple shield may facilitate a latch with large nipples.

Cracked nipples. Whenever the mother complains of nipple pain on nursing, the nipple should be examined in good light to look for cracks or subepithelial petechiae, which may be the precursor to cracking. Taking a thorough history about care of the breast is important to identify the use of soaps, oils, ointments, or other self-prescribed treatments. Watching the nursing process may identify abnormal positioning at the breast. The position of the crack also may identify the problem (Box 8-4).

Cracks straight across the tip of the nipple are caused by excessive dryness following original irritation of the nipple tip by poor nipple positioning against the infant's palate (see Fig. 8-16A). Pain may be eased by correct positioning, and healing may be promoted by application of therapeutic ointments such as A and D, purified lanolin, or a synthetic hydrocorticoid (Elocon ointment), followed by a "butterfly" bandage that brings the edges of the crack together between feedings in extreme cases in which the crack is wide. Local

anesthetics are not appropriate, nor are nipple shields, which draw and pull the nipple. Star-shaped cracks respond to similar treatment (see Fig. 8-16B). Cracks at the base of the nipple (see Fig. 8-16C) are usually caused by sucking of the lower lip and biting, which originate with poor positioning but require checking the lower lip. Mother can gently pull it out with her thumb or relatch the infant.

Therapy is indicated for true cracks. In the pre-cracked stage, letting the milk dry on the skin for a few moments and applying a cream between nursing are most effective. When true fissures have developed, opening both sides of the nursing brassiere at feedings and beginning to nurse on the less painful side first will permit the initial let-down to occur "atraumatically"; then the infant can be put carefully to the affected breast. When nursing must be stopped on a given breast, it sets up a chain reaction of engorgement, reduced flow, and plugging of the ducts. Changing the infant's position, such as using a football hold or cross-cradle, may help healing.

Hewat and Ellis[62] conducted a study comparing lanolin with dried-on milk. Mothers used one treatment on one nipple and the other treatment on the opposite breast. The authors found no correlation between pain and frequency of feedings or the mother's hair and skin color. The women reported no difference in soreness between the two treatments. Many dermatologists believe that applying two treatments to different parts on the same patient may lead to mixture of therapies and noncompliance rates higher than normal. A study of antiseptic sprays by Herd and Feeney[60] produced controversial results. Antiseptic sprays are rarely justified and may cause problems because the physiologic normal flora of the nipple and areola should not be artificially altered unless a culture has been done.[73]

In women with severe nipple cracking, the physician may prescribe synthetic topically applied corticoids, which are preferred by dermatologists. When position has been corrected and bacterial and fungal infections ruled out, application of Elocon 0.1% cream or ointment, which is antiinflamma-

---

BOX 8-4   Management of sore, painful, or cracked nipples

1. Examine the breast, nipple, and nursing scene.
2. Recommend manual expression before feeding and softening of areola.
3. Check for infant position on breast.
4. Suggest nursing on unaffected breast first with affected side exposed to air.
5. Let expressed breast milk dry on skin between feedings.
6. Recommend appropriate ointment.
7. Rarely, temporarily stop nursing on affected side and replace it with manual expression or pumping.
8. If necessary, give acetaminophen, ibuprofen, or codeine (for serious pain unresponsive to milder drugs) in short-acting preparations just before nursing (see Chapter 11).

tory, antipruritic, and vasoconstrictive, can be rapidly healing. Less than 0.5% of a dose of corticoids topically is absorbed. Ultravate (halobetasol propionate) 0.05%, another synthetic corticoid ointment, is also available by prescription. Usually a 2-day treatment is adequate, and the ointment does not need to be removed before feeding. It is important to treat the underlying cause of the original trauma to the nipple.

The application of any ointment that must be removed before nursing has disadvantages because removal is traumatic. A and D ointment, which does not have to be removed, is occasionally effective. A and D ointment contains vitamins A and D from fish liver oils in a petrolatum base. An individual would have to consume several large tubes of it at one sitting even to approach toxicity. The indiscriminate use of ointment, however, can be the cause of nipple pain, and as with many dermatologic problems, the initial treatment prescribed may be to discontinue previous treatments. Some ointments suggested as breast creams contain antibiotics, astringents, bismuth subnitrate, or petrolatum, all of which are contraindicated. These creams are available over the counter without a prescription; thus, the physician should inquire about their use as self-medication.

Premoistened towelettes that contain benzalkonium chloride 1:750 in 20% alcohol should not be used on a nipple or areola with or without soreness or cracks or used to cleanse. The infant could accumulate benzalkonium chloride by suckling. The infant might reject the breast because of the flavor or burning sensation in the mouth. Also, benzalkonium is usually painful for the mother.

Infant in the hospital
Feeding characteristics

Infants have been aptly classified by their feeding characteristics by Barnes and colleagues[15] as "barracudas," excited "ineffectives," procrastinators, gourmets or mouthers, and resters. These descriptions serve to demonstrate that infants are different and the management of the nursing experience will vary accordingly. Herein lies the secret to appropriate counseling: recognizing the differences among infants and developing management that fits each situation.

Barracudas. When put to the breast, barracudas vigorously and promptly grasp the nipple and areola and suck energetically for 10 to 20 minutes. There is no dallying. Occasionally, this type of infant puts too much vigor into the nursing and hurts the nipple at first, but this passes.

Excited ineffectives. Some infants become so excited and active at the breast that they alternately grasp and lose the breast. Then they start screaming. The nurse or mother often must pick up and quiet the infant first, then put the infant back to the breast. After a few days the mother and infant usually become adjusted. Having some expressed milk ready on the nipple and areola helps to focus the infant.

Procrastinators. Procrastinators often seem to put off until the fourth or fifth postpartum day what they could just as well have done from the start. They wait until the milk "comes in." They show no particular interest or ability in sucking in the first few days. It is important not to prod or force these infants when they seem disinclined. They do well once they start. The mother would do well to pump after each feeding so that her supply is building.

Gourmets or mouthers. Gourmets insist on mouthing the nipple, tasting a little milk, and then smacking their lips before starting to nurse. If hurried or prodded, the infant will become furious and start to scream. Otherwise, after a few minutes of mouthing the infant settles down and nurses very well.

Resters. Resters prefer to nurse a few minutes and then rest a few minutes. If left alone, they often nurse well, although the entire procedure will take much longer. They cannot be hurried.

Weight loss

Newborns usually lose some weight, which tends to be a function of whether they are appropriate, large, or small for gestational age as well as how many kilocalories they ingest in the first few days. Breastfeeding infants of multiparas often lose little weight because the milk "comes in" so quickly.

Conversely, the normal primipara may not have a full supply for 72 to 96 hours. If the weight loss is more than 5% (150 g in a 3-kg infant), evaluate the process to identify any problems before they become serious. A 7% loss is maximum, and weight should plateau by 72 hours. A 10% weight loss is acceptable only if all else is going well and the physical examination is negative, but it should be justified in the record, and the infant should be seen shortly after discharge from the hospital to ensure resolution of the problem. If discharge home has taken place in 48 hours or less, it is imperative that the pediatrician's office keep in touch with the mother. Many have a nurse practitioner who makes the follow-up telephone calls or a home visit.

Newton and Newton[109-112] described a simple observation of breastfeeding mothers that was an accurate predictor of ultimate lactation success (Table 8-2). All the observations were related to the milk-ejection reflex (i.e., uterine pain, milk dripping on sight of baby, and relief of nipple discomfort on initiation of sucking). Successful breastfeeders had significantly more uterine pain during suckling on day 2 post partum (afterpains), more dripping of opposite breast, more dripping on sight of infant, and cessation of nipple discomfort.[109] As a further evaluation, Newton and Newton compared the amount of milk left in the breast after feeding that was available with a dose of Pitocin (synthetic oxytocin) and pumping. Successful breastfeeders had only 27% left, and unsuccessful breastfeeders had 47% left. This technologic measurement is no better measure of success than the simple observations of the let-down reflex (see Table 8-2). This observation parallels the observations by ultrasound of Hartmann on storage capacity of the breast, which varies from woman to woman.[57]

Provision of early formula supplementation in the hospital was also associated with less successful lactation. A strong predictor of the need for supplementation was excessive time from delivery to first breastfeeding. When water and sugar water were routinely provided, there was greater weight loss in the infant and lower lactation success rate.[86]

Weighing the infant before and after feedings produces tremendous anxiety in the mother and affords little information if it is inaccurate. Weighing has been improved, however, by the introduction of electronic digital readout scales that are accurate to 1 g and are especially helpful in the intensive care nursery for infants under 1000 g.[26] Most newborn nurseries use these extremely accurate scales. Test weighings can be done when medically indicated. With development of similar

TABLE 8-2   Percentage of women reporting symptoms of milk ejection with significant difference between successful and unsuccessful breastfeeders

Symptoms	Successful breastfeeders (%)	Unsuccessful breastfeeders (%)	Probability (p)
Uterine pain (cramps) during suckling: day 2	64	38	<0.05
Dripping from opposite breast during suckling: day 6	95	67	<0.01
Dripping before suckling (as oxytocin is triggered by sight or expectation of baby or other times): day 5	78	56	<0.05
Cessation of nipple pain (as milk flow counteracts negative pressure produced by suckling):			
Day 4	89	69	<0.05
Day 5	87	52	<0.01
Day 6	92	70	<0.05
All symptoms: all days	59	48	<0.01

From Newton N: The quantitative effect of oxytocin (Pitocin) on human milk yield. Ann NY Acad Sci 652:484, 1992.

equipment, scales are practical for home use. Their accuracy in before-and-after weighings has been verified by several investigators using comparison techniques.[168] When ordinary balance scales are used, the margin of error has been shown to be greatest with the smaller volumes. In volumes of milk less than 60 mL, the error can be ± 20%.

Sequential breast volume measurements have been used to study short-term rates of milk synthesis.[35] Using a rapid, computerized breast measurement system, a close correlation was established between amount of milk the infant consumed and change in breast volume. The volumes measured varied between 11 and 58 mL/hour.[35] At some point this technique may be applied to clinical assessment of milk production.

This technology and the work of others have led to new insights into lactation physiology.[124] Mothers know that the breasts fill gradually to a certain degree between feedings. When feedings are delayed or missed, breasts can be very uncomfortable, with relief achieved when the infant nurses.[13] The rate of synthesis appears constant, as confirmed by topographic imaging. A factor has been identified by Prentice and associates[124] that is released into the milk space and inhibits milk synthesis locally by direct action. The action of this local inhibitory factor imposes a more phasic pattern of milk production, having its greatest effect when the breast has the least milk and slowing to a minimum as the breast fills.[13,124] "Empty breast" is a misnomer and is physiologically untenable.[176]

Vomiting blood

A breastfed baby who vomits blood should have the blood evaluated for fetal or adult hemoglobin by the Apt test (blood suspended in small amount of saline solution and equal amount of 10% sodium hydroxide added; adult hemoglobin turns brown; fetal hemoglobin stays pink). If it is adult hemoglobin, the nipple may be bleeding. Sometimes this bleeding is painless and unknown to the mother, and sometimes she is afraid to report it. If it is fetal hemoglobin, the infant needs evaluation. Breastfeeding can continue with pink milk if the infant retains it and the cause has been addressed.

Greenish or brown milk is occasionally described in the first few days if the mother is pumping or her infant vomits. It usually results from old blood in the ducts, a residual of rapid growth and vascularization during pregnancy. This milk is usually harmless and clears spontaneously in a day or two. If being pumped, it may be discarded. Breastfeeding does not need to be interrupted. This has been referred to as rusty pipe syndrome.

Let-down reflex

The most important single function that affects the success of breastfeeding is the let-down reflex. A mother may produce the milk, but if she does not excrete it, further production is suppressed. Much has been written on this single reflex by physiologists, endocrinologists, biochemists, pathologists, anatomists, psychologists, psychiatrists, obstetricians, and pediatricians. It is a complex function that depends on hormones, nerves, and glands, which can be inhibited most easily by psychological block (Fig. 8-18).[111]

The hormonal mechanism of milk ejection is described in Chapter 3. The reflex stimulation of milk ejection was meticulously studied by Caldeyro-Barcia[29] while he studied intramammary pressures. The more efficient stimulus for the milk-ejection reflex is suckling the nipple. The frequency of suckling is 70 to 120 strokes per minute, and the mean pressure is −50 to −150 mm Hg. The maximum recorded was −220 mm Hg. Within 1 minute of the onset of suckling, the first contraction of the mammary myoepithelium is recorded, but it may take 2 or more total minutes for full response.

Further research by Cobo and associates[32] has shown that, as in other species, the human response is undulating or spurtlike in release, although the level of oxytocin tends to reach a peak and plateau at 6 to 10 minutes during a feeding.[166] Some studies show no episodic secretion. When oxytocin levels are measured before the feeding, there is a response to the baby's crying or other anticipation of feeding. No prolactin response occurs before actual suckling (Fig. 8-19). A second release of oxytocin occurs when suckling begins.[38] No direct correlation exists

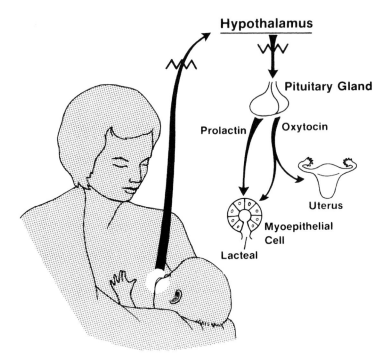

Figure 8-18.   Diagram of ejection reflex arc. When infant suckles breast, mechanoreceptors in nipple and areola are stimulated, which sends a stimulus along nerve pathways to hypothalamus, which stimulates posterior pituitary gland to release oxytocin. Oxytocin is carried via the bloodstream to breast and uterus. Oxytocin stimulates myoepithelial cells in breast to contract and eject milk from alveolus. Prolactin is responsible for milk production in alveolus. Prolactin is secreted by anterior pituitary gland in response to suckling. Stress such as pain and anxiety can inhibit let-down reflex. Sight or cry of infant can stimulate release of oxytocin but not prolactin.

between levels of oxytocin and the volume of milk released at a given feeding.[102] The average pituitary gland contains 1000 mU of oxytocin, and only 0.5 mU is required for the let-down reflex.

Uterine contractions are also stimulated by suckling, because the oxytocin released into the bloodstream also affects the target receptors in the uterine myoepithelial cells.[115] Amplitude and frequency may increase over time during nursing. Mechanical stimulation of the nipple can produce the same effect on the breast and uterus. The milk-ejection reflex is inhibited centrally by cold, pain, and emotional stress. Ejection response can be elicited by seeing the infant or hearing the infant cry. Also, overwhelming evidence indicates that the neuropeptide oxytocin is centrally involved in

activating maternal behavior at the appropriate time and plays a significant role in sustaining maternal behavior during lactation.[121]

The milk-ejection reflex can be at least partially blocked by large amounts of alcohol, which seems to have a central effect preventing the release of oxytocin, because the mammary gland and uterine response to injected oxytocin are not changed by alcohol. Studies on mothers with diabetes insipidus suggest that the patient retains the ability to synthesize and release oxytocin despite being unable to produce antidiuretic hormone (ADH, vasopressin) in response to stimuli. Artificial cervical dilatation post partum will also cause milk ejection. Vaginal stimulus also initiates let-down in all species.

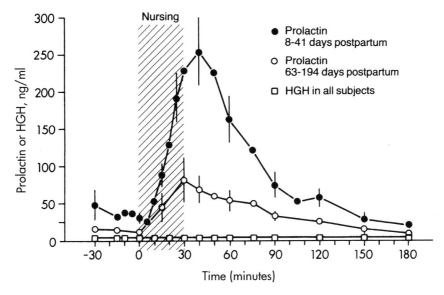

Figure 8-19. Plasma prolactin and growth hormone concentrations during nursing in postpartum women. Eight women were studied 8 to 41 days post partum and six women 63 to 194 days post partum. Prenursing prolactin levels in the latter group were within normal range. Plasma growth hormone showed no change in any subjects during nursing. (From Noel GL, Suh HK, Frantz AG: Prolactin release during nursing and breast stimulation in postpartum and non-postpartum subjects. J Clin Endocrinol Metab 38:413, 1974.)

Injection of oxytocin reproduces the effect of suckling. A rapid series of injections of 1 to 10 mU intravenously will simulate suckling. A continuous drip is less effective. Use of Pitocin as a snuff or nasal spray is the best method for home use of oxytocin to initiate let-down. The oxytocin concentration in the blood rises with suckling, which supports the hypothesis that suckling elicits the release of oxytocin.

The data on the question of ADH release during suckling are contradictory, but it would seem that release of oxytocin and of ADH are independent.

The mammary myoepithelium is stimulated to contract by oxytocin, and the milk-ejection reflex results in the contraction of the myoepithelium and the release, or let-down, of milk (see Fig. 8-18). In the first weeks of lactation, the threshold dose of oxytocin to cause let-down is very low, averaging 0.65 mU from the fifth day. Thirty days after weaning it is 100 mU. Vasopressin is not as effective and requires 100 times the dosage of oxytocin

to produce the same effect during lactation. Deaminooxytocin is 1.5 times as potent as oxytocin on the third postpartum day, but the difference disappears over time, probably because of the rapid breakdown of natural oxytocin by oxytocinase early in the postpartum period.

An objective assessment of milk ejection can be obtained by using ultrasound as described by Hartmann and associates.[57] The diameter of the milk ducts just below the nipple area can be visualized. In term mothers, there is an acute increase in milk duct diameter in the free breast while the infant feeds from the other (Fig 8-20). The same is true if one breast is pumped. The visualization of the increase in diameter Hartmann indicates is positive evidence of the effect and the let-down reflex.

Prostaglandins (PGs) have been shown to have a number of physiologic effects, including an effect on mammary epithelium to increase mammary duct pressure.[157] In a blind crossover study, oxytocin, intravenous (IV) PG, and nasal PG were given and

Milk Duct before Let-down　　　　　**Milk Duct after Let-down**

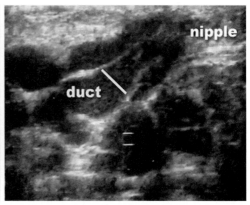

Figure 8-20.　Ultrasonography of breast before (*left*) and during (*right*) let-down, demonstrating the filling of the duct system with milk. Before milk ejection the ducts near the nipple are 2 to 8 mm in basal diameter. (Courtesy of Peter Hartmann, PhD, University of Western Australia, Perth, Australia)

the intraductal pressures measured. The most effective IV PGs were 16-phenoxy-PGE$_2$ and PGF$_2\alpha$, which were then tried nasally, but only PGF$_2\alpha$ was effective nasally. The potential of nasal PGF$_2\alpha$ treatment in engorgement and failure of let-down is possible but is as yet unexplored clinically.[22]

Practical aspects of milk-ejection reflex

When the nipple is stimulated, the receptors in the nipple and areola are stimulated, and nervous impulses are transmitted to the hypothalamus via the somatic afferent nerves. The hypothalamus stimulates the pituitary gland to secrete prolactin, which induces the alveoli in the breast to produce and secrete milk. The cell membranes release fat globules and protein into the lumen. This produces the hind milk, which has a higher protein and fat content. Part of the foremilk has been present since the previous nursing and is released first. It is a more dilute, less fatty solution that empties into the lactiferous sinuses awaiting the next suckling. The ejection reflex induces the holocrine excretion of milk from the cells. The posterior pituitary gland secretes oxytocin, which stimulates the myoepithelial cells to contract and eject the milk from the ducts.[159]

Early in lactation, if there is marked engorgement, the ejection reflex may be inhibited by the congested blood flow to the target organ, the myoepithelial cell. Therefore, when suckling is initiated and oxytocin is released into the bloodstream, it is delayed in reaching the myoepithelial cell with the message because of vascular congestion. Preparing the breast with warm soaks, gentle massage, and manual expression of a little milk may facilitate let-down.

Newton[111] has studied the milk-ejection reflex and clearly shows the effect of distraction on the let-down reflex. Distractions included immersing feet in ice water (reported to be the worst); being asked mathematic questions in rapid series, which resulted in electric shock if a wrong answer was given; or having painful traction on the big toe (Table 8-3). In practice, pain, stress, and mental anguish interfere with let-down in some mothers. When simple adjustments such as making the mother more comfortable, playing soft music, or leaving the mother in a quiet room do not work, other techniques should be tried.

Gentle stroking of the breast may help to decrease anxiety and stimulate flow. Use of tactile warmth as opposed to cold may improve release. Ice should not be used to make the nipple erect because it interferes with let-down. Cold is known to interrupt the neuropathway and cause vasoconstriction.[112]

TABLE 8-3	Milk-ejection reflex*
Maternal disturbance	**Mean amount of milk obtained by infant (g)**
No distractions (no injection)	168
Distraction (saline injection)	99
Distraction (oxytocin injection)	153

*Interrupted milk flow can be restarted with hormone injection.
Modified from Newton M, Newton N: The let-down reflex in human lactation. J Pediatr 91:1, 1977.

Hyperactive letdown can produce such a flood of milk that the infant is overwhelmed and often chokes and coughs. This overactivity occurs in the early days of lactation and gradually diminishes. The best approach is to have mother express and save the first 5 to 10 mL of milk before putting the infant to the breast. The expressed milk can be frozen for later use. If the second breast is exposed when the infant latches on, it too will let down and then will be defused when the infant attempts to latch on.

Excessive milk supply is more common in primiparas and is characterized by continued dripping between feedings, excessive amounts released dur-ing a feeding, and let-down at the slightest stimulus. Treatment is a firm well-constructed brassiere. If necessary, a Velcro binder and cool packs can be applied between feedings. Dripping between feedings can be reduced by folding the nipple over before applying the breast pads. If it persists beyond 2 to 3 weeks, the mother should be evaluated for hyperprolactinemia or hyperthyroid or hypothyroid state.

A rapid computerized breast measurement system has been developed by Hartmann and his laboratory for the determination of breast volume. Using patterns of 64 horizontal light stripes (moiré topography) projected onto the breast and chest wall allowed the calculation of volume by a digitalized camera image analysis (Fig. 8-21). The technique was verified by before and after test weighing of both the infant and the mother. Using this technology, they have been able to measure the amount of milk present, the storage capacity, and the amount of milk removed.

The average milk yield was in excess of 1100 mL/24 hours for the first 6 months according to Hartmann and Prosser[57] compared to previous estimations of 700 to 900 mL/24 hours reported by other investigators. They also noted acute changes in the concentrations of lactose, glucose, sodium,

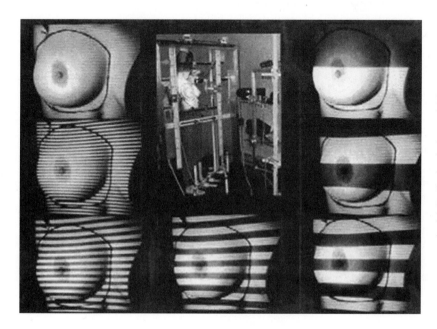

Figure 8-21. The computerized breast measurement system (CBM). Mother is positioned in the ultrasound machine. The breast images demonstrate the use of moiré patterning to measure change in breast volumes. (Courtesy of Peter Hartmann, PhD, University of Western Australia, Perth, Australia)

potassium, and chloride 5 to 6 days before and 6 to 7 days after ovulation.

Studies of women to determine short-term rates of milk synthesis revealed that there was a close relationship between the removal of milk by the infant and the change in breast volume. The rates of synthesis in this study varied from 11 to 58 mL/hour. The amount of milk available in the breast was not necessarily a determinant of the amount removed by the infant at a feeding.[35]

The use of ultrasound by experienced mammographers can be useful in evaluating mammary response to let-down as well as to determine the presence of abnormality of the ductal system. Ultrasound is a noninvasive, objective technique that can measure milk duct diameter and milk duct flow. A significant increase in milk duct diameter is seen when let-down occurs (see Fig. 8-20). When mother sensed let-down or infant swallowing increased, there was corresponding duct diameter change. Following initial let-down, subsequent surges were observed by ultrasound as ducts intermittently dilate. Pulses of oxytocin occurred every 45 seconds or so. The number of milk ejections influenced the amount of milk consumed.[126] There appears to be a maximum duct expansion regardless of pressure or oxytocin release. Milk intake is not related to the degree of dilation or the maximum duct diameter in these studies but to the number of milk ejections.

Ultrasound has also been used for treating plugged ducts (see Chapter 16).

Drug-enhanced lactation

The most direct therapy to enhance let-down is oxytocin. When simple supportive measures fail, oxytocin can be prescribed at home as a nasal spray. Oxytocin is no longer available as a packaged nasal spray and must be obtained by prescription as Pitocin, a synthetic oxytocin. Oxytocin is a polypeptide hormone of the posterior pituitary gland; the synthetic preparation avoids the risk of contamination with vasopressin (ADH). The hormone is destroyed by gastric juices and is not effective orally. The available preparation is intended for intramuscular (IM) or IV use and contains 10 units

of oxytoxic hormone per milliliter. It is packaged in 10-mL multidose vials containing a total of 100 U. The original nasal spray, Syntocinon, contained 40 U/mL. The prescription is for a 10-mL nasal spray or nasal dropper. The dose is 1 or 2 sprays or 2 to 4 drops in the naris, followed by feeding or pumping within 2 to 3 minutes. The dose may be repeated in the other naris if let-down falters or the infant is nursed on the other breast. In most cases it is effective within one or two feedings, and the prescription rarely needs refilling. Let-down usually will continue without medication.

Aono and associates[8] have suggested that sulpiride be given orally to mothers who produce less than 50 mL of total milk yield in the first 48 hours of lactation. Sulpiride is known to stimulate secretion of prolactin. In a control study of 96 normal primiparas and multiparas with poor lactation, half were given 50 mg sulpiride twice daily from the fourth to the seventh day post partum, and half received a placebo. There was no difference in milk production in the multiparas but a significant difference in the primiparas, who had higher milk yield, higher prolactin levels, and higher percentage still breastfeeding at 1 month in the treated group. Although such medication should not be given unless routine techniques for increasing milk production have failed, occasional indications exist.

Other studies[24,43] have shown the efficacy of metoclopramide in enhancing milk production in women pumping for infants unable to nurse or in women whose infants have significant failure to thrive because of inadequate milk supply. The dose is metoclopramide 10 mg three times a day until milk volume increases (i.e., 4 to 6 days, then taper over 4 to 6 days). When the infant is actively suckling, this stimulus is usually adequate. Mothers who are pumping for a premature or ill infant may find the effect totally disappears when the drug is discontinued. The original studies did not explore long-term use. Metoclopramide is used in adults for various forms of reflux for 4 to 12 weeks. It is also used for reflux in infants, especially premature newborns (0.1 to 0.5 mg/kg body weight/day). The amount transferred to the infant through breast milk is reported as only 28 to 157 μg/L (1 to 13 μg/kg/day). Side effects are uncommon but tend to be dose related (i.e., greater than 40 mg/day in adults). Mothers may experience diarrhea, sedation, or nausea, but no symptoms have been observed in neonates. The extrapyramidal tract symptoms are associated with large or chronic doses of metoclopramide. Caution should be used in hypertensive women. It is not recommended for long-term use. Domperidone, which is not approved in the United States, is available in Canada and other countries under the names Motilidone and Motilium. It has been reported anecdotally that 10 to 20 mg three to four times a day will increase prolactin levels and increase milk production. Women have taken it for months. Many herbal preparations have been credited as galactogogues but there are no controlled studies even though many of these preparations have been known for centuries. Fenugreek is probably the best known. As an herb, it is used as a "maple syrup" substitute. As a galactogogue, large amounts (3 capsules three times a day) are required. It has a cross-allergy to peanuts and may cause colic in the infant. Further discussion can be found in Chapter 11.

Side effects and let-down

The let-down reflex has been associated with headache, which occurs transiently at time of initial let-down and then on changing breasts, related to surges in oxytocin.

Nausea has also been associated with let-down and specifically with release of oxytocin. Women compare it with the waves of nausea of pregnancy. Treatment is taking food before initiating the let-down and breastfeeding. Dry crackers work well. The symptom is more effectively prevented than cured. Usually the symptom disappears in 3 to 4 weeks. Wearing pressure wrist bands which are effective for motion sickness can be effective if applied before starting to nurse.

Marshall and associates[100] used thermal probes on the mother and infant to document hot flashes. Skin conductance increased, followed by increased skin temperature. Women also experienced night sweats and hot flashes during lactation, especially in the early weeks post partum. They were most notable during night feedings. The phenomenon is also associated with oxytocin releases.

POSTNATAL PERIOD

Hospitals have gradually returned to "rooming-in" or birthing centers for uncomplicated deliveries.[90,135] Easy access of an infant to the mother has been shown to facilitate lactation success. The value of a well-trained, knowledgeable, empathetic nursing staff should not be underestimated. The knowledge and attitude of the staff have been two of the most important variables in successful breastfeeding. This style of postpartum care better prepares the parents for discharge, as they know their infants' cues.

The family's transition from hospital to home can be stressful.[164] The parents hear the infant, who has been passive and content, wake up and cry for the first time. Because of all the procedures necessary to discharge an infant from the hospital (discharge physical examinations, blood tests, etc.), the well-planned discharge is often delayed and everyone is frantic, including the infant. The mother should be reassured about this and not be alarmed if she has to feed the infant frequently the first day at home.

The role of the clock

Many women today who work in demanding careers live by the clock and have trouble when advised to let a new baby give the cues. Anthropologist Millard[103] examined pediatric advice on breastfeeding and noted that major textbooks on pediatrics focus on timing. She points out that "once the clock is seen as inherent in human behavior, adherence to the timetable becomes a standard for judging competence, adequacy, and normality." The clock is a central touchstone in our cultural system. Pediatric literature reinforces pressures on women regarding their infants and leads pediatricians to a role of shaping public views of infancy, motherhood, and humanity in general. In breastfeeding, the pediatrician can help the mother break her bonds to timing and move to the central issues of successful breastfeeding, responding to infant cues.

Feeding frequency

Many hospital schedules are on a 4-hour feeding program based on the feedings of bottle fed infants, whose slow emptying time of the stomach with formulas requires up to 4 hours. The emptying time for breast milk is about 1½ hours; thus, frequent feedings are not unusual. Pediatric textbooks at the beginning of the 20th century described 10 to 12 feedings a day as normal.[81] Comparison of mammalian care patterns and composition of their milk shows an inverse relationship between protein content and frequency of feedings. From this it might be deduced that the human infant might need to be fed more frequently than every 4 hours (Table 8-4).[95] Infants who sleep 5 to 6 hours at a stretch at night may make up for skipped feedings during the day. Fewer than 8 feedings per 24 hours in the first month of life is rarely associated with successful lactation.

When milk intake and feeding patterns of thriving, exclusively breastfed infants were documented from birth for the first 4 months of life by Butte and associates,[27] two feeding patterns emerged. In one, the authors describe the feedings as distributed throughout the 24-hour day. In the other, feedings were excluded from midnight to 6 AM, although all infants were feeding ad lib. Total intake was the same in 24 hours. Milk intake per feeding decreased over the day. Frequency and duration declined over the 4-month period. Weight gain was similar in the two groups.

The pattern of intake during a feeding is different between breastfed and bottle fed infants. A bottle feeding infant sucks steadily in a linear pattern, receiving 81% of the feed in 10 minutes. Howie and associates[70] showed that a breastfed infant has a biphasic pattern, which includes the first 4 minutes on the first breast and the first 4 minutes on the second breast (between 15 and 19 minutes into the feed). The infant receives 84% of the total volume in those 8 minutes. In another study, 50% of the feed on each breast was consumed in 2 minutes and 80% to 90% by 5 minutes.[96] Milk flow was minimal during the last 5 minutes. All these observations were made on the fifth to seventh day of life (Fig. 8-22).

Switch nursing is often suggested to increase total intake of an infant when milk production needs stimulating, especially if the infant is not gaining adequately (Fig. 8-22), but this may be counterproductive. When mothers fed 10 minutes on each breast (10 + 10), they produced the same amount of milk as they did nursing 5 minutes on a side and switching back (5 + 5 + 5 + 5). The suckling-induced prolactin is similar with both patterns as well. A major concern of switch nursing is not feeding long enough on either breast to obtain the full calories of hindmilk. Even if volume is improved by

TABLE 8-4	**Mammalian care patterns and composition of species milk**						
	Pinnipedia: seal, sea lion	**Tree shrew**	**Rabbit**	**Rat**	**Black rhinoceros**[*]	**Chimpanzee**	**Human**
Infant care pattern	Return to ocean after birth	—	Cache	Carry, hibernate	—	Carry	?
Feeding interval	Once a week	48 hr	24 hr	Continuous	—	Continuous	?
Composition of milk							
Total solids (%)	62–65	20	33–40	21	8.1	11.9	12.4
Protein (%)	8–14	11	14–23	10	0.0	3.7	3.8
Fat (%)	53	6.5	18	8	1.4	1.2	1.2
Carbohydrate (%)	0–0.90	3.2	2.0	2.6	6.1	7.0	7.0

[*]The rhinoceros has an anatomic variation in the stomach that provides four pouches that fill during a feeding and provide a constant trickle of milk to the central groove leading to the small intestine, thus creating a constant feed.

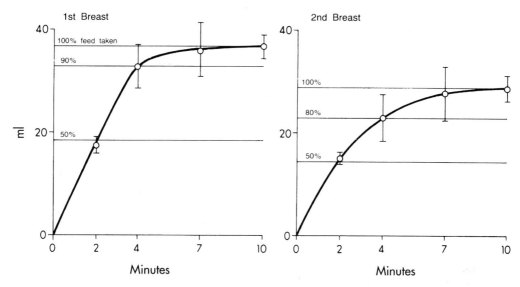

Figure 8-22. Mother-infant pattern of milk flow. (From Lucas A, Lucas PJ, Baum JD: Pattern of milk flow in breast-fed infants. Lancet 2:57, 1979.)

this, total calories may be decreased. The infants do not nurse for a full 20 minutes in some cases, and the nutritive feeding time is under 15 minutes. The duration of the feeding should be determined by the infant's response and not by time. Enough time must be spent on a single breast to assure getting the fat-rich, calorie-rich hindmilk.

The wide range in breast milk volume in well-nourished mothers was shown by Dewey and Lönnerdal[39] to be caused by a variation in infant "demand" rather than an inadequacy of milk production. They stimulated milk production with postfeeding pumping for 2 weeks, but the infants failed to continue to take more than previously. Although milk production was augmented by pumping, the infants regulated their own intake. It is difficult to overfeed a breastfeeding infant.

New mothers are often most insecure and most concerned about lack of scheduling, especially if an ad lib program of feeding has been suggested. Other mothers seem to thrive on random scheduling. Some physicians continue to instruct mothers rigidly about adhering closely to a schedule designed for the bottle fed infant. This can lead to

failure of lactation unless the mother is sufficiently confident to follow her infant's demands and feed more frequently and on demand.[81]

Breastfed infants do not differ from bottle fed infants at 3 and 5 months of age in terms of the number of night feedings. At 3 months, breastfed infants spend about 20 minutes less time at night sleeping and 20 minutes less time during the day, according to Alley and Rogers.[3]

When a mother expresses concerns about frequent feedings and worries about the adequacy of her milk (she is often disturbed that it looks so thin and blue after the luxurious color of colostrum), Jackson suggests she keep a record of feeding times and duration, as well as sleep and wakeful times.[15] If a chart is kept, the mother is usually surprised to find how quickly her infant develops a schedule. Often the infant is sleeping longer than she thought. The chart is also reassuring to the physician, especially if weight gain is marginal. In some cases it will highlight a problem not previously identified, such as a poor gainer who sleeps all night, missing several feedings. This approach serves to refocus attention on the infant and cues and not on the clock.

Milk production is influenced by the frequency, intensity, and duration of suckling by the infant, especially in the early postpartum period. Infant weight has been associated with the volume of milk intake. Greater suckling strength, frequency, and duration of feedings apparently play a part, according to cross-cultural studies by Prentice and associates.[124] Self-regulation of milk intake has been studied by several investigators with similar conclusions. When mothers increased their milk supply by pumping after a feed, infants took a little extra milk for a few days but gradually dropped back to their previous intake. Residual milk volumes were noted by Dewey and Lönnerdal[39] to average about 100 g/day when women compared the amount extracted by pump with the infant's intake. The volume available in the second breast in a given feeding is about 60% of the volume of the first breast.

The mother's age and parity have little effect on milk production once full lactation is established. The data available from adolescent women are sparse, but healthy well-nourished adolescents produce adequate milk for normal growth of their infants. Stress and acute illness have been associated with decreased volumes, especially in relationship to poor let-down.

One-breast/two-breast feedings

The dogma of over 50 years had been that an infant should feed at both breasts at each feeding until the case report of Woolridge and Fisher[179] concerning an infant who failed to thrive when fed both breasts at each nursing. The authors demonstrated that this mother did not produce high-fat milk until well into the feeding; thus, switching to the second side deprived the infant of fat-rich, calorie-rich milk. Confining the feeding to a single breast solved the problem. The authors also pointed out that consuming volumes of low-fat milk meant relatively high-lactose milk, which caused diarrhea and further calorie loss.

When a study compared the two patterns of feeding in 12 mother-infant pairs, Woolridge and

associates[181] found that the two patterns led to different milk volumes and mean feed-fat concentrations. The mean fat intake in 24 hours, however, was the same. Infants appeared to regulate their fat intake quickly; thus, the authors recommended "baby-led" feeding. In other words, the mother should initiate feeding at one breast and continue until the infant discontinues feeding. If, after burping, the infant wants more, the mother offers the second side. The next feeding time is started on the opposite breast. Other investigators report similar findings.[136]

These studies and observations were done after the infants were 1 month of age.[136,179] When a mother is establishing her milk supply in the first days and weeks, switching to the second breast for each feed allows frequent, short stimuli to both the breasts. If an infant drifts to sleep after the first side and will not latch on the second side, the infant should be started on the "second side" when waking for the next feeding. Most successful nursing mothers adapt to their own infants' cues instead of following arbitrary rules. Switching prevents full hindmilk fat production and lowers energy content. More high-calorie milk may be produced by nursing at only one breast per feeding.

The identification of a factor that exerts a direct and local inhibitory action on further milk synthesis may explain why some women nurse only on one breast as a cultural mode. In situations in which the infant rejects one breast,[124] some inhibition of milk production may precipitate the rejection. The inhibitory factor decreases the production in the "abandoned" breast while the other breast continues to function and totally sustain the infant's growth. There is no reason a woman cannot continue nursing on one breast indefinitely. This has been suggested in cases of recurrent mastitis in one breast that is unresponsive to repeated antibiotic therapy or after lumpectomies for cancer.

Van Geddren and Goosen[160] describe two cases of unilateral breastfeeding. A 41-year-old woman had nursed seven infants only on the left breast following an abscess in the right breast early with the first child. A mammogram while nursing her youngest, an 18-month-old infant, showed the left breast apparently lactating and the unused right breast normal and nonlactating. A 27-year-old mother was breastfeeding her second child, 2 years old, when mammography was done. The feeding breast appeared to be lactating, and the unused breast was larger and cystic. She had also nursed only on the left breast for 4 years with the first child.

Adequate rest

If nursing is not going well, a common cause of problems is maternal fatigue. The mother may need to be ordered by her physician to nap and rest. She must learn to nap when the infant is napping. This becomes more difficult when she has other young children, but a simultaneous nap for all the little ones and mother may have to be planned. Otherwise, she may have to go to bed with the children at night and just concentrate on resting and feeding the infant. When the need for rest is acute, the father should be assigned infant care, with the possible inclusion of bottle or cup feeding in extreme cases, while the mother sleeps undisturbed for a few hours.

Sore breasts and plugged ducts

Tender lumps in the breasts in a mother who is otherwise well are probably caused by plugging of a collecting duct. Some women on high-calcium diets have excreted grains of white sand that are thought to be calcium stones plugging a duct. The best treatment is to continue nursing. Manually massaging the area to initiate and ensure complete drainage should be recommended. Hot packs before feedings may help. If the breast is especially tender, initiating nursing on the opposite breast first permits the affected breast to let-down without the pressure of suckling. The affected breast should be completely emptied by nursing or manual expression. The brassiere may be cutting off an alveolus because of pressure from a narrow strap. Changing the infant's position may also help. Gentle persistent massage to relieve the lump usually clears the problem.

Repeated plugging

When plugging is recurrent, one needs to look for a major cause, such as exhaustion and fatigue. Several women have come to the lactation center's attention who have had repeated lumps in their breasts with poor flow of milk, often as if the ducts were plugged. The condition responded fairly well to manual expression before each feeding, often with the expulsion of small plugs. These plugs were fatty, in contrast to the hard white "grains of sand." The condition dramatically improved by limiting the mother to polyunsaturated fats and adding lecithin to the diet. It was also necessary for subsequent pregnancies in all three cases. Lecithin, a lipid constituent of human milk, is an oily substance that can be used as an oil on salads or taken by spoon, 1 tablespoon per day. It is also available in capsule form. An additional suggestion from a lactation consultant who had success with rubbing the lethicin into the nipple and areola with each feeding is supported.

Galactocele

Milk-retention cysts are uncommon and, when found, are almost exclusively a problem in lactating women. The contents at first are pure milk. Because of fluid absorption, they later contain thick, creamy, cheesy, or oily material. The swelling is smooth and rounded, and compression of it may cause milky fluid to exude from the nipple. Galactoceles are believed to be caused by the blockage of a milk duct. The cyst may be aspirated to avoid surgery but will fill up again. It can be removed surgically under local anesthesia without stopping the breastfeeding. Its presence does not require cessation of lactation. A firm diagnosis can be made by ultrasound; a cyst and milk will appear the same, whereas a tumor will be distinguishable. If it is recurrent or persistent, it can be surgically removed after weaning is over.

Figures 8-23 and 8-24 illustrate mammography of the lactating breast.

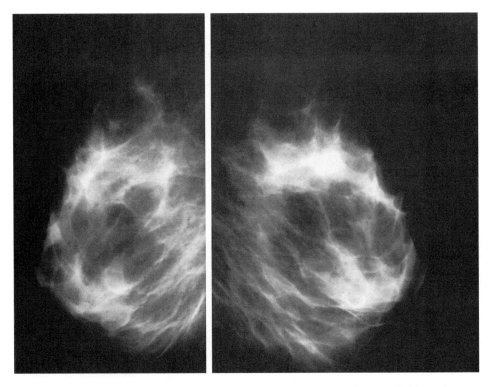

Figure 8-23. Normal breast tissue visualized by mammography. Tissue is one third fat and appears cystic in nature. (Courtesy of Dr. Wende Logan-Young, MD, University of Rochester School of Medicine, Rochester, NY)

White bleb on nipple (white dot)

Often described as a "white dot," a white bleb on the nipple has frequently been a source of considerable discomfort for the mother and concern for the health professional. The solitary bleb appears on the surface of the nipple, usually at the opening of a duct; has a shiny, smooth surface; and is a millimeter or less in diameter. The mother usually describes exquisite pinpoint pain when the baby nurses. The bleb does not break or disappear with proper grasp and suckling. It may be "cured" or disappear when the health professional opens it with a sterile needle. It may reappear and have to be opened again. A home treatment for a bleb is reported to be used in some cultures (Hmong). It involves taking a human hair, doubling it on itself, and rolling it until it forms a stiff fine rope. It is then inserted into the duct until the plug is freed (courtesy of the International Board of Lactation Consultant Examiners [IBLCE] network). A more sterile adaptation of this would be to take a strand of sterile heavy (0-00) suture and cannulate the duct threading the suture up the duct until the plug is released. Sterile suture is available in the average medical office (Fig. 8-25). The bleb probably represents a small pressure cyst formed at the end of the duct from milk seeping into this very elastic tissue. The bleb is different from the sucking blister that appears early in lactation associated with vigorous suckling or malposition. The blister covers a larger area and is not associated with a duct or exquisite pain. The bleb also should be distinguished from thrush, especially if there is more than one. Although a nipple with thrush usually is pink and painful with suckling, a nipple can have

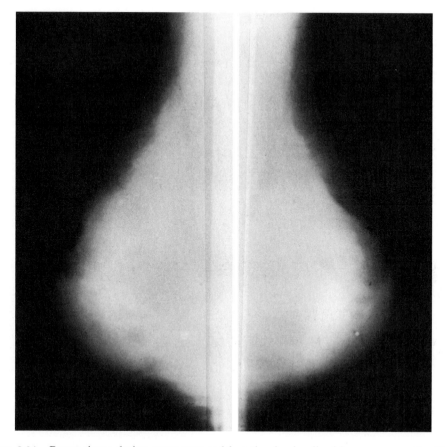

Figure 8-24. Breast tissue during pregnancy and lactation is visualized by mammography. Fat is replaced by lactation tissue and presents a solid appearance. Tumors would be easily distinguished by this procedure in the lactating breast. Mammography is a safe, noninvasive technique that does not interfere with nursing. (Courtesy of Dr. Wende Logan-Young, MD, University of Rochester School of Medicine, Rochester, NY)

small caseous lesions similar to oral thrush. This requires specific treatment for *Candida albicans.*

This painful white bleb is the end of a plugged duct. If "needling" has not cured it, rubbing lethicin into the nipple after each feeding may be effective here as well as with frank plugged ducts. A lactation consultant reports curing white blebs with multiple applications of lethicin. If it is a buildup of cells like seborrheic dermatitis or cradle cap, lethicin works. The best treatment for cradle cap is oil or greasy ointment and rarely is salicylic acid needed.

Breast rejection

Infants have been observed to reject the breast intermittently, most often at 3 to 4 months, and then to go back after several feedings or a day or so. A bottle can be substituted, or cup feedings as described in Chapter 14. Total rejection of both breasts may follow the return of menstruation. A mother will notice that the infant will reject the breast for a day or so with each period. Other infants seem unaffected. Strong foods in the diet may cause rejection of milk, which usually occurs 8 to 12 hours after

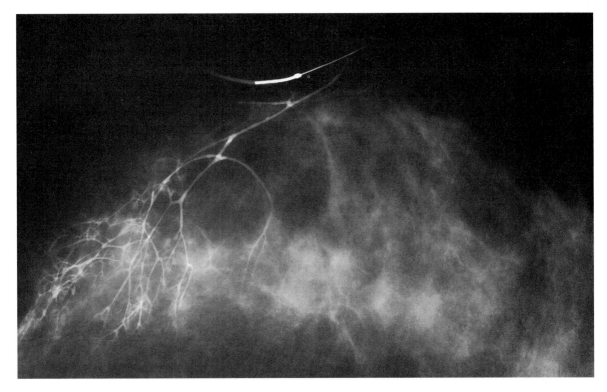

Figure 8-25. This 38-year-old patient's craniocaudal mammography view shows segmental duct draining a lobe in medial aspect of right breast. Ductal patterns differ among women. (From Logan-Young W, Hoffman NY: Breast Cancer: A Practical Guide to Diagnosis, Vol. 1. Procedures. Rochester, NY, Mt. Hope, 1994.)

ingestion and disappears by 24 hours after ingestion. Occasionally, one breast is permanently rejected so that the milk supply dwindles. One-breast nursing is done, as noted previously.

Refusal to nurse may not be a nursing strike or abrupt weaning. It may be a change in milk flavor. Onions and garlic have been cited as culprits and vindicated by research, but a case was reported of refusal to nurse after maternal ingestion of mint candies in especially large quantity.[48] Strong flavors may pass into the milk. A dietary history including beverages and herbs is an important part of searching out problems. (Nursing strikes are discussed in Chapter 10.)

Unilateral breast rejection

Some infants prefer one breast and even refuse the other. When this occurs, manual expression or softening the nipple for easier grasp may help, thus enticing the infant to suckle. Holding the infant in the same position (i.e., on same side in same direction, so-called cross cradle hold) for the other breast may lead the infant to take the second breast. Sometimes applying syrup to the rejected nipple will help. Unilateral breastfeeding is a custom in some parts of China. Sodium and chloride levels may rise in milk after mastitis. It is wise to taste the milk or have sodium and chloride levels measured in milk from both breasts if the problem persists to be sure no reason exists for the rejection.

Goldsmith[53] reported five cases of lactating women whose infants suddenly rejected a single breast. Weeks or months later the mother noted a mass, and biopsy revealed a malignancy. It would be wise to examine any patient who complains of unilateral breast rejection that does not respond to simple measures to rule out a tumor. Ultrasound followed by a mammogram, if necessary, can be performed without discontinuing lactation.

Other causes of nipple and breast pain

Classification of mastalgia, or breast pain, includes *cyclic* causes (67% of cases), *noncyclic* causes (i.e., not related to menstrual cycle, 26% of cases), and *Tietze syndrome* (painful lateral costochondral junction, 7%). Mastalgia in young women may spontaneously disappear with pregnancy. This has been associated with higher basal levels of prolactin (unrelated to lactation) and low plasma levels of essential fatty acid α-linolenic acid and its metabolites, which are important components of cell membranes. Administration of α-linolenic acid improves the pain, according to Gateley and Mansel.[50] Evening primrose oil (Efamast) is a rich source of α-linolenic acid. This is a safe, even nutritious solution to the problem and a safe herbal treatment.

Ankyloglossia

The common causes of nipple pain associated with lactation include poor position, nipple sucking, nipple tipped up too much because of finger pressure on the breast above nipple, infant's lower lip sucked in and irritating the underside of nipple, and taking the infant off the breast without first breaking the suction. These should be ruled out as possible causes of breast pain. Then the infant should be checked. Although rare, tongue-tie or tight-tongue frenulum may be a cause. If the infant cannot protrude the tip of the tongue over the gums and the tip

is tied to the floor of the mouth by a tight cord of a thick frenulum, and the tongue becomes heart-shaped when effort is made to extend it, it is known as *ankyloglossia*. When the infant tries to draw the teat into the mouth, it will not be possible, and nipple biting results. The physician should consider cutting the frenulum once the diagnosis of ankyloglossia (short lingual frenulum) is confirmed by oral examination (Box 8-5).[74,116] The procedure is simple, but the cut should be carefully placed to avoid the artery, nerve, and other anatomic sites. It is usually bloodless, and the infant can be nursed immediately, now in the correct position.

Eczema

Eczema of the nipple and sometimes also the areola and breast presents as a red, dry, sore, even burning, flaking rash, the flakes often appearing as "oily potato chips." Common causes are washing nipples with soap or applying ointments that have irritants. Some creams contain peanut oil, which should be avoided by those allergic to peanuts (the most common food allergy); lanolin, for those allergic to wool; and cocoa butter, for those allergic to chocolate. The physician should instruct the mother to remove all irritants, including breast shields and plastic-backed breast pads. Lesions usually clear quickly with proper treatment and avoiding the irritant. A short course of halobetasol propionate ointment (Ultravate) rubbed sparingly into the area after feeding will clear the persistent case.

BOX 8-5   Identification of ankyloglossia (tongue-tie)

---

1. When tongue protrudes, tip is anchored behind alveolar ridge.
2. When infant cries, tongue remains anchored.
3. Tongue is notched or heart-shaped when protruded.
4. Tongue cannot be manually extended by examiner.
5. Frenulum is short (less than 1 cm [½ inch]), and inelastic.
6. Tongue is attached close to alveolar ridge.

Nipple blanching

Blanching of the nipples may cause burning pain during suckling. A vigorous "barracuda baby" can cause blanching of the nipple from pressure. Later in lactation (i.e., after 4 months, when teething begins), infants may bite down to relieve gum pain and cause nipple blanching and burning pain. The mother should be instructed to keep her finger ready to break the suction if pain becomes extreme.

Blanching of the nipple to pure white with no apparent mechanical cause can also occur. This has been associated with some maternal medications, such as theophylline and terbutaline. Other medications that cause vasoconstriction may be associated.

Factors that control vasomotor tone in the mammary gland have not been well studied. Mammary blood vessels are exquisitely sensitive to epinephrine and norepinephrine, as well as serotonin and PGF_{20C}, as vasoconstrictive agents.

Other causes of nipple blanching are cold, especially when ice is applied, and maternal smoking. Nicotine is a vasoconstrictor, as is caffeine, especially in sensitive individuals.

In some women, warm compresses to the areola before nursing will prevent the reaction and thus the pain. Not all cases of nipple blanching have been relieved by heat; some have been relieved by cold, which is actually contrary to usual physiologic theory (see Chapter 16 for discussion of Raynaud's disease).

Supplementary feedings

To supplement-feed a breastfed infant continues to be controversial in pediatric circles. For the normal full-term infant it is not necessary. Evaluation of serial blood glucose levels in breastfed and bottle fed infants from birth reported by Heck and Erenberg[59] demonstrated a significant number of bottle fed infants with hypoglycemia, presumed to be a rebound phenomenon from dextrose and water feeding early in life. Some breastfed infants had a value less than 40 mg/dL on the second day. No significant differences were found in serum bilirubins and weight loss between supplemented and

unsupplemented breastfed infants in Herrara's study.[61] At age 3 months a significant number of supplemented infants were no longer breastfeeding (still breastfeeding, 81% unsupplemented versus 53% supplemented). Even in hot, dry climates, water supplements were not found to be necessary.[4,12,52] Urine osmolarity remained within physiologic ranges in unsupplemented breastfed infants studied by Goldberg and Adams.[52] This has been demonstrated by a number of other investigators. The supplementation with water did not influence the "coming-in" of mother's milk, according to Schutzman and associates.[143] They did observe, however, that infants in the group being supplemented took very little water after nursing (less than 4 oz total in the first 3 days).

Many physicians suggest to mothers that a supplementary bottle can be added any time. Actually, when lactation is going well, it is not needed, and when it is not going well, a bottle may aggravate the problem. During hospitalization, giving a substitute bottle may confuse a new infant, who may be having trouble sucking at first. Infants who are given water or glucose water in the hospital do less well and usually lose more weight. A significant relationship exists between supplements in the hospital and early discontinuation of breastfeeding. It is a marker of impending trouble and of insufficient milk production, which is best treated with frequent feedings at the breast and some intervention from an experienced lactation consultant.

In a study by Gray-Donald and associates[54] the effect of formula supplementation on outcome of breastfeeding was observed in two nurseries, one used as a control and the other supplemented. Mothers could request supplements in either group, and any baby put to the breast only twice was called "breastfed." It was clear that mothers who requested formula in the hospital and requested a going-home formula package were more likely to discontinue breastfeeding. They considered this early behavior a marker of high risk for failure. These patients,[54] therefore, should have received follow-up and considerable support when identified as high risk.

In a study by Cronenwett and associates,[33] when infants were randomly selected to receive one bottle feeding per day between 2 weeks and 6 weeks of age, there was little difference compared to those exclusively breastfed. The study group received five bottles a week and the control group two. At 6 months, 59% of the five-bottle group were still breastfeeding, compared with 69% of the two-bottle group. These infants had no trouble switching back and forth. The authors[33] believed their study justified a casual approach to the bottle in breastfed infants and suggested that the difference between two bottles per week and five bottles was insignificant and proved that nipple confusion did not happen. There was no group that was unsupplemented.

However, the use of complementary bottles, that is, those given after a breastfeeding to "top off" the feeding, is the beginning of a downhill course that may doom lactation to failure. It would be better to take the infant to breast more often or switch back to the first breast if the baby is hungry. If the mother must be away at feeding time, she can pump a feeding ahead of time and save it in the refrigerator or freezer for someone else to give by bottle. If this is not practical, a bottle of formula can be given. It can be made up from a formula powder more economically one feeding at a time, and there is no waste. Powder preparations have a long shelf life even when open and are better tolerated by the infant because lower temperatures are required to manufacture powders; thus, there is no caramelizing of the sugars or denaturing of the proteins as there is in liquid formula. A powder goes quickly into solution if the water is warm when mixing is attempted. (Prepare formula powder as follows: one scoop of powder to 2 oz of warm water gives 20 kcal/oz.) Mothers can pump and store milk in the freezer to be used in place of an occasional bottle of formula, however.

Solid foods

Successful nursing mothers are rarely impatient to start the baby on solid foods, as bottle feeding mothers frequently are. Milk, and especially human milk, supplies the appropriate nutrients. At about 6 months a normal infant begins to deplete iron stores, and this is probably an appropriate time to start solid foods, especially iron-containing ones. This permits the entire process of weaning to cup and solid foods to be gradual. An infant does not need teeth to eat baby food and, conversely, does not have to be weaned from the breast because teeth have erupted. By 6 months the number of feedings usually has decreased, and the timing and volume are beginning to cycle to a schedule that resembles three meals a day and some snacks.

Exclusive breastfeeding for 6 months

There is no objective evidence that solids are needed prior to 6 months according to a WHO/UNICEF meta-analysis.[83] Solids do not solve any problems. There was a reduced morbidity rate due to gastrointestinal infections in infants breastfed exclusively for 6 months or more and no observable deficits in growth. No benefits of introducing solids between 4 and 6 months have been identified, except for iron needs in a special infant, which are best treated by iron drops. A breastfed infant usually starts some solids by 6 months of age.[83]

Carrying and holding

Carrying and holding young infants have been considered by some in the era of peak bottle feeding as predisposing to spoiling the infants. In many cultures around the world, infants are carried with the mother night and day.[99] In Western cultures, infants are tightly swaddled, that is, wrapped up like a package, and put down. In a randomized controlled study of primiparous breastfeeding women, Hunziker and Barr[72] showed that increased carrying reduces infant crying and colicky behavior. The authors concluded that lack of carrying predisposes to crying and colic. A study among young mothers in New York City who were given infant carriers showed that carrying the infant was more apt to influence infant crying than was breastfeeding in that population.[72]

Sleeping

Sleeping through the night has been assumed to be an important developmental milestone dependent on maturation. Twenty-six first-time parents of exclusively breastfed infants were randomly assigned to a treatment or control group.[122] The treatment group was instructed to offer a "focal feed" between 10 PM and midnight and then offer reswaddling, diapering, walking, and rocking to postpone the next feeding to 5 AM, minimizing light and sound. By 3 weeks the treated group was sleeping significantly longer. By 8 weeks, 100% of the treated group, compared with 23% of control infants, was sleeping at least from midnight to 5 AM. They fed more frequently during the day, especially early morning. Milk intakes for 24 hours between the two groups were not different. The authors[122] concluded that parents can teach their breastfed infants to lengthen nighttime sleep periods. Parents should be encouraged to develop management plans that they find most comfortable. Whether they share the family bed or keep the newborn in the same room or in the next room is their decision. Continuing night feeds is associated with longer duration of breastfeeding and more abundant milk supply.

Milk composition influences infant sleep latency. Tryptophan concentrations are higher in human milk than in formula. Tryptophan is known to increase sleep in adults. When breastfed and formula fed infants were compared using formulas with different levels of tryptophan, they had shorter sleep latency with high levels of tryptophan.[151]

Colic and crying

By definition, colic is spasmodic contractions of smooth muscle causing pain and discomfort. It can be experienced in many organs, such as the gastrointestinal or genitourinary tract, and at all ages. When the term *colic* is used in reference to infants, it usually means a syndrome in which the young infant has unexplained paroxysms of irritability, fussing, and crying for a prolonged period, often at the same time of day, in the early months of life. The infant usually draws the legs up as if in pain. Myriad remedies are directed at various possible causes, including allergy, hypertonicity, and hormone withdrawal. It may be a matter of parenting style, however, and expectations that brings a par-

ent to complain about colic. Colic does occur in premature infants but usually not until they reach 42 weeks' adjusted gestation.[63]

Infantile colic has been reported to occur equally among breastfed (20%), formula fed (19%), and mixed breastfed and formula fed (21%) infants in a study of almost 1000 infants.[1] The fecal α-antitrypsin and fecal hemoglobins were not different in colicky infants. There was no evidence of dietary protein hypersensitivity in this series.[155]

Characteristically, the infant will cry and scream as if in pain from 3 to 4 hours at a stretch, often between 6 PM and 10 PM. The infant will nurse frequently, then scream and pull away from the breast as if in pain, only to cry out a few minutes later. Sometimes the infant can be comforted by another adult such as the father or grandmother. The infant will respond to gentle rocking when held against a warm shoulder. If the infant is put down, the screaming starts again. If the nursing mother holds the infant, he or she is frantic unless nursed and yet does not need to be fed. This may disturb a new mother, who wonders why she cannot console her infant. (Is her milk weak? Does it disagree with her infant? Is she an inadequate mother?) None of these is true, but smelling the mother's milk makes the infant behave as if it needs to nurse. Anyone who is not nursing can quickly quiet the infant. Picking up the infant does not spoil the child, and rocking and cuddling are appropriate. Warm pressure is usually palliative; a warm hot water bottle or warm shoulder with some pressure or massage is comforting. The use of rhythmic incessant sounds or lights (e.g., vacuum cleaner, TV out of focus so it is a changing pattern) has variable success.

A carefully taken history and physical examination are always in order to rule out other pathologic conditions, such at otitis media, anal fissure, hair tourniquet, or hernia before a diagnosis of colic is made. Hunger should be ruled out. Sometimes an infant who was just fed needs to be fed again. True colic, however, is characterized by an inconsolable infant who continues to fret, fuss, and cry out. If true colic is diagnosed because of the consistency of the screaming for several hours each day at the same time, treatment is in order.[79]

Influence of cow milk in maternal diet

The literature is not straightforward on the issue of the effect of cow milk in the maternal diet and infantile colic. Talbot[153] first published information on congenital sensitization to food, especially eggs and cow milk, in humans in 1918, which was manifested as clinical allergy in the breastfed infant. Research techniques are far superior today, and information is accumulating. Gerrard and Shenassa[51] report sensitization caused by substances in breast milk thought to be due to two types of food allergy; one is immunoglobulin E (IgE) mediated and triggered by trace amounts of antigen, and the other is not IgE mediated and is triggered by large amounts of antigen. Gastrointestinal (GI) transport of macromolecules in the pathogenesis of food allergy is under investigation, as is T-cell-mediated immunity in food allergy. However, the present state of scientific knowledge has not resolved the issue of colic and cow milk for the clinician.

Clinical studies have been done to test the association of dairy products in the mother with colic in some breastfed babies. Jakobsson and Lindberg[75] described a cause-and-effect relationship in a group of 18 mothers in 1978, which was criticized because it was not a double-blind study. Evans and associates[46] then reported that they found no such relationship when they did a double-blind crossover study in which mothers received cow's milk protein for 2 days and then a placebo for 2 days. Jakobsson and Lindberg[76] have repeated their work using a double-blind crossover study design in the mother-baby pairs in which the infants had colic; 35% of the infants improved on maternal diets free of cow milk. A torrent of mail to the journals confirmed these conclusions in small clinical practice trials as well.

Jakobsson and associates[77] found bovine β-lactoglobulin in the milk of 18 of 38 mothers chosen at random. Three mothers had very high amounts, and their infants had colic that was relieved by a maternal diet free of bovine milk products. Dietary modification with a low-allergen diet should be considered in the mothers of healthy breastfed infants with colic, according to Hill and associates,[64] who reported a community-based study. They also restricted the diet by eliminating artificial color, preservatives, and milk, eggs, wheat, and nuts.[64]

Colic has been investigated in breastfed and formula fed infants by measuring breath hydrogen (H_2) production, a product of lactose metabolism.[105] H_2 levels were significantly higher at both 6 weeks and 3 months of age in infants who developed colic. The authors suggest that increased lactose malabsorption may be related to colic. Studies that used lactase to minimize the effect of lactose did not cause an improvement. Nursing long enough to obtain high-fat hindmilk and relatively less lactose could improve colic, however.

Lothe and associates[94] reported macromolecular absorption using human α-lactalbumin as a marker. Breastfed infants with colic had significantly higher levels of macromolecules than infants without colic. The authors conclude that gut mucosa is affected in infants with colic. Further study by this laboratory reported that there were increased levels of motilin from the first day of life in infants who later developed colic, indicating the GI tract is affected even before symptoms appear.[93]

No type of crying should go untended in a young infant. Holding and rocking do not spoil infants. Crying levels normally increase from birth to 6 to 8 weeks. Most infants spend 2 to 2 ½ hours a day crying at this age.[150]

With a clinical picture of colic, a history of allergy in the family, especially to cow milk, is suggestive. A diet free of cow milk should be tried for at least a week (2 days rarely produces significant improvement) for any case of severe colic. Usually a mother eliminates drinking milk, and for some babies that is enough. If not, all milk products are then eliminated. If mild improvement results with elimination of dairy products, elimination of all bovine protein (i.e., beef) may make a difference. For the group of infants who have a cow milk allergy, the treatment is impressive. However, not all colic is caused by cow milk. It may be associated with other dietary items, such as eggs or chocolate, or it may be totally unrelated to maternal food intake.

Acute 24-hour colic in a breastfed infant may result from particular items in the maternal diet. If a strong vegetable (e.g., beans, onions, garlic, rhubarb) is taken for the first time and the infant starts to cry within a few hours and continues for 20 to 24 hours, this may be transient colic. This colic is self-limited and needs no treatment. The colic-inducing foods are different for different infants. Mailed questionnaires to 272 mothers, when their infants were about 4 months old, asked about symptoms related to colic. A high correlation was found between 24-hour colic and the mother's consumption of cruciferous vegetables, onions, cow milk, and chocolate and less so with beans, legumes, spicy foods, and caffeine.[98]

Management of colicky behavior

During the period of colic the infant may need frequent small feedings and much cuddling. Sometimes the infants overfeed, then vomit, and settle down and go quietly to sleep, just as an overfed bottle infant does.

The distress or discomfort may be caused by tension, and "colic" has been noted to be more common in the first infants of high-strung mothers.[149] Colic has been associated with hormone withdrawal and has been treated with progesterone. In the breastfed baby this is a less likely cause because of the presence of hormones in breast milk. Colicky breastfed infants who are weaned to formula are usually much worse. Weaning is not an appropriate treatment for the colicky breastfed infant in most cases. Colic usually diminishes in the third month of life, when the infant's GI tract matures.

Type A behaviors during pregnancy were measured by a self-selected cohort of 72 primiparas.[119] After delivery their infants were assessed at 48 hours and 3 months of age. The women who were type A had infants who cried more during neurobehavioral assessment compared with infants of type B women. At 3 months the infants were more intense and less predictable in their responses to the environment. Type A women, however, were more likely to be still breastfeeding.[119]

In a thorough review of infantile colic, Miller and Barr[104] conclude colic is still poorly under-stood. Causes in the GI tract include sensitivity to dietary components, excessive gas, hypermotility, and hormonal factors. Social causes include normal crying behavior, atypical parenting, and problems of parent-infant interaction. The authors conclude that colicky infants are not a homogeneous group and that it is a variation of normal behavioral and biologic factors and not pathology.[104] The breastfeeding mother needs to know it is not her fault. Appropriate remedial advice should be provided.

Weizman and associates[167] studied a herbal tea preparation and found it improved colic in 57% of infants, compared with only 26% of infants who received the placebo of warm glucose-flavored water. The herbal tea, however, contained chamomile, verbain (*Verbena officinalis*), licorice, fennel, and balm mint, several of which are not recommended for infants (see Chapter 11). Unfortunately, the dose of active ingredient is never predictable in herbal preparations, even when obtained from a reliable source.

Another explanation for colic and failure to thrive has been suggested by Woolridge and Fisher,[179] who note that when an infant is taken from the first breast and switched to the second, this may decrease the amount of fat and energy received. In addition, it will take the infant more volume to receive enough calories, which may cause symptoms of hunger with crying and fretfulness. The increased lactose and less fat causes increased gas.

When mothers were randomly assigned to use only one breast or both breasts at a feeding, Evans and associates[45] found that one-sided breastfeeding was associated with less colic and less postpartum engorgement. Later, most mothers felt they needed to feed on the second side to satisfy their infants' hunger.

Lower fat causes rapid gastric emptying with less digestion of lactose, thus producing diarrhea. It may be appropriate for such an infant to empty the first breast before switching. Colicky infants are often given more to eat, first one breast, then the other, which will increase volume but will also increase lactose and discomfort.

The *sleep tight* method of calming crying and colicky infants was developed by Karp, who produced an illustrative video demonstrating the technique. He compares the first few months of life to the fourth trimester and suggests that creating a "womb-like" atmosphere is very calming. His "five S" system consists of the following:

Swaddling—Tight swaddling provides the continuous touching and support the fetus experienced while still in mother's womb.

Side/stomach position—Place the baby, while holding her, either on her left side to assist in digestion or on her stomach to provide reassuring support. Once the baby is happily asleep, you can safely put her in her crib, on her back.

Shushing sounds—These sounds imitate the continual whooshing sound made by the blood flowing through arteries near the womb. This white noise can be in the form of a vacuum cleaner, a hair dryer, or a fan.

Swinging—Newborns are used to the swinging motions that were present when they were still in utero. Rocking, car rides, and other swinging movements all can help.

Sucking—"Sucking has its effects deep within the nervous system and triggers the calming reflex and releases natural chemicals within the brain."[79] This "S" can be accomplished with breast, bottle, pacifier, or even a finger.

All or some of these steps can be incorporated into the infant's management.

Esophageal reflux

Although less common than in bottle fed infants, esophageal reflux can occur in breastfed infants and may be a cause of colic. The pattern of colic may be different. Crying begins at the end of the feeding, or the infant falls asleep and is put down, only to wake up crying inconsolably. Esophageal reflux also tends to occur around the clock with little relief. The diagnosis can be confirmed by an esophageal probe test for reflux or by a trial of therapy with metoclopramide. Sleeping in a semi-upright position is often palliative.

Pacifiers

Pacifiers have become the subject of much controversy for full-term healthy infants. A bottle fed infant may have nonnutritive sucking with a pacifier and avoid overeating. Pacifiers in breastfed infants risk interfering with proper suckling at the breast. Conversely, some breastfed infants go back and forth with artificial nipples without a problem. Infants are born with some self-comforting mechanisms, including resuming the fetal position and sucking a thumb, finger, or fist.

When 354 children in Brazil were studied,[163] it was found that when a pacifier was used, there was a greater probability of early weaning. Mothers had introduced pacifiers to decrease crying. Victora and associates[163] followed an additional 650 infants for 6 months; 85% of infants had pacifiers by 1 month of age, and some started and abandoned them. Mothers seemed anxious to introduce them to increase the interval between feeding. Intense pacifier use was associated with weaning by 6 months. Nonwhite mothers and those with infant girls seemed more confident and less concerned about feeding difficulties. The authors concluded that epidemiologic and ethnographic factors influenced the complex relationship between pacifier use and breastfeeding.

In a positive approach to pacifiers, Anderson[6] concluded that they reduced stress in the infant and did not negatively influence feeding. In another study, 602 healthy newborns in 10 centers were randomly assigned to a UNICEF group with restrictive fluids, no bottles, and no pacifiers during the first 5 days or to a control group liberalized to have bottles and pacifiers.[142] Fluid supplements by bottle, with or without use of pacifiers, were not associated with lower frequency or shorter duration of breastfeeding in the first 6 months of life. When Righard[133] studied 52 healthy mother-infant pairs with breastfeeding problems, however, he noted a clear relationship between a faulty nursing pattern and introduction of bottle feedings and pacifier use when compared with a control group who were successfully breastfeeding.

In a randomized clinical trial of pacifier use and bottle feeding or cup feeding and their effect on breastfeeding, Howard and associates studied 700 breastfed newborns for 52 weeks. Cup feeding for those needing early feeding made no difference in long-term outcome except in cases in which multiple feedings were given. Introduction of pacifiers, however, early in the neonatal period was detrimental to exclusive breastfeeding, shortening overall duration. Findings support the recommendation to avoid exposing breastfeeding infants to artificial nipples in the neonatal period.[69]

Clearly, pacifiers are a parental decision. A pacifier should not be introduced by hospital staff unless the mother requests it. Exclusion of pacifiers is part of Baby Friendly Hospital Initiative, a program initiated by UNICEF.

Stool patterns for breastfed infants

In the first week of life the pattern of an infant receiving adequate colostrum, which has a cathartic effect on the gut, is to have a stool with most feedings. All the meconium will be passed in 48 hours, and after a few transitional stools (24 hours), the stool becomes yellow. The stools are loose and seedy in consistency. Breastfed infants have a strong gastrocolic reflex and continue to have stools with feedings, with a minimum of four seedy yellow stools per day. Over the next month, a breastfed baby should have a stool every day. When this does not happen, the physician needs to confirm that all is really well. This means a check of urine output (six to eight wet diapers a day and at least one really soaked) and urine specific gravity as well as a review of breastfeeding patterns. The purpose is to identify the potential failure-to-thrive situation before it becomes serious. Many wet diapers and no stool can indicate "low-calorie, low-fat milk." This requires a minor adjustment in breastfeeding to increase the amount of high-fat hindmilk by allowing the infant to nurse until satisfied on the first breast. Ultraabsorbent diapers make assessing voiding patterns difficult and should be avoided in breastfed infants in the first few weeks of life. Alternatively, tissue can be placed in the diaper to confirm voiding (Table 8-5).

Weight gain after the first week of life should be 15 to 30 g daily (½ to 1 oz). Birth weight should be regained in 2 weeks. The mother will observe milk leaking from her breasts, especially from the opposite breast while nursing. Feedings should occur every 2 to 3 hours for 8 to 12 per day. Length of

TABLE 8-5	Patterns in the Breastfed Infant			
	First 24 hours of life	Second 24 hours of life	Third 24 hours of life	First 30 days of life
Weight	Loss	Loss 27%	plateau	regain birth weight by 10–14 days
Stools	1x	2x	3x	minimum of 3x daily
Voids	1x	2x	3x	6–8x daily
Feeds	8–12x	8–12x	8–12x	at least 8/day

feedings will vary throughout the day, from very short and "businesslike" to dawdling and prolonged or a series of snacks. Mother and infant are symbiotic in this relationship. In most cases, the infant's cues guide the schedule. Successful breastfeeding is an infant-led process.

Insufficient milk syndrome

Perceived lack of milk is the most common reason women report for early termination of lactation.[107] As with all health problems, it is preferable to prevent a problem than to have to cure it. The medical care of infants and children is based on prevention. How can we prevent lactation problems, especially with early discharge from the hospital? Anticipatory care includes encouraging parents to attend breastfeeding classes prenatally and a breast examination by the obstetrician to identify any anatomic issues that might interfere with breastfeeding and need remedial care. The delivery service should have breastfeeding policies and practices that support and promote breastfeeding (rooming-in) and the trained staff to provide one-on-one care. Good hospital quality breast pumps should be readily available for the mother who cannot nurse her infant immediately. Schedule appropriate follow-up for pediatric care within 48 hours of discharge and offer peer support group referrals.

Several screening instruments have been developed. Presented in Box 8-6 is a simple screening tool for mothers as developed by The Health One Alliance Lactation Program, Denver, Colorado. Neifert recommends providing this at discharge from the hospital, to be completed by all breast-feeding mothers when infants are 4 to 6 days of age, following the initial follow-up visit (further discussion in Chapter 12).

Office practice of breastfeeding management

Breastfeeding health supervision during well child visits

The pediatrician's role is to create a breastfeeding atmosphere in the office including the acceptance of breastfeeding in the waiting room or providing special space for a mother to relax and feed her infant. The pediatrician should provide accurate information and realistic options for solutions when problems arise. If accurate information is not immediately available, the physicians should know where to look and whom to consult. Opening questions should target breast-feeding: How is breastfeeding going? Are there any questions? Is help needed with any aspect of breast-feeding? Age (of infant)-appropriate discussion should be initiated on the usual issues encountered at this age. If the physician is too busy for in-depth dis-cussion of these issues, the office should have a nurse practitioner available who is trained and certified in lactation and who can discuss a variety of issues (e.g., sore nipples, family support, preparing to return to work).

A model overview of breastfeeding health super-vision for the mother and infant from the prenatal period to 18 months post partum for office practice has been developed by Black.[18] The outline can be found in Appendix M. It identifies appropriate assessment, guidance, and interventions.

BOX 8-6   Early breastfeeding screening form

Please complete this screening form when your baby is 4 to 6 days old. If you circle any answers in the right-hand column, call your baby's doctor to arrange for further evaluation. The earlier problems are identified, the easier they are to correct. Your doctor may refer you to a lactation consultant who can observe your breastfeed-ing technique and provide assistance.

1. Do you feel breastfeeding is going well for you so far?	Yes	No
2. Has your milk come in yet? (That is, did your breasts get firm and full between the second and fourth postpartum days?)	Yes	No
3. Is your baby able to latch on to both breasts without difficulty?	Yes	No
4. Is your baby able to sustain rhythmic sucking for at least 10 minutes total per feeding?	Yes	No
5. Does your baby usually demand to feed? (Answer "No" if you have a sleepy baby who needs to be awakened for most feedings.)	Yes	No
6. Does your baby usually nurse at both breasts at each feeding?	Yes	No
7. Does your baby nurse approximately every 2 to 3 hours, with no more than one longer interval of up to 5 hours at night? (At least eight nursings each 24 hours?)	Yes	No
8. Do your breasts feel full before feedings?	Yes	No
9. Do your breasts feel softer after feedings?	Yes	No
10. Are your nipples extremely sore? (for example, causing you to dread feedings?)	No	Yes
11. Is your baby having yellow, seedy bowel movements that look like cottage cheese and mustard?	Yes	No
12. Is your baby having at least four good-size bowel movements each day? (That is, more than a stain on the diaper?)	Yes	No
13. Is your baby wetting his/her diaper at least six times each day?	Yes	No
14. Does your baby appear hungry after most feedings?	No	Yes
15. Do you hear rhythmic suckling and swallowing while your baby nurses?	Yes	No

Copyright © The HealthONE Alliance Lactation Program, Denver, CO.

REFERENCES

1. Adams LM, Davidson M: Present concepts of infant colic. Pediatr Ann 16:817, 1987.
2. Alexander JM, Grant AM, Campbell MJ: Randomised controlled trial of breast shells and Hoffman's exercises for inverted and non-protractile nipples. Br Med J 304:1030, 1990.
3. Alley JM, Rogers CS: Sleep patterns of breast-fed and non breast-fed infants. Pediatr Nurs 12:349, 1986.
4. Almroth SG: Water requirements of breastfed infants in a hot climate. Am J Clin Nutr 31:1154, 1978.
5. Amatayakul K, Vutyavanich T, Tanthayaphinant O, et al: Serum prolactin and cortisol levels after suckling for varying periods of time and the effect of a nipple shield. Acta Obstet Gynecol Scand 66:47, 1987.
6. Anderson GC: Pacifiers: The positive side. Matern Child Nurs 11:122, 1986.
7. Anderson GC, McBride MR, Dahm J, et al: Development of sucking in term infants from birth to four hours post birth. Res Nurs Health 5:21, 1982.
8. Aono T, Aki T, Koike K, et al: Effect of sulpiride on poor puerperal lactation. Am J Obstet Gynecol 143:927, 1982.
9. Aono T, Shioji T, Shoda T, et al: The initiation of human lactation and prolactin response to suckling. J Clin Endocrinol Metab 44:1101, 1977.
10. Ardran GM, Kemp FH, Lind J: A cineradiographic study of bottle feeding. Br J Radiol 31:11, 1958.
11. Ardran GM, Kemp FH, Lind J: A cineradiographic study of breast feeding. Br J Radiol 31:156, 1958.
12. Armelini PA, Gonzalez CF: Breastfeeding and fluid intake in a hot climate. Clin Pediatr 18:424, 1979.
13. Arthur PG, Jones TJ, Spruce J, et al: Measuring short-term rates of milk synthesis in breastfeeding mothers. Q J Exp Physiol 74:419, 1989.
14. Bader AM, Fragneto R, Terui K: Maternal and neonatal fentanyl and bupivacaine concentrations after epidural infusion during labor. Anesth Analg 81:829, 1995.
15. Barnes GR, Lethin AN, Jackson EB, et al: Management of breast feeding. JAMA 151:192, 1953.
16. Belfrage P, Berlin A, Raabe N, et al: Lumbar epidural analgesia with bupivacaine in labor. Am J Obstet Gynecol 123:839, 1975.
17. Bentovim A: Shame and other anxieties associated with breastfeeding: A systems theory and psychodynamic approach. In Ciba Foundation Symposium: Breast Feeding and the Mother, No 45. Amsterdam, Elsevier Scientific, 1976.
18. Black LS: Incorporating breastfeeding care into daily newborn rounds and pediatric office practice. Pediatr Clin North Am 48:299, 2001.
19. Blass EM, Teicher MH: Suckling. Science 210:15, 1980.
20. Bowen-Jones A, Thompson C, Drewett RF: Milk flow and sucking rates during breastfeeding. Dev Med Child Neurol 24:626, 1982.
21. Brazelton TB: Psychophysiologic reactions in the neonate. II. Effect of maternal medication on the neonate and his behavior. J Pediatr 58:513, 1961.
22. Bremme K, Eneroth P, Kindahl H: 15-Keto-13,14-dihydroprostaglandin F2α, and prolactin in maternal and cord blood during prostaglandin E2 or oxytocin therapy for labor induction. J Perinat Med 15:143, 1987.
23. Brenman HS, Pierce L, Mackowiak R, et al: Multisensor nipple recording oral variables. J Appl Physiol 26:494, 1969.
24. Budd SC, Erdman SH, Long DM, et al: Improved lactation with metoclopramide. Clin Pediatr 32:53, 1993.
25. Burke PM: Swallowing and the organization of sucking in the human newborn. Child Dev 48:523, 1977.
26. Butte NF, Garza C, Smith EO, et al: Evaluation of the deuterium dilution technique against the test-weighing procedure for the determination of breast milk intake. Am J Clin Nutr 37:996, 1983.
27. Butte NF, Wills C, Jean CA, et al: Feeding patterns of exclusively breast-fed infants during the first four months of life. Early Hum Dev 12:291, 1985.
28. Cadwell K, Turner-Maffei C: Case Studies in Breastfeeding: Problem-Solving Skills and Strategies. Boston, Jones & Bartlett Publishers, 2004.
29. Caldeyro-Barcia R: Milk ejection in women. In Reynolds M, Folley SJ (eds): Lactogenesis. Philadelphia, University of Pennsylvania Press, 1969.
30. Chayen B, Tejani N, Verma U: Induction of labor with an electric breast pump. J Reprod Med 31:116, 1986.
31. Christensen S, Dubignon J, Campbell D: Variations in intra-oral stimulation and nutritive sucking. Child Dev 47:539, 1976.
32. Cobo E, DeBernal MM, Gaitan E, et al: Neurohypophyseal hormone release in the human. II. Experimental study during lactation. Am J Obstet Gynecol 97:519, 1967.
33. Cronenwett L, Stukel T, Kearney M, et al: Single daily bottle use in the early weeks postpartum and breastfeeding outcomes. Pediatrics 90:760, 1992.
34. Cross BA: Comparative physiology of milk removal. Symp Zool Soc 41:193, 1977.
35. Daly SEJ, Kent JC, Huynh DQ, et al: The determination of short-term breast volume changes and the rate of synthesis of human milk using computerized breast measurement. Exp Physiol 77:79, 1992.
36. Da Silva OP, Knoppert DC, Angelini MM, et al: Effect of domperidone on milk production in mothers of premature newborns: A randomized, double-blind, placebo-controlled trial. Can Med Assoc J 164:17, 2001.
37. Davis HV, Sears RR, Miller HC, et al: Effects of cup, bottle, and breast feeding on oral activities of newborn infants. Pediatrics 2:549, 1948.
38. Dawood MY, Khan-Dawood FS, Wahi RS, et al: Oxytocin release and plasma anterior pituitary and gonadal hormones

in women during lactation. J Clin Endocrinol Metab 52:678, 1981.

39. Dewey KG, Lönnerdal B: Infant self-regulation of breast milk intake. Acta Paediatr Scand 75:893, 1986.

40. Dewey KG, Nommsen-Rivers LA, Heinig MJ, et al: Risk factors for suboptimal infant breastfeeding behavior, delayed onset of lactation, and excess neonatal weight loss. Pediatrics 112:607, 2003.

41. Drewett RF: Returning to the suckled breast: A further test of Hall's hypothesis. Early Hum Dev 6:161, 1982.

42. Edwards JE Jr: Should all patients with candidemia be treated with antifungal agents? Clin Infect Dis 15:422, 1992 (editorial).

43. Ehrenkranz RA, Ackerman BA: Metoclopramide effect on faltering milk production by mothers of premature infants. Pediatrics 78:614, 1986.

44. Elliott JP, Flaherty JF: The use of breast stimulation to ripen the cervix in term pregnancies. Am J Obstet Gynecol 145:553, 1983.

45. Evans K, Evans R, Simmer K: Effect of method of breast feeding on breast engorgement, mastitis and infantile colic. Acta Paediatr 84:849, 1995.

46. Evans RW, Fergusson DM, Allardyce RA, et al: Maternal diet and infantile colic in breast-fed infants. Lancet 1:1340, 1981.

47. Fisher SE, Painter M, Milmor G: Swallowing disorders in infancy: Symposium on pediatric otolaryngology. Pediatr Clin North Am 28:845, 1981.

48. Font L: "Incidental" maternal dietary intake and infant refusal to nurse. J Hum Lact 6:9, 1990.

49. Frantz K: Techniques for successfully managing nipple problems and the reluctant nurser in the early postpartum period. In Freier S, Eidelman A (eds): Human Milk: Its Biological and Social Value. Amsterdam, Excerpta Medica, 1980.

50. Gateley CA, Mansel RE: Management of the painful and nodular breast. Br Med Bull 47:284, 1991.

51. Gerrard JW, Shenassa M: Sensitization to substances in breast milk: Recognition, management and significance. Ann Allergy 51:300, 1983.

52. Goldberg NM, Adams E: Supplementary water for breast-fed babies in a hot and dry climate—Not really a necessity. Arch Dis Child 58:73, 1983.

53. Goldsmith HS: Milk-rejection sign of breast cancer. Am J Surg 127:280, 1974.

54. Gray-Donald K, Kramer MS, Munday S, et al: Effect of formula supplementation in the hospital on the duration of breastfeeding: A controlled clinical trial. Pediatrics 75:514, 1985.

55. Hafström M, Lundquist C, Lindecrantzk, et al: Recording non-nutritive sucking in the neonate: Description of an automatized system for analysis. Acta Paediatr 86:82, 1997.

56. Hall B: Changing composition of human milk and early development of an appetite control. Lancet 1:779, 1975.

57. Hartmann PE, Prosser CG: Physiological basis of longitudinal changes in human milk yield and composition. Fed Proc 43:2450, 1984.

58. Hauben DJ, Mahler D: A simple method for the correction of the inverted nipple. Plast Reconstr Surg 71:556, 1983.

59. Heck LJ, Erenberg A: Serum glucose levels in term neonates during the first 48 hours of life. J Pediatr 110:119, 1987.

60. Herd B, Feeney JG: Two aerosol sprays and nipple trauma. Practitioner 230:31, 1986.

61. Herrara AJ: Supplemented versus unsupplemented breastfeeding. Perinatol Neonatol 8:70, 1984.

62. Hewat RJ, Ellis DJ: A comparison of the effectiveness of two methods of nipple care. Birth 14:41, 1987.

63. Hide DW, Guyer BM: Prevalence of infant colic. Arch Dis Child 57:559, 1982.

64. Hill DJ, Hudson IL, Sheffield LJ, et al: A low allergen diet is a significant intervention in infantile colic: Results of a community-based study. J Allergy Clin Immunol 96:886, 1995.

65. Hill PD, Humenick SS: The occurrence of breast engorgement. J Hum Lact 10:79, 1994.

66. Hodgkinson R, Bhatt M, Wang CN: Double-blind comparison of the neurobehavior of neonates following the administration of different doses of meperidine to the mother. Can Anaesth Soc J 25:405, 1978.

67. Hoffmann JB: A suggested treatment for inverted nipples. Am J Obstet Gynecol 66:346, 1953.

68. Horowitz M, Higgins GD, Graham JJ, et al: Effect of modification of fluid intake in the puerperium on serum prolactin levels and lactation. Med J Aust 2:625, 1980.

69. Howard CR, Howard FM, Lanphear B, et al: A randomized clinical trial of pacifier use and bottle or cupfeeding and their effect on breastfeeding. Pediatrics 111:511, 2003.

70. Howie PW, McNeilly AS, McArdle T, et al: The relationship between suckling-induced prolactin response and lactogenesis. J Clin Endocrinol Metab 50:670, 1980.

71. Humenick SS, Hill PD, Anderson MA: Breast engorgement: Patterns and selected outcomes. J Hum Lact 10:87, 1994.

72. Hunziker UA, Barr RG: Increased carrying reduces infant crying: A randomized controlled trial. Pediatrics 77:641, 1986.

73. Inch S, Fisher C: Antiseptic sprays and nipple trauma. Practitioner 230:1037, 1986.

74. Jain E: Tongue-tie (ankyloglossia). Presented at First Annual International Meeting, Academy of Breastfeeding Medicine: Physicians and Breastfeeding: A New Alliance. Rochester, NY, October 1996.

75. Jakobsson I, Lindberg T: Cow's milk as a cause of infantile colic in breast-fed infants. Lancet 2:437, 1978.

76. Jakobsson I, Lindberg T: Cow's milk proteins cause infantile colic in breast-fed infants: A double-blind crossover study. Pediatrics 71:268, 1983.

77. Jakobsson I, Lindberg T, Benediksson B, et al: Dietary bovine β-lactoglobulin is transferred to human milk. Acta Paediatr Scand 74:342, 1985.

78. Johnson P, Salisbury DM: Breathing and sucking during feeding in the newborn. In Bosma JF, Showacre J (eds): Development of Upper Respiratory Anatomy and Function. Bethesda, MD, National Institutes of Health, 1975.

79. Karp H: The Happiest Baby on the Block: The New Way to Calm Crying and Help Your Newborn Baby Sleep Longer. New York, Bantam, 2003.

80. Kesaree N, Banapurmath CR, Banapurmath S, et al: Treatment of inverted nipples using a disposable syringe. J Hum Lact 9:27, 1993.

81. Klaus MH: The frequency of suckling. Obstet Gynecol Clin North Am 14:623, 1987.

82. Klaus MH, Kennell JH: The doula: An essential ingredient of childbirth rediscovered. Acta Pediatr 86:1034, 1997.

83. Kramer MS, Kakuma R: The Optimal Duration of Exclusive Breastfeeding: A Systematic Review. World Health Organization, Department of Nutrition for Health and Development, Geneva, Switzerland, 2002. http://www.who.int/inf-pr-2001/en/note2001-07.html

84. Kron RE, Stein M, Goddard KE: Newborn sucking behavior affected by obstetric sedation. Pediatrics 37:1012, 1966.

85. Kuhnert BR, Zuspan KJ, Kuhneet PM, et al: Bupivacaine disposition in mother, fetus and neonate after spinal anesthesia for cesarean section. Anesth Analg 66:407, 1987.

86. Kurinij N, Shiono PH: Early formula supplementation of breastfeeding. Pediatrics 88:745, 1991.

87. Lavergne NA: Does application of tea bags to sore nipples while breastfeeding provide effective relief? J Obstet Gynecol Neonatal Nurs 26:53, 1997.

88. Leonard EL, Trykowski LE, Kirkpatrick BV: Nutritive sucking in high-risk neonates after perioral stimulation. Phys Ther 60:299, 1980.

89. L'Esperance CM: Pain or pleasure: The dilemma of early breastfeeding. Birth Fam J 7:21, 1980.

90. Lindenberg CS, Artola RC, Jimenez V: The effect of early postpartum mother-infant contact and breastfeeding promotion on the incidence and continuation of breastfeeding. Int J Nurs Stud 27:179, 1990.

91. Lipitz S, Barkai G, Rabinovici J, et al: Breast stimulation test and oxytocin challenge test in fetal surveillance: A prospective randomized study. Am J Obstet Gynecol 157:1178, 1987.

92. Loftus JR, Hill H, Cohen SF: Placental transfer and neonatal effects of epidural sufentanil and fentanyl administered with bupivacaine during labor. Anesthesiology 83:300, 1995.

93. Lothe L, Ivarsson S-A, Ekman R, et al: Motilin and infantile colic. Acta Paediatr Scand 79:410, 1990.

94. Lothe L, Lindberg T, Jakobsson I: Macromolecular absorption in infants with infantile colic. Acta Paediatr Scand 79:417, 1990.

95. Lozoff B, Brittenham GM, Trause MA, et al: The mother-newborn relationship: Limits of adaptability. J Pediatr 91:1, 1977.

96. Lucas A, Lucas PJ, Baum JD: Differences in the pattern of milk intake between breast and bottle fed infants. Early Hum Dev 5:195, 1981.

97. Lucas A, Morley R, Cole TJ: Randomized trial of early diet in preterm babies and later intelligence quotient. BMJ 317:1481, 1998.

98. Lust KD, Brown JE, Thomas W: Maternal intake of cruciferous vegetables and other foods and colic symptoms in exclusively breast-fed infants. J Am Diet Assoc 96:47, 1996.

99. Maekawa K, Nara T, Hoashi E: Influence of breastfeeding on neonatal behavior. Acta Paediatr Jpn 27:608, 1985.

100. Marshall WM, Cumming DC, Fitzsimmons GW: Hot flushes during breastfeeding? Fertil Steril 57:1349, 1992.

101. Mashini IS, Devoe LD, McKenzie JS, et al: Comparison of uterine activity induced by nipple stimulation and oxytocin. Obstet Gynecol 69:74, 1987.

102. McNeilly AS, Robinson ICA, Houston MJ, et al: Release of oxytocin and prolactin in response to suckling. Br Med J 286:257, 1983.

103. Millard AV: The place of the clock in pediatric advice: Rationales, cultural themes, and impediments to breastfeeding. Soc Sci Med 31:211, 1990.

104. Miller AR, Barr RG: Infantile colic: Is it a gut issue? Pediatr Clin North Am 38:1407, 1991.

105. Moore DJ, Robb TA, Davidson GP: Breath hydrogen response to milk containing lactose in colicky and noncolicky infants. J Pediatr 113:979, 1988.

106. Murray AD, Dolby RM, Nation RL, et al: Effects of epidural anesthesia on newborns and their mothers. Child Dev 52:71, 1981.

107. Neifert MR: Prevention of breastfeeding tragedies. Pediatr Clin North Am 48:273, 2001.

108. Neifert MR, Seacat JM: A guide to successful breastfeeding. Contemp Pediatr 3:16, 1986.

109. Newton N: Nipple pain and nipple damage: Problems in the management of breast feeding. J Pediatr 41:411, 1952.

110. Newton N: The quantitative effect of oxytocin (Pitocin) on human milk yield. Ann NY Acad Sci 652:481, 1992.

111. Newton N: The relation of the milk-ejection reflex to the ability to breastfeed. Ann NY Acad Sci 652:484, 1992.

112. Newton M, Newton NR: The let-down reflex in human lactation. J Pediatr 33:698, 1948.

113. Newton M, Newton NR: The normal course and management of lactation. Clin Obstet Gynecol 5:44, 1962.

114. Nikodem VC, Danziger D, Gebka N, et al: Do cabbage leaves prevent breast engorgement? A randomized controlled study. Birth 20:61, 1993.

115. Nissen E, Lilja G, Widström A-M, et al: Elevation of oxytocin levels early postpartum in women. Acta Obstet Gynecol Scand 74:530, 1995.

116. Notestine GE: The importance of the identification of ankyloglossia (short lingual frenulum) as a cause of breastfeeding problems. J Hum Lact 6:113, 1990.

117. Nowlis GH, Kessen W: Human newborns differentiate differing concentrations of sucrose and glucose. Science 191:865, 1976.

118. Nysenbaum AN, Smart JL: Sucking behavior and milk intake of neonates in relation to milk fat content. Early Hum Dev 6:205, 1982.

119. Parker SJ, Barrett DE: Maternal type A behavior during pregnancy, neonatal crying and early infant temperament: Do type A women have type A babies? Pediatrics 89:474, 1992.

120. Paul K, Dittrichová J, Papousek H: Infant feeding behavior: Development in pattern and motivation. Dev Psychobiol 29:563, 1996.

121. Pedersen CA: Oxytocin control of maternal behavior: Regulation by sex steroids and offspring stimuli. Ann NY Acad Sci 807:126, 1997.

122. Pinilla T, Birch LL: Help me make it through the night: Behavioral entrainment of breastfed infants' sleep patterns. Pediatrics 91:436, 1993.

123. Pollitt E, Consolazio B, Goodkin F: Changes in nutritive sucking during a feed in two-day and thirty-day-old infants. Early Hum Dev 5:201, 1981.

124. Prentice A, Addey CV, Wilde CJ: Evidence for local feedback control of human milk secretion. Biochem Soc Trans 17:489, 1989.

125. Pugh LC, Buchko BL, Bishop BA, et al: A comparison of topical agents to relieve nipple pain and enhance breastfeeding. Birth 23:88, 1996.

126. Ramsay DT, Kent JC, Owens RA: Ultrasound imaging of milk ejection in the breast of lactating women. Pediatrics 113:361, 2004.

127. Raphael D: The Tender Gift: Breast Feeding. New York, Schocken, 1976.

128. Rayner CR: The correction of permanently inverted nipples. Br J Plast Surg 33:413, 1980.

129. Reiff MI, Essock-Vitale SM: Hospital influences on early infant-feeding practices. Pediatrics 76:872, 1985.

130. Renfrew M, Fisher C, Arms S: Breastfeeding: Getting Breastfeeding Right for You. Berkeley, CA, Celestial Arts, 1990.

131. Renfrew MJ, McCandish R: With women: New steps in research in midwifery. In Roberts H (ed): Women's Health Matters. London, Routledge, 1992.

132. Report of the Second Surgeon General's Workshop on Breastfeeding and Human Lactation. Washington, DC, National Center for Education in Maternal and Child Health, 1991.

133. Righard L: Are breastfeeding problems related to incorrect breastfeeding technique and the use of pacifiers and bottles? Birth 25:40, 1998.

134. Righard L, Alade MO: Effect of delivery room routine on success of first breastfeed. Lancet 336:1105, 1990.

135. Righard L, Alade MO: Sucking technique and its effect on success of breastfeeding. Birth 19:185, 1992.

136. Righard L, Flodmark C-E, Lothe L, et al: Breastfeeding patterns: Single and two-breast principles vis à vis infant behavior. Birth 20:182, 1993.

137. Riordan J, Auerbach KG: Breastfeeding and Human Lactation, 2nd ed. Boston, Jones and Bartlett, 1998.

138. Robert KL: A comparison of chilled cabbage leaves and chilled gelpaks in reducing breast engorgement. J Hum Lact 11:11, 1995.

139. Rosen AR, Lawrence RA: The effect of epidural anesthesia on infant feeding. J Univ Roch Med Ctr 6(1):3, 1994.

140. Rosier W: Cool cabbage compresses. Breastfeed Rev 12:28, 1988.

141. Salisbury DM: Bottle-feeding: Influence of teat hole size on suck volume. Lancet 1:655, 1975.

142. Schubiger G, Schwarz U, Tönz O, et al: UNICEF/WHO Baby Friendly Hospital Initiative: Does the use of bottles and pacifiers in the neonatal nursery prevent successful breastfeeding? Eur J Pediatr 156:874, 1997.

143. Schutzman DL, Hervada AR, Branca PA: Effect of water supplementation of full-term newborns on arrival of milk in the nursing mother. Clin Pediatr 25:78, 1986.

144. Second Surgeon General's Workshop on Breastfeeding and Human Lactation, Washington, DC, National Center for Education in Maternal and Child Health, 1991.

145. Sharp DA: Moist wound healing for sore or cracked nipples. Breastfeeding Abstracts 12(2):19, 1992.

146. Skoog T: Surgical correction of inverted nipples. J Am Med Wom Assoc 20:931, 1965.

147. Smith WL, Erenberg A, Nowak A: Imaging evaluation of the human nipple during breastfeeding. Am J Dis Child 142:76, 1988.

148. Smith WL, Erenberg A, Nowak A, et al: Physiology of sucking in the normal term infant using real-time US. Radiology 156:379, 1985.

149. Ståhlberg M-R, Savilahti E: Infantile colic and feeding. Arch Dis Child 61:1232, 1986.

150. St. James-Roberts I: Persistent infant crying. Arch Dis Child 66:653, 1991.

151. Steinberg LA, O'Connell NC, Hatch TF, et al: Tryptophan intake influences infants' sleep latency. J Nutr 122:1781, 1992.

152. Süsswein J: Zur Physiologie des Trinkens beim Säugling. Arch Kinder Heilkd 40:68, 1905.

153. Talbot FB: Eczema in childhood. Med Clin North Am 1:985, 1918.

154. Taylor RN, Green JR: Abruptio placentae following nipple stimulation. Am J Perinatol 4:94, 1987.

155. Thomas DW, McGilligan K, Eisenberg LD, et al: Infantile colic and type of milk feeding. Am J Dis Child 141:451, 1987.

156. Thomsen AC, Mogensen SC, Jepsen FL: Experimental mastitis in mice induced by coagulase-negative staphylococci isolated from cases of mastitis in nursing women. Acta Obstet Gynecol Scand 64:163, 1985.

157. Toppozada MK, El-Rahman HA, Soliman AY: Prostaglandins as milk ejectors: The nose as a new route of administration. Adv Prost Thrombox Leukotr Res 12:449, 1983.

158. Uvnäs-Moberg KU: The Oxytocin Factor. Cambridge, MA, DaCapo Press, 2003.

159. Uvnäs-Moberg K, Widström A-M, Werner S, et al: Oxytocin and prolactin levels in breastfeeding women. Acta Obstet Gynecol Scand 69:301, 1990.

160. Van Gelderen WF, Goosen A: Mammographic features of unilateral breastfeeding. Clin Radiol 5:134, 1996.

161. Vestermark V, Hogdall CK, Birch M, et al: Influence of the mode of delivery on initiation of breastfeeding. Eur J Obstet Gynecol Reprod Biol 38:33, 1990.

162. Victora CG, Behague DP, Barros FC, et al: Pacifier use and short breastfeeding duration: Cause, consequence or coincidence? Pediatrics 99:445, 1997.

163. Victora CG, Tomasi E, Olinto MTA, et al: Use of pacifiers and breastfeeding duration. Lancet 341:404, 1993.

164. Waldenstrom U, Sundelin C, Lindmark G: Early and late discharge after hospital birth: Breastfeeding. Acta Paediatr Scand 76:727, 1987.

165. Weber F, Woolridge MW, Baum JD: An ultrasonographic study of the organization of sucking and swallowing by newborn infants. Dev Med Child Neurol 28:19, 1986.

166. Weitzmen RE, Leake RD, Rubin RT, et al: The effect of nursing on neurohypophyseal hormone and prolactin secretion in human subjects. J Clin Endocrinol Metab 51:836, 1980.

167. Weizman Z, Alkrinawi S, Goldfarb D, et al: Efficacy of herbal tea preparation in infantile colic. J Pediatr 122:650, 1993.

168. Whitfield MF, Kay R, Stevens S: Validity of routine clinical test weighing as a measure of the intake of breast-fed infants. Arch Dis Child 56:919, 1981.

169. Widstrom A-M, Thingström-Paulsson J: The position of the tongue during rooting reflexes elicited in newborn infants before the first suckle. Acta Paediatr 82:281, 1993.

170. Widström A-M, Wahlberg V, Matthiesen A-S, et al: Short-term effects of early suckling and touch of the nipple on maternal behavior. Early Hum Dev 21:153, 1990.

171. Wight NE: Management of common breastfeeding issues. Breastfeeding 2001. Part I: The evidence for breastfeeding. Pediatr Clin North Am 48:321, 2001.

172. Wolff PH: Sucking patterns of infant mammals. Brain Behav Evol 1:354, 1968.

173. Wolff PH: The serial organization of sucking in the young infant. Pediatrics 42:943, 1968.

174. Woolridge MW: Aetiology of sore nipples. Midwifery 2:172, 1986.

175. Woolridge MW: The "anatomy" of infant sucking. Midwifery 2:164, 1986.

176. Woolridge MW, Baum JD: Recent advances in breastfeeding. Acta Paediatr Jpn 35:1, 1993.

177. Woolridge MW, Baum JD, Drewett RF: Does a change in the composition of human milk affect sucking patterns and milk intake? Lancet 2:1292, 1980.

178. Woolridge MW, Baum JD, Drewett RF: Effect of a traditional and of a new nipple shield on sucking patterns and milk flow. Early Hum Dev 4:357, 1980.

179. Woolridge MW, Fisher C: Colic, "overfeeding," and symptoms of lactose malabsorption in the breast-fed baby: A possible artifact of feed management. Lancet 2:382, 1988.

180. Woolridge MW, How TV, Drewett RF, et al: The continuous measurement of milk intake at a feed in breast-fed babies. Early Hum Dev 6:365, 1982.

181. Woolridge MW, Ingram JC, Baum JD: Do changes in pattern of breast usage alter the baby's nutrient intake? Lancet 336:395, 1990.

182. Work Group on Breastfeeding, American Academy of Pediatrics: Breastfeeding and the use of human milk. Pediatrics 100:1035, 1997.

9

Diet and dietary supplements for the mother and infant

Lactation is the physiologic completion of the reproductive cycle. The maternal body prepares during pregnancy for lactation not only by developing the breast to produce milk, but also by storing additional nutrients and energy for milk production. The transition to fully sustaining the infant should not be complex or require major adjustments for the mother. After delivery, mothers usually note an increase in appetite and thirst and a change in some dietary preferences. In simple cultures, anthropologists have noted that tradition prescribes on the birth of a baby bringing gifts of special foods—usually high in protein, nutrients, and calories—for the mother to ensure she will make good milk for the infant. This tradition may have affected some early studies in which relatively malnourished women were noted to produce milk comparable to that produced by well-nourished women in industrialized countries.

The Subcommittee on Nutrition During Lactation of the Committee on Nutritional Status during Pregnancy and Lactation of the Food and Nutrition Board of the Institute of Medicine at the National Academy of Sciences[167] published its first report in 1991 following an exhaustive study of the world's literature and current scientific evidence. The subcommittee stated that breastfeeding is recommended for all infants in the United States under ordinary circumstances. Women living under a wide variety of circumstances in the United States and elsewhere are capable of fully nourishing their infants by breastfeeding them. Furthermore, exclusive breastfeeding is preferred for the first 4 to 6 months. The report further stated that mothers with less than perfect diets could make good milk.

Throughout the course of its investigation,[167] the subcommittee was impressed by the overwhelming evidence indicating that women are able to "produce milk of sufficient quantity and quality to support growth and promote the health of infants—even when the mother's supply of nutrients is limited." Nonetheless, the depletion of mother's nutrient stores is a risk if efforts to achieve adequate food intake are not made to replace maternal stores.

Most writings for the nursing mother regarding maternal diet during lactation set up complicated "rules" about dietary intake that fail to consider the mother's dietary stores and normal dietary preferences and cultural patterns. Thus, one barrier to breastfeeding for some women is the "diet rules" they see as being too hard to follow or too restrictive.[57] Therefore, the physician and nutritionist must understand the simple requirements and widely acceptable variations so that dietary

317

guidelines make minimal demands on a woman's lifestyle. All over the world, women produce adequate and even abundant milk on very inadequate diets.[84] Women in primitive cultures with modest but adequate diets produce milk without any obvious detriment to themselves and none of the fatigue and loss of well-being that some well-fed Western mothers experience.[185,187] Insufficient milk is a problem in Western cultures and rarely in developing countries.

IMPACT OF MATERNAL DIET ON MILK PRODUCTION

Although much has been learned about dietary requirements for lactation by studying women from many cultures[85] and various levels of poor nutrition, some of the information is conflicting, principally because of varying sampling techniques and the improvement over time in laboratory analysis. Extensive reviews of the current literature on various nutrients in human milk and the influence of maternal dietary intake have been referenced.[50,71,96,100,104,184,185] Those readers needing access to the original studies are referred to the bibliographies from these reviews, which include hundreds of items, a listing beyond the scope of this text.

Milk volume

The volume of milk produced varies over the duration of lactation from the first few weeks to 6 months and beyond but is remarkably predictable except during extreme malnutrition or severe dehydration. In periods of acute water deprivation, manifested in the healthy mother by an acute bout of vomiting and diarrhea, the volume of milk will diminish only after the maternal urine output has been significantly compromised (10% dehydration).

Malnutrition, however, is complex, and single-nutrient deficiencies are rare. Malnutrition does seem to have an effect on the total volume of milk produced. In the extreme, when famine occurs, the milk supply dwindles and ceases, with ultimate starvation of the infant. The classic study is the report of Smith[151] on the effects of maternal undernutrition on the newborn infant in the Hunger Winter in Holland in 1944–1945. It was reported that the volume of milk was slightly diminished, but the duration of lactation was not affected. The latter is a testimony to courage rather than diet. Analysis of milk produced showed no significant deviations from normal chemical structure. Milk was produced at the expense of maternal tissue.

These data from the Dutch famine in the 1940s during World War II were reexamined by Stein and associates,[162] who pointed out that the women who had conceived during the famine did develop some maternal stores in anticipation of lactation that were not accounted for by the fetus, placenta, or amniotic fluid, even though the fetus was a pound lighter at birth. They reported fetal weight down by 10% but maternal weight down by only 4%. This demonstrates the maternal body's strong biologic commitment to preparing for lactation during pregnancy.

There is a wide range of volume of milk intake among healthy breastfed infants, averaging 750 to 800 g/day and ranging from 450 to 1200 g/day.[18] Any factor that influences the frequency, intensity, or duration of sucking by the infant influences the volume. In a study of wet nurses in the 1920s, Macy and associates[107] reported human capacity at 3500 mL/day compared to the 800 mL from mothers with singletons. Studies of mothers producing for multiples done by Saint and associates[146] confirmed production of 2 to 3 L/day for twins and triplets. At 3 months of age for all populations, the volume averages 770 g/day (range 500 to 1200 g/day).[87,120] The self-regulation of milk supply by the infant has been confirmed by studies by Dewey and associates[38] in which additional milk was pumped after each feeding for 2 weeks, thus increasing the milk supply. The infants, however, quickly went back to baseline consumption after the pumping ceased. The residual milk supply of healthy women (i.e., that which can be extracted after a full feeding) is about 100 g/day, even when an infant consumes comparatively low volumes of milk.[38,119,120]

Topographic computer imaging has been used to study breast production and storage capacities in the laboratory of Hartmann.[9,118] Using moiré patterns projected onto the breast, it has been possible to calculate the volume of milk produced. As the breast expands with increasing milk, the moiré patterns change. By correlating the maternal weights before and after a feeding and the imagery patterns, data were converted to accurate milk volumes. This technique has remarkable potential for clinical use. Hartmann reports the normal range of milk production from 1 to 6 months post partum to be between 440 and 1220 g/day for term mothers.

Prentice and Prentice[136] described "energy sparing adaptations" that were associated with normal lactation when energy intake is limited. These were decreases in basal metabolic rate, thermogenesis, and physical activity.

When well-nourished mothers reduced their intake by 32% for 1 week, consuming no less than 1500 kcal/day, there was no reduction in milk volume, although plasma prolactin levels increased. Those mothers who consumed less than 1500 kcal/day for a week did experience decreased milk volumes compared with those of the control group and the group consuming more than 1500 kcal.

Exercise, manual labor, and losing weight do not usually alter an established milk volume. Milk production will increase with infant demand, but infant demand will only increase with growth, which depends on sufficient nourishment.[87] Supplementing the mother could improve production and stimulate the infant's appetite. Milk may contain appetite inhibitors and possibly appetite stimulants.

Energy supplementation and lactation performance

In one study, when women received supplements during the last trimester of pregnancy, no effect was noted in their milk production. This suggests that short-term supplementation may be ineffective.[173] Other studies that provided supplementation of up to 900 kcal/day for 2 weeks resulted in an increase in milk production (662 to 787 g/day).[167] There was no increase in infant weight compared with the control group's infants in this period (2 weeks).

The problem of insufficient milk supply for the baby is reported in well-nourished as well as poorly nourished populations, but in cross-cultural studies it appears to be unrelated to maternal nutrition status.[171] The effect of supplementation may be more psychological than physiologic.

In countries where food supplies vary with the season, milk supplies drop 1 dL/day during periods of progressively greater food shortages. Studies continue on lactation performance of poorly nourished women around the world, including Burma, The Gambia, Papua New Guinea, and Ethiopia as well as among the Navajo. Results continue to reflect an impact on quantity, not quality, of milk.[17,32,93,128,149]

The interrelationship of milk volume, nutrient concentration, and total nutrient intake by the infant must be considered.[36] The reason for low protein content in a given sample may be lack of protein stores, lack of total energy content, or lack of vitamin B_6, a requirement of normal protein metabolism.

Of great concern, however, is the report of dietary supplementation of Gambian nursing mothers in which the lactational performance was not affected by increased calories (700 kcal/day).[138] The supplement produced a slight initial improvement in maternal body weight and subcutaneous fat but not in milk output. Whether the mothers utilized the increased energy to work harder farming or whether the infants did not stimulate increased milk production is unresolved. The Subcommittee on Nutrition during Lactation concluded that food supplementation of lactating women in areas where malnutrition is prevalent has generally had little, if any, impact on milk volume.[167] They believed, however, that such supplementation improves maternal health and is more likely to benefit the mother than the infant except where milk composition had been affected by specific deficiencies.

Protein content

Since the work of Hambraeus[70] has reestablished the norms for protein in human milk to be 0.8 to 0.9 g/dL in well-nourished mothers, figures from previous studies will have to be recalculated to consider that all nitrogen in human milk is not protein; 25% of the nitrogen is nonprotein nitrogen (NPN) in human milk, and only 5% of the nitrogen is NPN in bovine milk. The protein content of milk from poorly nourished mothers is surprisingly high, and malnutrition has little effect on protein concentration. An increase in dietary protein increases volume but not overall protein content, given the normal variations seen in healthy, well-nourished women.[45]

Observations made over a 20-month period of continued lactation showed that milk quality did not change, although the quantity decreased slightly, which Von Muralt[175] attributed to the decreasing demand of a child who is receiving other nourishment. Therefore, the total protein available with the decreased volume of milk and increased weight of the child decreased from 2.2 g/kg of body weight to 0.45 g/kg. The need for additional protein sources from other foods for the child after 1 year of age becomes obvious.

In its painstaking review of the literature, the Subcommittee on Nutrition during Lactation[167] determined that the composition of human milk is maintained even with less-than-recommended dietary intake of macronutrients. The concentrations of major minerals, including calcium, phosphorus, magnesium, sodium, and potassium, are not affected by diet. Maternal intakes of selenium and iodine, however, are positively affected by diet: an increase in the diet increases the level in the milk. The proportion of different fatty acids in human milk varies with the maternal dietary intake.

Eighty-three lactating Zairian mothers with protein malnutrition were given 500 kcal (2093 kilojoules, kJ) and 18 g of protein as a cow milk supplement for 2 months, after which their nutritional status improved significantly.[41] The volume of milk did not change (607 versus 604 mL). Their breastfed infants, however, did show significant improvement in their mean serum albumin levels, and their growth matched that of healthy infants of the same age.

The effect of very-low-protein (8% of energy) and very-high-protein (20% of energy) diets on the protein and nitrogen composition of breast milk in three healthy Swedish women "in full lactation" was significant.[67] High-protein diets produced higher production and greater concentrations of total nitrogen, true protein, and NPN. The increased NPN was caused by increased urea levels and free amino acids. The 24-hour outputs of lactoferrin, lactalbumin, and serum albumin were not significantly higher.

When marginally nourished women were provided a mixed-protein diet predominantly from plant sources up to 1.2 g/kg/day, equilibrium was achieved at a protein intake of 1.1 g/kg. In a study of healthy women given marginal protein intakes, Motil and associates[116] reported that maternal milk production and the protein nitrogen, but not the NPN, fraction of human milk were relatively well preserved in the short term.

The practical significance, except as related to fad diets, of these results is limited because the diets were extreme and were maintained for only 4 days. The impact on human nutritional physiology, however, is significant.[67]

Taurine, an amino acid found only in animal products, is the second most abundant free amino acid in human milk. Even milk of women who have no animal foods in their diet contains some taurine at levels (35 mg/dL) that are lower than those in women who consume animal products (54 mg/dL).[141]

Of practical significance for counseling the healthy woman in the industrialized world is the work of Butte and associates[18] investigating the effect of maternal diet and body composition on lactational performance. Forty-five healthy lactating women were followed for 4 months from delivery with detailed measurements of milk production, dietary intake, and maternal body composition. The overall mean energy intake was 2186 (± 463) kcal/day. Milk production averaged 751, 725, 723, and 740 g/day for months 1, 2, 3, and 4. Average maternal weight reduction was from 64.6 kg to 59.3 kg. Energy was calculated to be sufficient for maintenance and activity, yet the mothers achieved gradual weight reduction. The authors conclude that energy intakes of approxi-

TABLE 9-1	Milk production over first 4 months of lactation							
	Mo 1 (*n* = 37)		Mo 2 (*n* = 40)		Mo 3 (*n* = 37)		Mo 4 (*n* = 41)	
Human milk* (g/day)	751	(130)†	725	(131)	723	(114)	740	(128)
Feedings (no/day)	8.3	(1.9)	7.2	(1.9)	6.8	(1.9)	6.7	(1.8)
Total nitrogen (mg/g)	2.17	(0.30)	1.94	(0.24)	1.84	(0.19)	1.80	(0.21)
Protein nitrogen (mg/g)	1.61	(0.24)	1.42	(0.17)	1.34	(0.15)	1.31	(0.17)
Nonprotein nitrogen (mg/g)	0.56	(0.28)	0.52	(0.20)	0.50	(0.13)	0.48	(0.14)
Fat (mg/g)	36.2	(7.5)	34.4	(6.8)	32.2	(7.8)	34.8	(10.8)
Energy (kcal/g)	0.68	(0.08)	0.64	(0.08)	0.62	(0.09)	0.64	(0.10)

*At the onset of the study, milk was estimated by deuterium dilution, a technique that was later determined to be inaccurate. For this reason, data are missing at 17 time points during the first 3 months.
†Mean (SD).
From Butte NF, Garza C, Stuff JE, et al: Effect of maternal diet and body composition on lactational performance. Am J Clin Nutr 39:296, 1984.

mately 15% less than those currently recommended are compatible with full lactation, full activity, and gradual weight reduction to prepregnant weight (Tables 9-1 and 9-2). Diets otherwise contained recommended daily allowances for lactation.[52] Other investigators studying the impact of weight loss noted that the rate of postpregnancy weight loss affected the level of elaidic acid in milk and of *trans* fatty acid level.[22] This is explained by the mobilization of fatty acids from maternal adipose tissue.

Fat, cholesterol, and omega-3 fatty acids

Mature human milk contains about 50% of its energy as fat. This fat is necessary for the tremendous growth of the newborn and is essential to the structural development of the brain, retina, and other tissues. Both n-6 and n-3 fatty acids are essential components of the phospholipids of cell membranes. They are critical to the fluidity, permeability, and activity of membrane-bound

TABLE 9-2	Anthropometric changes in mothers during lactation									
Parameter	Postpartum		Mo 1		Mo 2		Mo 3		Mo 4	
Wt (kg)	64.6	(9.1)*	61.3	(9.5)	60.7	(10.0)	60.2	(10.4)	59.3	(10.5)
Wt/ht (kg/cm)†	0.40	(0.04)	0.37	(0.05)	0.37	(0.05)	0.37	(0.05)	0.36	(0.06)
Wt/prepregnancy wt‡	1.16	(0.06)	1.08	(0.05)	1.07	(0.05)	1.06	(0.05)	1.05	(0.07)
Wt change (kg/mo)			−3.83	(2.26)	−0.59	(1.20)	−0.62	(1.12)	−0.80	(1.86)
Triceps (mm)	16.3	(5.1)	16.9	(4.6)	17.0	(4.7)	17.3	(5.3)	17.2	(5.2)
Subscapular (mm)	18.2	(7.1)	16.8	(6.4)	16.4	(7.4)	15.7	(7.2)	15.1	(7.3)
Biceps (mm)	7.8	(3.9)	6.9	(3.2)	6.9	(3.3)	7.3	(4.6)	6.8	(3.4)
Suprailiac (mm)	26.1	(8.5)	25.7	(6.9)	25.2	(7.6)	23.1	(8.1)	22.2	(8.0)
Sum skinfolds (mm)	68.4	(20.2)	66.3	(18.9)	65.5	(20.6)	63.4	(22.9)	61.7	(21.8)
Midarm circumference (cm)	26.9	(3.5)	26.7	(2.6)	26.8	(3.2)	26.6	(2.9)	26.7	(3.6)

*Mean (SD).
†Maternal height (ht) = 163.0 cm (6.3 cm).
‡Prepregnancy weight (wt) gain = 14.4 kg (3.3 kg).
From Butte NF, Garza C, Stuff JE, et al: Effect of maternal diet and body composition on lactational performance. Am J Clin Nutr 39:296, 1984.

enzymes and receptors. During the first 4 to 6 months of life, an infant accumulates 1300 to 1600 g of lipids.[76]

Considerable attention has been focused on the impact of dietary fat and cholesterol on the composition of human milk. Fat is the main source of kilocalories in human milk for the infant. The fatty acid composition of the triglycerides, which make up more than 98% of the lipid component of human milk, can be affected by maternal diet. Diets with different lipid composition, caloric content, proportion of calories from fat, and fatty acid composition have been studied.

In a classic work that was carefully controlled, Insull and associates[82] fed lactating women in a metabolic ward diets that differed in caloric content, proportion of calories from fat, and fatty acid composition. Neither milk volume nor total milk fat was affected by diet. When the high-calorie, no-fat diet was fed, milk triglycerides were higher in fatty acids 12:0 and 14:0 and lower in 18:0 and 18:1, which indicated that when fatty acids were synthesized from carbohydrate, there were more intermediate-chain fatty acids. When the low-calorie, no-fat diet was fed, the fatty acid composition of the milk resembled the maintenance diet and the depot fat. When corn oil was the fat source, milk levels of 18:2 and 18:3 were higher, with a major increase in linoleic acid, than when lard or butter was used. Multiple studies have shown that medium-chain fatty acids, lauric and myristic acid (12:0 and 14:0), are not affected by diet, indicating synthesis by the mammary gland.[48,100,104]

Trans fatty acids are produced in hydrogenation reactions and appear in human milk as a reflection of dietary intake, so that women who eat margarine rather than butter have high levels in their milk.[95] Elaidic acid (18:1 *trans*) is found in margarine, for instance. Because of the high level of *trans* fatty acids in hydrogenated vegetable oils such as margarine, the milk of U.S. women is high in *trans* fatty acids, whereas the milk of West German women who do not use margarines is low in *trans* fatty acids.[48] Considerable controversy surrounds the biologic effects. The recommendations for substituting margarines were reversed in 1997. In mammals, *trans* isomers have been noted to alter permeability and fluidity of membranes, inhibit a number of enzyme reactions of lipid metabolism, and impair synthesis of arachidonic acid and prostaglandins.

The concern about fat composition in terms of the polyunsaturated fatty acid (PUFA) to saturated fatty acid ratio (P/S ratio) and the high level of cholesterol normally found in breast milk have led to monitoring mothers on altered lipid intakes. Potter and Nestel[131] studied lactating women who were placed on one of two experimental diets after a period of a study of their normal Australian diet, which includes 400 to 600 mg of cholesterol per day and fat that is rich in saturated fatty acids. Following this baseline study, the mothers were given either diet A, with 580 mg cholesterol and a high level of saturated fats, or diet B, with 110 mg cholesterol and a higher level of polyunsaturated fats from vegetable oils. A second study was carried out with the two diets high in either saturated or unsaturated fats, but the cholesterol remained the same, 345 to 380 mg/day.

The low-cholesterol diets lowered the maternal blood cholesterol but not the triglyceride levels. The cholesterol level of the milk, however, was unaffected in any diet combination.[100,101] The increase in PUFA in the diet rapidly increased the levels of linoleate in the milk to twice the previous level at the expense of myristate and palmitate. Protein levels remained the same in the milk throughout the study. Infant plasma cholesterol levels decreased in response to an increase in the concentration of linoleate in the milk. The significant dietary change seemed to depend on the consumption of high PUFA and low cholesterol to alter the levels in the milk and thus in the infant's plasma (Table 9-3).[131]

Cholesterol levels remain relatively stable throughout at least 16 weeks of lactation. The presence or absence of phytosterols influences both the accuracy of analysis (i.e., overestimate level of cholesterol) and the physiologic significance of cholesterol. *Phytosterols* are those sterols derived from plant sources. They are distinguishable from cholesterol, which is of animal origin. During a

TABLE 9-3	**Lipid concentrations of mature human milk**					
	Diet			Lipid concentration in milk		
Study	Plan	Saturation of fat*	Cholesterol (mg/day)	Cholesterol (mg/dL)	Triglyceride (g/dL)	Phospholipid (mg P/dL)
I ($n = 7$)	A	S	580	$18.1 \pm 2.7^{\dagger}$	3.42 ± 0.61	4.04 ± 0.71
	B	P	110	19.3 ± 3.6	3.57 ± 0.82	4.18 ± 0.91
II ($n = 3$)	C	S	380	23.3 ± 2.3	4.11 ± 0.42	
	D	P	345	21.3 ± 2.4	4.12 ± 0.56	

*S, rich in saturated fatty acids (P/S ratio ~0.07); P, rich in polyunsaturated fatty acids (P/S ~1.3).
†Mean ± SEM.
From Potter JM, Nestel PJ: The effects of dietary fatty acids and cholesterol on the milk lipids of lactating women and the plasma cholesterol of breast-fed infants. Am J Clin Nutr 29:54, 1976.

given feeding, the concentration of cholesterol in the milk may increase over 60%, although the total for the feeding is constant. The effect of maternal diet on cholesterol and phytosterol levels in human milk was measured by Mellies and associates,[110] who reported no change in cholesterol but a dramatic increase in phytosterols on high-cholesterol and phytosterol diets. The level of phytosterol in infant plasma did not change, however. These observations further confirm that cholesterol is synthesized at least in part in the mammary gland, whereas phytosterol is not.

Thus, there is no evidence that concentrations of cholesterol and phospholipid can be changed by diet. Milk cholesterol is stable at 100 to 150 mg/L even in hypercholesterolemic women and increases only in severe cases of pathologic hypercholesterolemia, according to Jensen.[86] The fat globule membrane contains both cholesterol and phospholipids, and their secretion rates are related to the total quantity and are not influenced by diet. This supports the conclusion that cholesterol is essential to the diet of the infant.

Where maternal undernutrition is commonplace, the percentage of maternal body fat may influence the concentration of fat in the milk.[136] Milk fat concentrations in Gambian women were positively correlated with maternal skinfold thickness and decreased over the course of lactation. In lactation beyond 6 months, similar correlations have been noted in the United States by Nommsen and associates.[121] Women with parity of 10 and above appear to have a decreased capacity to synthesize milk fat and thus have lower milk fat concentrations in their milk.

The synthesis of fatty acids up to the carbon number of 16, as well as the direct desaturation of stearic acid into oleic acid, can take place in the mammary gland, whereas longer-chain fatty acids come directly from plasma triglycerides (see Chapter 4). The intake of both carbohydrate and fat must be taken into account when evaluating maternal diet, because high-carbohydrate diets increase lauric acid and myristic acid and moderate levels of carbohydrate influence linoleic acid.

When serum lipids are measured in African women accustomed to a low fat intake, the levels are relatively low and the women are virtually free of coronary heart disease.[3,132] Among long-lactating (1 to 2 years minimum) African mothers, the amount of fat in their daily milk is of the same order as that ingested in their habitual diet.[178] Despite this, they are not significantly hypolipidemic when compared with nonlactators.

Human milk samples obtained from women living in five different regions of China showed the great diversity of milk fatty acids.[24] The docosahexaenoic acid (DHA) concentrations in women from the marine region were twice as high as those from rural areas.[127] The milk concentrations of

DHA varied greatly (0.44 ± 0.29 to 2.78 ± 1.20 g/100 g total fat), with pastoral regions being lowest and the marine region highest. Seafood consumption was high in the marine group. Similarly, arachidonic acid (AA), when stated as a ratio (AA/DHA, g/g), was 2.77 in pastoral areas and 0.42 in the marine region. AA has been associated with infant growth and DHA with brain and retinal growth. Similar findings are reported in Alaskan Eskimos who had a diet high in fish and fish oil. When women's diets were supplemented with fish and fish oils, the blood concentrations of DHA in the maternal plasma and red blood cells (RBCs) were increased.[26] Infants showed a 35% DHA increase in RBCs and 45% increase in plasma, which supports the concept that maternal diet can influence the DHA levels in the newborn.

Guthrie and associates[68] have provided data on the fatty acid patterns of human milk in correlation with the current American diet, which has a high P/S ratio. Compared with studies conducted in 1953, 1958, and 1967, there was a shift toward higher levels of $C_{18:2}$ fatty acids, linoleic acid, and $C_{18:3}$ linolenic acid. *Depot fat* reflects dietary fatty acid patterns and thus the pool for mammary gland synthesis of milk fats. The mammary gland can dehydrogenate saturated and monosaturated fatty acids.

Using newer methodologies of stable isotopes, Hachey and associates[69] confirmed the work of early investigators showing that diet composition affects milk fat synthesis. They demonstrated that when a woman is in energy balance, the fatty acids from the diet account for about 30% of the total fatty acids in her milk.

The habitual diet of healthy primiparas in Finland was associated with breast milk containing 3.8% fat.[176] Their diet was 16% protein, 39% fat, and 45% carbohydrate. Half the fatty acids of the diet and the milk were saturated, and one third were monoenoic. PUFAs were 15% of the diet and 13% of the breast milk, with a P/S ratio of 0.3 for both. The maternal diet had no effect on total fat content of the milk except for the low level of oleic acid, which is apparently peculiar to Finnish breast milk.

A word of caution on the lowering of fats in the diet inordinately: evaluation of the effects of a low-fat maternal diet on neonatal rats by Sinclair and Crawford[150] is pertinent. They made the distinction between two types of lipid in animals: storage and structural. This is correlated with histologic findings of visible and invisible fats. *Visible (storage) fats* are triglycerides found in body depots. *Invisible (structural) fats* include phosphoglycerides, sphingolipids, and some neutral lipids, including cholesterol. The structural fats are key constituents of cellular membranes, certain enzymes, and myelin. The brain contains more structural lipids than protein.

Sinclair and Crawford[150] found that neonatal rats born to mothers raised on low-fat diets had a higher mortality rate, and survivors had smaller body, brain, and liver weights than control rats. The lipid content of the body, brain, and liver was significantly lower than that in the control group. During life, the rat pups had depended entirely on their mother's milk for nutrition.

DHA, a long-chain fatty acid (22:6, ω-3), has attracted attention because deficiency has been associated with visual impairment in offspring of rhesus monkeys.[104] Human milk contains consistent levels; formulas historically contained little or none. DHA can be synthesized from linoleic acid, but high levels of linoleic acid suppress production. Fish oil is an excellent dietary source of DHA, and women who consistently eat fish have higher levels in their milk. In a study, Finley and as found that vegetarians have higher DHA levels in their milk than omnivore control subjects.[48] Many formulas have been supplemented with synthetically derived DHA in an effort to mimic human milk. They do not, however, contain cholesterol, and there are no data to support the concept that synthetically derived DHA is as effective as natural DHA is in human milk.

A strong association exists between body fat of the mother and lipid in her milk. Lovelady and associates found that the best predictor of milk lipids was overall "fatness" rather than the distribution of that fat. Dietary fat was not associated with milk fat in the "fat" women (27% or more body fat) but was positively correlated with diet in lean women (less than 27% body fat).[106]

When healthy pregnant women are supplemented with fish oil capsules from the 30th week of gestation, the fatty acid compositions of the phospholipids isolated from umbilical plasma and umbilical vessel walls differ from those of unsupplemented mothers, with more n-3 and less n-6 fatty acids.[172] This suggests that DHA status can be altered at birth.

A group of lactating women were given supplements of different doses of fish oil concentrates rich in omega-3 (ω-3) fatty acids, including DHA.[73] Receiving 5 g/day for 28 days, 10 g/day for 14 days, and 47 g/day for 8 days, each experienced significant dose-dependent increases in DHA in their milk and plasma. Baseline levels in milk were 0.1% of total fatty acids, and levels rose from 0.8% to as high as 4.8% on the 47 g/day diet. This suggests that relatively small supplements of DHA can enhance levels in the milk. Preformed dietary DHA is known to be better synthesized into nervous tissue than that synthesized from linolenic acid, and other essential fatty acids can inhibit this transformation to DHA.[73]

Studies of linoleic acid supplementation from 20 weeks' gestation in normal women showed that levels increased in those with low linoleic acid levels to match those with high levels.[1] The neonatal linoleic acid status did not change. Linoleic acid supplementation did result in slightly but significantly higher total amounts of n-6 long-chain polyenes in umbilical plasma. Linoleic acid (18:2, n-6) is essential to the maintenance of the epidermal water barrier and is the ultimate dietary precursor of eicosanoids, which include leukotrienes, prostaglandins, and thromboxanes. Linoleic acid is not synthesized by humans and must be supplied by diet.

A diet deficient in ω-3 fatty acids leads to a triad of signs in the rhesus monkey: visual impairment, electroretinographic abnormalities, and polydipsia. Profound biochemical changes in fatty acid composition of the membranes of the retina, brain, and other organs are seen experimentally. Low concentrations of ω-3 fatty acids occur at birth in the placenta, RBCs, and neural tissues when the mothers are fed deficient diets. Studies in monkeys confirm that the most critical period of life for providing ω-3 fatty acids is during pregnancy and during lactation in early infancy.[26] In humans, supplementation of the maternal diet with fish and fish oils has increased the levels of ω-3 fatty acids, especially DHA. Humans can synthesize DHA from linolenic acid, but this is limited in both infants and adults. Supplementing with linolenic acid does not significantly increase DHA in the blood.[24] There is no evidence to suggest that supplements in normal women with good diets are beneficial. Excesses of DHA affect AA levels and interfere with the AA/DHA ratio.

Lactose

In human milk the principal carbohydrate is lactose, present at about 70 g/L and second only to water as a major constituent. The milk of all species is isotonic with maternal plasma, and 60% to 70% of the osmotic pressure is created by lactose. Lactose provides twice the energy value per molecule or unit of osmotic pressure. Because milk volume is driven by available lactose, its concentration is very stable.[38] Changes in the carbohydrate levels in the diet have been studied. Comparison of mothers on diets with three different levels of carbohydrate shows that the amounts of protein, fat, and carbohydrate in their milk are similar. The Subcommittee on Nutrition during Lactation believes there is no evidence to indicate that dietary manipulations affect lactose.[167]

Water

No data support the assumption that increasing fluid intake will increase milk volume, and restricting fluids has not been shown to decrease milk volume.[80,124] Forcing fluids, however, has been shown by Dusdieker and associates[43] to affect milk production negatively in a controlled crossover-design study of breastfeeding mothers. Thus, women taking excessive fluids produced less milk, suggesting that drinking to thirst and heeding body cues is more physiologic than prescribing a specific amount of fluid a day. This observation was first demonstrated in a 1939 study by Olsen,[124] who concluded, "Forced, excessive drinking is therefore neither necessary nor beneficial as far as the nursing is concerned and may even be harmful." He had studied great variations in quantity of fluids taken and also noted that "hypogalactia cannot be arrested by forced drinking beyond the natural dictates of thirst." Urine output in these studies was proportional to intake. Illingworth and Kilpatrick[81] did a similar study in 210 postpartum mothers, half of whom drank ad lib, taking an average of 69 oz daily; the other half were forced to take 6 pints and averaged 107 oz daily. The mothers forced to drink beyond thirst produced less milk, and their babies gained less well.

From a practical standpoint, mothers have an increased thirst, which usually maintains a need for added fluid intake. When fluids are restricted, mothers will experience a decrease in urine output, not in milk. Sharply decreasing fluids to prevent engorgement in the mother who is not lactating is ineffectual, however, and only adds another inconvenience and discomfort.[42]

Kilocalories

The caloric content, sample by sample, of milk from well-nourished mothers does vary somewhat but averages about 75 kcal/dL. Because fat is the chief source of kilocalories, the fat content has the greatest impact on total kilocalories, with lactose and protein also contributing to the total. Thus, in malnourished mothers with low fat stores the caloric content may be reduced.

Body fat increases during pregnancy and decreases during lactation. Changes in the adipose depot primarily result from a change in fat cell size, not number. Adipose tissue fatty acid synthesis remains low throughout lactation, as does lipoprotein lipase activity. Conversely, mammary lipoprotein lipase activity increases and remains high during lactation.[164]

How does this correlate with the caloric needs of the mother to produce milk? The calculations for energy requirements have been made by comparing the energy intakes of nursing mothers and nonnursing mothers who were matched for other variables. English and Hitchcock[46] found that nursing mothers consumed 2460 kcal daily and nonnursing mothers consumed 1880 kcal, a net difference of 580 kcal.

Lactation will not produce a net drain on the mother if the amount of energy available and the requirement of any given nutrient are replaced in the diet. There is a small energy cost of milk production, because the breast does work at remarkable efficiency. During pregnancy, fat and other nutrients are stored for the fetus and in preparation for lactation. Lactation is subsidized, as is fetal growth, by maternal stores, even though the diet on any given day may be relatively deficient in a specific nutrient. This can be clarified by Figure 9-1, which shows that diet and stores are available for milk, as well as for maintenance of the mother. To determine if nutrient availability during gestation and early life modifies the effects of subsequent dietary intake on reproductive and lactation performance, McGuire and colleagues[109] fed restricted rats. Then using pre- and postweaning diets, they determined that past or current food restriction impairs reproductive success and decreases milk yield in rats.

A study of 26 healthy, normotensive, nonsmoking, euthyroid women—12 of whom were breastfeeding, 7 bottle feeding, and 7 nonpregnant, nonlactating control subjects—was reported by Illingworth and associates.[78] Energy expenditure at rest and in response to a meal and to an infusion of

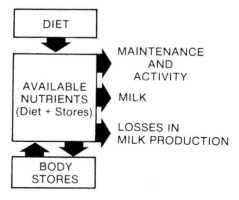

Figure 9-1. Energy utilization during lactation, showing availability of body stores and dietary sources.

noradrenaline was measured. During lactation the resting metabolic rate was unaltered, but there was a reduced response to infusion of noradrenaline and to a meal. These responses returned to normal control values in these women post lactation. Bottle feeders were similar to control subjects. The woman's metabolic efficiency is greatly enhanced during lactation and results in a reduction in the nonlactational component of maternal energy expenditure (Fig. 9-2).

When comparing dietary intake during lactation at 6 weeks post partum to the intake of a comparable group of nonpregnant women and a group of nonlactating but postpartum women using a 7-day food diary and questionnaire, total daily intakes and meal patterns were not different between body weight-matched lactators and nonlactators. The lactating women, however, consumed a significantly smaller percentage of the recommended dietary allowances (RDAs) per day and were much more calm both before and after meals. Because the lactating women did not increase their daily intake over their prepregnancy diet, Heck and deCastro[74] suggest that they catabolize the weight gain during pregnancy faster or increase their metabolic efficiency.

The Subcommittee on Nutrition during Lactation[167] stated that "the total amount of nutrients that the lactating mother secretes in her milk are directly related to the extent and duration of lactation." Furthermore, lactating women who consume a well-balanced diet with adequate calories (2700 kcal/day) also meet the RDAs for all nutrients with the exception of calcium and zinc, according to assessments of the average American diet for young women. The subcommittee based its assumption on nutrient density (nutrient intake per 1000 kcal) of the average woman's diet in the United States (see Appendix B). Nutrient densities for proteins, minerals, and vitamins were determined from nationally representative samples of women aged 19 to 50 years of age. The nutrient values at three different levels of energy have been calculated (nutrient density × kcal of energy = total intake). The levels of energy used are 2700 kcal, the recommendation for lactating women; 2200 kcal, as reported by lactating women as actual consumption; and 1800 kcal, the minimal level a lactating woman should consider in a restricted diet. The relative nutrient deficiencies are identified next.

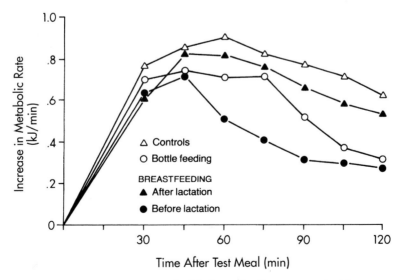

Figure 9-2. Metabolic response to test meal while breastfeeding compared with response of bottle feeders and nonpregnant control subjects. (From Illingworth PJ, Jung RT, Howie PW, et al: Diminution in energy expenditure during lactation. Br Med J 292:437, 1986.)

For the lactating woman, a 2700-kcal diet may be deficient in calcium and zinc; the 2200-kcal diet is deficient in calcium, magnesium, zinc, thiamin, vitamin B_6, and vitamin E; and the 1800-kcal diet is deficient in all the previously mentioned nutrient levels plus riboflavin, folate, phosphorus, and iron unless special attention is paid to intake of these nutrients (see Table 9-8).

The subcommittee[167] recommends that women be encouraged to follow dietary guidelines, especially in terms of fruits, vegetables, and whole grains; calcium-rich dairy products; and protein-rich foods. Vitamin and mineral supplements are not recommended for lactating women. If, however, dietary review suggests intake is lower than recommended, the woman should be encouraged to consume more foods rich in those nutrients. A woman with serious dietary problems leading to low intake of one or more nutrients should be encouraged by counseling to correct her dietary deficiencies. Nutrient supplements are recommended only as a last resort.

Diets of adolescents have been noted to be low in iron and vitamin A (1500 IU/1000 kcal instead of 1950 IU/1000 kcal). Black women consume 30% less calcium, 20% less magnesium, and 20% less vitamin A than white women. Appendix B lists recommendations for culturally acceptable diets, and Table 9-4 suggests measures for improving nutrient intake of women with restrictive eating patterns. Overt signs of deficiency are rare in the United States, even for the nutrients with small safety margins.

TABLE 9-4 Suggested measures for improving nutrient intake of women with restrictive eating patterns

Type of restrictive eating pattern	Corrective measures
Excessive restriction of food intake, i.e., ingestion of less than 1800 kcal of energy per day, which ordinarily leads to unsatisfactory intake of nutrients compared with amounts needed by lactating women	Encourage increased intake of nutrient-rich foods to achieve energy intake of at least 1800 kcal/day; if mother insists on curbing food intake sharply, promote substitution of foods rich in vitamins, minerals, and protein for those lower in nutritive value; in individual cases, it may be advisable to recommend a balanced multivitamin-mineral supplement; discourage use of liquid weight loss diets and appetite suppressants
Complete vegetarianism, i.e., avoidance of all animal foods, including meat, fish, dairy products, and eggs	Advise intake of regular source of vitamin B_{12}, such as special vitamin B_{12}–containing plant food products or a 2.6-μg vitamin B_{12} supplement daily
Avoidance of milk, cheese, or other calcium-rich dairy products	Encourage increased intake of other culturally appropriate dietary calcium sources, such as collard greens for blacks from southeastern United States; provide information on appropriate use of low-lactose dairy products if milk is being avoided because of lactose intolerance; if correction by diet cannot be achieved, it may be advisable to recommend 600 mg of elemental calcium per day taken with meals
Avoidance of vitamin D–fortified foods, such as fortified milk or cereal, combined with limited exposure to ultraviolet light	Recommend 10 μg of supplemental vitamin D per day

From the Subcommittee on Nutrition during Lactation. Committee on Nutritional Status during Pregnancy and Lactation. Food and Nutrition Board, Institute of Medicine. National Academy of Science: Nutrition during Lactation. Washington, DC, National Academy Press, 1991.

Vitamins

Water-soluble vitamins

Water-soluble vitamins move with ease from serum to milk; thus their dietary fluctuation is more apparent. Levels of water-soluble vitamins in milk are raised or lowered by change in the maternal diet. The body's requirement for vitamin C increases under stress, including lactation. Furthermore, the vitamin C content of human organs at autopsy is much higher in the neonate than at any other time of life. This is true of all the major organs, including the brain.

The influence of maternal intake of vitamin C on the concentration of vitamin C in human milk and on the intake of vitamin C by the infant was carefully measured by Byerley and Kirksey[19] in 25 well-nourished lactating women. Supplements ranged from 0 to 1000 mg (more than 10 times the RDA) vitamin C daily. Concentrations in milk ranged from 44 to 158 mg/L and were not correlated significantly with maternal intakes, which ranged from 156 (0 mg supplement) to 1123 (1000 mg supplement). Dietary vitamin C had no effect on the volume of milk produced. Maternal excretion of vitamin C in urine was correlated with maternal intake. Regardless of the level of maternal intake of vitamin C, the mean vitamin C concentration in breast milk was twice that recommended for infant formula. Vitamin C levels in milk did not increase in response to increasing maternal intake despite 10-fold increases, whereas urinary excretion did suggest that mammary tissue becomes saturated.

The investigators[19] postulate a regulatory mechanism to prevent an elevation in concentration of vitamin C beyond a certain level in milk. Vitamin C levels were at the same or higher levels in exclusively breastfed infants at 6 months and 9 months of age as compared with levels of supplemented bottle fed control infants.[147] Levels were dependent on maternal nutrition and vitamin C levels in milk. Byerley and Kirksey[19] found 6% of well-nourished healthy mothers had low levels of vitamin C. In malnourished women, tissue stores may take time to replenish, which explains why 35 mg/day supplementation failed to increase low plasma levels.[152]

Data from multiple studies suggest that there is a level above which further vitamin C supplementation will not affect milk vitamin C levels.[104]

The level of *B vitamins*, also water soluble, reflects dietary intake. The levels are affected acutely by maternal diet. Infantile beriberi is not unheard of in seemingly normal infants nursed by apparently well-nourished mothers with thiamin-deficient diets. The influence of maternal diet has been pointed out dramatically in reported cases of megaloblastic anemia and methylmalonic aciduria and homocystinuria in the breastfed infants of strict vegetarians. *Vitamin B_{12}* exists in all animal protein but not in vegetable protein. A strict vegetarian would require vitamin B_{12} supplements during pregnancy and lactation.[59,77,114] Vitamin B_{12} deficiency in infants has also been seen in New Delhi, where malnourished mothers produced vitamin B_{12}–deficient milk. These infants also had megaloblastic anemia.[32]

Specker and associates[156] have noted that infants of vegetarians who have low vitamin B_{12} serum and milk levels have methylmalonic acid in their urine inversely proportional to their vitamin B_{12} levels, even though they are asymptomatic. Other authors[59,77,114] have concluded that the current RDA for infants provides little margin of safety: 0.3 μg/day or 0.05 μg/kg body weight is close to the intake below which infant urinary methylmalonic acid measures are elevated.

Thiamine (vitamin B_1) has been studied infrequently, but maternal supplementation does not increase milk levels beyond a certain limit. Urinary excretion of thiamine is significantly higher in supplemented compared with unsupplemented women. In malnourished women, evidence indicates that supplementation does increase thiamine levels in milk. The Subcommittee on Nutrition during Lactation[167] recommends that thiamine intake be at least 1.3 mg/day (the RDA for nonpregnant, nonlactating women of 1.1 mg/day plus an increment for milk secretion of 0.2 mg/day) when the calorie intake is less than 2200 kcal/day.

Riboflavin (vitamin B_2) requirements of lactating women in a controlled study in The Gambia showed the minimum to be 2.5 mg/day to maintain normal biochemical status in the mother and adequate levels of vitamin B_2 in her milk.[14] This level is higher than that recommended in the United States and the United Kingdom.

Niacin (vitamin B_3) content of human milk has been reported to parallel dietary intake. In unsupplemented diets, low vitamin B_3 levels usually parallel low levels of other B vitamins and low protein intakes.

Pyridoxine (vitamin B_6) intake and milk levels were studied in healthy lactating women by West and Kirksey.[184] They found marked diurnal variations of vitamin B_6 levels, with peaks occurring in those mothers taking supplements 3 to 5 hours after a dose. Those taking less than 2.5 mg/day had much lower milk levels (129 μg/L). Vitamin B_6 concentrations in human milk change rapidly with maternal intake.[7] When supplemented, the level in the milk is a direct reflection of amount ingested. Plasma pyridoxal-5′-phosphate (PLP) levels and birth weight are the strongest predictors of infant growth.[91,166]

When lactating mothers in a subsequent study by Andon and associates[6] received supplements of vitamin B_6 ranging from 0 to 20 mg pyridoxine hydrochloride, the levels of vitamin B_6 measurable in the milk paralleled the intake, with levels peaking 5 hours after ingesting the supplement. When maternal intakes of vitamin B_6 approximated 2.0 mg/day, breastfed infants were unlikely to receive the current RDA of 0.3 mg vitamin B_6 per day when intake was calculated from morning vitamin B_6 levels in milk and daily volume was assumed to be 850 mL. The American Academy of Pediatrics (AAP) Committee on Nutrition[25] recommends a minimum of 0.35 mg vitamin B_6/100 kcal milk from birth to 12 months. The RDA for vitamin B_6 for lactating women is 0.5 mg daily. Vitamin B_6 is the vitamin in milk that is most likely to be deficient, because pyridoxine levels in milk are closely influenced by dietary intake.[7,91] Supplementing with an additional 2.5 mg/day results in levels twice as high as in unsupplemented women. As reported in two studies, however, infants of unsupplemented lactating women in the United States had no clinical symptoms of vitamin B_6 deficiency, although infant plasma PLP levels were lower than those in comparable bottle fed infants. None of the women in the study had used oral contraceptives in the previous 5 years.[7] The increment in the RDA for vitamin B_6 in lactation is more than five times the estimated secretion of this vitamin in milk,[167] which varies between 0.01 and 0.02 mg/L early in lactation to 0.10 to 0.25 mg/L in mature milk. The recommendation is to advise diets rich in vitamin B_6, such as poultry, meat, fish, and some legumes, and reserve supplementation for special-risk cases.

Pantothenic acid levels in milk are strongly correlated with maternal intake for the preceding day. Johnston and associates[89] have suggested that some pantothenic acid is stored in the body. Studies of malnourished women show increased levels in milk after supplementation. The pantothenic acid content of human milk does not vary appreciably with dietary variations in well-nourished mothers, but the overall intake over time does influence milk levels.[89]

Biotin is reported in few studies, but the findings are consistent that levels range from 5 to 12 μg/L, with supplementation even up to 250 μg/day having little effect except when levels are significantly below this range.[138]

Pregnant and lactating women are at risk for suboptimal *folate* status because of the increased dietary requirement to facilitate enhanced anabolic activity. Until megaloblastic anemia develops, no validated quick, nonintrusive tests exist to assess functional folate status. Milk folate levels are maintained at the expense of maternal reserves, thereby protecting the nursling. O'Connor[122] provides an extensive review of the issues.

Folate supplementation in well-nourished women does not affect the level of folate in the milk, although studies involving women with low folate (less than 60% RDA) show they responded to supplementation with an increased level in their milk. Differences in assay methods have produced inconsistencies among studies. Milk levels normally range between 40 and 70 μg/L and increase slightly in the early weeks of lactation. Supplementation should be 0.8 to 1.0 mg/day in those with chronic deficiency.[104]

TABLE 9-5   Water-soluble vitamins in human milk

Vitamin	Recognizable clinical deficiency in infant	Effect of maternal supplements		Effect of dietary intake on milk content
		In malnourished	In well-nourished	
Ascorbic acid (C)	Rare	Yes	Minimal	Limited at 50 mg/L
Thiamin (B_1)	Yes	Yes	Limited	Yes, up to 200 µg/L
Riboflavin (B_2)	Yes	Yes	Yes	Yes
Niacin (B_3)	Unknown	Yes	Yes	Yes
Pantothenic acid	Unknown	Yes	No	Yes
Pyridoxine (B_6)	Yes	Yes	Yes	Yes
Biotin	Yes	Yes	No	Limited
Folate	Unknown	Yes	No	No
Cyanocobalamin (B_{12})	Rare	Yes	No	Yes

Prepared from Subcommittee on Nutrition during Lactation. Committee on Nutritional Status during Pregnancy and Lactation. Food and Nutrition Board. Institute of Medicine. National Academy of Sciences: Nutrition during Lactation. Washington, DC, National Academy Press, 1991.

Deodhar and Ramakrishnan[32] studied the effect of the stage of lactation on levels of vitamins B_1, B_2, B_3, B_6, and B_{12} and ascorbic acid. The values remained fairly constant throughout, except for those of vitamin B_3, which increased slightly over time. The relationship to socioeconomic group showed an increase in vitamin B_3 and B_6 levels with increased status. Vitamin B_1 was higher in poorer mothers. Tables 9-5 and 9-6 summarize the effect of diet on vitamin levels in maternal milk.

Fat-soluble vitamins

Fat-soluble compounds are generally transported into milk via the fat, and levels are less easily improved by dietary change. Because vitamins A and D are stored in tissues, the impact of dietary supplementation is more difficult to measure. Milk levels do not change until a certain level is achieved in the stores. High dietary levels of β-carotene do not appear to result in excessive levels of either vitamin A or β-carotene. Increase in vitamin A in the diet of undernourished women does increase its level in milk.

Vitamin A. When malnourished mothers were given a single oral megadose of 209 µmol of vitamin A and the control subjects were given none, serum retinol (vitamin A_1) levels increased in the supplemented mothers and remained significantly higher for at least 3 months.[145] Breast milk levels were higher (11.3 µmol/L versus 2.9 µmol/L) and

TABLE 9-6   Fat-soluble vitamins in human milk

Vitamin	Recognizable clinical deficiency in infant	Effect of maternal supplements		Effect of dietary intake on milk content
		In malnourished	In well-nourished	
D	Yes	Yes	Yes	Yes
K	Yes	Yes	Variable	Probable
A	Unknown	Yes	Minimal	Yes
E	Unknown	Unknown	Yes	Unknown

Prepared from Subcommittee on Nutrition during Lactation. Committee on Nutritional Status during Pregnancy and Lactation, Food and Nutrition Board. Institute of Medicine, National Academy of Sciences: Nutrition during Lactation. Washington, DC, National Academy Press, 1991.

remained so for 6 months. An associated observation was the reduction in the duration of respiratory tract infections and febrile illnesses in the infants of the supplemented mothers. This observation was confirmed by Stoltzfus and associates, who did a randomized double blind study giving women 312 μmol of vitamin A as retinyl palmitate or placebo orally. Maternal levels in the supplemented group were significantly higher at 6 months than in the group given the placebo. Among the infants at 6 months, 36% of the placebo group and 15% of the vitamin A group had low retinol concentrations. Their relative dose response demonstrating low vitamin A stores was 23% in the placebo group and 10% in the treated group. This confirmed the value of high-single-dose vitamin A in lactating women.[165]

Vitamin D. Most women have adequate *vitamin D* levels.[167] Vitamin D was considered to be at a stable level in milk that was unaffected by diet. However, studies involving maternal supplementation have demonstrated increased milk levels.[78] When mothers were given 0, 500, and 2500 IU ergocalciferol daily, they produced milk with 39, 218, and 3040 mg/mL vitamin D. The effect on levels of 25-hydroxyvitamin D (25-OHD) was less dramatic. The physiologic significance to the infant is disputed, however, because the major source of antirachitic sterols seems to be sunlight, not milk. The role of water-soluble vitamin D in human milk has not been confirmed.[155,157] Infants born to mothers with inadequate vitamin D stores need a regular supply of vitamin D through diet, supplements, and exposure to ultraviolet light.[169]

Because of the report of clinical rickets in breastfed infants in a sunny climate, the American Academy of Pediatrics and the Centers for Disease Control (CDC) have determined that breastfed infants should be supplemented regardless of maternal vitamin D status and exposure to sunlight. This mandate has been supported by dermatologists who have recommended no sun exposure and the use of sunscreen in infancy. The best estimate of adequate exposure to sunlight for white infants is 30 minutes per week clothed only in a diaper or 2 hours per week fully clothed with head and hands exposed.

Multiple studies have demonstrated that maternal 25-OHD levels can be raised by supplementation.[29] In women at risk, this supplementation should begin in pregnancy and continue through lactation to ensure adequate levels in their milk. Supplementing mothers is preferred to supplementing the breastfed infant because the mother is also in deficit.[126,154]

Vitamin D deficiency is not breast milk deficiency but the deficiency of sunlight. Societal changes have diminished infant sun exposure including the avoidance of sunlight, the use of sunscreen, the migration to northern latitudes by dark-skinned individuals, and the use of total body clothing for religious reasons by individuals migrating to northern climates. Replacing this natural source of vitamin D has been a challenge.

While recommending vitamin D supplementation across the board, the AAP and the CDC have not considered maternal supplementation partially because of possible toxicity, although doses of 4000 IU/day for up to 5 months have been shown to be safe in a wide population of adults. To achieve normal vitamin D status in breastfeeding mother-infant pairs, high-dose maternal vitamin D was utilized by Wagner and associates.[177] A dose of 1600 IU vitamin D per day for 3 months has minimal effect on vitamin D levels in mother or her infant; 3600 IU/day provided clinically relevant increases in the nutritional vitamin D_2 status of both mother and her infant. In the absence of sunshine or in dark-skinned individuals, 4000 IU/day appears to be the minimal maternal dose to achieve clinical results. The authors are continuing this study to establish the optimal maternal supplementation as a function of latitude, cultural practices, and race.[177]

Dark-skinned infants reared in climates where sunlight is minimal may be at significant risk for rickets when breastfed unless attention is given to the possible need for supplements of vitamin D.[12] Although rickets was considered a disease of the past, the disease has reemerged since the 1980s partially because of the high risk of premature infants, especially micropremature infants, but also because of the increase in breastfeeding, especially by women who avoid dairy products, which are the major food source of vitamin D supplementation.[29]

The emphasis has been on the rare cases of deficiency in breastfed infants, but accidents of over-supplementation with vitamin D have appeared since mass supplementation has been mandated as a public health policy. A recent report of a dairy adding 70 to 600 times the recommended amount of vitamin D resulted in exposure to a large population, with variable subclinical effects.[148]

The recommendation is for all breastfed infants, and any infant receiving less than 500 mL of fortified formula per day, to receive 200 units of vitamin D daily beginning at 2 months of age.[4]

Vitamin E. *Vitamin E* has not been the focus of study of maternal dietary supplements except in the report by Kramer and associates[96] that sunflower oil replacing lard in the diet resulted in a 50% increase in vitamin E levels in the milk. Liberal use of vitamin E creams by health enthusiasts may well expose an infant to large doses by maternal absorption as well as directly when the creams are applied to the breast. Alpha-tocopherol levels are highest in the colostrum, when the neonate is most dependent on its physiologic effect as an antioxidant and in the prevention of hemolytic anemia attributed to vitamin E deficiency. Maternal vitamin E intake can influence the levels of vitamin E in the milk. However, no evidence indicates that vitamin E deficiency occurs in individuals with normal fat absorption.[167]

Vitamin K. The most critical need for *vitamin K* for the infant is during the birth process and in the first few days of life, when the risk of bleeding, especially intracranial bleeding, is greatest.[65] Maternal dietary intake is most critical during the last trimester. Transplacental passage of vitamin K is slow. Cord blood levels are almost imperceptible. The synthesis of menaquinones by bacteria in the breastfed infant gut is minimal because lactobacilli do not synthesize them. Studies on supplementation of lactating women have shown that small doses are inadequate to raise the maternal level. Greer and associates[62] have shown that the average woman's intake is now 0.8 to 1.03 μg/kg/day. The content of human milk is 0.1 to 0.2 μg/dL, which does not supply the daily requirement of 1 μg/kg/day. Maternal supplements of 5 mg/day of vitamin K increase breast milk concentration to 4.5 to 6.0 μg/dL, thus increasing serum concentrations in exclusively breastfed infants.

Following the intramuscular injection of 1 mg of vitamin K at birth, no further recommendations for vitamin K supplements are made for healthy breastfeeding infants and their mothers. If the infant receives an oral preparation at birth, the dose of 2 mg should be repeated at 7 and 28 days of age.

PIVKA (undercarboxylated prothrombin produced in the absence of vitamin K) levels are a marker of K deficiency. The cord blood of full-term infants often has high PIVKA levels (0.1 AU/mL) correlating with low vitamin K. Levels in the infant are undetectable at 4 weeks after intramuscular (IM) vitamin K administration at birth, but in some infants they become elevated by 8 weeks. This has led to the recommendation that mothers be supplemented with 5 mg of vitamin K daily through the first 3 months of lactation.[62]

The consensus is that late vitamin K deficiency bleeding should be prevented by prophylaxis (Box 9-1). After a study of different oral schedules in Australia, Germany, the Netherlands, and Switzerland, it was confirmed that oral doses of 1 mg vitamin K for the infant are less effective than IM dosing. Further, Cornelissen and associates[28] reported that the most effective regimen was an initial dose of 1 mg followed by 25 μg vitamin K orally for breastfed infants. The new mixed micellar preparation remains under investigation. The least invasive method would be to increase the milk levels by supplementing the mother. In the 1950s, efforts to increase vitamin K and prothrombin levels at birth by giving mothers a large dose of vitamin K in labor failed to change the incidence of hemorrhagic disease in newborns. However, maternal supplementation during lactation is effective for the mother.

Although the amount of vitamin K available in infant formulas is very high, no toxicity has yet been demonstrated.

BOX 9-1   Administration of vitamin K to newborns

Because parenteral vitamin K prevents a life-threatening disease of the newborn and the risks of cancer are unproved and unlikely, the American Academy of Pediatrics recommends the following:
1. Vitamin K₁ should be given to all newborns as a single, intramuscular dose of 0.5 to 1 mg.
2. Further research on the efficacy, safety, and bioavailability of oral formulations of vitamin K is warranted.
3. An oral dosage form is not currently available in the United States but ought to be developed and licensed. If an appropriate oral form is developed and licensed in the United States, it should be given at birth (2.0 mg) and should be administered again at 1 to 2 weeks and at 4 weeks of age to breastfed infants. If diarrhea occurs in an exclusively breastfed infant, the dose should be repeated.

From American Academy of Pediatrics Committee on Nutrition: Pediatric Nutrition Handbook, 5th ed. Elk Grove, Ill, 2004.

Summary

Although dietary supplements improve the milk quality and quantity in malnourished women, a balanced diet without excessive supplementation is the most physiologic and economic way to ensure good milk. Nutrients, especially vitamins, are excreted in the urine only when taken in excess. The AAP Committee on Nutrition recommends 200 mg vitamin D for breastfeeding infants beginning at 2 months of age in the absence of adequate sun exposure. Maternal supplementation is under study.

Minerals

Calcium

Calcium has been associated with bone growth, and concern has been expressed because the total calcium in breast milk is low. The available information is inadequate to determine the true requirement for lactation. Studies with radioactive calcium in the nonpregnant adult have shown that losses occur into the gut and through the kidney. Absorption and retention also depend on the reserves in the body. Long-term shortage causes economy of utilization, and the apparent requirement is lower.[20] During lactation the absorption and retention are greater.

Serum calcium and phosphorus concentrations are greater in lactating women compared with nonlactating women.[90] Lactation stimulates increases in fractional calcium absorption and serum calcitrol. This is most apparent after weaning. Alterations in absorption, metabolism, and excretion may conserve calcium during lactation. Women with low calcium intakes have no direct benefit from supplementation as a protective mechanism to maintain breast milk calcium or maternal bone mineral content.[134,135] Urinary calcium was found to be higher in the supplemented group. Of significance, however, is the presence of risk factors: positive family history of osteoporosis, fair complexion, lower body mass and height, not breastfeeding their infants, smoking, and fat deposits have greatest predictability for osteoporosis.[90]

Atkinson and West[11] showed by scanning transmission techniques that lactating women mobilize about 2% of their skeletal calcium over 100 days of nursing. The calcium content of milk appears to be maintained despite greatly deficient intake, probably because of skeletal stores. The milk calcium levels are the same in mothers of rachitic and nonrachitic infants. This is most important for women under age 25 because the calcium content of bones is expected to increase until age 25.[103] Peak bone mass is achieved during the childbearing years.

Estradiol concentrations are related to bone mineral density (BMD) because estradiol stimulates osteoblastic proliferation and enhances collagen gene expression. The relatively low estrogen levels during lactation increase bone mobilization. Prolonged amenorrhea is associated with increased mobilization, and the greatest reduction in bone mass occurs early in lactation. Prolactin has a synergistic effect on mobilization. The ratio of dietary calcium to dietary protein has also been identified as important; that is, women with high-protein diets must also have high calcium intake. Recovery after weaning is reported to be negatively affected by parity.[99]

The RDI (Reference Dietary Intake) for calcium is higher for women under age 18, even when prepregnant, than for older women (1300 mg calcium compared with 1000 mg recommended for nonpregnant women over age 18).[52] Calcium status is only one of many possible factors in the etiology of osteoporosis. Dietary guidance during lactation should include recommendations for the replacement of stores. Women who have lactated are not more prone to osteoporosis than nonlactators or nulliparas, and they may be less prone.[20,37,164] Postweaning bone regeneration is accelerated for the first 4 to 6 months. Bone density is then often greater than prepregnancy.

There is no additional requirement for calcium while lactating as noted in the 1998 RDIs. Note that the requirement of 1000 mg/day is adequate intake (AI). When dietary calcium intake is greater than the RDA for lactating women, bone mineral content is not diminished during at least the first 6 weeks of lactation.

Sodium, potassium, and chlorine

The concentration of sodium is the most variable of all the minerals, fluctuating as much as 10-fold during normal lactation and diurnally, separate from the effects of mastitis, emotional stress, or involution. Maternal sodium or potassium intake has no immediate influence, either high or low, on postprandial milk sodium or potassium concentrations.[47] Dietary potassium may influence milk potassium more significantly. With increasing numbers of women with cardiac and renal disease choosing to lactate, potassium levels in the diet would be of significance, in addition to concerns about necessary medications[92] that are known to deplete potassium levels.

Chlorine level in the breast milk is not believed to be affected by maternal diet. Chlorine deficiency reported in a breastfed infant was associated with normal maternal serum and dietary intake[10] but with deficit levels in the milk (less than 2 mEq/L). Normal is greater than 8 mEq/L. This deficit in the milk was assumed to be a defect of breast function.

The concentration of electrolytes (sodium, potassium, chloride) in milk is determined by an electrical potential gradient in the secretory cell rather than by maternal nutritional status.[164]

Iron

The iron content of milk is not readily affected by the iron content of the diet or the maternal serum iron level. Increases in dietary iron that increase serum levels do not increase iron in the milk. It is important, however, for the mother to replace her iron stores post partum.[129] It has not been established that increases in tissue iron are advantageous. Iron that is added to human milk will bind to lactoferrin and may interfere with its function. Infants exclusively breastfed for 7 months or longer were not found to be anemic at 12 or 24 months.[130] Half the infants breastfed for a shorter period were anemic at 12 months if additional dietary iron from solids was not provided.

Iron supplementation appears safe according to Friel and associates,[49] who conducted a double-masked, randomized control trial of iron supplementation in early infancy in a total of 77 healthy term breastfed infants using 7.5 mg/day of elemental iron as ferrous sulfate or placebo from 1 to 6 months of age. Iron supplementation produced higher hemoglobin and mean corpuscular volume at 6 months of age as well as higher visual acuity and psychomotor development index at 13 months of age. The authors suggest that iron supplementation in selected infants might be beneficial.

Phosphorus, magnesium, zinc, and copper

Phosphorus, magnesium, zinc, and copper levels in milk are not affected by dietary administration of these elements.[97] Again, however, it is important for the mother to replenish her stores.[129]

According to the RDA, many lactating women are receiving marginal amounts of magnesium.[110] The amount recommended for lactation is two to three times the amount estimated to be in the milk.

Zinc has an RDA increment during lactation 4 to 13 times higher than the amount estimated to be in the milk on the basis that it is poorly absorbed (20%).[51] Studies done with stable isotopes in lactating women show that absorption was 59% to 84% of intake. Zinc absorption during pregnancy increases dramatically and during lactation decreases slightly but is double the prepregnant rates, presumably in response to the demand by the breast for milk synthesis.[56] Milk levels are unaffected by supplementation and gradually decline over time from 2 mg/day.[98] Supplementation does result in increased maternal absorption and increased plasma levels. Although no major health risks have been associated with low zinc intakes, zinc is known to be important to immune function.[83] RDA for zinc is 34 mg/day during pregnancy and lactation. Recommended intake for infants 0 to 6 months of age is 4 mg/day.

Iron supplementation has no significant effect on levels of copper, selenium, and zinc in mother's serum and breast milk.[8]

Selenium

A correlation exists between selenium in human milk and maternal dietary intake.[102] Maternal plasma levels vary with the form of selenium supplementation (selenomethionine or selenium-enriched yeast).[108] The original source of selenium is the soil, and levels vary geographically. It is transferred to plants and works up the food chain. Breastfed infants are known to have higher intake and utilization than infants fed formula or cow milk because of the bioavailability.[2] Many seleno-proteins have been identified, but glutathione peroxidase is involved with producing a variety of organic hydroperoxides or reactive oxygen radicals in the liver. Although selenium toxicity is possible, deficiency from low intake is a problem.[102] Two diseases described are Keshan disease and Kashin-Beck disease, which are associated with accumulation of lipid peroxides. Dietary studies have shown that intake can affect the mother's plasma and milk levels.[2]

Chromium

Breast milk levels of chromium are reported to be 3.54 ± 40 nmol/L (0.18 ng/mL) and independent of dietary intake.[5] Total absorption for lactating

women was 0.79 ± 0.08 μmol/dL, which was greater than that of nonlactators. Serum levels were correlated with urinary chromium excretion, a good indicator of serum levels. The estimated RDA for breastfed infants is 10 μg, which is much greater than the levels measured in the study by Anderson and associates. The RDA for adults is 50 μg; most adults achieve 50% to 60% of this level. RDAs for chromium may need to be reevaluated.[51]

Iodine

Iodine in milk does depend on dietary content. The breast is able to raise the concentration of iodine in the milk above that in the blood, and thus, there is an increased danger in giving radioactive iodine to the lactating woman. With iodized salt, bread dough conditioners, and common use of iodine-containing cleansers, there is actually a risk of excessive iodine intake. Milk iodine concentrations are higher now than were reported in the 1930s. Mean breast milk iodide levels ranged from 29 to 490 ng/L, averaging 178 ng/L, above the RDA for infants.[67]

Fluorine

Human milk contains 16 ± 5 μg fluoride per liter and reflects to some degree the level in the water supply. The risk of excessive fluoride has been pointed out by Walton and Messer,[183] who report dental mottling and milk fluorosis in supplemented breastfed infants. The AAP Committee on Nutrition therefore has stated, "It may not be necessary to give fluoride supplements to breastfed infants who are living in an area where water is adequately fluoridated."[25] If the water is not fluorinated or mother drinks fluoride-free bottled water, she should be supplemented.

Fluoride concentrations of infant foods and drinks have been found to vary widely, ranging from 0.01 to 0.72 mg/kg, so that no need exists for supplementation when solid foods are initiated if the diet is well balanced.[174]

Summary

Table 9-7 summarizes constituent levels in human milk and changes over time.

TABLE 9-7	Representative values for constituents of human milk[*]	
Constituent (per liter)[*]	Early milk (< 28 d post partum)	Mature milk (≥28 d post partum)
Energy (kcal)		650–700
Carbohydrate		
Lactose (g)	20–30	67
Glucose (g)	0.2–1.0	0.2–0.3
Oligosaccharides (g)	22–24	12–14
Total nitrogen (g)	3.0	1.9
Nonprotein nitrogen (g)	0.5	0.45
Protein nitrogen (g)	2.5	1.45
Total protein (g)	16	9–12.6
Total casein (g)		
β-casein (g)	3.8	5.7
κ-casein (g)	2.6	4.4
Whey proteins		6.7
α-Lactalbumin (g)	3.62	3.26
Lactoferrin (g)	3.53	1.94
Serum albumin (g)	0.39	0.41
sIgA (g)	2.0	1.0
IgM (g)	0.12	0.2
IgG (g)	0.34	0.05
Amino acids (g)[†]		
Alanine	0.65–1.71	0.26–0.42
Arginine	1.16–1.42	0.25–0.40
Aspartic acid	1.18–3.52	0.54–0.92
Cystine	0.47–1.41	0.11–0.23
Glutamic acid + glutamine	2.03–4.75	1.26–1.97
Glycine	0.36–1.42	0.10–0.27
Histidine	0.41–0.67	0.15–0.25
Isoleucine	0.43–1.27	0.33–0.57
Leucine	1.48–2.80	0.82–0.94
Lysine	0.72–2.06	0.30–0.90
Methionine	0.16–0.45	0.09–0.19
Phenylalanine	0.50–1.52	0.26–0.36
Proline	0.93–2.51	0.57–1.05
Serine	1.27–2.59	0.42–0.62
Threonine	0.65–1.94	0.32–0.42
Tryptophan	0.25–0.42	0.09–0.17
Tyrosine	0.76–0.54	0.31–0.47
Valine	0.88–1.66	0.35–0.51
Total lipids (%)	2	3.5
Triglyceride (% total lipids)	97–98	97–98
Cholesterol[‡] (% total lipids)	0.7–1.3	0.4–0.5
Phospholipids (% total lipids)	1.1	0.6–0.8

(Continued)

TABLE 9-7   Representative values for constituents of human milk*—cont'd

Constituent (per liter)*	Early milk (< 28 d post partum)	Mature milk (≥ 28 d post partum)
Fatty acids (weight %)	88	88
Total % saturated fatty acids	43–44	44–45
C12:0		5
C14:0		6
C16:0		20
C18:0		8
Total % monounsaturated fatty acids		40
C18: 1ω-9	32	31
Total % polyunsaturated fatty acids (PUFA)	13	14–15
Total ω-3	1.5	1.5
C18: 3ω-3	0.7	0.9
C20: 5ω-3	0.2	0.1
C22: 6ω-3	0.5	0.2
Total ω-6	11.6	13.06
C18: 2ω-6	8.9	11.3
C20: 4ω-6	0.7	0.5
C22: 4ω-6	0.2	0.1
Water-soluble vitamins		
Ascorbic acid (mg)		80–100
Thiamin (μg)	20	200
Riboflavin (μg)		400–600
Niacin (mg)	0.5	1.8–6.0
Vitamin B_6 (mg)		0.09–0.31
Folate (μg)		80–140
Vitamin B_{12} (μg)		0.5–1.0
Pantothenic acid (mg)		2.0–2.5
Biotin (μg)		5–9
Fat-soluble vitamins		
Retinol (mg)	2	0.3–0.6
Carotenoids (mg)	2	0.2–0.6
Vitamin K (μg)	2–5	2–3
Vitamin D (μg)		0.33
Vitamin E (mg)	8–12	3–8
Major minerals		
Calcium (mg)	250	200–250
Magnesium (mg)	30–35	30–35
Phosphorus (mg)	120–160	120–140
Sodium (mg)	300–400	120–250
Potassium (mg)	600–700	400–550
Chloride (mg)	600–800	400–450
Trace minerals		
Iron (mg)	0.5–1.0	0.3–0.9
Zinc (mg)	8–12	1–3
Copper (mg)	0.5–0.8	0.2–0.4

TABLE 9-7   Representative values for constituents of human milk*—cont'd

Constituent (per liter)*	Early milk (< 28 d post partum)	Mature milk (≥ 28 d post partum)
Trace minerals—cont'd		
Manganese (mg)	5–6	3
Selenium (mg)	40	7–33
Iodine (mg)		150
Fluoride (mg)		4–15

*All nutrient values except for amino acids are adapted from Picciano MF: Appendix: Representative values for constituents of human milk. Pediatr Clin North Am 48:263, 2001.

The values are expressed per liter of milk as a percentage on the basis of milk volume or weight of total lipids. Values as mean values or ranges of means.

†Adapted from George DR, De Francesca BA: Human milk in comparison to cow milk. In Lebenthal E (ed): Textbook of Gastroenterology and Nutrition in Infancy and Childhood, 2nd ed. New York, Raven Press, 1989, pp 242–243.

‡The cholesterol content of human milk ranges from 100 to 200 mg/L in most samples of human milk after day 21 of lactation.

MATERNAL NUTRITION: IMMUNOLOGIC SUBSTANCES AND LEUKOCYTE ACTIVITY

Substances in colostrum and mature milk confer important infection protection on the breastfed infant. Maternal malnutrition was associated with lower levels of immunoglobulins G and A (IgG, IgA) in a group of Colombian women studied by Miranda and associates.[115] The colostrum contained only one third the normal levels of IgG and less than half the normal albumin. Significant reductions in IgA and complement C4 were observed in colostrum, but lysozyme, C3, and IgM were normal. Titers against respiratory syncytial virus were unaffected by nutritional status. The protective deficiencies improved in mature milk over time and with improvement of nutritional status. The total leukocyte concentrations as well as their bactericidal capacity were similar in well-nourished and undernourished women.[15]

Prentice and associates[137] measured breast milk antimicrobial factors of rural Gambian mothers. The concentrations and daily secretions of all immunoproteins, except lysozyme, decreased during the first year and then remained steady. Compared with those in Western women, levels of IgG, IgM, C3, and C4 were higher in Gambian women; IgA and lactoferrin were similar; and lysozyme was lower. Dietary supplement in Gambian women did not raise the breast milk immunoproteins in this study.

The Subcommittee on Nutrition during Lactation has concluded that the effects of maternal nutritional status on the immunologic system in human milk are controversial.[167] Some studies suggest that malnutrition decreases the production and secretion of some components of the immunologic system, but further investigation clearly is necessary.

RECOMMENDATIONS FOR NUTRITIONAL SUPPORT DURING LACTATION

The previous section noted that the quantity, protein content, and calcium content of milk are relatively independent of maternal nutritional status and diet. Amino acids lysine and methionine, certain fatty acids, and water-soluble vitamin contents vary with intake. It is important to point out that stores of calcium, minerals, and fat-soluble vitamins need to be replenished.[187] Much of the data collected have varied, depending on the method used in collection. The daily intakes believed necessary for infants were determined by feeding infants processed human milk in a bottle, which is not a physiologic standard.

It is known, for example, that putting the entire sample in one container removes the natural variation in fat from beginning to end of the feeding.

The Subcommittee on Nutrition during Lactation[53,167] has recommended a balanced diet comparable to one for the nonlactating postpartum mother, with a few additions. Although the calculated caloric cost of producing 1 L of milk is 940 kcal, during pregnancy most women store 2 to 4 kg of extra tissue in the physiologic preparation for lactation. Thus, it is probably necessary to add only 500 kcal to the diet, except in women with known high metabolic rates.

Preparation for lactation begins in pregnancy, if not before. The major daily increases for pregnancy are 300 kcal; 20 g of protein; a 20% increase in all vitamins and minerals except folic acid, which is doubled; and a 33% increase in calcium, phosphorus, and magnesium. In comparing the RDAs[51,52] for lactating women with those for nonlactating adult women, the increases suggested should provide ample nutrition and replace stores (Table 9-8).

When dietary supplements are suggested (Table 9-9), concern arises about increased costs. Cost increases are modest for the standard diet and minimal for the low-budget diet, as demonstrated by Worthington-Roberts.[188] Although one rarely chooses breastfeeding or bottle feeding on the basis of cost, the price of a few extra maternal kilocalories versus the cost of formula feeding makes a reassuring comparison. Hypoallergenic formulas are even more costly, estimated to be more than $5 per day.

Following the report of the Subcommittee on Nutrition during Lactation,[167] an additional report was prepared, Nutrition during Pregnancy and Lactation: an Implementation Guide. Its purpose is to offer practical guidance to the primary care provider by including a sample nutrition screening questionnaire, indications for supplementation, nutritional assessment guidelines, and how and when to refer to a registered dietitian.[168]

The subcommittee did not propose a food guide because it recognized that diverse ways are available to meet nutrient needs and that culturally appropriate foods are important, especially in the perinatal period. It did offer the following recommendations[168]:

- Avoid diets and medications that promise rapid weight loss.
- Eat a wide variety of breads and cereal grains, fruits, vegetables, milk products, and meats or meat alternates each day.
- Consume three or more servings of milk products daily.
- Make a greater effort to eat vitamin A-rich vegetables or fruits often. Examples of foods high in vitamin A include carrots, spinach or other cooked greens, sweet potatoes, and cantaloupe.
- Be sure to drink when thirsty. Lactation requires more fluid than usual.
- If you drink coffee or other caffeinated beverages, such as cola, do so in moderation. Two servings daily are unlikely to harm the infant. Caffeine passes into the milk.

Malnutrition: special supplementation for the lactating woman

It has been suggested that supplementing the diet of malnourished mothers with a special formula would be the best way to achieve ideal nourishment for mother and child. The infant will then gain the additional advantages of human milk, such as protection against infection.[94] Such formulas have been devised. Sosa and associates[153] successfully tried this approach in Guatemala in 1976. When nutritional supplements are recommended, ideally they are given to the mother. Such studies have been repeated in many geographic areas. The results all confirm that the provision of supplemental food improves milk production and the duration of exclusive breastfeeding among undernourished women. In contrast, well-nourished women do not show any benefits from supplementation.[61,186]

With the ready availability of well-balanced nutrition supplements today in both supermarkets and drugstores in the form of stable powders, it should not be difficult to initiate a high-protein, vitamin-enriched diet supplementation that is also palatable for the occasional mother who is at nutritional risk. With the inclusion of breastfeeding as a goal in the Women, Infants, and Children (WIC) program, dietary counseling and supplementation are available for mothers at poverty level to encourage these mothers to breastfeed and give them nutritional support while doing so. Infants in the WIC programs will receive the greatest benefit from being breastfed. Present WIC supplements focus on improved diet.

Because studies have revealed a negative effect of malnutrition on infection protection

properties as well as on galactopoietic hormones (corticosteroids are greatly increased and prolactin decreased), nourishing the mother is the most effective way of benefiting the infant rather than supplementing the infant to meet growth standards.[104]

The impact of dietary supplementation on lactating women with restricted diets has been reported to be inconsistent with respect to lactational amenorrhea.[36] Most recently, a study in Sri Lankan women did not show an effect on menstruation or ovulation with supplementation. However, the study did result in a longer duration of full breastfeeding in the

TABLE 9-8   Estimated mean nutrient intakes by U.S. women at three age groups compared with the dietary reference intakes (DRIs) for lactation

A.   Protein and fat-soluble vitamins

Lactating mother's age	Protein (g/d)	Vitamin A (μg/d)	Vitamin D (μg/d)	Vitamin E (mg/day)	Vitamin K (μg/d)
≤18 years	60	980	5* (200 IU/d)	16	75*
19–30 years	60	900	5* (200 IU/d)	16	90*
31–50 years	60	900	5* (200 IU/d)	16	90*

B.   Water-soluble vitamins

Lactating mother's age	Vitamin C (mg/d)	Thiamin (mg/d)	Riboflavin (mg/d)	Niacin (mg/d)	Vitamin B$_6$ (mg/d)	Folate (μg/d)	Vitamin B$_{12}$ (μg/d)
≤18 years	96	1.2	1.6	17	1.7	450	2.4
19–30 years	100	1.2	1.6	17	1.7	450	2.4
31–50 years	100	1.2	1.6	17	1.7	450	2.4

C.   Minerals

Lactating mother's age	Calcium (mg/d)	Phosphorus (mg/d)	Magnesium (mg/d)	Iron (mg/d)	Zinc (mg/d)	Iodine (μg/d)	Selenium (μg/d)
≤18 years	1300*	1250	360	10	13	290	70
19–30 years	1000*	700	310	9	12	290	70
31–50 years	1000*	700	320	9	12	290	70

These data are taken from the DRI reports from the National Academy of Sciences. The data marked with an asterik (*) represent adequate intake (AI). All other data represent the recommended dietary allowances (RDAs). RDAs are set to meet the needs of almost all (97 to 98%) individuals in a group.
Sources for data: Dietary Reference Intakes for Vitamin A, Vitamin K, Arsenic, Boron, Chromium, Copper, Iodine, Iron, Manganese, Molybdenum, Nickel, Silicon, Vanadium, and Zinc (2002); Dietary Reference Intakes: Applications in Dietary Planning (2003); Dietary Reference Intakes: Applications in Dietary Assessment (2001). These reports can be accessed via www.nap.edu.

TABLE 9-9	Extra daily nutrient allowances for lactation over baseline values		
Nutrient	Nonpregnant, nonlactating	Lactating	Increase
Energy (kcal)	2100	2700	500
Protein (g)	40	65	25
Retinol (µg)	800	1300	500
Vitamin D (µg)	7.5	10	3
Vitamin E (mg)	8	11	3
Vitamin C (mg)	60	100	40
Riboflavin (mg)	1.3	1.8	0.5
Nicotinic acid (mg)	14	20	6
Vitamin B_6 (mg)	2.0	2.5	0.5
Folate (µg)	40	280	240
Thiamin (mg)	1.1	1.6	0.5
Calcium (mg)	800	1200	400
Iron (mg)	18	18	18
Zinc (mg)	15	25	10

From Food and Nutrition Board, National Research Council: Recommended Dietary Allowances, 11th ed. Washington, DC, National Academy Press, 1994.

supplemented women, which may have had an effect in suppressing ovulation. No difference was seen between supplemented and unsupplemented women in regard to lactational amenorrhea.[169]

Allergy

In families with a strong history of allergy, a hypoallergenic diet avoiding the common allergens such as wheat and eggs should be recommended. Interest in the transfer of cow milk proteins to the infant via breast milk has increased as case reports appear of breastfed infants' reaction to cow protein. β-Lactoglobulin has been identified in breast milk and appears to be related to long-term exposure to cow milk products.[54] Controlling intake has also been reported to reverse the presence of β-lactoglobulin in the milk. Ovalbumin has been identified in human milk in only a fraction of mothers tested, although the average intake was four eggs per week (see Chapter 18).

Vegetarian diet

The growing interest in vegetarianism has necessitated a better understanding of the several types of diets and their potential for adequate nutrients and growth as well as the motivation for these diets (Table 9-10). In general, serious vegetarians usually have a greater knowledge of and commitment to good nutrition.[23]

Reports of malnutrition among breastfed infants of vegetarians usually focus on the very strict groups such as vegans and those on macrobiotic diets. The dietary risks involved are chiefly with the B vitamins because these vitamins are usually associated with protein, which is also proportionally lower from vegetable sources.[140] An additional concern is the availability of various amino acids in specific concentrations to utilize them for protein synthesis. The *net protein utilization* (NPU) of a food may be considerably lower than total protein content; therefore, it is important when using vegetable sources of protein to use foods with "complementary protein" at the same meal. Vegetarian cookbooks emphasize this.[143] Throughout history, culturally traditional meals have ensured complementary proteins. Concentrations of PCBs (polychlorinated biphenyls) are lower in milk of vegetarians.

Vitamin B_{12} deficiency has been described in vegans because of the absence of animal protein.[189] It is

TABLE 9-10	Vegetarianism and associated risks		
Type of vegetarian	Diet includes	Diet avoids	Risks
Semivegetarian	Vegetables, milk products, seafood, poultry	Red meat	Minerals[*]
Ovolactovegetarian	Vegetables, milk products, eggs	Flesh foods (meat, seafood, poultry)	Minerals,[*] esp. zinc
Lactovegetarian	Vegetables, milk products	Flesh foods, eggs	Minerals,[*] esp. zinc, protein[†]
Ovovegetarian	Vegetables, eggs	Flesh foods, milk products	Minerals,[*] esp. iron and zinc, protein,[†] riboflavin, vitamin D, vitamin B_{12}
Vegan	Only vegetables	Flesh foods, milk products, eggs	Minerals,[*] protein,[†] riboflavin, vitamin D, vitamin B_{12}
Macrobiotic	Gradual progression to a diet of only cereals		Advanced stage nutritionally inadequate

[*]Excessive dietary phytates and dietary fiber inhibit absorption of minerals such as iron, zinc, and calcium. *Phytates* are organic chemicals present in many vegetables and unleavened bread that bind with minerals.

[†]Diets not using complementary proteins may be deficient in net protein because the net protein utilization (NPU) is low.

advisable in these cases to supplement diets of the pregnant or lactating woman, as well as of an infant or growing child, with up to 4 mg/day of vitamin B_{12}. It has been shown that fermented soybean foods do contain vitamin B_{12}, as do the single-cell proteins such as yeast because even single cell animal species contain small amounts of vitamin B_{12}. In a study of vegetarian mothers and their infants, a large proportion of the infants had elevated methylmalonic acid levels, indicative of vitamin B_{12} deficiency.[155] A significant number of vegetarian women, both lactators and nonlactators, had elevated methylmalonic acid levels and low vitamin B_{12} levels.

As noted previously, vegetarians had lower levels of DHA.[142] Comparison of umbilical cord blood of infants born to South Asian vegetarian women showed less DHA in the plasma and cord artery phospholipids than in infants born to omnivores.[142] Early onset of labor, incidence of cesarean birth, lower birth weight, head circumference, and length, after adjusting for maternal height, duration of gestation, parity, smoking, and gender of infant were also related to DHA levels

Reports of growth curves in vegetarian children over the first few years show them to be shorter and leaner than standard, with the greatest effect among those on the most restricted diets.[44] Studies of children from birth to 10 years in the Netherlands reared in macrobiotic tradition showed the greatest growth retardation with fat and muscle wasting and slower psychomotor development between 6 and 18 months of age.[30] Breast milk of their mothers, who breastfed an average of 13.6 months, contained less vitamin B_{12}, calcium, and magnesium compared with matched omnivorous control subjects.[31] Breastfed vegetarian infants are usually on the norms for growth with the exception of those receiving minimal vitamin D and calcium, as reported in dark-skinned mothers in cloudy climates. The mean serum 1,25-dihydroxyvitamin D (1,25-OH_2D) concentrations were 37% higher in lactating vegetarian women than nonvegetarian women.[157] The serum parathyroid hormone was elevated in all lactators compared with the nonlactators. It is postulated that the low calcium in the vegetarian diet stimulates the elevated 1,25-OH_2D level, and this in turn stimulates the increased absorption of calcium to meet the needs of milk production.[156]

A study of the milk from vegetarian mothers compared with that from nonvegetarian mothers looked at fat and fatty acid composition.[31] Those fats and fatty acids produced de novo by the breast were not different.[160] The precursors of AA were higher in the vegetarians, yet the AA level in the milk was lower and continued to decrease the longer the vegetarian diet was maintained. Linoleic acid was greater among vegetarians. The amounts of DHA were not different. Among 34 breastfed infants at 7 months in the Tufts study, 3 were below the 10th percentile for height and weight, 1 had low weight for length, and 3 had high weight for length, whereas of the 51 who were not breastfed, 6 were below the 10th percentile, 2 had low weight for length, and 4 had high weight for length.[55]

Four vegetarian children between 8 months and 24 months of age were reported by Hellebostad and associates[75] to have vitamin D–deficient rickets (three with tetany and seizures) and vitamin B_{12} deficiency. All the infants were initially breastfed by mothers whose diets were low in vitamin D, high in fiber and phytate (which interferes with enterohepatic circulation of vitamin D), and low in calcium and phosphate.

General recommendations for lactating vegetarian women are as follows[167]:

1. Supplement with soy flour, molasses, and nuts.
2. Use complementary protein combinations.
3. Avoid excessive phytates and bran.
4. Watch protein and iron intake. Calcium should be supplemented if bone mineralization decreases, as the milk levels will be adequate.
5. Supplement with 10 µg vitamin D plus adequate sunshine.
6. Know that vitamins B_{12} and B_2 (riboflavin) are low in vegetarian diets and should be supplemented. If the mother does not supplement herself, the infant must be supplemented.

Supplementation of the breastfed infant's diet

For the newborn infant, human milk is the ideal food containing all the necessary nutrients. In establishing dietary norms for infants fed cow milk, many nutrients identified as being needed in the diet were found to exist in greater amounts in cow milk than in human milk. This does not consider the probability that the nutrient may be in a more bioavailable form in human milk. The specific items in question are protein, sodium, iron, vitamin D, and fluorine.

When a breastfed infant must be supplemented with formula, it is preferable that a formula low in iron be used to avoid providing excessive iron that will bind with lactoferrin and interfere with its infection protective activity.

The AAP Committee on Nutrition[25] has noted that iron deficiency is rare in breastfed infants and attributes this to increased absorption and the absence of microscopic blood loss into the gastrointestinal tract, which is seen in bottle fed infants. The Section on Breastfeeding of the AAP recommends a source of iron in solid foods (fortified infant cereal) at 6 months of age for breastfed infants (the Committee on Nutrition for the AAP recommends 4 to 6 months).

The AAP no longer recommends fluoride supplements in all breastfed infants.[25] Many breastfed infants have done without fluorine supplementation and have had no adverse dental problems, but the decision should be based on individual determinants, including family dental history and level of fluoride in the water supply, which is ideally between 0.7 and 1.0 ppm. If the level is less than 0.3 ppm, 0.25 mg of daily fluoride should be given. Maternal supplementation may be the better choice in this case.

The AAP now recommends 200 IU vitamin D daily for all breastfed infants by 2 months of age unless they are supplemented with at least 500 mL fortified formula daily. Maternal supplementation is a viable alternative. The Section on Breastfeeding of the AAP, however, tailors the recommendation to the dyad, using supplements of vitamin D as a last resort.

Exercise while breastfeeding

There are usually no contraindications to exercise in moderation during lactation. The greatest obstacle usually is having sufficient time. The availability of home exercise equipment does offer an option for home programs. Exercise baby carriages, which have large wheels for greater speed and rough terrain, are another option. Because they tip somewhat easily, the infant may need a helmet and a safety strap. A safety strap that attaches to the runner's wrist prevents the vehicle from getting away. These carriages are excellent for brisk walks as well.

The impact of programmed exercise on milk volume, milk composition, and ultimately milk acceptability has been studied.[34] Women who exercise excessively, especially those who jog, may have trouble maintaining their milk supply. This difficulty has been attributed to any activity that results in persistent motion of the breasts and excessive friction of clothing against the nipples. A firm athletic brassiere made of cotton will reduce this effect. No data are available on the impact of jogging with or without support on later breast sagging.

The production of lactic acid during exercise has been studied in relation to lactation by Wallace and associates,[180,182] who had mothers report whether their infants refused to nurse or fussed when breastfed after exercise. The study demonstrated that seven healthy lactating women who normally spent more than 30 minutes in aerobic activity (jogging, running, swimming, biking, and aerobics), as well as some who did calisthenics and racket sports, had an increase in their blood lactic acid levels after exercise. When a standardized treadmill exercise was used to maximal voluntary effort, blood lactic acid level increased at 10 minutes compared with that of the resting sample, but the level at 30 minutes had returned almost to the resting level. Milk samples at 10 and 30 minutes continued to have elevated lactic acid, although wide variation was seen among subjects.[182]

In a larger sample, when 26 women between 2 and 6 months post partum who normally exercised during pregnancy and post partum were exercised on a standardized treadmill to maximal voluntary effort, the levels of lactic acid were correlated to infant acceptance of the milk.[180] The breast was wiped with a dry towel before milk col-

lection. Milk samples collected before exercise and at 10 and 30 minutes after exercise revealed an increase in lactic acid levels over baseline at both 10 and 30 minutes. In a double-blind order of samples, the infants were offered milk by dropper and were less likely to accept samples with high lactic acid. The authors[180] noted that the levels of lactic acid were high enough for adults to detect when offered water solutions at the same concentrations (1.6 mmol). Human milk is very sweet, but lactic acid is known to be bitter/sour. Infants have been noted to make a puckering facial expression to a sour taste as early as a few hours of age.[163] Studies of sucking in newborns have shown more rapid rates with sweet than sour, with some change in heart rate, respiratory rate, and sucking patterns.[88] The lactic acid level can remain elevated in the milk for as long as 90 minutes, according to Wallace and Rabin.[182]

When exercise studies were undertaken by Wallace and associates[179,181] comparing the effects of a typical workout and a standard maximal exercise regimen, significant differences were noted. The milk lactate level before exercise was 0.61 ± 0.14 mM and after typical exercise was 1.06 ± 33 mM. After maximal exercise in the same women, the level was 2.88 ± 0.80 mM. Seventeen percent of the subjects had lactate levels above the reported adult taste threshold of 1.5 mM.[181] Milk rejection probably is a function of lactate concentration in the milk and the infant's sensitivity to taste. Women who exercised with full breasts developed a peak postexercise lactate concentration at 10 minutes, whereas women who exercised with empty breasts did not peak until 30 minutes.[179] Many of the studies reported may have not measured peak lactate when samples were collected only at 10 minutes.

Mothers have reported that their infants may reject their milk after the mother had exercised. Women have reported to the Lactation Study Center that their infants have been fussy and colicky for as long as 4 to 6 hours after the mother's strenuous exercise. Exercise generates sweat high in sodium and chloride, and lactic acid may change the pH. While these studies are being expanded, the following precautions might be recommended when breastfeeding after strenuous exercise:

- Shower, or at least wash the breast of perspiration.
- Manually express 3 to 5 mL of milk from each breast and discard.
- If infant displays puckering facial expression, postpone feeding or replace feeding with previously pumped milk.

Levels of prolactin and adrenal activation have been studied in eumenorrheic and amenorrheic women who exercise regularly. Prolactin levels following exercise are elevated for 20 to 40 minutes.[34] The effect appears to be unrelated to anaerobiosis. The hypothalamic-pituitary-adrenal (HPA) axis is known to be activated under the influence of various forms of stress, including exercise. How this activation might affect milk production or oxytocin-stimulated milk let-down after exercise has yet to be determined.

Serum prolactin and growth hormone increased severalfold during prolonged acute exercise in normal women and runners with and without menses, demonstrating that a threshold of exercise intensity must be reached for this reaction to occur.[21] There was no correlation to menstrual dysfunction.

When the lactation performances of eight physically fit, exercising women were compared with those of sedentary control subjects, there were no significant differences in milk volume or composition despite wide variations in energy intake and expenditure.[105] Exercising women compensated by increasing energy intake; thus, no net difference was seen between the groups. It has been reported that lactating women exercising on a regular basis expend an average of 2630 kcal/day exclusive of milk energy output, compared with the 1800 to 1900 kcal/day expenditures of women who did not exercise.[167]

Dewey and associates[39] studied the impact of regular exercise on the volume and composition of breast milk and further confirmed that breastfeeding women can safely exercise. Whereas previous studies were done on exercising fit women, this study randomly assigned sedentary women to exercise with supervised aerobic exercise to 60% to 70% of the heart rate reserve for 45 minutes per day, 5 days a week for 12 weeks. The control group remained breastfeeding but sedentary. Measurements of energy expended, dietary intake, body composition, and milk volume and composition were collected at 6 to 8 weeks, 12 to 14 weeks, and 18 to 20 weeks post partum. Maximum oxygen uptake and plasma prolactin response over 2 hours after nursing were measured at the first and last assessment times. No significant differences were seen in maternal weight and fat losses, volume or composition of milk, infant weight gain, or plasma prolactin response between exercising and sedentary women. No women reported difficulty nursing after moderate exercise. The authors[39] did note that the 300 kcal/day mean extra energy expenditure of the exercise group at midpoint in the study decreased toward the end as they cut back on other activities to compensate. This suggests that high levels of energy expenditure may be difficult to sustain while lactating because of fatigue and time limitations (Figs. 9-3 and 9-4).

Lovelady and associates[105] further evaluated this same study group, randomly assigned to exercise or remain sedentary. Exercise marginally increased high-density lipoprotein (HDL) cholesterol levels but did not affect other lipid concentrations. Further, resting metabolic rate did not change over time. Weight and body fat percentage declined similarly in both groups. No difference was found between exercising and sedentary groups regarding insulin, glucose, or thermal response. The authors concluded that sedentary women can initiate moderate exercise programs during lactation but that exercise does not increase weight loss or fat loss without dietary control, that is, avoiding compensatory increased intake. In a similar randomized study of 33 women, Prentice[133] reported that moderate exercise sufficient to improve cardiovascular fitness without marked changes in energy expenditure, dietary intake, and body weight and composition does not jeopardize lactation performance.

Dieting while breastfeeding

The Subcommittee on Nutrition during Lactation[167] stated in its report that the average rate of weight

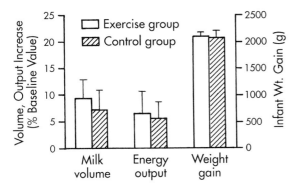

Figure 9-3. Percent increase in breast milk volume and energy output and absolute increase in infants' weight in exercise and control groups during a 12-week study. Values shown are means ± SE. To convert kilocalories to megajoules, multiply by 0.004186. None of the differences between the groups was significant. The 95% confidence intervals were as follows: for the percent change in milk volume, 2% to 17% for the exercise group and −1% to 16% for the control group (p = 0.66); for the percent change in energy output in breast milk, −2% to 15% for the exercise group and −1% to 12% for the control group (p = 0.85); and for infant weight gain, 1871 to 2279 g for the exercise group and 1733 to 2355 g for the control group (p = 0.86). (Modified from Dewey KG, Lovelady CA, Nommsen-Rivers LA, et al: A randomized study of the effects of aerobic exercise by lactating women on breast-milk volume and composition. N Engl J Med 330:449, 1994.)

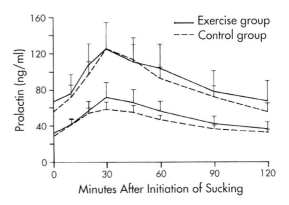

Figure 9-4. Plasma prolactin response to nursing in control and exercise groups at beginning and end of study. Values shown are mean ± SE. Study began 6 to 8 weeks post partum and ended 18 to 20 weeks post partum. Change in the area under the curve from beginning to end of the study was not significantly different between the two groups (p = 0.38). (Modified from Dewey KG, Lovelady CA, Nommsen-Rivers LA, et al: A randomized study of the effects of aerobic exercise by lactating women on breast-milk volume and composition. N Engl J Med 330:449, 1994.)

loss post partum while maintaining adequate milk volume is 0.5 to 1.0 kg (1 to 2 lb) per month. In individuals who are significantly overweight, a weight loss of up to 1 to 2 kg (about 4 to 5 lb) per month should not affect milk volume, although weight gain and feeding pattern in the infant should be monitored. The subcommittee[167] considers rapid weight loss, that is, more than 2 kg per month after the first month, unadvised. In addition, because no data exist about curtailing maternal energy intake during the first 2 to 3 weeks post partum, dieting immediately post partum is not recommended and could be associated with poor milk supply. Energy intake must be balanced with the level of physical activity. The subcommittee does not recommend intakes less than

1500 kcal/day; however, brief fasts, perhaps for religious reasons, of less than a day are unlikely to affect milk supply. Liquid diets or weight loss medications are not recommended. In studies of food-deprived rats, a clear correlation exists between adequate milk production and adequate food intake. This finding was amplified if diet was also restricted during pregnancy.[109]

Studies of weight loss during lactation are scarce. Many women in developed countries experience an appetite surge with lactation and may experience no weight loss in the first months beyond that lost with the first weeks. They may not return to prepregnancy weight for 6 months. Women who are prone to gaining weight may be more apt to gain on an unregulated diet. Maternal nutrition status in the United States, as measured by anthropometric indices prenatally and post partum, is unrelated to milk volume, according to studies of Butte and associates[18] and Dewey and associates.[38] Total energy expenditure of sedentary women, including those housebound with a new baby, averages 1800 kcal/day, exclusive of the energy put into the milk produced.[104]

No consistent relationship was reported in a study of 411 postpartum women between mode of feeding and postpartum weight loss.[132] Despite the energy deficiency of breastfeeding women, the trend was to greater weight loss in nonlactators. Women who gained more during pregnancy lost more post partum regardless of their pregnancy weight. No dietary intake was recorded because the data were collected retrospectively.

The Stockholm Pregnancy and Weight Development Study prospectively investigated trends in eating patterns, physical activity, and sociodemographic factors in relation to postpartum body weight development, following 1423 pregnant women.[123] Weight retention 1 year post partum was greater in women who increased their energy intake during and after pregnancy. Weight retention also increased in those who not only increased their snacking to three or more times a day but also decreased their lunch frequency. Sedentary lifestyle was correlated with 5 kg or more weight gain over prepartum weight. The authors summarized their findings as being related most closely to a change in lifestyle after pregnancy.[123]

The tremendous variability in women's responses to the stress of reproduction and lactation suggests that there is very low stress per unit time. Thus, many different variables exist during the perinatal period to rebalance the energy equation, according to Prentice and Prentice.[136] Some women are energy sparing and some energy profligate. Although generally beneficial, the interaction between exercise and skeletal integrity is influenced by hormonal status and many exercise variables.

During lactation, many women do not need additional dietary supplements as often recommended according to work by Hartmann and associates.[72] They reported considerable variation among individual women for the energy output in milk and the energy actually mobilized from maternal stores for milk synthesis and recommend

that energy should be calculated for each mother depending on her energy stores and milk demands. Even a low-fat diet could be appropriate to maximize the de novo synthesis of fatty acids for milk triacylglycerols, if one were sure there was adequate intake of long-chain polyunsaturated fatty acids as well as basic nutrients. Further, they demonstrated that perceived inability to make milk was usually a function of inappropriate suckling, scheduled feeds, and other lactation management issues, not lack of substrate.

Weight loss during lactation is greatest between 3 and 6 months.

Dietary advice for women who choose to diet while lactating should include the following[167]:

- Diet must include balanced, varied foods rich in calcium, zinc, magnesium, vitamin B_6, and folate.
- Minimum energy intake should be 1800 kcal.
- Calcium and multivitamin-mineral supplements may be necessary to replace stores if diet is marginal.

Foods to avoid

The concern about foods causing gas in the breast-fed baby has no scientific basis. The normal intestinal flora produce gas from the action on fiber in the intestinal tract. Neither the fiber nor the gas is absorbed from the intestinal tract, and they do not enter the milk, even though they may cause the mother some discomfort. The acid content of the maternal diet also does not affect the milk because it does not change the pH of the maternal plasma. Essential oils are present in such foods as garlic, and some spices that have characteristic odors and flavors may pass into the milk, and an occasional infant objects to their presence.

Studies by Mennella and Beauchamp[111] show that the diet of the lactating woman alters the sensory qualities of her milk. They found that garlic ingestion significantly and consistently increased the intensity of the milk odor as perceived by blinded adult panelists. The odor was not apparent at 1 hour, peaked at 2 hours, and decreased thereafter. Similar observations have been made in other species. Garlic is one of the most potent of the volatile sulfur-containing foods (onions, broccoli, etc.). Garlic consumption by the mother increased the length of time spent suckling and the rate of suckling of the next feeding.[111] This behavior is usually associated with a tendency of the breast to make more milk. The authors suggest that the mouth movements made during sucking facilitated the retronasal perception of the garlic volatile oils in the milk. This study reports only the first 4 hours postingestion and makes no reference to the period between 4 and 24 hours after ingestion, a time occasionally associated with colic in the breastfed infant after ingestion of certain foods by the mother (often called 24-hour colic).

When these mothers and infants were tested over an 11-day period, those infants who had garlic previously showed no response to reexposure; that is, suckling pattern and volume ingested were unchanged.[112] Garlic odor of amniotic fluid has been noted when the mother consumed garlic. These investigators also report that alcohol, mint, and cheese flavors are transmitted to milk. When mothers were fed carrot juice while lactating, the infant subsequently preferred cereal mixed with carrot juice rather than with plain formula or milk.[113]

Animal studies show that odors in utero and early in life are associated with a preference for them after birth. Breastfed infants experience a wide variety of odors and flavors during maternal lactation, which may enhance their weaning to solid foods. This suggests that infants fed standard formulas experience a constant set of flavors, thus missing significant sensory experiences. In experiments with rats, Galef and Sherry[58] found a mother's milk contains gustatory cues reflecting the flavor of the mother's diet and that these cues are sufficient to influence dietary preferences at weaning.

Extensive clinical experience suggests, however, that some infants do not tolerate certain foods in the mother's diet, particularly specific vegetables and fruits. Garlic and onions may cause 24-hour colic in some infants. Cabbage, turnips, broccoli, or beans may also bother others, making them colicky for 24 hours. The same has been said of rhubarb, apricots, and prunes. If a mother questions the effect of a food, she should avoid it or document its effect carefully by watching for colic in the 24 hours following ingestion. In the summer, a heavy diet of melon, peaches, and other fresh fruits may cause colic and diarrhea in the infant. Chocolate rarely lives up to its reputation and can be consumed in moderation without causing colic, diarrhea, or constipation in most infants.

Red pepper, which contains capsaicin and related compounds, has been reported to cause dermatitis in the breastfed infant within an hour of milk ingestion.[27] The rash can last 12 to 48 hours and differs from the contact dermatitis known to occur from capsaicin applied directly. When hot peppers are prepared with bare hands, an intensely painful reaction can occur. In countries where red pepper dishes such as gimchee are common (Korea), a perianal rash has long been seen in breastfed infants whose mothers ingested these hot dishes.

Food additives

Artificial sweeteners are the most common food additives. Saccharin and cyclamate are not known to be tetratogenic, but the remote relationship to cancer in rats has led to the recommendation that they be used in moderation. The same pertains during lactation. Cyclamate is a cyclohexylamine, an indirectly acting sympathomimetic amine that has been banned from use.

Aspartame is a dipeptide sweetener, aspartylphenylalanine methyl ester, that metabolizes to phenylalanine and aspartic acid. Thus, it poses a risk to those with phenylketonuria. Normal individuals can consume 50 mg/kg/day without adverse effects. In large doses of 75 mg/kg/day, individuals increase their excretion of formate and methanol. When given aspartame, lactating women were noted to have phenylalanine levels four times the normal in their plasma.[161] Milk levels of phenylalanine and tyrosine were only slightly elevated. Aspartame in moderation during lactation is presumed safe.

Color of milk and maternal diet

The color of mature human milk is bluish white (foremilk), initially changing to creamy white (hindmilk). The color of colostrum is yellow to yellow-orange. Mothers occasionally report changes in the color of their milk. Most of these changes can be traced to pigments consumed in the diet, medications, or herbal remedies. The infant's urine may also turn color.

Pink or pink-orange milk

Pink-orange milk was traced to Sunkist orange soda, which contains red and yellow dyes. A case of a breastfed infant with pink to orange urine was reported by Roseman.[144] This combination of food dyes is also used in other brands of soda, fruit drinks, and gelatin desserts. Even fresh beets can change the urine of both mother and infant to a red-pink hue.

Green milk

Several cases of green milk have been reported to our study center. A careful search of the diet for the offending substance was made in each case. The effect of ingestion of the identified culprit and its avoidance were then tested to confirm the association with the milk's color. Several items have been clearly identified. Gatorade (the green beverage), kelp and other forms of seaweed (especially in tablet form), and natural vitamins from health food sources each have been associated with one or more cases of green milk and usually green urine.

Black milk

Minocycline hydrochloride therapy was associated with black milk galactorrhea in a 24-year-old woman who had received the compound for pustulocystic acne for 4 years.[11] Examination of the fluid revealed that the macrophages contained hemosiderin, thus causing the black color. This drug is known to cause black pigmentation of the skin. A second case was reported in a 29-year-old female who had weaned but could express black milk 3 weeks after beginning oral minocycline therapy. Hunt and associates[79] found iron-staining pigment particles in the macrophages and suggested it was an iron chelate of minocycline.

SUMMARY

Supplements recommended during lactation for mothers are unnecessary unless the mother's diet is deficient. Finishing up the prenatal vitamin supply post partum is more than adequate. Having adequate vitamin D stores during pregnancy and lactation is important. Continued studies are being conducted to determine the efficacy of large doses of vitamin D for the mother so that supplementing the infant can be avoided.

Supplements for breastfeeding infants are ordinarily unnecessary in exclusively breastfed infants unless a deficiency is identified. The AAP does recommend vitamin D 200 mg beginning at 2 months of age. Iron needs should be taken care of with appropriate solid foods after 6 months of exclusive breastfeeding. Fluoride supplementation is unnecessary if the mother is adequately resourced.

REFERENCES

1. Al MD, Houwelingen AC, Badart-Smook A, et al: Some aspects of neonatal essential fatty acid status are altered by linoleic acid supplementation of women during pregnancy. J Nutr 125:2822, 1995.
2. Alaejos MS, Romero CD: Selenium in human lactation. Nutr Rev 53:159, 1995.
3. Alexander RP, Walker BF, Bhamjee D: Serum lipids in long-lactating African mothers habituated to a low-fat intake. Atherosclerosis 44:175, 1982.
4. American Academy of Pediatrics Committee on Nutrition: Pediatric Nutrition Handbook, 5th ed. Elk Grove, Ill, American Academy of Pediatrics, 2004.
5. Anderson RA, Bryden NA, Patterson KY, et al: Breast milk chromium and its association with chromium intake, chromium excretion, and serum chromium. Am J Clin Nutr 57:519, 1993.
6. Andon MB, Howard MP, Moser PB, et al: Nutritionally relevant supplementation of vitamin B6 in lactating women: Effect on plasma prolactin. Pediatrics 76:769, 1985.

7. Andon MB, Reynolds RD, Moser-Veillon PB, et al: Dietary intake of total and glycosylated vitamin B6 and the vitamin B6 nutritional status of unsupplemented lactating women and their infants. Am J Clin Nutr 50:1050, 1989.

8. Arnaud J, Prual A, Preziosi P, et al: Effect of iron supplementation during pregnancy on trace element (Cu, Se, Zn) concentrations in serum and breast milk from Nigerian women. Ann Nutr Metab 37:262, 1993.

9. Arthur PG, Jones TJ, Spruce J, et al: Measuring short-term rates of milk synthesis in breastfeeding mothers. Q J Exp Physiol 74:419, 1989.

10. Asnes R, Wisotsky DH, Migel PF, et al: The dietary chloride deficiency syndrome occurring in a breastfed infant. J Pediatr 100:923, 1982.

11. Atkinson PJ, West RR: Loss of skeletal calcium in lactating women. J Obstet Gynecol Br Commonw 77:555, 1970.

12. Bachrach S, Fisher J, Parks JS: An outbreak of vitamin D deficiency rickets in a susceptible population. Pediatrics 64:871, 1979.

13. Basler RS, Lynch PJ: Black galactorrhea as a consequence of minocycline and phenothiazine therapy. Arch Dermatol 121:417, 1985.

14. Bates CJ, Prentice AM, Watkinson M, et al: Riboflavin requirements of lactating Gambian women: A controlled supplementation trial. Am J Clin Nutr 135:701, 1982.

15. Bhaskaram P, Reddy V: Bactericidal activity of human milk leukocytes. Acta Paediatr Scand 70:87, 1981.

16. Blaauw R, Albertse EC, Beneke T, et al: Risk factors for development of osteoporosis in a South African population. South Afr Med J 84:328, 1994.

17. Butte NF, Calloway DH, Van Duzen JL: Nutritional assessment of pregnant and lactating Navajo women. Am J Clin Nutr 34:2216, 1981.

18. Butte NF, Garza C, Stuff JE, et al: Effect of maternal diet and body composition on lactational performance. Am J Clin Nutr 39:296, 1984.

19. Byerley LO, Kirksey A: Effect of different levels of vitamin C intake on the vitamin C concentration in human milk and vitamin C intakes of breastfed infants. Am J Clin Nutr 41:665, 1985.

20. Byrne J, Thomas MR, Chan GM: Calcium intake and bone density of lactating women in their late childbearing years. J Am Diet Assoc 87:883, 1987.

21. Chang FE, Dodds WG, Sullivan M, et al: The acute effects of exercise on prolactin secretion: Comparison between sedentary women and women runners with normal and abnormal menstrual cycles. J Clin Endocrinol Metab 62:551, 1986.

22. Chappell JE, Clandinin MT, Kearney-Volpe C: Trans fatty acids in human milk lipids: Influence of maternal diet and weight loss. Am J Clin Nutr 42:49, 1985.

23. Christoffel K: A pediatric perspective on vegetarian nutrition. Clin Pediatr 20:632, 1981.

24. Chulei R, Xiaofang L, Hongsheng M, et al: Milk composition in women from five different regions of China: The great diversity of milk fatty acids. J Nutr 125:2998, 1995.

25. Committee on Nutrition, American Academy of Pediatrics: Pediatric Nutrition Handbook, 5th ed. Elk Grove, Ill, American Academy of Pediatrics 2004, pp 6, 71, 307, 793.

26. Connor WE, Lowensohn R, Hatcher L: Increased docosahexaenoic acid levels in human newborn infants by administration of sardines and fish oil during pregnancy. Lipids 31:5183, 1996.

27. Cooper RL, Cooper MN: Red pepper-induced dermatitis in breast-fed infants. Dermatology 193:61, 1996.

28. Cornelissen M, vonKries R, Loughnan P, et al: Prevention of vitamin K deficiency bleeding: Efficacy of different multiple oral dose schedules of vitamin K. Eur J Pediatr 156:126, 1997.

29. Daaboul J, Sanderson S, Kristensen K, et al: Vitamin D deficiency in pregnant and breastfeeding women and their infants. J Perinatol 17:10, 1997.

30. Dagnelie PC, van Staveren WA: Macrobiotic nutrition and child health: Results of a population-based, mixed-longitudinal cohort study in the Netherlands. Am J Clin Nutr 59(suppl):1187S, 1994.

31. Dagnelie PC, van Staveren WA, Roos AH, et al: Nutrients and contaminants in human milk from mothers on macrobiotic and omnivorous diets. Eur J Clin Nutr 46:355, 1992.

32. Deodhar AD, Ramakrishnan CV: Studies on human lactation. II. Effect of socioeconomic status on vitamin content of human milk. Indian J Med Res 47:352, 1959.

33. DeSantiago S, Villalpando S, Ortiz N, et al: Protein requirements of marginally nourished lactating women. Am J Clin Nutr 62:364, 1995.

34. DeSouza MJ, Maguire MS, Maresh CM, et al: Adrenal activation and the prolactin response to exercise in eumenorrheic and amenorrheic runners. J Appl Physiol 70(6):2378, 1991.

35. Dewey KG: Does maternal supplementation shorten the duration of lactational amenorrhea? Am J Clin Nutr 64:377, 1996.

36. Dewey KG, Finley DA, Lönnerdal B: Breast milk volume and composition during late lactation (7–20 months). J Pediatr Gastroenterol Nutr 3:713, 1984.

37. Dewey KG, Finley DA, Strode MA, et al: Relationship of maternal age to breastmilk volume and composition. In Hamosh MH, Goldman AS (eds): Human Lactation: Maternal and Environmental Factors. New York, Plenum, 1986.

38. Dewey KG, Heinig MJ, Nommsen LA, et al: Maternal vs infant factors related to breast milk intake and residual milk volume: The Darling Study. Pediatrics 87:829, 1991.

39. Dewey KG, Lovelady CA, Nommsen-Rivers LA, et al: A randomized study of the effects of aerobic exercise by lactating women on breast-milk volume and composition. N Engl J Med 330:449, 1994.

40. Domellof M, Lonnerdal B, Dewey KG, et al: Iron, zinc, and copper concentrations in breast milk are independent of maternal mineral status. Am J Clin Nutr 79:111, 2004.

41. Donnen P, Brasseur D, Dramaix M, et al: Effects of cow's milk supplementation on milk output of protein deficient

lactating mothers and on their infants' energy and protein status. Trop Med Int Health 2:38, 1997.

42. Duckman S, Hubbard JF: The role of fluids in relieving breast engorgement without the use of hormones. Am J Obstet Gynecol 60:200, 1950.

43. Dusdieker LB, Booth BM, Stumbo PJ, et al: Effect of supplemental fluids on human milk production. J Pediatr 106:207, 1985.

44. Dwyer JT, Palombo R, Thorne H, et al: Preschoolers on alternate lifestyle diets. J Am Diet Assoc 72:264, 1978.

45. Edozien JC, Khan MAR, Waslien CI: Human protein deficiency: results of a Nigerian village study. J Nutr 106:312, 1976.

46. English RM, Hitchcock NE: Nutrient intakes during pregnancy, lactation and after the cessation of lactation in a group of Australian women. Br J Nutr 22:615, 1968.

47. Ereman RR, Lönnerdal B, Dewey KG: Maternal sodium intake does not affect postprandial sodium concentrations in human milk. J Nutr 117:1154, 1987.

48. Finley DA, Lönnerdal B, Dewey KG, et al: Breast milk composition: Fat content and fatty acid composition in vegetarians and non-vegetarians. Am J Clin Nutr 41:787, 1985.

49. Friel JK, Aziz K, Andrews WJ, et al: A double-masked randomized control trial of iron supplementation in early infancy in healthy term breast-fed infants. J Pediatr 143:582, 2003.

50. Fomon SJ: Breastfeeding and evolution. J Am Diet Assoc 86:317, 1986.

51. Food and Nutrition Board, National Research Council: Recommended Dietary Allowances, 11th ed. Washington, DC, National Academy Press, 1994.

52. Food and Nutrition Board, National Research Council: Dietary Reference Intakes (RDIs). Washington, DC, National Academy Press, 1998.

53. Forsum E, Lönnerdal B: Effect of protein intake on protein and nitrogen composition of breast milk. Am J Clin Nutr 33:1809, 1980.

54. Fukushima Y, Kawata Y, Onda T, et al: Consumption of cow milk and egg by lactating women and the presence of β-lactoglobulin and ovalbumin in breast milk. Am J Clin Nutr 65:30, 1997.

55. Fulton JR, Hutton CW, Sitt KR: Preschool vegetarian children. J Am Diet Assoc 76:260, 1980.

56. Fung EB, Ritchie LD, Woodhouse LR, et al: Zinc absorption in women during pregnancy and lactation: A longitudinal study. Am J Clin Nutr 66:80, 1997.

57. Gabriel A, Gabriel KR, Lawrence RA: Cultural values and biomedical knowledge: Choices in infant feeding: Analysis of a survey. Soc Sci Med 23:501, 1986.

58. Galef BG, Sherry DF: A medium for transmission of cues reflecting the flavor of mother's diet. J Comp Physiol Psychol 83:374, 1973.

59. Gambon RC, Lentze MJ, Rossi E: Megaloblastic anaemia in one of monozygous twins breast fed by their vegetarian mother. Eur J Pediatr 145:570, 1986.

60. Gartner LM, Greer FR: Prevention of rickets and vitamin D deficiency: New guidelines for vitamin D intake. Pediatrics 111:908, 2003.

61. Gonzalez-Cossio T, Habicht JP, Rasmussen KM, Delgado HL: Impact of food supplementation during lactation on infant breast-milk intake and on the proportion of infants exclusively breast-fed. J Nutr 128:1692, 1998.

62. Greer FR, Marshall SP, Foley AL, et al: Improving the vitamin K status of breastfeeding infants with maternal vitamin K supplements. Pediatrics 99:88, 1997.

63. Greer FR, Marshall SP, Severson RR, et al: A new mixed-micellar preparation for oral vitamin K prophylaxis: Comparison with an intramuscular formulation in breast-fed infants. Arch Dis Child 79:300, 1998.

64. Greer FR, Marshall SP, Suttle JW: Improving the vitamin K status of breast-feeding infants with vitamin K supplements. Pediatrics 99:88, 1997.

65. Greer FR, Tsang RC, Levin RS, et al: Increasing serum calcium and magnesium concentrations in breast-fed infants: Longitudinal studies of minerals in human milk and in sera of nursing mothers and their infants. J Pediatr 100:59, 1982.

66. Griffin IJ, Abrams SA: Iron and breastfeeding. Pediatr Clin North Am 48:401, 2001.

67. Gushurst CA, Mueller JA, Green JA, et al: Breast milk iodide: reassessment in the 1980s. Pediatrics 73:354, 1984.

68. Guthrie HA, Picciano MF, Sheehe D: Fatty acid patterns of human milk. J Pediatr 90:39, 1977.

69. Hachey DL, Thomas MR, Emken EA, et al: Human lactation: Maternal transfer of dietary triglycerides labeled with stable isotopes. J Lipid Res 28:1185, 1987.

70. Hambraeus L: Proprietary milk versus human breast milk in infant feeding: A critical approach from the nutritional point of view. In Neumann CG, Jelliffe DB (eds): Symposium on nutrition in pediatrics. Pediatr Clin North Am 24:17, 1977.

71. Hanafy MM, Morsery MRA, Seddick Y, et al: Maternal nutrition and lactation performance. J Trop Pediatr Environ Child Health 18:187, 1972.

72. Hartmann P, Sherriff J, Kent J: Maternal nutrition and the regulation of milk synthesis. Proc Nutr Soc 54:379, 1995.

73. Harris WS, Connor WE, Lindsey S: Will dietary omega-3 fatty acids change the composition of human milk? Am J Clin Nutr 40:780, 1984.

74. Heck H, deCastro JM: The calorie demand of lactation does not alter spontaneous meal patterns, nutrient intakes, or moods of women. Physiol Behav 54:641, 1993.

75. Hellebostad M, Markestad T, Halvorsen KS: Vitamin D deficiency rickets and vitamin B12 deficiency in vegetarian children. Acta Paediatr Scand 74:191, 1985.

76. Hernell O: The requirements and utilization of dietary fatty acids in the newborn infant. Acta Paediatr Scand Suppl 365:20, 1990.

77. Higginbottom MC, Sweetman L, Nyhan WL: A syndrome of methylmalonic aciduria, homocystinuria, megaloblastic anemia and neurologic abnormalities in a vitamin B12 deficient breastfed infant of a strict vegetarian. N Engl J Med 299:317, 1978.

78. Hollis BW, Pittard III WB, Reinhardt TA: Relationships among vitamin D, 25-hydroxyvitamin D, and vitamin D-binding protein concentrations in the plasma and milk of human subjects. J Clin Endocrinol Metab 62:41, 1986.

79. Hunt MJ, Salisbury ELC, Grace J, et al: Black breast milk due to minocycline therapy. Br J Dermatol 134:943, 1996.

80. Illingworth PJ, Jung RT, Howie PW, et al: Diminution in energy expenditure during lactation. Br Med J 292:437, 1986.

81. Illingworth RS, Kilpatrick B: Lactation and fluid intake. Lancet 2:1175, 1953.

82. Insull W, Hirsch J, James T, et al: The fatty acids of human milk. II. Alterations produced by manipulation of caloric balance and exchange of dietary fats. J Clin Invest 38:443, 1959.

83. Jackson MJ, Giugliano R, Giugliano LG, et al: Stable isotope metabolic studies of zinc nutrition in slum dwelling lactating women in the Amazon valley. Br J Nutr 59:193, 1988.

84. Jelliffe DB, Jelliffe EFP: Human Milk in the Modern World. New York, Oxford University Press, 1978.

85. Jelliffe EFP: Maternal nutrition and lactation. In Ciba Foundation Symposium, no 45. Breast Feeding and the Mother. Amsterdam, Elsevier Science, 1976.

86. Jensen RG: The Lipids of Human Milk. Boca Raton, Fla, CRC, 1989.

87. Jensen RG: Miscellaneous factors affecting composition and volume of human and bovine milks. In Jensen RG (ed): Handbook of Milk Composition. San Diego, Academic Press, 1995.

88. Johnson P, Salisbury DM: Preliminary studies on feeding and breathing in the newborn. In Weiffenbach JM (ed): Taste and Development: The Genesis of Sweet Preference. Bethesda, Md, Public Health Service, National Institutes of Health, Department of Health, Education and Welfare Publication (NIH), 1977.

89. Johnston L, Vaughn L, Fox HM: Pantothenic acid content of human milk. Am J Clin Nutr 34:2205, 1981.

90. Kalkwarf HJ, Specker BL, Herbi JE, et al: Intestinal calcium absorption of women during lactation and after weaning. Am J Clin Nutr 63:526, 1996.

91. Kang-Yoon SA, Kirksey A, Giacoia G, et al: Vitamin B6 status of breastfed neonates: Influence of pyridoxine supplementation on mothers and neonates. Am J Clin Nutr 56:548, 1992.

92. Keenan BS, Buzek SW, Garza C, et al: Diurnal and longitudinal variations in human milk sodium and potassium: Implications for nutrition and physiology. Am J Clin Nutr 35:527, 1982.

93. Khin-Maung-Naing, Tin-Tin-Oo, Kywe-Thein, et al: Study on lactation performance of Burmese mothers. Am J Clin Nutr 33:2665, 1980.

94. Kliewer RI, Rasmussen KM: Malnutrition during the reproductive cycle: Effects on galactopoietic hormones and lactational performance in the rat. Am J Clin Nutr 46:926, 1987.

95. Koletzko B, Gwosdz M, Bremer HJ: Trans isomeric fatty acids in human milk lipids in West Germany. In Schaub J (ed): Composition and Physiological Properties of Human Milk. Amsterdam, Elsevier Science, 1985.

96. Kramer M, Szöke K, Lindner K, et al: The effect of different factors on the composition of human milk and its variations. III. Effect of dietary fats on the lipid composition of human milk. Nutr Diet 7:71, 1965.

97. Krebs NF, Hambidge KM, Jacobs MA, et al: The effects of a dietary zinc supplement during lactation on longitudinal changes in maternal zinc status and milk zinc concentrations. Am J Clin Nutr 41:560, 1985.

98. Krebs NF, Reidinger CJ, Hartley S, et al: Zinc supplementation during lactation: Effects on maternal status and milk zinc concentrations. Am J Clin Nutr 61:1030, 1995.

99. Krebs NF, Reidinger CJ, Robertson AD, et al: Bone mineral density changes during lactation: maternal, dietary, and biochemical correlates. Am J Clin Nutr 65:1738, 1997.

100. Lammi-Keefe CJ, Jensen RG: Lipids in human milk: A review. II. Composition and fat-soluble vitamins. J Pediatr Gastroenterol Nutr 3:172, 1984.

101. Lammi-Keefe CJ, Jensen RG, Clark RM, et al: Alpha tocopherol total lipid and linoleic acid contents of human milk at 2, 6, 12, and 16 weeks. In Schaub J (ed): Composition and Physiological Properties of Human Milk. Amsterdam, Elsevier Science, 1985.

102. Levander OA, Moser PB, Morris VC: Dietary selenium intake and selenium concentrations of plasma, erythrocytes, and breast milk in pregnant and post partum lactating and non-lactating women. Am J Clin Nutr 46:694, 1987.

103. Lipsman S, Dewey KG, Lönnerdal B: Breastfeeding among teenage mothers: Milk composition, infant growth, and maternal dietary intake. J Pediatr Gastroenterol Nutr 4:426, 1985.

104. Lönnerdal B: Effects of maternal dietary intake on human milk composition. J Nutr 116:499, 1986.

105. Lovelady CA, Lönnerdal B, Dewey KG: Lactation performance of exercising women. Am J Clin Nutr 52:103, 1990.

106. Lovelady CA, Nommsen LA, McCrory MA, et al: Effects of exercise on plasma lipids and metabolism of lactating women. Med Sci Sports Exerc 27:22, 1995.

107. Macy IG, Huncher HA, Donelson E, et al: Human milk flow. Am J Dis Child 6:492, 1930.

108. McGuire MK, Burgent SL, Milner JA, et al: Selenium status of lactating women is affected by the form of selenium consumed. Am J Clin Nutr 58:649, 1993.

109. McGuire MK, Littleton AW, Schulze KJ, Rasmussen KM: Pre- and postweaning food restrictions interact to determine reproductive success and milk volume in rats. J Nutr 125:2400, 1995.

110. Mellies MJ, Ishikawa TT, Gartside P, et al: Effects of varying maternal dietary cholesterol and phytosterol in lactating women and their infants. Am J Clin Nutr 31:1347, 1978.

111. Mennella JA, Beauchamp GK: Maternal diet alters the sensory qualities of human milk and nursling's behavior. Pediatrics 88:737, 1991.

112. Mennella JA, Beauchamp GK: The effects of repeated exposure to garlic-flavored milk on the nursling's behavior. Pediatr Res 34:805, 1993.

113. Mennella JA, Beauchamp GK: The early development of human flavor preferences. In Capaldi ED (ed): Why We Eat What We Eat: The Psychology of Eating. Washington, DC, American Psychological Association, 1996.

114. Michaud JL, Lemieux B, Ogier H, et al: Nutritional vitamin B12 deficiency: Two cases detected by routine newborn urinary screening. Eur J Pediatr 151:218, 1992.

115. Miranda R, Saravia NG, Ackerman R, et al: Effect of maternal nutritional status on immunological substances in human colostrum and milk. Am J Clin Nutr 37:632, 1983.

116. Motil KJ, Thotathuckery M, Bahar A, et al: Marginal dietary protein restriction reduced nonprotein nitrogen, but not protein nitrogen components of human milk. J Am Coll Nutr 14:184, 1995.

117. National Academy of Sciences: Dietary Reference Intakes, 2000, 2001, 2002, 2003. Accessed at www.nap.edu.

118. Nelson TR, Pretorius DH, Schiffer LM: Menstrual variation of normal breast NMR relaxation parameters. J Comput Assist Tomogr 9:875, 1985.

119. Neville MC: Anatomy and physiology of lactation. In Schanler RJ (ed): Breastfeeding 2001, Part I. The evidence for breastfeeding. Pediatr Clin North Am 48(1):13, 2001.

120. Neville MC: Volume and caloric density of human milk. In Jensen RD (ed): Handbook of Milk Composition. San Diego, Academic Press, 1995, p 99.

121. Nommsen LA, Lovelady CA, Heinig MJ, et al: Determinants of energy, protein, lipid and lactose concentrations in human milk during the first 12 mo of lactation: The Darling Study. Am J Clin Nutr 53:457, 1991.

122. O'Connor DL: Folate status during pregnancy and lactation. Adv Exp Med Biol 352:157, 1994.

123. Ohlin A, Rossner S: Trends in eating patterns, physical activity and sociodemographic factors in relation to postpartum body weight development. Br J Nutr 71:457, 1994.

124. Olsen A: Nursing under conditions of thirst or excessive ingestion of fluids. Acta Obstet Gynaecol Scand 20:313, 1940.

125. Olson CM: Promoting positive nutritional practices during pregnancy and lactation. Am J Clin Nutr 59(suppl):525S, 1994.

126. Park MJ, Namgung R, Kim DH, et al: Lower serum 25-hydroxyvitamin D, but similar bone mineral content by DEXA in human milk-fed versus cow milk-based formula-fed infants. Pediatr Res 35:205A, 1994.

127. Parkinson AJ, Cruz AL, Heyward WL, et al: Elevated concentrations of plasma ω-3 polyunsaturated fatty acids among Alaskan Eskimos. Am J Clin Nutr 59:384, 1994.

128. Paul AA, Muller EM, Whitehead RG: The quantitative effects of maternal dietary energy intake on pregnancy and lactation in rural Gambian women. Trans R Soc Trop Med Hyg 73:686, 1979.

129. Picciano MF: Nutrient composition of human milk. Pediatr Clin North Am 48:53, 2001.

130. Pisacane A, DeVizia B, Vallante A, et al: Iron status in breast-fed infants. J Pediatr 127:429, 1995.

131. Potter JM, Nestel PJ: The effects of dietary fatty acids and cholesterol on the milk lipids of lactating women and the plasma cholesterol of breast-fed infants. Am J Clin Nutr 29:54, 1976.

132. Potter S, Hannum S, McFarlin B, et al: Does infant feeding method influence maternal postpartum weight loss? J Am Diet Assoc 91:441, 1991.

133. Prentice A: Should lactating women exercise? Nutr Rev 52:358, 1994.

134. Prentice A: Maternal calcium requirements during pregnancy and lactation. Am J Clin Nutr 59(suppl):477S, 1994.

135. Prentice A, Jarjou LM, Cole TJ, et al: Calcium requirements of lactating Gambian mothers: Effects of a calcium supplement on breast milk calcium concentration, maternal bone content, and urinary calcium excretion. Am J Clin Nutr 62:58, 1995.

136. Prentice AM, Prentice A: Energy costs of lactation. Annu Rev Nutr 8:63, 1988.

137. Prentice A, Prentice AM, Cole TJ, et al: Breast milk antimicrobial factors of rural Gambian mothers. I. Influence of stage of lactation and maternal plane of nutrition. Acta Paediatr Scand 73:796, 1984.

138. Prentice AM, Roberts SB, Prentice A, et al: Dietary supplementation of lactating Gambian women. I. Effect on breast milk volume and quality. Hum Nutr 37C:53, 1983.

139. Prentice AM, Whitehead RG, Roberts SB: Dietary supplementation of Gambian nursing mothers and lactational performance. Lancet 2:886, 1980.

140. Rana SK, Sanders TAB: Taurine concentrations in diet, plasma, urine, and breast milk of vegans compared with omnivores. Br J Nutr 56:17, 1986.

141. Rassin DK, Sturman JA, Gaull GE: Taurine and other free amino acids in milk of man and other mammals. Early Hum Dev 2:1, 1978.

142. Reddy S, Sanders TAB, Obeid O: The influence of maternal vegetarian diet on essential fatty acid status of the newborn. Eur J Clin Nutr 48:358, 1994.

143. Robertson L, Flinders C, Godfrey B: Laurel's Kitchen: A Handbook for Vegetarian Cookery and Nutrition. Petaluma, Calif, Nilgiri, 1976.

144. Roseman BD: Sunkissed urine. Pediatrics 67:443, 1981 (letter).

145. Roy SK, Islam A, Molla A, et al: Impact of a single mega-dose of vitamin A at delivery on breastmilk of mothers and morbidity of their infants. Eur J Clin Nutr 51:302, 1997.

146. Saint L, Maggione P, Hartmann PE: Yield and nutrient content of milk in eight women breastfeeding twins and one woman breastfeeding triplets. Br J Nutr 56:49, 1986.

147. Salmenpera L: Vitamin C nutrition during prolonged lactation: Optimal in infants while marginal in some mothers. Am J Clin Nutr 40:1050, 1984.

148. Scanlon KS, Blank S, Sinks T, et al: Subclinical health effects in a population exposed to excess vitamin D in milk. Am J Publ Health 85:1418, 1995.

149. Schutz Y, Lechtig A, Bradfield RB: Energy expenditures and food intakes of lactating women in Guatemala. Am J Clin Nutr 33:892, 1980.

150. Sinclair AJ, Crawford MA: The effect of a low-fat maternal diet on neonatal rats. Br J Nutr 29:127, 1973.

151. Smith CA: Effects of maternal undernutrition upon newborn infants in Holland (1944–1945). J Pediatr 30:229, 1947.

152. Sneed SM, Zane C, Thomas MR: The effects of ascorbic acid, vitamin B6, vitamin B12 and folic acid supplementation on the breast milk and maternal nutritional status of low socioeconomic lactating women. Am J Clin Nutr 34:1338, 1981.

153. Sosa R, Klaus M, Urrutia JJ: Feed the nursing mother, thereby the infant. J Pediatr 88:668, 1976.

154. Specker BL: Do North American women need supplemental vitamin D during pregnancy or lactation? Am J Clin Nutr 59(suppl):484S, 1994.

155. Specker BL: Nutritional concerns of lactating women consuming vegetarian diets. Am J Clin Nutr 59(suppl):1182S, 1994.

156. Specker BL, Black A, Allen L, et al: Vitamin B12: Low milk concentrations are related to low serum concentrations in vegetarian women and to methylmalonic aciduria in their infants. Am J Clin Nutr 52:1073, 1990.

157. Specker BL, Tsang RC, Ho M, et al: Effect of vegetarian diet on serum 1,25-dihydroxyvitamin D concentrations during lactation. Obstet Gynecol 70:870, 1987.

158. Specker BL, Tsang RC, Hollis BW: Effect of race and diet on human milk vitamin D and 25-hydroxyvitamin D. Am J Dis Child 139:1134, 1985.

159. Specker BL, Valanis B, Hertzberg V, et al: Sunshine exposure and serum 25-hydroxy vitamin D concentration in exclusively breastfed infants. J Pediatr 107:372, 1985.

160. Specker BL, Wey HE, Miller D: Differences in fatty acid composition of human milk in vegetarian and nonvegetarian women: Long-term effect of diet. J Pediatr Gastroenterol Nutr 6:764, 1987.

161. Stegnink LD, Filer LJ, Baker GL: Plasma erythrocyte and human milk levels of free amino acids in lactating women administered aspartame or lactose. J Nutr 109:2173, 1979.

162. Stein ZA, Susser MW, Saenger G, et al: Famine and Human Development: The Dutch Hunger Winter of 1944–45. New York, Oxford University Press, 1975.

163. Steiner JE: Facial expressions of the neonate indicating the hedonics of food-related chemical stimuli. In Weifferbach JM (ed): Taste and Development: The Genesis of Sweet Preference. Bethesda, MD, Public Health Service, National Institutes of Health, Department of Health, Education and Welfare Publication (NIH), 1977.

164. Steingrimsdottir L, Brasel JA, Greenwood MRC: Diet, pregnancy, and lactation: Effects on adipose tissue, lipoprotein lipase, and fat cell size. Metabolism 29:837, 1980.

165. Stoltzfus RJ, Hakimi M, Miller KW, et al: A supplementation of breast-feeding Indonesian mothers: Effects on the vitamin A status of mother and infant. J Nutr 123:666, 1993.

166. Styslinger L, Kirksey A: Effects of different levels of vitamin B6 supplementation on vitamin B6 concentrations in human milk and vitamin B6 intakes of breastfed infants. Am J Clin Nutr 41:21, 1985.

167. Subcommittee on Nutrition during Lactation, Committee on Nutritional Status during Pregnancy and Lactation, Food and Nutrition Board, Institute of Medicine, National Academy of Sciences: Nutrition during Lactation. Washington, DC, National Academy Press, 1991.

168. Suitor CW, Olson C, Wilson J: Nutrition care during pregnancy and lactation: New guidelines from the IOM. J Am Diet Assoc 93:478, 1993.

169. Tennekoon KH, Karunanayake EH, Seneviratne HR: Effect of skim milk supplementation of the maternal diet on lactational amenorrhea, maternal prolactin and lactational behavior. Am J Clin Nutr 64:238, 1996.

170. Tomashek KM, Nesby S, Scanlon KS, et al: Commentary: Nutritional rickets in Georgia. Pediatrics 107:e45, 2001.

171. Tully J, Dewey KG: Private fears, global loss: A cross-cultural study of insufficient milk syndrome. Med Anthropol 9:225, 1985.

172. Van Houwelingen AC, Sorensen JD, Hornstra G, et al: Essential fatty acid status in neonates after fish-oil supplementation during late pregnancy. Br J Nutr 74:723, 1995.

173. vanSteenbergen WM, Kusin JA, VanRems MM: Lactation performance of Akamba mothers, Kenya breastfeeding behavior, breast milk yield, and composition. J Trop Pediatr 27:155, 1981.

174. Vlachou A, Drummond BK, Curzon MEJ: Fluoride concentrations of infant foods and drinks in the United Kingdom. Caries Res 26:29, 1992.

175. Von Muralt A: Maternal nutrition and lactation. In Ciba Foundation Symposium, no 45. Breast Feeding and the Mother. Amsterdam, Elsevier Scientific, 1976.

176. Vuori E, Kiuru K, Makinen M, et al: Maternal diet and fatty acid pattern of breast milk. Acta Paediatr Scand 71:959, 1982.

177. Wagner CL, Hulsey TC, Howard CR, et al: Efficacy of maternal vitamin D (vit D) supplementation during lactation. ABM News Views 9:17, 2003 (abstract).

178. Walker ARP, Walker BF, Bhamjee D, et al: Serum lipids in long-lactating African mothers habituated to a low fat intake. Atherosclerosis 44:175, 1982.

179. Wallace JP, Ernsthausen K, Inbar G: The influence of the fullness of milk in the breasts on the concentration of lactic acid in post exercise breast milk. Int J Sports Med 13:395, 1992.

180. Wallace JP, Inbar G, Ernsthausen K: Infant acceptance of post exercise breast milk. Pediatrics 89:1245, 1992.

181. Wallace JP, Inbar G, Ernsthausen K: Lactate concentrations in breast milk following maximal exercise and a typical workout. J Women's Health 3:91, 1994.

182. Wallace JP, Rabin J: The concentration of lactic acid in breastmilk following maximal exercise. Int J Sports Med 12:328, 1991.

183. Walton JL, Messer LB: Dental caries and fluorosis in breast-fed and bottle-fed children. Caries Res 15:124, 1981.

184. West KD, Kirksey A: Influence of vitamin B6 intake on the content of the vitamin in human milk. Am J Clin Nutr 29:961, 1976.

185. Whitehead RG: Pregnancy and lactation: Nutrition and growth, aging and physiologic stress. In Shils ME, Young VR (eds): Modern Nutrition in Health and Disease, 7th ed. Philadelphia, Lea & Febiger, 1988.

186. Winkvist A, Habicht JP, Rasmussen KM: Linking maternal and infant benefits of a nutritional supplement during pregnancy and lactation. Am J Clin Nutr 68:656, 1998.

187. World Health Organization: Handbook on Human Nutritional Requirements. Geneva, World Health Organization, 1974.

188. Worthington-Roberts BS: Lactation, human milk, and nutritional considerations. In Worthington-Roberts BS, Williams SR (eds): Nutrition in Pregnancy and Lactation, 6th ed. Madison, WI, Browne Benchmark, 1997.

189. Zmora E, Gorodischer R, Bar-Ziv J: Multiple nutritional deficiencies in infants from a strict vegetarian community. Am J Dis Child 133:141, 1979.

10

*W*eaning

What does *weaning* mean? The textbooks on pediatrics and the mother's manuals all imply that it is the process by which one changes from one method of feeding to another. Raphael[58] states that the very first introduction of solid foods is the true beginning of weaning. The term *weaning* is derived from the Anglo-Saxon *wenian*, which means "to become accustomed to something different." It does not mean the total cessation of breastfeeding but the addition of other things.[60] If one consults the dictionary, however, one learns that to *wean* is to transfer the young of any animal from dependence on its mother's milk to another form of nourishment or to estrange from former habits or associations. A *weanling* is a child or animal who is newly weaned. If one likens breastfeeding to the continuation of intrauterine life, weaning is a "second birth."

Weaning from a physiologic point of view is a complex process involving nutritional, microbiologic, immunologic, biochemical, and psychological adjustments. Boys tend to be weaned earlier than girls, possibly because the energy intakes of boys at all ages are greater and male growth rate is more rapid. Psychosocial pressures also trend toward the earlier weaning of male infants.[13]

INFANT'S NEED

When discussing the process of weaning the human infant, one might say it is the transfer of the infant from dependence on mother's milk to other sources of nourishment. If one were to determine the appropriate time for this to take place, it would be based on nutritional needs and developmental goals. Observations among other mammals suggest that achievement of a degree of maturity that allows the pup to forage for food is a trigger for initiating weaning by the mother.

Search for the appropriate weaning time for the human infant has produced a number of extremes, from the regimen of J. R. Sackett in 1953 of introducing solids on the second day of life to withholding all solid foods until the infant had sufficient teeth to chew thoroughly, a method described by Bartholomaus Mettinger, a German physician, in 1473.[11] The birth of the infant food industry began with German chemist Justis von Leitbig in 1867. He marketed "the perfect infant food" to the public at the turn of the 20th century, a mixture of wheat flour, malt flour, and cow milk. Jacobi, the father of modern pediatrics, advised no solids for a year and no vegetables before 2 years of age. Thus, the winds of weaning varied by culture, ethnic group, medical intervention, and financial resources.

Acknowledging that humans are primates, Dettwyler[13] recognized that lactation and weaning occur according to certain regular patterns in nonhuman primates. She searched for a natural age of weaning for the human infant uninfluenced by culture and trends. Evaluating various "rules of thumb" for determining weaning age by biologic references, she found them inappropriate. Breastfeeding from an anthropologic point of view is both a biologic process and a culturized activity. In primitive cultures, age of weaning from the breast is between 2 and 5 years, averaging 3 to 4 years.

If the definition of weaning is used to mean the cessation of all feedings at the breast, the age at weaning in nonhuman primates and other mammals is a function of genetics and instinct. Primates have a longer gestation, greater infant dependency, longer life spans, and larger brains per unit of body size than other mammals. Dettwyler[13] suggests that a possible formula for weaning is the ratio of present weight to birth weight as 4 to 1; that is, the offspring weans when four times the birth weight is achieved, usually between 2 and 3 years for well-fed healthy human infants.

If weaning according to attainment of one third the adult weight is used as the rule of thumb, Dettwyler[13] notes the variations in size of human adults by ethnic and cultural groups. With averaging, adult female weight is 54 kg (119 lb), then one third is 18 kg (39½ lb), a weight achieved between 4 and 7 years for girls; 59 kg (130 lb) is average for adult males, and one third is 19.3 kg (42½ lb). This would mean boys would be nursed longer. The present tendency for obesity in the developed world would accentuate these calculations. The average female weight in the United States is 55 kg (121 lb). Harvey and Clutton-Brock[29] suggest the following equation for calculation of weaning age:

Weaning age (days) = 2.71 × adult female weight (kg)

Thus, a modern infant whose mother weighed 55 kg would be weaned at 1228 days, or 3.36 years. Calculating for small, medium, and large women, this period would range from 2.8 to 3.7 years.

When length of gestation is used as the determinant for weaning time, the weaning/gestation ratio can be determined. According to the work of Harvey and Clutton-Brock,[29] the ratio across primate species varies from 0.41 in the *Galago demidovii,* a small-bodied primate, to 6.40 in the *Pan troglodytes* (chimpanzee). The former nurses less than half the length of pregnancy (11 of 45 days), whereas the chimpanzee nurses 1460 days (228-day gestation). The gorilla nurses for 1583 days

(256-day gestation). Because the human is closest to the chimpanzee and gorilla, six times the gestation period might be a more physiologic norm: 54 months, or 4½ years.

When the eruption of the first permanent molar is used as the indicator for complete weaning, it estimates weaning at 5½ to 6 years in humans.[13] Tooth eruption is genetically controlled and comparatively unaffected by diet or disease. Six years is also identified as the time of achieving adult level of immunocompetence in the human.

The range of calculated ages for weaning derived from these formulations ranges from 2.3 years to 6 or 7 years. Before the widespread availability of foods suitable for infants and of artificial formulas, infants were traditionally breastfed for 3 to 4 years (Fig. 10-1).

Other species gradually introduce other foods and teach their offspring how to obtain them on their own. Usually the mothers in most species make the determination for final termination and no longer permit the young to nurse. Studies on the milk-borne factors that might cue the initiation of weaning in other species have not shown any cause and effect. The rat undergoes a "weaning crisis" during which the anatomy of the gut changes; some enzymes appear and others disappear. Chapter 3 discusses the enzymatic adaptations of the human infant.

Among humans, many cultural influences mandate weaning time and process. Public and social pressures have influenced weaning for some families in industrialized society. Very few traditional societies wean before 1 year of age, and some do not begin until 2 years of age (Fig. 10-2).[32] In ancient Hebrew tradition (c. 536 BC), breastfeeding duration according to the Talmud was at least 3 years. Aristotle had suggested that women should breastfeed while no menstruation was occurring, failing to recognize that one influences the other (lactation suppresses menstruation). The Romans recommended breastfeeding at least to the age of 3. In the Muslim world, especially Africa and the Sudan, however, weaning of children is by the Islamic teaching of the Koran, which advises breastfeeding until at least 2 years of age, with

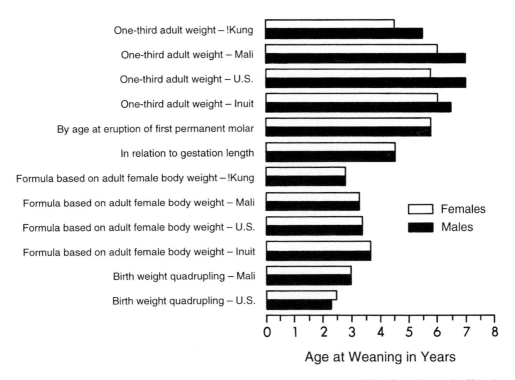

Figure 10-1. Natural age at weaning according to technique used. (Modified from Dettwyler KA: A time to wean. In Stuart-MacAdam P, Dettwyler KA (eds): Breastfeeding: Biocultural Perspectives. New York, Aldine de Gruyter, 1995.)

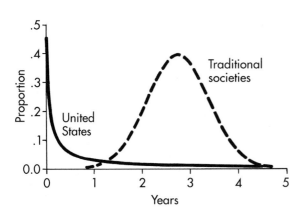

Figure 10-2. Comparison of age at weaning in United States and 64 traditional societies. (Modified from Dettwyler KA: A time to wean. In Stuart-MacAdam P, Dettwyler KA (eds): Breastfeeding: Biocultural Perspectives, New York, Aldine de Gruyter, 1995.)

many breastfeeding to age 4 or 5. Before 1979 the average time of complete cessation worldwide was 4.2 years. Hervada and Newman[32] provide a historic review of weaning that also presents recent concerns about iron deficiency and other problems more common to formula fed infants.

Breastfeeding benefits for an older infant have also been evaluated. In the developing world, breastfeeding continues for at least 1 to 2 years after introduction of solid foods. Major benefits include not only the nutrients but also protective, digestive, and trophic agents that extend the period of infertility in the mother[61] and reduce the incidence and severity of infectious diseases for the infant. A review of middle-class breastfed infants between the ages of 16 and 30 months in the United States revealed a decrease in the number of infections and improved overall health compared with those children no longer breastfed.[25]

Nutritionally, it is appropriate to begin iron-containing foods at 6 months, the time the stores from birth are being diminished. The requirement at this age exceeds that supplied by human milk. An additional source of protein becomes necessary toward the end of the first year of life because the grams of protein needed per kilogram of body weight can no longer be supplied by milk alone as the infant grows heavier. The content of protein in the milk begins to drop slightly after 9 months of lactation. A human infant also needs bulk, or roughage, in the diet. The exact time this need becomes apparent is not known, but it may well be by the end of the first year.[60]

Developmentally, the infant is ready to learn to chew solids instead of suckle liquids at about 6 months.[4] Illingworth and Lister[38] have suggested a "critical period of development" during which infants can and must learn to chew. Chewing is an entirely different motion of the tongue and mouth from sucking. The sucking fat pads in the cheeks begin to disappear at the end of the first year. The rooting reflex has been lost. Even though the teeth are not all in, the development of good dentition requires chewing exercise.

ROLE OF DEVELOPMENT IN INITIATION OF WEANING

Although the developmental milestones of infant behavior are noted to influence the introduction of weaning foods, the development of the gastrointestinal tract plays an equal role. Even the taste buds, which can be identified at the seventh week of fetal life as collections of elongated cells on the dorsal surface of the tongue, are fully innervated over the next weeks. The fetus is known to suck and swallow in utero[51]; sucking is discussed in Chapter 8.

When taste becomes a factor in feeding is not known, although a lack of discrimination has been noted in the first weeks of life: infants have consumed formula with high salt or absence of chloride with morbid results.[19] Because of the variation in the composition of mother's milk over a feeding, over a day, and from time to time according to maternal dietary intake, the breastfed infant has had a richer range of experience in tasting than the formula fed infant. Breastfed infants are therefore more accustomed to new taste experiences. Similarly, feeding problems in infants are rare in breastfed infants.

Both sucking and chewing are complex movements, having reflexive as well as learned components. The development of the chew-swallow reflex is necessary for the successful introduction of solids. Schmitz and McNeish[60] hypothesized that this skill develops sequentially with neuronal development, and then is a learned behavior conditioned by oral stimulation. Before this point, when a spoon is introduced, the infant purses the lips and pushes the tongue against the spoon. By 4 to 6 months, the tongue is depressed in response to the spoon and the food accepted, and by 7 to 9 months, rhythmic biting movements occur regardless of the presence of teeth. Biting and masticatory strength and efficiency progress throughout infancy. If a stimulus is not applied when the neural development is taking place, Merchant[51] believes that the chewing reflex will not develop and the infant will always be a poor chewer. There is a relationship between prolonged sucking without solids and poor eating. The clinical model for this is the child sustained on parenteral feedings or gastrostomy beyond a year who has tremendous difficulty accepting solids.

For the human infant, nursing also plays a role as a comfort and emotional support, a mechanism often referred to as "comfort nursing." Inadequate nipple contact may lead to thumb sucking or the substitute use of a pacifier. Young monkeys and apes in the wild do not suck their thumbs, but they do in captivity when bottle fed.[29] Infants of the !Kung tribe in Africa do not suck their thumbs.[13] They are carried and breastfed in frequent short bursts.

In summary, the infant is ready to explore new feeding experiences at around 6 months. Feeding is an important social as well as nutritional encounter. Eating solids and learning to drink from a cup are important social achievements as well. This readiness does not mean the infant is taken from the breast, but that the diet is expanded and now includes solid foods, other liquids, and breast milk. Although there are a range of qualitative, quantitative, and temporal practices, the optimal approach matches the needs and requirements of a given child with the functions and capacities of the body.

Introduction of solids

The World Health Organization (WHO), the Canadian Pediatric Society, the Paediatric Society of New Zealand, and similar groups in England and Scotland[7,74] emphasize that weaning is not the termination of breastfeeding but the addition of solids while continuing breastfeeding. The key recommendation on length of exclusive breastfeeding reads as follows:

> to strengthen activities and develop new approaches to protect, promote and support exclusive breastfeeding for six months as a global public health recommendation, taking into account the findings of the WHO expert consultation on optimal duration of exclusive breastfeeding, and to provide safe and appropriate complementary foods, with continued breastfeeding for up to two years of age or beyond, emphasizing channels of social dissemination of these concepts in order to lead communities to adhere to these practices.[74]

The Subcommittee on Nutrition during Lactation of the National Academy of Sciences[66] points out that the intake of supplementary foods may add nutrients in a less bioavailable form, decrease the bioavailability of nutrients in human milk, and decrease the intake of other important factors in human milk. Investigators have shown that when solid foods are introduced in the diet of breastfed infants, energy intake per kilogram of body weight does not increase.[54] Solid foods displaced energy intake from human milk in 6-month-old infants even though they were breastfed on demand.

The duration for which exclusive breastfeeding is adequate was studied in a cohort of infants in Amman, Jordan, a well-nourished community.[33] The norms used for comparison were those determined by Fomon in the United States in 1974 using well-nourished formula fed infants and indicated 4 to 6 months as the maximum time for exclusive breastfeeding. If these data are compared with information collected by Dewey and associates[14] in 1994 on well-nourished breastfed infants, no "faltering" in growth pattern would be identified. In a review of protein and energy during weaning, Axelsson and Räihä[2] conclude that 1.65 g/kg/day from 5 to 9 months and 1.48 g/kg/day from 9 to 12 months are appropriate. Dewey and associates[16] reported that growth of exclusively breastfed infants from 4 to 6 months of age matched or exceeded that of randomly selected breastfed infants given 20% added protein. The exclusively breastfed group received 0.98 g/kg/day, whereas the supplemented group received 1.18 g/kg/day. Thus, protein intake is not a limiting factor with respect to growth that would mandate weaning from the breast. On review of protein requirements for infants and children established by WHO in 1985, Dewey and associates[16] determined they were higher than necessary for the breastfed infant. Formula fed infants require more protein because of comparatively poor utilization.[10]

Recommendations for the optimal time to introduce complementary foods to the breastfed infant remain controversial. The Section on Breastfeeding of the American Academy of Pediatrics (AAP) supports the introduction of solids at 6 months in concert with the WHO and UNICEF. This choice was in response to a systematic review of all published reports in developed and underdeveloped countries conducted by Kramer and Kakuma[44] that included controlled clinical trials and observational studies in all languages. From a total of 2668 reports, only 36 citations met criteria of an internal comparison group. Rigorous assessment of health outcomes included growth, iron and zinc status, infectious morbidity, atopic disease, neuromotor development, rate of maternal weight loss, and duration of lactational amenorrhea.

In summary, exclusive breastfeeding for 6 months supported appropriate gain in weight and length, adequate iron and zinc status when mother is well nourished, reduced infection rates, some reduction in atopy, and a significant advantage in achieving some developmental milestones. The important conclusion reached by WHO-UNICEF is the recommendation of exclusive breastfeeding for 6 months. In a report to be published in *Pediatrics* in 2005, the Committee on Breastfeeding of the AAP continues to recommend 6 months.[47]

The duration for which the iron endowment at birth remains adequate varies, so some infants will benefit from additional iron at 4 to 6 months.[15] The data on zinc are meager. The concentrations of zinc in milk decline after the first few months of lactation and are independent of maternal zinc intake.[45] Hepatic stores will sustain levels in the infant, but exogenous zinc will be required and is most readily obtained from meat.

Breastfed infants self-regulate their total energy intake when other foods are introduced, reported Cohen and associates,[9] who further comment that there is no advantage to introducing complementary foods before 6 months and that there may even be disadvantages. A review by Foote and Marriott[20] expresses the concern that some infants might need additional nutrients. They point out that the energy density of the food should exceed that of breast milk (4.2 kJ/g or 0.55 to 0.80 kcal/g). They also warn that foods with high phytate levels can interfere with mineral absorption and recommend the avoidance of juices and other drinks. Giving infants solids by 4 months is associated with less positive health outcomes such as increased body fat, higher body mass index, and a greater incidence of wheezing and respiratory illness in childhood, according to Fewtrell and associates.[18]

When iron was added to the diet at 4 months by giving iron-rich solids to infants who did not have iron deficiency anemia, the length growth was less than in unsupplemented control infants. Head growth was also slower in iron-supplemented infants. There was no improvement in weight gain, and the treated infants had more diarrhea if their hemoglobin levels were normal.[15] More boys than girls had iron deficiency anemia at 9 months according to Dewey and associates.[15]

In the study of nutrient intakes and food choices of 3000 infants and toddlers participating in the Feeding Infants and Toddlers Study (FITS), there were 450 Women, Infants and Children nutrition program (WIC) participants. It was observed that WIC infants were less likely to have ever been breastfed and were more likely to be taking formula.[55] The mean usual intake of nutrients exceeded adequate intakes. Mean energy intake was excessive with little consumption of fruits and vegetables. In the entire study of 3000 infants, 76% were fully or partially breastfed at birth, dropping to 30% at 6 months and to 16% at 1 year. Average duration of breastfeeding was 5.5 months. From 4 to 6 months, over 65% had been given solids, not all of which were nutrient dense. Sweetened juices, French fries, hot dogs, potato chips, popcorn, pizza, and candy were reported in up to 9% of infants aged 7 to 8 months old.

The infant's first flavor experiences probably occur in utero. When garlic was ingested by mothers before amniocentesis or delivery, the amniotic fluid smelled of garlic.[50] The normal fetus ingests amniotic fluid in utero and thus experiences those flavors. When breastfed, the infant continues to experience those flavors as a bridging experience to solid foods.[49] Not surprisingly, breastfed infants consume cereal prepared with their mother's milk more eagerly and in greater volume than when it is prepared with water. In a carefully controlled experiment, infants were fed the cereals by their mothers, who wore facial masks but no perfume to avoid affecting the infant's interest in the food.[50] The infant's interest was reflected in opening of the mouth sooner, fewer negative facial expressions, and greater intake. Mennella and Beauchamp[50] suggest that from the perspective of flavors, weaning means "to accustom," which actually describes what occurs with breastfeeding: The flavors in the milk accustom the infant to new flavors in the transition to solid foods. Putting mother's milk in the bland cereal is part of the bridging. Infants whose mothers have a more varied diet during pregnancy and lactation tend to adapt to solid foods more readily, according to these investigations.

Weaning to a cup is a natural transfer because infants learn to drink from a cup by 7 to 9 months. The use of fruit juice in the cup was originally encouraged for its vitamin C content. Fruit juice may be replacing milk, however, in the diets of young children.[12] This is a concern because milk is an important source of protein and calcium, whereas nutrients in fruit juices are limited predominantly to carbohydrates, calories, and varying amounts of vitamin C. Juices are also replacing fruit in the diet. Excessive fruit juice consumption reportedly leads to short stature and failure to thrive in some infants, chronic diarrhea in some, and obesity in others.[48] The trend often begins when fruit juice is put in a nursing bottle. The pediatrician should be alert to the exact content of the weaning foods, ensuring adequate protein, calcium, vitamins, and fiber, as well as the development of feeding skills, including feeding from a cup and from a spoon.

MOTHERS' RIGHTS

In practice, human mothers are often the determinants of weaning time, as is true for other species. Some mothers want to nurse for a few weeks and wean to a bottle to go to work. Other mothers wean at 3 months to be free again.[52,53] Certainly any time spent breastfeeding is to the infant's advantage. The critical point in weaning is to make it a gradual adjustment for both mother and infant. The year 2010 health goals for the United States recommend that mothers nurse exclusively for at least 6 months,[70] continuing while adding weaning foods until 1 year and then for as long thereafter as mother and child wish.

A study of the psychosocial factors influencing weaning time in primigravidas was conducted when the 81 participants were 8 months post partum.[37] Maternal worries about the demands of breastfeeding had a negative effect on the duration. If mothers worried about the demands of breastfeeding, they were more likely to perceive problems with scheduling breastfeeding when they returned to work. Mothers who worried about lack of family support to breastfeed were more apt to worry about the demands of breastfeeding. Those women who saw the practical advantages of breastfeeding did not perceive returning to work as presenting a problem and nursed longer. Medical

illness, sore nipples, fatigue, or breast infections were not influential in weaning. Work and scheduling have a larger role in most mothers' decision to wean.[32]

WEANING PROCESS

Gradually replacing one feeding at a time with solids or a bottle or cup, depending on the infant's age and stage of development, is usually preferable.[3] After the adjustment has been made to one substitute feeding, a second feeding is replaced with a substitute, usually at the opposite time of day. This process is continued until only the morning and night feedings remain. Then these two are gradually stopped. The morning and night feedings can be maintained for some months, and often an infant is nursed well beyond the second year, especially at these times. Mothers who wish to wean partially as early as 3 months may continue the morning and night nursing. This schedule is especially suited to the working mother. The decline in lactation and the regression of the mammary gland occur slowly with gradual weaning.

When an infant is fully breastfeeding and solids are initiated, a feeding of solids is given during the day and breastfeeding continues on demand. As solids are increased and a three-meals-a-day schedule is reached, breastfeeding still continues on demand, although nursings may be fewer or briefer. No nursings need be intentionally omitted in this scheme, although it is important to give the scheduled solids before breastfeeding the infant.

The composition of milk during abrupt weaning, carefully analyzed by Hartmann and Kulski,[28] revealed that the secretory capability of the mammary gland of women changed dramatically after complete cessation of breastfeeding but that the involuting gland remained partially functional for 45 days. After termination that occurred in 1 day, sample collections were attempted for each breast by manual expression at the same time on days 1, 2, 4, 8, 16, 21, 31, 42, and 45. The concentrations of lactose and potassium decreased, while sodium, chloride, fat, and total protein increased progressively over 42 days. The milk becomes notably salty. Infants continue to drink the salty fluid.[19] The increase in protein was related to increases in the concentrations of lactoferrin, immunoglobulin A (IgA), IgG, IgM, albumin, lactalbumin, and casein. Concentrations from each breast were similar throughout. One woman in the study breastfed for 39 days; six women fully lactated an average of 332 days (range of 251 to 443 days).

The involution in other species is rapid. For example, complete reabsorption occurs in 7 days in cows. Caldeyro-Barcia[6] showed that the threshold dose of oxytocin required to elicit milk ejection increased progressively for at least 30 days after termination of breastfeeding. It is believed that a psychological nursing stimulus contributes to this effect in humans because they continue contact with their infants, whereas other species are separated. Experimental animals given oxytocin after weaning also show a delay in involution.

Weaning ages and techniques in a sample of American women who practiced extended breastfeeding were reported by Sugarman and Kendall-Tackett.[67] Women were recruited from La Leche League meetings in the area and nationally utilizing survey forms (closed-end, self-administered 96-item questionnaires originally trialed in 1974). The weaning age (representing 134 mothers and 211 children) ranged from 1 month to 7 years 4 months. For those who weaned three children, as well as the entire sample, the tendency was to nurse the youngest the longest, perhaps because it was not supplanted by a sibling.

Reasons for weaning were predominantly child-led for about 60% of children, but weaning was the mother's decision in up to 15.8% in the youngest child (Table 10-1). Those who were still nursing responded to the question, "Have you thought about weaning this child?" predominantly with a "no" (Table 10-2).[67]

TABLE 10-1   Reasons for weaning and types of methods

	Child A* (*n* = 25)	Child B* (*n* = 125)	Child C* (*n* = 69)
Reasons for weaning (%)			
Lack of information	5.3	4.2	8.7
Lack of support or opposition	2.6	4.2	8.7
Next pregnancy affected taste or supply of milk	7.9	14.3	8.7
Next pregnancy affected mother's motivation	5.3	21.8	24.6
Illness or separation from child	5.3	5.9	11.6
Child-led, happened naturally	63.2	57.1	52.2
Mother's decision that child was ready	158.0	13.4	10.1
Mother's decision based on family circumstance	7.9	5.0	4.3
Other	0.0	5.9	1.4
How weaning was accomplished (mean %)			
Sudden	12.8	7.6	8.8
Gradual	56.4	60.2	45.6
Child-led	53.3	56.7	54.1
Mother deliberately weaned	2.6	11.0	13.2
Mother encouraged weaning by talking to child	23.1	31.4	20.6
Substituted thumb, pacifier	2.6	3.4	1.5
Other	1.7	1.8	1.7
Number of reasons (mean)	1.8	1.8	1.7

*A, B, and C represent three consecutive children, child A being the youngest.

From Sugarman M, Kendall-Tackett KA: Weaning ages in a sample of American women who practice extended breastfeeding. Clin Pediatr 34:642, 1995.

TABLE 10-2 Reasons for weaning or not weaning ("Have you thought about weaning this child?")

Response	Frequency (%)
No, weaning should be child-led	75.9
No, enjoy the nursing relationship	72.3
Yes, for a specific reason (pregnancy, returning to work)	4.8
Yes, child is ready/child is biting	7.8
Yes, due to social pressure	3.6
Yes, child is nursing too frequently for age	3.6

From Sugarman M, Kendall-Tackett KA: Weaning ages in a sample of American women who practice extended breastfeeding. Clin Pediatr 34:642, 1995.

The normal, well-adjusted mother may experience some depression and sadness at the reality of the last feeding.[59] It may be very difficult to face this experience. It is important to recognize this as a physiologic phenomenon as well as an emotional one. If a mother is forced by circumstances beyond her control to wean early, she may need much understanding and encouragement to cope with the disappointment. If she has had pressure from friends or relatives to breastfeed, she may need to face what she considers failure and recognize that one can bottle feed and still mother very well.

Historically, weaning has varied from strict to permissive schedules depending upon cultural norms.[11] Rigid feeding schedules were associated with early weaning.[7] Weaning has varied from early strict denial to slow and gentle withdrawal. In the 20th century the time considered proper for weaning gradually shortened from 2 or 3 or 4 years to as soon as 6 to 8 months, or less for some mothers and infants. Public opinion has overlooked the infant's needs in favor of what are considered the mother's rights. It is not necessary to have clearly in mind a specific plan for weaning in the early weeks of nursing unless there are some constraints on the mother's time. Weaning should be done with the infant's needs as a guide.[25] If an infant under 1 year

of age rejects the breast, it is unusual but not abnormal and should not be considered by the mother as a personal rejection. Some bottle fed infants throw down the bottle at 9 months as well.

Studies of weaning practices are few. In a study of primigravidas, they introduced solids because their infant seemed hungry and less satisfied and woke more frequently. The average time to introduce nonmilk food in bottle fed infants was 3 months and in breastfed infants, 5 months. Most observations are done on duration of feeding when the success rate is low. Jackson and associates[40] studied weaning times in mothers participating in a rooming-in project from 1942 to 1951 as compared with mothers who received traditional postpartum care at the New Haven Hospital during the same period. Rooming-in meant mother and infant were together in a special postpartum unit designed to accommodate both mothers and infants who were managed as a pair by the same nursing staff. Infants were with their mothers as much as each mother wished. The rooming-in mothers nursed significantly longer.[39] They averaged 3.5 to 3.8 months, whereas the control mothers weaned at 1.8 to 2.5 months post partum. The incidence of breastfeeding decreased as the difficulty of the delivery increased. The number who breastfed their infants did not differ by age, education, or race. Older mothers, better-educated mothers, and black mothers who breastfed, however, nursed longer in this study in 1950.

The reasons given why women in Dunedin, New Zealand, elected to wean their infants early included concern about their milk supply and other maternal problems.[34] One of the most significant factors in lactation termination was mismanagement of breastfeeding by health professionals. A similar study in Sweden reported that 66% of the mothers weaned because they thought their milk was drying up.[63]

Sousa and associates[64] studied the patterns of weaning in southern Brazil. Brazil was also experiencing a decline in breastfeeding. The study was undertaken to understand the causes of early weaning to develop better means of encouraging longer breastfeeding and delaying weaning. The bottle was introduced at birth by 24% of women, at 2 months by 72.6%, and at 6 months by 88.0%.

Table 10-3 lists the main reasons given for weaning. A third of the mothers believed their milk was weak. Gunn[28] believed these data supported the hypothesis that the mothers did not understand the value of human milk and were influenced by advertisements about formulas and therefore compared their milk with formulas. In general, most studies of weaning practices indicated that most weaning is mother initiated, most often because she thinks her milk is no longer adequate. The primary cause of failing milk supply reported by most investigators is inadequate help or instructions about milk production from medical personnel. In a study of 750 mother-baby dyads, Howard and associates[35] showed a clear relationship to early weaning and decreased exclusive breastfeeding and the early introduction of a pacifier. In most studies, those who breastfeed longer tend to be older than 25 years, well-educated, middle class, and self-educated about lactation and to enjoy breastfeeding.[26]

The problem of recall bias when reporting breastfeeding duration was investigated by Huttly and associates,[37] who compared responses given at 11, 23, and 47 months post partum by the mothers of 1000 children; 24% misclassified weaning time at 23 months and 30% at 4 years. Those in the better-educated, higher socioeconomic group were more apt to report longer breastfeeding.

In worldwide epidemiologic studies, Edmonston[17] pointed out that interruption of breastfeeding because of pregnancy may play a significant role. He estimated the mean monthly bias introduced was to reduce breastfeeding by 2 months. In Third World countries, infant death also lowers the duration of breastfeeding inversely to the mother's education; that is, the less educated the mother, the greater the risk of infant death from infection and accident.

Why women wean

Using the National Survey of Family Growth to analyze breastfeeding behaviors of a national probability sample of 6733 first-time U.S. mothers from 15 to 44 years of age, Taylor and associates found 3267 women who breastfed.[68] Among these women 46%, 68%, 78%, and 85% had weaned by 3, 6, 9, and 12 months, respectively. The reason 1091 women stopped was because their infant was "old enough to wean." This reason was claimed by 15%, 34%, and 78% at the same 3-month intervals. White and Hispanic women had similar weaning patterns. For black women who stopped because their child was "old enough to wean," greater numbers weaned sooner (22%, 46%, 68%, and 86% stopped at 3, 6, 9, and 12 months, respectively).

Physical and medical problems were the next most common reasons (26.9%), followed with "job or schedule" (only 17.9%), and "preferred to bottle feed" (15.3%) (Table 10-4). Differences by race revealed black women stopped because they "preferred to bottle feed." Hispanic women had a few more infants who refused the breast (3.7%) compared to black women (0.5%) and white women (2.1%).

Infant-initiated weaning

Infant-initiated weaning in the first year of life was investigated by Clarke and Harmon,[8] who studied 50 healthy breastfed infants who were totally

TABLE 10-3 **Main reasons for premature weaning**

Reason	N	%
Not enough, inadequate, or "weak" milk	307	30.9
Child refused breast	177	17.8
Illness of child	159	16.0
Mother needed to go to work	149	15.0
"Correct age for bottle feeding"	139	14.0
Other reasons	64	6.3
Total	995	100.0

From Gunn TR: The incidence of breastfeeding and the reasons for weaning. NZ Med J 97:360, 1984.

TABLE 10-4 Reasons women stopped breastfeeding their first child ($n = 3267$)*

Reason	Race/ethnicity				Hispanic vs. white		Black vs. white	
	Total sample (%)	Hispanic (%)	Black (%)	White (%)	Unadjusted OR (95% CI)†	Adjusted OR (95% CI)†‡	Unadjusted OR (95% CI)†	Adjusted OR (95% CI)†‡
Baby old enough to wean	35.7	34.7	30.4	37.0	1.00	1.00	1.00	1.00
Job/schedule	17.9	14.9	17.5	19.0	0.70 (0.52–0.94)	1.04 (0.77–1.42)	1.01 (0.70–1.47)	1.10 (0.74–1.65)
Physical/medical problem	26.9	25.6	23.6	27.9	0.87 (0.66–1.15)	0.61 (0.44–0.85)	0.97 (0.68–1.38)	0.75 (0.52–1.08)
Preferred to bottle feed	15.3	20.2	25.8	11.8	1.62 (1.20–2.18)	1.17 (0.85–1.62)	2.80 (1.96–3.99)	2.18 (1.55–3.05)
Baby refused	2.2	3.7	0.5	2.1	1.86 (1.00–3.46)	1.86 (1.05–3.30)	0.18 (0.04–0.86)	0.16 (0.03–0.82)

CI, confidence interval; NSFG, National Survey of Family Growth; OR, odds ratio.

*The 90 women who were still breastfeeding at the time of the interview and the 131 women who categorized their race as "other" (211 in total, as 10 women were in both groups) were not included in the analyses. The 25 women (0.8%) who answered "other" as a reason for not breastfeeding (including the baby's father or someone else discouraged breastfeeding, fears about breastfeeding, and other) were not included in the analyses. The reference group is always women who stopped breastfeeding because the baby was "old enough to wean" (final $n = 3000$).

†NSFG sampling weights applied.

‡Adjusted for maternal demographics (age, race, marital status, education, poverty level).

weaned; 46% of the group of infants initiated the weaning. This is often mistakenly referred to as "self-weaning." The onset was usually between 5 and 9 months of age, with a median age of 6 months. Mothers described the behavior as an increased interest in exploring the environment and in other foods and a decreased interest in breastfeeding. Brazelton[4] described a similar phenomenon and reported three stages in the first year during which the infant exhibits a lagging interest in breastfeeding as a direct or indirect result of developmental events: 4 to 5 months, 7 months, and 9 to 12 months.

The duration of infant-initiated weaning is about 1 month and is an interactive process that requires "at a minimum maternal complicity." It can lead to relatively easy mutual weaning. It can usually be reversed, however, by the mother's efforts to continue breastfeeding.

Emergency weaning

Occasionally, sudden weaning is necessary because of severe illness in the mother or some prolonged separation of mother and infant. (Sudden illness in the infant does not require weaning, and, in fact, weaning, would be contraindicated.) This is difficult for both. After abrupt weaning the mammary glands remain partially functional for more than a month.

Depending on the infant's age and flexibility, a patient "surrogate mother" may need to provide a feeding or two by bottle to switch the infant to a bottle in abrupt weaning, as the nursing mother will be unsuccessful. In other cases the infant may take only solids and refuse other liquids for days. The mother in the meantime may have considerable discomfort. Engorgement may be significant if it is only 4 to 6 weeks post partum. The mother may experience *milk fever* at any time there is abrupt weaning. This illness is characterized by fever, chills, and malaise, resembling a flulike syndrome. It is believed to be caused by the sudden reabsorption of milk products into the system. Milk fever usually lasts 3 to 4 days and should not be confused with more serious illness.

The hormonal change resulting from sudden weaning early in lactation is more definitive because the prolactin levels from suckling are higher immediately post partum (see Chapter 3). The hormone-withdrawal syndrome may be more marked with early weaning. Prolactin has been associated with a feeling of well-being; thus, its decrease may be associated with relative depression. Patients with psychiatric disorders have been observed to cope post partum until they wean the infant from the breast. It is important to provide an adequate social and medical support system during weaning for the mother who is prone to depression or psychiatric problems.

Refusal to breastfeed: "nursing strike"

Sudden onset of refusal to nurse can occur at any time and often is taken as a personal rejection by the mother, who promptly follows through by weaning completely. Often these mothers consider the refusal to mean that they do not have enough milk or that something is wrong with their milk. This behavior has been called "nursing strike" and has been noted to be temporary.[20] The various causes associated with this abrupt behavior include the following:

1. Onset of menses in the mother
2. Dietary indiscretion by the mother
3. Change in maternal soap, perfume, or deodorant
4. Stress in the mother
5. Earache or nasal obstruction in the infant
6. Teething
7. Episode of biting with startle and pain reaction by the mother

If a reason is identified that is possibly associated and can be changed, nursing should resume. It may take extra effort to reestablish the relationship. Suggestions that may be made to the mother include the following:

1. Make feeding special and quiet, with no distractions and no other people in the room.
2. Increase amount of cuddling, stroking, and soothing the baby. Walk with the infant cradled in the arms or an infant sling.

3. Offer the breast when the infant is very sleepy.
4. Do not starve the child into submission.
5. If simple remedial steps do not result in a return to nursing, the physician should see the child to rule out otitis media, fever, infection, thrush, and so on.
6. If biting was the associated event, keep finger ready to break suction should it occur again to avoid startling the infant.

Weanling diarrhea and malnutrition

Most writings on weaning refer to the problems in underdeveloped countries when infants are weaned early to overdiluted cow milk or to artificial formulas that do not contain the antiinfective properties of human milk for the human infant.[62] Weanling diarrhea is well described by Gordon and associates[24] as the clinical syndrome (weanling diarrhea is a collection of diseases) associated with weaning from the breast. In 1900 in New York City, the death rate from dysentery, diarrhea, and enteritis in children in the first year of life was 5603 in 100,000 infants. This was largely attributed to weaning from the breast. Diarrheas are strongly associated with weaning not only because of the introduction of other foods but also because of the loss of the protective properties of human milk.

The diarrheas contribute to the malnutrition seen in underdeveloped countries because of the resultant lack of appetite and increased metabolic losses. In Third World countries, morbidity and mortality rates in infancy rise sharply at the time of weaning from human milk because of the rapid onset of infections. Malnutrition is also a major threat to the weanling in the developing world.[57] Rickets, iron deficiency, and protein energy malnutrition are the three major threats. Close behind are the risks of zinc deficiency, allergy, and obesity, which affect a wider group of children.[71]

In well-nourished mothers and their infants, diarrhea does not occur from controlled gradual weaning unless the infant has a cow milk allergy or metabolic disorder.

Changes in milk composition during gradual weaning

Changes in the nutrient composition of human milk during gradual weaning were studied by Garza and associates[22] in six fully lactating women recruited at 5 to 7 months post partum (Table 10-5). The weaning consisted of decreasing the frequency and duration of breastfeeding by one third each month for a period of 3 months. Milk was collected at 2-week intervals. Volume decreased to 67%, 40%, and 20% of baseline each month. The concentrations of protein and sodium were increased to 142% and 220% of baseline, respectively, by the

TABLE 10-5	Nutrient density (mg/100 kcal) of milk during weaning								
	Week								
	0	**2**	**4**	**6**	**8**	**10**	**12**	**PTM***	**R†**
Protein	1.5	1.2	1.3	1.0	1.3	1.2	1.9	1.8	2.7
Na	24.0	17.0	20.0	13.0	24.0	25.0	46.0	25.0	53.0
Ca	38.0	30.0	33.0	21.0	30.0	26.0	38.0	34.5	140.0
Zn	0.21	0.17	0.19	0.09	0.10	0.10	0.11	3.8	0.5

PTM, preterm milk; R, rate

*Nutrient densities of milk from women who deliver premature infants.

†Nutrient densities calculated to achieve intrauterine growth rates assuming that the caloric requirement of low-birth-weight infants is 130 kcal/kg.

From Garza C, Johnson CA, Smith E, et al: Changes in the nutrient composition of human milk during gradual weaning. Am J Clin Nutr 37:61, 1983.

12th week of weaning. Changes in fat composition were linear through the 10th week but at the 12th week were similar to baseline. Iron was increased 172%, calcium was unchanged, and zinc fell to 58%. Similar observations have been made in bovine milk. Milk produced during either rapid or gradual weaning is characterized by a decreasing concentration of lactose. Fat accounts for an increasing percentage of calories (up 80%) and protein remains stable at 6% of calories.

The immunologic components in human milk were also measured, and the concentrations of certain components of the immunologic system are maintained during gradual weaning.[23] The effect of gradual weaning differs from that of abrupt weaning, in which the concentrations of all components rise dramatically. Measurements at 4 weeks, 8 weeks, and 12 weeks showed a decrease in the milk volume of 67%, 40%, and 20% as the levels of IgA and secretory IgA rose slightly. Lysozyme and lactoferrin rose slightly. The total intake of protective factors is stable temporarily (increased concentration in spite of decreased volume).

Lipase activities in human milk during weaning were studied by Freed and associates.[21] Bile salt-stimulated lipase (BSSL) slowly decreased throughout weaning, whereas lipoprotein lipase (LPL) became substantially lower or absent as compared with colostrum. Lipase activity continues but decreases with the decrease in milk volume.

Studies in other species suggest that gut maturation observed at normal weaning time is not dependent on components in the milk but is triggered by thyroxine and corticosterone in the plasma of the offspring.[31] The anatomic changes in the breast during weaning are discussed in Chapter 2.

The caloric needs for infants have been overestimated in the past. Continued growth occurs on lower volumes of human milk than formula, with breastfed infants refusing additional milk even when a woman increases her volume by pumping.[56] The energy requirement is 115 kcal/kg/day in the first 2 months of life, after which requirements decline rapidly, reaching a low of 85 kcal/kg/day at 6 months. Between 6 and 12 months of age, requirements gradually increase with increased activity to 100 kcal/kg/day. These figures are a radical departure from those recommended in the past.[73] Most studies of energy intakes show, at all ages, that boys have greater intake and greater rates of growth than girls and are usually weaned sooner.[69] Further, the effects of infection and social deprivation are important to consider; children in supportive, loving environments have been noted to grow on fewer calories than the deprived child.

Physician's role

The physician's responsibility in weaning is to advise the mother concerning the initiation of the appropriate solid foods, which probably should begin at 6 months of age and usually not before.

Introduction of a cup as a developmental step should usually begin by 7 months.

Eating finger foods and learning self-feeding are the next steps for the child.

None of the above means the termination of breastfeeding but rather the gradual developmental progression of feeding. Breastfeeding continues "on demand." As other foods are introduced and feeding begins to cluster into three meals and some "snacks," breastfeedings will be decreased eventually to two or three per day in the second year.

The nourishment value is not a key issue of continued nursing after 1 year if other foods are adequate, although very valuable nutrition and immunoprotection continue to be provided.[62] The physician's role is to ensure adequate nutrition and be available for advice for as long as breastfeeding continues.

There is no known detriment to nursing, and some indication that nursing a few times a day or during times of stress is beneficial to the mother-infant relationship, when the child is over a year of age. The objections raised are usually based on custom or personal taste. It is important for the clinician to avoid judgmental counseling based only on personal biases. Lay publications on the subject may help guide the mother who is nursing a toddler.

The physician may need to help the mother work through her own feelings about nursing her infant beyond the first year. Many women have been overwhelmed by friendly advice from lay experts about the infant who nurses for several years. Beyond a year, weaning is rarely child initiated until age 4. The child may not lose interest, so that the final steps in termination may require maternal intervention if weaning is desired sooner. A mother is not a poor parent if she begins to feel resentful toward nursing. Planning appropriate alternatives to the breastfeeding session that is to be eliminated is helpful in turning the child's attention toward the new event instead of toward the loss of an old and cherished one, a feeding at the breast. The mother may need to be helped to see how to avoid situations that easily predispose to nursing. She needs to know that it is acceptable to set some rules and to have some limitations and control over the breastfeeding.

If the mother becomes pregnant, she should decide when she wants to wean or whether she will continue to nurse through pregnancy and then tandem-nurse the new baby (see Chapter 19). For the child, it is important to avoid abrupt weaning or weaning to make room for the new baby, who will now take the child's place. Weaning well before delivery is usually less traumatic for the child than at delivery time. At delivery, however, the new infant is fed first to assure that the newborn receives adequate colostrum.

Motivation to wean

The motivation to wean the infant may be multifactorial and often is suggested by the father, grandmother, or members of the mother's social circle. The physician should not initiate the plan to wean except for medical reasons but may initiate discussion about it, to ensure that the mother has given it some thought.

Reasons for weaning have been analyzed by a number of investigators.[57] Factor analysis of a longitudinal database was done by Kirkland and Fein.[43] Mother's concern about her milk supply, wanting to leave the infant, and wanting someone else to feed the infant were the major reasons for weaning in this group from 6 to 12 months post partum. Concern about the appropriate age for breastfeed-

ing cessation was a prominent concern toward the later months. Parents may find nursing an older baby or a toddler distasteful. Mothers are encouraged to anticipate and plan for weaning; it can be gradual, taking advantage of developmental progress and new interests of the toddler. It is wise to avoid associating sleeping with a feeding as the time to wean approaches, or it may be more difficult to make the break. The father can play a vital role in nonnutritive cuddling, beginning from birth, and can be especially helpful in easing an infant through weaning, particularly when night feedings have become the custom. Not all parents perceive weaning, night feedings, and bringing an infant to the parents' bed in the same light. Not all physicians view these matters equally, but they should avoid imposing personal views on patients. The family bed and co-sleeping practices are discussed in Chapter 6.

With regard to weaning in developing countries, the decision was thought to be made on the basis of traditional beliefs, nutritional status of the child, or similar reasons. When the reasons for termination were studied in West Africa, however, illness in the child, a new pregnancy, and illness in the mother were found to be the most common precipitating events.[41] Health workers should be aware of this in order to counsel mothers appropriately.

CLOSET NURSING

The physician should be fully informed about breastfeeding physiologically and psychologically. The trusted physician communicates well with patients and is kept informed by the parents. Unfortunately, many mothers are driven to "closet nursing" by insensitive, uninformed relatives and friends and even health care providers. Closet nursing is nursing privately at home in secret. The practice propagates ignorance about breastfeeding duration and influences not only other mothers but also physicians who are unaware and custody court judges who are led to believe extended nursing is abnormal. Thousands of normal, healthy children are breastfed until they are 3 or 4 years old. The benefits of human milk continue. Research documents health protection and improved development for at least 2 years. It has not been evaluated beyond that except for the positive emotional and bonding experience associated with long-term nursing.[42,57,59,67] Although not necessarily common in the United States, worldwide, breastfeeding a child beyond 2 years is in no way abnormal.

WORKING MOTHERS

Some mothers return to work. Whether the reason is money, career, or personal satisfaction is not relevant to management. It takes tremendous commitment to work and breastfeed, but it can be done, it has been done, and it will be done. Usually the biggest problem a mother faces is coping with people who do not understand why she bothers. An understanding physician who provides the reassurance and support necessary to manage is a great asset. A mother may go home for a feeding in the middle of the day, pump milk to leave for the infant to have from a bottle, or give a substitute bottle. If there are occasional bottles of formula, the powder preparations are more economical and require only warming the water before adding the powder to ensure rapid solution. Chapter 21 offers suggestions for collecting milk.

Some infants quickly learn the mother's schedule and will sleep while she is away and feed more frequently during the evening and night to make up for it. It takes some personal adjustment to plan ahead and a babysitter who is patient and cooperative. Many infants are tended in daycare centers, which requires packing up and transporting the infant to other surroundings.

A mother needs to be alert to the infant's needs as well and can plan to leave feedings ready when she is away, even if she had hoped the infant would sleep through the day. If a mother works long hours or has an inflexible schedule, it may be necessary to wean the infant to morning and night feedings at the breast. This arrangement still provides the special benefits of human milk as well as the closeness

that an infant needs; thus, it is worth the effort. Chapter 13 discusses maternal employment.

LEGAL ISSUES

In the present turmoil of family life in which parents are separating when the children are still young, several custody cases have been based on weaning times or, more accurately, on the time breastfeeding is totally terminated. A number of cases in the United States have come to the attention of the Study Center in which the father has sought custody on the basis of prolonged breastfeeding, when the child nursed for comfort to about age 4. In most cases the judge found in favor of the mother. In one case in Rochester, NY, the judge found in favor of the father when an expert witness, a local psychologist, declared that "you have to be crazy to nurse that long." No amount of scientific evidence could counter this inappropriate remark.

Other issues of parental rights have surfaced in cases of child custody and visitation rights when the child is under 2 years of age and breastfeeding. Usually the argument over separation of mother from her breastfeeding infant is part of a larger problem. Physicians called on to give expert testimony need to review carefully all the issues because rarely is the breastfeeding question the only problem. Right and wrong have not been established for all circumstances. It would seem appropriate also that judges review the entire case and qualifications of the respective parents and refrain from basing their decision on personal biases and emotional testimony. It is also advisable for expert witnesses to be fully informed on a subject about which they will testify and to avoid extending their comments beyond their area of expertise.

Developmental psychologist Ainsworth[1] has studied the maturation of the child and summarized the literature, which shows that infants with a strong attachment to their mothers through breastfeeding are psychologically independent at 2 years of age. These children have more mastery of themselves at age 5 and less anxiety entering school than bottle fed children.

WHY DON'T SOME WOMEN BREASTFEED?

Given the tremendous benefits to mother and infant of breastfeeding, why do some women choose not to breastfeed? Studies in our laboratory in the 1990s among young WIC women prenatally indicated that although they knew that mother's milk was best and why, they did not plan to breastfeed because there were too many rules. Prenatal classes about infant feeding given at WIC made formula feeding look easy and breastfeeding complicated. These complications began with dietary restrictions, moved to hand grips and body positions, and ended with all the limitations about alcohol, caffeine, and medications. They found it overwhelming and certainly not physiologic or natural.

Taking the data from the National Survey of Family Growth to analyze the breastfeeding behaviors of a national probability sample of 6733 first-time mothers, aged 15 to 44 years, Taylor and associates measured the reasons for never breastfeeding.[68] The most common reason mothers gave was "preferred to bottle feed" (66.3%). The next most common reason was a "physical or medical problem" (14.9%). For women giving physical or medical problem as the reason, no one problem was significant, and most were probably surmountable. Job or schedule was a distant third as a reason (9.8%). "Did not know how to breastfeed" was given by 4.7% women even though over 97% had received prenatal care. According to the survey, 1.8% of the babies refused the breast. The authors stated that provider encouragement increased breastfeeding initiation among women of all social and ethnic backgrounds. They found that most women have decided about breastfeeding by the third trimester; thus, providers of prenatal care should have a significant role in breastfeeding promotion. "Preferred to bottle feed" was interpreted by Taylor and associates as representing an intrinsic decision on the part of the mother or an amalgam of many indistinct social and cultural pressures.

REFERENCES

1. Ainsworth MA: The development of infant-mother attachment. In Caldwell BM, Ricciuti HN (eds): Review of Child Development Research. Chicago, University of Chicago Press, 1973.
2. Axelsson IEM, Räihä NCR: Protein and energy during weaning. Adv Pediatr 39:405, 1992.
3. Barnes GR, Lethin AN, Jackson EB, et al: Management of breast feeding. JAMA 151:192, 1953.
4. Brazelton TB: Infants and Mothers: Differences in Development. New York, Delacorte, 1969.
5. Briefel RR, Reidy K, Karwe V, Devaney B: Feeding infants and toddlers study: Improvements needed in meeting infant feeding recommendations. J Am Diet Assoc 104:S31, 2004.
6. Caldeyro-Barcia R: Milk ejection in women. In Reynolds M, Folley SJ (eds): Lactogenesis: The Initiation of Milk Secretion at Parturition. Philadelphia, University of Pennsylvania Press, 1969.
7. Canadian Pediatric Society Nutrition Committee: Infant feeding: A statement. Can J Publ Health 70:376, 1979.
8. Clarke SK, Harmon RJ: Infant-initiated weaning from the breast in the first year. Early Hum Dev 8:151, 1983.
9. Cohen RJ, Brown KH, Canahuati J, et al: Effects of age of introduction of complementary foods on infant breast milk intake, total energy intake, and growth: A randomized intervention study in Honduras. Lancet 344:288, 1994.
10. Committee on Nutrition, American Academy of Pediatrics: Pediatric Nutrition Handbook, 5th ed. American Academy of Pediatrics, Elk Grove Village, IL, 2004.
11. Cone TE Jr: History of American Pediatrics. Boston, Little, Brown, 1979.
12. Dennison BA: Fruit juice consumption by infants and children: A review. J Am Coll Nutr 15:45, 1996.
13. Dettwyler KA: A time to wean: The hominid blueprint for the natural age of weaning in modern human populations. In Stuart-MacAdam P, Dettwyler KA (eds): Breastfeeding: Biocultural Perspectives. New York, Aldine de Gruyter, 1995.
14. Dewey KG, Beaton G, Fjeld C, et al: Protein requirements of infants and children. Eur J Clin Nutr 50(suppl 1):S119, 1996.

15. Dewey KG, Cohen RJ, Brown KH, Rivera LL: Age of introduction of complementary foods and growth of term, low-birth-weight, breast-fed infants: A randomized intervention study in Honduras. Am J Clin Nutr 69:679, 1999.

16. Dewey KG, Cohen RJ, Rivera L, et al: Do exclusively breast-fed infants require extra protein? Pediatr Res 39:303, 1996.

17. Edmonston B: Interruption of breastfeeding by child death and pregnancy. Soc Biol 37:233, 1990.

18. Fewtrell MS, Lucas A, Morgan JB: Factors associated with weaning in full term and preterm infants. Arch Dis Child Fetal Neonatal Ed 88:F296, 2003.

19. Finberg L, Kiley J, Luttrell CN: Mass accidental salt poisoning in infancy. JAMA 184:121, 1963.

20. Foote KD, Marriott LD: Weaning of infants. Arch Dis Child 88:488, 2003.

21. Freed LM, Neville MC, Hamosh M: Lipase activities in human milk during weaning. Pediatr Res 25(pt 2):290A, 1989.

22. Garza C, Johnson CA, Smith E, et al: Changes in the nutrient composition of human milk during gradual weaning. Am J Clin Nutr 37:61, 1983.

23. Goldman AS, Goldblum RM: Immunologic components in human milk during weaning. Acta Paediatr Scand 72:133, 1983.

24. Gordon JE, Chitkara ID, Wyon JB: Weanling diarrhea. Am J Med Sci Prev Med Epidemiol 245:345, 1963.

25. Gulick EE: The effects of breastfeeding on toddler health. Pediatr Nurs 12:51, 1986.

26. Gunn TR: The incidence of breastfeeding and reasons for weaning. N Z Med J 97:360, 1984.

27. Hall RT, Mercer AM, Teasley SL, et al: A breast-feeding assessment score to evaluate the risk for cessation of breast-feeding by 7 to 10 days of age. J Pediatr 141:659, 2002.

28. Hartmann PE, Kulski JK: Changes in the composition of the mammary secretion of women after the abrupt termination of breastfeeding. J Physiol 275:1, 1978.

29. Harvey PH, Clutton-Brock TH: Life history variations in primates. Evolution 39(3):559, 1985.

30. Helsing E, King FS: Breast-feeding Practice. New York, Oxford University Press, 1980.

31. Henning SJ: Role of milk-borne factors in weaning and intestinal development. Biol Neonate 41:265, 1982.

32. Hervada AR, Newman DR: Weaning: Historical perspective, practical recommendations, and current controversies. Curr Probl Pediatr 22:223, 1992.

33. Hijazi SS, Abulaban A, Waterlow JC: The duration for which exclusive breastfeeding is adequate. Acta Paediatr Scand 78:23, 1989.

34. Hood LJ, Faed JA, Silva PA, et al: Breast feeding and some reasons for electing to wean the infant: A report from the Dunedin Multidisciplinary Child Development Study. N Z Med J 88:273, 1978.

35. Howard CR, Howard FM, Lanphear B, et al: A randomized clinical trial of pacifier use and bottle or cupfeeding and their effect on breastfeeding. Pediatrics 111:511, 2003.

36. Huggins K, Ziedrich L: The Nursing Mother's Guide to Weaning. Boston, Harvard Commons Press, 1994.

37. Huttly SRA, Barros FC, Victora CG, et al: Do mothers overestimate breastfeeding duration? An example of recall bias from a study in southern Brazil. Am J Epidemiol 132:572, 1990.

38. Illingworth RS, Lister J: The critical or sensitive period, with special reference to certain feeding problems in infants and children. J Pediatr 65:839, 1964.

39. Jackson EB: Pediatric and psychiatric aspects of the Yale Rooming-In Project. Conn State Med J 14:616, 1950.

40. Jackson EB, Wilkins LC, Auerbach H: Statistical report on incidence and duration of breast feeding in relation to personal-social and hospital maternity factors. Pediatrics 17:700, 1956.

41. Jacobsen MS, Sodemann M, Molbak K, et al: Reason for termination of breastfeeding and the length of breastfeeding. Int J Epidemiol 25:115, 1996.

42. Kendall-Tackett KA, Sugarman M: The social consequences of long-term breastfeeding. J Hum Lact 11:179, 1995.

43. Kirkland VL, Fein SB: Characterizing reasons for breastfeeding cessation throughout the first year postpartum using the construct of thriving. J Hum Lact 19:278, 2003.

44. Kramer M, Kakuma R: The optimal duration of exclusive breastfeeding: A systematic review. Geneva, World Health Organization, 2001.

45. Krebs NF, Reidinger CJ, Hartley S, et al: Zinc supplementation during lactation: Effects on maternal status and milk zinc concentrations. Am J Clin Nutr 61: 1030, 1995.

46. La Leche League: The Womanly Art of Breastfeeding, 7th ed. Schaumberg, IL, La Leche League, 2004.

47. Lanigan JA, Bishop JA, Kimber AC, Morgan J: Systematic review concerning the age of introduction of complementary foods to the healthy full-term infant. Eur J Clin Nutr 55:309, 2001.

48. Lifshitz F: Weaning foods: The role of fruit juice in the diets of infants and children. J Am Coll Nutr 15:15, 1996.

49. Mennella JA, Beauchamp GK: Maternal diet alters the sensory qualities of human milk and the nursling's behavior. Pediatrics 88:737, 1991.

50. Mennella JA, Beauchamp GK: Mother's milk enhances the acceptance of cereal during weaning. Pediatr Res 41:188, 1997.

51. Merchant SM: Neural development for sucking, swallowing and chewing. In Ballabriga A, Rey J: Weaning: Why, What and When? Workshop Series, Vol. II. New York, Vevey/Raven, 1987.

52. Newton N: Breast feeding. Psychol Today 98:68, 1971.

53. Newton N: The role of the oxytocin reflexes in three interpersonal reproductive acts: Coitus, birth and breastfeeding.

In Carenza L, Pancheri P, Zichella L (eds): Clinical Psychoneuroendocrinology in Reproduction. Proceedings of the Serono Symposia, Vol. 22. London, Academic Press, 1978.

54. Nommsen LA, Lovelady CA, Heinig MJ, et al: Determinants of energy, protein, lipid and lactose concentrations in human milk during the first 12 months of lactation: The Darling Study. Am J Clin Nutr 53:457, 1991.

55. Ponza M, Devaney B, Ziegler P, et al: Nutrient intakes and food choices of infants and toddlers participating in WIC. J Am Diet Assoc 104:S71, 2004.

56. Poskitt EME: Energy needs in the weaning period. In Ballabriga A, Rey J (eds): Weaning: Why, What and When? New York, Vevey/Raven, 1987.

57. Prentice A: Breastfeeding and the older infant. Acta Paediatr Scand Suppl 374:78, 1991.

58. Raphael D: The Tender Gift: Breastfeeding. New York, Schocken, 1976.

59. Reamer SB, Sugarman M: Breastfeeding beyond six months: Mothers' perceptions of the positive and negative consequences. J Trop Pediatr 33:93, 1987.

60. Schmitz J, McNeish AS: Development of structure and function of the gastrointestinal tract: Relevance for weaning. In Ballabriga A, Rey J (eds): Weaning: Why, What and When? Workshop Series, Vol. 11. New York, Vevey/Raven, 1987.

61. Short RV: The biological basis for the contraceptive effects of breastfeeding. In Jelliffe DP, Jelliffe EFP (eds): Advances in International Maternal and Child Health, Vol. 3. Oxford, Oxford University Press, 1983.

62. Short RV: Breastfeeding. Sci Am 250(4):35, 1984.

63. Sjölin S, Hofvander Y, Hillervik G: Factors related to early termination of breastfeeding. Acta Paediatr Scand 66:505, 1977.

64. Sousa PLR, Barros FC, Pinheiro GNM, et al: Patterns of weaning in South Brazil. J Trop Pediatr Environ Child Health 21:210, 1975.

65. Stuff JE, Nichols BL: Nutrient intake and growth performance of older infants fed human milk. J Pediatr 115:959, 1989.

66. Subcommittee on Nutrition during Lactation, Committee on Nutrition Status during Pregnancy and Lactation, Food and Nutrition Board, Institute of Medicine, National Academy of Sciences: Nutrition during Lactation. Washington, DC, National Academy Press, 1991.

67. Sugarman M, Kendall-Tackett KA: Weaning ages in a sample of American women who practice extended breastfeeding. Clin Pediatr 34:642, 1995.

68. Taylor JS, Risica RM, Cabral HJ: Why primiparous mothers do not breastfeed in the United States: A national survey. Acta Paediatr 92:1308, 2003.

69. Underwood BA, Hofvander Y: Appropriate timing for complementary feeding of the breastfed infant. Acta Paediatr Scand Suppl 294:5, 1982.

70. U.S. Department of Health and Human Services: Healthy People 2010 (Conference Edition, in two volumes). Washington, DC, Department of Health and Human Services, 2000.

71. Wharton BA: Food for the weanling: The next priority in infant nutrition. Acta Paediatr Scand Suppl 323:96, 1986.

72. Whitehead RG: Infant physiology, nutritional requirements, and lactational adequacy. Am J Clin Nutr, 41:447, 1985.

73. Widdowson EM: Mental contentment and physical growth. Lancet 1:1316, 1952.

74. World Health Organization: Joint WHO/UNICEF Meeting, Global Strategy for Infant and Young Child Feeding. Document No. A54, Information Document/4. Geneva, WHO, 2001.

$\mathcal{D}$rugs in breast milk

Despite the overwhelming advantages of human milk and the advantages of being breastfed, at times the physician must consider the risk of a maternal medication to the nursing infant. Even when the data about the medication include the milk/plasma ratio, the physician has to consider several factors related to each infant and each situation before deciding if breastfeeding can be initiated or continue. The more complicated the mother's medical problems, the greater is the possibility that the infant also has complications of prematurity or illness that will alter the ability to excrete medication. This situation requires scientific information and experienced clinical judgment to appraise the problems and determine the therapeutic regimen. The clinician must determine the risk/benefit ratio of continued breastfeeding. The data are still meager and sometimes conflicting, yet maternal medication is the single most common medical problem in managing breastfeeding patients.

There are a number of general reviews of drugs in breast milk and hundreds of articles about the effect of a specific medication in a particular infant.* The American Academy of Pediatrics (AAP) Committee on Drugs[28,29] has published a list of drugs and other chemicals that transfer into human breast milk. The list, which is continually updated, is divided into those that are contraindicated, those that require temporary interruption of breastfeeding, and those that are compatible with breastfeeding. Concern about this issue of drugs in breast

milk has spread. The U.S. Department of Health and Human Services (DHHS) and Food and Drug Administration (FDA) have proposed a standard warning on all nonprescription drugs that are absorbed by the body: "As with any drug, if you are pregnant or nursing a baby, seek professional advice before using this product." Because studies of pregnant women have shown that they take five to eight medications on their own during pregnancy and post partum, the clinician's education of these patients needs to continue.

A study of more than 14,000 pregnant women in 148 hospitals in 22 countries revealed that 79% of women received an average of 3.3 drugs.[27] The drugs most often given were analgesics and anesthetics. Of the 91% of women who initiated breastfeeding, 36% received methylergonovine and 5% antibiotics. Another study of 885 women 3 to 5 months post partum in Oslo showed that breastfeeders took fewer medications (daily dose/1000 women/day) than nonbreastfeeders.[100] The most common medication in the latter group was oral contraceptives. Colds, dyspepsia, hemorrhoids, and breast infections were the disorders that precipitated the use of albuterol (Salbutamol), clemastine fumarate (Tavist), dexchlorpheniramine maleate (cold preparations), phenylpropanolamine hydrochloride (Comtrex, Dimetane), cromolyn sodium, and methotrimeprazine hydrochloride (levomepromazine).[100]

No substitute exists for specific knowledge. It is equally inappropriate to discontinue breastfeeding when it is not medically necessary as it is to

---

*See references 6, 19, 20, 29, 60, 68, 84, 108, 112, 120, 174.

continue breastfeeding while taking contraindicated drugs.

Consideration of the pharmacokinetics contributes to the understanding of the problems involved. Some data reported have been extrapolated from experiments performed on cows, goats, and rodents. Bovine experiments have been conducted using continuous infusions, which provide data on the passage of a drug into milk under certain pH and plasma levels. In an effort to explain and clarify the issues involved, the literature has oversimplified the problem so that individuals lacking a background in pharmacology or pediatrics have misused the published data in drawing unwarranted conclusions.

Factors that influence the passage of a drug into the milk in humans include the size of the molecule, its solubility in lipids and water, whether it binds to protein, the drug's pH, and diffusion rates. The following outline summarizes these factors:

I. Drug
   A. Route of administration
     1. Oral (PO)
     2. Intravenous (IV)
     3. Intramuscular (IM)
     4. Transdermal drug delivery system (TDDS)
   B. Absorption rate
   C. Half-life or peak serum time
   D. Dissociation constant
   E. Volume of distribution
II. Size of molecule
III. Degree of ionization
IV. pH of substrate
   A. Plasma 7.4
   B. Milk 6.8
V. Solubility
   A. In water
   B. In lipids
VI. Protein binding more to plasma than to milk protein

Passive diffusion is the principal factor in the passage of a drug from plasma into milk. The drug may appear in an active form or as an inactive metabolite.

Finally, a most important factor that has received relatively little attention is the infant. Will the infant absorb the chemical from the intestinal tract? If the infant absorbs the chemical, can the infant detoxify and excrete it, or will minimal amounts in the milk build in the infant's system? Is the infant premature, small for gestational age, or high risk because of complications of the pregnancy or delivery? Is the drug a material that could be safely given to an infant directly, and at what risk? What dosages and blood levels are safe? These latter two questions are more critical than the pharmacokinetic theory. The ultimate question faced by the physician is, Can this infant be safely exposed to this chemical as it appears in breast milk without a risk that exceeds the tremendous benefits of being breastfed? Almost any drug present in mother's blood will appear to some degree in her milk.

CHARACTERISTICS OF DRUGS

Protein binding

Drugs entering the circulation become protein bound or remain free in the circulation. The protein-bound component of the drug serves as an inactive reservoir for the drug that is in equilibrium with the free drug. Most drugs enter the mammary alveolar cells in the unbound form (Fig. 11-1).

At term, plasma proteins may be reduced and the fatty acid and hypoprotein fraction slightly increased in the mother, which results in the displacement of some drugs from plasma proteins.[42] During the early postpartum period for 5 to 7 weeks the free fraction of some drugs increases and therefore more readily crosses into milk (e.g., salicylate, phenytoin, diazepam).

For most drugs, more drug will be found in the plasma than in the milk. Only the small free fraction of drug can cross the biologic membrane. The total concentration in milk is only minimally influenced by binding of drugs in milk proteins (milk protein concentration is 0.9% in mature milk). Only those drug molecules that are free in solution can pass through the endothelial pores, either by diffusion or by reverse pinocytosis. *Pinocytosis* is the process whereby drug molecules dissolved in the interstitial

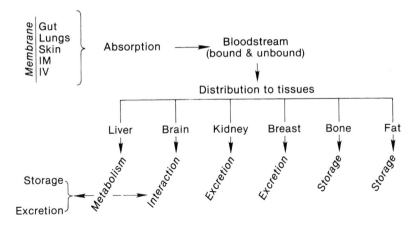

Figure 11-1. Distribution pathways for drugs, once absorbed during lactation. (Modified from Rivera-Calimlim L: The significance of drugs in breast milk. Clin Perinatol 14:51, 1976.)

fluid attach to receptors located at the surface of the cell membrane.[127,128] The cell membrane invaginates at the site of the drug attachment, bringing the drug into the cell. The membrane is pinched off, and the drug, surrounded by membrane, remains in the cell. Then the membrane is dissolved, leaving the drug molecule free in the cell.

Reverse pinocytosis is the process by which the apical membrane evaginates after fusion of the intracellular membrane-bound secretion granules with the plasma membrane. The granules include lipids, proteins, lactose, drug molecules, and other cellular constituents. The evagination of the plasma membrane is pinched off and released into the alveolar lumen. Within the extravascular space the drug may be bound to proteins in the interstitial fluid. Some agents in free solution can pass into the alveolar milk directly by way of the spaces between the mammary alveolar cells. These paracellular areas account for a major portion of the fluid changes across the epithelium. These spaces between adjacent alveolar cells serve to carry water-soluble drugs from the tissue into the milk.

The intercellular junctions are "open" at delivery as lactation is being established and gradually "tighten" over the next few days. The amount of drug passed into milk on day 1 is greater than on day 3 or later. The composition of the milk changes

as well from colostrum to mature milk, altering the amount of protein and fat, which could also influence drug levels in the milk. It is always important to know when plasma and milk samples were measured in relationship to the onset of lactation. Furthermore, some studies have been done on nonlactating women by pumping enough milk to measure the drug. These "weaning samples" provide only misinformation.

Ionization

Drugs that are nonionized are excreted in the milk in greater amounts than are ionized compounds. Depending on the pH of the solvent and the drug *dissociation constant* (pK_a), many weak electrolytes are more or less ionized in solution. Blood plasma and interstitial fluid are slightly alkaline (pH 7.4). Drugs that are weak acids are ionized to a greater extent in alkaline solution and are more extensively bound to protein. The amount of drug excreted from plasma (pH 7.4) to milk (pH 6.8 to 7.3, average 7.0) depends on the pH of the compound. Thus a weakly acidic compound has a higher concentration in plasma than in milk. Conversely, weakly alkaline compounds are in equal or higher levels in the milk than in the plasma.

The degree of drug ionization changes with the pH of the plasma and milk. Weak bases become more ionized with decreasing pH; thus the ionized component will increase in milk. The concentration in plasma and milk for the nonionized fraction will be the same, but the total amount of drug in the milk will be greater than in plasma. The sulfonamides demonstrate the effect of the pK_a on the concentration of drug that reaches the milk. Sulfacetamide, with a low pK_a (5.4), has a low milk/plasma (M/P) ratio (0.08), whereas sulfanilamide has a pK_a of 10.4 and an M/P ratio of 1.00 (Table 11-1).

The studies done in cows and goats with constant infusions demonstrate this principle more dramatically because the pH of bovine plasma is 7.4 to 7.5 and the pH of bovine milk is 6.5. Under normal circumstances, however, concentrations of drugs are rarely constant, and there is a delay in achieving a new equilibrium. During periods of rapidly decreasing blood levels, some back diffusion occurs into the plasma.

Molecular weight

The passage of molecules into the milk also depends on the size of the molecule, or the molecular weight (mol wt, in daltons). Water-filled membranous pores permit the movement of molecules of less than 100 mol wt. Because of action similar to the limitation of transport of certain large-molecular-weight chemicals across the placenta, insulin and heparin are not found in human milk either, presumably because of the molecule's size.

Solubility

The alveolar epithelium of the breast is a lipid barrier that is most permeable in the first few days of lactation, when colostrum is being produced. The solubility of a compound in water and in lipid is a determining factor in its transfer. Nonionized drugs, which are lipid soluble, usually dissolve and descend in the lipid phase of the membrane. The solubility is closely linked to the manner in which the drug crosses the membranes (Table 11-2). The membrane of the alveolar epithelial cells is composed of lipoprotein, glycolipid, phospholipid, and free lipids, as described in Chapter 3. The transfer of water-soluble drugs and ions is inhibited by this hydrophobic barrier. Water-soluble materials pass through pores in the basement membrane and paracellular spaces. Low lipid solubility of a nonionized compound will diminish its excretion into milk.

Lipid solubility affects the profile of the drug in the milk and plasma. A drug with high lipid solubility will have parallel elimination curves in the plasma and the milk. A drug with low lipid solubility will clear the plasma at a constant rate, but the clearance curve for the milk will peak lower and later, and the drug will linger in the milk. A

TABLE 11-1   Association between milk/plasma (M/P) ratios and dissociation constants (pK_a) of sulfonamides

Sulfonamide	Milk/plasma ratio	pK_a
Sulfacetamide	0.08	5.4
Sulfadiazine	0.21	6.5
Sulfathiazole	0.43	7.1
Sulfamethazine	0.51	7.4
Sulfapyridine	0.85	8.4
Sulfanilamide	1.00	10.4

Modified from Gaginella TS: Drugs and the nursing mother-infant. US Pharm 3:39, 1978.

TABLE 11-2   Predicted distribution ratios of drug concentrations in milk and plasma

General drug type	Milk/plasma (M/P) ratio
Highly lipid-soluble drugs	~1
Highly protein-bound drugs in maternal serum	<1
Small (mol wt <200) water-soluble drugs	~1
Weak acids	≤1
Weak bases	≥1
Actively transported drugs	>1

Modified from Gaginella TS: Drugs and the nursing mother-infant. US Pharm 3:39, 1978.

prolonged terminal elimination phase may exist when time between feedings is long.[42]

Mechanisms of transport

Drugs pass into milk by simple diffusion, carrier-mediated diffusion, or active transport, as follows:

Simple diffusion: concentration gradient decreases

Carrier-mediated diffusion: concentration gradient decreases

Active transport: concentration gradient increases

Pinocytosis

Reverse pinocytosis

Pharmacokinetic principles relate to the specific variation with time of the drug concentration in the blood or plasma as a result of its absorption, distribution, and elimination. Ultimately, by extrapolation of these factors, one determines the effect of the drug. The most elementary kinetic model is based on the body as a single compartment. Distribution of the drug in the compartment is assumed to be uniform and rapidly equilibrated. In the single-compartment model, the volume of distribution of a drug is considered to be the same as that of the plasma, assuming a rapid uniform distribution.[50] The volume of distribution (V_d) is calculated as follows:

$$V_d = \text{Total amount of drug in body / Concentration of drug in plasma}$$

The absorption and elimination are considered to be exponential or first-order kinetics. A two-compartment model of drug kinetics takes into account the phase of decreasing drug concentration as the drug distributes into the tissues. Initially, concentrations fall rapidly as the drug distributes, then first-order elimination follows. When considering the pharmacokinetics of drugs in breast milk, one must also consider that elimination in the breast is then by two potential routes: excreted with the milk to the infant and back diffusion into the plasma to reequilibrate with the falling level in the plasma.

With access to the volume of distribution of the drug in question, the amount of the dose, and the weight of the mother, the concentration of drug in breast milk could be theoretically calculated as follows:

$$\text{Concentration in breast milk} = \text{Dose / Volume of distribution}$$

Other models have been developed for measuring the amount of drug that reaches the infant when the M/P ratio is not known. Using a stepwise linear regression for acidic and basic drugs, based on the drug's pK_a, the plasma protein binding value, and the octanol/water partition coefficient, an M/P ratio can be calculated. In a study of several proposed equations, Begg and associates[9] demonstrated that the error is lowest for the drugs with the highest M/P ratio, that protein binding is the most important single predictor, and that the M/P ratios for basic drugs are more accurately predictable.

The concentration of the drug in the circulation of the mother depends on the mode of administration: PO, IV, IM, or TDDS. Absorption through the skin, the lungs (inhalants), or vaginally may also need to be considered.

The *transdermal drug delivery system* (TDDS) depends on absorption of the drug through the skin at a steady rate; it has become a significant route of administration for certain medications. The delivery rate is determined by diffusion of drug from the reservoir matrix through the epidermis. This method offers some advantages, including convenience of dosing, reduced dosing frequency, ease of reaching a steady state, increased patient compliance, avoidance of first-pass hepatic biotransformation, and reduction of side effects through heightened selectivity of drug action.[139] The level in the plasma remains constant during the drug's anticipated life span while the patch is in place. TDDS patches are available for scopolamine, nicotine, clonidine, fentanyl, and other drugs (Table 11-3).

The levels in the blood depend on the route of administration. The curves produced by bolus IV medication peak high and early and taper sharply, thus making avoiding peak plasma levels more feasible. Absorption from IM dosing is less rapid but follows a similar but less sharp curve. PO dosing

TABLE 11-3   Representative transdermal drug delivery systems (TDDS)

Drug	Total amount in patch (mg)	Delivery rate (duration of use)	Approximate postuse drug residue (mg)	Pediatric dose
Scopolamine	1.5	0.5 mg/D (3 D)	0	Therapeutic[*]: 6 µg/kg
Nicotine				
Habitrol 30 cm²	52.5	29 µg/cm²/h (24 h)	21.5	**Toxic[†] (mg/kg)**
				Severe (1.4–1.9)
Nicoderm 22 cm²	114.0	40 µg/cm²/h (24 h)	83.0	**Mild** (0.2–1.8)
Prostep 7 cm²	30.0	130 µg/cm²/h	8.0	
Clonidine				
Catapres-TTS-1	2.5	0.1 mg/24 h (7 days)	0.5–1.9	**Toxic[‡]**: 0.025 to 3 mg
Catapres-TTS-3	10.5	0.3 mg/24 h (7 days)	2.1–7.9	
Fentanyl				
Duragesic-75	10.0	100 µg/h (24 h)	6.5	Surgery: 1–3 µg/kg[§]

[*]IM, IV, or SC.
[†]PO, based on nicotine content of cigarettes.
[‡]PO.
[§]IM or IV.
From Sangalli BC: The hazard (potential hazard) with transdermal drug delivery systems (TDDS), a.k.a. drug patches. Hudson Valley Poison Center Toxicol Newslett 2:1, 1992.

depends on other factors, such as whether the medication is taken between or during meals. Depending on the curve of uptake and removal of drug from the plasma, the area under the curve varies. Single doses are simple area-under-the-curve calculations, but calculations for multiple doses or chronic use vary with the steady state of the drug in the body.

Nonelectrolytes such as ethanol, urea, and antipyrine enter the milk by diffusion through the lipid membrane barrier and may reach the same concentrations in the milk as in the plasma, regardless of the pH. The main entrance site of molecules is at the basement laminal membrane, where water-soluble materials pass through the alveolar pores. Nonionized drugs cross the membrane more easily than ionized ones because of the structure of the membrane. The nonionized drugs pass through the membrane by diffusion. When simple diffusion takes place, the M/P ratio is 1.0. Passive diffusion provides the same ratio regardless of the plasma concentrations of the drug or the volume of milk secreted. Different

M/P ratios depend on the binding to protein and are a measure of the protein-free fraction. The dissimilar ratios for the sulfa drugs (see Table 11-1) partly result from the difference in protein binding, and partly from ionization.

Large molecules depend on their lipid solubility and ionization to cross the membrane, because they pass in a lipid-soluble nonionized form. The M/P ratio is determined when there is equilibrium in the amount of nonionized drug in the aqueous phase on both sides of the membrane. When drugs are only partially ionized, the nonionized fraction determines the concentration that crosses the membrane. The drugs whose nonionized fraction is not very lipid soluble will pass only in limited degree into breast milk.

Passive drug transport may occur in the form of *facilitated diffusion*. The active compound is transported across the cell membrane by a carrier enzyme or protein. The gradient is toward a lesser or equal concentration in both simple diffusion and facilitated diffusion and is controlled by chemical activity gradients. Facilitated diffusion usually involves a water-soluble substance too large to pass through the membrane pores.

Active transport mechanisms provide a process whereby the gradient is "uphill," or higher, in the milk. The process is similar to facilitated diffusion except that metabolic energy is required to overcome the gradient. Examples of substances actively transported include glucose, amino acids, calcium, magnesium, and sodium. Pinocytosis and reverse pinocytosis, as described previously, are involved in the transport of very large molecules and proteins. Chloride ions are secreted into milk via an active apical membrane pump, whereas sodium and potassium are diffused by electrical gradient. Because the level of sodium is kept low, an active return of sodium may occur into the plasma, referred to as a *reverse pump*.

A summary of the steps in the passage of drugs into breast milk follows:

1. Mammary alveolar epithelium represents a lipid barrier with water-filled pores and is most permeable for drugs during colostral phase of milk secretion (first week post partum).
2. Drug excretion into milk depends on the drug's degree of ionization, molecular weight, solubility in fat and water, and relation of pH of plasma (7.4) to pH of milk (7.0).
3. Drugs preferably enter mammary cells basally in the nonionized, non-protein-bound form by diffusion or active transport.
4. Water-soluble drugs of mol wt below 200 pass through water-filled membranous pores.
5. Drugs leave mammary alveolar cells apically by diffusion or active transport.
6. Drugs may enter milk via spaces between mammary alveolar cells.
7. Most ingested drugs appear in milk; drug amounts in milk usually do not exceed 1% of ingested dosage, and levels in the milk are independent of milk volume.
8. Drugs are bound much less to milk proteins than to plasma proteins.
9. Drug-metabolizing capacity of mammary epithelium is not understood.

EFFECT ON NURSING INFANT

Absorption from gastrointestinal tract

Although concern surrounds the amount of a given agent in the breast milk, of greater importance is the amount absorbed into the infant's bloodstream. No accurate way exists to measure this because other factors also affect the level in the infant's bloodstream. The tolerance of the chemical to the pH of the stomach and the enzymatic activity of the intestinal tract are significant. The volume of milk consumed is a factor as well. Some drugs are not well absorbed with food (see later discussion of food-drug interactions). Oral bioavailability of a compound is a major factor in risk to the infant.

Infant's ability to detoxify and excrete agent

Any drug given to an infant by any route has to be evaluated according to the infant's ability to detoxify or conjugate the chemical in the liver and excrete it in the urine or stool. Some compounds that appear in milk in very low levels are not well excreted by the infant and therefore accumulate in the infant's system to the point of toxicity.

Drugs that depend on the liver for conjugation, such as acetaminophen, are theoretic risks because of the limited reserve of the neonatal hepatic detoxification system. When actual measurements were made of neonates given acetaminophen, they were noted to handle it well because they conjugate it in the sulfhydryl system as an alternative pathway used only to a small extent in adult metabolism of acetaminophen. When a single dose of a drug is given to a mother and the level is measured in her milk and in her infant, it does not give a clear picture of the potential for accumulation in the infant's system. The competition for binding a drug to protein is also important. Some drugs, such as sulfadiazine, compete for binding sites that might normally bind bilirubin in the first week or so of life. This puts the infant in jeopardy of kernicterus at a given bilirubin level because of an increase in the fraction of bilirubin left unbound for lack of binding sites. The indirect bilirubin level may even appear to be below the dangerous level. Some other compounds that displace bilirubin from albumin-binding sites include salicylic acid (aspirin or acetylsalicylic acid breaks down to salicylic acid), furosemide, and phenylbutazone.

The maturity of the infant at birth is an extremely important factor during the first few months of life; thus the gestational age at birth should be established. Clearly, the less mature the infant, the less well tolerated is the drug, not only because of the immaturity of the organ systems but also because of differences in body composition (Fig. 11-2). The less mature the infant, the greater are the water content of the body and the proportion of extracellular water. Although the percentage of body weight taken up by protein is similar for all newborns (i.e., 12%), the absolute amount of protein for binding is less the smaller the infant. The amount of body fat is also low, by percentage of body weight and in absolute values. The distribution of highly lipid-soluble drugs therefore will be more apt to deposit in the brain of a 1000-g infant with 3% body fat by weight than in a 3500-g full-term infant with 12% body fat. This may explain the more sedating effect of a drug on the central nervous system of a younger and less mature infant. The relative lack of plasma protein-binding sites in the small premature infant compared with the more mature and older infant results in more free (unbound) active drug in circulation. Complications of premature birth such as acidosis and hypoxia also contribute to the unavailability of albumin-binding sites and thus result in more unbound drug.

The inability of the liver to metabolize drugs effectively results in the accumulation of some compounds that might be readily cleared by an older infant. At about 42 weeks' conceptual age, an infant's liver is able to metabolize most drugs competently. Renal clearance similarly is less effective with decreasing maturity, which increases the risk

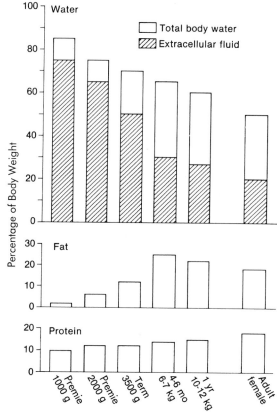

Figure 11-2. Comparative body composition of infants and adults. (Redrawn from Pencharz PB: In Walker WA, Watkins JB (eds): Nutrition in Pediatrics: Basic Science and Clinical Application. Boston, Little, Brown, 1985.)

of drug accumulation. The need to dose a premature infant only once or twice a day is common to many drugs, such as antibiotics, caffeine, and theophylline, and confirms that a small premature infant does not clear drugs well.

Special problems in the neonate in addition to the presence of jaundice or low serum albumin may require special consideration. Low Apgar scores at birth signifying some degree of stress, hypoxia, or acidosis may alter binding-site availability but may also alter metabolism and excretion of a drug. Continuing respiratory distress requiring ventilatory support, sepsis, and renal failure demand special consideration when determining if a sick neonate can receive the mother's milk when she is being treated with certain medications. Prescribing for such a mother should be done in consultation with the neonatologist if the woman is providing her milk for her infant.

The age of the infant makes a difference in the total volume of milk consumed; in the older child, the diet includes other items so that milk does not compose the total intake. Age makes a difference because the more mature infant can metabolize drugs more effectively; thus sulfa drugs, for instance, can be given to infants after the first month of life.

If the agent is fat soluble, the fat content of the milk may be a significant variable. The fat content at any feeding increases over time; thus, the so-called foremilk is low in fat and the hindmilk is four to five times richer in fat toward the end of a feeding. The total amount of fat in a given feeding is less in the morning, peaks at midday, and drops off in the evening even though the total amount of fat will be about the same in each 24-hour period. The coefficient of lipid solubility for a nonionized drug determines both its penetration of the biologic membrane to gain entrance to milk and its concentration in milk fat. Sulfonamides with low fat solubility are in the aqueous and protein fraction of milk, whereas many barbiturates are in the lipid fraction. An inverse relationship exists between a drug's lipid solubility and the amount that appears in the skim fraction. The concentrations in fat differ for each member of the barbital family. Pentobarbital and secobarbital are found in the lipid phase, whereas phenobarbital is found in the aqueous phase.

The agent may appear in low levels in a mother's serum, but mammary blood flow during lactation is 500 mL/minute and a mother produces between 60 and 300 mL of milk/hour. The agent that appears in minimal concentrations in the milk may present a significant problem when one considers that 1000 mL of milk may be consumed in a day by an infant. Even though the volume is low, during the colostral phase of lactation, the breast is more permeable to drugs.

BREAST MILK/PLASMA RATIO FOR DRUGS

The M/P ratio for drugs has been measured and reported for many medications. This ratio can be helpful to the clinician in making a decision about a medication during lactation.[174] By definition, M/P ratio is the concentration of the drug in the milk versus the concentration in maternal plasma (serum) at the same time. It presumes that the relationship between the two concentrations remains constant, which in most cases it does not. If it were a constant, it would allow the estimation of the amount of drug in the milk from any given plasma level in the mother.

An inaccurate ratio or one determined under variable circumstances produces erroneous estimates of the amount of drug in the milk, as pointed out by Wilson and associates,[174] who state that a pharmacokinetic model is a requisite foundation for studies of drugs in breast milk. A single-point-in-time M/P ratio or an average ratio calculated with single-dose, area-under-the-curve data does not work for all drugs. Neither ratio accounts for the importance of time-dependent variations of drug concentration in milk.

The M/P ratio is most valuable if obtained when the infant would be nursed. If the ratio is 1:0, it means only that the levels are equal. If the level is minimal in the mother's plasma because of the large volume of distribution, and if the milk level is also low, the M/P ratio is 1:0. If levels are drawn at peak plasma level and are equal, the M/P is still 1:0, but the infant receives a large dose. Thus, the M/P ratio is valuable only when the time of the measurement is known in relationship to dosing of the mother. Dose strength, duration of dosing, maternal variation in drug disposition, maternal disease, drug interactions and competition of additional drugs for metabolism or binding sites, and racial variations in drug metabolism all influence the M/P interpretation. The characteristics of the drug and the dosing pattern are essential to the interpretation of the M/P ratio.[174]

EVALUATING DRUG DATA

The paucity of carefully controlled studies on large enough samples to validate the results when such a large number of variables are active has been lamented by many authors. Some data collected are not pharmacokinetically sound. The clinician needs to understand these variables as well as pharmacokinetic principles to make a reasonable judgment about a given case.

Interethnic and racial differences in drug responsiveness are well established. The increased heterogeneity of national populations has brought increased awareness of genetic diversity. Plasma binding, especially with drugs dependent on glycoproteins for binding, often varies greatly between Caucasian and Chinese subjects, for example.[182] Such differences contribute to the differences in drug disposition and pharmacologic response.

It should be theoretically possible to determine how much of a specific drug reaches the infant in the mother's milk by knowing all the properties of the drug, including its volume of distribution, ionization, pK_a, lipid solubility, protein-binding activity, and rate of detoxification in the maternal system. Sufficient variation in the levels that reach the infant and in how the infant deals with the agent, however, makes it necessary to have specific data about a specific drug. Thus, a few simple questions in the decision-making process are helpful in determining risk.

Safety for infant

Is this a drug that can be given to the infant directly if necessary? Antibiotics (e.g., penicillin) that one could give the infant are in this category, whereas an antibiotic such as chloramphenicol, which one would not give the infant under ordinary circumstances, should be avoided in the nursing mother. The toxicity of chloramphenicol in the infant is dose related and associated with an unpredictable accumulation of the drug. Also, an idiosyncratic reaction occurs with chloramphenicol, which is unrelated to dose but is capable of causing pancytopenia.

If the drug in question can be given to the infant, is there any risk to the infant in the amount in the milk? Phenobarbital can be given to infants for various reasons; thus the question is whether enough will reach the infant to cause difficulty. The infant should be watched for symptoms of lethargy or sleepiness, such as a change in feeding or sleeping pattern. If the infant is sleeping long periods and feeding less than usual (specifically, fewer than five or six times a day), the medication may be at fault. Phenobarbital is a significant drug for the mother with seizures; therefore, a careful review of the risk/benefit ratio to the mother as well as to the infant should be undertaken. Barbiturates vary in their effect in young infants. The newborn does not handle the short-acting barbiturates well because they are dependent on detoxification in the liver, whereas phenobarbital depends more on the kidney for excretion.

If the drug was taken during pregnancy, as in epilepsy, the infant already has the drug in his system via the placenta at a steady state and will have to begin to excrete it on his or her own after delivery.[118] Enzyme induction may have taken place in the neonate because of exposure to the drug in utero, however; phenobarbital hastens maturation of the fetal liver.[129] Enzyme induction of the hepatic oxygenase system by phenobarbital, phenytoin, primidone, and carbamazepine is well established. Valproate, however, does not induce enzyme activity.

If one can safely give the drug to an infant, administration becomes a question of watching for any symptoms of excessive accumulation that might develop. The age of the infant affects the ability to clear the drug.

When the drug in question is one not normally given to an infant at that particular age, weight, or degree of maturity, decision making is more difficult. Specific information about the amount of the drug that appears in the milk is essential in decision making. Often, conflicting information is available. Many lists of drug-milk levels have perpetuated the same errors in calculation; thus, having more than one reference report the same information may not provide confirmation as to its accuracy.

If the medication will have to be taken for weeks or months, as with cardiovascular drugs, the drug has greater potential impact than when taken only for a few days. If the drug exposure has gone on for 9 months in utero already, some think it is less of a problem; it also may compound the problem.

To determine the dose delivered to the infant, the following formula is used:

Dose/24 hours = Concentration of drug in milk × Weight (kg) of infant × Volume of milk per kg ingested in 24 hours

Dose/24 hours = C_{milk} × Weight × Volume/kg/24 hr

Sensitization

Is there risk of sensitization, even in the small dosages of a drug that might pass into the milk? This question arises most frequently with the use of antibiotics, and use of penicillin is most frequently questioned. Certainly, if the family has a strong history of drug sensitization, it should be considered. In that case, however, it should be questioned for the mother as well. Whether infants are put at risk of developing resistant strains of bacteria in their systems by small amounts of antibiotic in their feedings is a serious question. It also is pertinent for the dairy and meat industries as well as for the humans who consume those food products that have a small amount of antibiotic because of administration to livestock.

Correlation of drug safety in pregnancy and lactation

Very rarely is valid information on the appearance of a drug in breast milk available on the package insert, because the pharmaceutical companies usually merely indicate that it should not be taken during pregnancy and lactation. Agents that may be safe during pregnancy may not be so during lactation. During pregnancy the maternal liver and kidney are serving as detoxification and excretion resources for the fetus via the placenta, whereas during lactation the infant has to handle the drug

totally on his own once it has reached his circulation. The infant in utero receives the drug in greater quantity via the circulation, whereas the nursing infant receives only what reaches the milk. One should be cautious about translating data pertaining to these two states back and forth.

Oral bioavailability

The dose of a drug delivered via the milk to the infant is significantly affected by the oral bioavailability, which is the percentage of the drug absorbed into the infant's system via the gut.[132]

Oral bioavailability is the rate and extent to which an active drug is absorbed and enters the general circulation. Absolute oral bioavailability compares the oral route with the IV route. To reach the general circulation, the oral dose must pass through the wall of the gut, liver, or lungs.[147] First-pass metabolism or elimination in the tissues of these three organs may reduce the drug's bioavailability. It is possible for a drug to be absorbed 100% and be destroyed or eliminated and have 0% bioavailability, because it is so rapidly metabolized.

These values are provided in Table D-1, Appendix D. If a compound is poorly absorbed, it is of less concern than one with 100% bioavailability. Most drugs administered by injection (e.g., insulin, heparin) only are not orally bioavailable.

Food-drug interactions

When drugs are taken with meals, numerous opportunities exist for food-drug interactions to occur.[116] Because the breastfed infant receives all maternal medications excreted in the milk "with food," this is an important consideration in the discussion of drugs in milk. The effects of food may reduce gastrointestinal irritation. Mechanisms of food-drug interactions can be summarized as follows[116]:

Physiologic
1. Changes in gastric emptying
2. Increased intestinal motility
3. Increased splanchnic blood flow

4. Increased bile, acid, and enzyme secretion
5. Induction and inhibition of drug metabolism
6. Competition in active transport

Physiochemical
1. Food as a mechanical barrier to absorption
2. Altered dissolution of drugs
3. Chelation and adsorption

Pharmacodynamic
1. Altered enzyme activity
2. Changes in homeostasis

MINIMIZING EFFECT OF MATERNAL MEDICATION

If a mother needs a specific medication and the hazards to the infant are minimal, the following important adjustments can be made to minimize the effects:

1. Do not use the long-acting form of the drug because the infant has even more difficulty excreting such an agent, which usually requires detoxification in the liver. Accumulation in the infant is then a genuine concern.
2. Schedule the doses so the least amount possible gets into the milk. Check the usual absorption rates and peak blood levels of the drug. Having the mother take the medication immediately after breastfeeding is the safest time for the infant with most, but not all, drugs.
3. Watch the infant for any unusual signs or symptoms, such as change in feeding pattern or sleeping habits, fussiness, or rash.
4. When possible, choose the drug that produces the least amount in the milk (see Tables 11-1 and 11-2).

Classification systems

A drug classification system for information regarding drug use during pregnancy and breastfeeding was devised in 1978 by the National Swedish Board of Health with the help of the drug manufacturers' trade organizations.[11,140] The system classifies drugs into categories regarding pregnancy (Categories A, B, C, or D) and the following four groups to describe drugs during lactation:

Group I: Active ingredients do not enter the milk.

Group II: Active ingredients enter the milk but in such small amounts that there is no risk to the infant.

Group III: Active ingredients enter the milk in sufficient quantities to represent a risk to the child even at therapeutic levels.

Group IV: Not known whether active ingredients enter the milk.

Of 960 drugs registered and reviewed, 5% were in Group I, 32% in Group II, 12% in Group III, and 50.8% in Group IV.

The transfer of drugs and other chemicals into human milk also has been detailed in a statement by the AAP Committee on Drugs in 1983, 1989, 1994, and 2001.[29] The list includes only those drugs about which there is published information, and it does not provide the pharmacologic properties of the compounds. The 2001 list is divided into the same seven categories as the earlier lists, grouping drugs by their risk factors in relationship to breastfeeding. The categories are the following:

1. Cytotoxic drugs that may interfere with cellular metabolism of the nursing infant
2. Drugs of abuse
3. Radioactive compounds that require temporary cessation of breastfeeding
4. Drugs for which the effect on nursing infants is unknown but may be of concern
5. Drugs that have been associated with significant effects on some nursing infants and should be given to nursing mothers with caution
6. Maternal medications usually compatible with breastfeeding
7. Food and environmental agents: effect on breastfeeding

The list of more than 300 items is not inclusive. Further, the committee encourages physicians to report adverse effects in the infant consuming milk of a mother taking a specific drug to the committee at the American Academy of Pediatrics.[29] Other rating systems have been suggested, but this system has been used consistently since 1983.

As new texts regarding drugs in lactation are published, many authors have chosen their own scales to describe the status of a given drug, although AAP had established one in 1983. Briggs, Freeman, and Yaffe[20] use the AAP classification. Hale[55] designed a new system: L_1 safest, L_2 safer, L_3 moderately safe, L_4 possibly hazardous, and L_5 contraindicated, which is the reverse of the AAP system. Weiner and Buhimschi[167] have published an additional system with only three categories: S, safe; NS, not safe; and U, unknown, as categories. This text will continue to use the AAP scale to facilitate consistency.

The Breastfeeding and Human Lactation Study Center at the University of Rochester continually updates its database on drugs, medications, and contaminants in human milk. More than 3000 references pertain to drugs in the database. The tables in Appendix D have been prepared from this information. In addition to information gleaned from reports of specific levels in breast milk, the tables include the ratings by the AAP, Hale, and Weiner. In addition, other drugs typically used by women in their childbearing years about which there are no specific milk levels are listed with their oral bioavailability for the infant, peak serum time in the mother, volume of distribution for the drugs, and other pharmacologic information (pH, solubility, protein binding, metabolism) obtained from a host of resources. With this information, the physician should be able to determine relative risk and thus select the best compound and adjust the dose and the time of and association to the breastfeeding.

Further information is available from the Finger Lakes Regional Poison and Drug Information Center, which has a specially equipped "Lactation Line" to deal with questions about toxicity and lactation, at 585-275-3232. For hearing-impaired persons, TDD (585-273-3854) services are available 24 hours a day every day. This service is staffed by physicians, nurses, pharmacists, and clinical toxicologists. The Breastfeeding and Human Lactation Center is available during limited hours (8 AM to 4 PM EST, Monday to Friday) for more complex questions (585-275-0088).

SPECIFIC DRUG GROUPS

Analgesics

Drugs such as heroin have been known for decades to appear in milk, and at one time withdrawal symptoms in the neonate were prevented or treated by breastfeeding and then gradual weaning. Codeine and meperidine (Demerol) appear in milk at low levels. The pharmacokinetics of IV *meperidine* in neonates and infants under 5 months has shown great interindividual variability in elimination half-life, median clearance, and volume of distribution.[108,123] For example, a breastfed newborn was transferred to the special care nursery at Rochester because of unusual floppiness and poor muscle tone. His mother was taking dextropropoxyphene (Darvon) every 4 hours. Temporarily stopping the nursing until the mother's drug level dropped and discontinuing use of the drug produced dramatic improvement, which persisted when the infant went back to nursing.

Diazepam (Valium) taken in multiple doses has caused sleepiness, mild depression, and decreased intake in some infants and tends to accumulate in the neonate, especially in the first weeks of life. However, an occasional dose of diazepam is not contraindicated.

The dose schedule for analgesics is usually single dose, especially in the postpartum period. A mother should not be subjected to great discomfort when a dose or two of analgesics would improve her well-being.[48] *Aspirin* on a single-dose schedule is quite safe, although it is known to pass into her milk. The case of metabolic acidosis reported in a nursing infant occurred when the mother took 10 grains of aspirin every 4 hours for arthritis.[25] A serum salicylate level in the infant on the third day of hospitalization with no breastfeeding was still 24 mg/dL. This demonstrates the tendency of salicylate to accumulate in the neonate. Acetylsalicylic acid, not the metabolite salicylate, is responsible for the platelet aggregate abnormalities, so there should be no concern about aspirin in this regard, because it is the metabolite salicylate that appears in the milk. *Acetaminophen* is remarkably well tolerated by the neonate and can be given to a nursing mother. Although it does reach the milk in small amounts, the neonate metabolizes it well.

Prescription *ibuprofen* has been extensively used in 600- to 800-mg doses as an antiinflammatory agent, especially in the treatment of arthritis. Since it became available in over-the-counter preparations of 200-mg tablets, ibuprofen has become widely used by the public for pain. Pediatricians are using it liberally for fever and myalgia and generalized aches and pains. It is widely used for postpartum pain of episiotomy or cesarean birth.

Because of the initial concern about adverse effects of prostaglandin synthetase inhibiting drugs on the neonate, as well as a report of negligible (less than 0.05 µg/mL) levels in the milk of a woman after 17 days of therapy (400 mg twice a day), a careful study of ibuprofen was undertaken.[163,164] Twelve postcesarean birth women had serum and milk samples collected at intervals for 34 hours following 400 mg ibuprofen every 6 hours for five doses. Serum half-life was 1.5 hours. No measurable amounts (capable of detecting 1 µg/mL) of ibuprofen were found in breast milk. The authors concluded that under normal dosing, a nursing infant would be exposed to less than 1 mg of ibuprofen per day.[164]

Fentanyl citrate is frequently used to provide analgesia or anesthesia to women during the postpartum period. It is a potent synthetic phenylpiperidine with extremely high lipid solubility and high pK_a but a large volume of distribution, suggesting a predisposition to appear in breast milk but clear rapidly. In a study of postpartum lactating women receiving fentanyl, concentrations were higher in colostrum than in the serum, probably due to the open cell junctions, peaked at 45 minutes after administration, and were undetectable 6 to 10 hours later. The oral bioavailability of less than 50% is reduced by food, which makes the risk to the infant minimal via the mother's milk, especially if peak serum time is avoided.

The use of *epidural anesthesia* during delivery and its continuation postcesarean birth for pain has provided considerable relief to parturient women. Despite epidurals during labor having become commonplace; the effects of this procedure on the neonate's ability to breastfeed are still disputed. The obstetric literature clearly shows that epidurals in early labor result in an increased rate of interventions, including forceps use, vacuum extraction, and cesarean delivery.[110] These in turn result in increased postpartum complications and an increase in the length of hospital stay. When women who had cesarean delivery were followed prospectively, those who had epidural anesthesia breastfed sooner and continued longer than those women who had general anesthesia.[90] The challenging question, however, is whether an epidural affects the infant's ability to suckle and initiate breastfeeding in women who have a vaginal delivery (see infant suckling discussion in Chapter 8).

Although labor pain relief is superior with epidural analgesia compared with meperidine, labor is prolonged, uterine infection increased, and the number of operative deliveries increased, all of which interfere with successful initiation of suckling in the neonate.[110] Meperidine is no longer used during labor, but other short-acting analgesics such as nalbuphine (Nubain) are.[114,115] A study of butorphanol and nalbuphine demonstrated that receiving no medication or receiving a dose less than 1 hour before delivery was associated with earlier initiation of breastfeeding and establishment of effective feeding significantly earlier compared with mothers who received the drug more than an hour before delivery.[126] Righard and Alade[131] also observed the impact of meperidine on neonatal behavior. When they observed infants left on the maternal abdomen to find the breast and latch on, the nonmedicated infants were suckling in 20 minutes, but the medicated infants were unable to locate the breast and latch on and, in several cases, were unable to locate the breast after 40 minutes of trial.

Ketorolac tromethamine has been used for maternal pain in the first few days post partum, especially in cesarean delivery patients. The concern has been the safety of breastfeeding during that time because ketorolac is an acidic pyrrolo-pyrrole prostaglandin synthetase inhibitor with a pK_a of

3.54 and 99.2% plasma protein binding. Would the drug get into the milk and interfere with the physiologic closing of the infant's ductus arteriosus? Wischnik and associates[175] examined this question in 10 women who received the drug 2 to 6 days after delivery. The mothers were pumping and discarding the milk because of illness in both mother and baby. Ketorolac 10 mg was given four times a day for 2 days. Plasma and milk samples were collected and levels measured; limits of detection were 10 μg/mL. The range was 5.9 μg/L to 7.9 μg/L in milk, although four patients never had measurable amounts in the milk. The M/P ratio was 0.015 to 0.037. The authors estimated that a maximum dose for an infant would be 3.16 to 7.9 μg/day. They assumed 400 to 1000 mL of milk was consumed, an improbable amount in the first few days. At maximum, the ketorolac level in milk was 0.16% to 0.40% of total daily maternal dose. Clinically, the authors concluded that significant sequelae from ketorolac are unlikely. The AAP rates ketorolac a category 6 drug, usually compatible with breast-feeding.[175]

Antibiotics

Levels of antibiotics in milk vary with the concentration of the drugs in plasma and their pK_a. The risks vary among groups of antibiotics. *Penicillins* are not usually toxic but theoretically can cause sensitivity. *Sulfa drugs* should not be used in the first month of life because they can interfere with the binding of bilirubin to protein. The risk diminishes with age, and infants are given sulfa drugs directly at 4 to 6 weeks of age. Infants with glucose-6-phosphate dehydrogenase (G6PD) deficiency should never receive sulfa drugs directly or via the breast milk. *Chloramphenicol* is contraindicated in nursing very young infants because of the risk of accumulation of the drug even from small amounts in milk and the potential for idiosyncratic reaction.

Tetracycline causes staining of teeth and abnormalities of bone growth when given directly to children for a week or more. Infants breastfed by mothers taking tetracycline for mastitis may have stained and mottled first and second teeth when therapy exceeds 10 days. The amount in milk is half that in the mother's plasma. Tetracycline should be given to mothers only for life-threatening infections.

Erythromycin appears in higher amounts in milk than in plasma. When given intravenously to the mother, the levels are 10 times higher. When the infant is old enough to receive erythromycin directly, the mother can take it as well. The major concerns regarding erythromycin pertain to its cross-effects with other medications, especially the potential to increase terfenadine (Seldane) levels, possibly resulting in increased QT intervals. Terfenadine pharmacokinetics has been studied in breast milk.[20] Seldane has been removed from the market. Erythromycin also has the potential for decreasing the clearance of carbamazepine, cyclosporine, digoxin, triazolam, theophylline, anticoagulants, and drugs metabolized by the P-450 system.

Aminoglycosides are common constituents of postpartum antibiotic therapy and are given parentally. They readily appear in the milk but, as with kanamycin, are not readily absorbed from the gastrointestinal (GI) tract; therefore, under usual circumstances they pose no problem to the neonate, who will not absorb them. Newborns are given aminoglycosides directly.

Metronidazole (Flagyl) does appear in milk at levels equal to those in serum. Most researchers consider the risk to the infant sufficient to suggest alternative therapy for the mother. Symptoms include decreased appetite and vomiting and, occasionally, blood dyscrasia.

An alternative treatment regimen is 2 g metronidazole in a single dose. When milk concentrations are measured with a 2-g dose, the highest concentrations are found at 2 and 4 hours postingestion and decline over the next 12 hours to 19.1 μg/mL and to 12.6 μg/mL at 24 hours.[40,58] The dose to the infant is calculated to be 21.8 mg over the first 24 hours and only 3.5 mg in the second 24 hours. It has been recommended that the single-dose regimen be used in nursing mothers, which necessitates that a mother pump and discard milk for only 24 hours. Metronidazole in gel or cream form contains only 0.75% of the medication and is poorly absorbed because the purpose is to work on tissues locally. As a result, maternal plasma levels are $\frac{1}{50}$ of levels from comparable oral dosing. Use of the drug in this form would probably result in undetectable amounts in the milk. Normally the gel or cream is applied in small amounts twice daily. Peak absorption could be avoided. Metronidazole is often the only drug that works in a serious trichomoniasis, giardiasis, or amebiasis infection[40] when all other treatments have failed. It has also been used directly in infants.

Amoxicillin, cephalexin, and cefadroxil, when given orally in a single dose, peak in the milk at 4 to 6 hours.[70] Cephalothin, cephapirin, and cefotaxime, when given in a bolus IV injection, peak at 2 hours. Cefadroxil reached the highest levels (1.64 ± 0.73 μg/mL) at 6 hours. Little gets into the milk. These drugs are also given to children.

Cephalosporins are weak acids with variable protein binding. Third-generation cephalosporins may affect the flora of the gut. Sterilization of the gut often leads to diarrhea. In general, cephalosporins are considered safe during lactation.[30] Breastfed infants rapidly recolonize the gut with lactobacillus. Oral absorption is poor and little reaches the milk so they usually are considered safe.

The serum half-lives of parenterally administered cephalosporins are three to four times longer in the neonate than the serum half-lives in the mother. The half-life of ceftriaxone in the milk is 12 to 17 hours, compared with the maternal serum half-life of 6 hours. The M/P ratio at 8 hours was 0.05 and at 24 hours, 0.1. The neonate can be given cephalosporins directly. Ceftriaxone is given IM to infants once a day.

Chloroquine, gentamicin, streptomycin, and rifampin (only 0.05%) are reported by AAP[29] to be safe because they are not excreted in milk. Additional antibiotics are listed in Appendix D.

Because antibiotics are the most frequent medication prescribed for lactating women, it is noteworthy that the compliance is low. Maternal noncompliance was measured by Ito and associates[66] in 203 breastfeeding women who consulted the Motherisk Program for information about antibiotics. Despite reassuring advice, one in five women either did not initiate therapy or did not continue breastfeeding. This has serious implications for recurrent infections, especially mastitis. Mastitis represents another situation in which termination of breastfeeding is not indicated.

Anticholinergics

Anticholinergic drugs include atropine, scopolamine (hyoscine), and synthetic quaternary ammonium derivatives, some of which are available in over-the-counter medications. Some *atropine* does enter the milk. Infants are particularly sensitive to this drug; therefore, the infant involved should be watched for tachycardia and thermal changes, which are more easily measured in infants. The most important consideration is that milk secretion may decrease in the mother. Constipation and urinary retention may occur in the infant with repeat doses. The *quaternary anticholinergics* should not appear in milk to any degree because, as anions, they do not pass into the acidic milk. Both O'Brien[118] and Gaginella[47] have reported that mepenzolate methylbromide (Cantil) does not appear in milk.

Scopolamine is available by dermal patch for motion sickness and causes maternal mucous membrane dryness, which could affect milk production. Only a small amount appears in milk. The AAP rates it and atropine as category 6 drugs, usually compatible with breastfeeding, although the scopolamine patch, which provides a constant level, has not been tested per se. Pressure point wristbands are reported to be effective for motion sickness in pregnancy and lactation and contain no medication.

Gastrointestinal medications

Cimetidine (Tagamet), a potent H_2-receptor antagonist, is used for conditions associated with acid peptic digestion in the GI tract, especially elevated gastric acidity. Cimetidine excretion into breast milk has resulted in concentrations higher than in the corresponding plasma sample.[151] Levels were highest at 1 hour after a single dose. Chronic-dose studies revealed variable M/P ratios, all of which were higher than the single-dose ratio. The authors suggest an active transport mechanism for this medication. The maximum amount of cimetidine ingested by an infant was calculated at 6 mg for 1 L of milk (or 1.5 mg/kg). It is rated 6 by the AAP.

The neonatal dose is 10 to 20 mg/kg/24 hours for severe gastroesophageal reflux or gastric ulcer, conditions that are rare in a breastfed infant. The half-life in a neonate is 1.1 to 3.4 hours. It is contraindicated when either infant or mother is receiving cisapride because of the risk of precipitating cardiac arrhythmias.[151] Caution is recommended with nursing when taking cimetidine until more is known of its side effects, especially antiandrogenic features.[42] Although previously rated as contraindicated during breastfeeding and put in category 1 by the AAP, cimetidine is now category 6, compatible with breastfeeding, although levels may be higher in milk than in serum.[29] Cimetidine does interfere with several drugs, including phenytoin, propanolol, warfarin, and tricyclic antidepressants.

Sulfasalazine treatment of ulcerative colitis and Crohn's disease during breastfeeding has been widely discussed on theoretic grounds because the compound splits to sulfapyridine and 5-aminosalicylic acid (5-ASA). The sulfapyridine is absorbed from the colon and is metabolized in the liver. The 5-ASA is partly absorbed and rapidly excreted in the urine, so serum concentrations are low (although AAP rates it 5). The sulfapyridine and its metabolites do appear in the milk in lower concentrations than in the serum. A dose of 2 g/day of drug to the mother would produce 4 mg/kg of sulfapyridine in the milk, about 40% of maternal levels. The oral absorption from the milk is low, so the actual amount in the infant's plasma is minimal. The risk of recurrent ulcerative colitis if medication is withdrawn outweighs the risk of sulfasalazine to the infant.[75] The AAP rates it a 6 (in 2001 list).[29]

Famotidine (Pepcid-AC) reduces gastric acidity. Its milk levels are low and it has poor oral bioavailability so is of little risk, although not listed by AAP. Omeprazole (Prilosec), which also reduces gastric acidity, has milk levels that are also low. It is highly protein bound and only 40% orally bioavailable so should be safe, although it is not listed by AAP.

Anticoagulants

Heparin, regular or unfractionated, is a large-molecular-weight molecule that does not pass into breast milk. Because it is not absorbed from the GI tract, its use in the breastfeeding mother is acceptable.

Low-molecular-weight (LMW) heparins are glycosaminoglycans consisting of chains of alternating residues of D-glucosamine and uronic acid. The regular or unfractionated heparin is a heterogeneous mixture of polysaccharide chains ranging from 3000 to 30,000 mol wt. LMW heparin has a mean mol wt of about 5000 daltons (2000 to 8000), with slight variation among brands: ardeparin (Normiflo), dalteparin (Fragmin), enoxaparin (Lovenox), nadroparin (Fraxiparine), reviparin (Clivarin), and tinzaparin (Innohep). Both unfractionated and LMW heparins cause anticoagulation by activating antithrombin. LMW heparins produce a more predictable anticoagulant response because of their better bioavailability, longer half-life, dose-independent clearance, and decreased tendency to bind to plasma proteins and endothelium. They are less likely to interfere with platelets. They are considered safer and more effective in the treatment of venous thromboembolism, can be given subcutaneously without laboratory monitoring, carry less risk of thrombocytopenia and osteoporosis, and can be given at home.[168]

No studies are reported of LMW heparin use in pregnancy or lactation. Because mol wt is greater than 2000 and only a molecule of less than 1000 mol wt crosses the placenta or into the milk, these molecules are unlikely to cross. These LMW compounds are not orally bioavailable and would not be absorbed by the infant. They are considered safe during lactation.

Analysis of the milk of mothers using *warfarin* by Orme and associates[120] did not reveal any drug in the milks or in the infants. The infants' prothrombin times remained normal. This has been further confirmed by McKenna and associates,[102] who followed two breastfed infants whose mothers were anticoagulated before delivery and maintained on warfarin post partum. They found no immediate or delayed biologic effect on coagulation in 56 and 131 days of follow-up. From this, it has been suggested that warfarin is the drug of choice in the lactating mother who requires anticoagulant therapy and wants to continue breastfeeding. If surgery is contemplated or unusual trauma occurs, a review of the infant's coagulation status is indicated as a precautionary measure, and 1 mg vitamin K can be given orally or intramuscularly if there is concern.

Antithyroid drugs

Iodide has been known for generations to pass into the milk in levels higher than in the maternal plasma. It has been reported to cause symptoms in infants when used not only for hyperthyroidism but also in asthma preparations and cough medicines. Iodides have been noted to be goitrogenic and to sensitize the thyroid gland to other drugs, such as lithium, chlorpromazine, and methylxanthines.

Thiouracil is actively transported into the milk and appears in higher concentration in milk than in blood or urine, being reported at levels 3 to 12 times higher in milk than in blood. It has the potential of causing goiter-suppressing thyroid activity or agranulocytes. Thiouracil is contraindicated during lactation but is labeled category 6 by the AAP.

Methimazole (Tapazole) presents risks to the nursing infant similar to those seen with thiouracil (i.e., thyroid suppression, goiter). Giving 0.125 grain of thyroid extract may not adequately protect the infant, and careful monitoring of neonatal thyroid function is mandatory. Measurements of amounts of methimazole in milk and serum when a mother received 2.5 mg every 12 hours were found to be similar. Tegler and Lindström[159] found 7% to 16% of the maternal dose in the milk; thus, a dose of 5 mg four times daily might provide the infant with 3 mg daily. Studies of carbimazole using ^{38}S-labeled compound show a similar trend, with 0.47% of the dose appearing in the milk. Studies were done on a single dose of 10 mg carbimazole.

Propylthiouracil (PTU) has been investigated by several groups with similar results reported, showing that little of the compound is excreted in the milk (0.025% to 0.077% of total dose) in single-dose studies.[71] An infant followed 5 months on maternal doses of 200- to 300-mg PTU daily showed no neonatal thyroid symptoms and normal triiodothyronine (T_3), thyroxine (T_4), and thyroid-stimulating hormone (TSH). On the strength of these reports, others have proceeded to use PTU and permit breastfeeding. The availability of microdeterminations for T_3, T_4, and TSH improves the quality of monitoring, and all infants given PTU via the milk should be followed closely. The AAP lists PTU in category 6, compatible with breastfeeding.[29]

Caffeine and other methylxanthines

Caffeine ingestion has been singled out for discussion because it is a frequent concern, but the data provided in most reviews are misleading. With a given dose of caffeine that is comparable to that in a cup of coffee, the level in the milk is low (1% of level in mother), and the level in the infant's plasma is also low. However, caffeine does accumulate in the infant.

Before the availability of the laboratory test for caffeine, cases were managed on clinical symptoms alone. Many clinicians recognized and the Rochester series[132] of nursing mothers documented that wakeful, hyperactive infants were often the victims of caffeine stimulation. If a mother drank more than 6 to 8 cups of any caffeine-containing beverage in a day's time, her infant could accumulate symptomatic amounts of caffeine. Soft drinks such as colas and other carbonated drinks (e.g., Mountain Dew) often contributed to the caffeine buildup. When the situation was identified—a wide-eyed, active, alert infant who never slept for long—it was suggested that the mother try caffeine-free beverages, both hot and cold. Often the infant settled down to a reasonable sleep pattern after a few days with no caffeine.

Since information on milk and plasma levels has become available, researchers have identified three cases of caffeine excess in breastfed infants, one of which Rivera-Calimlim[132] reported. The infants all had measurable levels of caffeine in the plasma, which disappeared over a week's time after the caffeine was discontinued. The corresponding milk levels were as previously reported, about 1% of the mother's level, which supports the hypothesis that caffeine accumulates in the infant. The infants do not need to be hospitalized, and verification of blood caffeine levels is helpful but not mandatory because a clinical trial will suffice. Smoking has been observed to augment the caffeine effect.

With an increasing number of women with asthma wanting to breastfeed, a question arises about the impact of theophylline. The methylxanthines have also been used in apnea of prematurity, so information has been generated regarding dose, clearance, and toxicity in the neonate.[12] In addition, microdeterminations of blood levels are readily available.

Several studies of *theophylline* in mothers receiving regular doses have shown that the serum levels are lowest just before the oral dose and that M/P ratio is 0.60 to 0.73, with milk levels paralleling serum levels.[136,152,181] The infant receives an estimated 1% of the maternal dose. Data on IV and PO medication are similar in terms of M/P ratio. Maximum exposure was estimated at 7 to 8 mg/24 hours.

Dyphylline is a compound introduced clinically as a bronchodilator because of its lack of side effects.[67] It is excreted renally with little biotransformation. The M/P ratio was determined to be 2.08 ± 0.52, and the biologic half-life was 3.21 hours. Although this is considerably greater than that of theophylline, it is not yet known how this would affect the infant.

Theobromine, which occurs in chocolate and cocoa, has been studied as well to evaluate its possible cumulative effects when taken with caffeine or theophylline.[12] A very small amount was detected in the milk, with a potential dose to the infant after one chocolate bar (1.2 oz) of 0.44 to 1.68 mg. No theobromine was found in the infant's urine.[13]

The management of asthma has shifted in recent years to steroids, antibiotics, and inhalants. *Steroids*

are excreted in the milk in low doses that have not presented a problem to the nursling, who is automatically weaned as the mother is weaned. Antibiotics are well tolerated, as discussed previously. *Inhalants* are unique because they act at the level of the bronchial mucosa and are poorly absorbed. *Albuterol* (Proventil, Ventalin) is a β_2-adrenergic agonist that is rapidly effective when inhaled, peaking within 30 minutes. The potential for drug levels in the milk is minimal, as less than 10% of inhaled drug is absorbed, and no adverse reactions have been reported in nurslings. The PO albuterol dose for infants with asthma is 0.1 to 0.3 mg/kg every 6 to 8 hours.

Fluticasone (Flovent inhaled and Flonase nasally) by inhalation so that systemic levels are less than 2% nasally and 30% by inhalation and plasma levels is almost undetectable, and given the usual dosing schedule, there should be no buildup. Use during lactation is considered safe, although AAP did not rank either form.

Drugs of abuse and alcohol

The AAP Committee on Drugs[29] has assigned a special category to drugs of abuse: category 2, which they consider contraindicated during breastfeeding. The list is short: amphetamine, cocaine, heroin, marijuana, and phencyclidine hydrochloride (angel dust, PCP). They strongly state further that these compounds and all other drugs of abuse are hazardous not only to the nursing infant, but also to the mother's physical and emotional health. Obviously, the latter is also true for bottle feeding mothers. (See Chapter 16 for further discussion of nicotine and smoking.) Nicotine's inclusion in category 2 was controversial, especially because the data are clear that children of smoking mothers do better if breastfed in regard to general health, respiratory illness, and risk of sudden infant death syndrome (SIDS). Nicotine no longer appears in any AAP category.

The epidemiologic evidence of the impact of maternal smoking on breastfeeding was studied by Amir and Donath.[3] They concluded that psychosocial factors are largely responsible for the lower rates of breastfeeding found in women who smoke compared to those who do not. Fewer smokers intend to breastfeed in the first place. The duration of breastfeeding in smokers is inversely related to the number of cigarettes smoked per day.[62]

The consumption of alcohol during lactation also deserves careful consideration because of the wide range of effects and the wide range of dosages.[74] Beer and wine are standard beverages in many parts of the world and have been recommended to enhance lactation, especially when the mother is stressed with worldly chores. Some forms of alcohol have also been used as an aperitif to encourage a woman to eat heartily while lactating. The AAP listing is category 6.[29]

Alcohol is one of the most rapidly absorbed compounds. Maximum blood levels are achieved in 15 minutes in adults. Lactating and nonlactating women handle alcohol differently. Lactators tend to peak at lower levels and clear the drug more quickly. Alcohol passes quickly between blood and milk, however, with peak levels in milk at 30 to 60 minutes and at 60 to 90 minutes when taken with food. Studies in males and nonlactating women show an increase in serum prolactin with alcohol.[32,105] This has not been tested in lactators. The impact of alcohol on oxytocin is dose related. No effect is seen on ingesting 0.5 g/kg or less, and varying effects are reported in different women as dose is increased.[32] At least a partial decrease in milk let-down is seen at 1.0 to 1.5 g/kg, and all women have significant to complete block in milk ejection at 1.5 to 2.0 g/kg.[26] Alcohol blocks the release of oxytocin rather than blocking the response of the breast. The amount of alcohol excreted into milk with doses less than 1 g/kg of absolute alcohol usually does not affect the infant.[86]

Experimental prolactin studies in lactating rats show that acutely administered alcohol does not affect basal plasma prolactin but does inhibit suckling-induced prolactin for about 2 hours. This effect is manifest at a blood alcohol level of 0.65%.[157] When alcohol levels were 0.20% (inebriated), extended suckling overcame the effect. The amount of milk consumed in experimental and control rats was the same in 3 hours, and growth rate over 21 days did not differ.

Many investigations have measured the pharmacologic impact of alcohol consumption.[23,45,69,74,104,174] Alcohol appears quickly in both foremilk and hindmilk at a level equivalent to or higher than corresponding maternal blood samples. Although levels are high in the blood, no acetaldehyde is found in the milk. Levels in milk drop in parallel to those in the blood because alcohol is not stored in the breast. In a study by Lawton,[86] milk levels were very low despite that the participating mothers drank as much as they could as quickly as possible, averaging between 43 and 90 mL of absolute alcohol. Levels were drawn every half hour for 4 hours in this study.

When women served as their own controls in an experiment to observe feeding behavior and volume of milk consumed by the infant with and without maternal alcohol, there was significant and uniform intensity of odor to their milk, peaking between 30 and 60 minutes after ingestion.[104] The odor paralleled the concentration of alcohol (0 to 32 mg/dL). Infants sucked more frequently but consumed less milk in the presence of alcohol (120.4 ± 9.5 mL vs. 156.4 ± 8.2 mL). When a similar study was done with beer and nonalcohol beer, the findings were similar: the infants sucked less well with the alcohol beverage.[23] Mothers, however, were unaware of the differences and felt they had experienced let-down and their infants had nursed well. This work has precipitated considerable response because of the belief that a little beer or wine enhances mother's release of milk.

Although this work suggests that a little alcohol may not enhance milk volume received by the infant, the alcohol was taken in a research setting and consumed in 10 minutes. When the mother takes a little wine socially, it is usually to create a different ambience and help her relax and improve her ejection reflex. In addition, many women who enjoy sipping an occasional beer or wine may well be discouraged from breastfeeding if they think wine or beer would be forbidden.

The report of Little and associates[93] regarding the effect of alcohol on the nursing infant implies that alcohol causes developmental delay. The drinking would be classified as heavy in this group, whose infants had slight gross motor delay at 1 year. Furthermore, the infants were subjected to the alcohol in utero as well. Heavy drinking should not be condoned; however, it will be very important to follow the children in all the cohorts for at least 7 years until their higher learning centers are testable.

Infants spent significantly less time sleeping during the 3.5 hours after consuming alcohol-flavored breast milk by bottle (56.8 minutes) compared with plain breast milk by bottle (78.2 minutes). The authors concluded that short-term exposure to small amounts of alcohol in breast milk produces distinctive changes in the infant's sleep-wake pattern.[105]

A study in Mexico following 32 infants born to mothers who drank a mild Mexican alcoholic beverage called *pulque* (3% alcohol, up to 2 L/day) throughout pregnancy produced no infants with fetal alcohol syndrome, but there was a higher incidence of low birth weight (less than third percentile).[45] Relative risk was 3.39. The infants were followed during lactation as well. Ethanol found in the milk accounted for 40 mg/day available to the infant. Postnatal growth was similar in both groups at 6 months. Developmental studies were not reported.

The recommendation regarding alcohol requires the physician to avoid prescribing or proscribing it and assist the mother in appropriately adjusting her alcohol consumption in both timing and volume.

When a nursing mother does have "a drink or two," she should avoid breastfeeding for at least 2 hours. Pumping and discarding milk does not hasten the removal from the milk because the level in the milk matches that in the plasma at the time of the feeding.

Herbs and herbal teas

Herbal medicine is the use of plants or plant parts in their natural state without chemical processing. Natural is not a synonym for safe. Because herbals are considered dietary supplements, they are not controlled by the Food and Drug Administration,

although the FDA has spoken out on the dangers of comfrey and ephedra (Table 11-4). Herbal products contain many chemicals in each, some of which may have pharmacologic properties. The major concerns are quality control, unknown additives, unknown side effects, and no placebo controlled studies regarding efficacy and toxicity. Labels in the United States must say: "This product is not intended to diagnose, treat, cure, or prevent any disease."

Use of herbs and herbal teas has increased, especially among those interested in natural foods.[146] As is well known to all students of pharmacology, many effective medications originated from these natural products. In the early part of the 20th century, many compounds were still being dispensed in their natural form, including foxglove leaves for digitalis. The natural product was unpredictable because one leaf or plant contains more or less active principle than another, so careful dose control was impossible and results were often unpredictable. Much of the interest in herbal teas has evolved as individuals seek a beverage that does not contain caffeine; what they receive is another compound instead, often one more potent and frequently one about which considerably less is known (Table 11-5). Contamination, adulteration, and misidentification contribute to the problems associated with use.

Herbal teas are available that are prepared carefully, using herbs only for essence (e.g., Celestial Seasonings brand tea) and avoiding heavy doses of herbs with active principles. However, the strength of any tea depends on how it is made. An ordinary teabag with hot water run over it will contain little caffeine and theobromine; however, when the tea is steeped for 5 minutes, the potency is increased 10-fold. Some of the preparations are benign or even nutritious, such as rose hips tea, which contains a large amount of vitamin C. Other teas are made from plants known to the toxicologist as poisonous. Isolated reports of toxicity from these preparations are appearing in the medical literature; many others probably go undiagnosed.[143] Use of these preparations is certainly an important part of a medical and dietary history.

TABLE 11-4   Clinically important effects and perioperative concerns of 8 herbal medicines and recommendations for discontinuation of use before surgery

Herb: common name(s)	Relevant pharmacologic effects	Perioperative concerns	Preoperative discontinuation
Echinacea: purple coneflower root	Activation of cell-mediated immunity	Allergic reactions; decreased effectiveness of immunosuppressants; potential for immunosuppression with long-term use	No data
Ephedra: ma huang	Increased heart rate and blood pressure through direct and indirect sympathomimetic effects	Risk of myocardial ischemia and stroke from tachycardia and hypertension; ventricular arrhythmias with halothane; long-term use depletes endogenous catecholamines and may cause intraoperative hemodynamic instability; life-threatening interaction with monoamine oxidase inhibitors	At least 24 hours before surgery
Garlic: ajo	Inhibition of platelet aggregation (may be irreversible); increased fibrinolysis; equivocal antihypertensive activity	Potential to increase risk of bleeding, especially when combined with other medications that inhibit platelet aggregation	At least 7 days before surgery
Ginkgo: duck foot tree, maidenhair tree, silver apricot	Inhibition of platelet-activating factor	Potential to increase risk of bleeding, especially when combined with other medications that inhibit platelet aggregation	At least 36 hours before surgery
Ginseng: American ginseng, Asian ginseng, Chinese ginseng, Korean ginseng	Lowers blood glucose; inhibition of platelet aggregation (may be irreversible); increased PT-PTT in animals; many other diverse effects	Hypoglycemia; potential to increase risk of bleeding; potential to decrease anticoagulation effect of warfarin	At least 7 days before surgery
Kava: awa, intoxicating pepper, kawa	Sedation, anxiolysis	Potential to increase sedative effect of anesthetics; potential for addiction, tolerance, and withdrawal after abstinence unstudied	At least 24 hours before surgery
St. John's wort: amber, goat weed, hardhay, Hypericum, klamatheweed	Inhibition of neurotransmitter reuptake, monoamine oxidase inhibition is unlikely	Induction of cytochrome P450 enzymes, affecting cyclosporine, warfarin, steroids, protease inhibitors, and possibly benzodiazepines, calcium	At least 5 days before surgery

channel blockers, and many other drugs; decreased serum digoxin levels

Valerian: all heal, garden heliotrope, vandal root	Sedation	Potential to increase sedative effect of anesthetics; benzodiazepine-like acute withdrawal; potential to increase anesthetic requirements with long-term use	No data

Herbal medicine and other dietary supplement-related sites on the World Wide Web

Organization	Web address	Site information
Center for Food Safety and Applied Nutrition, Food and Drug Administration	http://vm.cfsan.fda.gov/~dms/supplmnt.html	Clinicians should use this site to report adverse events associated with herbal medicines and other dietary supplements. Sections also contain safety, industry, and regulatory information.
National Center for Complementary and Alternative Medicine, National Institutes of Health	http://nccam.nih.gov	This site contains fact sheets about alternative therapies, consensus reports, and databases.
Agricultural Research Service, United States Department of Agriculture	http://www.ars-grin.gov/duke	The site contains an extensive phytochemical database with search capabilities.
Quackwatch	http://www.quackwatch.com	Although this site addresses all aspects of health care, there is a considerable amount of information covering complementary and herbal therapies.
National Council Against Health Fraud	http://www.ncahf.org	This site focuses on health fraud with a position paper on over-the-counter herbal remedies.
HerbMed	http://www.herbmed.org	This site contains information on more than 120 herbal medications, with evidence for activity, warnings, preparations, mixtures, and mechanisms of action. There are short summaries of important research publications with MEDLINE links.
ConsumerLab	http://www.consumerlab.com	This site is maintained by a corporation that conducts independent laboratory investigations of dietary supplements and other health products.

PT-PTT, prothrombin time-partial thromboplastin time.
From Ang-Lee MK, Moss J, Yuan CS: Herbal medicines and perioperative care. JAMA 286(2):213, 214, 2001.

TABLE 11-5 Psychoactive substances used in herbal preparations

Labeled ingredient	Botanical source	Pharmacologic principle	Suggested use and reported effects
African yohimbé bark; yohimbine	*Corynanthe yohimbé*	Yohimbine	Smoke or tea as stimulant; mild hallucinogen
Broom; scotch broom	*Cytisus spp.*	Cytisine	Smoke for relaxation; strong sedative-hypnotic
Buckthorn	*Hiptothae rhamnoides*	Anthraquinones	Tea; cathartic toxin, severe watery diarrhea
Burdock root	*Arctium minus*	Atropine	Tea; anticholinergic blockade, anaphylactic shock
California poppy	*Eschscholtzia californica*	Alkaloids and glucosides	Smoke as marijuana substitute; mild euphoriant
Catnip	*Nepeta cataria*	Nepetalactone	Smoke or tea as marijuana substitute; mild hallucinogen
Chamomile	*Chamomilla recutita* *Chamaemelum nobile*	Antigens of Compositae family	Tea; contact dermatitis (in patients sensitive to ragweed, asters, chrysanthemum)
Cinnamon	*Cinnamonum camphora*	?	Smoke with marijuana; mild stimulant
Comfrey	*Symphytum officinale*	Pyrrolizidine alkaloids	Tea; venoocclusive disease, hepatic failure, ?hepatocarcinogen
Foxglove tea	*Digitalis purpurea*	Digitalis	Tea; malignant arrhythmias, cardiac arrest
Gordolobo, groundsel	*Senecio longilobus* *Senecio vulgaris* *Senecio spartoides*	Pyrrolizidine alkaloids	Tea, venoocclusive disease, hepatic failure
Hops	*Humulus lupulus*	Lupuline	Smoke or tea as sedative and marijuana substitute; none
Hydrangea	*Hydrangea paniculata*	Hydrangin, saponin, cyanogens	Smoke as marijuana substitute; stimulant
Jimson tea	*Datura stramonium*	Atropine, scopolamine, hyoscyamine, stramonium	Tea; ?PNH-like defect, anticholinergic blockade; CNS intoxication, hallucinations, ataxia, blurred vision
Juniper	*Juniper macropoda*	?	Smoke as hallucinogen; strong hallucinogen
Kavakava	*Piper methysticum*	Yangonin, pyrones	Smoke or tea as marijuana substitute; mild hallucinogen
Kola nut; gotu kola	*Cola spp.*	Caffeine, theobromine, kolanin	Smoke, tea, or capsules as stimulant; stimulant
Lobelia	*Lobelia inflata*	Lobeline	Smoke or tea as marijuana substitute; mild euphoriant
Mandrake	*Mandragora officinarum*	Scopolamine, hyoscyamine	Tea as hallucinogen
Maté	*Ilex paraguensis*	Caffeine, pyrrolizidine	Tea as stimulant; ?stimulant, venoocclusive disease
Mormon tea	*Ephedra nevadensis*	Ephedrine	Tea as stimulant; stimulant
Nutmeg	*Myristica fragrans*	Myristin	Hallucinogen, MAD inhibitor; hallucinogen, CNS intoxicant
Oleander	*Nerium oleander*	Myristin	?Hepatic damage
		Cardiac glycosides	Malignant arrhythmias, cardiac arrest

Passion flower	Passiflora incarnata	Digitogenin Nerioside Oleandroside Harmine alkaloids	Smoke, tea, or capsules as marijuana substitute; mild stimulant
Periwinkle	Catharanthus roseus	Indole alkaloids	Smoke or tea as euphoriant; hallucinogen
Pokeroot, pokeweed	Phytolacca americana Phytolacca decandra	Saponins Pokeweed mitogen	Gastroenteritis, bloody diarrhea ?Respiratory depression, ?mitogenic alterations
Prickly poppy	Argemona mexicana	Protopine, berberine, isoquinilines	Smoke as euphoriant; narcotic-analgesic
Sassafras	Sassafras albidum	Safrole	Tea or cold beverage; hepatocarcinogen
Senna	Cassia acutifolia Cassia angustifolia	Antraquinones	Tea; cathartic toxin, severe watery diarrhea
Snakeroot	Rauwolfia serpentina	Reserpine	Smoke or tea as tobacco substitute; tranquilizer
Thorn apple	Datura stramonium	Atropine, scopolamine	Smoke or tea as tobacco substitute or hallucinogen; strong hallucinogen
Tobacco	Nicotiana spp.	Nicotine	Smoke as tobacco; strong stimulant
Valerian	Valeriana officinalis	Chatinine, valerine alkaloids	Tea or capsules as tranquilizer
Wild lettuce	Lactuca sativa	Lactucarine	Smoke as opium substitute; mild narcotic-analgesic
Woodruff	Galium odoratum	Coumarin	Hemorrhagic diathesis, prolonged prothrombin time
Wormwood	Artemisia absinthium	Absinthin	Smoke or tea as relaxant; narcotic-analgesic
Yohimbé bark	Corynanthe yohimbé	Yohimbine	α_2-Sympathetic (presynaptic) blockade

PNH, Paroxysmal nocturnal hemoglobinuria; CNS, central nervous system; MAD, major affective disorder.
Modified from Siegel RK: Herbal intoxication: Psychoactive effects from herbal cigarettes, tea, and capsules. JAMA 236:473, 1976; copyright © 1976, American Medical Association; and Ridker PM: Toxic effects of herbal teas. Arch Environ Health 42:135, 1987.

Box 11-1 lists herbal teas that are thought to be safe for the infant and mother during lactation when used as flavorings and not in therapeutic doses.

In some sense, safety is a matter of dose. In studies of herbs that will safely eliminate the nausea and emesis of pregnancy, ginger and peppermint are reported to be more effective than placebo. Dosing, however, was by capsule of powdered plant (1 g/day) for ginger and oil of peppermint, with no dose provided. It is of concern that ginger in large doses is known as an emmenogogue, which is a promoter of menstruation because it increases the blood flow to the uterus and inhibits platelet aggregation. In literature reviews, 7% consider peppermint unsafe and 16% consider ginger unsafe in pregnancy.[173] There are no data for lactation. Any herbal tea consumed in large volumes (32 oz) daily could be a problem.

Mother's milk tea

Mother's milk tea is a blend of plants handed down for many generations as a galactagogue; it contains a mixture of fennel seeds, coriander seeds, chamomile flowers, lemon grass, borage leaves, blessed thistle leaves, star anise, comfrey leaves, and fenugreek seeds (Table 11-6).[156] It is promoted as containing no caffeine. Although not all the constituents have pharmacologic actions, several do and were used medicinally for centuries. These popular teas have the same potential for problems as do the common popular beverages coffee and cola. The euphoric effects are the most prominent.[146]

BOX 11-1 Herbal teas considered safe during lactation

Tea	Origin/use
Chicory	Root/caffeine-free coffee substitute
Orange spice	Mixture/flavoring
Peppermint	Leaves/flavoring
Raspberry	Fruit/flavoring
Red bush tea	Leaves, fine twigs/beverage
Rose hips	Fruits/vitamin C

Comfrey and pyrrolizidine alkaloids

Considerable concern is mounting over the use of comfrey leaves *(Symphytum officinale)* in the United States, and they have been banned in Canada and Germany. The leaves have been used in teas, salads, and poultices. The use of comfrey has been associated with venoocclusive disease and hepatotoxicity. Comfrey is also rich in hepatotoxic pyrrolizidine alkaloids.[63,130] The highest level of toxin occurs in the roots, which can be obtained in powder form in capsules. Comfrey has been recommended for use to cure various pregnancy, labor, and postpartum symptoms and appears in many home remedy handbooks. It has the greatest potential for toxicity in the fetus and the suckling infant, with fatal fetal venoocclusive disease reported.[1] It is also known to have carcinogenic properties. All credible references caution against its use topically, orally, or in any form.[37,165]

Another herb associated with venoocclusive disease and even death is *Senecio longilobus,* commonly known as *thread-leafed groundsel.*[63,130] As with comfrey, it contains hepatotoxic pyrrolizidine alkaloids. Seven cases of hepatitis have been reported resulting from use of *Teucrium chamaedrys* (germander), a member of the mint family. Botanical identification is essential; sometimes the packet contains substances other than those the label indicates.

Pyrrolizidine alkaloids have been identified in an herbal tea used in the Southwest that was responsible for deaths of several children who were given the tea when they were ill. The alkaloid is excreted within 24 hours, but symptoms may not appear for several days or weeks. Death results from liver failure.

Sassafras and coumarins

Sassafras contains an aromatic oil, safrole, which has been shown to cause cancer in mice; it is therefore no longer permitted as a commercial flavoring, but it appears in herbal teas. It causes central nervous system (CNS) symptoms in mice, including ataxia, ptosis, and hypothermia.[143] It is also thought to interfere with the action of other medications.

TABLE 11-6   **Possible ingredients and effects of mother's milk tea**

Plant	Constituents	Effects	Toxicity
Fennel seed	Volatile oil, anisic acid	Weak diuretic stimulant	CNS disturbances
Coriander seed	Volatile oil, coriandrol	Increases flow of saliva and gastric juice	
Chamomile flower	Volatile oil, bitter glycoside	Sudorific, antispasmodic, used to lighten hair	Vomiting, vertigo
Lemongrass	Lemon flavor		
Borage leaf	Volatile oil, tannin, mineral acids	Diuretic, sudorific, euphoric	Possible
Blessed thistle leaf	Volatile oil, bitter principle	Aperitif, galactagogue, diaphoretic	Strongly emetic
Star anise	Volatile oil, anethole, resin, tannin	Stimulant, mild expectorant	
Comfrey leaf (*Symphytum officinale*)	Protein, vitamin B_{12}, tannin, allantoin, choline, pyrrolizidine alkaloids	Used as mucilage to knit bones, weak sedative, demulcent, astringent	Venoocclusive disease Hepatotoxic
Fenugreek seed (Greek hayseed) (coffee substitute and natural dye)	Mucilage, trigonelline, physterols, celery flavor	Digestive tonic, galactagogue, uterine stimulant, reduces blood sugar	Hypoglycemia, can induce labor
Other beverages			
Coffee plant	Volatile oil, caffeine, tannin	Stimulant, diuretic, coloring	Insomnia, restlessness
Blue cohosh	Saponin, glucoside that affects muscles	Oxytocic, potent, acts on voluntary and involuntary muscles	Irritant, causes pain in fingers and toes

Noted herbalists state that sassafras has no really significant medical or therapeutic use.[37,165] The oil, along with many other volatile oils, does have mild counterirritant properties on external application. It has a pleasant flavor but many harmful qualities. Although banned by the FDA, sassafras appears in other natural food products. Belladonna alkaloids are common in some teas used to create euphoria or ease pain.

A hemorrhagic diathesis was described in a woman who drank quarts of herbal tea that contained tonka beans, melilot (sweet clover), and woodruff, all of which contain natural coumarins.[61] She narrowly avoided gynecologic surgery for excessive hemorrhaging before the history was obtained. The tea also included hawthorn, which contains cardioglucosides that cause hypotension.

Licorice

Licorice, the dry root of *Glycyrrhiza glabra,* has been used for medicinal purposes for millennia; stores of licorice were found in the tombs of Egyptian pharaohs, including that of King Tut. Its history is carefully reviewed by Davis and Morris.[33] The active principle is a glycoside of a triterpene called *glycyrrhizic acid.* Licorice continues to be used as a flavoring agent in drinks, drugs, and candies. In addition to its universal role as an expectorant and demulcent and in ointments for various skin disorders, it has been used for peptic ulcers. Its most perplexing properties are those that cause the retention of water, sodium, and chloride and the increased excretion of potassium, mimicking the effects of large doses of desoxycorticosterone. Because licorice is used to flavor chewing tobacco, chewing has been associated with hypertension, sodium retention, and hypokalemia. Licorice derivatives have been found to reroute the metabolism of aldosterone, desoxycorticosterone, and glucocorticoids.[33] Excessive amounts of licorice should be avoided by the lactating woman. Its use to lose weight should be discouraged. Some licorice candy contains little or no licorice, and the flavor is provided by anise, which is probably harmless. An occasional stick of licorice should not be a risk.[137,162]

Echinacea

Echinacea (coneflower) is used for the common cold and when "immune system enhancement is desired."[165] A lipophilic fraction of the root and leaves contains the most potent immunostimulating compounds, some yet to be identified. It is used topically to stimulate wound healing and orally to enhance immune response. The public seeks it out for the common cold. No data exist about its entry into milk. It has no known side effects, however, even when injected in high doses. Placebo controlled studies have indicated it is not effective to take echinacea for long periods prophylactically, but echinacea does appear to minimize cold symptoms when taken as symptoms begin. Taking it for over 8 weeks has been associated with immunosuppression. It is also important to note that it is a member of the daisy/chrysanthemum family, and can cause allergy in those prone to pollen allergies. It is also reported to have caused asthma, atopy, and anaphylaxis. Its entry into milk is unknown. It is not rated by the AAP.

Use in children has not been effective and has a greater risk of allergic response. Echinacea may even be safer in modest amounts than the polypharmacy available for the common cold (see Table 11-4).

Ginseng

Ginseng is one of the oldest, most widely recognized, and most documented Oriental herbs. It enjoys a reputation for increased capacity for mental work and physical activity and also "antistress" effects. The plant of origin is *Panax schinseng* (Chinese) or *P. quinquefolius* (American), two species of the Araliaceae family. *Panax* is derived from the Greek, meaning "all healing."[85] It has been called an "adaptogen" since it is believed to protect the body against stress and restores homeostasis or provides nonspecific resistance.[4]

The root contains dozens of steroidlike glycosides (ginsenosides), which vary with the species, age, location of growth, and harvest time. It contains sterols, coumarins, flavonoids, and polysaccharides. Although animal studies suggest increased strength and stamina, Engels and Wirth[39] reported that in a carefully blinded and controlled study of 31 healthy men randomized to take 200 mg/day, 400 mg/day, or a placebo, no difference was found in any physiologic or psychological parameter. They measured oxygen consumption, blood lactic acid, and heart rate while the subjects worked at maximum effort on stationary bikes. It does lower blood sugar and can cause hypoglycemia. It has some effect on coagulation pathways and on platelet coagulability which may be irreversible (see Table 11-4).

Products available are numerous and variable, and more than half are worthless according to independent studies, and 25% contain no ginseng, which is extremely expensive ($20 per ounce). It is reported to have estrogen-like effects on some women, with mastalgia common with extended use and mammary nodularity also reported. Although animal experimentation has been considerable, there are no extensive human data, no reliable or standardized preparations, no information on dosage, and no accurate recording of side effects. Ginseng is a medical enigma with no proven efficacy for humans, according to Tyler.[165] General side effects include excitement, nervousness, inability to concentrate, hypertension, hypoglycemia, and skin rash. A case of ginseng use during pregnancy and lactation is reported because the infant showed excessive hirsutism and androgen effect, which cleared when breastfeeding was discontinued at 2 weeks of life.[72] Because of the reported breast effects and occasional reports of vaginal bleeding, it is considered problematic during lactation.

St. John's wort

St. John's wort is being touted in Europe and the United States as an antidepressant and anxiolytic and is now sold in supermarkets as well as health food stores. It comes from an aggressive perennial weed in meadows and roadsides noted for its spotted leaves and numerous yellow-orange flowers with black spots and the capsular fruit. It contains 10% tannin and hypericin, a reddish dianthrone pigment, and other hypericum-like substances (0.2% to 0.5%) as well as a number of volatile oils. The extract is sold as tablets, capsules, drops, transdermal patches, oils, and teas.

The pharmacology of the extract includes inhibition of the neurotransmitters serotonin, norepinephrine, and dopamine; it also binds to γ-aminobutyric acid (GABA) receptors in vitro. When the extract is taken orally, hypericin peaks in serum in 5 hours and reaches steady state with continued dosing in 4 days. The half-life in plasma is 25 hours.[85]

Studies of varying quality abound, and some are reported on the hypericum home page on the Internet. Some are carefully controlled and include standardized testing of depression and mood before and after 3 to 6 weeks of treatment with St. John's wort versus placebo or treatment versus standard antidepressant medication. In their overview and meta-analysis, Linde and associates[92] conclude evidence indicates that extracts of hypericin are more effective than placebo and equally effective as standard antidepressants for mild to moderately severe depressive disorders. Side effects of dry mouth, dizziness, constipation, and confusion occurred in about 20% of subjects receiving hypericin and in 53% taking standard antidepressants. The doses, duration, and assessment tools varied widely in these 23 studies and 1757 outpatients.

Adverse effects with chronic high doses (more than 30 mg/day) include photosensitivity, abdominal symptoms, rarely tachycardia, tachypnea, fever, and fatigue. Because hypericin inhibits dopamine β-hydroxylase, which leads to increased dopamine, increased prolactin inhibitory factor, and suppression of prolactin, it could decrease lactation. No clinical study has investigated this pharmacologic potential. "Better, longer studies are needed to establish the effectiveness and safety of St. John's Wort for treatment of depression. The active ingredients, potency and purity of preparations sold in the USA are all unknown."[103] It is licensed in Germany but is considered a dietary supplement in the United States and has not been evaluated by the FDA (see Table 11-4).

Product identification

The clinician needs to inquire about all foods and beverages when taking a history. If the mother is consuming an excessive amount of any herbal product, its contents should be checked. The regional poison control center may be able to identify active principles if the plant constituents of the food or beverage are known (Table 11-7).

Galactogogues

A galactogogue is a material or action that stimulates milk production. When trying to increase milk supply, the action of increased pumping is the best "galactogogue." When careful lactation management has not produced adequate results, as in the case of a mother pumping for her sick premature infant, various medications and herbs have been recommended. Unfortunately, there are no random blinded placebo controlled studies of efficacy or safety.

Metaclopramide has been studied in small series in which mothers took 10 mg three times daily with an increase in milk supply that in most cases dwindled when the drug was tapered after 10 days, which is the recommended limit because of possible maternal side effects. Metaclopramide has been used in infants for reflux; however, when plasma levels were studied, the less mature the infant, the less good the clearance, and it accumulated.[166] There is a risk for extrapyramidal side effects in some individuals.[38] AAP lists it as a 4 (may be of concern).

Sulpiride, an antidepressant and antipsychotic, is no longer available in the United States and Canada because of its drug interactions and risk of dyskinesia and neuroleptic malignant syndrome. It

TABLE 11-7	**Herbal teas and their side effects**		
Herb/parts used	**Common uses**	**Method of application**	**Side effects**
Aconite (monkshood, wolfsbane)	Aconitine, hypaconitine, aconine, mesaconitine	Tea	Nausea, vomiting, hypersalivation Perioral paresthesia, progressing rapidly to neuromuscular weakness, seizures, coma Cardiac effects: Bradycardia and hypotension (most common), supraventricular or ventricular tachycardia, ventricular fibrillation, asystole
Aloe vera/pure gel from leaves	Burns Constipation Ulcers Canker sores Immunostimulant HIV infections	Gel applied topically or taken internally several times daily Doses not standardized	Diarrhea, gastric cramping when taken internally Contact dermatitis from related species, *Aloe arboresce*
Chamomile/flowers	Calming, sedating Aromatherapy Antispasmodic Colic Antiinflammatory Soothe diaper rash, chickenpox, poison ivy	Tea (in infants) or tinctures Essential oil used in aromatherapy or added to bath	Allergic reactions One case of botulism in infant given tea from homegrown plant
Comfrey	Pyrrolizidine Demulcent Sedative Astringent	Tea Poultice Ointment	Hepatic venoocclusive disease marked by severe abdominal pain and vomiting, which may be followed by hepatomegaly and abdominal distention with ascites Hepatic necrosis leading to cirrhosis *Not recommended*
Echinacea/leaves, stalks, roots	Immunostimulant Colds, ear and sinus infections HIV infections	Tincture, capsules, or tablets taken internally as immunostimulant Doses not standardized	None reported
Ephedra (ma huang)/leaves, stalks	Decongestant Asthma, allergy Weight loss "Natural high"	Generally taken internally	Hypertension, tachycardia Toxic psychosis Death *Not recommended*
Feverfew/fresh or dried leaves	Migraine prophylaxis Rheumatoid arthritis Insect repellent Menstrual pain	1–3 fresh leaves, 25–50 mg capsules, or crushed, dried leaves twice a day to prevent migraine	Allergic reactions Mouth ulcers Rebound headache if discontinued abruptly
Goldenseal/roots	Diarrhea Antiseptic,	¼–½ tsp of tincture or ⅛ tsp of fluid extract	Hypotension, hypertension Local irritation

TABLE 11-7   Herbal teas and their side effects—cont'd

Herb/parts used	Common uses	Method of application	Side effects
	antimicrobial for acne, conjunctivitis, eczema, ear infections Possible immuno-stimulator Antiarrhythmic	three or four times a day for diarrhea Can be mixed with 4 oz water or juice	Nausea, vomiting, diarrhea Displaces bilirubin from albumin *Not recommended for infants*
Pennyroyal	Pulegone	Tea Oil	Hepatotoxicity, hepatic failure, nausea, vomiting, abdominal pain Renal failure Delirium, confusion, restlessness, dizziness, seizures, alternating lethargy and agitation Abortion *Not recommended*
Tea tree oil/ essential oil from leaves	Minor skin infections Fungicide Acne Vaginitis	Applied topically two to four times a day	Contact dermatitis if applied to broken or irritated skin As little as 10 mL PO can affect CNS function and cause muscle weakness *Not for internal use*

HIV, Human immunodeficiency virus: CNS, central nervous system.

Modified from Mack RB: "Something wicked this way comes"—herbs even witches should avoid. Contemp Pediatr 15:49, 1998; and O' Hara MA, Kiefer D, Farrell K, et al: A review of 12 commonly used medicinal herbs. Arch Fam Med 7:523, 1998.

does increase prolactin levels as a dopamine agonist. Even small doses have maximum effect. It does pass into milk. It is not rated by AAP.

Domperidome (Motilium) also increases prolactin as a dopamine antagonist. A randomized double-blind placebo-controlled trial of domperidome on milk production in mothers of premature newborns showed an increase in milk production, 49.5 ± 29.4 mL/day compared to 8.0 ± 39.5 mL/day in the control group (44.5% increase with the drug and 16.6% with the placebo). The prolactin levels rose significantly with domperidome. A small amount was found in the milk.[31]

A thorough review of the pharmacology of domperidome is available in Drugdex, a product of Micromedix, available by subscription to poison centers and medical libraries. Domperidone has a long history with many trials for nausea and vomiting and postprandial dyspepsia. It undergoes extensive first pass hepatic and gut wall metabolism which results in oral bioavailability of 13% to 17%. After IV administration, the half-life is 7.5 hours and after oral dosing the half-life is 14 hours with time to peak serum levels of 30 to 110 minutes. The volume of distribution is 440. It is metabolized in the liver. Reported adverse effects include arrhythmias, extrapyramidal tract effects, and dystonic reactions more common in children and in patients on antipsychotic medication. Side effects include dry mouth, headache, and abdominal cramps. Galactorrhea is a secondary effect that is not universal. It occurs in both males and females along with mastalgia and gynecomastia. The augmentation of preexisting lactation in a breast that has been primed by pregnancy may well be different. It has been suggested as an aid to induced or relactation efforts. Dosage is 10 to 20 mg three to four times a day for 3 to 8 weeks. There are cases of longer term usage. Withdrawal symptoms have been described of gastric irritability and nausea.

Herbs listed as galactagogues are numerous and known by hearsay and historic usage but not by scientific study. Most prominent on the list are fenugreek, fennel, milk thistle (not blessed thistle, which is an entirely different species), lemongrass, goat's rue, and anise.

Fenugreek (*Trigonella foenum graecen*) is a member of the Leguminosae family of plants, which includes peanuts and chick peas. Fenugreek is the dried ripe seeds of a small southern European herb known as *Greek hayseed,* which contains about 40% mucilage. In addition to being used for poultices and ointments, it is used in teas and syrups and has a faint flavor similar to maple syrup. It is soothing, flavorful, and possibly nutritious. It is available as a spice, flavoring, and tea. It is used as a galactogogue and goes back to ancient times. It is generally regarded as safe (GRAS) by the FDA, although it has been noted to cause colic in the infants of mothers using it similar to that caused by peanuts and chickpeas and other allergic symptoms in individuals with asthma.[121] It has been noted to lower cholesterol in normal individuals and also produce hypoglycemia in diabetics. Several cases of mistaken diagnosis of maple syrup urine disease have been reported as case reports in which the infant was found to smell of maple syrup.

In moderate use, fenugreek is considered harmless. As with all things in pregnancy and lactation, moderation is appropriate. Transport into milk is not documented, but the milk might smell like maple syrup. Fenugreek has been touted as a galactagogue, but no scientific reports support or refute this claim. Because it is in the same botanical family as peanuts and chick peas, a potential for allergy exists. It is also recognized to aggravate symptoms of allergy.

The dose is 2 to 3 capsules four times a day recognizing that varieties differ, as dose potency will change with variations in plant products.

Fennel seed (*Foeniculum vulgere*) is a common spice with estrogenic properties that has a reputation as a galactagogue but has no supporting evidence.[122]

Milk thistle (*Silybum marianum*) also has a reputation as a galactagogue with no scientific evidence. It is taken as a tea two or three times a day. It is also used as an antispasmodic and has many other uses. Milk thistle is a member of the family Asteraceae but should not be confused with blessed thistle, which is *Cnicus benedictus*, an entirely different plant. The active parts of the milk thistle plant are the small hard fruits known as achenes (they are not seeds). The leaves have no therapeutic efficacy. The usable material silymarin is an extract of the fruits. It has been credited with inhibiting oxidative damage to liver cells and stimulating regenerative capacity of liver cells. It has no acknowledged effect on lactation. There is known toxicity to the milk thistle teas.

Lemon grass (*Cymbopogon citratus*) is used for its dried leaves and oil of citronella. The latter is used as an insect repellent in the United States. It is used for joint pains and gastrointestinal discomforts. Herbal references do not mention lactation.[122]

Grapefruit seed extract (GSE) has been noted in animal experimentation to be an antiinfective, antiviral, antibacterial, and antifungal. Grapefruit itself has been known to contain quinine, especially in the bitter skin and section fibers. GSE has been recommended as an extract for use by direct application on sore nipples. If it has antiinfectious properties, it should be effective when traumatized nipples have become infected.

Laboratory studies have been reported on the Internet claiming that GSE inactivated herpes simplex (HSV-1), influenza A, and other viruses (see Nutri Team: support@nutriteam.com).

Neem oil (*Antelaea azadirachta*) is obtained from neem, a plant whose bark, leaves, branches, seeds, and latex are used as an antiinflammatory and antipyretic prevalent in India and other tropical countries. It is being used in the West by herbalists for many problems, sometimes placed directly on the breast or on the infant. It has caused severe dermatitis, gastrointestinal irritation, and CNS depression. Fruits are known to be toxic, containing some ricin. It should not be used during lactation or in infants and children.[85,161]

An illustration of the problems associated with herbals, that there are no guarantees regarding contamination or accuracy of labeled amounts, was the tryptophan (another amino acid) withdrawal. The eosinophilia-myalgia syndrome (EMS) had been noted in over 1500 patients taking L-tryptophan supplements. Characteristics included severe, incapacitating myalgia and eosinophilia. This outbreak was exclusively linked to L-tryptophan manufactured by a single Japanese manufacturer, and thus, a contaminant was suspected; however, the identity of the contaminant is still unknown.

Further concern regarding herbals, especially those from Asian sources, is the possible contamination with toxic heavy metals or even, in some cases, that they may be laced with prescription medications. Lead is the most common contamination identified. *Pay-loo-ah* is a powder containing lead that is used to treat headaches, muscle aches, and abdominal pain and is widely marketed.

Lactation suppression

Pseudoephedrine is widely used as a nasal mucous membrane and sinus decongestant and has a rating of 6 from the AAP. Its effects on milk production were measured by Aljazaf and associates,[2] who found it had no effect on breast blood flow or temperature. The mean change in prolactin compared to placebo was minimal. The milk production, however, was reduced by 24% with a single dose. Little drug was found in the milk. This confirms the standard advice that breastfeeding women should not take decongestants and should rely instead on saline nose drops and moisture (vaporizers) for relief of upper respiratory symptoms.

Sage has one major physiologic effect—it is antisudorific in cases of excessive sweating, and it also is said to reduce lactation. Considering the similarity between sweat glands and alveolar cells of the breast, this cross relationship is not surprising. No references are found regarding lactation, although there are many references to confirm the antisudorific effect.

The sage family is a large group of horticulturally important plants consisting of over 750 species distributed throughout the world. Some are of culinary use and others medicinal. There is even a Central American species that is a powerful hallucinogen traditionally used in religious and magical rites. The best known is *Salvia officinalis,* which has been cultivated for thousands of years. The name salvia is from the Latin word *salvus,* meaning to be in good health. It is also used as an antiseptic and a gargle and for many other symptoms. It is specifically contraindicated during pregnancy.

The literature supports the use of sage to decrease milk supply, treat engorgement, or hasten weaning. From that standpoint, it would be unwise to use it on nipples themselves in spite of the fact that it has antibacterial, astringent, and disinfectant properties according to most herbal references.

Cardiovascular drugs and diuretics

Digitalis is given to infants, but only for serious reasons. Measurements of digitalis in the milk in mothers maintained on digitalis throughout pregnancy and lactation showed concentrations of 0.825 nmol/L, which was 59% of the maternal plasma level in one study[24] and 75% in another.[43] If one calculates the predicted level of digitalis using the higher volume of distribution, 7.5 L/kg, the infant would receive 1.1 ng/mL in the milk of a 60-kg (132-lb) mother receiving a 0.5-mg dose of digoxin. Authors agree that digoxin levels would be low and the dosage to the infant low, but the long-range effects are not known.[24,43,96] There is sufficient experience accumulated to date, however, to conclude that mothers taking sustaining doses of digitalis preparations may nurse their infants without any harm to the infant. The AAP rates digitalis a 6, compatible with breastfeeding. Peak plasma levels occur 1.5 to 3 hours after ingestion, so breastfeeding should be avoided during that time.

Propranolol, a beta-blocker, was found in the milk of mothers but does not appear to accumulate in the infant. Thus, experienced cardiologists have permitted mothers taking propranolol to nurse their infants without any ill effect observed in the infants. In 1973, Levitan and Manion[89] reported significant quantities of propranolol in breast milk. Propranolol and its major metabolites were measured in milk and found by Smith and associates[149] to provide the infant with a maximum dose of less than 0.1% of the maternal dose or approximately 7 μg/dL. The half-life of elimination from the milk was 3 to 5 hours.[8] Beta-adrenergic blockade effects, including hypoglycemia, have been described in an infant breastfed by a mother taking propranolol. Because the reports are conflicting, it is necessary to monitor the breastfed infant carefully when the mother is taking propranolol. Monitoring plasma levels of the infant may be helpful if there is any question. It is 6 on AAP scales, considered safe for breastfeeding.

The antihypertensive drugs atenolol (Tenormin), metoprolol tartrate (Lopressor), and nadolol (Corgard, Corzide) have been evaluated in human milk.[34,35,91] *Metoprolol* had a peak level in blood of 713 ng/dL at 1.1 hours and in milk of 4.7 ng/dL at 3.8 hours. The data suggest that metoprolol appears minimally in milk and is probably safe for breastfeeding neonates.[35] *Nadolol* appears in serum at 77 ng/dL and in milk at 357 ng/dL.[34] *Atenolol* levels in milk are also higher than in the maternal serum.[104] Of this group, metoprolol would be the safest. These drugs are rated 6 (AAP). Serum levels of atenolol in one breastfed infant reached 0.16 μmol/L. It is rated 5 by AAP, give with caution. Acetobutolol is rated 6 by AAP but the dose must be at or below 400 mg/day.[18]

A number of effective antihypertensive medications are available. The clinician should review the properties and amount excreted in breast milk when choosing the best drug for the mother.

Reserpine has been reported to cause nasal stuffiness, bradycardia, and respiratory difficulty with increased tracheobronchial secretion and is contraindicated in both pregnancy and lactation, because safer drugs are available.[118]

Most *diuretics* are weak acids and little passes into milk. Use of diuretics, however, requires careful observation because they have the potential for causing a diuresis in the neonate that could be extremely dehydrating.[5] Although diuretics such as furosemide (Lasix) are given to neonates, this is done only when fluid and electrolyte levels can be followed closely. Oral diuretics were used to suppress lactation in a study by Healy[57] in 40 postpartum women who chose not to breastfeed. *Bendroflumethiazide* (Naturetin) was used, 5 mg twice daily for 5 days. He found it more effective than estrogens, with fewer side effects. Milk volume may be reduced by the thiazides.

Reports document the interaction of three diuretics with bilirubin-albumin complexes.[169] *Chlorothiazide* presented the greatest risk for producing free bilirubin, with ethacrynic acid and furosemide producing considerably less. The latter two are clinically effective in lower doses as well. The levels of chlorothiazide and hydrochlorothiazide in milk are less than 100 ng/mL.[106,111] For most infants, these are safe; however, these findings certainly suggest caution is necessary if the infant is jaundiced or very immature.

Chlorthalidone (Hygroton) appears in milk.[170] A term baby might receive 180 μg/day. The half-life is 60 hours. Although it is rated 6 by AAP, it can reduce milk production, especially early in lactation.

Furosemide has been shown by several techniques not only to displace bilirubin from albumin in the newborn, but also to be slowly excreted by the newborn, with only 84% excreted in 24 hours when given to the infant directly. Mofenson and Caraccio[108] reported that furosemide is not excreted into breast milk and is poorly absorbed orally; thus, it would be safe for the lactating mother. It is not rated by AAP.

A mother who is lactating may actually require substantially less medication, particularly diuretics. Close monitoring of the mother during lactation to try to reduce her medications may provide a therapeutic balance that is good for the mother and safe for the infant. With the short half-life of most diuretics in the adult, dosing can be timed to avoid peak plasma levels during feedings.

Central nervous system drugs

Phenobarbital can be given to infants and is usually safe, but careful observation of the infant for variation in sleeping and feeding habits is important.[81]

Phenytoin in the breast milk has been associated with vomiting, tremors, rash, blood dyscrasia (rarely), and methemoglobinemia, but not with drowsiness and lethargy. Many mothers have nursed without apparent incident while taking phenobarbital and phenytoin.[153] Phenytoin levels in milk of mothers treated for epilepsy have been measured, and levels in the infant have been calculated to provide less than 5% of the therapeutic dose for infants.[115] *Valproic acid* in maternal milk is low (3% of maternal serum concentrations), but the mean half-life is 47 hours, four times that in adults, so there is risk of accumulation (Table 11-8).[116,153] The AAP rating for valproic acid and phenytoin is 6.

A single case of *carbamazepine* exposure during pregnancy and breastfeeding is reported to have caused cholestatic hepatitis, diagnosed when the infant was 3 weeks of age.[46] The mother did not develop hepatic symptoms and continued the drug. Breastfeeding was discontinued, and the hepatitis resolved. Diagnosis was confirmed by liver function studies and liver biopsy. Carbamazepine hepatitis has been described in children and adults as a rare complication of therapy.

Poor weight gain after birth of infants whose mothers received antiepileptic medication during pregnancy has been reported by Kaneko and associates.[72] They also report inadequate suckling and high incidence of vomiting immediately after birth with difficulty establishing lactation. The drug continues to be provided through the milk, and the poor suckling becomes protracted. Table 11-8 lists levels of drug in the milk. When newborn levels are high, the authors suggest giving mixed feedings for the first few days post partum until the level of drug in the infant drops and the infant is able to clear the drug that was in the system transplacentally prior to birth. The clinician should observe these infants closely to be sure they receive adequate calories until they can suck vigorously. The mother should supplement the infant's suckling stimulus to the breast with a breast pump. With proper management in the first few days, the adjustment can be smooth and the infant can go on to nurse effectively and safely.[17] When infant plasma level determinations are available, it might be advisable to check the plasma level after 1 or 2 weeks of nursing, providing an opportunity to evaluate possible accumulation.

Psychotherapeutic agents

Lithium is the one drug in the psychotherapeutic group with a clear risk of toxicity in the neonate and clear evidence that it reaches the breast milk. Lithium is contraindicated in pregnancy but has been used cautiously in lactation. Infants have been reported to be hypotonic, flaccid, and "depressed" when the nursing mother is taking lithium. Although rated a 6 by AAP at one time, it is now a 5, use with caution.

TABLE 11-8	Anticonvulsant concentrations in maternal serum and milk				
Drug (half-life in neonate)	Maternal serum (µg/mL)	Milk (µg/mL)	Day 1	Milk/serum day 7	Day 30
Diphenylhydantoin (9–56 h)	3.0	0.7	18 ± 15	19 ± 4	13 ± 6
Phenobarbital (156 ± 29 h)	12.0	5.0	30 ± 16	36 ± 7	30 ± 5
Primidone (23 ± 8 h)	4.0	2.1	141 ± 9	56 ± 15	46 ± 7
Carbamazepine (13–36 h)	4.0	1.8	41 ± 16	38 ± 8	—
Valproic acid (47 h)	123 µmol/L	3 µmol/L	0.01 to 0.16	—	—

Modified from Kaneko S, Suzuki K, Sato T, et al: The problems of antiepileptic medication during the neonatal period: Is breastfeeding advisable? In Janz D, Dam M, Richens A, et al (eds): Epilepsy, Pregnancy, and the Child. New York, Raven, 1982.

After a careful review of the clinical data, Schou[141] states that accumulating evidence points strongly to the beneficial effects of breastfeeding while taking lithium for both infant and mother, mentally and physically. Lithium concentrations in the breastfed infant have been measured at one tenth to one half of the concentration in the mother's blood.[142] Such concentrations are considered harmless in adults, but their risk is unknown in a child. Schou[141] also states that, supported by husband and physician, the mother should make her own choice. Initiating lithium therapy after delivery or when the breastfeeding infant is several months old greatly minimizes the theoretic risks. The Lactation Study Center has been contacted about several infants being breastfed by mothers taking lithium with the psychiatrist's and pediatrician's consent. No symptoms were apparent. No long-term follow-up is yet available on these children.

Chlorpromazine or *phenothiazine* appears in the milk in small amounts, even at doses of 1200 mg, but apparently does not accumulate.[7] Doses of 100 mg/day do not appear to cause symptoms in the infants. It is usually taken once a day, peaking in plasma 1 to 2 hours after dose, and breastfeeding should be timed to avoid peak. *Diazepam* (Valium) has been detected in milk and in breastfed infants' serum and urine. It has caused depression and poor feeding with weight loss in the infant. In a single dose it should not present a problem. Shorter acting lorazepam is safer for multiple dose therapy. *Chlordiazepoxide* (Librium) and *clorazepate* (Tranxene) do reach the milk and may cause drowsiness and poor suckling. These substances' metabolites are also active, and therefore the half-life of therapeutic activity is prolonged. *Meprobamate* (Miltown, Equanil) has an M/P ratio greater than 1 and has been identified in milk. Infants whose mothers are taking meprobamate may become drowsy, but dosage adjustment may be indicated if there is significant benefit for the mother to breastfeed.[7] Usual dosing is three to four times a day, which makes avoiding peak plasma times difficult.

Tricyclic antidepressants such as imipramine are lipid soluble and have been identified in the breast milk; thus, cautious use may be appropriate.[29] In an extensive study of tricyclic antidepressants in pregnancy and lactation, Misri and Sivertz[107] found that an attitude of informed and cautious encouragement regarding the growing information suggests it is safe to breastfeed while taking such medication. It is rated 4 by the AAP, effect on nursing infants is unknown but may be of concern.

When Yoshida and associates[179] investigated the pharmacokinetics and possible adverse effects in infants exposed to tricyclic antidepressants in breast milk, they found no reason to prevent mothers who are taking established tricyclic antidepressants from breastfeeding. The drugs were imipramine, amitriptyline, clomipramine, and dothiepin. They had compared infants breastfed by mothers medicated with a tricyclic antidepressant with infants bottle fed by medicated mothers. In addition, they measured the drugs in all maternal plasma and urine and in foremilk and hindmilk of the lactators. Infant plasma and urine levels were also measured. Levels in the mother and her milk were correlated with the dose. The daily dose of drug via the breast milk was about 1% of the maternal dose per kilogram of weight. Amounts were barely detectable in the infant's plasma and urine. The 30-month follow-up detected no differences in growth and development.[179]

The *selective serotonin reuptake inhibitors* (SSRIs) are a class of drugs developed as antidepressants and also used in the treatment of panic attacks, obsessive-compulsive disorder, obesity, substance abuse, sleep disorders, chemotherapy-induced nausea and vomiting, migraine, and appetite suppression. Serotonergic dysfunction has been implicated in these illnesses. This group of drugs has antidepressant actions and selectively blocks the reuptake of serotonin into presynaptic neurons (Box 11-2).

These agents undergo extensive metabolism to clinically inactive compounds, have large volumes of distribution, and are highly bound to maternal plasma proteins, suggesting little transfer into milk. The elimination half-lives in the mother range from 15 to 26 hours. Reports of isolated cases have recorded maternal plasma and milk

BOX 11-2   Serotonin (5-HT) reuptake inhibitors (brand names)

Fenfluramine (Ponderax, Pondimin)
Fluoxetine (Prozac)
Fluvoxamine (Faverin)
Nefazodone (Serzone)
Paroxetine (Paxil, Seroxat)
Sertraline (Lustral, Zoloft)
Trazodone (Desyrel)
Venlafaxine (Effexor)

levels of a few of the compounds, but no long-term follow-up of the nurslings. In general, no symptoms have been reported in the infants. One case of severe colic and crying in a 6-week-old infant was reported to clear when the infant was weaned when the mother was taking fluoxetine (Prozac) (see Box 11-2).[88] The available pharmacology can be found in Appendix D.

The clinician must weigh the risk/benefit ratio of each drug, keeping in mind that being cared for by a depressed mother is not beneficial for the infant. Some mothers have been medicated with antidepressants during their pregnancies, and the withdrawal experienced when the infant is not breastfed may go undiagnosed and be attributed to colic, fussiness, or other disorders. If a mother is to begin medication during lactation, a baseline for the infant should be established by the pediatrician so that any effects of the medication received via the milk can be detected. The age of the infant and the feeding pattern are very important issues in the decision.

Fluoxetine (Prozac), a common and usually effective therapy for depression and other neuropsychiatric disorders, is reported to have few side effects. Pharmacologically, it is chemically unrelated to the antidepressants, has few autonomic effects, and is considered an alternative to standard antidepressant therapy. Its peak plasma time is 6 to 8 hours, and it is highly protein bound.[21,65] Case studies on lactating women taking fluoxetine have reported no changes in the infant. Maternal blood and milk samples have one fifth to one quarter as much drug (i.e., M/P = 0.20 to 0.25) when fluoxe-

tine and the active metabolite norfluoxetine are measured.[65] Total ingestion by the infant per day was no more than 15 to 20 μg/kg, a low exposure when mother had received 20 mg at bedtime for 53 days. The reported levels in milk depend on sampling and lipid content of the milk and range from 47 to 469 ng/mL.[21] Hale[55] reports a case in which a mother took fluoxetine throughout pregnancy and while breastfeeding. At 11 days, infant was somnolent, then unresponsive. Levels were measurable in milk and in infant.

The AAP considers the psychotropic drugs to be of special concern because they are taken for a long time. Although no adverse effects have been published, the drugs do appear in milk and could conceivably alter short-term and long-term CNS function. These drugs clearly require the physician's careful consideration of the benefits of breastfeeding and the therapeutic risks in each case.[109] The peak plasma time varies from 1½ to 12 hours, so avoiding a peak is difficult. Giving a feeding of formula once daily would dilute the impact. Other SSRIs such as sertraline (Zoloft), paroxetine (Paxil), and citalopram (Celexa) may be better choices. Neonatal paroxetine withdrawal syndrome has been described in four term infants who presented with jitteriness and necrotizing enterocolitis after paroxetine exposure in utero. Neonatal withdrawal from paroxetine in infants who did not breastfeed is 10 times higher (0.3/1000) than with sertraline and fluvoxamine and 100 times higher than with fluoxetine (0.002).[155]

Citalopram exposure in breastfeeding infants was examined prospectively in three groups: (a) depressed women treated with citalopram; (b) depressed women not treated with citalopram; and (c) normal women. The infants were no different in the three groups in feeding, medication, or adverse events.[87]

In a study of 78 infants[87] who were exposed to antidepressants through breast milk, mother's mood status was evaluated along with infants' weight gain.[59] Weights were not significantly different from the population of normal infants. The infants, however, whose mothers relapsed to significant depression did gain less weight. The authors concluded that the drugs did not decrease weight gain but maternal depression may influence behaviors that over 2 months could affect infant's weight gain.

Methadone maintenance and risks of breastfeeding

Methadone maintenance treatment for heroin and other addictions has had a significant impact on the recovery of many addicts. When first introduced, it was hoped it would be an ideal treatment for neonatal withdrawal syndrome. It was not. It was also hoped that withdrawal from methadone for the infant born to a woman receiving maintenance therapy would be negligible, but it is not. When pregnant women were maintained on 25 mg/day or less, neonatal withdrawal rarely required treatment. Present regimens during pregnancy typically are for maternal doses over 100 mg/day. Neonatal withdrawal from this level is substantial, requiring treatment with tincture of opium (Paregoric) for 6 to 8 weeks.

The therapeutic use of methadone in opiate addiction has become a common concern in the childbearing years, especially during pregnancy and lactation. The recommended daily dose has been increased sharply from 25 mg/day to as high as 150 mg/day. Neonatal abstinence syndrome has become more common, often requiring 6 to 8 weeks of hospitalization for the neonate. The question of breastfeeding is frequently asked.

Geraghty and associates[49] present two cases with multiple maternal blood and milk samples. At a single daily dose of 73 mg, plasma levels peaked at 1 hour and milk levels peaked at 1 to 5 hours. The M/P ratio varied over time and reflected the slow drop in the plasma level and slower drop in the milk level, but the differences as a ratio are negligible. A second mother took 30 mg at 9 AM and 30 mg at 6 PM. Her plasma levels were steady over time while milk levels dropped from a high of 0.25 mg/L to 0.11 mg/L at 14 hours, giving an M/P ratio of 1.53 at peak milk level 2 hours after the second dose and the lowest ratio of 0.91 at 14 hours. This demonstrates that an M/P ratio is of little value unless levels are known. It does suggest that peak plasma level is at about 1 to 2 hours and peak milk level is under 5 hours. Ranges were not different between a total of 60 mg and 73 mg.

Ten women were studied by Blinick and associates,[15,16] who collected milk and plasma for 3 to 10 days after delivery. Their doses varied from 10 to 80 mg/day. Levels in the breast milk ranged from 0.05 to 0.57 μg/mL, with an average M/P ratio of 0.83. Higher doses resulted in higher levels, but the relationship was not linear. Pond and associates[124] reported two women who had M/P ratios that remained constant at 0.32 and 0.61, and the infants received a calculated 0.01 to 0.03 mg of methadone per day. Kreek[79] estimated daily infant intake from a mother taking 50 mg daily, assuming consumption of almost a liter of breast milk a day, as a maximum of 0.112 mg/day. Kreek and associates[80] also noted peak levels in the milk at 4 hours after dosing. Pumping and discarding the milk at 3 to 4 hours after dosing has been suggested as a method of reducing exposure.

A study of eight mother-baby pairs in which mothers were on at least 40 mg/dL methadone daily showed the infants received 2.8% of mother's dose, not sufficient to prevent neonatal abstinence syndrome.[10] In a second study[101] of mothers on methadone who were receiving 25 to 180 mg/day the methadone levels ranged from 27 to 260 ng/mL with a mean of 95 ng/mL. There were no adverse events associated with breastfeeding or weaning. It was estimated the infant received 0.05 mg/day, which parallels other estimates.[176] If the infant is weaned from the breast gradually, there should be no withdrawal, and breastfeeding should not be withheld. The AAP now rates methadone 6 (Table 11-9).

Pesticides and pollutants

Human milk has been used as a biomonitoring tool for assessing mothers' and infants' exposures to environmental chemicals since 1950. Since that time a solid database has been created on DDT, dioxins, furans, and PCBs in various geographic areas. Consistency of analytical methods, sampling techniques, timing post partum, and reporting chemical concentrations has been lacking.

TABLE 11-9   **Maternal methadone dose, milk methadone levels, and infant age**

Patient	Maternal dose, mg/day	Breast milk level (ng/mL)	Infant age (days)
A	25	102	202
B1	96	100	60
B2	96	85	67
B3	96	82	68
C1	130	142	22
C2	130	91	22
C3	110	85	85
D	90	79	34
E	120	141	27
F	110	260	110
G1	80	19	3
G2	80	27	21
G3	80	83	33
H	180	32	173
Mean	102	95	66
SD	42	60	

From McCarthy JJ, Posey BL: Methadone levels in human milk. J Hum Lactation 16:115, 2000.

A technical workshop on Human Milk Surveillance and Research on Environmental Chemicals in the United States was held in 2002 and a published report appeared in the *Journal of Toxicology and Environmental Health*.[14] In increasing numbers, human milk is being used as the biologic marker of environmental exposures. The disturbing backlash is that the public interprets this to mean that breast milk is contaminated and the problem is getting worse.

Monitoring chemical exposure in the breastfed infant is at the mercy of the epidemiologist and the chemist.[148] Human milk has been known to contain insecticides. *Chlorinated hydrocarbons* such as DDT and its metabolites dieldrin, aldrin, and related compounds are the best known. The major reason these compounds appear in breast milk is that they are deposited in body lipid stores and move with lipid. The fetus receives the greatest dose in utero, and adult body fat has approximately 30 times the concentration in milk.

Polychlorinated biphenyls (PCBs) in heavily contaminated pregnant Japanese women produced small-for-gestational-age infants who had transient darkening of the skin ("cola babies"). *Polybrominated biphenyls* (PBBs) are similar compounds associated with a heavy exposure to farm animals and contaminated cattle fed in the lower Michigan peninsula. The women in the United States who have the greatest risk of high exposure to PCBs or PBBs are those who have excessively worked with or eaten the fish caught by sport fishing in contaminated waters.

Studies have refuted earlier observations of concern. No information is available in the United States on the levels of polychlorinated dibenzodioxins (PCDDs) or dibenzofurans (PCDFs) in anglers who consume a great deal of fish.[76] Others at high risk are those who live near a waste disposal site or have been involved in environmental spills. Unless there is heavy exposure, however, no contraindication exists to breastfeeding. The state health department can be consulted for specific advice or to measure plasma and milk levels. The epidemiologists are usually aware of the risks in a given geographic area and whether it is necessary to measure milk levels once lactation is fully established. If this sampling is planned in advance during the pregnancy, little time need be lost. Unless there is a unique and excessive exposure, the infant can breastfeed until levels are returned from the laboratory. Risk has diminished as environmental cleanups continue.

In most cases the levels of pesticides in human milk have been less than those in cow milk. The accumulated amounts have not usually exceeded safe allowable limits. Several extensive reviews explore the dilemma of pollutants in human milk.[134,135,172,177] In a 1997 review of world reports on occurrence and toxicity, Rogan[133] has reaffirmed that breastfeeding should be recommended despite the presence of chemical residues. He further states that the benefits of breastfeeding outweigh the risks of pollutants. It has been suggested that the body burden at birth can be added to by exposing the infant to small levels in the milk that may indeed exceed the exposure limits allowable for daily intake set by the World Health Organization (WHO).[154] Human milk levels are used epidemiologically as markers of human exposure in a community exposure because of a close correlation between milk levels and the levels in fat stores. Unselected mothers in the Great Lakes region were tested by the State of New York in 1978, and no chemical (PCB, PBB) was found in any milk in random sampling of residents. Thus, unless the circumstances are unusual, breastfeeding should not be abandoned on the basis of insecticide contamination.

Chemicals that are lipophilic, biologically stable, nonionized at a physiologic pH, and of low molecular weight transfer easily into maternal milk. Ten to 20 times more of the mother's body burden of persistent organohalogens are transferred via the milk than via the placenta, according to Jensen and Slorach,[68] who have published an extensive review of chemical contaminants in human milk. They further caution that the absolute amount transferred depends on the structure of the chemical. PCBs, for instance, are highly chlorinated and transfer more easily than less chlorinated PCBs. There is no difference in placental and milk transfer of heavy metals.

If extractable fat is measured, the levels of persistent organohalogens are about the same in milk, blood, adipose tissue, and muscle. Mobilization from fat stores is greater than that from dietary intake during lactation.[68]

Agent Orange, the best known of the dioxins, was identified in Vietnam as a powerful teratogen. *Dioxin* has been found in human milk from pooled samples from high-risk women with known exposure. No evidence suggests that the population at large is at risk. Women working in dry-cleaning plants, viscose rayon plants, photographic laboratories, and chemical industries where proper precautions are not taken have been noted to absorb tetrachloroethylene, carbon disulfide, and bromides.[51]

Flame retardants, polybrominated diphenylethers (PBDEs), which are found in upholstery, electronics, automotive interiors, and plastics, have been banned in several states because of rising body burdens as reflected in several studies in breast milk. A 40-fold increase is recorded since 1972. In high levels, PBDEs cause cognitive and behavior disorders. The risk is in utero. There is minimal risk from breastfeeding, so it is recommended that breastfeeding should take place.[53]

Heavy metals that have been found in milk include lead, mercury, arsenic, and cadmium.[119] Whenever maternal exposure occurs, the breastfed infant and the milk should be tested. The intake of lead and cadmium by breastfed infants, as reported by the WHO study, is the same as or somewhat lower than that of infants fed formula mixed with local water.[83] Levels of these heavy metals, in milk however, are lower than would be predicted from maternal levels (see Appendix D). Most common air pollutants are not found in human milk.

Although removal of lead from gasoline has been associated with a drop in blood lead levels in children from 15 µg/dL in 1978 to 2 µg/dL in 1999,[136] *lead* has become a significant issue because of the number of mothers testing positive for lead on routine screens for lead in family members of young infants.[160] Release of lead from bone in pregnancy and lactation was studied by Manton and associates,[97] who concluded that the whole skeleton undergoes resorption and blood lead levels of nursing mothers continue to rise, reaching maximum at 6 to 8 months post partum. They also noted that lead levels fall from pregnancy to pregnancy, suggesting that the greatest risk is with the first pregnancy.[97] The Centers for Disease Control and Prevention (CDC) has revised the standards for treatment downward (Table 11-10). Meta-analysis reflects a 2.6 to 5.8 point decline in IQ for an increase in lead level from 10 to 20 µg/dL.[136] Blood lead concentrations below 10 µg/dL are inversely associated with children's IQ scores at 3 to 5 years of age according to studies by Canfield.[22] The first step is always to clean up the environment and identify the source. The level of lead in milk depends on its ionization and tight binding to the red blood cells. The M/P ratio is 0.2. A lead level of 40 µg/dL or lower in a nursing mother is considered below the level of transfer through the breast milk (Fig. 11-3). In addition to environmen-

TABLE 11-10		Classes and management of lead levels in blood

Blood lead level (μg/dL)	Class	Management
<10	I	Not considered lead poisoning
10–14	IIA	Many children (or large proportion of children) with blood lead levels in this range should trigger community-wide childhood lead poisoning prevention activities. Children in this range may need to be rescreened more frequently.
15–19	IIB	Nutritional and educational interventions and more frequent screening; if level persists in this range, environmental investigation and intervention recommended
20–44	III	Environmental evaluation and remediation and a medical evaluation; possible pharmacologic treatment of lead poisoning
45–69	IV	Both medical and environmental intervention, including chelation therapy
>69	V	Medical emergency; immediate medical and environmental management

Modified from Centers for Disease Control and Prevention: Blood levels—United States, 1988–1991. MMWR 43(30):545, 1994.

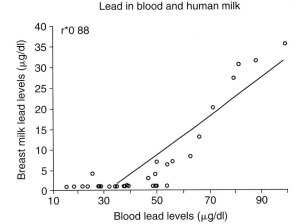

Lead in blood and human milk

Figure 11-3. Graph showing regression line between blood lead levels and milk lead levels. (From Namihira D, Saldivar L, Pustilnik N, et al: Lead in human blood and milk from nursing women living near a smelter in Mexico City. J Toxicol Environ Health 38:225, 1993.)

tal sources of lead (e.g., old paint, contaminated ground, lead batteries), diet should be reviewed. In some cities the water supply is a significant source, especially in formula making. Herbs and herbal teas may also be a source.

Organic mercury is another heavy metal that is being increasingly identified in food around the world. Fish is a major source, as are herbs and tonics. Levels of mercury in mother's blood are about three times higher than levels in milk. Two major forms of mercury enter milk. Methylmercury is attached to red blood cells and so has limited access, although it is easily absorbed by the infant. Inorganic mercury enters milk easily but is poorly absorbed by the infant. When the source of the methylmercury is from breast milk, the developmental scores exceed those of formula fed infants, suggesting that the advantages of breastfeeding are significant in a study in the Faroe Islands by Grandjean and associates.[52] A similar, more extensive study in the Seychelles Islands of mothers and children from birth followed over 5 years suggests that the value of a fish diet over time and during breastfeeding is significant despite measurable mercury levels.[99] Almost all the infants in the Seychelles are breastfed for at least 6 months and meet or exceed international developmental scores.[98] Acute exposures to methylmercury from industrial or environmental sources should be evaluated on a case-by-case basis, although it appears breastfeeding is safe.

Well water

Drinking well water has been a concern because of varying levels of minerals and especially of *nitrate*. More than 18% of wells in the state of Iowa are reported to exceed the maximum contaminant level of 45 mg of nitrate/L or 10 mg NO_3/L. Infants under 6 months of age are especially susceptible to *methemoglobinemia*, which can lead to anoxic injury and death. It reportedly occurs at nitrate concentrations greater than 100 mg/L. Although this is a major issue for formula fed infants, Dusdieker and associates[36] explored the question, Does increased nitrate ingestion elevate nitrate levels in human milk? Carefully studying 20 healthy mothers with breastfeeding infants over 6 months old subjected to 47, 168, and 270 mg of nitrate per day, they found that urine spot tests rose from 36 mg on day 1 to 66 mg on day 2 and 84 mg on day 3. Nitrate concentrations of their milk on days 1, 2, and 3 were 4.4, 5.1, and 5.2 mg/L, respectively. The authors concluded that "women who consume water with a nitrate concentration of 100 mg/L or less do not produce milk with elevated nitrate levels."[36]

Chemicals in the workplace

An increasing number of women return to the workplace after birth of an infant, and an increasing number are breastfeeding their infants. The need for information regarding the transfer of chemicals in the workplace to human milk is an increasing problem.

Volatile chemicals in the workplace represent an important but little understood hazard, especially in paint shops, repair shops, garages, and the chemical industry. Fisher and associates[44] developed a physiologically based pharmacokinetic model for a lactating woman to estimate the amount of chemical that the nursing infant ingests for a given nursing schedule and maternal occupational exposure. The two major factors are the blood/air partition coefficient, a thermodynamic factor that governs the body burden that may be achieved from inhalation of a chemical, and the pharmacokinetics of the chemical, which determines the length of time a chemical remains in the

systemic circulation and is available to transfer into milk. Because milk fat is available, preferential uptake of lipophilic chemicals occurs. Of the 19 chemicals simulated in the study, the authors consider bromochloromethane, perchloroethylene, and 1,4-dioxane exposure at highest risk for the infant based on U.S. Environmental Protection Agency (EPA) drinking water guidelines (Table 11-11). Protective gear is the most practical way of minimizing exposure to both mother and infant.

The Occupational Health and Safety Act of the province of Quebec has mandated the establishment and maintenance of a *Toxicological Index* that provides information on chemical and biologic contaminants potentially present in the workplace.[51] Information can also serve as a basis for the protective reassignment of pregnant or breastfeeding employees. The *Infotox* database has information about 5500 chemicals. Of the substances in the database, 2.2% (153 of 5736) show evidence of milk transfer and pose relative risks to the breastfed infant (see Appendix D).[51]

Psychological impact of toxin in milk

The psychological reactions of a group of nursing mothers from the lower Michigan Peninsula whose breast milk was contaminated with a toxic fire-retardant chemical, PBB, were studied.[56] Every 10th woman who had had her milk tested for PBB was contacted for the study (a sample of 200 women); 139 responded and received a questionnaire, and 97 (70%) filled out the questionnaire. The subjects knew their own level and that the range for all mothers was from undetected to 0.46 ppm with an average of 0.1 ppm. The testing was voluntary and cost $25. Of those tested, 96% had measurable amounts.

The data were collected in a six-page questionnaire. Two modes of coping emerged: denial and mastery. In general, the findings indicated that the greater the level of toxic contamination of PBB reported in a mother's milk, the greater the denial, to the point of not having correct information, even about her own level. Ambivalence toward nursing

TABLE 11-11 Predicted amount of chemical ingested by nursing infant (AMILK) over 24-hour period and EPA drinking water health advisory values

Chemical	Threshold limit value (TLV) (ppm)	AMILK (mg)	EPA health advisory intake* (mg/day)
Benzene	10	0.053	0.20[†]
Bromochloromethane	200	2.090	1.00
Carbon tetrachloride	5	0.055	0.07
Chlorobenzene	10	0.229	—
Chloroform	10	0.043	0.1
Methylchloroform	350	3.51	40.0
Diethylether	400	1.49	—
1,4-Dioxane	25	0.559	0.4[†]
Halothane	50	0.232	—
n-Hexane	50	0.052	4.0
Isoflurane	50[‡]	0.336	—
Methylene chloride	50	0.213	2.0[†]
Methyl ethyl ketone	200	12.08	—
Perchloroethylene	25	1.36	1.0
Styrene	50	0.650	2.0
Trichloroethylene	50	0.496	0.6[§]
1,1,1,2-Tetrachlorothane	100[‡]	4.31	0.9
Toluene	50	0.460	2.0
o,p,m-Xylenes	100	6.590	40.0

*Modified from EPA Health Advisory values for chronic ingestion of contaminated water by 10-kg (22-lb) children, assuming ingestion of 1 L of water per day. These Health Advisory concentrations for chemicals in water are thought to be protective of adverse health effects for chronic exposure.
†Modified from 10-day Health Advisory values for ingestion of contaminated water by 10-kg children, assuming ingestion of 1 L of water per day. These Health Advisory values for contaminated water are thought to be protective of adverse health effects for a 10-day period.
‡No TLV; concentration value was assigned.
§Lifetime Health Advisory value for ingestion of 2 L water per day in adults.
From Fisher J, Mahle D, Bankston L, et al: Lactation transfer of volatile chemicals in breast milk. Am Ind Hyg Assoc J 58:429, 1997.

was correlated with guilt in both groups (only 15% discontinued breastfeeding). The "draw-a-baby" test showed an unusual amount (94%) of distortion and expressions of anguish. These findings were consistent throughout all the test modalities; thus, they were not thought to be a function of personality.[56]

Radioactive materials

Because of the increasing number of diagnostic tests that use radioactive materials, a nursing mother may have such a procedure done.

Radioactive iodine (^{125}I and ^{131}I) passes into milk at levels as high as 5% of the dose. When this is used for diagnostic purposes, breastfeed-ing should be discontinued until milk is clear. The excretion by the breast may alter the validity of the test result. If radioactive iodine is to be used therapeutically, breastfeeding must be discontinued until the iodine has cleared the system, which may be 1 to 3 months. A carefully collected sample of milk can be tested for radioactivity so that the period that the infant is off the breast is not unnecessarily long. If a 30 µCi dose of ^{131}I is used, 24 hours may be adequate to pump and discard. If the infant is older and receiving other foods, time can be altered accordingly. A lung scan (300 µCi dose) requires 7 days and renography requires 2 days of pumping and discarding the milk.[73]

Gallium-67 citrate appears in significant amounts in the milk. It does clear the body quickly and is relatively safe for use in patients. Breastfeeding should be discontinued for at least 72 hours.

Technetium-99m (^{99m}Tc) is reported to clear the milk in 6 to 48 hours. The stage of lactation, whether the breast is emptied before receiving the dose, and the method of clearing the breast may be responsible for the inconsistent results. Discontinuing breastfeeding for at least 24 hours is advisable.

The amount of radioactivity excreted in breast milk after administration of ^{99m}Tc hexakis 2-methoxyisobutyl isonitrile (MIBI) in a single dose was reported by Rubow and associates.[138] The measurement was highest in the first sample at 3.3 hours, 0.488 kilobecquerel (kBq)/mL, with negligible amounts thereafter (less than 0.180 kBq/mL). Less than 2.96 kBq/mL is considered safe. Only the first sample needs to be discarded.[138]

With the advent of ultrasound examination, computed tomography scanning, magnetic resonance imaging, and other techniques, alternatives exist in many situations to use of radioactive material during lactation (see Appendix E).

IMMUNIZATIONS

Immunizing the breastfed infant

Questions often arise as to whether a breastfed infant should be immunized on a different schedule because of the protective maternal antibodies that might interfere with the infant's response to antigen stimulation. Following are some brief guidelines on the more common situations of concern[30]:

1. All infants should be vaccinated on the regular schedule regardless of the mode of feeding (AAP).
2. Vaccinations for diphtheria-pertussis-tetanus (DPT) are not altered by breastfeeding, and the regular schedule should be followed for the infant.
3. Because oral poliovirus vaccine (OPV) is a live virus vaccine, there was concern that the maternal antibodies would inactivate the live virus. However, the CDC recommendation is that the same schedule be followed. The current scientific literature indicates that for infants older than 6 weeks, which is the earliest age of vaccination recommended, no indication exists for withholding breastfeeding in relationship to OPV administration, and no need exists for extra doses of vaccine. Furthermore, antibody responses to parenteral and oral vaccines are better in breastfed than formula fed infants. The same is true for diphtheria and tetanus toxoid.[183]
4. Rubella, mumps, and measles vaccines should be given at the regularly scheduled times.[30]
5. A *Haemophilus influenzae* type B vaccine is available for infants. The *H. influenzae* type B conjugate vaccines should be given at 2 months of age or as soon as possible thereafter, following the AAP *Red Book* guidelines in the Report of the Committee on Infectious Disease. No modification of the immunization schedule is necessary for breastfed infants. Furthermore, data suggest breastfed infants ultimately have higher antibody titers than formula fed infants.

Immunizing the nursing mother

There is no reason for concern about the potential presence of live viruses from vaccines in mother's milk if she is vaccinated during the postpartum period. Breastfeeding women may follow the same schedule for adults that is followed for other adults for measles, mumps, rubella, tetanus, diphtheria, influenza, *Streptococcus pneumoniae* infection, hepatitis A, hepatitis B, and varicella. When traveling to an endemic area, inactivated poliovirus vaccine can be given.[30]

Smallpox

Smallpox vaccination is inadvisable for the mother of any infant under 1 year of age, nursing or not. The personal contact, not the breastfeeding, causes the risk; therefore, no advantage exists to weaning if vaccination is necessary. This vaccination is not given routinely and is rarely indicated.

Rh immune globulin

Only rare trace amounts of anti-Rh are present in colostrum and none is found in mature milk of women given large doses of Rh immune globulin immediately post partum. No adverse response was noted, even with these high dosages. Any Rh antibodies in the mother's milk are thought to be inactivated by the gastric juices. Rh immune globulin or Rh sensitization is not a contraindication to breastfeeding.

Rubella

Following are the recommendations with respect to rubella[30]:

1. Approximately 85% to 90% of the adult female population are thought to have a high level of naturally acquired immunity, and only 10% to 15% are considered to be susceptible to rubella infection.
2. Vaccination of pregnant women is contraindicated under all circumstances.
3. No woman of childbearing age should be vaccinated without having been first tested for immunity.
4. If the test is negative, the woman may be vaccinated if there is reasonable assurance that she will not become pregnant for at least 2 months.

The rubella virus was found in the milk of 69% of the women immunized with live attenuated rubella (HPV-77 DE5 or RA 27/3 strains).[94,95] A virus-specific immunoglobulin A (IgA) antibody response was seen in milk of all the women. Infectious rubella virus or virus antigen was recovered from the nasopharynx and throat of 56% of the breastfed infants and none of the non-breastfed infants. No infant had disease in this study, but 25% of the breastfed group had seroconversion transiently.[95] Infants given early strains of the virus via the milk were reported to develop mild symptoms.[19,77,82,95] Although the attenuated virus may appear in the milk, this should not dissuade one from vaccinating a breastfeeding mother at the safest time, that is, immediately post partum.

REFERENCES

1. Abbott PJ: Comfrey: Assessing the low-dose health risk. Med J Aust 149:678, 1988.
2. Aljazaf K, Hale TW, Ilett KF, et al: Pseudoephedrine: Effects on milk production in women and estimation of infant exposure via breastmilk. J Clin Pharmacol 56:18, 2003.
3. Amir LH, Donath SM: Does maternal smoking have a negative physiological effect on breastfeeding? The epidemiological evidence. Breastfeeding Rev 11:L19, 2003.
4. Ang-Lee MK, Moss J, Yuan C-S: Herbal medicines and perioperative care. JAMA 286:208, 2001.
5. Aranda JV, Lambert C, Perez J, et al: Metabolism and renal elimination of furosemide in the newborn infant. J Pediatr 101:777, 1982.
6. Arena JM: Drugs and breast feeding. Clin Pediatr 5:472, 1966.
7. Ayd F: Excretion of psychotropic drugs in human breast milk. Int Drug Ther Newslett 8:33, 1973.
8. Bauer JH, Pape B, Zajicek J, et al: Propranolol in human plasma and breast milk. Am J Cardiol 43:860, 1979.
9. Begg EJ, Atkinson HC, Duffull SB: Prospective evaluation of a model for the prediction of milk: Plasma drug concentrations from physicochemical characteristics. Br J Clin Pharmacol 33:501, 1992.
10. Begg EJ, Malpas TJ, Hackett LP, et al: Distribution of R- and S-methadone into human milk during multiple, medium to high oral dosing. J Clin Pharmacol 52:681, 2001.
11. Berglund F, Flodh H, Lundborg P, et al: Drug use during pregnancy and breastfeeding. Acta Obstet Gynecol Scand Suppl 126:1, 1984.
12. Berlin CM: Excretion of methylxanthines in human milk. Semin Perinatol 5:389, 1981.
13. Berlin CM, Daniel CH: Excretion of theobromine in human milk and saliva. Pediatr Res 15:492, 1981.
14. Berlin CM, LaKind JS, Selevan SG: Human milk monitoring for environmental chemicals: Guidance for future research. J Toxicol Environ Health 66(22):1829, 2002.
15. Blinick G, Inturrisi C, Jerez E, et al: Methadone assays in pregnant women and progeny. Am J Obstet Gynecol 121:617, 1975.
16. Blinick G, Wallach R, Jerez E, et al: Drug addiction in pregnancy and the neonate. Am J Obstet Gynecol 125:135, 1976.

17. Bossi L: Neonatal period including drug disposition in newborns: Review of the literature. In Janz D, Dam M, Richens A, et al (eds): Epilepsy, Pregnancy and the Child. New York, Raven, 1982.

18. Boutroy MJ, Bianchetti G, Dubruc C, et al: To nurse when receiving acebutolol: Is it dangerous for the neonate? Eur J Clin Pharmacol 30:737, 1986.

19. Bowes WA Jr: The effect of medications on the lactating mother and her infant. Clin Obstet Gynecol 23:1073, 1980.

20. Briggs GG, Freeman RK, Yaffe S: Drugs in Pregnancy and Lactation, 5th ed. Baltimore, Williams & Wilkins, 1998.

21. Burch KJ, Wells BG: Fluoxetine/norfluoxetine concentrations in human milk. Pediatrics 89:676, 1992.

22. Canfield RL, Henderson CR, Cory-Slechta DA, et al: Intellectual impairment in children with blood lead concentrations below 10 µg per deciliter. N Engl J Med 348:1517, 2003.

23. Carlson HE, Wasser HL, Reidelberger RD: Beer-induced prolactin secretion: A clinical and laboratory study of the role of salsolinol. J Clin Endocrinol Metab 60:673, 1985.

24. Chan V, Tse TF, Wong V: Transfer of digoxin across the placenta and into breast milk. Br J Obstet Gynecol 85:605, 1978.

25. Clark JH, Wilson WG: A 16-day-old breastfed infant with metabolic acidosis caused by salicylate. Clin Pediatr 20:53, 1981.

26. Cobo E: Effect of different doses of ethanol on milk-ejecting reflex in lactating women. Am J Obstet Gynecol 115:817, 1973.

27. Collaborative Group on Drug Use in Pregnancy: Medication during pregnancy: An intercontinental cooperative study. Int J Gynaecol Obstet 39(3):185, 1995.

28. Committee on Drugs, American Academy of Pediatrics: Psychotropic drugs in pregnancy and lactation. Pediatrics 69:241, 1982.

29. Committee on Drugs, American Academy of Pediatrics: The transfer of drugs and other chemicals into human milk. Pediatrics 72:375, 1983; 84:924, 1989; 93:137, 1994; 108:776, 2001.

30. Committee on Infectious Disease: Report of the Committee on Infectious Disease. In The Red Book, 25th ed. Elk Grove, IL, American Academy of Pediatrics, 2000.

31. daSilva OP, Knoppert DC, Angelini MM, et al: Effect of domperidone on milk production in mothers of premature newborns: A randomized, double-blind, placebo-controlled trial. Can Med Assoc J 164:17, 2001.

32. daSilva VA, Malheiros LR, Moraes-Santos AR, et al: Ethanol pharmacokinetics in lactating women. Braz J Med Biol Res 26:1097, 1993.

33. Davis EA, Morris DJ: Medicinal uses of licorice through the millennia: The good and plenty of it. Mol Cell Endocrinol 78:1, 1991.

34. Devlin RG, Duchin KL, Fleiss PM: Nadolol in human serum and breast milk. Br J Clin Pharmacol 12:393, 1981.

35. Devlin RG, Fleiss PM: Captopril in human blood and breast milk. J Clin Pharmacol 21:110, 1981.

36. Dusdieker LB, Stumbo PJ, Kross BC, et al: Does increased nitrate ingestion elevate nitrate levels in human milk? Arch Pediatr Adolesc Med 150:311, 1996.

37. Ellenhorn MJ: Ellenhorn's Medical Toxicology: Diagnosis and Treatment of Human Poisoning, 2nd ed. Baltimore, Williams & Wilkins, 1997.

38. Ehrenkranz RA, Ackerman BA: Metoclopramide effect on faltering milk production by mothers of premature infants. Pediatrics 78:614, 1986.

39. Engels HJ, Wirth JC: No ergogenic effects of ginseng during graded maximal aerobic exercise. J Am Diet Assoc 97(10):1110, 1997.

40. Erickson SH, Oppenheim GL, Smith GH: Metronidazole in breast milk. Obstet Gynecol 57:48, 1981.

41. Ernst E: Toxic heavy metals and undeclared drugs in Asian herbal medicines. TRENDS Pharmacol Sci 23:136, 2002.

42. Feldman S, Pickering LK: Pharmacokinetics of drugs in human milk. In Howell RR, Morris FH, Pickering LK (eds): Human Milk, Infant Nutrition and Health. Springfield, IL, Thomas, 1986.

43. Finley JP, Waxman MB, Wong PY, et al: Digoxin excretion in human milk. J Pediatr 94:339, 1979.

44. Fisher J, Mahle D, Bankston L, et al: Lactational transfer of volatile chemicals in breast milk. Am Ind Hyg Assoc J 58:425, 1997.

45. Flores-Huerta S, Hernández-Montes H, Argote RM, et al: Effects of ethanol consumption during pregnancy and lactation on the outcome and postnatal growth of the offspring. Ann Nutr Metab 36:121, 1992.

46. Frey B, Schubiger G, Musy JP: Transient cholestatic hepatitis in a neonate associated with carbamazepine exposure during pregnancy and breastfeeding. Eur J Pediatr 150:136, 1990.

47. Gaginella TS: Drugs and the nursing mother-infant. US Pharm 3:39, 1978.

48. George DI, O'Toole TJ: A review of drug transfer to the infant by breastfeeding: Concerns for the dentist. J Am Dent Assoc 106:204, 1983.

49. Geraghty B, Graham EA, Logan B, et al: Methadone levels in breast milk. J Hum Lact 13:227, 1997.

50. Gilman AG, Rall TW, Nies AS, et al (eds): Goodman and Gilman's The Pharmacological Basis of Therapeutics, 8th ed. New York, Macmillan, 1990.

51. Giroux D, Lapointe G, Baril M: Toxicological index and the presence in the workplace of chemical hazards for workers who breastfeed infants. Am Ind Hyg Assoc J 53:471, 1992.

52. Grandjean P, Wiehe P, White RF: Milestone development in infants exposed to methyl mercury from human milk. Neurotoxicology 16:27, 1995.

53. Greater Boston Physicians for Social Responsibility (GBPSR): In Harm's Way: Toxic Threats to Child Development. May 2000. Accessed at http://ww.igc.org/psr/.

54. Grigg J: Environmental toxins: Their impact on children's health. Arch Dis Child 89:244, 2004.

55. Hale TW, Shum S, Grossberg M: Fluoxetine toxicity in a breastfed infant. Clin Pediatrics 40:681, 2001.

56. Hatcher SL: The psychological experience of nursing mothers upon learning of a toxic substance in their breast milk. Psychiatry 45:172, 1982.

57. Healy M: Suppressing lactation with oral diuretics. Lancet 1:1353, 1961.

58. Heisterberg L, Branebjerg PE: Blood and milk concentrations of metronidazole in mothers and infants. J Perinat Med 11:114, 1983.

59. Hendrick V, Smith LM, Hwang S, et al: Weight gain in breastfed infants of mothers taking antidepressant medications. J Clin Psychiatry 64:410, 2003.

60. Hervada AR, Feit E, Sagraves R: Drugs in breast milk. Perinat Care 2:19, 1978.

61. Hogan RP III: Hemorrhagic diathesis caused by drinking an herbal tea. JAMA 249:2679, 1983.

62. Horta BL, Kramer MS, Platt RW: Maternal smoking and the risk of early weaning: A meta-analysis. Am J Publ Health 91:304, 2001.

63. Huxtable RJ: The myth of beneficent nature: The risks of herbal preparations. Ann Intern Med 117:165, 1992.

64. Illingworth RS, Finch E: Ethyl discoumacetate (Tromexan) in human milk. J Obstet Gynecol Br Empire 66:487, 1959.

65. Isenberg KE: Excretion of fluoxetine in human breast milk. J Clin Psychiatry 51:169, 1990.

66. Ito S, Koren G, Einarson TR: Maternal noncompliance with antibiotics during breastfeeding. Ann Pharmacother 27:40, 1993.

67. Jarboe CH, Cook LN, Malesic I, et al: Dyphylline elimination kinetics in lactating women: Blood to milk transfer. J Clin Pharmacol 21:405, 1981.

68. Jensen AA, Slorach SA: Chemical Contaminants in Human Milk. Boca Raton, CRC, 1991.

69. Jones AW: Alcohol in mother's milk. N Engl J Med 326:766, 1992.

70. Kafetzis DA, Siapas CA, Georgakopoulos PA, et al: Passage of cephalosporins and amoxicillin into breast milk. Acta Paediatr Scand 70:285, 1981.

71. Kampmann JP, Johansen K, Hansen JM, et al: Propylthiouracil in human milk. Lancet 1:736, 1980.

72. Kaneko S, Suzuki K, Sato T, et al: The problems of antiepileptic medication during the neonatal period: Is breastfeeding advisable? In Janz D, Dam M, Richens A, et al (eds): Epilepsy, Pregnancy, and the Child. New York, Raven, 1982.

73. Karjalainen P, Penttilä IM, Pystynen P: The amount and form of radioactivity in human milk after lung scanning, renography and placental localization by ^{131}I labelled traces. Acta Obstet Gynecol Scand 50:357, 1971.

74. Kesäniemi YA: Ethanol and acetaldehyde in the milk and peripheral blood of lactating women after ethanol administration. J Obstet Gynecol Br Commonwealth 81:84, 1974.

75. Khan AKA, Truelove SC: Placental and mammary transfer of sulphasalazine. Br Med J 2:1533, 1979.

76. Kimbrough RD: Consumption of fish: Benefits and perceived risk. J Toxicol Environ Health 33:81, 1991.

77. Klein EB, Byrne T, Cooper LZ: Neonatal rubella in a breast-fed infant after postpartum maternal infection. J Pediatr 97:774, 1980.

78. Koren G, Randor S, Martin S, et al: Maternal ginseng use associated with neonatal androgenization. JAMA 264:2866, 1990.

79. Kreek MJ: Methadone disposition during the perinatal period in humans. Pharmacol Biochem Behav 11:7, 1979.

80. Kreek MJ, Schecter A, Gutjahr CL, et al: Analyses of methadone and other drugs in maternal and neonatal body fluids: Use in evaluation of symptoms in a neonate of mother maintained on methadone. Am J Drug Alcohol Abuse 1:409, 1974.

81. Kuhnz W, Koch S, Helge H, et al: Primidone and phenobarbital during lactation period in epileptic women: Total and free drug serum levels in the nursed infants and their effects on neonatal behavior. Dev Pharmacol Ther 11:147, 1988.

82. Landes RD, Bass JW, Millunchick EW, et al: Neonatal rubella following postpartum maternal immunization. J Pediatr 97:465, 1980.

83. Larsson B, Slorach SA, Hagman U, et al: WHO Collaborative Breastfeeding Study. II. Levels of lead and cadmium in Swedish human milk, 1978-1979. Acta Paediatr Scand 70:281, 1981.

84. Lawrence RA, Friedman LR: Drugs and contaminants in human milk. In Jensen RG (ed): Handbook of Milk Composition. San Diego, Academic Press, 1995.

85. Lawrence RA: Review of Natural Products, Facts and Comparisons. St Louis, Wolters Kluwer, 1980.

86. Lawton ME: Alcohol in breast milk. Aust NZ J Obstet Gynaecol 25:71, 1985.

87. Lee A, Woo J, Ito S: Frequency of infant adverse events that are associated with citalopram use during breast-feeding. Am J Obstet Gynecol 190:218, 2004.

88. Lester BM, Cucca J, Andreozzi L, et al: Possible association between fluoxetine hydrochloride and colic in an infant. J Am Acad Child Adolesc Psychiatry 32:1253, 1993.

89. Levitan AA, Manion JC: Propranolol therapy during pregnancy and lactation. Am J Cardiol 32:247, 1973.

90. Lie B, Jurel J: Effect of epidural versus general anesthesia on breastfeeding. Acta Obstet Gynaecol Scand 67:207, 1988.

91. Liedholm H, Melander A, Bitzen PO, et al: Accumulation of atenolol and metoprolol in human breast milk. Eur J Clin Pharmacol 20:229, 1981.

92. Linde K, Ramirez G, Mulrow CD, et al: St. John's wort for depression: An overview and meta-analysis of randomised clinical trials. Br Med J 313:253, 1996.

93. Little RE, Anderson KW, Ervin CH, et al: Maternal alcohol use during breastfeeding and infant mental and motor development at one year. N Engl J Med 321:425, 1989.

94. Losonsky GA, Fishaut JM, Strussenberg J, et al: Effect of immunization against rubella on lactation products. I. Development and characterization of specific immunologic reactivity in breast milk. J Infect Dis 145:654, 1982.

95. Losonsky GA, Fishaut JM, Strussenberg J, et al: Effect of immunization against rubella on lactation products. II. Maternal-neonatal interactions. J Infect Dis 145:661, 1982.

96. Loughnan PM: Digoxin excretion in human breast milk. J Pediatr 92:1019, 1978.

97. Manton WI, Angle CR, Stanek KL, et al: Release of lead from bone in pregnancy and lactation. Environment Res 92:139, 2003.

98. Marsh DO, Clarkson TW, Cox C, et al: Fetal methylmercury poisoning. Arch Neurol 44:1017, 1987.

99. Marsh DO, Clarkson TW, Myers GJ, et al: Seychelles study of fetal methylmercury exposure and child development: Introduction. Neurotoxicology 16(4):583, 1995.

100. Matheson I, Kristensen K, Lunde PKM: Drug utilization in breastfeeding women: A survey in Oslo. Eur J Clin Pharmacol 38:453, 1990.

101. McCarthy JJ, Posey BL: Methadone levels in human milk. J Hum Lactation 16:115, 2000.

102. McKenna R, Cole ER, Vasan U: Is warfarin sodium contraindicated in the lactating mother? J Pediatr 103:325, 1983.

103. Medical Letter on Drugs and Therapeutics: St. John's wort. Med Lett Drugs Ther 36(1014):107, 1997.

104. Mennella JA, Beauchamp GK: The transfer of alcohol to human milk. N Engl J Med 325:981, 1991.

105. Mennella JA, Gerrish CJ: Effects of exposure to alcohol in mother's milk on infant sleep. Pediatrics 101:e2, 1998.

106. Miller ME, Cohn RD, Burghart PH: Hydrochlorothiazide deposition in a mother and her breast-fed infant. J Pediatr 101:789, 1982.

107. Misri S, Sivertz K: Tricyclic drugs in pregnancy and lactation: A preliminary report. Int J Psychiatry Med 21:157, 1991.

108. Mofenson HC, Caraccio TR: Drugs, breast milk and infants. Pediatr Ther Toxicol 2(suppl):S1, 1988.

109. Mortola JF: The use of psychotropic agents in pregnancy and lactation. Psychiatr Clin North Am 12:69, 1989.

110. Morton SC, Williams MS, Keeler EB, et al: Effect of epidural analgesia for labor on the cesarean delivery rate. Obstet Gynecol 83:1045, 1994.

111. Mulley BA, Parr GA, Pau WK, et al: Placental transfer of chlorthalidone and its elimination in maternal milk. Eur J Clin Pharmacol 13:129, 1978.

112. Nation RL, Hotham N: Drugs and breastfeeding. Med J Aust 146:308, 1987.

113. Namihira D, Saldivar L, Pustilnik N, et al: Lead in human blood and milk from nursing women living near a smelter in Mexico City. J Toxicol Environ Health 38:225, 1993.

114. Nau H, Rating D, Hauser I, et al: Placental transfer at birth and postnatal elimination of primidone and metabolites in neonates of epileptic mothers. In Janz D, Dam M, Richens A, et al (eds): Epilepsy, Pregnancy, and the Child. New York, Raven, 1982.

115. Nau H, Rating D, Koch S, et al: Valproic acid and its metabolites: Placental transfer, neonatal pharmacokinetics, transfer via mother's milk and clinical status in neonates of epileptic mothers. J Pharmacol Exp Ther 219:768, 1981.

116. Neuvonen PJ, Kivistö KT: The clinical significance of food-drug interactions: A review. Med J Aust 150:36, 1989.

117. Nissen E, Matthiesen LG, Ransjo-Arvidsson A-S, et al: Effects of maternal pethidine on infant's developing breastfeeding behavior. Acta Paediatr 84:140, 1995.

118. O'Brien TE: Excretion of drugs in human milk. Am J Hosp Pharm 31:844, 1974.

119. Ong CN, Phoon WO, Law HY, et al: Concentrations of lead in maternal blood, cord blood and breast milk. Arch Dis Child 60:756, 1985.

120. Orme ML, Lewis PJ, DeSwiet M, et al: May mothers given warfarin breast-feed their infants? Br Med J 1:1564, 1977.

121. Patil SP, Niphadkar PV, Bapat MM: Allergy to fenugreek (Trigonelia foenum graecum). Ann Allergy Asthma Immunol 78:297, 1997.

122. Physician's Desk Reference for Herbal Medicnes, 2nd ed. Montvale NJ, Medical Economics Co., 2000.

123. Pokela M-L, Olkkola KT, Koivisto M, et al: Pharmacokinetics and pharmacodynamics of intravenous meperidine in neonates and infants. Clin Pharmacol Ther 52:342, 1992.

124. Pond SM, Kreek MJ, Tong TG: Altered methadone pharmacokinetics in methadone-maintained pregnant women. J Pharmacol Exp Ther 233:1, 1985.

125. Primal Health Research Centre: Mercury exposure during the primal period. 11(3), 2003. Accessed at http://www.birthworks.org/primalhealth.

126. Ramin SM, Gambling DR, Lucas MJ, et al: Randomized trial of epidural versus intravenous analgesia during labor. Obstet Gynecol 86:783, 1995.

127. Rasmussen F: Mammary excretion of benzylpenicillin, erythromycin and penethamate hydroiodide. Acta Pharmacol Toxicol (Kbh) 16:194, 1959.

128. Rasmussen F: Mammary excretion of antipyrine ethanol and urea. Acta Vet Scand 2:151, 1961.

129. Rating D, Jäger-Roman E, Koch S, et al: Enzyme induction in neonates due to antiepileptic therapy during pregnancy. In Janz D, Dam M, Richens A, et al (eds): Epilepsy, Pregnancy, and the Child. New York, Raven, 1982.

130. Ridker PM: Toxic effects of herbal teas. Arch Environ Health 42:133, 1987.

131. Righard L, Alade MO: Effect of delivery room routines on success of first breast-feed. Lancet 336(8723):1105, 1990.

132. Rivera-Calimlim L: The significance of drugs in breast milk. Clin Perinatol 14:51, 1987.

133. Rogan WJ: Pollutants in breast milk. Arch Pediatr Adolesc Med 150:981, 1997.

134. Rogan WJ, Bagniewska A, Damstra T: Pollutants in breast milk. N Engl J Med 302:1450, 1980.

135. Rogan WJ, Gladen B: Monitoring breast milk contamination to detect hazards from waste disposal. Environ Health Perspect 48:87, 1983.

136. Rogan WJ, Ware JH: Exposure to lead in children—How low is low enough? N Engl J Med 348: 1515, 2003.

137. Rosti L, Nardini A, Bettinelli ME, et al: Toxic effects of an herbal tea mixture in two newborns. Acta Paediatr 83:683, 1994.

138. Rubow SM, Ellmann A, LeRoux J, et al: Excretion of technetium 99m hexakis methoxyisobutyl isonitrile in milk. Eur J Nucl Med 18:363, 1991.

139. Sangalli BC: The hazard (potential hazard) with transdermal drug delivery systems (TDDS), a.k.a. drug patches. Hudson Valley Poison Center Toxicol Newslett 2:1, 1992.

140. Sannerstedt R, Berglund F, Flodh H, et al: Medication during pregnancy and breastfeeding: A new Swedish system for classifying drugs. Int J Clin Pharmacol Ther Toxicol 18:45, 1980.

141. Schou M: Lithium treatment during pregnancy, delivery and lactation: An update. J Clin Psychiatry 51:410, 1990.

142. Schou M, Amdisen A: Lithium and pregnancy. III. Lithium ingestion and children breastfed by women on lithium treatment. Br Med J 2:138, 1973.

143. Segelman AB, Segelman FP, Karliner J, et al: Sassafras and herb tea. JAMA 236:477, 1976.

144. Sewell, AC, Mosandl A, Bohles H: False diagnosis of maple syrup urine disease owing to ingestion of herbal tea. N Engl J Med 341:769, 1999.

145. Siddiqui S, Siddiqui BS, Ghiasuddin, et al: Neem tree (*Azadirachia indica*). J Nat Prod 54:408, 1991.

146. Siegel RK: Herbal intoxication: Psychoactive effects from herbal cigarettes, tea and capsules. JAMA 236:473, 1976.

147. Sietsema WK: The absolute oral bioavailability of selected drugs. Int J Clin Pharmacol Ther Toxicol 27:179, 1989.

148. Sim MR, McNeil JJ: Monitoring chemical exposure using breastmilk: A methodological review. Am J Epidemiol 136:1, 1992.

149. Smith MT, Livingstone I, Hooper WD, et al: Propranolol, propranolol glucuronide, and naphthoxylactic acid in breast milk and plasma. Ther Drug Monit 5:87, 1983.

150. Solomon GM, Weiss PM: Chemical contaminants in breast milk: Time trends and regional variability. Environment Health Perspectives 110:A339, 2002.

151. Somogyi A, Gugler R: Cimetidine excretion into breast milk. Br J Clin Pharmacol 7:627, 1979.

152. Stec GP, Greenberger P, Ruo TI, et al: Kinetics of theophylline transfer to breast milk. Clin Pharmacol Ther 28:404, 1980.

153. Steen B, Rane A, Lonnerholm G, et al: Phenytoin excretion in human breast milk and plasma in nursed infants. Ther Drug Monit 4:331, 1982.

154. Stephens RD, Rappe C, Hayward DG, et al: World Health Organization International Intercalibration Study on dioxins and furans in human milk and blood. Anal Chem 104:3109, 1992.

155. Stiskal JA, Kulin N, Koren G, et al: Neonatal paroxetine withdrawal syndrome. Arch Dis Child Fetal Neonatal Ed 84:F134, 2001.

156. Stuart M (ed): The Encyclopedia of Herbs and Herbalism. New York, Crescent, 1979.

157. Subramanian MG, Chen XG, Bergeski BA: Pattern and duration of the inhibitory effect of alcohol administered acutely on suckling-induced prolactin in lactating rats. Clin Exp Res 14:771, 1990.

158. Taylor L, Willies LJ: The culturally competent pediatrician: Respecting ethnicity in your practice. Contemp Pediatr 20:83, 2003.

159. Tegler L, Lindström B: Antithyroid drugs in milk. Lancet 2:591, 1980.

160. Tellier L, Aronson RA: Lead in breast milk: Should mothers be routinely screened? Wis Med J 71:257, 1994.

161. The Review of Natural Products by Facts and Comparisons. St. Louis, Wolters Kluwer, 1999.

162. Thorley V: Breastfeed Rev 4:82, 1996 (letter).

163. Townsend RJ, Benedetti TJ, Erickson SH, et al: A study to evaluate the passage of ibuprofen into breast milk. Drug Intell Clin Pharm 16:482, 1982.

164. Townsend RJ, Benedetti TJ, Erickson SH, et al: Excretion of ibuprofen into breast milk. Am J Obstet Gynecol 149:184, 1984.

165. Tyler VE: The New Honest Herbal. Philadelphia, Stickley, 1987.

166. Vauzelle-Kervroedan F, Rey E, D'Athis P, et al: Metoclopramide plasma concentration in neonates. Int J Clin Pharmacol Ther 35:519, 1997.

167. Weiner CP, Buhimschi C: Drugs for Pregnancy and Lactating Women. New York, Churchill-Livingston, 2004.

168. Weitz JI: Low-molecular-weight heparins. N Engl J Med 337:688, 1997.

169. Wennberg RP, Rasmussen LF, Ahlors CE: Displacement of bilirubin from human albumin by three diuretics. J Pediatr 90:647, 1977.

170. Werthmann MW, Krees SV: Excretion of chlorothiazide in human breast milk. J Pediatr 81:781, 1972.

171. Westfall RE: Use of anti-emetic herbs in pregnancy: Women's choices, and the question of safety and efficacy. Complementary Ther Nurs Midwifery 10:30, 2004.

172. Wickizer TM, Brilliant LB: Testing for polychlorinated biphenyls in human milk. Pediatrics 68:411, 1981.

173. Wilkenson JM: What do we know about herbal morning sickness treatments? A literature survey. Midwifery 16:224, 2000.

174. Wilson JT, Brown RD, Hinson JL, et al: Pharmacokinetic pitfalls in the estimation of the breast milk/plasma ratio for drugs. Annu Rev Pharmacol Toxicol 25:667, 1985.

175. Wischnik A, Manth SM, Lloyd J, et al: The excretion of ketorolac tromethamine into breast milk after multiple oral dosing. Eur J Clin Pharmacol 36:521, 1989.

176. Wojnar-Horton RE, Kristensen JH, Yapp P, et al: Methadone distribution and excretion into breast milk of clients in a methadone maintenance programme. Br J Clin Pharmacol 44:543, 1997.

177. Wolff MS: Occupationally derived chemicals in breast milk. Am J Ind Med 4:259, 1983.

178. Wright P: Learning experiences in feeding behaviour during infancy. J Psychosom Res 32:613, 1988.

179. Yoshida K, Smith B, Craggs M, et al: Investigation of pharmacokinetics and of possible adverse effects in infants exposed to tricyclic antidepressants in breast-milk. J Affect Disord 43:225, 1997.

180. Young TE, Mangum OB: Neofax A: Manual of Drugs Used in Neonatal Care, 10th ed. Raleigh, NC, Acorn, 1997.

181. Yurchak AM, Jusko WJ: Theophylline secreted into breast milk. Pediatrics 57:518, 1976.

182. Zhou H-H, Adedoyin A, Wilkinson GR: Differences in plasma binding of drugs between Caucasians and Chinese subjects. Clin Pharmacol Ther 48:10, 1990.

183. Zoric-Hahn M, Fulconis F, Minoli I, et al: Antibody responses to parenteral and oral vaccines are impaired by conventional and low protein formulas as compared to breast-feeding. Acta Paediatr Scand 79:1137, 1990.

$\mathcal{N}$ormal growth, failure to thrive, and obesity in the breastfed infant

NORMAL GROWTH

The growth of exclusively breastfed infants has become the focus of much interest among pediatricians, researchers, and nutritionists.[14] A number of long-range follow-up studies have been initiated to address the issues of growth during the critical first year of life, when brain growth is greater than it ever will be again in postnatal life. An interest in height and weight increments and ratios is only part of the concern about obesity and the long-range issues of adiposity. Does breastfeeding protect against adult obesity? Does human milk protect against cholesterol "intolerance" in adult life? The questions are clear, but the answers are not unless one assumes the teleologic approach: human milk is ideal for the human infant with its low protein, controlled calories, and persistent unchangeable cholesterol.

The questions are actually, "Is it safe to overfeed an infant with formula?," Is it safe to deprive an infant of cholesterol during a period of critical brain growth when brain growth depends on cholesterol?," and "When infants are deprived of cholesterol in early infancy, are they less able to tolerate it later?"

Antiquated data and anthropometric standards have led to the belief that the growth curves and tables of normal height and weight do not reflect the growth of most healthy, well-fed breastfeeding infants.[95] Reliability of weight gain as a measure of growth has developed because it is a measurement easily obtained.[87] Measurement of length, however, is considered a better standard.[100] Weight gain and linear growth are not always correlated. Furthermore, during infancy and childhood the lower leg grows at a higher rate than the rest of the body. Knee-heel length can be expressed as a percentage of total length increases with age: 25% at birth, 27% at 12 months, and 31% in adult life. During several decades of formula feeding, "normal" growth curves were developed based only on formula fed infants. Furthermore, whole cow milk is fortunately almost totally abandoned, and the recommendations for introduction of solid food beyond 4 or even 6 months have been universally adopted by nutrition-conscious physicians and parents. WHO and UNICEF have reconfirmed that breastfeeding should be exclusive for the first 6 months. New growth curves are being developed based on breastfed or formula fed infants on delayed solids.

Bottle fed infants gain more rapidly in weight and length during the first months of life than do breastfed infants.[31] Therefore, evaluating an infant's physical growth by standards set by bottle fed infants predisposes one to the diagnosis of failure to thrive. Fomon and associates[39] reported a longitudinal study of breastfed and bottle fed infants during the first few months of life that demonstrated the 10th and 90th percentile values for weight and length of the two groups were similar at birth, and the 10th percentile values of the two groups were similar at age 112 days. The significant difference was in the values for the 90th percentile. Bottle fed infants were above this percentile in substantially greater numbers. These differences were attributed to caloric intake rather than the difference in composition of the diet. Fomon and associates[39] have shown that the bottle fed infant not only gains more in weight and length, but also gains more weight for a unit of length. This gain reflects the overfeeding of the bottle fed infants. Whether this contributes to subsequent obesity is an important issue.

Most studies of growth in breastfed infants have been plagued with the problem of variation in supplementation and the occurrence of partial weaning. The growth of the exclusively breastfed infant was investigated in 1980 by Ahn and MacLean,[1] who conducted a retrospective study of enthusiastic and successful La Leche League mothers and their infants in the Baltimore–Washington, DC, area. Mothers who had exclusively breastfed their infants for 6 months or longer were randomly selected, and all agreed to participate. They were educated, middle-income, married women. Growth records were obtained from the mothers and from their pediatricians' records. The weight and length curves of these infants remained above the National Center for Health Statistics (NCHS) 50th percentile through at least the sixth month.[95] In those infants who were exclusively breastfed longer, all were above the 25th percentile through the 9th and 10th months of life. Vitamin and mineral supplements were taken by 75% of all mothers and given to 35% of the infants. This study does demonstrate that under optimal circumstances, exclusive breastfeeding does support growth in the first 6 months or longer that matches norms set by formula fed infants.

When the growth of healthy, exclusively breastfed infants was evaluated in the first 6 months of life in Australia, the weight increments in the first 3 months compared favorably with standards from the Ministry of Health in Great Britain.[60] The weight increment for the second 3 months was significantly less. The data from Great Britain have been accumulated from a mixed sample of breastfed and bottle fed infants in the 1950s, when most infants were fed cow milk with a high solute load.

The growth pattern of full-term infants in the United States followed prospectively from birth showed no significant differences in mean growth measurements (weight, crown-rump length, head circumference, skinfold thickness) between infants fully breastfed and those fed whey-predominant formula. Plasma amino acid concentrations, including those for taurine, were similar at 3 days and 2, 8, and 16 weeks of age in both groups.[116]

The effects on growth of specific protein and energy intake in 4- to 6-month-old infants who were either breastfed or formula fed with high and low protein were measured by Axelsson and associates.[5] No significant differences were found in the growth rate of crown-heel length and head circumference or weight gain. The authors concluded that the differences in protein intake between breastfed and formula fed infants without differences in growth indicate that the formulas may provide a protein intake in excess of the needs. When milk intake and growth in 45 exclusively breastfed infants were carefully documented in the first 4 months by Butte and associates,[14] energy and protein intakes were substantially less than current nutrient allowances. Infant growth progressed satisfactorily when compared with NCHS standards, despite that energy dropped from 110 ± 24 kcal/kg/day at 1 month to 71 ± 17 kcal/kg/day at 4 months.[14] Similarly, protein intake decreased from 1.6 ± 0.3 g/kg/day at 1 month to 0.9 ± 0.2 g/kg/day at 4 months. Axelsson and associates[5] urge reevaluation of protein and energy requirements stating they are currently set too high.

Weight-for-length and weight gain were significantly correlated with total energy intake but not with activity level during the first 6 months of life in breastfed infants studied by Dewey and associates.[25-27,30] Energy intake was considerably lower than recommended, 85 to 89 kcal/kg/day, when compared with the 115 kcal/kg/day recommended dietary allowances (RDAs) of the National Academy of Sciences in 1980.[19] Those infants who consumed the most breast milk became the fattest.

The physical growth of normal, healthy, breastfed and formula fed infants from birth to 2 years was reported by Czajka-Narins and Jung[21] in 1986 at a university hospital in the Midwest. Although breastfed males were lighter at 6 and 12 months, at 24 months the differences were not significant. Using height-to-weight indices, fewer infants who were breastfed longer were categorized as obese. These data suggest that longer breastfeeding affects weight but not length. Pomerance[104] followed 128 breastfed and 3084 formula fed infants from birth through infancy and again from 3 to 12 years and reported in 1987. A comparison of the two groups, both given additional foods with similar timing, revealed no significant differences in growth velocity for weight or for length/height, either during the first 3 years or from age 3 to age 12.

When patterns of growth are examined in the infants of marginally nourished mothers, weight gain is comparable to a reference population but does not permit recovery of weight differential at birth, which was significantly small for gestational age.[11] The intakes of energy and protein by individual infants were reflected in their weight gain but were below internationally recommended norms. Maternal milk alone, when produced in sufficient amounts, can maintain normal growth up to the sixth month of life. Exclusive breastfeeding in Chilean infants of low-middle and low socioeconomic families produced the highest weight gain and practically no illness or hospitalization.[67]

In the Copenhagen Cohort Study in 1994, exclusively breastfed term infants had a mean intake of 781 and 855 mL/24 hours at 2 and 4 months, respectively.[88] The median fat concentration of human milk was 39.2 g/L and was positively associated with maternal weight gain during pregnancy. This supports the concept that maternal fat stores laid down during pregnancy are easier to mobilize

during lactation than other fat stores. This may limit milk fat when pregnancy fat stores are exhausted.

The effect of prolonged breastfeeding on growth has been an issue of concern, especially in developing countries.[41] In a review of 13 studies, Grummer-Strawn[48] pointed out in 1993 that eight reported a negative relationship, two had a positive relationship, and three had mixed results. Grummer-Strawn identified the flaws in study design and suggested that until better information is available, women should nurse as long as possible because the benefits to infant health exceed the risks in these geographic areas. Pomerance[104] studied a breastfed and formula fed group of infants who were given solids at 6 months. No significant difference was found in growth velocity for weight or length/height, either during the first 3 years or during the period from 3 to 12 years.

In addition to recognizing the importance of genetic, metabolic, and environmental influences in producing significant differences in growth patterns, Barness[7] suggests that recommendations for nutrition of healthy neonates may be too high for some and too low for others. However, the benchmark for nutritional requirements of the full-term infant remains milk from the infant's healthy, well-nourished mother. Dietary energy intakes are substantially lower than most recommendations, according to Whitehead and Paul[119] and Whitehead and associates,[120] who reviewed infant feeding practices. Both studies indicate that diet-related growth faltering in breastfed infants rarely occurs in developing countries until later than would be suggested by growth standards currently in use.

Gain in physical growth is not as critical as gain in brain growth, but measurements of brain growth are only indirectly implied from growth of the head. In evaluating any infant's progress, head circumference is an important consideration, especially in the first year of life. Deceleration in the rate of increase in head circumference occurs over the first year. The head circumference increases about 7.5 cm (3 inches) in the first year of life and another 7.5 cm in the next 16 years of life. When growth failure includes failure of head growth, the failure is severe. However, many other factors independent of body growth influence head growth.

A weight loss of 5% is usually accepted as the norm for bottle fed infants in the first week of life, although information in pediatric textbooks is meager.[103] A loss of 7% is average for breastfed infants, but when this occurs in the first 72 hours of life, the clinician should be alert to breastfeeding problems and should review the process. A loss of 10% is the maximum for a breastfed infant. The clinician should confirm that positioning and latch-on are correct and that the breasts have responded with some engorgement and milk production. The mother-infant dyad with this problem will need close observation and support. Referral to a licensed certified lactation consultant may be appropriate if the pediatric office does not have a trained staff member available (nurse practitioner with lactation training).

Initially after birth, the normal infant loses 5% of body weight before starting to gain, whether breastfed or bottle fed. In a study of infants at the University of Rochester, breastfed infants who were given added water or added formula to force fluids in the first few days of life lost more weight and were less likely to start gaining by the fourth day than infants who were exclusively breastfed or who were bottle fed.

The time at which an infant regains birth weight is equally unclear. In their extensive study of breastfed and formula fed infants, Nelson and associates[98] summarize weight at 8 days for 1139 infants by stating, "Most formula fed but not most breastfed infants have exceeded their birth weights by age 8 days." They also report that gains in weight and length were greater by males than by females in the age intervals of 8 to 42 days, 42 to 112 days, and 8 to 112 days. These authors provide weights and lengths for the critical first 112 days. These data and the gains in grams per day are provided in Appendix J. The mean values are provided in Tables 12-1 and 12-2.

According to the NCHS, birth weight is doubled between the 50th and 75th percentiles at 4 months of age and tripled at 12 months.[54] When doubling and tripling times were studied by type of feeding as well as birth weight, gender, and race by Czajka-Narins and Jung,[21] they concurred with doubling time but found tripling time to be 412 days for black males and 484 days for white females, with no significant difference between breastfeeders or bottle feeders. They found obese infants with higher weight/length ratios tripled their weight sooner, suggesting that rapid tripling time may be an indicator of obesity. Black infants in general doubled and tripled their weights sooner, but more blacks were bottle fed in this study.[21]

Growth charts for breastfed infants

Dewey and associates[25-27, 30] have suggested that new, separate growth charts are needed for breastfed infants. The DARLING (Davis Area Research on Lactation, Infant Nutrition, and Growth) Study collected data prospectively on growth patterns, nutrient intake, morbidity, and activity levels of matched cohorts of infants who were either exclusively breastfed or bottle fed during the first 12 months of life. Measurements were followed beyond 12 months to 18, 21, 24, and 36 months as well. Growth in length and head circumference did not differ significantly between the two groups; however, weight gain was slower among breastfed infants after about 3 months of age. These weight gain differences continued even after solid foods were added at 6 months in both groups. Breastfed infants were leaner than their counterparts. The slower growth rates and lower energy intake of the breastfed infants were associated with normal or accelerated development and less morbidity from infectious illnesses. The authors[25,26] concluded that it is normal for breastfed infants to gain at this pace, which is less rapid than that indicated by the scales developed for bottle fed infants.

When the growth patterns of a large sample of breastfed infants were pooled from the United States, Canada, and Europe, Dewey and associates[24] reported that results were consistent across studies. Breastfed infants grew more rapidly in weight during the first 2 months and less rapidly during 3 to 12 months. Head circumference was well above the

TABLE 12-1   Weights and lengths of breastfed and formula fed infants at selected ages

| | Breastfed | | | | Formula fed | | | |
| | 203 males | | 216 females | | 380 males | | 340 females | |
Age (days)	Mean	SD	Mean	SD	Mean	SD	Mean	SD
Weight (g)								
8	3457	425	3355	406	3585	437	3396	387
14	3660	434	3545	413	3790	438	3575	390
28	4245	493	4058	453	4393	460	4081	396
42	4780	524	4504	496	4940	487	4529	430
56	5237	562	4879	534	5426	526	4935	461
84	5956	622	5512	593	6248	597	5642	536
112	6559	677	6085	661	6920	685	6262	607
Length (mm)								
8	512	18	506	17	514	18	504	17
14	521	18	515	17	523	18	513	17
28	539	18	533	18	542	18	530	17
42	556	18	549	17	559	19	546	17
56	570	18	562	17	576	19	562	17
84	598	19	588	18	605	19	589	18
112	623	20	611	18	631	20	612	18

SD, Standard deviation.
From Nelson SE, Rogers RR, Ziegler EE, et al: Gain in weight and length during early infancy. Early Hum Dev 19:223, 1989.

World Health Organization/Centers for Disease Control and Prevention (WHO/CDC) median throughout the first year. Length for age did not decline as did the weight for age and weight for length scores as breastfeeding increased in duration.

Since 1983 the reference standard for growth has been the WHO/CDC report *Measuring Change in Nutritional Status*.[123] This report used the anthropometric indications of nutritional status proposed by the WHO working group. When Garza and associates[43] reviewed growth patterns of breastfed infants, breastfed infants clearly consumed less energy than recommended by WHO in the second 3-month period by choice and not because the mother could not produce more milk.[123] Dewey and Lönnerdal[28] first pointed this out when they had mothers pump to increase their

production, and the infants self-regulated to the original intake measured before the pumping program in spite of the fact that the mother was producing more milk.[28]

Tables 12-1 and 12-2 provide the growth charts that are currently used as the standard for following breastfed infants. Close monitoring of length measurements, which should match the current growth charts, is a very important parameter.

Impact of weaning foods on growth

The timing of initiation of weaning foods before 6 months of age has shown that as energy intake increases from solid foods, energy intake from breast milk decreases. The downward trend of

TABLE 12-2   **Gains in weight and length during selected age intervals in relation to gender and type of feeding**

| | Breastfed | | | | Formula fed | | | |
| | 203 males | | 216 females | | 380 males | | 340 females | |
Gain	Mean	SD	Mean	SD	Mean	SD	Mean	SD
Weight (g/day)								
8–42	38.9	9.7	33.8	9.3	39.8	7.7	33.3	7.4
42–112	25.4	6.2	22.6	6.3	28.5	6.4	24.7	5.2
8–112	29.8	5.8	26.2	5.6	32.2	5.6	27.5	4.9
Length (mm/day)								
8–42	1.29	0.22	1.24	0.22	1.33	0.22	1.25	0.19
42–112	0.96	0.17	0.89	0.13	1.03	0.12	0.94	0.11
8–112	1.07	0.12	1.01	0.11	1.13	0.11	1.04	0.09

SD, Standard deviation.
From Nelson SE, Rogers RR, Ziegler EE, et al: Gain in weight and length during early infancy. Early Hum Dev 19:223, 1989.

weight/age and weight/length ratios continues with the addition of solids, which would not be expected if growth faltering were the basis for the decline.[43] Breastfed infants apparently self-regulate when offered solids and also leave some solids uneaten. When breastfed infants were given solids between 4 and 7 months, their weight for age and weight for length were consistently lower than those for infants introduced to solids at 8 months or older. Length for age was similar between the two groups.

Does the growth rate of exclusively breastfed infants reflect a need for higher protein?[57] This question has challenged the wisdom of exclusive breastfeeding. A group of exclusively breastfed infants were matched with a second group who received preprepared solid foods, including egg yolk, beginning at 4 months of age.[29] Neither weight gain nor length gain from 4 to 6 months differed between the groups. The solid-food group received 20% higher protein intake as well as higher intakes of iron, zinc, calcium, vitamin A, and riboflavin. The authors concluded that protein intake is not a limiting factor in the growth of breastfed infants.[57]

Similarly, Cohen and associates[18] demonstrated that breastfed infants given solids at 4 months self-regulated so that the energy intake and protein intake were the same in both the supplemented group and the unsupplemented group. Furthermore, when Motil and associates[92] calculated the gross efficiency of nutrient utilization for each infant in a longitudinal study of breastfed and bottle fed infants, length and weight gains and lean body mass and body fat accretion during the first 24 weeks of life were similar. The formula fed infants had received significantly higher nitrogen and energy. The gross efficiency of dietary energy utilization for lean body mass deposition was two times greater in breastfed than bottle fed infants. No association was found between lean body mass deposition and dietary protein intake. This confirms previous studies that human milk protein does not limit growth.[92]

Prolonged breastfeeding

Considerable controversy surrounds the question of prolonged breastfeeding. Although the value of prolonged breastfeeding has not been challenged in industrialized countries, it has in developing countries. Some studies showed that small, undergrown infants are breastfed longer.[16,65] Careful assessment reveals that larger infants are weaned earlier. A cautious review of available studies suggests that prolonged breastfeeding does not cause malnutrition; rather, the small and undergrown infants are kept at the breast longer. Child size appears to be related to the decision to wean so that, in general, large healthy infants are weaned completely from the breast earlier.[16] Thus, smaller infants being breastfed longer is not the cause of the undergrowth.

Catch-up growth in small-for-gestational-age infants

Small-for-gestational-age (SGA) infants have been identified as being at risk for continued growth failure in extrauterine life, learning difficulties, and behavioral problems. Lucas and associates[80] explored the influence of early nutrition on growth in the first year of life in full-term SGA infants, comparing those receiving breast milk and those receiving formula. This was a subset of a study on early carnitine supplementation. An equal number of breastfed and formula fed infants received carnitine. Additional demographic, social, clinical, and anthropometric data were collected. Breastfeeding was associated with a greater increase in weight at 2 weeks and 3 months of age, which persisted beyond the actual breastfeeding period. The authors reported greater catch-up growth in head measurement and a greater increase in body length in the breastfed infant. They suggest that breastfeeding promotes faster catch-up growth, and breastfed infants have the potential for improved catch-up growth in developmental parameters as well.[80]

In a study designed to examine the role of zinc supplementation in catch-up growth in SGA infants, Castillo-Duran and associates[15] reported that infants who were exclusively breastfed had increased growth over those who were formula fed and supplemented with zinc.

Cognitive and motor development

Cognitive development in the first 7 years of life was related to breastfeeding practices of a birth cohort in New Zealand.[35] The researchers took into account maternal intelligence, maternal education, maternal training in child rearing, childhood experiences, family socioeconomic status, birth weight, and gestational age. The breastfed children had slightly higher test scores on the Peabody Picture Vocabulary Test, the 5-year measure on the Stanford Binet Intelligence Scale, and the 7-year measure on the Weschler Child Intelligence Scale. Measures of language development were equally influenced. This very small improvement in scores persisted when all variables were taken into account. The scores were also influenced by length of breastfeeding less than and longer than 4 months.

An additional study on the same birth cohort was done to assess breastfeeding and subsequent social adjustment in 6- to 8-year-old children. Fergusson and associates[36] studied prospectively 1024 children who were part of the Christ Church Child Development Study. They used the maternal and teacher ratings of childhood conduct disorders. There was a statistically significant tendency for conduct disorder scores to decline with increasing duration of breastfeeding; that is, breastfed children were less prone to conduct disorders than bottle fed children. Breastfed children, however, tended to come from slightly more socially advantaged, economically privileged homes that were more stable. The analysis failed to examine early mother-infant interaction patterns.

This cohort of 1000 individuals has now been reported as an 18-year longitudinal study by Horwood and Fergusson.[63] There continued to be a small but detectable increase in child cognitive and educational achievement in the children who had been breastfed as infants. The results were confirmed in standardized tests, teacher ratings, and academic outcomes in high school and young adulthood.

De Andraca and Uauy[22] reviewed the factors in human milk and the breastfeeding process that affect optimal mental and visual development. The complex relationships point to a clear advantage to breastfeeding.

Another group of children was followed in New Zealand to evaluate the effects of infant feeding, birth order, paternal occupation, and socioeconomic status on speech in 6-year-old children. Controlling for the demographic effects, the association of breastfeeding with clear speech was different for the genders, being negligible for girls and strongly positive for boys.[35]

The relationship of infant-feeding practices and dependent variables to the subsequent cognitive abilities were reported by Young and associates[126] from the Yale Harvard Research Project in Tunisia. Within the underprivileged group they found that breastfeeding promoted not only physical growth but also sensorimotor development as assessed by Bayley motor and mental scales. There were no great differences in the ability to sit alone or to take first steps, but especially among males in the lower socioeconomic group, there was significant superiority of breastfed infants at 8, 14, and 16 months of age in Bayley mental scales. In this study, all infants were from the same social and intellectual strata.

The question of whether breastfeeding influences a child's developmental outcome has appeared in modern literature since Hoefer and Hardy[61] first reported that breastfed infants were more active and achieved their motor milestones earlier than bottle fed infants in 1929. These authors described enhanced learning ability and higher intelligence quotient (IQ) scores at 7 to 13 years of age, as well as in children exclusively breastfed for 4 to 9 months. Although socioeconomic status and mother's education were not reported, it is an interesting historic note that it was the well-educated, higher socioeconomic mothers who could afford to bottle feed in the 1920s and 1930s and into the 1940s. In an attempt to clarify the relationship to maternal status, Taylor and Wadsworth[115] took the negative hypothesis but were unable to eliminate the possibility that breastfeeding had a positive effect on intellectual development at 5 years of age.

In a national study of 13,135 children in England, Scotland, and Wales, a positive correlation between duration of breastfeeding and performance in tests of vocabulary and visuomotor coordination was found; these behavior scores remained steady when tested against intervening social and biologic variables. This British 1946 cohort study has continued. In 2002, Richards and Wadsworth used meta-analysis to show that breastfeeding conferred a 3.2-point increment in cognitive function through adolescence. They further showed that breastfeeding was significantly and positively associated with educational attainment and cognition at age 15 years and also with adult social class. Breastfeeding did not affect verbal memory independently at 53 years of age. Breastfeeding clearly has long-term potential impact across life's course according to the authors.[107]

The advantage of human milk for at-risk infants has been investigated by Lucas and associates,[81,82] who raised public awareness when their results were reported in newspapers internationally in 1992. The initial cohort of 771 infants whose birth weight was less than 1850 g were given their mother's milk; these infants had a mean 8-point advantage on the Bayley Mental Developmental Index over infants of mothers choosing not to do so.[81] Both groups received nutrition by feeding tube for the first month of life. A 4.3-point advantage remained when outcome was adjusted for demographic and perinatal factors. The same advantage was found using an IQ equivalent test, which is a fundamentally different test. The same group of infants was tested regularly, and results at age 7½ to 8 years showed a 10-point advantage in IQ testing even when controlled for maternal social class and education.[125]

This report precipitated a torrent of responses from other investigators,[64,90,101] who provided support for and against the conclusion that breast milk is effective in improving the outcome of high-risk infants.

Breastfeeding and cognitive development were studied prospectively between 1978 and 1982 by Rogan and Gladen.[109] They followed 788 children longitudinally through early school. There were small but statistically significant increases in scores on the Bayley and McCarthy tests among breastfed infants at all times. The infants were 95% white and all came from similar middle-class families, so the study population was a homogeneous one. There were higher scores with increasing length of breastfeeding.

To determine the effect of breastfeeding on optimal visual development, Birch and associates[9] studied term and preterm infants fed human milk or corn oil–based formula with no ω-3 essential fatty acids. Visual testing using visual-evoked potential and forced-choice preferential looking activity was performed at 4 months' adjusted age; infants given human milk scored better. This was confirmed at 36 months using random dot stereo acuity and letter-matching ability. Results correlated with a measure of dietary ω-3 sufficiency index from the infants' red blood cells (RBCs) at 4 months.

FAILURE TO THRIVE

Definition

Failure to thrive is a symptom and not a diagnosis. The causes of failure to thrive in children have been associated with malfunctions of many organ systems as well as with nutritional, environmental, social, and psychological factors. Failure to thrive while breastfeeding has often been inappropriately considered in the same terms as failure associated with other sources of nourishment and involving other age groups. Failure to thrive while breastfeeding is a phenomenon associated with the first year of life and more likely under 6 months. Exclusive breastfeeding is appropriate for the first 6 months, and then solids should be added, along with the gradual addition of other liquids by cup after 7 months. Therefore, the symptom is no longer exclusively associated with lactation, except in rare cases in which the infant is breastfed beyond 9 months with no solids added.

The term *failure to thrive* has been loosely used to describe all infants who show some degree of growth failure. It is a syndromic classification that has been used to describe infants whose gain in weight or length or both fails to occur in a normal progressive fashion. For the breastfed infant, it may be a matter of comparing a slower gainer to the excessive weight-gain patterns of the bottle fed infant. The definition offered by Fomon[38] states that "failure to thrive [should] be defined as a rate of gain in length and/or weight less than the value corresponding to two standard deviations below the mean during an interval of at least 56 days for infants less than five months of age and during an interval of at least three months for older infants." Fomon further suggests that infants gaining in length and weight at rates less than the 10th percentile values be suspected of failing to thrive.[38] Certainly in managing the breastfed infant, more careful and frequent medical evaluation should be provided for the infant who drops to the 10th percentile for weight, fails to gain weight, or continues to lose after the 10th day of life, rather than waiting for 56 days to establish the trend unquestionably.

The disorder is now defined as failure to thrive when the infant continues to lose weight after 10 days of life, does not regain birth weight by 3 weeks of age, or gains at a rate below the 10th percentile for weight gain beyond 1 month of age. Unlike the bottle fed infant, who can then be placed in the hospital where professionals can feed him, the breastfed infant needs to be evaluated in the home setting, nursing at the breast, unless it is an emergency. If the infant requires hospitalization, then the breastfeeding mother is part of the workup, including examination of the breasts for signs of milk production and response to pumping.

A more serviceable measure of failure to thrive than percentiles is proposed by Frank and associates,[42] who suggest the use of a percentage of the median values for the age on the growth chart. Thus, normal is greater than 90% of median weight, mild malnutrition is 75% to 90% of median, moderate is 60% to 74% of median, and severe is less than 60% of median weight. Similar percentages are applied to height and weight for height. Thus, a 1-month-old infant whose median weight for age would be 5000 g and who is only 3800 g is 75% of median, or mildly malnourished (Table 12-3).

Human growth has been considered a continuous process, characterized by changing velocity

TABLE 12-3 Daily weight gain and recommended allowances

Age	Median daily weight gain (g)	Recommended daily allowance (kcal/kg/day)
0–3 mo	26–31	108
3–6 mo	17–18	108
6–9 mo	12–13	98
9–12 mo	9	98

From National Research Council, Food and Nutrition Board, National Academy of Sciences: Recommended Dietary Allowances, 10th ed. Washington, DC, US Government Printing Office, 1989.

with age. Lampl and associates[71] made serial measurements of normal infants weekly, semiweekly, and daily during their first 21 months. They show clearly that growth in length occurs by discontinuous, aperiodic, saltatory spurts. Furthermore, these bursts were 0.5 to 2.5 cm (⅕ to 1 inch) during intervals separated by no measurable change (2 to 63 days duration). The authors suggest that 90% to 95% of normal development during infancy is growth free.[71] Length accretion is distinctly a saltatory process of incremental bursts punctuating background stasis. Thus, evaluation of length requires more than one measurement and the careful consideration of an experienced physician familiar with growth parameters.

As more and more women breastfeed, increasing numbers of cases of failure to thrive appear in the literature, although it is a rare phenomenon. No statistical data on incidence rates are available because no large prospective study has been done.[74] Only in extreme cases are infants hospitalized, but the number of these cases is increasing as well, partly because of a failure to recognize the disorder and refer the infant to medical care promptly.

Diagnosis

The problem of slow or inadequate weight gain has confounded even the physicians most committed to breastfeeding. It should be approached with the same orderly diagnostic process used to attack any medical problem. Thus, a complete history, including the details of the breastfeeds, a physical examination of the infant, an examination of the maternal breast, observation of the feeding, and appropriate laboratory work are indicated. Organizing the data amassed by this process will help identify the facts that do appear under maternal and infant causes separately.

Slow gaining versus failure to thrive

Some helpful distinctions exist between the breastfed infant who is slow to gain weight and the infant who is failing to thrive while breastfeeding.[72,73] These parameters should be included in the routine "well baby" evaluation of all breastfed infants, beginning with the first visit (Table 12-4). With early discharge often occurring less than 48 hours after birth, the first visit may need to be within 48 hours of discharge from the hospital, depending on the infant's gestational age, weight loss before discharge, history of jaundice, and the mother's experience. The pediatric office or clinic should have a fail-safe system of follow-up for all newborns that includes access by telephone. In the absence of a telephone in the home, visiting nurse involvement may be appropriate. Although many hospitals provide breastfeeding warm lines that mothers can call for information and help, the family must make the transition from the birthplace to the primary care provider promptly, especially for parents of a first baby who have no previous office contact.

The feeding pattern of the infant with slow weight gain is usually frequent feedings with evidence of a good suck. The mother's breasts are full before feeding, and she can describe a let-down during the feeding. There are at least six wet diapers a day, urine is pale and dilute, and stools are loose and seedy. Weight gain is slow but consistent. If the infant is gaining extremely slowly but is alert, bright, and responsive and developing along the appropriate level, the infant is a "slow gainer." In contrast, the infant with true failure to thrive is usually apathetic or weakly crying with poor tone and poor turgor. There are few wet diapers (none is ever

TABLE 12-4   **Parameters for evaluation of breastfed infants**

Infant who is slow to gain weight	Infant with failure to thrive
Alert healthy appearance	Apathetic or crying
Good muscle tone	Poor tone
Good skin turgor	Poor turgor
At least six wet diapers/day	Few wet diapers
Pale, dilute urine	"Strong" urine
Stools frequent, seedy (or if infrequent, large and soft)	Stools infrequent, scanty
Eight or more nursings/day, lasting 15–20 minutes	Fewer than eight feedings, often brief
Well-established let-down reflex	No signs of functioning let-down reflex
Weight gain consistent but slow	Weight erratic; may lose

soaked) and "strong" urine. Stools are infrequent and scanty. Feedings are often by schedule but always fewer than eight per day and brief. There are no signs of a good let-down reflex. True failure to thrive is potentially serious; early recognition is essential if the integrity of both brain growth and breastfeeding is to be safely preserved.

Although slow gaining may be familial or genetic (small parents), it is always appropriate to be sure the process of breastfeeding is optimized.[12] Attention to adequate fat in the milk is important, especially because mothers have often been encouraged to "switch nurse," that is, switch back and forth between breasts to build up an adequate milk supply. The switch-nursing process interrupts the release of fat and the production of fat-rich hindmilk. If the mother is interrupting the feeding to go to the other side, a period of feeding exclusively on one breast during each feeding may change the gaining pattern. If necessary, the level of fat in the milk can be checked by doing a "creamatocrit," comparing milk before and after the timing change (see Chapter 21). By weighing the infant before and after a feeding with a digital readout scale, an accurate measurement of breast milk intake can be recorded. A slower gainer will have good intake.

In a schema for classifying failure to thrive at the breast, the causes associated with infant behavior and problems are distinguished from those related to maternal problems (Fig. 12-1). The causes in the infant can be further evaluated by looking at net intake, which may be associated with poor feeding, poor net intake from additional losses, or high energy needs. The maternal causes can be divided into poor production of milk and poor release of milk. When a poor let-down reflex continues long enough, it will eventually cause a decrease in milk production. Several factors may affect the outcome, and more than one management change may be indicated.

Evaluation of infant

Examination of the infant should suggest any underlying physical problems, such as hypothyroidism, congenital heart disease, mechanical abnormalities of the mouth (e.g., cleft palate), or major neurologic disturbances.[8] The infant's ability to root, suck, and coordinate swallowing should be observed. There is a greater risk today of missing subtle structural problems because infants spend much of their hospital life out of the newborn nursery away from the watchful eyes of experienced nurses and then are discharged before problems become manifest.

The routine observation of a feeding by the infant's physician should be part of the discharge examination from the hospital. If this is not practical, such an examination should be incorporated into the first office or clinic visit within the first week of life. The focus should be the positioning of the mother and the infant, placement of the

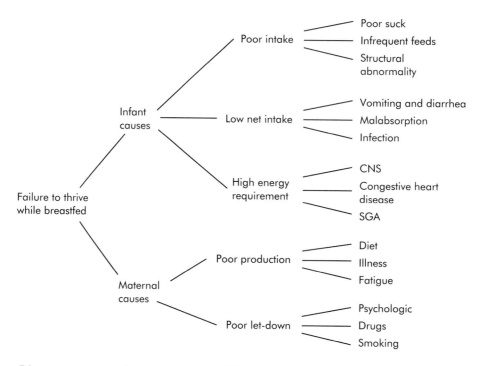

Figure 12-1. Diagnostic flowchart for failure to thrive. CNS, central nervous system; SGA, small for gestational age.

mother's hands, and initiation of latch-on (see Chapter 8). A small number of infants will be identified with physical abnormalities that need medical attention (Table 12-5).

Lukefahr[83] identified 38 infants under 6 months of age in a suburban pediatric practice as having failure to thrive while breastfeeding. Only 2 of 28 infants (7.1%) who presented in the first 4 weeks had underlying illnesses (salt-losing adrenogenital syndrome and congenital hypotonia), whereas 5 of the 10 brought in between 1 and 6 months had underlying disease (all of whom actually presented with a problem by 4 months). This report stresses the importance of ruling out underlying disease and the urgency of having the pediatrician evaluate the child when the symptom of poor weight gain is first suspected, thus avoiding the serious complications of dehydration and metabolic disorders that may result when "home remedies" for lactation problems are used.

Oral motor problems: feeding skills disorder. *Growth failure secondary to feeding skills disorder* is the terminology proposed by Ramsay and associates[106] to replace nonorganic failure to thrive (NOFTT). The authors describe a series of children who were referred for NOFTT who had displayed subtle problems since birth. The criteria include early abnormal feeding-related symptoms present shortly after birth, such as impaired oral function, suggesting the infants are minimally neurologically abnormal, sometimes associated with borderline low Apgar scores. Difficulties during earlier stages of feeding development not only may interfere with the development of more mature feeding skills, but also may contribute eventually to difficulties in mother-infant interaction. The common finding among all infants with failure to thrive was underlying feeding-related symptoms that were neurophysiologic but manifest in different degrees of oral sensorimotor (and pharyngeal) impairment. The neurologic impairment may vary from obvious

TABLE 12-5 Conditions associated with or causing disorders of sucking and swallowing		
Absent or diminished suck	**Mechanical factors interfering with sucking**	**Disorders of swallowing mechanism (not including esophageal abnormalities)**
Maternal anesthesia or analgesia	Macroglossia	Choanal atresia
Anoxia or hypoxia	Cleft lip	Cleft palate
Prematurity	Fusion of gums	Micrognathia
Trisomy 21	Tumors of mouth or gums	Postintubation dysphagia
Trisomy 13-15	Temporomandibular ankylosis or	Palatal paralysis
Hypothyroidism	hypoplasia	Pharyngeal tumors
Neuromuscular abnormalities		Pharyngeal diverticula
Kernicterus		Familial dysautonomia
Werdnig-Hoffmann disease		
Neonatal myasthenia gravis		
Congenital muscular dystrophy		
Central nervous system infections		
Toxoplasmosis		
Cytomegalovirus infection		
Bacterial meningitis		

From Behrman RE, Driscoll JM Jr, Seeds AE (eds): Neonatal-Perinatal Medicine: Diseases of the Fetus and Infant, 2nd ed. St Louis, Mosby, 1977.

cerebral palsy to symptoms that are inapparent on casual observation but lead to abnormal feeding-related symptoms in early life. When the mother copes and adapts, the disorder goes unnoticed until solid foods are added. Diagnosis requires oral sensorimotor assessments and a neurologic examination sensitive enough to measure minimal neurologic impairment in an apparently healthy child who is failing to gain. Early history is also critically important.

Small-for-gestational-age infant. The SGA infant will be identified if gestational age and birth weight are scrutinized. This infant is small at birth despite full gestation time in utero. The SGA infant has a large nutritional deficit to make up from intrauterine failure to grow. The cause of the intrauterine problem should be assessed: placental insufficiency, maternal disease, toxemia, heavy smoking, or intrauterine infection such as toxoplasmosis.

SGA infants are difficult to feed initially by any method and often require tube feedings for a few days. Their caloric needs parallel the needs of an infant of appropriate weight for gestation rather than their actual low weight. SGA infants should be placed on frequent feedings, every 2 to 3 hours by day and every 4 hours at night. They should be awakened for feedings if they sleep long periods. If they have not been nursing well, the breast has not been stimulated to produce to its full capability. The mother may need to express milk manually or mechanically pump milk to enhance her production. Her milk may then be given by a passive means such as a tube, a small cup, or the lactation supplementing device, which provides additional stimulus to the breast while providing the extra calories needed (see Appendix F and Chapter 19).

An infant who is sufficiently starved in utero may have a degree of inanition that prevents active suckling at first, predisposing to further starvation. The successful nursing of an SGA infant may require extended efforts by the mother to ensure adequate growth. Such efforts are well worth the trouble if one considers the impact of intrauterine growth failure on the central nervous system (CNS). It would be to the infant's advantage to have the critical amino acids such as taurine and the lipids of human milk with which to "catch up" brain growth. As noted earlier, SGA infants are more likely to close the growth gap more rapidly if breastfed.

Jaundice. An infant with an elevated bilirubin level from any cause may be depressed and lethargic and therefore may not nurse well. If the infant appears jaundiced, laboratory evaluation to determine the cause and its appropriate treatment should be undertaken. Visible jaundice under 24 hours of age requires a full evaluation and is not related to breastfeeding. When an infant is taken from the breast at 2 or 3 days of age because of jaundice, this interferes with the establishment of lactation at a critical time, especially for a primipara. Management of the jaundiced infant depends on adequate calories and the active passage of stools, which is the means by which the body excretes the bilirubin in meconium and stools.

"Breastfeeding jaundice," which is related to underfeeding or starvation, does not develop until the infant is 3 or more days old, so other causes must be sought. In addition, care must be taken to help the mother continue to stimulate production with manual expression or pumping to avoid inducing iatrogenic lactation failure. (See Chapter 15 for discussion of hyperbilirubinemia.)

Metabolic screen. Most hospitals provide, often because the law mandates it, screening for metabolic disorders, including galactosemia, phenylketonuria (PKU), maple syrup urine disease, and disorders of metabolism of other amino acids. If these simple screening tests were not performed or their validity is in doubt, they should be done again. Usually the service is available in the state or county laboratory. Thyroid screening for abnormal thyroxine (T_4) or thyroid-stimulating hormone (TSH) should also be performed. Mass screening programs for neonatal thyroid disease have identified cases of deficiency that, even in retrospect, were not in evidence; the infant showed none of the characteristic findings of hypothyroidism, such as thick coarse features, hoarse cry, slow pulse,

macroglossia, umbilical hernia, and jaundice. In the neonate, hypothyroidism is often associated with failure to thrive, if undiagnosed.

Galactosemia. Galactosemia, which is a hereditary disorder of the metabolism of galactose-1-phosphate, is manifest by renal disease and liver dysfunction after ingestion of lactose. The lack of galactose-1-phosphate uridyltransferase activity may be relative or partial. The clinical symptoms may be fulminating, with severe jaundice, hepatosplenomegaly, weight loss, vomiting, and diarrhea, or may be more subtle. Cataracts are not invariably present. In mild cases, failure to thrive may be the presenting symptom. A urine screen for reducing substances (by Clinitest and not Dextrostix, which will only identify glucose) should be done on all infants who fail to thrive, especially if there is hepatomegaly or jaundice.

The definitive diagnosis is the identification of absence or near absence of galactose-1-phosphate uridyltransferase activity in RBC hemolysates. A urine screen should be considered even though an initial metabolic screen for galactosemia was done on the second or third day of life by hospital routine. The treatment is a lactose-free diet, which would mandate prompt weaning from breast milk to prevent further insult to the liver, kidneys, and brain. This is one of the few indications for prompt weaning from human milk. A formula free of lactose (e.g., Isomil, Nutramigen) is indicated. No medical indications exist, however, to use a lactose-free formula for a normal breastfeeding infant either to supplement or to wean from breast milk, which contains lactose. (Refer to pediatric texts on neonatal metabolic disorders for a full description of galactosemia; see also Chapter 15.)

Vomiting and diarrhea. Vomiting and diarrhea are very unusual in a breastfed infant. Spitting up small amounts of milk after feedings is sometimes observed in otherwise normal infants and is of no consequence if it does not affect overall weight gain. Although pyloric stenosis is reportedly less common in breastfed infants, this phenomenon should be ruled out in any infant who vomits consistently after feeding, has diminished urine and stools, shows no weight gain or actually loses weight, and has reverse peristalsis. Usually these infants do well initially and then the vomiting becomes progressive.

Vomiting may be a presenting symptom for various metabolic disorders. Thus, metabolic disorders should be considered in the differential diagnosis. Not all possible metabolic disorders, such as congenital adrenal hyperplasia, are routinely screened. These infants may present with vomiting and weight loss in the first week or two of life or with an acute episode of sepsis. The usual causes of vomiting, as well as the causes peculiar to breast milk, should be considered. Maternal diet should be checked for unusual foods. In families at high risk for allergy, intake by the mother of known family food allergens may cause symptoms in the infant. Diarrhea may be caused by foods in the mother's diet or her use of cathartics such as phenolphthalein.

Chronic infections. Chronic fetal infection in utero, which predisposes an SGA infant to intrauterine growth failure, may continue to cause growth problems in the presence of adequate kilocalories. Chronic viral infections include cytomegalovirus (CMV), hepatitis, acquired immunodeficiency syndrome (AIDS), or other less common viruses (see Chapter 17).

Acute infections. An infant who is not growing well may have an infection in the gastrointestinal tract; therefore, the nature of the stools is important. The urinary tract may be another site of infection not readily identified. If, however, the initial evaluation includes a urinalysis with microscopic evaluation and a white blood cell (WBC) count and differential count, this can usually be ruled out.

High energy requirements. When the metabolic rate of the infant is increased, the weight gain will be diminished or absent. When the infant is hyperactive with a strong startle reflex and sleeps poorly, consideration should be given to stimulants present in the milk as well as to neurologic disorders. When a mother drinks coffee, tea including herbal teas, cola, or other carbonated beverages with added caffeine, the accumulated caffeine may be sufficient to make the infant very irritable and

hyperactive. The best treatment is to replace the caffeine-containing beverages (see Chapter 11). Some CNS disorders are associated with hyperactivity. Infants with severe congenital heart disease are constantly exercising to breathe and oxygenate and have greatly increased metabolic rates. For management of these special infants at the breast, see Chapter 15.

Observation of nursing process

In addition to establishing that no obvious physical or metabolic reasons exist for the failure to gain weight, the infant should be observed suckling at the breast. Does the infant get a good grasp and suck vigorously? If not, what interferes? A receding chin, a weak suck, lack of coordination, the breast obstructing breathing, and mouthing of the nipple or other ineffectual sucking techniques are some of the possibilities. If the problem is the suckling process, the infant may need assistance. This cause is more common with infants who have had some experience with bottles or rubber nipples or who use a pacifier. Small or slightly premature infants who were started on bottle feedings have trouble relearning the proper sucking motion with the tongue (see Figs. 8-7 to 8-12).

Bottle feedings and pacifiers may have to be discontinued until the infant is more experienced at the breast. This will require a program of manually expressing milk to soften the areola, having milk at the nipple to entice the infant, and gently offering the nipple and areola well compressed between two fingers. If the infant has a receding chin or a relaxed jaw, it may help to have the mother hold the lower jaw forward by supporting the angle of the jaw with her thumb. The physician should examine the infant carefully to be sure the jaw is not dislocated, especially if a vertex delivery was done in the posterior position ("sunny side up"). The physician can easily move the jaw forward to relocate it.

Positioning infants for the breast so they directly face the breast, straddling the mother's leg in a semi-upright position, may work best. This is the position twins may assume when nursing simultaneously when they are 3 to 4 months old. Although it is not recommended routinely, for an infant with a receding chin or a cleft, having the mother lean slightly forward for latch-on may help. She should then bring infant upward as she sits back for the feeding.

It may be necessary to assist both mother and baby. If the infant by 2 weeks of age cannot maintain the breast in the mouth without the mother holding it there, it is an indication of improper suckling. In that situation the infant may need to be repositioned with the ventral surface squarely facing the mother's chest wall, that is, tummy to tummy, and the breast presented by the mother with her hand positioned with thumb on top and fingers below the breast. (See discussion in Chapter 8.) Mother may have to maintain the support throughout the feeding. Failure to maintain the breast in the mouth has neurologic implications for long-term follow-up.

A good check of adequate let-down is to observe the opposite breast as the baby nurses to see if milk flows. It can also be tested by seeing if milk is flowing when nursing is interrupted abruptly. If there has been a good let-down, milk will continue to flow, at least drop by drop, for a few moments from the breast being suckled. The mother can also be trained to listen for the infant's swallowing. During proper sucking, the masseter muscle is in full view and is contracting visibly and rhythmically. Swallowing can be seen and heard. The ratio of suck to swallow is 1:1 or 2:1. Occasionally, infants do not suck vigorously at the breast but occasionally use rapid shallow sucks called "flutter sucking" with little or no swallowing. These infants can be gradually taught to suck effectively. Correct positioning of the breast directly in the infant's mouth and holding the breast firmly in position with all the fingers under the breast and only the thumb above allow the infant to grasp properly without sucking the tongue or lower lip. Nipple shields usually make the situation worse.

The most productive part of the diagnostic workup is often observation of the baby at the breast. For this reason, this critical responsibility should not be passed on to others but should be performed personally by the physician as well as a board certified lactation consultant (IBCLC).

The five general types of nursing patterns described in Chapter 8 should be kept in mind. If the mother understands that it is acceptable for the infant to drop off to sleep and snack later, she may not hesitate to follow this lead, thus providing a more adequate feeding.

Some infants will not settle down and nurse well if there is too much activity or noise. Some need to be tightly swaddled; others fall asleep and need to be unwrapped and stimulated to provide adequate suckling time. Frequent feedings, using both breasts, may be the answer in some cases. In others, there may be too many ineffective feedings, which are wearing the mother out; a change that lengthens the time between feedings but also lengthens the time at the breast may help, especially if it is quiet and the chair allows mother to nap while feeding. Concentrating on using one breast at a feeding to increase the fat content may be the most effective change.

Nonorganic failure to thrive

In the study of undernutrition in bottle fed infants and infants beyond the suckling age, terminology has received more attention than the underlying issues. Thus the emphasis has been on "organic" versus "nonorganic" failure to thrive. Unfortunately, the term *nonorganic failure to thrive* (NOFTT) has been equated with a disorder of maternal/infant bonding and has become synonymous with maternal deprivation. *Reactive attachment disorder* has been the term substituted for NOFTT and essentially suggests the mother is guilty until proved innocent. In most cases, utilizing the approach of most "failure-to-thrive" management teams is rarely appropriate in cases associated with breastfeeding in the early months of life. It is important to involve a source of breastfeeding experience as well as an expert in failure to thrive.

When an infant does not have an organic disorder that explains the growth failure, the patient is diagnosed as having NOFTT. The typical psychosocial and nutritional pattern reported in NOFTT includes evidence of a chaotic family life, emotional deprivation, and inadequate nutrition, as pointed out by Weston and associates.[118] These authors reported four children ages 13 to 19 months with NOFTT who were breastfeeding. They had exclusively breastfed for at least 12 months, reportedly refusing solid foods. Failure to gain was noted at 9 months, followed by weight loss increasing at 12 months. Children were all from middle-class families, and parents had at least high school educations or more. The children all were first born and scored "advanced" on the Bayley scales. They were active and alert but difficult to control. They all separated only briefly from their mothers in the clinic and initiated nursing for comfort when anxious. Total dietary energy intakes were below levels for growth. These children were not typical NOFTT in any of their demographics but had missed a critical developmental task of learning to eat. The authors interpreted this as being part of these mothers' need to keep the child close. Treatment included having someone else teach these children to eat solids.

Prolonged exclusive breastfeeding may occasionally result in a unique deficit in the developmental process of eating.[118] Exclusive breastfeeding is not nutritionally adequate in the second half of the first year, especially beyond 12 months, although nursing can safely continue for several years when combined with adequate solids that provide protein, iron, and zinc.[102]

The syndrome of the breastfed infant in the second 6 months of life with very frequent breastfeedings, poor intake of complementary foods, and poor growth has been labeled a manifestation of "vulnerable child syndrome" by O'Connor and Szekely.[99] These children are described to have good weight gain for 5 to 6 months of age, and by 8 months their weight/height score has decreased dramatically. The intake of solid foods is minimal. These infants refuse solids, aggressively spitting food out. The breastfeeding pattern is usually every 1 to 2 hours during the day and frequently at night. Further investigation revealed numerous household stressors and usually the mother's need to maintain control by breastfeeding.

Parental misconception and health beliefs concerning what constitutes a normal diet for infants have been reported by Pugliese and associates[105] as a cause for NOFTT as well. They report seven infants from 7 to 22 months of age with poor weight gain and linear growth who received only 60% to 90% of minimum caloric intake for their age and gender. The parents explained that they wanted to avoid obesity, atherosclerosis, or junk food habits. It has also been shown that parental health beliefs and expectations have led to short stature and delayed puberty in older children.

Fruit juice excess

The custom of excess use of fruit juices in recent decades has replaced the use of water for additional fluids after 6 months of life when the infant is learning to drink from a cup or a straw. The attractive packaging has contributed to this trend. Excessive fruit juice diminishes appetite, resulting in decreased dietary intake of nutrient-dense foods and a decrease in weight gain and ultimately in linear growth. An excess of fruit juice may be a cause of failure to thrive in older infants. Decrease in total high energy intake is combined with malabsorption of fructose and diarrhea from sorbitol, thus compounding the problem.[111] Excessive fruit juice intake in infancy is a major nutrition problem. The American Academy of Pediatrics (AAP) has developed a guideline with restrictions.

Maternal causes

Questions about the mother's health, dietary habits, sleep pattern, smoking habits, medication intake, the events that occur during nursing, and the psychosocial atmosphere in the home are an important part of the history (Fig. 12-2).

Anatomic causes

Lactation failure from insufficient glandular development of the breast has been described by Neifert and Seacat[96] and Neifert and associates,[97] who report three cases in which the breast tissue was asymmetric. Transillumination confirmed a minimally active gland. One family showed a history of

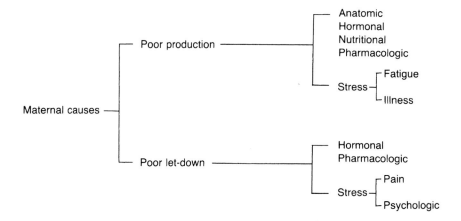

Figure 12-2.   Maternal causes of failure to thrive.

similar failure. All three women benefited psychologically from the diagnosis and chose to continue to breastfeed and supplement. The authors have since identified 14 more women who had anatomic deficiency but normal prolactin levels and failed to respond to a thorough team approach to lactation support.[96] Retained placenta is also a cause of early lactation failure that is quickly identified by a complete history of postpartum breast change and patterns of lochia that the obstetrician associates with retained tissue (see Chapter 16). If prolactin response to stimulus is adequate, ultrasonography can determine the presence of adequate mammary tissue and ductal arborization.

One-breast versus two-breast feeding

After an initial report by Woolridge and associates[122] describing an infant whose failure to thrive was traced to inadequate fat intake associated with using both breasts, each feed resulting in low fat (and relatively high lactose by comparison), the debate regarding using one or two breasts during each feeding has rekindled. When this infant was fed at one breast per feeding, the low-density feeding changed to high-fat feeding, resulting in decreased stooling and increased weight gain. Since that time the authors have continued to investigate the hypothesis that some women require

longer time to release fat into the milk and that limiting the feed to one breast enhances fat content. In some cases this is true, and it is further verified by the infant fed at both breasts having many loose stools because of the high lactose and considerable gassy discomfort that also resolves with the change to single-breast feeds. No report of reducing substances in the stools has been published.

In early lactation, when milk supply is being established, mothers are encouraged to nurse on both breasts at each feed to provide frequent stimulus. The case report[122] in favor of one breast does not change that recommendation. The clinician, however, should obtain a thorough history of feeding frequency and distribution between breasts, especially when the infant is well hydrated, has many stools, and may or may not be fussy but fails to gain weight, remaining under birth weight for several weeks. The need for higher fat content in the feeding may be a consideration in the slow-gaining baby as well. An adjustment in feeding to enhance the fat content should be tried. Usually limiting each feeding to one breast will do that (see Chapter 8). However, some women have smaller storage capacity than others, as demonstrated with ultrasound imagery by Hartmann.[56] These women need to feed from both breasts at each feed. Storage capacity ranges from 100 to more than 250 mL per breast.[56]

Poor milk production

Diets. Although it has been demonstrated that malnourished mothers can produce milk for their infants, marginal diets in Western cultures do affect some mothers' ability to nourish an infant. A case is reported of failure to thrive in a breastfed infant associated with maternal dietary protein and energy restriction.[91] The mother at 8 months post partum independently reduced her dietary energy to 20 kcal/kg/day and her protein to 0.7 g/kg/day to treat cholecystitis medically and avoid surgery. At 12 months her infant's growth curves had fallen below the fifth percentile in both weight and length, although the infant had been receiving solid foods since 24 weeks of age. The authors concluded the failure to thrive was directly related to severe maternal restriction.[91]

Dietary analysis and maternal anthropometry showed that women who gained adequate weight and skin thickness during pregnancy had increased milk production and weight gain in their infants for the first 6 months of life.[34]

If the mother is restricting intake deliberately or inadvertently, she should be instructed to meet the dietary requirement for lactating women (a minimum of 1800 kcal per day for adequate nutrient intake) (see Chapter 9). She does not have to drink milk, but the necessary dietary constituents should be in the diet through cheese, eggs, ice cream, or other sources of calcium and protein. It may not be the nutrition itself but the calming effect of a nourishing beverage while breastfeeding that facilitates nursing. Studies of hormones triggered while eating have shown that more milk is produced if a mother eats just before or during breastfeeding. Prescribing brewer's yeast as a dietary supplement has been observed to provide improvement in milk production beyond that accounted for by mere addition of the same nutrients. Some mothers report a feeling of well-being from taking yeast that they do not obtain from taking daily vitamins. Concern has been expressed regarding the effect of increased vitamin B_6 on prolactin production, but doses that suppress lactation are 60 times the therapeutic dose.

Maternal illness. The presence of infection or other illness in the mother may affect milk production, and the cause of the illness should be identified and treated. Urinary tract infection, endometritis, or upper respiratory infection may need treatment with antibiotics. The antibiotic prescribed should be appropriate for the infant as well because it will pass into the milk. Metabolic disorders such as thyroid disease should also be considered. Postpartum hypothyroid disease is increasingly being recognized as screening tests of T_4 and TSH are being done when a mother complains of severe "baby blues" or fatigue. Adequate treatment will result in increased milk supply.

Fatigue. The most common cause of inadequate milk supply is fatigue. Fatigue may be caused by lack of sleep because the infant demands considerable attention at night, but generally it is more subtle. The pressures of the rest of the family for meals or services or the self-inflicted demands of a job, career, or social commitments may be the cause. The mother must be placed on a medically mandated strict rest regimen that is respected by family and friends. In the first month, while lactation is being established, fatigue is devastating to milk production. The infant then becomes hungry more often, cries, and demands more frequent feeding; thus, the vicious circle is established. In later months of lactation, a mother becomes quickly aware of the impact of protracted fatigue on the nursing experience and usually will take steps to increase her rest.

Poor release of milk. Interference with the let-down reflex may cause a well-nourished lactating mother to fail to satisfy her infant. The collecting ducts may be full, but if the let-down or ejection reflex is not triggered, the process will be at a standstill. The infant becomes frustrated and pulls away crying or screaming. Interference with the ejection reflex is predominantly iatrogenic and rarely hormonal (see Fig. 8-18).

Smoking may interfere with the let-down reflex. Mothers should be discouraged from ever smoking in the same room with the infant because of the occurrence of early and frequent respiratory infections in infants of smokers. Smokers are less likely to breastfeed, and if they do choose to breastfeed, they tend to wean earlier because of insufficient milk. Trouble with milk production may be related to the nicotine itself. Extensive studies of smoking mothers have demonstrated a clear relationship between smoking and the amount of milk produced.[62] The infants of these mothers grow more slowly. Avoiding smoking for 2 hours before a feeding will improve the let-down reflex and minimize the amount of nicotine in the milk. Given the value of breastfeeding to the infant, especially in reducing the risk of sudden infant death syndrome (SIDS), it is important that smokers try to reduce the smoke exposure but still breastfeed (see Chapter 16).

Experimentally, *alcohol* has been shown to interfere with oxytocin release in laboratory animals, but the dosage used correlates with moderate to heavy drinking in humans. Studies following the offspring of women who drink heavily have shown some delay in gross motor activity at 1 year using the Bayley developmental scales.[79] Other studies have suggested that alcohol changes the flavor of the milk and that infants nurse less well at a feeding immediately after the mother has had a drink.[75,86] This is contrary to observations over the years in countries where wine and beer are common beverages and are considered galactagogues (see Chapter 11).

The clinician should consider the impact of smoking or alcohol use in the context of reviewing inadequate milk production.

Medications that the mother may be taking should be evaluated. Although L-dopa and ergot preparations are known to inhibit prolactin release, other medications less well identified may have the same effect (see Chapter 11).

The most common cause for the failure of the ejection reflex is *psychological inhibition*. In a few cases the cause of the psychological stress may be obvious, such as a husband or mother who openly disapproves of breastfeeding, but in most cases the nursing mother has already considered this possibility and reassures the physician that she is relaxed and calm. It will require carefully assessing the mother's history to "tease out" the source of stress. This is the time when a home visit by the nurse practitioner from the physician's office or an experienced public health nurse will be valuable. The nurse may observe what is overlooked by the mother: construction of a new building next door, incessant barking from the neighbor's dog, or marital discord. Home observation may lead to the key to the problem.

No obvious cause

Even though no obvious cause for failure to thrive is identified, the treatment may have to include establishing a positive attitude. Jelliffe and Jelliffe[66] have often referred to nursing as a "confidence game." It becomes necessary to instill confidence rather than fear in the mother. Threatening the mother with stopping breastfeeding and switching to formula does not instill confidence. The physician should prescribe a positive plan for number and length of feedings, suggest diet and rest for the mother, and set reachable goals for infant growth.

If the let-down reflex is the crux of the problem and simple adjustments have not changed the ejection quality, oxytocin as a nasal spray (Pitocin) can be prescribed (see Chapters 8 and 19). It is available only by prescription and should be used under the physician's guidance because of possible side effects in some women (e.g., headache, vasoconstriction), although it is not dangerous. Oxytocin nasal spray does not affect the milk or the infant. It is contraindicated only in pregnancy or hypersensitivity.

Seven mothers whose breastfed infants were contented but starving were given metoclopramide (or chlorpromazine in one) in various dosages.[51] Only one mother thought it was not helpful. The authors did not describe how effective appropriate supportive breastfeeding management was and when the medication was started or how long it was maintained. All the infants gained weight, and breastfeeding was continued for 2 to 12 months.

Other authors have reported the recovery from lactation failure by mothers taking metoclopramide (10 mg three times a day).[12] Gupta and Gupta[50] report a 67% success rate in those with no milk and 100% recovery in those with an inadequate supply.

The effect continued after the drug was discontinued. Such a medication is useful only when accompanied by appropriate instructions for proper breastfeeding and assistance in using a breast pump for additional stimulus to increase the supply of milk mechanically. A medication should be prescribed only when routine methods fail. Effect of the drug may dissipate if the infant is still unable to go to the breast. Domperidone (Motilium), a peripheral dopamine antagonist, has been reported to enhance milk production, although clinical experience in blinded controlled studies is absent. Available internationally but not in the United States, it has to be ordered by prescription. It is antidotally reported to enhance milk production with a dosage of 10 to 20 mg orally three to four times a day.[52]

Measurement of prolactin levels is readily available in most laboratories, but the appropriate clinical protocol has not been confirmed by controlled study. Given the information about baseline and response to stimuli (see Chapter 3), it would be advisable to obtain a baseline level, which should be above normal for the laboratory, and a second value after 10 minutes of breastfeeding. Using a heparin lock with venous line placed well before the baseline specimen is drawn and before feeding ensures the least disturbance to lactation. The intrafeeding value should show a significant increase over baseline (twice baseline).

A group of women diagnosed with lactational insufficiency by history were given thyrotropin-releasing hormone (TRH).[52] Four received 5 mg every 12 hours for 5 days. There was a consistent 50% increase in prolactin concentrations. Both milk production and let-down were increased. Nine women received 20 mg twice a day, and baseline prolactin was significantly elevated. The women all reported subjective and objective increases in breast engorgement and milk let-down, and all returned to full nursing. Two women were given 40 mg TRH daily for 5 days and developed clinical signs of thyrotoxicosis by the seventh day, which disappeared by the tenth day. The investigators[53] had previously given TRH to fully lactating women in a controlled study to demonstrate prolactin response, which did occur within 60 minutes. There was no change in the milk volume or quality in these fully lactating women and no side effects. When Hall and Kay[53] gave 200 μg TRH and followed prolactin and milk production for 6 hours, there were no dramatic changes in milk production, although the prolactin levels rose. There is no indication that the mothers received more than 1 day's dose.

The rare infant who does not respond to management adjustment may have a malabsorption or metabolic disease as yet undiagnosed that will not become overt until formula or cow milk is introduced. Infants with a strong family history of cystic fibrosis, milk allergy, or malabsorption should have a careful diagnostic workup before abandoning human milk, which may be the most physiologic feeding available for the infant. Neonatal metabolic screening tests should be repeated.

Dehydration, hypernatremia, or hypochloremia

A few cases of severe disease have been reported in the literature.[2,4,17,46,47,58,102] These infants have been hospitalized because of dehydration and evidence of more severe metabolic disturbance. They serve to illustrate the outcome if anticipatory care or palliative home management is unsuccessful. The mothers are usually but not always primiparas, new at breastfeeding and child rearing. When the record is reviewed, one often sees that the early danger signs were present at discharge from the hospital. The mother may have a history of difficult delivery or taking medication for pain that leads to a less vigorous baby and, secondarily, inadequate stimulus for lactation. Supplementary bottles of water or milk are initiated in the hospital instead of directing attention toward the lactation process.

As a precautionary measure, the physician should see all breastfeeding dyads promptly. At this visit, review of the weight, feeding history, number of wet diapers, stool pattern, and physical findings should alert the physician to impending difficulties. Observation of the infant at the breast should be part of the assessment. A problem in monitoring breastfed infants is the use of ultraabsorbent diapers, which makes it impossible to detect the number of voidings or volume of urine passed. No specimen can be wrung from the diaper for specific gravity or other analysis. It is recommended that parents of infants younger than 2 months not use ultraabsorbent diapers, especially when the infant is breastfed, until a better monitoring device is developed or until breastfeeding is well established. If, on the other hand, the patient is not seen in the office until there is significant dehydration, it is urgent that laboratory studies, including those for sodium, chloride, potassium, pH, blood urea nitrogen (BUN), and hematocrit (bilirubin when indicated), be obtained. An assessment of the degree of dehydration should be made based on skin and tissue turgor and tone and urinary findings.

When the breastfed infant has abnormal electrolyte levels, the physician should also obtain levels of sodium, chloride, and potassium from mother's milk, being certain to sample each breast separately. Collecting a few milliliters at the beginning and the end of the feeding and mixing the two samples from a single breast is a good technique. The infant may have occult loss of electrolytes, such as that seen in abnormal renal wasting or retention, cystic fibrosis, hyperaldosteronism, or pseudohyperaldosteronism. The simplest approach is to measure milk electrolytes and infant urine levels to rule out high milk sodium as a cause of the infant's hypernatremia.

In reported cases, infants with hypernatremic failure to thrive are no different at initial presentation from infants with normal sodium levels.[17,73] They may even have a negative neonatal history. At home they develop a poor suck, sleep for long intervals, cry infrequently, and feed infrequently. When observed at the breast, they may be labeled as having a sucking disorder. On examination, however, the lethargy, dehydration, and malnutrition are obvious to the skilled clinician. In the extreme, the infant may have cardiovascular collapse with hypothermia and hypoglycemia. Elevated serum BUN, creatinine, and hematocrit and urinary specific gravity confirm the diagnosis. Hypernatremia has been observed in approximately half the reported cases of severe dehydration in breastfed infants.[108,110] Although milk

sodium levels were not reported in all cases, several cases of elevated milk sodium are reported. Sodium, chloride, and lactose are the prime constituents that control the osmolarity of the milk. Because the sodium, chloride, and lactose have a reciprocal relationship, inadequate lactose production ultimately results in elevated sodium levels.

Elevated sodium in the milk may be a cause or an effect of insufficient milk. When the breast is inadequately stimulated, it begins to involute and produces "weaning milk," which is high in sodium. Milk pumped from nonlactators in the postpartum period has high sodium. Maternal sodium intake excesses do not result in elevated sodium levels in the milk, however.[32] Sodium enters the milk by a controlled mechanism independent of maternal levels in normal women. Milk sodium is much lower than serum sodium, whereas milk potassium is much higher than serum levels.

Hypernatremic dehydration is an emergency that requires hospitalization.[72,73] The mother should room-in if at all possible. Most pediatric units provide this option. It is preferable to maintain lactation in most cases. The treatment of the illness after the dehydration has been treated with intravenous (IV) fluids depends on the etiology of the hypernatremia. The sodium of the infant's serum and mother's milk should be followed until normal. Increasing maternal milk output with appropriate lactation counseling, including mechanical pumping between feedings to increase volume, usually normalizes the sodium. The oral feedings for the infant should be limited to breastfeeding once milk sodium is normal while the IV fluids are tapered. To provide increased caloric resources to the infant and an appropriate sodium load, the Lact-Aid supplementer (see Chapter 19 and Appendix F) may also be used to stimulate the breast and to avoid bottle feeding and inadequate intake until the breast increases production.

Chloride deficiency has received attention because of a highly publicized formula-manufacturing error. This syndrome is characterized by failure to thrive with anorexia, hypochloremia, and hypokalemic metabolic alkalosis. Chloride deficiency syndrome has also been reported in an infant whose mother had only 2 mEq/L chloride in her milk (normal 8 mEq/L).[58] The mother had successfully nourished her previous five infants. The infant had done well until 3 months of age and then had gradually slipped below the third percentile for weight at 6 months. The infant was severely dehydrated and hypotonic with plasma sodium of 123 mEq/L, chloride of 72 mEq/L, potassium of 2.9 mEq/L, and blood pH of 7.61. There were no abnormal urinary losses. When the breastfeeding infant has clinical dehydration, it is important to check not only the sodium but also the chloride content of the infant's serum and urine and the mother's milk.

Human infants younger than 3 weeks of age do not respond to inappropriate solutions by not suckling. This finding is also observed in studies in other species in which pups continue to suck when the solution is unphysiologic.[10] A natural experiment occurred in a newborn nursery in the 1960s, when six infants died of hypernatremia after receiving many feedings of formula made from salt rather than sugar.[37] The infants who were less than 1 week old did not reject the feedings.

Lactation failure

Occasionally, failure to thrive is actually caused by lactation failure. Historically, sudden complete cessation of lactation was described in the late 1800s after horse-drawn carriage accidents and other great trauma. Advocates of breastfeeding have tended to dismiss this as a possibility and struggle frantically to reverse the situation. Some women who cannot make milk have primary hypoprolactinemia, and others have secondary hypoprolactinemia, as in Sheehan's syndrome (see Chapter 16). Because it is now possible to identify these women by obtaining prolactin levels that confirm the diagnosis,[117] when reasonable efforts at stimulation are ineffective and the mother is unable to do without the Lact-Aid providing almost a full feeding volume, evaluation of the mother is appropriate. Some mothers prefer to discontinue efforts to breastfeed before they have been completely stripped of their egos by total failure.

If one explores the animal literature, one finds no similar situations in other species. Lactation failure in nursing animals is rare—it is not a trait that is transmitted from generation to generation, because the offspring do not survive. Interferences with milk ejection can be identified and treated in some mammals. A syndrome in sows involves agalactia associated with mastitis and metritis.[20] Mammalian lactation failure is attributed to nutritional, pharmacologic, and "emotional stress" causes in animals. Aside from gross dietary deficiency, there is depression or inhibition of the anterior pituitary gland, which is responsible for synthesis in the alveolar cells, and inhibition of transport and discharge of synthesized products from alveolar cells to the lumen. Certain plant alkaloids have been noted in other species to inhibit lactation. Ergot derivatives are best known, but colchicine, vincristine, and vinblastine are also causative. Some plant lectins such as concanavalin interfere with transport and discharge phases of milk production.

Understanding lactation failure is increasing among clinicians as the diagnostic resources expand.[117] Some herbs may inadvertently suppress lactation. A thorough history of herbal use is always appropriate in any clinical assessment.

MATERNAL AND INFANT OBESITY AND BREASTFEEDING

It is generally recognized that women who breastfeed return to their prepregnancy weight more quickly and in greater numbers than do bottle feeding mothers.[113] In studies in rats, pregnancy without subsequent lactation results in increased adipose tissue stores and increased fat cell numbers. Studies in humans date back to 1949 and 1952 but do not include relevant variables or the duration and degree of lactation.[89]

When lactation performance was examined, Hilson and associates[59] reported that overweight or obese women had less success initiating breastfeeding than their normal-weight counterparts. The rates of discontinuance of exclusive breastfeeding in overweight and obese women were also higher, even when socioeconomic status and maternal education were controlled. The population was predominantly white. When the study was conducted on a minority population in Rochester, New York, the Hispanic obese women were poor lactators but black women's lactation was not affected by obesity.[70] The authors conclude that excessive fatness in the reproductive period may inhibit lactational performance.

Discussion of the impact of adiposity is rarely undertaken without including a discussion of cholesterol levels. Obesity and atherosclerosis in developed societies constitute a major public health issue. Does breastfeeding in infancy protect against obesity and atherosclerosis in adult life? This remains an open question. Energy requirements for infants receiving formula have been overestimated.[14] Breastfed infants require and receive 110 kcal/kg/day at 1 month and 70 kcal/kg/day at 4 months. The low energy intakes are not caused by limitations in maternal milk production as previously assumed but represent physiologically regulated intakes. Breastfed infants deposit less fat than formula fed infants despite the fact that the two diets appear similar on paper. Although the breastfed infant appears protected against obesity in infancy, the effect appeared to be lost after 3 years of age according to Hamosh.[55]

A prospective cohort study of 462 healthy full-term infants observed from birth to 12 months was done by Kramer and associates.[69] Their goal was to overcome methodologic defects in previous studies of the etiologic determinants of childhood obesity that failed to control for confounding factors. At 6 and 12 months, measurements of height, weight, body mass index (BMI, weight/height^2), and skinfold were taken and correlated with duration of breastfeeding, introduction of solids, and parental heights and weights. Significant determinants of BMI were birth weight, duration of breastfeeding, and introduction of solid foods. Breastfeeding and delayed introduction of solid foods offered some protective effect against obesity at 1 year in this study.

The effect of breastfeeding on plasma cholesterol and weight in young adults was studied longitudinally by Marmot and associates[84] in a sample of people born in 1946. The infant-feeding history was obtained. At age 32, women who had been breastfed had significantly lower mean plasma cholesterol than women who had been bottle fed. The difference for men was smaller, and the breastfed male had higher mean weight and skinfold thickness (Fig. 12-3). Multiple studies, both short- and long-range, with small populations and conflicting results have been reported in humans, although animal studies strongly suggest that species-specific milk reduces the risk of obesity and elevated cholesterol.

McGill[85] reviewed dietary cholesterol effects on serum cholesterol and atherosclerosis in humans, as did the report of the Conference on Blood Lipids in Children: Optimal Levels for Early Prevention of Coronary Artery Disease.[121] Indices of fatness and serum cholesterol at age 8 years in relation to feeding and growth during early infancy were reported by Fomon and associates[40] from their detailed longitudinal nutrition project involving 469 children born between 1966 and 1971. In infancy the formula fed children had more rapid gains in height and weight, which were attributed to greater food intake. At age 8, there were no differences in indices of fatness related to mode of feeding during infancy and no significant differences in serum cholesterol concentrations. Fomon and associates[40] suggested that childhood and adolescence are too early to detect possible beneficial effects of breastfeeding on cholesterol homeostasis in later life in the human.

Serum cholesterol may be too insensitive a quantitation to detect early changes and classify lipoprotein classes, and apoprotein concentrations may be necessary.[55] The effects of breastfeeding versus formula feeding are not attributable to differences in cholesterol intake. According to Mott and associates,[94] varying the cholesterol content of infant formulas, which normally contain no cholesterol, has not reduced long-lasting differences in serum cholesterol or lipoprotein concentrations or in cholesterol metabolism. Lack of control of genetic differences and sampling under uncontrolled dietary conditions have limited the interpretation of

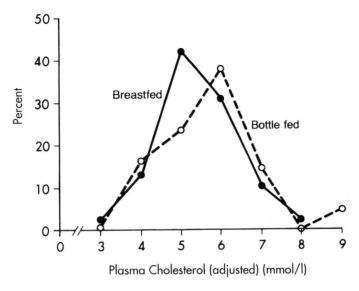

Figure 12-3.   Plasma cholesterol in adults according to type of infant feeding. (From Marmot MG, Page CM, Atkins E, et al: Effect of breastfeeding on plasma cholesterol and weight in young adults. J Epidemiol Community Health 34:164, 1980.)

many human studies. Mott and associates[92,93] performed a long-term study with 83 baboons to determine the effects of infant diet (breastfeeding versus formula feeding and the level of cholesterol in the formula). The type of dietary fat and level of dietary cholesterol as well as gender and heredity were reviewed. The progeny of 6 sires and 83 dams were randomly assigned to diet groups of breastfeeding or formula with 2, 30, or 60 mg/dL, respectively, of cholesterol. The 30 mg/dL milk resembled baboon milk. They were weaned to controlled juvenile diets. The differences in cholesterol content of the formula did not lead to later differences in serum cholesterol, lipoprotein concentrations, or cholesterol metabolism. Breastfeeding (species-specific milk), however, affected the subsequent cholesterol metabolism, with absorption of a higher percentage of cholesterol and lower cholesterol production rates as juveniles. The baboons were bred for high or low serum cholesterol concentrations, and in both groups the breastfed animals had higher very-low-density lipoprotein (VLDL) and low-density lipoprotein (LDL) cholesterol levels from 6 months

to 3 years than formula fed animals and higher serum cholesterol from 6 months to 2 years (Fig. 12-4). Baboons are vegetarian, however, and the weaning diet was not, which may have altered the results.

Overfeeding was a variable in a study of preweaning food intake influences on the adiposity of young adult baboons reported by Lewis and associates.[76] Overfeeding did not have a major effect on the fat cell number. Overfed male baboons had a greater fat mass in 4 of 10 fat depots at necropsy at age 5. Overfed female baboons had significantly greater fat depot mass in general primarily because of fat cell hypertrophy. Underfeeding in the preweaning period did not affect body weight or adipose mass in either gender in the juveniles.

In guinea pigs, stimulation of cholesterol catabolism by feeding cholestiramine rather than cholesterol after birth can influence the response to dietary cholesterol in the adult.[77] The efficient handling of dietary cholesterol in the cholestiramine-fed guinea pigs is directly associated with

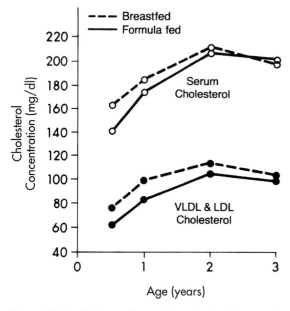

Figure 12-4. Cholesterol, very low density lipoprotein (VLDL), and low-density lipoprotein (LDL) in baboons: Breastfed vs. formula fed. Open circle, Serum cholesterol; closed circle, VLDL plus LDL cholesterol; solid line, formula fed; dashed line, breastfed. (From Mott GE: Deferred effects of breastfeeding versus formula feeding on serum lipoprotein concentration and cholesterol metabolism in baboons. In Report of 91st Ross Conference on Pediatric Research: The Breastfed Infant: A Model Performance. Columbus, Ohio, Ross Laboratories, 1986.)

significantly higher levels of cholesterol 17α-hydroxylase as sensitive to high dietary cholesterol during lactation.[58] Mott[93] suggests that the long-term effects of breastfeeding on cholesterol metabolism are not likely to result from the differences in neonatal cholesterol intake but rather from other components of breast milk, such as fatty acid composition, immunoglobulins, and hormones that might affect cholesterol metabolism.[93]

The definition of obesity should be based on the percentage of body weight accounted for by fat. Fomon[38] suggested that a clinical definition that circumvents clinical impressions would be useful and suggested that "values greater than +2 standard deviation value for triceps and subscapu-lar skin-fold thickness be considered evidence of obesity" (Table 12-6).

A more practical measure of obesity is body mass index (BMI).[113] Using the chart (Fig. 12-5), the BMI can be determined by plotting for an individual adult the point where the height and the weight intersect. That is the BMI. It can be mathematically calculated as follows:

$$\frac{\text{weight (kg)}}{\text{height (m)}^2} = \text{BMI (metric)}$$

$$\frac{\text{weight (lb)}}{\text{height (in)}^2} = \text{BMI (English)}$$

A normal BMI is 19.8 to 26, overweight is 26.1 to 29.0, obese is over 29, and underweight is 19.8 and under. This measurement is a more useful and universal index of obesity (Table 12-7).

The infant with a heavy bone structure and musculature but without excessive fat may appear to be obese based on the categories in Table 12-6. Infants who are overfed also grow in height and may be in an advanced percentile for height. The infant who is born with a weight in the 80th percentile (weight for age) and remains there may not be obese, but the infant who is born with a weight in the 50th percentile and crosses percentiles over time to the 80th percentile may be at risk for long-term obesity. Therefore, some discretion is advised when using percentiles for determining obesity.

Restraint of growth and development during critical periods of fetal life and infancy has an important effect on the development of cardiovascular disease, as reported by Barker[6] in a long-range study of 6500 men born between 1911 and 1930 in England. Ninety-five percent of the men were breastfed, 20% of these for more than a year. Barker notes the significance of fetal growth and growth in the first year of life being unrelated to social class and cardiovascular disease in adult life when most infants had the advantage of breastfeeding.

Serum cholesterol levels (total and LDL) at ages 60 and 70 were higher in those men who had been bottle fed or exclusively breastfed beyond 1 year. These data and other studies were reviewed by Fall,[33] who also concludes that adult serum choles-

TABLE 12-6   **Tentative definition of infant obesity**

Age (mo)	Males		Females	
	Length (cm) less than	Weight (kg) more than	Length (cm) less than	Weight (kg) more than
1	51.8	4.2	51.5	4.0
	53.0	4.5	52.2	4.3
	54.2	4.7	53.5	4.6
	55.2	5.1	54.6	4.8
3	58.0	6.0	57.1	5.6
	59.2	6.4	58.0	5.9
	60.2	6.9	59.2	6.2
	61.5	7.3	60.5	6.6
6	65.6	7.7	63.3	7.5
	66.5	8.2	65.2	8.0
	67.8	9.0	66.3	8.4
	69.2	9.6	67.8	8.9
9	70.0	9.1	68.2	8.9
	70.9	9.7	69.5	9.4
	72.3	10.7	71.1	9.9
	73.6	11.2	73.1	10.4
12	73.6	10.2	72.5	9.9
	74.7	10.9	73.2	10.5
	76.4	11.6	75.1	11.1
	78.0	12.5	76.9	11.6
18	80.0	11.6	78.7	11.1
	81.7	12.6	80.2	11.8
	83.2	13.3	82.0	12.7
	85.3	14.4	84.2	13.2
24	85.0	12.8	84.2	12.3
	87.3	13.9	85.8	13.1
	88.8	14.5	87.5	14.2
	90.9	16.0	90.3	14.9
36	93.4	14.8	92.1	14.3
	95.3	15.7	94.2	15.3
	97.3	16.8	96.2	17.0
	100.6	18.6	99.0	17.7

At each age, values for length for each gender are the 10th, 25th, 50th, and 75th percentiles, and values for weight are the 50th, 75th, and 90th percentiles, with the mean +2 standard deviations. From Fomon SJ: Infant Nutrition. 2nd ed. Philadelphia, WB Saunders, 1974.

terol concentrations and death rates from ischemic heart disease are related to method of infant feeding and age at weaning. Exclusive breastfeeding (i.e., no weaning foods or solids until the infant is older than 1 year) is not recommended.

In a 7-year longitudinal study of children at the Slovak Academy of Sciences, the obesity rates in children breastfed for less than 3 months were substantially higher than those in children who had been breastfed longer.[112] Total serum cholesterol increased with age at weaning. The atherogenic index in 6-year-old children was best in those who were breastfed more than 1 month but not more than 3 months. The authors also report breastfeeding advantages for respiratory disease, gastrointestinal disease, and thyroid levels.[112]

In a study of adiposity in 4-year-old Anglo- and Mexican-Americans, genetic and environmental factors other than infant feeding practices had the greater influence.[127] Before age 4, breastfeeding and delayed introduction of solids to 6 months appeared to be associated with normal lean body mass and skinfold thickness.

No benefits are derived from infantile obesity. The concern for obesity rests with the long-range outcome as an obese adult. The problem is that obesity in infancy predisposes the child to immobility and inactivity; thus, an obese infant lags on the developmental curve or at least has delayed gross motor skills. The question of whether obesity in infancy predisposes the child to obesity in adult life has not been resolved satisfactorily. Retrospective studies support both sides of the question. A prospective study of 403 newborns in Canada was done measuring weight, length, and subcutaneous fat, but an infant was considered "breastfed" if the infant received any breastfeeding for 2 months and early solids.[68] Food feeding was defined as beginning solids by 2 months of age. Kramer[68] believed the 18-month follow-up refuted the hypothesis of bottle fed obesity. Most students of this subject would question the population definitions. A study of adolescents retrospectively tested the question of whether breastfeeding and delayed introduction of solids protect against subsequent obesity. Yeung and associates[125]

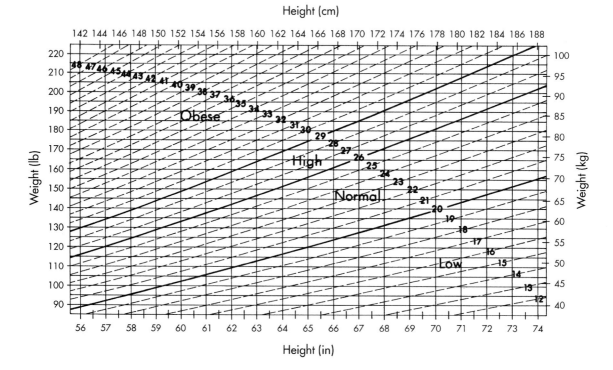

Figure 12-5. Chart for estimating body mass index (BMI) category and BMI. To find BMI category (e.g., obese), find point where woman's height and weight intersect. To estimate BMI, read bold number on the dashed line that is closest to the point. (From Subcommittee on Nutrition during Lactation, Committee on Nutritional Status during Pregnancy and Lactation: Nutrition during Pregnancy and Lactation: An Implementation Guide. Washington, DC, National Academy Press, 1992.)

TABLE 12-7 Weight classification according to body mass index (BMI)

Relative weight classification	Prepregnant BMI
Underweight	<19.8
Normal	19.8–26.0
Overweight	26.1–29.0
Obese	>29.0

Nutrition during Pregnancy and Lactation: An Implementation Guide. Washington, DC, National Academy Press, 1992.

concluded that breastfeeding does, but delayed solids alone do not protect against obesity.

Breastfeeding is related to slower growth during the first 12 months of life. Breastfed infants also consume less protein in infancy. In a large study of 5- and 6-year-old children, a consistent, protective, and dose-dependent effect of breastfeeding on overweight and obesity was seen. Conversely, rapid growth during the first year of life is associated with increased BMI at the age of 6 years in both genders. In boys, high intake of protein in infancy could also contribute to childhood obesity.[49]

The growing epidemic of childhood obesity has become a major public health problem with both short- and long-term consequences, not the least of which is the increase in adolescent type 2 diabetes. A large number of studies have been carried out, and meta-analysis has wrestled with the merits of the dozens of these historical studies. There is a growing consistency of evidence supporting the conclusion that being breastfed lowers the risk of excess weight in childhood and may well lower the risk of excess weight in later life perhaps because it affects long-term energy metabolism.[44] A study of 32,200 Scottish children showed that the prevalence of obesity was significantly lower in breastfed children even after adjusting for socioeconomic status, birth weight, and gender. The conclusion was that breastfeeding is associated with a reduction in the risk of childhood obesity. Similar results were reported in a study of over 15,000 adolescents as part of the Growing Up Today Study in the United States.[45] Those who had been breastfed had a lower risk of being overweight during childhood and adolescence. More than 1000 preadolescent children followed in Germany also showed significantly decreased prevalence of being overweight.[78] On reviewing 11 studies of at least 100 participants, Dewey[23] found that 8 showed a lower risk of being overweight in children who had been breastfed. The three studies that did not make that conclusion lacked information on exclusivity and duration. Studies that include children "ever breastfed" dilute the impact of significant breastfeeding. Dewey suggests the effect may be due to learned self-regulation of energy intake, metabolic programming in early life, and residual confounding by parental attributes.

Butte[13] reviewed a number of studies published since 1945, many of which were retrospective, small, and using no definitions of breastfeeding. Many were inconclusive. Use of "ever breastfed" subjects contributed to the inconclusive results.

The preponderance of large studies have shown a clear impact on reduced risk of obesity in childhood and adolescence in breastfed infants, probably because large numbers reduce the impact of partial breastfeeding and short duration. There are no studies that demonstrate a null hypothesis.

Breastfed infants are rarely obese. The usual cause of obesity in these infants is the early addition of solids. Solids often provide excessive kilocalories. The obese breastfed infant should have the diet and feeding pattern scrutinized. If necessary, some restriction of prolonged feeding should be suggested. In the normal course of a breastfeeding, the fat content of the milk increases over the duration of the feeding and satisfies the infant after 10 to 15 minutes of nursing.

Because of general agreement that, once established, childhood obesity often becomes chronic and resistant to treatment,[84] it is appropriate to focus attention on prevention and early intervention. The physician can counsel a family whose breastfed infant meets the criterion for obesity (above the 85th percentile for weight for length). The routine use of skinfold measurements as part of well-baby care will increase the ability to diagnose obesity because it distinguishes the constitutionally larger body frame from the fat infant.

Recommendations that will help taper unusual weight gain include the following:

1. Limit excessive feedings that are being provided on the mistaken belief that all the infant's needs are nutritional.
2. Encourage nonnutritive cuddling. If feeding is a response to all distress signals, the infant may expect feeding inappropriately, causing dissociation between appetite and energy need.
3. Use exclusive breastfeeding, that is, no solids for 6 months.
4. Increase activity and energy utilization by encouraging movement rather than containing or restricting the infant in carriers or swaddlings. For the older infant, encourage play activity and crawling and minimize sitting.
5. If there is persistent growth excess, it is appropriate to obtain a sample of maternal milk to rule out the rare case of hyperlipidemia with a "creamatocrit" (see Chapter 21).

REFERENCES

1. Ahn CH, MacLean WC: Growth of the exclusively breast-fed infant. Am J Clin Nutr 33:183, 1980.
2. Anand SK, Sandborg C, Robinson RG, et al: Neonatal hypernatremia associated with elevated sodium concentration of breast milk. J Pediatr 96:66, 1980.
3. Armstrong J, Reilly JJ, Child Health Information Team: Breastfeeding and lowering the risk of childhood obesity. Lancet 359:2003, 2002.
4. Asnes RS, Wisotsky DH, Migel PF, et al: The dietary chloride deficiency syndrome occurring in a breastfed infant. J Pediatr 100:923, 1982.
5. Axelsson I, Borulf S, Righard L, et al: Protein and energy intake during weaning. I. Effects on growth. Acta Paediatr Scand 76:321, 1987.
6. Barker DJP: Symposium on "Impact of diet on critical events in development": The effect of nutrition of the fetus and neonate on cardiovascular disease in adult life. Proc Nutr Soc 51:135, 1992.
7. Barness LA: Nutrition for healthy neonates. In Gracy M, Falkner F (eds): Nutritional Needs and Assessment of Normal Growth. New York, Vevey/Raven, 1985.
8. Behrman RE, Driscoll JM Jr, Seeds AE (eds): Neonatal-Perinatal Medicine: Diseases of the Fetus and Infant, 2nd ed. St. Louis, Mosby, 1977.
9. Birch E, Birch D, Hoffman D, et al: Breastfeeding and optimal visual development. J Pediatr Ophthalmol Strabismus 30:33, 1993.
10. Blass EM, Teicher MH: Suckling. Science 210:15, 1980.
11. Brown KH, Robertson AD, Akhtar NA: Lactational capacity of marginally nourished mothers: Infants' milk nutrient consumption and patterns of growth. Pediatrics 78:920, 1986.
12. Budd SC, Erdman SH, Long DM, et al: Improved lactation with metoclopramide. Clin Pediatr 32:53, 1993.
13. Butte NF: The role of breastfeeding in obesity. Pediatr Clin North Am 48:189, 2001.
14. Butte NF, Garza C, Smith EO, et al: Human milk intake and growth in exclusively breastfed infants. J Pediatr 104:187, 1984.
15. Castillo-Duran C, Rodriguez A, Venegas G, et al: Zinc supplementation and growth of infants born small for gestational age. J Pediatr 127:206, 1995.
16. Caufield LE, Bentley ME, Ahmed S: Is prolonged breastfeeding associated with malnutrition? Evidence from nineteen demographic and health surveys. Int J Epidemiol 25:693, 1996.
17. Clarke TA, Markarian M, Griswold W, et al: Hypernatremic dehydration resulting from inadequate breastfeeding. Pediatrics 63:931, 1979.
18. Cohen RJ, Brown KH, Canahuah J, et al: Effects of age of introduction of complementary foods on infant breast milk intake, total energy intake, and growth: A randomised intervention study in Honduras. Lancet 343:288, 1994.
19. Committee on Dietary Allowances, Food and Nutrition Board, National Research Council: Recommended Dietary Allowances. Washington, DC, National Academy of Sciences, 1989.
20. Cowie AT, Forsyth IA, Hart IC: Hormonal control of lactation. In Monographs on Endocrinology. Heidelberg, Springer Verlag, 1980.
21. Czajka-Narins DM, Jung E: Physical growth of breastfed and formula fed infants from birth to age two years. Nutr Res 6:753, 1986.
22. De Andraca I, Uauy R: Breastfeeding for optimal mental development. In Simopoulos AP, Dutra DC, Olivena JE, et al (eds): Behavioral and Metabolic Aspects of Breastfeeding. Basel, Karger, 1995.
23. Dewey KG: Is breastfeeding protective against child obesity? J Hum Lact 19:9, 2003.
24. Dewey KG, Cohen RJ, Rivera LL, et al: Do exclusively breast-fed infants require extra protein? Pediatr Res 39:303, 1996.
25. Dewey KG, Heinig MJ, Nommsen LA, et al: Growth of breastfed and formula fed infants from 0 to 18 months: The DARLING study. Pediatrics 89:1035, 1992.
26. Dewey KG, Heinig MJ, Nommsen LA, et al: Breastfed infants are leaner than formula fed infants at one year of age: The DARLING study. Am J Clin Nutr 57:140, 1993.
27. Dewey KG, Heinig MJ, Nommsen LA, et al: Adequacy of energy intake among breastfed infants in the DARLING study: Relationships to growth velocity, morbidity, and activity levels. J Pediatr 119:538, 1991.
28. Dewey KG, Lönnerdal B: Infant self-regulation of breast milk intake. Acta Paediatr Scand 75:893, 1986.
29. Dewey KG, Peerson JM, Brown KH, et al: Growth of breast-fed infants deviates from current reference data: A pooled analysis of US, Canadian, and European data sets. Pediatrics 96:495, 1995.
30. Dewey KG, Peerson JM, Heinig MJ, et al: Growth patterns of breastfed infants in affluent (US) and poor (Peru) communities: Implications for timing of complementary feeding. Am J Clin Nutr 56:1012, 1992.
31. Duncan B, Schafer C, Sibley B, et al: Reduced growth velocity in exclusively breast-fed infants. Am J Dis Child 138:309, 1984.
32. Ereman RR, Lönnerdal B, Dewey KG: Maternal sodium intake does not affect postprandial sodium concentrations in human milk. J Nutr 117:1154, 1987.
33. Fall C: Nutrition in early life and later outcome. Eur J Clin Nutr 46(suppl 4):57, 1992.
34. Fawzi WW, Forman MR, Levy A, et al: Maternal anthropometry and infant feeding practices in Israel in relation to growth in infancy: The North African Infant Feeding Study. Am J Clin Nutr 65:1731, 1997.

35. Fergusson DM, Beautrais AL, Silva PA: Breastfeeding and cognitive development in the first seven years of life. Soc Sci Med 16:1705, 1982.

36. Fergusson DM, Horwood LJ, Shannon FT: Breastfeeding and subsequent social adjustment in six- to eight-year-old children. J Child Psychol Psychiatry 28:379, 1987.

37. Finberg L, Kiley J, Luttrell CN: Mass accidental salt poisoning in infancy: A study of a hospital disaster. JAMA 184:187, 1963.

38. Fomon SJ: Infant Nutrition, 2nd ed. Philadelphia, WB Saunders, 1974.

39. Fomon SJ, Filer LJ Jr, Thomas LN, et al: Growth and serum chemical values of normal breast fed infants. Acta Paediatr Scand Suppl 273:1, 1978.

40. Fomon SJ, Rogers RR, Ziegler EE, et al: Indices of fatness and serum cholesterol at age eight years in relation to feeding and growth during early infancy. Pediatr Res 18:1233, 1984.

41. Forman MR, Lewando-Hundt G, Graubard BI, et al: Factors influencing milk insufficiency and its long term health effects: The Bedouin Infant Feeding Study. Int J Epidemiol 21:53, 1992.

42. Frank DA, Silva M, Needleman R: Failure to thrive: Mystery, myth and method. Contemp Pediatr 10:114, 1993.

43. Garza C, Frongillo E, Dewey KG: Implications of growth patterns of breastfed infants for growth references. Acta Paediatr Suppl 402:4, 1994.

44. Gillman M: Breastfeeding and obesity. J Pediatr 141:749, 2002.

45. Gilliman MW, Rifas-Shiman SI, Camargo CA, et al: Risk of overweight among adolescents who were breastfeeding as infants. JAMA 285:2461, 2001.

46. Gilmore HE, Rowland TW: Critical malnutrition in breastfed infants. Am J Dis Child 132:885, 1978.

47. Ghishan FK, Roloff JS: Malnutrition and hypernatremic dehydration in two breast-fed infants. Clin Pediatr 22:592, 1983.

48. Grummer-Strawn LM: Does prolonged breastfeeding impair child growth? A critical review. Pediatrics 91:766, 1993.

49. Gunnarsdottir I, Thorsdottir I: Relationship between growth and feeding in infancy and body mass index at the age of 6 years. Int J Obesity 27:1523, 2003.

50. Gupta AP, Gupta PK: Metoclopramide as a lactagogue. Clin Pediatr 24:269, 1985.

51. Habbick BF, Gerrard JW: Failure to thrive in the contented breastfed baby. Can Med Assoc J 131:765, 1984.

52. Hale TW: Medications and Mothers' Milk, 10th ed. Amarillo, TX, Pharmasoft Publications, 2002.

53. Hall DMB, Kay G: Effect of thyrotrophin-releasing factor on lactation. Br Med J 1:777, 1977.

54. Hamill PVV, Drizd TA, Johnson CL, et al: Growth curves for children: Birth to 18 years. U.S. National Center for Health Statistics, Series 11, No. 165. Hyattsville, MD, U.S. Department of Health, Education and Welfare, 1977.

55. Hamosh M: Does infant nutrition affect adiposity and cholesterol levels in the adult? J Pediatr Gastroenterol Nutr 7:10, 1988.

56. Hartmann PE, Regan MD, Ramsav DT, et al: Physiology of lactation in preterm mothers: Initiation and maintenance. Pediatr Ann 32:351, 2003.

57. Heinig MJ, Nommsen LA, Peerson JM, et al: Energy and protein intakes of breastfed and formula fed infants during the first year of life and their association with growth velocity: The DARLING study. Am J Clin Nutr 58:152, 1993.

58. Hill ID, Bowie MD: Chloride deficiency syndrome due to chloride-deficient breast milk. Arch Dis Child 58:224, 1983.

59. Hilson JA, Rasmussen KM, Kjolhede CL: Maternal obesity and breast-feeding success in a rural population of white women. Am J Clin Nutr 66(6):1371, 1997.

60. Hitchcock NE, Gracey M, Owles EN: Growth of the healthy breast-fed infants in the first six months. Lancet 2:64, 1981.

61. Hoefer C, Hardy MC: Later development of breast-fed and artificially fed infants. JAMA 92:615, 1929.

62. Hopkinson JM, Schanler RJ, Fraley JK, et al: Milk production by mothers of premature infants: Influence of cigarette smoking. Pediatrics 90:934, 1992.

63. Horwood LJ, Fergusson DM: Breastfeeding and later cognitive and academic outcomes. Pediatrics 101:e9, 1998 (electronic article).

64. Jacobson SW, Jacobson JL: Breastfeeding and intelligence. Lancet 339:926, 1992.

65. Jakobsen MS, Sodemann M, Molbak K, et al: Reason for termination of breastfeeding and the length of breastfeeding. Int J Epidemiol 25:115, 1996.

66. Jelliffe DB, Jelliffe EFP: Human Milk in the Modern World. Oxford, Oxford University Press, 1978.

67. Juez G, Diaz S, Casado ME, et al: Growth pattern of selected urban Chilean infants during exclusive breastfeeding. Am J Clin Nutr 38:462, 1983.

68. Kramer MS: Do breast-feeding and delayed introduction of solid foods protect against subsequent obesity? J Pediatr 98:883, 1981.

69. Kramer MS, Barr RG, Leduc DG, et al: Determinants of weight and adiposity in the first year of life. J Pediatr 106:10, 1985.

70. Kugyelka JG, Rasmussen KM, Frongillo EA: Maternal obesity and breastfeeding success among black and Hispanic women. J Nutr 134:1746, 2004.

71. Lampl M, Veldhuis JD, Johnson ML: Saltation and stasis: A model of human growth. Science 258:801, 1992.

72. Lawrence RA: Successful breastfeeding. Am J Dis Child 135:595, 1981.

73. Lawrence RA: Infant nutrition. Pediatr Rev 5:133, 1983.

74. Lawrence R: Maternal factors in lactation failure. In Hamosh M, Goldman AS (eds): Human Lactation. II. Maternal and Environmental Factors. New York, Plenum, 1986.

75. Lawton ME: Alcohol in breast milk. Aust NZ J Obstet Gynaecol 25:71, 1985.

76. Lewis DS, Bertrand HA, McMahan CA, et al: Preweaning food intake influences the adiposity of young adult baboons. J Clin Invest 78:899, 1986.

77. Li JR, Bale LK, Kottke BA: Effect of neonatal modulation of cholesterol homeostasis on subsequent response to cholesterol challenge in adult guinea pig. J Clin Invest 65:1060, 1980.

78. Liese AD, Hirsch T, von Mutius E, et al: Inverse association of overweight and breastfeeding in 9 to 10 year old children in Germany. J Hum Lact 25:1644, 2001.

79. Little RE, Anderson KW, Ervin CH, et al: Maternal alcohol use during breastfeeding and infant mental and motor development at one year. N Engl J Med 321:425, 1989.

80. Lucas A, Fewtrell MS, Davies PSW, et al: Breastfeeding and catch-up growth in infants born small for gestational age. Acta Paediatr 86:564, 1997.

81. Lucas A, Morley R, Cole TJ, et al: Early diet in premature babies and developmental status at 18 months. Lancet 335:1477, 1990.

82. Lucas A, Morley R, Cole TJ, et al: Breast milk and subsequent intelligence quotient in children born premature. Lancet 339:261, 1992.

83. Lukefahr JL: Underlying illness associated with failure to thrive in breastfed infants. Clin Pediatr 29:468, 1990.

84. Marmot MG, Page CM, Atkins E, et al: Effect of breastfeeding on plasma cholesterol and weight in young adults. J Epidemiol Community Health 34:164, 1980.

85. McGill HC Jr: The relationship of dietary cholesterol to serum cholesterol concentration and to atherosclerosis in man. Am J Clin Nutr 32:2664, 1979.

86. Mennella JA, Beauchamp GK: The transfer of alcohol to human milk. N Engl J Med 325:981, 1991.

87. Michaelson KF: Nutrition and growth during infancy: The Copenhagen Cohort Study. Acta Paediatr 86(suppl 420):1, 1997.

88. Michaelson KF, Larsen PS, Thomsen BL, et al: The Copenhagen Cohort Study on Infant Nutrition and Growth: Breast-milk intake, human milk macronutrient content, and influencing factors. Am J Clin Nutr 59:600, 1994.

89. Moore BJ, Brasel JA: One cycle of reproduction consisting of pregnancy, lactation or no lactation, and recovery: Effects on fat pad cellularity in ad libitum-fed and food-restricted rats. J Nutr 114:1560, 1984.

90. Morley R, Cole TJ, Powell R, et al: Mother's choice to provide breast milk and developmental outcome. Arch Dis Child 63:1382, 1988.

91. Motil KJ, Sheng H-P, Montandon CM, et al: Case report: Failure to thrive in a breast-fed infant is associated with maternal dietary protein and energy restriction. J Am Coll Nutr 13:203, 1994.

92. Motil KJ, Sheng H-P, Montandon CM, et al: Human milk protein does not limit growth of breast-fed infants. J Pediatr Gastrenterol Nutr 24:10, 1997.

93. Mott GE: Deferred effects of breastfeeding versus formula feeding on serum lipoprotein concentration and cholesterol metabolism in baboons. In Report of the 91st Ross Conference on Pediatric Research: The Breastfed Infant: A Model Performance. Columbus, Ohio, Ross Laboratories, 1986.

94. Mott GE, Jackson EM, McMahan CA, et al: Cholesterol metabolism in juvenile baboons: Influences of infant and juvenile diets. Arteriosclerosis 5:347, 1985.

95. National Center for Health Statistics: Trends in breastfeeding: Advance data from vital and health statistics, DHHS Pub. No. 59. Washington, DC, U.S. Department of Health, Education and Welfare, 1980.

96. Neifert MR, Seacat JM: Mammary gland anomalies and lactation failure. In Hamosh M, Goldman AS (eds): Human Lactation. II. Maternal and Environmental Factors. New York, Plenum, 1986.

97. Neifert MR, Seacat JM, Jobe WE: Lactation failure due to insufficient glandular development of the breast. Pediatrics 76:823, 1985.

98. Nelson SE, Rogers RR, Ziegler EE, et al: Gain in weight and length during early infancy. Early Hum Dev 19:223, 1989.

99. O'Connor ME, Szekely LJ: Failure to thrive in breastfed 8-11 month olds: A manifestation of the "vulnerable child syndrome." ABM News Views 2(2):9, 1996.

100. Oliva-Rasbach J, Neville MC: Longitudinal growth patterns of a reference population of breastfed infants. Fed Proc 45:362, 1986.

101. Palmer MM, Crawley K, Blanco IA: Neonatal oral-motor assessment scale: A reliability study. J Perinatol 13:28, 1993.

102. Paneth N: Hypernatremic dehydration of infancy. Am J Dis Child 134:785, 1980.

103. Podratz RO, Broughton DD, Gustafson DH, et al: Weight loss and body temperature changes in breastfed and bottle fed neonates. Clin Pediatr 25:73, 1986.

104. Pomerance HH: Growth in breastfed children. Hum Biol 59:687, 1987.

105. Pugliese MT, Weyman-Daum M, Moses N, et al: Parental health beliefs as a cause of nonorganic failure to thrive. Pediatrics 80:175, 1987.

106. Ramsay M, Gisel EG, Boutry M: Non-organic failure to thrive: Growth failure secondary to feeding skills disorder. Dev Med Child Neurol 35:285, 1993.

107. Richards M, Hardy R, Wadsworth ME: Long-term effects of breast-feeding in a national birth cohort: Educational attainment and midlife cognitive function. Publ Health Nutr 5: 631, 2002.

108. Roddey OF, Martin ES, Swetenburg RL: Critical weight loss and malnutrition in breastfed infants. Am J Dis Child 135:597, 1981.

109. Rogan WJ, Gladen BC: Breastfeeding and cognitive development. Early Hum Dev 31:181, 1993.

110. Rowland TW, Zori RT, Lafleur WR, et al: Malnutrition and hypernatremic dehydration in breastfed infants. JAMA 247:1016, 1982.

111. Smith MM, Lifshitz F: Excess fruit juice consumption as a contributing factor in nonorganic failure to thrive. Pediatrics 93:436, 1994.

112. Strbák V, Skultétyová M, Hromadova M, et al: Late effects of breastfeeding and early weaning: Seven-year prospective study in children. Endocr Regulat 25:53, 1991.

113. Subcommittee on Nutrition during Lactation, Committee on Nutritional Status during Pregnancy and Lactation, Food and Nutrition Board, Institute of Medicine, National Academy of Sciences: Nutrition during Lactation. Washington, DC, National Academy Press, 1991.

114. Subcommittee on Nutrition during Lactation, Committee on Nutritional Status during Pregnancy and Lactation: Nutrition during Pregnancy and Lactation: An Implementation Guide. Washington, DC, National Academy Press, 1992.

115. Taylor B, Wadsworth J: Breastfeeding and child development at five years. Dev Med Child Neurol 26:73, 1984.

116. Volz VR, Book LS, Churella HR: Growth and plasma amino acid concentrations in term infants fed either whey-predominant formula or human milk. J Pediatr 102:27, 1983.

117. Weichert CE: Lactational reflex recovery in breastfeeding failure. Pediatrics 63:799, 1979.

118. Weston JA, Stage AF, Hathaway P, et al: Prolonged breastfeeding and nonorganic failure to thrive. Am J Dis Child 141:242, 1987.

119. Whitehead RG, Paul AA: Growth charts and the assessment of infant feeding practices in the Western world and in developing countries. Early Hum Dev 9:187, 1984.

120. Whitehead RG, Paul AA, Ahmed EA: Weaning practices in the United Kingdom and variations in anthropometric development. Acta Paediatr Scand 323 (suppl):14, 1986.

121. Wissler RW, McGill HC Jr (chairmen): Conference on blood lipids in children: Optimal levels for early prevention of coronary artery disease. Prev Med 12:868, 1983.

122. Woolridge MW, Ingram JC, Baum JD: Do changes in pattern of breast usage alter the baby's nutrient intake? Lancet 336:395, 1990.

123. World Health Organization/Centers for Disease Control: Measuring change in nutritional status: Guidelines for assessing the nutritional impact of supplementary feeding programmes for vulnerable groups. Geneva, WHO, 1983.

124. World Health Organization Working Group on Infant Growth: An evaluation of infant growth: The use and interpretation of anthropometry in infants. Bull WHO 73:165, 1995.

125. Yeung DL, Pennell MD, Leung M, et al: Infant fatness and feeding practices: A longitudinal assessment. J Am Diet Assoc 79:531, 1981.

126. Young HB, Buckley AE, Hamza B, et al: Milk and lactation: Some social and developmental correlates among 1000 infants. Pediatrics 69:169, 1982.

127. Zive MM, McKay H, Frank-Spohrer GC, et al: Infant feeding practices and adiposity in year old Anglo- and Mexican-Americans. Am J Clin Nutr 55:1104, 1992.

$\mathcal{M}$aternal employment

Maternal employment has been cited by many authors as the major reason for the decline in breastfeeding worldwide.[9,57] The international data do not actually support this contention. Year after year the Ross Laboratories Mothers Survey[62] in the United States confirms that the highest percentage of women initiating breastfeeding in the hospital is among women who plan to return to full-time employment, the next highest among women who plan to return to part-time employment, and the lowest among those who plan to remain at home.[63,65] In 2002, initiation in the hospital was 69% among women fully employed, 72.9% among those employed part-time, and 69% among those not employed. The duration, however, is affected by employment, with 36.8% of those employed part-time still breastfeeding at 5 to 6 months, 35.2% of nonemployed women still breastfeeding, and only 27.1% of those employed full-time still breastfeeding at 5 to 6 months (Fig. 13-1).[53,62] The individual mother who chooses to return to work and breastfeed is confronted by significant constraints, regardless of the statistical data. The physician should be knowledgeable about the principles and practice of this dual role when counseling about breastfeeding during maternal employment.[78]

Although economic, cultural, and political pressures often confound decisions about infant feeding, the American Academy of Pediatrics (AAP) firmly adheres to the position that breastfeeding ensures the best possible health and the best developmental and psychosocial outcomes for the infant.[3] Enthusiastic support and involvement of pediatricians in the promotion and practice of breastfeeding are essential to the achievement of optimal infant and child health, growth, and development.[5] The American College of Obstetricians and Gynecologists (ACOG) and the American Academy of Family Practice (AAFP) have made equally strong statements.[6]

HISTORICAL PERSPECTIVE

In modern cultures a stigma has been attached to a mother's earning money while her children are young, but no such stigma is associated with leaving her children for social interaction, personal reasons, or a volunteer job. All women work when work is defined as expending energy for a purpose, but not all women are employed when it is defined as earning money for labor. Before industrialization, the working mother was the rule and not the exception. Home and work were separated by industrialization, making parenting a separate role for women.

Sanday[66] has described women's work as domestic or productive, public or private, traditional or modern. Domestic work, when performed for the family, is unpaid and thus is undervalued and not counted as productive work. Domestic work is performed in the private domain, and "productive" work is associated with the public domain. Women

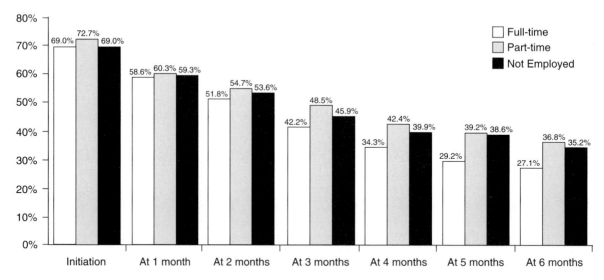

Figure 13-1. Comparison of breastfeeding duration rates during first 6 months post partum among mothers who are working full time, working part time, and not employed. (From Ross Products Division, Abbott Laboratories: Mothers Survey: Updated Breastfeeding Trends through 2002. Columbus, OH, Abbott Laboratories, 2002.)

had previously worked in agriculture and cottage industries as well as in small-scale marketing, whereas today they participate in formal work (i.e., they are *employees*), including clerical, factory, and professional jobs predominantly in urban settings.

More women are employed outside the home today than previously in the 20th century.[68-71] In 1900, 20% of the labor force was female; in 1950, 29%; in 1997, 56.6%; and in 2003 it was 57.5%. Women with children under 6 years old are the fastest-growing segment of the female work force; their numbers reached 59% in 1992 and more than 65% in 1996 but dropped to 59.4% in 2002. Even more critical is that the number of employed mothers with infants under age 1 year escalated to 48% of all women in 1985 and has continued to climb. Many more women facing the decision about infant feeding methods must include the early return to work. In 1998 at least 50% of women employed in the United States when they became pregnant returned to the labor force by the time their children were 3 months old. U.S. Department of Labor[68] statistics show that 54.3% of mothers with children under age 1 year were in the work force in 1996. This figure rises to 63.3% for women with children under 2 years of age. The fastest growing segment of the work force in the United States is women with infants and children. In Australia, about 27% of women with infants under 1 year return to work and 49% of women with children under age 5 are part of the paid work force. In the United States, 70% of employed women with children under age 3 work full time. One third of mothers return to work within 3 months after delivery and the rest return by 6 months.

Generations ago, the woman who worked violated the Victorian norms of role definition. Even when forced to work by sheer necessity, she was accused of neglecting her primary responsibility to her children. The new ethic proclaims work a cardinal virtue for the liberated woman, so that the woman who can and does stay home may begin to feel inadequate.

Why women enter the work force is important to understanding the trend.[37] Before 1970, the need to earn money motivated 3 million women either because the mother was a single parent or because husband-fathers were unable to earn an adequate income. For women whose husbands earned "enough," there was the need to provide a higher standard of living or provide the father with greater freedom of career choice.[78] Few women sought careers for careers' sake because need for income was the only socially acceptable, defensible reason for a mother to work outside the home.

Since that time many women have found that the full-time care of a home leads only to higher standards of cleanliness with no greater sense of achievement or completion.[29] Some believed that the exclusive investment of energy and emotion in the rearing of one to three children would involve a considerable hazard not only to a mother, but also to her children's ultimate achievement and ability to form a variety of responsive and satisfying personal relationships.[38,50] Women are responding to the pressures of an inflationary economy, to the costs of higher education, to the opportunities for personal fulfillment, and to the growing market for service occupations.[9,13] Married women continue to carry at least 70% to 80% of the child care and household duties when both parents work.

Women have reached the point where marriage in itself has relatively little effect on the labor supply, according to Cohen and Bianchi.[16] Educational differentials in the labor market have grown over time, widening the gap between the better and the less educated women, giving the former greater opportunities.

Children exerted less of a downward trend on the women's labor supply in the 1990s than they did in the 1970s. Having preschool-aged children still has a significant impact.

ATTITUDES OF PROFESSIONALS TOWARD WORKING MOTHERS

Professional[11] and lay[45] books alike on child rearing have viewed working negatively except for eco-nomic necessity, thus enhancing the working mother's guilt and providing little substantial advice about how to balance or how to continue breastfeeding.

The AAP Committee on Psychosocial Aspects of Child and Family Health[4] wrote in 1984: "Many mothers work outside the home and most have concerns about substitute child care. In addition to providing advice to individual parents, pediatricians can make an important contribution by supporting subsidized parental leaves after birth of a newborn infant, by encouraging the active participation of fathers in child and household care, and by having the knowledge to aid parents in access to high quality substitute child care." The AAP strongly stated in 1997 that pediatricians should "encourage employers to provide appropriate facilities and adequate time in the workplace for breast-pumping."[5]

The American College of Obstetricians and Gynecologists (ACOG)[6] has acknowledged the current trend to work throughout pregnancy and to return to work promptly after delivery by preparing a physician's guide to patient assessment and counseling, which has not been updated since 1987. ACOG also provides a patient occupational questionnaire for the practitioner. This forms a basis of discussion with the patient and provides an opportunity to counsel the patient and her husband about plans to maintain a healthy environment and any special needs for child care. With few exceptions, "the normal woman with an uncomplicated pregnancy and a normal fetus, in a job that presents no greater potential hazards than those encountered in normal daily life in the community, may continue to work without interruption until the onset of labor and may resume working several weeks after an uncomplicated delivery."[6] Frederick and Auerbach[25] put it in more practical terms when they suggest that the obstetrician has a role in facilitating continued breastfeeding after the return to work or school. This includes counseling regarding pumping and storing milk and avoiding exhaustion.

Attitudes of pediatricians toward mothers working outside the home have been measured by mail survey, because attitudes seem to determine advice given.[33] The majority of pediatricians responding thought that the children of working and nonworking women were similar, that the mother could return to work at any age of the child, and that it did not make any difference. Many respondents said they did not give advice about working (Tables 13-1 and 13-2). Only half the respondents provided special considerations, such as evening hours for employed mothers.

Some respondents, however, did express bias against employed mothers. Bias was related to the respondent's age and gender and to whether the respondent's spouse worked. Those whose spouses did not work outside the home, those in older age groups, and male pediatricians in general held more negative attitudes toward maternal employment. The researchers thought that a substantial number might give advice or cues that maternal employment might be detrimental to children, producing maternal conflict and guilt.

The physician plays an important role in guiding parents with information about quality and availability of child care facilities, as well as with advice about coping strategies.[23] As family counselor, the physician can help support mothers and fathers seeking to fulfill parental, occupational, and personal needs in a rapidly changing society. With

TABLE 13-2 Responses for reasons to recommend against working

Reason	Frequency	
	No.	%
Child's physical health	1724	24
Child's mental health	1445	20
Never recommend against work	1318	18
Inadequate child care	701	10
Child's age	591	8
Mother feels guilty	540	7
No economic need	459	6
Usually say, "Do not work"	72	1
Other	402	6
Total	7252	

From Heins M, Stillman P, Sabers D, et al: Attitudes of pediatricians toward maternal employment. Pediatrics 72:286, 1983; copyright © American Academy of Pediatrics, 1983.

the firm recommendation of the AAP to breastfeed throughout the first year and beyond, support from pediatricians will be critical.[5]

OUTCOME FOR CHILDREN OF EMPLOYED MOTHERS

Numerous studies since the early 1930s have looked at the effects of maternal employment. Assessment of infant behavior, school achievement and adjustment, children's attitudes, adolescence, and delinquency have all been used as outcome measures.[21] Annotated bibliographies covering the range of research in areas of medicine, psychology, sociology, and education are available. The four major considerations are the variables that facilitate or impede maternal employment, the effect of maternal employment on children during the four developmental stages, the effects on the family, and the effects on society in general. Society is far more accepting of the working mother now.

It has been emphasized that the presence of the mother in the home does not guarantee high-quality mothering.[29] It has also been shown that well-educated (college) mothers, including those

TABLE 13-1 Responses for reasons to recommend work

Reason	Frequency	
	No.	%
Economic	1709	25
Never recommend mother work	1566	22
Mother's emotional needs	1220	18
Mother's fulfillment	1059	15
Child is better off without mother	644	9
Reassure mother	270	4
Adequacy of child care	266	4
Child's age	170	2
Mother does important work	64	1
Total	6968	

From Heins M, Stillman P, Sabers D, et al: Attitudes of pediatricians toward maternal employment. Pediatrics 72:283, 1983; copyright © American Academy of Pediatrics, 1983.

who are employed, spend time with their children at the expense of their own personal needs.[39] Because employed mothers encompass a large group of women with different educations, different reasons for working, and different opportunities for employment, it is difficult to generalize about effects. Literature reviews have emphasized critical factors that are more important than maternal employment, such as good substitute care, maternal role satisfaction, family stability, paternal attitude toward maternal employment, and the quality of the time spent with the children.[36] Despite the abundance of research on school-age children, there is still little reported about preschoolers because no school records or test results are available to use in large-population analysis.

To date, there is no direct effect of nonexclusive mothering per se. Studies of infants of adolescent mothers have shown that the children do better socially and academically if there are multiple caregivers instead of the adolescent alone.[46] No uniformly harmful effects on family life or on the growth and development of children have been demonstrated. Maternal employment may jeopardize family life when the conditions of the mother's employment are demeaning to self-esteem, when others are strongly disapproving of her work away from the home, or when arrangements for child care are not adequate.[66]

Questions have been raised about the impact of separation of mother and infant and the timing of this separation.[13] Resumption of full-time employment when the child is under 1 year has sparked studies. Using the Ainsworth "strange situation" validated techniques, no relationship between maternal work status and the quality of the infants' attachment to their mothers is reported.[1,2] Early resumption of employment may not impede development of a secure infant-mother attachment.[15] A significantly higher proportion of insecure attachments to fathers in employed-mother families is reported for boys but not for girls. Boys are more insecurely attached than girls in most studies. It is believed that an infant's attachment relationship to mother emerges at about 7 months.[26] Other studies suggest that maternal employment can have a positive effect on girls but not boys. Whether breastfeeding accounts for some of the variability in these studies is not stated.[35-37,73] One of the strategies suggested is to advocate for infant care centers that provide breastfeeding facilities in the workplace, schools, and other locations serving working women.

BREASTFEEDING AND EMPLOYMENT

An important distinction must be made between work that separates the mother and infant for blocks of time and work that does not. In rural settings, women's work is usually compatible with all aspects of child care, including breastfeeding. Work in or around the home is usually flexible. If there are provisions for infants at the workplace, even formal urban work is compatible with child care and breastfeeding. The higher the education of the mother and the more advanced the job, the more opportunity exists for flexible arrangements that permit breastfeeding. Among the strategies available is pumping and saving milk while on the job to be fed to the baby by the babysitter the next day.

Overall, the breastfeeding rates for working women do not show that breastfeeding and employment are mutually exclusive.[78] In Finland the incidence of mothers breastfeeding at 1 month is 78% among nonworking and 80% among working mothers. The duration is also unaffected: 29% of nonworking and 32% of working mothers are breastfeeding at 3 months, and 8% and 7% at 6 months.[72] Similar statistics are reported from Nigeria, the Philippines, and Chile.

In 1987, Ryan and Martinez[65] conducted a study of the impact of employment on breastfeeding as part of the annual Ross Laboratories Mothers Survey, which explores infant feeding practices. Those mothers at 6 months who were employed full time numbered 22,316 (26.6%), part time 12,186 (14.5%), and not working 49,483 (58.9%). The same proportion of employed mothers (55%) as not employed were breastfeeding when they left the hospital. Only 10% of full-time employed mothers were breastfeeding at 6 months compared to 24% of those who were not employed, however. The highest incidence of breastfeeding at birth and at 6 months was among the over-30-year-old mothers who are well educated and in a higher socioeconomic group. The continuance rate* for all mothers was 18% breastfeeding among those employed and 44% among those not employed. Not surprisingly, working mothers also used more supplementary bottles. These trends are confirmed by more recent surveys.[43] In 2002, the duration of breastfeeding at 6 months was as follows: of those mothers employed full time, 27.1% were breastfeeding, of those employed part time, 36.8% were breastfeeding, and of those not employed 35.2% were breastfeeding, not a remarkable rate for those at home. At 6 months, 42.3% of women over 30 were still breastfeeding; those with a college education were at 44.6%.

Although there was no association between planning to be employed within the first 6 months and initiation of breastfeeding, Gielen and associates[28] found that there was a significant association with cessation of breastfeeding as early as 2 to 3 months post partum, even with adjustment for demographics. Among employed mothers, working 20 hours a week or less was protective for continuation of breastfeeding. When the factors influencing the duration of breastfeeding at 6 months were examined by West[74] by postal questionnaire in Edinburgh, only 5 of 116 mothers listed "return to work" as a reason for discontinuing.

A comparison by Martinez and Stahle[48] of low-income mothers who were receiving assistance from Women, Infants, and Children (WIC) Program showed that of the 38% who planned to work full time and left the hospital breastfeeding, only 8.8% were breastfeeding at 6 months, whereas of the 42.4% who had no plans for employment on leaving the hospital, 17.1% were still breastfeeding at 6 months in 1982.

Employment among black women around Johannesburg, South Africa, following the birth of a baby strongly influenced duration of breastfeeding (1990).[14] Although 97% had initiated breastfeeding, only 30% continued for 20 weeks; there was a direct association with return to work, because these women did not consider it feasible to do both. Similar findings were reported in Washington, D.C., where 80% of black women worked during pregnancy and those who planned to return to work only part time were more likely to breastfeed.[44] In this study, those who returned to a professional occupation had a longer duration of breastfeeding than those who returned to sales or technical jobs, regardless of whether the individual was black or white (1989).

Although work has been listed as the primary cause of early weaning, women seldom give employment as a reason for terminating breastfeeding. A review of the world literature documenting reasons for weaning, starting bottle feeding, or not initiating breastfeeding rarely mentioned employment.[72] In studies of the effect of mother's employment on the nutritional status of her children, poverty, not mother's work, was associated with poor nutrition.

The effect of employment on the duration of breastfeeding may be influenced by the fact that breastfeeding can be carried out while the mother performs other tasks around the house so that it is easier to breastfeed when she is home.[34] Many studies have found that employment has little or no effect on the duration of breastfeeding, especially where cottage industry was prevalent. The greatest problems are the difficulties encountered finding a place to pump and store the milk on the job. Those women who work outside the home must schedule and plan carefully and are motivated to continue once the complex schedule is established. They also are more able to accommodate themselves to the stresses involved.

A national study among women who responded to an advertisement in popular parenting magazines about working and breastfeeding found a relationship between work and breastfeeding success.[8] The timing of the return to work and the number of hours worked, not the type of work, influenced the duration of breastfeeding. Most of the respondents, however, were well educated and were motivated to respond to the advertisement and to fill out retrospectively a lengthy questionnaire.

---

*Continuance rate $= \dfrac{1.0 - \%\ \text{breastfed in hospital} - \%\ \text{breastfed at 6 months}}{\%\ \text{breastfed in hospital}}$

Results showed that mothers who pumped or hand-expressed milk (86% of the respondents) while at work continued to breastfeed longer than the small percentage who did not pump at work.

In times of economic downturn, work patterns are influenced by money. More women feel forced to return to work for economic reasons. Thus, more women with less flexible jobs find it impossible to handle the job, the home, the baby, and breastfeeding. As a result, returning to work or inability to combine work and breastfeeding appears as a reason for early weaning.

In a study by Morse and associates[56] in Canada, monthly semistructured interviews were conducted with 61 mothers who intended to continue breastfeeding after returning to work. Maternity leaves in Canada vary from 17 to 37 weeks. Mothers were hesitant to commit themselves to continuing to breastfeed because they believed too many factors were beyond their control despite elaborate plans and backup plans. The authors[55,56] concluded that financial constraints, increased education, and professional preparation were forcing women back to work in greater numbers, but few could manage to continue to breastfeed because there were no accommodations in the workplace. When the final results were reported, 36 mothers (of the 61) successfully combined breastfeeding and work for a mean of 18 weeks. Five different strategies for modifying feeding facilitated the transition from home to the workplace in this study: (1) breastfeeding on demand, (2) early introduction of a routine bottle, (3) transition to minimal breastfeeding, (4) transition to partial breastfeeding, and (5) transition to flexible breastfeeding (total breastfeeding on weekends, partial during the week). Only one mother expressed her milk at work; five expressed their milk at home to be given to the infant at daycare.[55,56]

The introduction of a bottle at 2 weeks of age for 4 weeks before returning to work was studied by Cronenwett and associates.[19] In a prospective study of 121 women who were committed to at least 6 weeks of breastfeeding, the mothers were randomly assigned to the "add-a-bottle" group or to the exclusive breastfeeding group. Some of the mothers pumped and gave their own milk by bottle.

The mean breastfeeding duration for both groups exceeded 6 months, although there was a slight difference in rates between the two groups at 12 weeks. The most important predictor of duration of breastfeeding was the mother's goal. The authors[19] saw no evidence that a single daily bottle in the early weeks was incompatible with prolonged breastfeeding in women committed to breastfeeding. Mothers who returned to work in the early postpartum period were likely to wean earlier. The conclusion in this study was that no evidence supports the "nipple confusion" hypothesis, because the infants went back and forth between breast and bottle without difficulty.

Impact of stress on milk supply

The stability of a milk supply is an individual matter. Some women can cope with extreme pressures and maintain an abundant milk supply, whereas other women find milk production to be very volatile. In the early weeks of lactation, the effect of external factors is much greater, but fatigue is consistently the most detrimental factor to milk production. In a study of the influence of commonplace stresses represented by academic stress and season of the year, 24-hour concentrations of growth hormone and prolactin were measured in 37 male first-year medical students during examination week.[47] Although measurements of perceived stress (perceived stress scale, PSS) rose sharply, there was no significant change in growth hormone or prolactin. This would suggest stress does not affect prolactin levels.

The workplace

Although working mothers are commonplace, companies who make working mothers comfortable are still uncommon. Efforts to increase parental leave, even unpaid leave, have not been widely established, although laws requiring minimal parental leave have been passed and have been applied to both parents. In the interest of equality, institutions have established family leave to provide for other family needs; care of elderly parents is an example.

Some major companies, however, have been recognized by *Working Mother* magazine's annual survey as making some efforts to support mothers in the workplace.[57,77] The yardstick includes everything from the number of female vice presidents to fair advancement and equal pay for equal work. No company has been nominated for its support of breastfeeding, although maternity leave policies are considered important. The 2003 report of the 18th Annual Survey named JFK Medical Center, King's Daughters Medical Center, Pittsburgh County Memorial Hospital, and St. Mary's Medical Center in the top 100 companies, but none were in the top 10, even though hospitals should be the model workplace. The top 10 included pharmaceutical houses Abbott Laboratories and Eli Lilly (best in the industry). Hospitals employ a number of professional women in their childbearing years as physicians, nurses, therapists, psychologists, laboratory technicians, and child life specialists.

A very significant contribution could be made by allocating space and providing staff for daycare centers. This would allow mothers to interact with their infants and breastfeed them during the work day. Small experiments providing daycare have shown a decrease in tardiness and absenteeism and a general increase in job satisfaction among employees who are mothers. For hospitals, where highly skilled and trained staff require as much as 6 months of costly on-the-job training, daycare has been shown to be very cost effective in eliminating excessive turnover.

In 1987 Moore and Jansa[54] sent surveys to 12 institutions known to support breastfeeding and to 100 of the Fortune 500 companies; only 29 were returned. Only two workplaces had breast pumps, and no documentable support of breastfeeding existed. Only an additional 14% of the 29 respondents even permitted breastfeeding in the workplace.

The Fortune 500 top companies so named in 1994 were contacted by Dusdieker and associates,[20] who received 242 (48%) responses to their four-item questionnaire. Five corporations (2.0%) had written policies regarding infant feeding or breastfeeding in the workplace; the policy was companywide for only two (0.8%). Less than 70%

of the 242 responding companies followed any infant feeding policy. A room or facility (other than a rest room) was provided to express milk in private by 64%, and the other 36% stated that no space was provided. Only 12% provided breast pumps, but 83% provided refrigerators for storage of breast milk. Most (76%) allowed flexible time schedules to allow for pumping; 7% had on-site daycare facilities. This represents a vast improvement in the 7 years since the previous survey.

Almost half the companies in Auerbach's study were unaware that an employee was breastfeeding.[7] The *Working Mother* survey considers compassion for the mother's regular day-to-day activities the "acid test."[57] Physicians who serve as consultants to large and small industries, unions, not-for-profit agencies, and daycare centers are in very important positions to influence corporate trends, which are changing very slowly. Companies that have been recognized by *Working Mother* for their corporate efforts to support breastfeeding include but are not limited to Amoco Corporation, Chicago; Dow Chemical Company, Midland, Michigan; General Motors, Detroit; Kodak, Rochester, New York; and the Los Angeles Department of Water and Power.[57]

In a study of Women, Infants and Children (WIC) program employees, it was hypothesized that WIC employees would initiate and continue breastfeeding at significantly higher rates than the national averages since there has been a major breastfeeding campaign at WIC in the past decade. Six Los Angeles WIC agencies participated; 99% of WIC employees began breastfeeding and 68.6% continued to 1 year. Key variables that contributed to the outcome were (1) intention to breastfeed for a year, (2) delayed use of formula, (3) breastfeeding support groups, and (4) availability of pumps at the worksite. Thus, it was proved that full-time employment and breastfeeding are compatible if the worksite is supportive.[76]

The welfare-to-work program, a central theme of welfare reform, requires recipients to engage in work, even mothers whose newborns are only a few months old, decreasing the incidence of breastfeeding. The negative consequences of these requirements were studied by Haider and associates.[31]

They indicate that the national breastfeeding rate would have been 5.5% higher at 6 months in 2000 without this mandate. They further suggest that the negative consequences of this policy should be considered because the potential benefits of breastfeeding these at-risk infants are so great.[31]

A comparison of maternal absenteeism and infant illness rates among breastfeeding and formula feeding women showed breastfeeding reduced absenteeism.[17,18] In two corporations with on-site lactation programs, one had 100 births among 2400, and the second had 30 births among 1200 female employees. Of the 101 mother-infant dyads studied, 59 were breastfed and 42 formula fed. The company provided lactation counseling as well as pumping and storing facilities. Of the 28% of the infants who had no illnesses, 86% were breastfed and 14% formula fed. Among mothers

who were absent because of infant illness, 75% were formula feeding and only 25% were breastfeeding (Fig. 13-2).

Following a mail panel questionnaire study in which questionnaires were sent in late pregnancy and 10 times during the first year, mothers' work patterns were clarified. Working full-time at 3 months decreased breastfeeding duration by 8.6 weeks relative to not working. Part-time work for 4 hours or less per day did not decrease duration of breastfeeding; part-time over 4 hours per day decreased breastfeeding duration only slightly. The authors concluded that part-time work is actually a good strategy to help mothers combine breastfeeding and work.

Planning to return to work prior to 6 weeks post partum reduced the likelihood of initiating breastfeeding in a study of over 10,000 mothers of singleton term infants.[58]

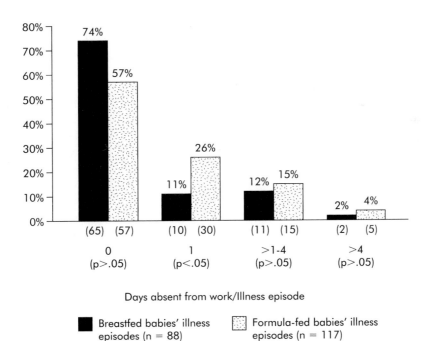

Days absent from work/Illness episode

■ Breastfed babies' illness episodes (n = 88)   ▨ Formula-fed babies' illness episodes (n = 117)

Figure 13-2. Distribution of illness episodes and maternal absenteeism by nutritional groups. (Modified from Cohen R, Mrtek MB, Mrtek RG: Comparison of maternal absenteeism and infant illness rates among breast-feeding and formula-feeding women in two corporations. Am J Health Promotion 10:148, 1995.)

Most of the studies concerning employment and breastfeeding were retrospective, relied on voluntary responses, and did not clearly define breastfeeding in terms of exclusivity or working in terms of part time or full time.[19,42] A prospective study reported by Kurinij and associates[44] involving over 1000 women confirmed the reports of others that women with professional occupations breastfeed longer than nonprofessionals and that part-time work is more conducive to longer duration than full-time jobs. Both groups of women found equal satisfaction from breastfeeding. The duration of breastfeeding was evaluated in a separate study in the same two corporations mentioned previously. Cohen and associates[17,18] reported that of the 187 participants, 75% who returned to work breastfed for 6 months or longer. The average duration for breastfeeding was 8.1 months. These rates were equal to the statistical norms for the region among women not employed outside the home.

In a provocative commentary, Furman[27] points out "the dilemma every woman faces, whether breastfeeding or bottle feeding, is leaving one's child." She further comments that mother's milk in a bottle given by any of several staff members at daycare is not equal to nursing at the breast. Her solution was part-time work, which is not a new idea but does depend on the nature of the mother's employment. The decision to work or not work is a very personal one and does not separate women into good and bad mothers. The role of the health professional is to discuss the mother's plans nonjudgmentally and then assist her in adjusting her infant and herself to the process.

Counseling breastfeeding mothers who choose to work

Part of the physician's counseling session before the birth of a baby should include inquiry about the mother's plan to work post partum. Open discussion about work, breastfeeding, child care arrangements, and general stress will be helpful. Most well-educated women who plan to return to a career have thought out the entire process carefully but may want some reassurance or alternative suggestions. The physician should know what services are available locally. It may be helpful to have a list of other working mothers who are willing to share experiences and knowledge of resources. It is often helpful for a woman to know another person who has experienced similar career choices.

Some women have no experience with newborns and are totally unrealistic about the new responsibility and what it entails. Even pediatricians in training may be unrealistic. The pediatrician may have to recommend a more realistic view of parenting and urge the parents to plan carefully and practically for working and parenting. The new mother needs to appreciate that events occur around children that cannot be totally controlled. Even when a woman has been an efficient career woman in total control of her destiny, an infant with normal needs may be overwhelming. Women who have jobs that are rigid from the standpoint of work hours and workplace will not find a few glib remarks in a pamphlet very helpful when they want to maintain their milk supply.

The physician may need to discuss specific issues of child care while the mother is working, as follows:

1. Child care arrangements should be sought that permit sufficient time for feeding an infant inexperienced with a bottle and sufficient time for extra cuddling of an infant who is used to a closer relationship with the "feeder." The child care specialist should be familiar with breastfeeding and sympathetic to the philosophy.

2. The advantages and disadvantages of child care in the infant's home, in the sitter's home, with or without the sitter's children, and with or without other children should be discussed. Is daycare a good arrangement for this family, and what centers take young infants and will work with breastfeeding mothers? Despite low cost, nursery "warehousing" should be avoided.

3. Are there child care facilities available close to the workplace so that the mother could leave work on her breaks to breastfeed?

Plans for feeding the infant while the mother is working depend on the infant's age and feeding pattern. If the infant is totally breastfed and under 6 months of age, the mother can breastfeed if she can leave work and go to the infant or if the infant can be brought to the workplace. If the mother cannot leave work to nurse, she may choose to pump her milk at work and save it for the following day. This necessitates having (1) a reasonably sanitary place to pump, such as a lounge or clean locker room, and (2) a means of storing the milk until she gets home, either in a refrigerator at work or in a portable refrigerator system. Mothers have used insulated containers with ice, reusable cold packs, or dry ice. If no such arrangement for chilling can be made, the milk can be stored in a sterile container for 8 hours without refrigeration if collected under clean conditions.

A woman who is away from her breastfeeding infant past feeding time may need to pump to maintain her milk supply. A mother may also anticipate the infant's needs before she returns to work. She can practice pumping and storing a small amount of her milk daily for several weeks in her home freezer so that a stockpile is available while she is at work (see Chapter 21).

The mother should be instructed to introduce the baby to the bottle and an alternate caregiver before the first day of work. Developing a plan of organization and practicing it before the first day of work may avoid initial disaster. Also, returning to work part time at first may help minimize the adjustment. In addition, starting back to work on Wednesday or Thursday allows the first week to be a short one.

No evidence indicates that it is necessary to introduce a bottle sooner than 10 days before returning to work. Unless a mother is returning to work immediately after delivery, a bottle should not be introduced before lactation is well established (at least 4 weeks for most primiparas) because it interferes with the mother's milk-making rhythm. Furthermore, it may confuse the infant. Although some infants readily go back and forth between breast and bottle, no way exists to identify the infant who will develop sucking difficulties and "nipple

confusion," resulting ultimately in preference for the bottle if it is introduced too early. Babies given a bottle well before 3 months may easily reject it after 3 months. For the infant who does not accept the bottle gracefully, the following techniques may facilitate the process:

1. Someone other than the mother should give the feeding.
2. The mother should be out of sight and hearing range, preferably out of the building, so the infant does not await her arrival.
3. The infant should be held by the "feeder" in the same position as for breastfeeding, that is, slightly elevated and close to the chest wall at about breast level. The bottle can be slipped down against the caregiver's chest wall.
4. Use a soft nipple and a small bottle at first for easy handling. A Volufeed, the clear plastic cylinder used for premature infants, allows a better view of the infant.
5. Create a soothing atmosphere; use a rocking chair, quiet music, and muted light.
6. The initial bottle feedings, if not all of them, should contain warm mother's milk to reduce the elements of change being introduced.

If the bottle feedings do not go well and alternate feedings are needed, milk can be provided by medicine cup feeding (see Chapter 15).

If the infant is over 6 months of age, the physician may consider introduction of other foods. The feeding given by the caregiver can be solids by spoon and liquids from a cup so that no breastfeeding is actually missed. The health professional can anticipate these issues and tailor feeding counseling accordingly. Some infants quickly learn the mother's schedule and may adjust their sleep pattern to allow a long stretch while mother is away. This may result in feedings during the night instead, but if the mother is informed of this phenomenon, she may be less anxious if it occurs.

Bottle fed infants have more infections and illnesses, which is another reason to encourage a mother to continue breastfeeding. This is especially important during the first weeks of adjustment to the transient, recurrent separation of mother and infant associated with the mother's return to work.

Maternal considerations

Counseling the breastfeeding family when the mother returns to work should also include attention to mothering the mother.[59] Fatigue is a significant problem for all postpartum women and many nursing mothers. It can easily become a major stress when the mother adds outside employment to her schedule. Several days or more of adjustment are necessary for a major change in one's schedule. If the mother can focus on a few essential concerns (infant, job, own well-being) as opposed to housework, fancy meals, or a social schedule, she will weather this transition without despair. The first casualty of fatigue may be breastfeeding unless some anticipatory action is taken.

Once the schedule has been adjusted and a routine established, breastfeeding may offer tremendous satisfaction for both mother and infant in terms of a sustained relationship as well as a reaffirmation for the mother of the quality of her parenting. One of the most difficult adjustments to motherhood is the need to set priorities and eliminate some chores of lesser urgency. The physician needs to reinforce this when the mother returns to work. Whether or not a mother continues to breastfeed, holding and cuddling her baby cannot become a lower priority. The mother's nourishment is also important and can be consumed during the time spent pumping. A mother should plan to have a beverage available every time she sits down to nurse or pump.

Daycare

Infants in daycare have created a special concern for parents, pediatricians, social scientists, and policymakers. The early published information did not discuss the impact of breastfeeding before or during the infant's involvement with daycare. Haskins and Kotch[32] first reviewed the literature (172 articles) and concluded, "Children in day care, especially those under three years old and sometimes their teachers and household contacts, have higher rates of diarrhea, hepatitis A, meningitis and possibly also otitis media than children not in day care." The data are less clear for respiratory illnesses and cytomegalovirus. Extremely valuable but unavailable data would be the relationship between breastfeeding and illness in and out of daycare. Revisions of state regulatory policy regarding health practices in daycare are necessary. Parents choosing daycare facilities for their children need to select them with consideration for health and safety. More than 60% of the children under 6 years of age of women who work are in out-of-home care, approximately 8 million U.S. children in 1995. In some situations, daycare may actually improve the infant's potential, especially when the mother is young, immature, depressed, overwhelmed, or without family support.

Concern about infant illness should result in pediatricians' involvement in ensuring quality daycare in the local community. For the infant age appropriate for breastfeeding, one possible preventive measure would be to encourage a continuation of breastfeeding when possible. Furthermore, daycare policy and procedure should encourage and facilitate breastfeeding. Mothers should inquire about daycare centers' policies toward breastfeeding. Physicians who consult for daycare centers should be well informed as well. Breast milk can safely stand at room temperature for 6 to 8 hours and need not be discarded if the first feeding attempt is incomplete. In contrast, formula must be refrigerated and discarded after the first feeding attempt because it contains no antibodies or infection protection factors. No infant feeding of any kind should be warmed in a microwave oven. Protective gloves are not necessary to feed breast milk. The accidental feeding of a different mother's milk is not cause for alarm, although it should be reported to the parents for public health reasons. One feeding of milk produced by a mother who is positive for human immunodeficiency virus (HIV) will probably not transmit the disease. Women who are HIV positive in developed countries, however, are discouraged from breastfeeding.

Resources for parents

The popular press has been inundated with books on child care and child rearing, with a significant number on breastfeeding, specifically breastfeeding and employment. These volumes can be extremely helpful to young parents, providing detailed information about how to manage. Many recognize that mothers, fathers, infants, jobs, child care arrangements, and support resources are all different. A disturbing number, however, are dogmatic and single-minded, giving the impression that the author's method is the only recipe for successful lactation. The pediatrician should become familiar with a few of these guidebooks and certainly not recommend any without reading them first. A few of these books have instilled guilt in the working woman about leaving her infant.

The brochure *Working and Breastfeeding: Can You Do It?* was prepared by the National Healthy Mothers, Healthy Babies Coalition and is available free by calling the coalition in Alexandria, Virginia, at 703-836-6110. It is also available through local WIC nutritional programs. It is simple and direct, providing directions for managing a job and breastfeeding as well as collecting and storing breast milk.

Women in health care head the list of authors, because many women physicians (especially residents), nurses, and hospital employees return to work while breastfeeding and then share their experiences in print.[30] Even the worst setup in a hospital may surpass the resources available to the women working in industry. Certainly hospitals and health care centers should provide models for other workplaces in supporting optimal daycare sources and making it possible for a mother-employee to return to work and maintain her milk supply.[41] Independent lactation practitioners provide an additional resource. Women should contact the International Lactation Consultants Association (ILCA) for consultants in the area (see Chapter 22). Some industries have hired certified lactation consultants to provide assistance to their employees in maintaining their milk supply. The company also usually provides "a pumping room" and equipment. As pointed out by Cohen and associates,[17,18] this also reduces absenteeism because the infant who is provided the mother's milk has fewer illnesses.

Responding to parental needs, Brazelton captured the quintessential challenge to parents in the title and the text *Working and Caring*.[12] It is possible for parents to both work and care! Freud and Dann[26] pointed out that the two most powerful requirements for human existence are "love" and "work." Our culture had suggested that men work and women love in relation to family obligations. Today it is possible not only for a mother to love her children and work, but also for a father to work and love his children. Although Brazelton's book was written for parents in his usual style of live reports of representative families, it also contains valuable guidance for the health care professional who counsels working parents.[12]

Surgeon General's Workshop

The *Report of the Surgeon General's Workshop on Breastfeeding and Human Lactation*[60] clearly enunciates that strategies need to be developed to reduce the barriers to breastfeeding while employed. All six categories of the report address the issue in some capacity. Category 1, The World of Work, states that a national breastfeeding promotion initiative directed to all those who influence breastfeeding decisions and opportunities of women involved in school, job training, professional education, and employment is needed. Along with data collection, education, and change in institutional policy, the report suggests that legislation related to federal, state, and local tax incentives might be provided for institutions that successfully implement breastfeeding programs at work or at school. It also recommends the development of appropriate support services in the world of work, such as prenatal care, social and nutritional services, paid maternity leave, child care, and alternative types of work arrangements such as flextime and job sharing.

The workshop report also states that successful initiation and continuation of breastfeeding will require a broad spectrum of support services involving families, peers, care providers, employers, and community agencies and organizations.[60] Although little has been accomplished toward these specific goals, the U.S. Breastfeeding Committee has been formed in concert with the Innocenti Declaration recommendations. The U.S. Breastfeeding Committee has undertaken as a major activity the improvement of the atmosphere for the breastfeeding working woman. The Committee's policy paper on the subject states the following benefits for employers to adopt a breastfeeding support program:

- Cost savings of $3 per $1 invested in breastfeeding support
- Less illness among the breastfed children of employees
- Reduced absenteeism to care for ill children
- Lower health care costs (an average of $400 per baby over the first year)
- Improved employee productivity
- Higher morale and greater loyalty
- Improved ability to attract and retain valuable employees
- Family-friendly image in the community

Each company or employer should tailor the program to its unique needs.

The Committee has suggested that several strategies are feasible, safe, and relatively easy to implement. They include developing a breastfeeding support program, distribution of support policy, consideration of flexible scheduling option, sufficient break time to feed or pump, and providing useful information. The full statement is available at http://www.usbreastfeeding.org.

Workplace kit

Women in Australia face the same challenges to working while breastfeeding as reported in many countries of the world. McIntyre and colleagues[49] report a project that promoted balancing breastfeeding and paid work through the development, distribution, promotion, and evaluation of suitable materials to workplaces, employers, and employees. Materials for employees were translated into Arabic, Chinese, Turkish, Spanish, and Vietnamese.

In this project targeting employers, women, and workplaces in Australia, 500,000 information kits were distributed with preference to places that had women of childbearing age and women of diverse cultural background. The project was widely publicized in all media.

The kit contained a poster to display key points and a booklet to provide more detailed information in an easy-to-read format. The contents had been tested in focus groups and evaluated by other key stakeholders, including a working mother and a lactation consultant.

The evaluation of the project included a simple survey sent via email or fax to 1571 organizations. Only 202 (12.8%) were returned. Those who responded thought it was excellent, over half thought it would be useful, and two thirds thought the kit would provide suitable solutions to support balancing breastfeeding and work at their organization. The authors recognize the need for further work to implement the policies and procedures to support breastfeeding in the workplace.

Maternal benefits

In 1919 the International Labor Organization established the Maternity Protection Convention for working women.[61] This document provided for two half-hour nursing breaks per day. It also recommended that employers provide crèches (day nurseries, especially European) or daycare when more than a given number of women are employed, but few countries hold to its tenets today. Maternity benefits vary from country to country and may include maternity leave with or without pay, nursing breaks, provision of daycare facilities, and prohibition of dismissal. Physicians who care for mothers and infants should take a leadership role in ensuring that mothers can continue breastfeeding even when the mother is employed.

Many women, especially when faced with coping with a second or third child, reexamine the working issue in light of the needs of their children, even though they may have previously managed to breastfeed and work at one time. No one else can or should decide for a woman how she will handle parenting, especially in the early years of a child's life. Furman[27] poignantly addresses some of the issues. No woman should be embarrassed to stay home or should apologize for working part time or not at all. Breast milk is not a substitute for good parenting, any more than quantity parenting is synonymous with quality parenting. It is possible to work and to care, however.

Physician's role

The primary role of the pediatrician is as an advocate for children. Physicians can help support fathers and mothers alike who are faced with fulfilling the roles of parent, employee, and citizen in a rapidly changing society. Physicians should be able to provide understandable information concerning the child's growth and development combined with a realistic view of the issues in parenting and family life. They should show an openness and willingness to discuss nonjudgmentally with the parents their specific situation, options, and choices for caring for their child.

If the physician is the medical consultant to the daycare program, the role can be to assure mothers who want to provide their milk that they will be supported by the staff. The physician should develop policies and procedures for the storage and use of the breast milk provided. In addition, space and facilities (at least a rocking chair and a screen) should be available for the mother to nurse the infant before leaving the child and on her return later before going home. If the physician is in the medical department of a large company or the pediatrician for a working breastfeeding mother, he or she can advocate for time and resources for pumping while at work as part of good preventive care.

The success of breastfeeding depends to a degree on ever-widening circles of support for the breastfeeding infant-mother dyad. Support should come first from the husband/father, then from other family members, other caregivers in the home, daycare facilities, employers and other employees, and community members to help the mother and family comfortably and safely breastfeed, work, and care for their child as they choose. Breastfeeding is not just a woman's issue. It is a family issue and a pub-

lic health issue as well. Articles abound in the medical and lay literature describing how one can achieve success in breastfeeding and returning to work. Most authors list pumps and milk storage as important items. Each mother has to plan her own approach based on her job requirements and her own resources and her support system, as well as her infant's needs. Although it is not easy to balance a job and breastfeed, it can be done, with adequate strategizing and planning, which is appropriate with or without breastfeeding and returning to work post partum.

The physician's role in achieving a successful return to work for the breastfeeding mother includes the following steps:

1. Discuss the mother's plans for returning to work in advance.
2. Recommend appropriate local child care facilities that are "breastfeeding friendly."
3. Suggest that the mother discuss breastfeeding with her employer or supervisor.
4. Have a lactation consultant available in the practice or office, or if not, know where one can be contacted.
5. Provide recommendations for collecting and storing breast milk, which can be included in an office handout.
6. When medical problems arise, seek adequate information so that an appropriate solution can be recommended that supports continued breastfeeding.

Reading for parents regarding breastfeeding and working outside the home

Mason D, Ingersoll D: Breastfeeding and the Working Mother, rev. ed. Griffin, NY, St. Martins/Griffin, 1997.

Meek JY (ed): New Mother's Guide to Breastfeeding. Bantam Books, NY (American Academy of Pediatrics, Elk Grove, Ill), 2002.

Eiger MS, Olds SW: The Complete Book of Breastfeeding. New York, Workman, 1999.

REFERENCES

1. Ainsworth MDS: The development of infant-mother attachment. In Caldwell BM, Ricciuti HN (eds): Review of Child Development Research. Chicago, University of Chicago Press, 1973.

2. Ainsworth MDS, Blehar MC, Waters E, et al: Patterns of Attachment. Hillsdale, NJ, Erlbaum, 1978.

3. American Academy of Family Physicians: AAFP Position Paper on Breastfeeding. Leawood, KS American Academy of Family Physicians, 2001.

4. American Academy of Pediatrics, Committee on Psychosocial Aspects of Child and Family Health: The mother working outside the home. Pediatrics 73:874, 1984.

5. American Academy of Pediatrics, Work Group on Breastfeeding: Breastfeeding and the use of human milk. Pediatrics 100:1035, 1997.

6. American College of Obstetricians and Gynecologists: Guidelines on Pregnancy and Work. Chicago, ACOG Publications, 1987.

7. Auerbach KG: Assisting the employed breastfeeding mother. J Nurse Midwifery 35:26, 1990.

8. Auerbach KG, Guss E: Maternal employment and breastfeeding: A study of 567 women's experiences. Am J Dis Child 138:958, 1984.

9. Baden C: Work and family: An annotated bibliography 1978–1980. Boston, Wheelock College Center for Parenting Studies, 1981.

10. Biagioli F: Returning to work while breastfeeding. Am Family Physician 68:2199, 2003 [electronic article accessed at www.aafp.org/afp].

11. Brazelton TB: Toddlers and Parents. New York, Delta, 1974.

12. Brazelton TB: Working and Caring. Reading, MA, Addison-Wesley, 1985.

13. Bronfenbrenner U, Crouter AC: Work and family through time and space. In Kamerman SB, Hayes CD (eds): Families that Work: Children in a Changing World. Washington, DC, National Academy Press, 1982.

14. Chalmers B, Ransome OH, Herman A: Working while breastfeeding among coloured women. Psychol Rep 67:1123, 1990.

15. Chase-Lansdale PL, Owen MT: Maternal employment in a family context: Effects on infant-mother and infant-father attachments. Child Dev 58:1505, 1987.

16. Cohen PN, Bianchi SM: Marriage, children, and women's employment: What do we know? U.S. Department of Labor Monthly Labor Review, December 1999, p 22.

17. Cohen R, Mrtek MB: The impact of two corporate lactation programs on the incidence and duration of breast-feeding by employed mothers. Am J Health Promotion 6:436, 1994.

18. Cohen R, Mrtek MB, Mrtek RG: Comparison of maternal absenteeism and infant illness rates among breast-feeding and formula-feeding women in two corporations. Am J Health Promotion 10:148, 1995.

19. Cronenwett L, Stukel T, Kearney M, et al: Single daily bottle use in the early weeks post partum and breastfeeding outcomes. Pediatrics 90:760, 1992.

20. Dusdieker LB, Losch ME, Dungy CI: Breastfeeding and the workplace: A survey of Fortune 500 industrial corporations. Pediatr Res 37:136A, 1995.

21. Easterbrooks MA, Goldberg WA: Effects of early maternal employment on toddlers, mothers and fathers. Dev Psychol 21:774, 1985.

22. Eiger MS, Olds SW: The Complete Book of Breastfeeding, 2nd ed. New York, Workman, 1987.

23. Eisenberg L: Caring for children and working dilemmas of contemporary womanhood. Pediatrics 56:24, 1975.

24. Fein SB, Roe B: The effect of work status on initiating and duration of breast-feeding. Am J Publ Health 88:1042, 1998.

25. Frederick IB, Auerbach KG: Maternal-infant separation and breastfeeding: The return to work or school. J Reprod Med 30:323, 1985.

26. Freud A, Dann S: An experiment in group upbringing. Psychoanal Study Child 6:127, 1961.

27. Furman L: A second look at breastfeeding and full-time maternal employment. Am J Dis Child 146:540, 1992.

28. Gielen AC, Faden RR, O'Campo P, et al: Maternal employment during the early postpartum period: Effects on initiation and continuation of breastfeeding. Pediatrics 87:298, 1991.

29. Ginzberg E: The changing pattern of women's work. Am J Orthopsychiatry 28:313, 1958.

30. Grams M: Breastfeeding success for working mothers. Carson City, National Capitol Resources, 1985.

31. Haider SJ, Jacknowitz A, Schoeni RF: Welfare work requirements and child well-being: Evidence from the effects on breastfeeding. Demography 40:479, 2003.

32. Haskins R, Kotch J: Day care and illness: Evidence, costs, and public policy. Pediatrics 77(suppl):951, 1986.

33. Heins M, Stillman P, Sabers D, et al: Attitudes of pediatricians toward maternal employment. Pediatrics 72:283, 1983.

34. Hirschman C, Sweet JA: Social background and breastfeeding among American mothers. Soc Biol 21:39, 1974.

35. Hock E: Working and nonworking mothers and their infants: A comparative study of maternal caregiving characteristics and infant's social behavior. Merrill-Palmer Q 46:79, 1980.

36. Hoffman LW: Effects of maternal employment on the child: A review of the research. Dev Psychol 10:204, 1974.

37. Hoffman LW: Increased fathering: Effects on mother. In Lamb M, Sagi A (eds): Fatherhood and Family Policy. Hillsdale, NJ, Erlbaum, 1983.

38. Howell MC: Employed mothers and their families. Pediatrics 52:252, 1973.

39. Hurst M, Zambrana RE: Determinants and Consequences of Maternal Employment. Washington, DC, Business and Professional Women's Foundation, 1981.

40. Jalilvand M: Married women, work, and values. U.S. Department of Labor Monthly Labor Review, August 2000.

41. Katcher AL, Lanese MG: Breastfeeding by employed mothers: A reasonable accommodation in the work place. Pediatrics 75:644, 1985.

42. Kearney MH, Cronenwett L: Breastfeeding and employment. J Obstet Gynecol Neonatal Nurs 20:471, 1991.

43. Krieger F: Ross Laboratories Mothers Survey: A Marketing Research Tool. Presented at the Editors Conference, New York, Sept 22, 1992.

44. Kurinij N, Shiono PH, Ezrine SF, et al: Does maternal employment affect breastfeeding? Am J Publ Health 79:1247, 1989.

45. La Leche League: The Womanly Art of Breastfeeding, 6th ed. Schaumburg, IL, La Leche League, 1997.

46. Lawrence RA: Early mothering by adolescents. In McAnarney ER (ed): Premature Adolescent Pregnancy and Parenthood. New York, Grune & Stratton, 1983.

47. Malarkey WB, Hall JC, Pearl DK, et al: The influence of academic stress and season on 24-hour concentrations of growth hormone and prolactin. J Clin Endocrinol Metab 73:1089, 1991.

48. Martinez GA, Stahle DA: The recent trend in milk feeding among WIC infants. Am J Publ Health 72:68, 1982.

49. McIntrye E, Pisaniello D, Gun R, et al: Balancing breast-feeding and paid employment: A project targeting employers, women and workplaces. Health Promotion International 17:215, 2002.

50. Mead M: A cultural anthropologist's approach to maternal deprivation. In Deprivation of Maternal Care. Public Health Papers No. 14. Geneva, World Health Organization, 1962.

51. Meek JY: Breastfeeding in the work place. Pediatr Clin North Am 48:461, 2002.

52. Meyers D: Breastfeeding and returning to work in the physician's office. Am Family Physician 68(11):2129, 2003.

53. Mizera J: Personal communication, Ross Laboratories Mothers Survey, 1997.

54. Moore JF, Jansa N: A survey of policies and practices in support of breastfeeding mothers in the work place. Birth 14:191, 1987.

55. Morse JM, Bottorff JL: Intending to breastfeed and work. J Obstet Gynecol Nurs 18:493, 1989.

56. Morse JM, Bottorff JL, Boman J: Patterns of breastfeeding and work: The Canadian experience. Can J Publ Health 80:182, 1989.

57. Moskowitz M: 100 best companies for working mothers. Working Mother, October 1997, p 18.

58. Noble S, ALSPAC Study Team: Maternal employment and the initiation of breastfeeding. Acta Paediatr 90:423, 2001.

59. Popkin BM: Time allocation of the mother and child nutrition. Ecol Food Nutr 9:1, 1980.

60. Report of the Surgeon General's Workshop on Breastfeeding and Human Lactation, Lawrence RA (chair), DHHS Pub. No. HRS-D-MC 84-2. Washington, DC, Department of Health and Human Services, 1984.

61. Richardson JL: Review of the international legislation establishing nursing breaks. J Trop Pediatr Environ Child Health 21:249, 1975.

62. Ross Products Division, Abbott Laboratories: Mothers Survey: Updated Breastfeeding Trend through 1996. Columbus, Ohio, Abbott Laboratories, 1998.

63. Ryan AS: The resurgence of breastfeeding in the United States. Pediatrics 99(4):e12, 1997 (electronic article).

64. Ryan AS, Wenjun Z, Acosta A: Breastfeeding continues to increase into the new millennium. Pediatrics 110:1103, 2002.

65. Ryan AS, Martinez GA: Breastfeeding and the working mother: A profile. Pediatrics 83:524, 1989.

66. Sanday P: Female status in the public domain. In Rosaldo M, Lamphere L (eds): Woman, Culture and Society. Stanford, Stanford University Press, 1974.

67. U.S. Breastfeeding Committee: Workplace breastfeeding support. Accessed at http://usbfg.org.

68. U.S. Department of Labor: Facts on women workers. Washington, DC, U.S. Government Printing Office Web Page, 1997, accessed at www.gpo.gov.

69. U.S. Department of Labor: Manpower report of the president. Washington, DC, U.S. Government Printing Office, 1974.

70. U.S. Department of Labor, Office of the Secretary: Facts on women workers. Washington, DC, Women's Bureau, 1980.

71. U.S. Department of Labor, Bureau of Labor Statistics: Employment status of the civilian population by sex and age. Accessed at www.bls.gov/news.release/empsit.t01. htm.

72. Van Esterik P, Greiner T: Breastfeeding and women's work: Constraints and opportunities. Stud Fam Plan 12:184, 1981.

73. Vaugh BE, Gove FL, Egeland B: The relationship between out-of-home care and the quality of infant-mother attachment in an economically disadvantaged population. Child Dev 51:1203, 1980.

74. West CP: Factors influencing the duration of breastfeeding. J Biosoc Sci 12:325, 1980.

75. Winikoff B, Baer EC: The obstetrician's opportunity: Translating "breast is best" from theory to practice. Am J Obstet Gynecol 138:105, 1980.

76. Whaley SE, Meehan K, Lange L, et al: Predictors of breast-feeding duration for employees of the Special Supplemental Nutrition Program for Women, Infants, and Children (WIC). J Am Diet Assoc 102:1290, 2002.

77. Working Mother Magazine: Working Mother—The 100 Best, 2003. Accessed at www.workingmother.com/oct03/100BestList.shtml 2003.

78. Zambrana RE, Hurst M, Hite RL: The working mother in contemporary perspective: A review of the literature. Pediatrics 64:862, 1979.

14

$\mathcal{B}$reastfeeding the premature infant

PREMATURE INFANTS

Research in the science of nutrition for the low-birth-weight infant and the micropremature infant has advanced tremendously as the technology to study the important questions has improved. Neonatologists meanwhile have spent the last decades studying the physiology of respiration. Their advances have contributed to the survival of smaller and smaller infants. The edge of viability is 24 weeks and a weight of 500 g; however, there are examples of survivors under these values. One of the key points learned retrospectively about survival, generation after generation, has been the critical impact of fluid and nutrition. Although human milk has gained prominence in these studies, the early use of unsupplemented drip milk and some donor milks produced poor growth patterns. Drip milk is very low in fat and therefore low in calories. The protein levels in donor milk from women late in lactation (i.e., beyond 6 to 8 months, when the levels have dropped) parallel the child's decreased biologic needs with the addition of solid foods. These factors contributed to the abandonment of human milk until supplements were developed and studies of the milk of women who had delivered prematurely sparked new investigations.

This discussion highlights only the important issues; the reader is referred to reviews such as the exhaustive summary of human milk for the premature infant and the extensive bibliography by Steichen, Krug-Wispe, and Tsang.[119] *Nutritional Needs of the Preterm Infant,* by Tsang and associates,[125] is an international collaboration that involved many major premature infant centers in discussions to create unity out of a tremendous disparity of practice and various recipes for nutritional support. This collaboration also produced a consensus on individual nutrient requirements for infants under 1000-g birth weight, for 1000-g to 1750-g infants, and for postdischarge management. Neonatologists, however, have not reached a consensus on the feeding of premature infants.[82] The absolute standard for evaluating the nutritional outcome of preterm infants remains undefined. A strategy to minimize mobilization of endogenous nutrient stores is moving away from a focus on intrauterine-based, short-term growth and nutrient retention rates to a system that considers long-term growth achievement.[113] The optimal time to initiate oral feedings in the smallest and sickest preterm infants is under revision.[112] Prolonged exclusive parenteral nutrition is being replaced with minimal amounts of oral feedings with parenteral nutrition to preserve and maintain intestinal function.[2,110] As nutritional markers shift, the preterm infant's own mother's milk may well be recognized, even by the most skeptical clinicians, as the "gold standard" to prevent short-term morbidities and enhance long-term outcome.[111] With this change may come the recognition that fortified donor milk is superior to artificial feeds.

No goal is universal, according to Gross and Slagle,[52] who define the task as (1) achieving well-defined, standard short-term growth, such as intrauterine growth curves or mimicking reference fetus composition; (2) preventing feeding-related morbidities, such as nosocomial infection and necrotizing enterocolitis; and (3) optimizing long-term neurodevelopmental and physical growth. This discussion addresses these goals. As the technology of ultrasound continues to advance, serial observations of fetuses that result in normal full-term infants are being assessed.[1] Intrauterine growth patterns so determined may come closer to a normal model than previous assessments done on infants delivered prematurely, which in itself is not normal.

A normal full-term infant can usually be breast-fed with only minor adjustment, even without the support of medical expertise. When the infant cannot nurse directly at the breast, is providing mother's milk appropriate? What is the overall prognosis for ever feeding at the breast or, perhaps, for survival itself? Parents are so awed by the med-ical staff of special and intensive care nurseries that they are often afraid to bring up the subject of breastfeeding. In addition, the nursery staff may be so busy balancing electrolytes and adjusting ventilators and monitors that they have not thought to ask what plans the mother might have had for feeding before the infant developed a problem.

The birth of an extremely low birth weight (ELBW) premature infant is a nutritional emergency. Even with parenteral nutrition from the first day, weight loss exceeds 10%, and it takes at least 10 days to regain birth weight. The long-term consequences of early nutrition have a great impact on neurodevelopment and may well reduce the risk of perinatal brain lesions. Fetal and postnatal events affect gut development.

The gastrointestinal tract is one of the first structures defined in the developing embryo. Gut length proceeds rapidly throughout fetal life and for the first years of life. The proton pump is present at 13 weeks of gestation. Intrinsic factor and pepsin are identifiable a few weeks later (Fig. 14-1). Even in ELBW premature infants, the gastric pH can be lowered to 4.0. Digestive enzymes are capable of intraluminal digestion of fat, protein, and carbohydrates.

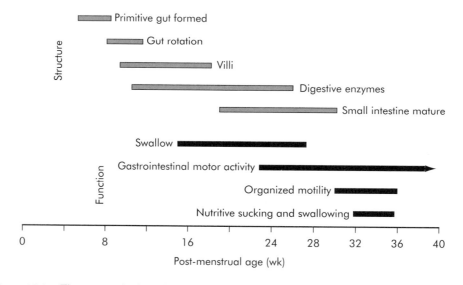

Figure 14-1. The ontogenic timetable showing structural and functional gastrointestinal development. (Modified from Newell SJ: Enternal feeding of the micropremie. Clin Perinatol 27:221, 2000.)

Although pancreatic lipase and bile salts are minimal in ELBW infants, the introduction of mother's milk will stimulate maturation and also provide lipases and other digestive enzymes.

The intestinal villae and cellular differentiation occur at about 10 to 12 weeks' gestation and begin a complex interrelationship with developing epithelium and the mesoderm according to Newell.[103] Lactase and other carbohydrate enzymes begin to appear. Gut motility is believed to appear first as irregular gastrointestinal activity at 23 weeks progressing to organized motility at about 28 weeks. Most studies of nutritive sucking and swallowing are done with artificial feeding with a bottle. Suckling at the breast, which begins with peristaltic motion of the tongue and continues down the esophagus, has been initiated by breastfeeding as early as 28 weeks.

Gastric emptying in the premature infant is slow, generating the impression that feedings are not tolerated. Gastric emptying is enhanced by human milk and slowed by formula and increased osmolarity (Table 14-1). Half emptying time with human milk is reported to be as rapid as 20 to 40 minutes.[72] Ultrasound studies have assessed small volume feeds. Some premature infants show delayed antral distention following a nasogastric feeding with emptying following a curvilinear pattern after an initial rapid phase.

Maturation of the small intestinal motility, and hence tolerance of feeds, is enhanced by previous exposure of the gut to nutrition. Early feeding precipitates preferential maturation and thus a more mature response to feeds. Total gut transit time in the premature infant varies from 1 to 5 days and is more rapid in those who have received food.[11] In those under 28 weeks, it takes 3 days to pass meconium. Breast milk feedings, however, increase motility and stool passage.[131]

When prematurity is complicated by intrauterine growth failure (IUGR), the resultant cascade of events includes decreased splanchnic circulation and oligohydramnios, poor gut perfusion, decreased growth of the small intestine and pancreas culminating in a fetal echogenic gut, and poor intestinal motility resulting in poor tolerance to milk feeds. It is not uncommon for this to result in necrotizing enterocolitis (NEC). These events require careful consideration, including the choice to use mother's milk, especially beginning with colostrum.

Although feeding regimens vary, there is almost universal agreement that mother's milk is preferred. The challenge is increasing the availability of mother's milk.

Initiation of enteral feeds

When feedings are delayed in any newborn, luminal starvation results in epithelial cell atrophy. Lung injury may aggravate this because of multiorgan system dysfunction, increasing the risk of intestinal mucosal injury and associated barrier

---

TABLE 14-1   Factors affecting gastric emptying

Faster gastric emptying	No effect	Slower gastric emptying
Breast milk	Phototherapy	Prematurity
Glucose polymers	Feed temperature	Formula milk
Starch	Nonnutritive sucking	Caloric density
Medium-chain triglycerides		Fatty acids
Prone position		Dextrose concentration
		Long-chain triglycerides
		Osmolality
		Illness

From Newell SJ: Enteral feeding of the micropremie. Clin Perinatol 27:221, 2000.

dysfunction. The ultimate injury would be the invasion of bacteria from the gut lumen.[18] Initiating feeds is a delicate balance between insufficient feeds that fail to trigger gut maturation and excessive feeds that overwhelm the digestive capacity. Excessive feeds too can result in bacterial overgrowth and injury to the brush border.[18]

In the words of Lucas,[81] "It is fundamentally unphysiological to deprive an infant of any gestation of enteral feeding since the deprivation would never normally occur at any stage." This statement is based on the fact that the fetus normally makes sucking motions and swallows amniotic fluid from early gestation. This may even have a trophic effect on the gut. By the third trimester, the infant is swallowing up to 150 mL/kg/day, which actually provides as much as 3 g/kg of protein per day. The secretion of gastrointestinal hormones is believed to occur in response to the first postdelivery feedings.[125] In animals, after only a few days of deprivation of enteral feeds, atrophic changes take place in the gut.[83] In human infants who have never received enteral feedings, there are no gut peptide surges, not even those of the trophic hormones enteroglucagon, gastrin, and gastric inhibitory polypeptide.[62] These hormones are believed to be key to the activation of the enteroinsular axis (Table 14-2).[83]

Although early enteral feedings are by no means universally accepted, a number of randomized controlled studies support the concept.[31,52] Berseth[10] reports that the response of the preterm infant's intestine to entire feedings at different postnatal ages showed significantly more mature motor patterns of the gut as well as higher plasma concentrations of gastrin and gastric inhibitory peptide. From a management standpoint, early-fed infants were able to tolerate full oral feeds sooner, had fewer days of feeding intolerance, and required shorter hospital stays.[93] Studies varied from infants who were fed under 24 hours of age at 1 mL/hour to infants who were fed full feeds starting at days 2 to 7 compared to infants on usual delayed protocols. All showed an advantage to early feeds.[83]

Requirements of the ELBW infant begin with water, the first great need, followed by energy requirements of 120 kcal/kg/day to meet metabolic and growth rates. Protein is key, as the ELBW infant missed the last trimester, when protein and fat are stored. To stop catabolism and promote protein accretion, Brumberg and LaGamma[18] recommend 3.5 to 4 g/kg/day of protein, presuming a daily loss of 1.1 to 1.5 g/kg of stored protein per day. Protein should start early either orally or by parenteral nutrition.

Human milk is the preferred feeding for all infants, including premature and sick newborns with rare exception according to the American Academy of Pediatrics (AAP) and the Institute of Medicine (IOM).

Gross and Slagle[52] pointed out that human milk is better than formula in early feeds, in establishing

---

TABLE 14-2 The biology of the gut in VLBW infants

- Swallows amniotic fluid daily, up to 150 mL/kg/day
- Potential for gut atrophy if not fed
- All of gastrointestinal track is immature
- Enzymes and nutrients in human milk enhance maturation
- Higher total body water, muscle mass, growth accretion rates, and oxygen consumption
- Higher evaporative water loss due to greater surface area
- Prone to hyperglycemia due to poor insulin response
- Lower brown fat reserves and glycogen stores
- Immature thyroid control of metabolic rate

VLBW, very low birth weight.

Modified from Brumberg H, LaGamma EF: Perspectives on nutrition: Enhance outcomes for premature infants. Pediatric Annals 32: 617, 2003.

enteral tolerance and discontinuation of parenteral nutrition, in long-term improved neurodevelopmental outcome, and in the psychological benefit to the mother. They found that human milk fell short after 4 to 6 weeks in the amount of protein, calcium, and phosphorus, a problem solvable with use of human milk fortifier. No substitute has been developed that replaces the many and varied advantages of human milk, however.

Many investigators have concluded that minimal enteral feedings with human milk can optimize growth, development, and progress for small premature infants, even if ventilator dependent.[2,62,83,118] In most studies the incidence of NEC has been similar with and without early feeds.[81] The presence of an umbilical catheter has long been a contraindication to feeding because of the risk of NEC. When Davey and associates[27] investigated this question, the incidence of NEC was comparable in infants with and without umbilical catheters.

Other advantages of early feeds include lower serum direct and indirect bilirubin and less phototherapy. Benefits from early feeds were measurable with raw maternal milk, pasteurized premature milk, and even infant formula.[62,118]

Low-birth-weight infants

All premature infants are not the same. Infants who are born weighing less than 2500 g are referred to as being *low birth weight* (LBW). If the infants are less than 37 weeks of gestation, they are *premature;* if they are full term and LBW, they are *small for gestational age* (SGA).

Very low birth weight (VLBW) refers to an infant weighing less than 1500 g. The probability of survival has changed dramatically in all weight ranges. With the availability of surfactant for respiratory distress, infants between 500 and 1000 g are surviving in greater numbers. The problems of nutrition, however, pose new challenges to the neonatologist. The feedings appropriate for a 2000-g premature infant vary only in volume and frequency from the full-term infant in most cases. Feedings for a VLBW infant must address the advantages and disadvantages of human milk at

this point in their growth curve. The composition of mother's milk varies in some constituents with the degree of prematurity (Box 14-1).[60]

The advantages of human milk for the LBW infant include the physiologic amino acid and fat profile,[16] the digestibility and absorption of these proteins and fats,[122] and the low renal solute load.[119] The presence of active enzymes enhances the maturation and supplements the enzyme activity of this underdeveloped gut. The antiinfective properties and living cells protect the immature infant from infection and may even protect against NEC. The psychological benefit to the mother who can participate in her infant's care by providing her milk is a less tangible but no less important advantage.

The disadvantages are the gap in certain nutrients that have been estimated to be required for adequate growth, which include the volume of total protein and macrominerals, especially calcium and phosphorus.[37-39] Much of the attention to the shortcomings has been based on work done using pooled milk samples collected from women whose infants are full term and many months old. The source of the human milk and processing—freezing or pasteurizing—are significant to the question of

---

BOX 14-1   Milk of mothers who deliver preterm

Level increased in preterm	Level unchanged in preterm
Total nitrogen	Volume
Protein nitrogen	Calories
Long-chain fatty acids	Lactose (? less)
Medium-chain fatty acids	Fat (?) by "creamatocrit"
Short-chain fatty acids	Linolenic acid
Sodium	Potassium
Chloride	Calcium
Magnesium (?)	Phosphorus
Iron	Copper
	Zinc
	Osmolality
	Vitamin B_{1-12}

nutritional adequacies. In the last decade, many laboratory and clinical scientists have studied the questions posed here and provided hundreds of reports regarding the nutrition and nurturance of the LBW and VLBW infant. Only a fraction of the resources can be referenced here.[41]

Optimal growth for premature infants

Optimal growth for infants born prematurely is considered to be the growth curve they would have followed had they remained in utero (Fig. 14-2 and Tables 14-3 and 14-4).[39] Achieving this goal utilizing the immature intestinal tract requires that the nutrients be digestible and absorbable and not impose a significant metabolic stress on the other immature organs, especially the kidney. Although human milk provides the ideal nutrients, it would require an inordinate nonphysiologic volume to achieve adequate amounts of some nutrients without calculated supplementation. To fill these growth needs, one can use an artificial or chemical formula or use human milk as a base, with all its advantages, and add the deficient nutrients to it.

Special properties of preterm milk

The identification of special quantitative differences in nutrients in the milk of mothers who delivered prematurely brought new interest in the use of human milk for premature infants (see Box 14-1). Many investigators have contributed to the pool of knowledge after the initial revelations in 1980 by Atkinson and associates, who reported the nitrogen concentration of milk from mothers of premature infants to be greater than that of milk from mothers delivering at term.[7,8,13,60]

Preterm milk is higher in protein content during the first months of lactation, containing between 1.8 and 2.4 g/dL. Preterm milk contains similar fat in quality and quantity,[53] although Anderson and associates[5] reported increased values for preterm milk over term milk. Lactose in preterm milk averages 5.96 g/dL and up to 6.95 g/dL at 28 days, whereas

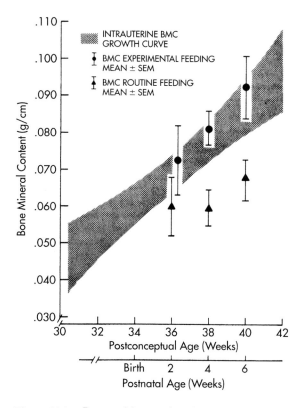

Figure 14-2. Postnatal bone mineral content (BMC) in 33- to 35-week-old appropriate-for-gestational-age/preterm infants compared with intrauterine bone mineralization curve (IUBMC). Regression curve and 95th-percentile confidence limits for regression for BMC of infants born at different gestational ages (30 to 42 weeks' gestational age) represent IUBMC. Infants fed routine cow milk formula (*solid triangles*) had significantly lower BMC than infants fed standard formula supplemented with calcium and phosphorus (*solid circles*). In these infants, BMC was not different from IUBMC at 4 and 6 weeks' postnatal age. (From Steichen JJ, Gratton TL, Tsang RC: Osteopenia of prematurity: the cause and possible treatment. J Pediatr 96:528, 1980).

the values in term milk are 6.16 and 7.26 g/dL, respectively. Preterm milk has higher energy than term milk, 58 to 70 kcal/dL, compared with 48 to 64 kcal/dL over the first month post partum (Fig. 14-3).

The macronutrients calcium and phosphorus are slightly higher in preterm milk (14 to 16 mEq/L vs. 13 to 16 mEq/L calcium and 4.7 to 5.5 mM/L vs.

TABLE 14-3   Estimated requirements and advisable intakes for protein by infant's weight as derived by factorial approach

Birthweight range	Tissue increment (per day)	Dermal loss (per day)	Urine loss (per day)	Intestinal absorption (% intake)	Estimated requirement (per day)	Advisable intake		
						Per day	Per kg[*]	Per 100 kcal[†]
800–1200 g	2.32 g	0.17 g	0.68 g	87 g[†]	3.64 g	4.0 g	4.0 g	3.1 g
1200–1800 g	3.01 g	0.25 g	0.90 g	87 g	4.78 g	5.2 g	3.5 g	2.7 g

[*]Assuming body weight of 1000 g and 1500 g for 800-g to 1200-g infant and 1200-g to 1800-g infant, respectively.
[†]Assuming calorie intake of 120 kcal/day.
From Ziegler EE, Biga RL, Fomon SJ: Nutritional requirements of the premature infant. In Suskind RM: Textbook of Pediatric Nutrition, New York, Raven, 1981, pp. 29–39.

4.0 to 5.1 mM/L phosphorus). Neither term nor preterm milk has adequate calcium and phosphorus for the VLBW infant. Magnesium levels in preterm milk are 28 to 31 mg/L, dropping to 25 mg/L at 28 days, and term milk levels are 25 to 29 mg/L. Zinc levels are higher in preterm milk, beginning at 5.3 mg/L and dropping to 3.9 mg/L, whereas term milk begins at 5.4 mg/L and drops to 2.6 mg/L. Sodium levels in preterm milk are higher (26.6 mEq/L, dropping to 12.6 mEq/L) whereas term milk is 22.3 mEq/L, decreasing to 8.5 mEq/L at 28 days.[115] Chloride has a similar average (preterm 31.6 mEq/L decreasing to 16.8 mEq/L and term 26.9 mEq/L decreasing to 13.1 mEq/L).

Requirements for growth in premature infants

The *whey protein* in human milk is an advantage for all infants but especially for the premature

TABLE 14-4   Accumulation of various components during last trimester of pregnancy

Component	Accumulation during various stages of gestation				
	26–31 wk	31–33 wk	33–35 wk	35–38 wk	38–40 wk
Body weight (g)[*]	500	500	500	500	
Water (g)	410	350	320	240	220
Fat (g)	25	65	85	175	200
Nitrogen (g)	11	12	12	6	7
Calcium (g)	4	5	5	5	5
Phosphorus (g)	2.2	2.6	2.8	3.0	3.0
Magnesium (mg)	130	110	120	120	80
Sodium (mEq)	35	25	40	40	40
Potassium (mEq)	19	24	26	20	20
Chloride (mEq)	30	24	10	20	10
Iron (mg)	36	60	60	40	20
Copper (mg)	2.1	2.4	2.0	2.0	2.0
Zinc (mg)	9.0	10.0	8.0	7.0	3.0

[*]Body weight of 26-week fetus is 1000 g and of 40-week fetus is 3500 g.
Modified from data of Widdowson, from Heird WC, Anderson TL: Nutritional requirements and methods of feeding low birth weight infants. In Gluck L et al (eds): Current Problems in Pediatrics, Vol. 7, No. 8, Chicago, Year Book, 1977, pp. 1–4.

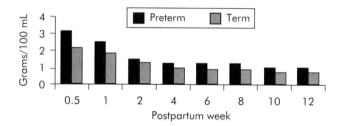

Figure 14-3. Protein content of human milk. (Data from Butte NF, Garza C, Johnson CA, et al: Longitudinal changes in milk composition of mothers delivering preterm and term infants. Early Hum Dev 9:153, 1984; Gross SJ, David RJ, Bauman L, Tomarelli RM: Nutritional composition of milk produced by mothers delivering preterm. J Pediatr 96:641, 1980.)

infant. It includes the nine amino acids known to be essential to all humans, as well as taurine,[122] glycine, leucine, and cystine, which are considered essential for the premature infant.[112] The premature infant lacks the necessary enzymes for metabolism and has been noted to accumulate nonphysiologic levels of methionine, tyrosine, phenylalanine, blood urea, and ammonia. The protein requirement for the LBW infant based on intrauterine accretion rates is 2.5 g/100 kcal or 325 mg/kg of body weight/day.[119] Metabolizable energy requirement is 109 kcal/kg/day.

A diurnal variation in the creamatocrits (see chapter 21) of expressed breast milk of mothers delivering prematurely was demonstrated in 23 mothers by Lubetsky and associates.[79] The creamatocrit was significantly higher in the evening, 7.2 ± 2.0% compared to first morning samples, 5.4% ± 1.2% ($p < 0.001$) regardless of gestational age or birth weight.

The requirement for fat is based on the *essential fatty acid* proportion as 3% of total caloric intake. Human milk has high levels of linoleic acid (9% of lipids) and adequately meets this requirement. Human milk fat is more readily absorbed in the presence of milk lipase and other enzymes in human milk. It is reported that infants under 1500 g absorb 90% of human milk fat and 68% of cow milk formula fats.[114]

Fat digestion is very efficient in LBW infants who receive their own mother's milk fresh and untreated. Fat absorption is decreased by calcium supplementation, however, and by sterilizing the

milk, which decreases lipase activity. If human milk is supplemented with lipids, it will change the vitamin E/polyunsaturated fatty acid (PUFA) ratio. Vitamin E may need to be added to keep the E/PUFA ratio greater than 0.6 (human milk E/PUFA is 0.9 normally).[58]

Special attributes of human milk for VLBW infants have been confirmed as investigators inspect the value of adding nutrients to formulas specifically for these infants.[128] In a study of omega-3 (ω-3) fatty acids on retinal function, using electroretinograms, human milk was associated with the best function, followed by formula supplemented with ω-3 fatty acids. This supports the concept that ω-3 fatty acids are essential to retinal development.[14]

Preterm and term milk do not contain sufficient calcium and phosphorus for bone accretion. *Rickets* has developed in LBW infants who are not supplemented, because the requirement for bone growth at this point in the growth curve is high. *Calcium* and *phosphorus* fetal accretion increases steadily over the last trimester. *Magnesium* accretion is unchanged in that period.

Mineral accretion is a complex phenomenon dependent on a number of variables beyond simple levels of calcium, phosphorus, magnesium, and vitamin D.[1] Absorption and retention are altered by the quantities of other minerals as well as other nutrients, including fat, protein, and carbohydrate. Although the calcium/phosphorus ratio in human milk is more physiologic than that of cow milk, the low levels of phosphorus may lead to loss of calcium in the urine.[117]

Even with optimal vitamin D and magnesium, the amount of calcium absorbed from preterm milk is not enough to meet intrauterine accretion rates without supplementation.[119] Because human milk phosphorus levels are low, even with high intestinal absorption and high renal tubular reabsorption, compared with the needs of the premature infant, supplementation is necessary to avoid depletion or deficiency.[19] Intrauterine accretion rates for calcium and phosphorus were achieved when Schanler and Abrams[112] fed human milk supplemented with calcium gluconate and glycerophosphate to VLBW infants. In their study, supplementation with magnesium was not included. The authors concluded that greater intakes of calcium and phosphorus and not improved bioavailability were responsible for the improved net retention.

Vitamin D requirements in this period of high skeletal development depend on maternal vitamin D status, because significant correlation exists between maternal serum and preterm infant cord serum 25-hydroxyvitamin D (25-OHD) values. LBW infants quickly become dependent on exogenous vitamin D because fetal storage is minimal. The recommended dietary allowance (RDA) of 400 units of vitamin D appears to be appropriate for all LBW infants, regardless of feedings, as well as for term infants. The 2004 American Academy of Pediatrics (AAP) Committee on Nutrition recommends 125 to 333 USP units of vitamin D for infants less than 1000 g and the same for more than 1000 g varying the absolute value by the actual weight—larger infants receive the larger dose.

Other vitamin needs of LBW infants depend on body stores, intestinal absorption, bioavailability of the vitamin, and rates of utilization and excretion.[40] Little information suggests that major differences exist in absorption between term and LBW infants, although fat-soluble vitamins depend on bile acids for absorption. (See Chapter 9 for vitamin requirements.) It is recommended that LBW infants receive daily vitamin supplements to address the increased need and borderline levels provided in the volume of human milk they can reasonably consume (Box 14-2).

BOX 14-2 Vitamin supplements for low birth weight infants fed human milk (HM)

Vitamin B_{12}: only if mother's diet deficient
Folic acid: HM usually adequate
Thiamin (B_1): borderline
Riboflavin (B_2): borderline
Vitamin B_6: HM usually adequate
Niacin: HM usually adequate
Vitamin A: 1000–1500 IU/day
Vitamin C: if infant receives supplementary protein up to 60 mg/day
Vitamin D: 400 IU/day
Vitamin K: all infants should receive 0.5–1.0 mg at birth; recommended 5 µg/kg/day; HM borderline
Vitamin E: 25 IU/day for first month; 5 IU/day after first month; HM adequate

Data from multiple sources.

The mineral supplementation required for LBW infants fed human milk is based on intrauterine accretion rates, which may not actually be achieved (Table 14-5). Not all premature infants fed human milk develop rickets, which occurs infrequently in infants greater than 1500 g. The VLBW infant does need supplementation, and cases of rickets are well documented in the literature for this group.[115] Supplements are usually not necessary when the infant reaches 40 weeks' postconceptual age. *Hypophosphatemia* is a sensitive biochemical indicator of low bone mineralization in VLBW infants fed human milk. Weekly measurements of serum phosphorus for the first month and biweekly until 2000 g or 40 weeks' gestation are recommended by Steichen and associates.[119] A level below 4 mg/dL should be followed by x-ray films of the wrists for osteopenia and rickets. Supplementation should be based on the infant's needs. Calcium levels should also be obtained weekly to evaluate levels above 11 mg/dL for too much calcium or too little phosphorus.[115] Supplements of calcium and phosphorus are incorporated in available human milk supplements (Tables 14-6, 14-7, and 14-8).

TABLE 14-5 **Required calcium (Ca), phosphorus (P), and magnesium (Mg) intake to meet fetal accretion rate of 27 and 30 weeks**[*]

	27 weeks			30 weeks		
	Ca	P	Mg	Ca	P	Mg
Accretion (mg/kg/day)	121	72	3.37	123	72	3.17
Retention (% intake)	50	89	59	50	89	59
Intake (mg/kg/day)	242	81	5.70	246	81	5.37

[*]Assuming a weight of 1000 g and 1250 g, respectively, in an infant fed human milk.
From Steichen JJ, Krug-Wispe SK, Tsang RC: Breastfeeding the low birth weight preterm infant. Clin Perinatol 14:131, 1987.

Trace minerals in general appear in physiologic amounts in human milk and are more bioavailable from human milk than artificial feedings. The minimum daily requirements for LBW infants are based on daily accretion rates as calculated from third-trimester data and calculated obligatory losses.

Zinc is known to be readily available in human milk, although zinc deficiency syndromes from hyperalimentation are well known in the literature and in neonatal intensive care units (NICUs). Zinc requirements are probably met by the mother's own milk, but pooled milk levels are lower because zinc levels drop from term birth through 6 months, and this milk will need supplementation.

Copper accretion requires 59 µg/kg/day, and absorption is thought to be 50% to 70%. Copper levels also decline in milk from term to 6 months post partum. It is recommended that VLBW infants receive an additional 30 to 40 µg/day of copper for the first 3 months.[119]

Manganese represents an apparent deficiency because the minimum daily requirement is calculated to be 7 µg/kg/day. The provision in human milk is 0.35 ng/mL or 0.5 µg/kg/day, but no information is available recommending supplementation.

The *selenium* suggested requirement is 1.5 to 2.5 µg/kg/day (1 µg minimum). Human milk provides 1 to 2 µg/dL and is stable throughout lactation so that no supplementation has been recommended.[49]

Iodine levels in human milk are sufficient to meet daily requirements in the LBW infant.

Chromium requirements are calculated to be 1.0 to 2.0 µg/kg/day based on an accretion rate of 0.1 to 0.2 µg/kg/day and only 10% absorption. Levels in human milk are reported to be 0.03 µg/dL, which with 150 mL/kg/day intake would supply 0.045 µg/kg/day. Supplementation is not usually provided, and absorption in human milk is probably greater than 10%.

Molybdenum levels in human milk are believed sufficient to meet LBW accretion rates (1 µg/kg/day).[119]

Iron requirements are a complex issue, and intrauterine accretion rates are not appropriate values on which to base requirements.[67,104] Iron stores partially enlarged by hemoglobin breakdown in early life will eventually be used up if no iron is provided. Providing iron, however, interferes with the immunologic properties of human milk, especially the bacteriostatic properties of lactoferrin in the gut.

The recommendations for iron supplementation for infants receiving human milk (either own mother's or donor milk, which are similar in iron) are based on age and weight of the infant. Supplementation should begin at 2 to 3 months or when birth weight has doubled. For birth weight under 1000 g, the infant should receive 4 mg elemental iron/kg/day; infants weighing 1000 to 1500 g should receive 3 mg/kg/day.[67,104]

It is necessary also to ensure adequate *vitamin C* and *vitamin E* supplementation (4 to 5 mg/day), even though human milk normally contains 5 mg/dL vitamin C and 0.25 mg/dL vitamin E.

TABLE 14-6 Composition of infant feeding using human milk with and without various supplements

	Preterm human milk*		Similac Natural Care*	50:50 Mix Similac Natural Care and preterm human milk*		Enfamil human milk fortifier (4 packets)	Enfamil human milk fortifier (4 packets) added to preterm human milk*	
Weeks post partum	1	4		1	4		1	4
Kilocalories	67	70	81	72	76	14	81	84
Protein (g)	2.44	1.81	2.1	2.27	1.96	0.7	3.14	2.5
Carbohydrate (g)	6.05	6.95	8.6	7.3	7.8	2.7	8.75	9.65
Fat (g)	3.81	4.00	3.6	3.7	3.8	0.04	3.85	4.04
Vitamin A (IU)[†]	330	230	550	440	390	780	1110	1010
Vitamin E (mg)[†]	0.9	0.25	3	2.0	1.61	3.4	4.3	3.65
Vitamin K (µg)[†]	NA	1.5	10	NA	5.8	9.1	NA	10.6
Vitamin D (IU)[†]	NA	2.5	120	NA	61	260	NA	262
Thiamin (µg)	5.4	8.9	200	103	104	187	192	196
Riboflavin (µg)	36.0	26.6	500	268	263	250	286	277
Niacin (mg)	0.11	0.21	4.0	2.1	2.1	3.1	3.2	3.3
Pyridoxine (µg)	2.6	6.2	200	101	103	193	196	199
Folate (µg)	2.1	3.1	30	16.1	16.6	23	25	26
Vitamin B_{12} (µg)	NA	0.1	0.45	NA	0.27	0.21	NA	0.3
Vitamin C (mg)[†]	7	5	30	19	18	24	31	29
Calcium (mg)	25	22	170	98	96	60	85	82
Phosphorus (mg)	14	14	85	50	50	33	47	47
Magnesium (mg)	3	2.5	10	6.5	6.3	4	7	6.5
Iron (mg)	0.1	0.1	0.3	0.2	0.2	0	0.1	0.1
Sodium (mEq)	2.2	1.3	1.7	2.0	1.5	0.3	2.5	1.6
Potassium (mEq)	1.8	1.7	2.9	2.4	2.3	0.4	2.2	2.1
Chloride (mEq)	2.5	1.6	2.0	2.3	1.8	0.5	3.0	2.1
Zinc (mg)	0.48	0.39	1.2	0.84	0.80	0.31	0.79	0.70
Copper (mg)	0.08	0.06	0.2	0.14	0.13	0.08	0.16	0.14
Manganese (µg)[†]	NA	0.4	NA	NA	NA	9	NA	9.4
Biotin (µg)	0.15	0.54	NA	NA	NA	0.8	NA	1.34
Pantothenic acid (mg)	0.16	0.23	1.5	0.83	0.87	0.79	0.95	1.02
Osmolality (mOsm/kg H_2O)[†]	302	305	300	301	303	+60	362	365

NA, Not available.

*Volume 100 mL (1 dL).

[†]Listed values for 1 and 4 weeks reflect reported values for full-term transitional and mature human milk, respectively.

TABLE 14-7   Protein, calcium, and sodium requirements by growing premature infants and composition of banked human milk

	Protein (g/100 kcal)	Calcium (mg/100 kcal)	Sodium (mEq/100 kcal)
Estimated requirements for hypothetic, growing premature infants[*]	2.54	132[†]	2.3
Composition of banked human milk	1.50	43	0.8

[*]Assumed body weight is 1200 g; weight gain, 20 g/day, energy intake, 120 kcal/kg/day. The basis for estimating requirements is described in the text.
[†]This estimate does not apply to infants fed formulas from which calcium absorption is less than 65% of intake.
From Fomon SJ, Ziegler EE, Vazquez HD: Human milk and the small premature infant. Am J Dis Child 131:463, 1977.

Brain growth and subsequent intelligence

Although physical growth and plasma levels of nutrients have been closely scrutinized by investigators following nutrition in LBW infants,[66] adequate measurement of brain growth is not currently possible except indirectly in long-range studies of neurodevelopment and intelligence. A carefully controlled, long-range study of preterm infants by Lucas and associates[87,88] over a 10-year period has produced some remarkable results. Mothers who provide their milk have a special desire to be good parents and embrace positive health behaviors, which has been suggested as the real cause of this study's measured differences. Several points deserve attention, however. LBW infants are born at a time of rapid brain growth. In fact, term infants have considerable brain growth in the first year of life, doubling the size of the brain by 1 year of age. Several nutrients in human milk have been associated with brain tissue growth, including taurine, cholesterol, ω-3 fatty acids, and amino sugars in the free and bound forms.[58] Amino sugars such as N-acetylneuraminic acid are important constituents of brain glycoproteins and gangliosides.

The Lucas study[87,88] included infants weighing less than 1850 g at birth, delivered at multiple centers, who were entered in four parallel trials of preterm feedings from 1982 to 1985. Mothers decided whether to provide their milk; the remaining infants were assigned to receive preterm formula. All feedings were by feeding tube the first 4 weeks. At both age 18 months and age 7½ to 8 years, when the children were tested by an examiner blinded to their feeding method, the children who had received their mother's milk scored better. At 18 months, they were more advanced on the Bayley Developmental Scales.[87] In a subset of the larger study, comparison groups of infants who received preterm formula were more advanced than infants who received regular formula. At the second point, 7½ to 8 years of age, using the Weschler Intelligence Scale for Children, the children who received their mother's milk had an 8.3 point

TABLE 14-8   Weight gain (g/day) supported by intake of 180 mL human milk/kg at selected body weights

	Weight gain (g/day)			
	800 g	1000 g	1500 g	2000 g
Calcium	4	5	6.7	8.4
Phosphorus	4	5	6.8	8.7
Nitrogen	10	12	16	21
Sodium	5	7	11	15
Magnesium	12	15	22	28
Chloride	22	30	48	68
Potassium	21	33	49	66

Data from Forbes GB: Nutritional adequacy of human breast milk for premature infants. In Lebenthal E (ed): Textbook of Gastroenterology and Nutrition in Infants. New York, Raven, 1981, pp 321–329.

advantage, even after adjustments for mother's education and social class ($p < 0.0001$).[88]

A subset of this large study was also reported in 1990 on infants who had been randomly assigned for 30 days to receive preterm formula, unfortified donor milk, or their mother's milk (with donor milk supplements as necessary).[87] The infants fed donor milk or those whose mothers produced less than 50% of the diet and were supplemented with donor milk were disadvantaged by 0.25 standard deviation (SD) on the developmental scales. This was not pronounced in infants with mental growth retardation. The method of collection of milk from the donors was by drip; that is, the mother fed her baby at the breast and collected milk by drip from the other breast.[87] Drip milk is low in fat and fat-soluble nutrients. Donor milk actively pumped has a higher fat and calorie content. An important feature of these studies was that they focused on the first month of life, a critical time to protect the brain and facilitate its growth.[86-88] The infants were all tube fed, thus removing the physical interaction of the breastfeeding mother. Impact of early diet on long-term neurodevelopment demands continued review and assessment. Unfortified human milk has been shown to have measurable impact on neurodevelopment, but investigation of these same parameters comparing fortification of human milk has not shown improvement over unfortified milk. Neurodevelopmental outcomes at 18 months were not affected by fortification.[85,86]

The effect of human milk on cognitive and motor development was compared to the effect of formula in a matched cohort of premature infants. Assessment at 3, 7, and 12 months corrected ages revealed higher motor scores at 3 and 7 months and higher cognitive scores at 12 months when adjusted for maternal vocabulary score on the Peabody Picture Vocabulary Tests. The improved development scores persisted.[12]

In a study of three groups of preterm infants matched for birth weight (mean 1308 g, range 640–1780 g), gestational age (mean 30.8 wk, range 26–35 wk), medical status, birth order, gender, parental age, and educational and socioeconomic level, grouped by (1) over 75% breast milk intake, (2) 25 to 75% breast milk, and (3) less than 25% breast milk, the group 1 infants scored highest, independent of whether mother's milk was given by bottle, tube, or breastfeeding. The more milk, the greater the score on the Brazelton (NBAS). The authors concluded that human milk enhances neurodevelopment quantitatively. The mothers who provided more milk were less depressed and had better interactive affiliative care styles.[33,36]

Visual function is improved in premature infants fed human milk. This is believed to be a result of the long-chain polyenic fatty acids and the antioxidant activity of human milk in β-carotene, taurine, and vitamin E.[85] The diagnosis of retinopathy of prematurity was 2.3 times greater in formula fed infants than in those fed human milk in a report by Hylander and associates.[64] Few infants fed human milk advanced to severe retinopathy, and none required cryotherapy. Results were similar in fortified and unfortified human milk feeds.

Mother's own milk has clear advantages. Donor milk is now regulated and requires pasteurization, which may destroy some valuable properties, but it is still advantageous.

Gastrointestinal characteristics of premature infants

The anatomic differentiation of the intestinal tract begins before 20 weeks' gestation, but the functional development is very limited before 26 weeks.[76] Different parts of the fetal gut develop at different times so that some nutrients are better tolerated than others (Tables 14-9 and 14-10). The present concentration of digestive enzymes determines the rate of digestion and absorption, along with the maturity of membrane carriers. (See Chapter 3 for impact of human milk on gut maturation.) The presence of active enzymes in the gut improves the digestion and absorption of human milk. As noted earlier, the gastric emptying time in preterm infants when given human milk is biphasic, with an initial fast phase in which 50% has left the stomach in the first 20 to 25 minutes.[20] After an hour, 25 mL of human milk has left the stomach. In contrast, the formula feeding follows a linear

TABLE 14-9	**Gastrointestinal tract in human fetus: first appearance of developmental markers**

Anatomic part	Developmental marker	Weeks of gestation
Esophagus	Superficial glands develop	20
	Squamous cells appear	28
Stomach	Gastric glands form	14
	Pylorus and fundus defined	14
Pancreas	Differentiation of endocrine and exocrine tissue	14
Liver	Lobules form	11
Small intestine	Crypt and villi develop	14
	Lymph nodes appear	14
Colon	Diameter increases	20
	Villi disappear	20
Stomach	Gastric motility and secretion	20
Pancreas	Zymogen (proenzyme) granules	20
Liver	Bile metabolism	11
	Bile secretion	22
Small intestine	Active transport of amino acids	14
	Glucose transport	18
	Fatty acid absorption	24
Enzymes	α-Glucosidases	10
	Dipeptidases	10
	Lactase	10
	Enterokinase	26
Functional ability		
Suckling	Mouthing only	24
Swallowing	Immature suck-swallow	26

Modified from Lebenthal E, Leung Y-K: The impact of development of the gut on infant nutrition. Pediatr Ann 16:215, 1987.

pattern, with half emptying in 51 minutes and a total of 19 mL in 1 hour.

Use of human milk for premature infants

A clear distinction must be made between an infant's own mother's milk and pooled human milk for the feeding of LBW infants. The mother's milk has some higher levels of nutrients but never lower levels than term milk. Mothers who donate to milk banks are also feeding their own infants, who may be any age from birth to 6 months (but no donor should be more than 6 months post partum). Donor milk must also be prepared by sterilization, and in

only a few milk banks is fresh or fresh-frozen donor milk ever available. An infant's own mother's milk may be fed fresh or fresh-frozen and is rarely heat treated. Chapter 21 discusses milk storage and milk banking.

When the volume of milk produced by the mother is not sufficient to meet the infant's needs each day, there is a clear need to provide additional nourishment by formula or donor milk.[48]

A 2001-g to 2500-g infant without complications may be weaned from the incubator to an open crib within 24 hours. Although the suck reflex may be poor, the infant can usually be breastfed. The infant is ready to breastfeed even if he takes a bottle poorly. If the infant can stimulate the breast briefly

TABLE 14-10 Digestion and absorption in human fetus and neonate

Factors	First detectable (week gestation)	Term neonate (% of adult)
Protein		
H$^+$ (hydrogen ion)	At birth	<30
Pepsin	16	<10
Trypsinogen	20	10–60
Chymotrypsinogen	20	10–60
Procarboxypeptidase	20	10–60
Enterokinase	26	10
Peptidases (brush border and cytosol)	<15	>100
Amino acid transport	?	>100
Macromolecular absorption	?	>100
Fat		
Lingual lipase	30	>100
Pancreatic lipase	20	5–10
Pancreatic co-lipase	?	?
Bile acids	22	50
Medium-chain triglyceride uptake	?	100
Long-chain triglyceride uptake	?	10–90
Carbohydrate		
α-Amylases		
Pancreatic	22	0
Salivary	16	10
Lactase	10	>100
Sucrase-isomaltase	10	100
Glucoamylase	10	50–100
Monosaccharide absorption	11–19	>100 (?)

From Lebenthal E, Leung Y-K: The impact of development of the gut on infant nutrition. Pediatr Ann 16:215, 1987.

and obtain the rich, antibody-containing, cell-filled colostrum, it will be protected against infection while receiving nutrition. Inadequate stimulation of the breast will require mechanical pumping after the feeding. If the infant cannot suck and must be tube fed, any colostrum the mother can manually express or pump from the breast can be given by gavage tube along with donor milk or the prescribed formula necessary for nourishment. Chapter 5 reviews the protective value of colostrum to the infant.

A study in Guatemala that was repeated in the special care nursery of the Rainbow Children's Hospital in Cleveland showed that the infection rate among sick and premature newborns was greatly diminished by providing 15 mL of human colostrum contributed by random donors daily.[28] These findings were especially dramatic in Guatemala, where the mortality rate from infection in the nursery is extremely high. It has been suggested that mixed feedings of an infant's own mother's milk and formula to necessary volume be calculated over a 24-hour period so that the infant receives some mother's milk at each feeding and a supplement of formula, in contrast to alternating feedings or using all mother's milk until it runs out and finishing the day with formula. The reasoning is based on the concept of "inoculating" every feeding with human milk to provide the enzymes and immunologic properties with each feeding. Generous levels of active enzymes in the milk will also assist in the digestion and absorption of the formula. The immunologic properties are less measurable, but the only known interference with function is the addition of iron, which blocks the effectiveness of lactoferrin. Therefore, the nutritional and infection-protective properties are also spread throughout each feeding around the clock.

The quantities of direct-acting antimicrobial factors in human milk vary according to the method of collection, processing, and storage. Donor milk's ability to protect against infection in the premature infant has not been tested in clinical studies.[42]

Supplementation of mother's own milk or pooled human milk

Although some banks can provide single-donor milk for a specific baby and resources are usually more than enough for the newborn recipient, no supplement to human milk is usually needed if the infant is over 1500 g at birth.

The options for supplementing an infant's own mother's milk depend on need for additional volume or for specific nutrients, especially protein, calcium, and phosphorus, based on birth weight and growth rates.[68,69,124]

The ideal supplementation is one using human milk nutrients and is referred to as *lactoengineering,* in which nutrient concentration is increased by adding specific nutrients derived from human milk.[41] Techniques involve use of donor milk and separating the cream and protein fractions, reducing the lactose content, and heat-treating the product by high-temperature short-time (HTST) process of pasteurization. This completely human milk product provides higher protein and energy needs so that weight gains and nitrogen retention are similar to intrauterine rates.

Using a feeding prepared from human milk protein and medium-chain triglyceride supplementation of human milk for VLBW infants was reported

by Rönnholm and associates.[107] Forty-four infants averaging 30 weeks' gestation with birth weights ranging from 710 to 1510 g were nourished by one of four protocols: plain human milk, human milk and protein, human milk and triglycerides, or human milk and protein and triglycerides. The triglycerides did not influence weight and length, but the two groups receiving added protein gained along a curve comparable with the intrauterine growth for their birth weight, gaining faster from 4 to 6 weeks than the unsupplemented infants. The protein-supplemented groups also grew more in length; however, head circumference growth was similar in all groups.[106]

Fortified mother's milk containing an infant's own mother's milk plus skim and cream components derived from mature donor milk was fed *fresh* during the first two postnatal months to 18 VLBW infants (birth weight of 1180 ± 35 g, gestation of 29 ± 0.2 weeks).[23] A comparison group of 16 VLBW infants (birth weight of 1195 g ± 30 g, gestation of 29 ± 0.1 weeks) were fed commercial formula with comparable nitrogen and energy distribution. Balance studies were performed on both groups. Growth measurements were similar in the two groups. Metabolizable energy was similar (109 kcal/kg/day) in both groups, as was fat absorption. The only recorded difference was a high serum calcium but lower serum phosphorus in the mother's milk group.

Total protein is usually calculated by determining the total nitrogen content (Kjeldahl method) and multiplying the number by the protein factor (6.25). Total protein corrected for nonprotein nitrogen (NPN), which is high in human milk, is true protein.[9] *True protein* is a heterogeneous mixture of casein and whey proteins. All caseins but not all whey proteins have nutritional value. Whey proteins include lactoferrin, immunoglobulins, and lysozyme. True protein minus those more or less indigestible proteins is called *digestible protein.* Analysis of preterm milk by Beijers and associates[9] demonstrated that NPN was dependent on the degree of prematurity and averaged 20% to 25%, increasing over the time of lactation. Only 30% to 60% of total protein is available for synthesis. However, in absolute amounts over lactation time, it remains stable.

Schanler and Garza[113] compared plasma amino acid levels in VLBW infants (mean age 16 days, mean birth weight 1180 g, mean gestation 29 weeks) fed either human milk fortified with human milk or whey-dominant cow milk formula. The infants received continuous enteral infusions of isonitrogenous, isocaloric preparations. Taurine and cystine were significantly higher in the human milk fed infants, and threonine, valine, methionine, and lysine were significantly higher in the formula fed infants.[108]

The authors[113] suggest that synthesis of specific functional proteins in the cow milk protein-based formula fed to VLBW infants requires further review. Human milk supplements for human milk may someday be commercially available and are ideal from most standards.[113-115]

Artificial fortification of human milk

Supplementing an infant's own mother's milk with specially prepared formula supplements is an alternative that still provides the riches of human milk.[127] Available commercial preparations for such supplementation are intended to complement human milk and not to be used as an exclusive formula. When multicomponent fortified human milk for promoting growth in preterm infants was examined in a Cochrane Review,[73] the authors found short-term increases in weight gain, linear growth, and head circumference. There was no effect on serum alkaline phosphatase levels, and the effect on bone mineral content was unclear. Nitrogen retention and blood urea levels were increased. Conclusions about long-term neurodevelopmental and growth outcomes were limited by insufficient data beyond 1 year. so adverse effects were confirmed, however. The significance of increased blood urea nitrogen and blood pH levels was unclear. The authors suggest that efforts should be directed at finding the best preparation and measuring both short-term and long-term outcomes. Preparations are different and are used differently (see Table 14-6). The powdered supplement is intended to add special nutrients to an adequate

volume of mother's own milk (Enfamil human milk fortifier or Similac human milk fortifier), or it can be used to enhance pooled donor human milk. Neither fortifier contains fat. Milk fortification extends the mother's milk and provides additional nitrogen, calcium, phosphorus, and vitamins for an LBW infant.[17] If an infant is fed the mother's milk, pooled donor milk, and a fortifier, the sum total should meet the infant's daily requirements (see Table 14-7).

Studies comparing fortified mother's milk with premature infant formulas have shown comparable growth in weight, length, and head circumference, making it possible to retain the many advantages of mother's milk while providing the additional nutrients for appropriate accretion rates.[120]

Trials have been conducted. When powdered fortifier was added to mother's milk, the supplemented infants had significantly greater weight gain, linear growth, and head circumference growth than those not supplemented.[44] The supplemented infants also had higher blood urea nitrogen levels (Table 14-11).[49]

When a preterm infant's own mother's milk was fortified with protein (0.85 g/dL), calcium (90

TABLE 14-11   Fortified vs. unfortified human milk

13 studies, 596 infants; randomized*

Growth	Fortified
❑ Weight gain	+ 3.7 g/kg/d
❑ Length	+ 0.13 cm/wk
❑ Head circumference	+ 0.12 cm/wk
Bone mineral content	+ 8.3 mg/cm
Nitrogen balance	+ 66 mg/kg/d
BUN	+ 5.8 mg/dL
Necrotizing enterocolitis	no significant difference
Feeding tolerance	no significant difference

*Some comparisons with partial supplements.
BUN, blood urea nitrogen
From Kuschel CA, Harding JE: Multicomponent fortified human milk for promoting growth in preterm infants (Cochrane Review). In Cochrane Library, Issue 4. Chichester, UK, John Wiley and Sons, 2004.

mg/dL), and phosphorus (45 mg/dL), the rate of weight gain was greater than that of the unfortified group and comparable with that of the Similac Natural Care formula group.[44-46] Bone mineralization improved over the 6 weeks of the study but did not reach the intrauterine accretion rate of 150 mg/kg/day. A relative phosphorus deficiency occurred in the human milk groups both with and without supplementation. Greer and McCormick[44] conclude that fortifying preterm mother's milk permits biochemically adequate growth comparable with that provided by special care formula. Similar results using fortified human milk have been obtained by other investigators (Table 14-12).[55]

The effect of calcium supplementation on fatty acid balance studies in LBW infants fed human milk or formula has been shown to be significant by Chappell and associates.[23] They showed a decrease in total fatty acid absorption both in LBW infants fed their own mother's milk and in formula fed infants when calcium was added. Fecal output of fat and fatty acid excretion were higher in the formula fed infants. In mother's milk–fed infants, total fat absorption and coefficient of absorption were higher.

Preterm milk with routine multivitamin supplementation (providing 4.1 mg of tocopherol) uniformly resulted in vitamin sufficiency in VLBW infants when they received iron, as well as when they were not iron supplemented, in a control study by Gross and Gabriel.[51] VLBW infants were fed preterm milk, bank milk, or formula, utilizing 2 mg/day of iron. Vitamin E content of preterm milk does not differ significantly from that of term human milk from days 3 to 36.[58]

Jocson and associates[70] studied the effects of nutrient fortification and varying storage conditions on host-defense properties of human milk. Total bacterial colony counts and immunoglobulin A (IgA) were not affected by the addition of fortifier.

A novel fortification scheme for human milk was compared with the traditional system of fortification and a group of infants receiving human milk fortifier. To achieve a better match between individual infant needs and actual intakes, Moro and associates[96] designed a regimen in which the amount of fortifier is based on the infant's metabolic response, which is monitored by frequent determinations of serum urea nitrogen (SUN). Twelve infants were studied with each of the three

TABLE 14-12   Comparison of selected fortifiers for human milk (prepared per 100 mL milk)

Fortifier	PrHM	EHMF	SNC	Eoprotin*	S-26/SMA HMF	FM85[†]	SHMF
Energy (kJ) (kcal)	298(71)	357(85)	319(76)	357(85)	361(86)	374(89)	357(85)
Fat (g)	3.6	3.6[‡]	4.0	3.6[‡]	3.65	3.6	4.0
Carbohydrate (g)	7.0	9.7	7.8	9.8	9.4	10.6	8.8
Protein (g)	1.8	2.5	2.0	2.6	2.8	2.6	2.8
Calcium (mg)	22	112	97	72	112	73	139
Phosphorus (mg)	14	59	50	48	59	48	81
Magnesium (mg)	2.5	3.5	6.3	5.3	4.0	4.5	9.5
Sodium (mEq)	0.7	1.0	1.1	1.9	1.1	1.9	1.35
Zinc (μg)	320	1030	760	320[‡]	450	320[‡]	1320
Copper (μg)	60	122	1045	60[‡]	60[‡]	60[‡]	230
Vitamins	Yes	Multi[§]	Multi[§]	A, C, E, K	Multi[§]	Multi[§]	Multi[§]

*Milupa, Friedrichsdorf, Germany.
[†]Nestle, Vevey, Switzerland.
[‡]Nutrient not contained in fortifier.
[§]Multivitamins: A, D, E, K, B_1, B_2, B_6, C, niacin, folate, B_{12}, pantothenate, and biotin.
PrHM, Preterm human milk; EHMF, Enfamil Human Milk Fortifier (Mead Johnson Nutritionals, Evansville, IN); SNC, Similac Natural Care (Ross Laboratories, Columbus, OH) mixed 1:1 (vol:vol) with PrHM; S-26/SMA HMF, SMA Human Milk Fortifier (Wyeth Nutritionals, Philadelphia, PA); SHMF, Similac Human Milk Fortifier (Ross Laboratories, Columbus, OH).
From Schanler RJ: The use of human milk for premature infants. Pediatr Clin North Am 48: 207, 2001.

regimens—traditional, adjusted fortification, and human milk protein fortification—for 3 weeks. Protein intake was generally higher and weight gain somewhat higher in the adjusted-fortification group. SUN was also higher in this group, as were calcium, phosphorus, and potassium. Plasma amino acid levels were also increased but not out of range. The authors conclude that adjustable fortification is feasible and safe but needs further work. In general the adjusted fortifier was equivalent to human milk fortifier.[96]

The effect of powdered human milk fortifiers on the antibacterial actions of human milk were explored by Chan.[21] Human milk inhibited the growth of *Escherichia coli* (EC), *Staphylococcus aureus* (SA), *Enterobacter sakazakii* (ES), and group B *Streptococcus* (GBS) when Enfamil and Similac human milk fortifiers (EHMF and SHMF) were mixed with human milk and medium-chain triglycerides (MCT) and 1.09 mg ferrous sulfate in 25 mL milk. The fortifiers containing iron and the iron alone inhibited the protective effect of human milk against the bacteria. The probable explanation is the interference of the iron with the protective action of lactoferrin in human milk. The ferrous iron in the fortifier is changed to ferric state in human milk and that readily binds with lactoferrin. The effect was strongest with EHMF with iron and iron alone.

Long-term follow-up of growth parameters in VLBW infants

Weight gain and growth in length and head circumference are similar in VLBW infants breastfed or given standard formula after discharge.[126] *Bone mineral content* (BMC) was also followed at 10, 16, and 25 postnatal weeks in those NICU graduates who had formerly received fortified human milk. At 16 and 25 weeks the breastfed infants had lower BMC and BMC/bone width ratio and serum phosphorus concentration and higher alkaline phosphatase activity than the formula fed group. These data suggest a need to monitor this select group of VLBW infants very carefully for suboptimal bone accretion while receiving their mother's milk.[59]

Reduced bone mineralization is common in preterm infants and has been associated with growth stunting at 18 months of age and dietary insufficiency of calcium and phosphorus. Bishop and associates[15] evaluated 54 children at a mean age of 5 years who were born prematurely and had been part of a longitudinal dietary growth study. The diets included were banked donor milk or preterm formula as a supplement to mother's own milk. Increasing human milk intake was strongly associated with better BMC. Those children who had the greater proportion of human milk had greater BMC than children born at term; that is, supplementing with donor milk produced a better outcome at age 5 years than supplementing with infant formula, even though the nutrient content of formula was greater. The authors[15] suggest that the early nutritional environment of the preterm infant could play an important role in determining later skeletal growth and mineralization.

Iron status has also been studied in LBW infants at 6 months' chronologic age. The incidence of iron deficiency was 86% in the breastfed group of LBW and only 33% in those receiving iron-fortified formula.[1] The breastfed group had significantly lower serum ferritin and hemoglobin values at 4 months of age. The authors[1] recommend that these special breastfed infants should receive iron from 2 months of age because they have a risk of developing iron deficiency not seen in term infants.

Late *hypertriglyceridemia* was detected in a group of VLBW infants fully breastfed at home after premature births (30 weeks) and with a mean birth weight of 1140 g.[45] Blood samples were collected at 31, 33, and 35 days postconceptual age and 6 weeks after hospital discharge. During hospitalization triglycerides averaged 153 to 166 mg/dL. The mean fat content of the mother's milk was 3.2 to 3.4 g/dL and mean fat intake 5.0 to 5.5 g/kg/day. At home the infants fed human milk received ad lib feedings at the breast, and the formula fed infants received standard 20 kcal/oz (81 kcal/dL) formula with 3.6 g/dL fat. Six of the 13 LBW infants fed human milk had serum triglyceride concentrations greater than 300 mg/dL, none of the formula fed infants had levels over 300 mg/dL, and only three were less than 200 mg/dL. Only 2 of 25 term breastfed infants had levels greater than 300 mg/dL. Three LBW infants had levels over 700 mg/dL and demonstrated hyperchylomicronemia. The meaning of these findings is unclear, but these parameters deserve watching.[45] The role of lipase and postheparin plasma lipolytic activity is undetermined.

The feeding of these special VLBW infants after discharge and for the next 6 to 9 months is an important consideration. Although no data yet exist on breastfeeding with added supplementation, there are some important results from a randomized double-blind trial of the effect of supplementary standard formula feedings.[82] Growth and clinical status of infants receiving nutrient-enriched "postdischarge" formula were significantly affected, without vomiting, gas, or stool problems. The group receiving the enriched formula ingested volumes similar to those receiving regular formula. The neurodevelopmental status of these infants is being studied.[82] Box 14-3 lists recommendations modified from the work of Steichen and associates[119] and Schanler and Hurst.[116]

Antimicrobial properties of preterm breast milk

The infection-protective properties of human milk have been considered a key reason to provide human milk to high-risk infants who are prone to devastating infections such as NEC, sepsis, meningitis, and viral infections such as respiratory syncytial virus (RSV) and rotavirus. The antimicrobial properties of milk produced by mothers who deliver preterm have been studied by several investigators.

The antiinfective factors in preterm human colostrum were studied by Mathur and associates,[91] who compared the colostrum values of a comparable group of postpartum mothers. The mean concentrations of IgA, lysozyme, and lactoferrin were significantly higher than in full-term colostrum. IgG and IgM were similar in both groups. The absolute counts of total cells, macrophages, lymphocytes, and neutrophils were significantly higher in preterm colostrum. The mean percentage of IgA

BOX 14-3   Feeding schedule for human milk in low-birth-weight infants

1. Use *refrigerated milk* from the preterm infant's mother when it is available and has been collected within 48 hours of feeding.
2. When fresh milk is not available, use *frozen human milk* from the infant's mother. This milk should be provided in the sequence that it was collected to provide the greatest nutritional benefit.
3. When the preterm infant is tolerating human milk at greater than 100 mL/kg/day, supplementation using a human milk *fortifier* is started.
   a. If it requires more than 1 week to reach 100 mL/kg/day intake, fortifier is added even though volume tolerance has not been achieved.
   b. Milk volumes should increase to 150 but not exceed 200 mL/kg/day. Weight gain is optimally 15 g/kg/day and length increment 1.0 cm/wk. Urinary excretion of calcium should be less than 6 mg/kg/day and phosphorus greater than 4 mg/kg/day.

   c. If weight gain is less than 15 g/kg/day, hindmilk is used if mother's milk production exceeds the infant's requirements by 30%.
4. If the mother's milk supply is inadequate to meet her infant's feeding needs, an *infant formula* designed for preterm feeding is used as described.
5. *Fortification of human milk* is recommended until the infant is taking all feedings from the breast directly or weighs 1800 g to 2000 g, depending on nursery policy on infant discharge weight. During the transition from feeding human milk by gavage or bottle and nipple to feeding at the breast, only those feedings given by gavage or bottle require fortification.
6. *Multivitamin supplementation* is started once feeding tolerance has been established. This supplementation varies depending on the composition of human milk fortifier.
7. *Iron supplementation* providing 2 mg/kg/day is started by the time the infant has doubled birth weight.

in the premature colostrum was also significantly higher. The degree of prematurity had no effect, although the study group ranged in gestation from 28 to 36 weeks (mean 33 ± 2.1 weeks) compared with the control infants, who were at 38 to 40 weeks (mean 39.1 ± 0.8 weeks). Colostrum of preterm mothers had even greater potential for preventing infection than term colostrum and is an additional reason to begin early enteral feeds with human colostrum.[91] Table 14-13 lists the specific antiinfective components.

The cells of preterm milk were compared with those of term milk and found to be similar in number and in capacity to phagocytose and kill staphylococci.[99] The ability of the preterm cells to produce interferon on stimulation with mitogens was marginally better than that of term cells. The cells survived 24 hours refrigerated at 4° C (39.2° F); at 48 hours, cell number, but not function, was reduced. Passing the milk through a feeding tube did not diminish the number or function of the cells. The levels of lactoferrin and lysozyme were greater in preterm milk than in term milk from the second to the 12th week post partum.[43]

Secretory IgA (sIgA) was the predominant form of IgA, and values increased from the sixth to the 12th week in preterm milk. The increase in IgA was not dependent on method of collection, rate of flow, or time of day, but the concentration varied inversely with the milk volume; thus, total production of IgA

in 24 hours is thought by some investigators to be comparable for the two groups.[22,50] When preterm (31 to 36 weeks' gestation) infants were fed human milk and compared with a matched group of premature infants fed infant formula, the serum levels of IgA at 9 to 13 weeks were higher in the formula fed infants.[109] Those infants who received at least 60% of their own mother's milk had higher IgA levels at 3 weeks of age than those receiving less than 30% of the feedings from their mother's milk.

Serum IgG levels were higher in the breast milk group, and serum IgM levels were similar in the two feeding groups. Samples of precolostrum collected from undelivered mothers were assayed and found to contain equal or greater amounts of IgA, IgG, IgM, lactoferrin, and lysozyme as mature colostrum.[78]

When the impact on actual prevention of infection among premature infants is reviewed, significantly less infection is found in infants receiving human milk as compared with those receiving formula (9 of 32 receiving breast milk, 28.1%; 24 of 38 receiving formula, 63.3%).[101] In a prospective evaluation of the antiinfective property of varying quantities of expressed human milk for high-risk LBW infants, infections were found to be significantly less in the groups that received human milk.[121]

NEC is a major cause of morbidity and death in preterm and other high-risk infants. The absolute

TABLE 14-13   Comparison of antiinfective properties in colostrum of preterm vs. term mothers

	Preterm colostrum	Term colostrum
Total protein (g/L)	0.43 ± 1.3	0.31 ± 0.05
IgA (mg/g protein)	310.5 ± 70	168.2 ± 21
IgG (mg/g protein)	7.6 ± 3.9	8.4 ± 1
IgM (mg/g protein)	39.6 ± 23	36.1 ± 16
Lysozyme (mg/g protein)	1.5 ± 0.5	1.1 ± 0.3
Lactoferrin (mg/g protein)	165 ± 37	102 ± 25
Total cells/ml^3	6794 ± 1946	3064 ± 424
Macrophages	4041 ± 1420	1597 ± 303
Lymphocytes	1850 ± 543	954 ± 143
Neutrophils	842 ± 404	512 ± 178

Modified from Mathur NB, Dwarkadas AM, Sharma VK, et al: Anti-infective factors in preterm human colostrum. Acta Paediatr Scand 79:1039, 1990.

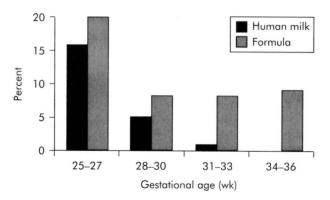

Figure 14-4. Effect of gestational age and human milk versus formula feeding on necrotizing enterocolitis (NEC). In infants fed formula, incidence of NEC decreases after 27 weeks, then remains the same. In infants fed human milk, incidence of NEC continues to decline. (From Lucas A, Cole TJ: Breast milk and neonatal necrotising enterocolitis. Lancet 336:1519, 1990.)

cause has eluded neonatologists, although many theories have been put forth and associations suggested.[84] When researchers investigate its prevention, the role of human milk is prominent. In a large prospective multicentered study of 926 infants, 51 (5.5%) infants developed NEC. Mortality rate was 26% (Fig. 14-4). In exclusively formula fed infants, the incidence was 6 to 10 times more common than in those who received human milk exclusively. In those who received human milk and formula, it was three times more common than in the exclusively breastfed group. Pasteurization did not diminish the effect of human milk. The comparison was more dramatic above 30 weeks' gestation, when formula fed infants were 20 times more apt to develop NEC than human milk fed infants. Early enteral feeding did not change the risk in those receiving breast milk, whereas delaying feedings of formula did lower the rate of NEC.[74] In a study of the prevention of NEC in LBW infants with feedings higher in IgA and IgG, none of the infants in the study group or the breastfeeding comparison group developed NEC, whereas six cases developed among the 91 infants in the untreated group.[32]

The intestinal flora in the second week of life in hospitalized preterm infants who had been treated previously with antibiotics and were fed stored frozen human milk was compared with the flora of those fed formula.[101] The flora was very different from term infants, and both groups contained Enterobacteriaceae predominantly. Human milk did not alter the flora in these antibiotic-treated infants. Studies have shown that the acidic pH in the stomach of the human milk fed LBW infants protects against the bacteria in the unpasteurized milk.[129] Although cultures of the milk (feeding sample) had grown both pathogens and nonpathogens, the 2-hour postfeeding cultures of the gastric contents had no growth and a pH less than 3.5. It is notable that human milk also affects the incidence of other infections in the premature infant, including upper respiratory infections (Fig. 14-5).

When stool colonization and incidence of sepsis in human milk fed (HMF) and formula fed (FF) infants were studied in an intensive care nursery, there was a protective effect against nosocomial sepsis, which was unrelated to gastrointestinal flora. It was concluded that human milk feeding is associated with significantly decreased incidence of nosocomially acquired sepsis that cannot be explained by the effect of human milk feeding on the GI flora.

In South Africa, where mothers remain with and help care for their premature babies, a study com-

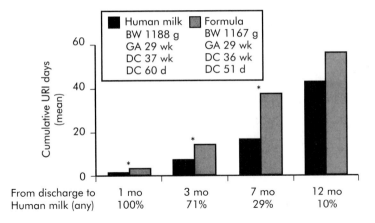

Figure 14-5. Effect of human milk on upper respiratory infection (URI) symptoms in premature infants during their first year. BW, birth weight; GA, gestational age. (Blaymore Bier J-A, Oliver T, Ferguson A, et al: Human milk reduces outpatient upper respiratory symptoms in premature infants during their first year of life. Perinatol 22:354, 2002.)

pared feeding an infant its own mother's milk with feeding pooled pasteurized breast milk. Birth weights were between 1000 and 1500 g. Nonventilator babies were begun on feedings by 96 hours of age. There was significantly greater weight gain using untreated mother's milk, both for regaining birth weight and reaching 1800 g sooner. The SGA and appropriate-for-gestational-age (AGA) infants both did better on their own mother's milk. This diet decreased hospital stays and decreased hospital-acquired infection. The authors attribute the advantages to milk being fed fresh with early initiation of feeding at the breast compared to pasteurization of the bank milk.[120]

The Committee on Nutrition at the American Academy of Pediatrics (AAP),[24] has published "Nutritional needs of low-birth-weight infants," in which they suggest that mother's own milk and new special formulas for those babies needing breast milk substitutes are promising alternatives. *Nutrition and Feeding of Preterm Infants* is published as a report of the Committee on Nutrition of the Preterm Infant, European Society of Paediatric Gastroenterology and Nutrition.[25] The report enthusiastically supports mother's own milk as the

preferred nourishment, recognizing the need to supplement certain nutrients for the VLBW infant. It recommends 180 to 200 mL/kg/day mother's milk as soon as possible, adding sodium, phosphate, and, in some cases, protein and calcium. The committee recommends heat treatment for donor milk.[25]

A joint effort of the AAP Committee on the Fetus and Newborn and the American College of Obstetricians and Gynecologists (ACOG) Committee on Obstetric Practice states that "human milk has a number of special features that make its use desirable in feeding preterm babies."[26]

Milk production by mothers of premature infants

The production of milk by a mother who is not actively nursing her infant, as is frequently the case in LBW infants and other neonates in NICUs, is a challenge to the resources of the NICU and the postpartum staff.[92] Insufficient milk production is a common problem that becomes more critical as time passes, as production continues to drop, and as the infant's needs increase. Evaluation of various protocols has been undertaken by investigators who looked at times of onset of pumping post partum, frequency of pumping, and duration in total minutes per day and length of time when no pumping occurred.

Thirty-two healthy mothers, 19 of whom had no previous breastfeeding experience, were entered into a study protocol by Hopkinson and associates.[61] Their infants were 28 to 30 weeks' gestation. All the mothers initiated pumping between days 2 and 6, and the day of initiation was correlated with the volume of milk at 2 weeks but not at 4 weeks with mothers who had nursed previously and initiated pumping sooner. Parity, gravidity, age, and prior nursing experience were not correlated with volumes at 2 weeks. Parity and prior nursing experience were associated with milk volume at 4 weeks, with multiparas producing 60% greater volumes. These investigators found no significant relationship between 24-hour milk volume and frequency, duration, or maximal night interval. The change in milk volume from 2 weeks to 4 weeks was correlated with frequency and duration of pumping but not to maximal night intervals. The range in number of pumpings per day was four to nine. The authors[61] concluded that optimal milk production occurs with at least five expressions per day and pumping durations that exceed 100 minutes/day.

The frequency of milk expression was evaluated by de Carvalho and associates[28] in a crossover design study of 25 mothers who delivered at between 28 and 37 weeks' gestation. Frequent expression of milk was significantly associated with greater milk production (342 ± 229 mL) than with infrequent expression (221 ± 141 mL). They compared three or less pumpings a day to four or more times. The mean number was 2.4 versus 5.7, neither number being the frequency with which a mother would usually feed her infant in the first few weeks.

Although minimum frequency and duration figures have been provided, it is advisable to increase the frequency of pumping as the need to raise production increases and as it comes closer to time for discharge and feeding the infant exclusively at the breast. Consideration for increasing nighttime pumpings is also important as discharge approaches.

Some mothers experience a dread of the pump when demands are increased for "more milk production." The management of the mother producing milk for her hospitalized infant should be coordinated by the neonatologist and primary care physician with the assistance of the primary care nurse and the unit's lactation coordinator to maximize support and minimize stress.

When the physiology of lactation is applied to the practical management of inducing a milk supply without benefit of the infant's participation, it is apparent that mimicking natural breastfeeding is more effective. Although some women succeed with manual expression, it is rare, and a good pump should be recommended. None of the hand pumps can truly duplicate the milking action of the infant, and all are essentially vacuum extractors. They should be used only as a stopgap measure when the electric pump is unavailable (see Chapter 21). A pump that is provided for pumping both breasts simultaneously saves time but may generate higher levels of prolactin and greater total milk volume compared with pumping each breast separately for the same length of time.[102] Subsequent studies have produced variable observations. Groh-Wargo and associates[47] studied 32 women randomly assigned to single or double pumping for 6 weeks. No difference was found in prolactin levels or total volume of milk produced, although the time-saving effect was considered important.

A randomized controlled trial to compare methods of milk expression after preterm delivery involved 36 women: 19 used simultaneous pumping and 17 used sequential pumping by random assignment. A crossover design was used to evaluate the effect of breast massage on milk volume and fat content (estimated by creamatocrit). The authors reported the results were unequivocal showing that pumping both breasts simultaneously produced more milk—125.1 g with massage and 87.7 g without compared to sequential volumes of 78.7 g with massage and 51.3 g without.

Pumping should be initiated as soon as the mother's condition permits, and offering this opportunity to the mother should be part of the supportive care offered by the postpartum staff. All the points of preparation for pumping should be included: comfortable position, tranquil atmosphere, preparation of the breast with gentle stroking and warmth, confidence, and reassurance of the staff. The obstetrician is in an important position to initiate the offer to pump by knowing during the mother's prenatal care that she wants to breastfeed. She may not know it is appropriate to ask about it. Providing knowledgeable, accurate, consistent, and sensitive support should be the rule in every perinatal center, especially for mothers of high-risk infants who choose to breastfeed.[98,102] The opportunity to pump should be offered to *all* women, regardless of previous feeding choice, as often a mother changes her mind when she learns that her high-risk infant would receive many benefits from her milk.

Nationwide, mothers who give birth to infants who are admitted to special care nurseries (SCN) are less likely to initiate lactation than mothers of healthy, term infants according to Meier.[94] The profile of mothers who give birth to these high-risk infants includes a higher percentage of low-income, low-education, young mothers, who do not breastfeed in great numbers. Postpartum and NICU staff should work to encourage these women.

Providing an appropriate room for pumping after the mother has been discharged is critical to individual success and is an expression of commitment to breastfeeding. This room should be clean, bright, and cheery and accommodate more than one mother and companion at a time unless several rooms are available. It should have a sink for washing hands and storage for equipment and supplies. A nurse call button or other alarm system is also essential. Additional conducive features are soft music, a telephone, and reading material. The hospital should have a supply of approved electric pumps and individual disposable attachment packets for each mother. A place should be available to store her properly labeled and dated milk in a freezer or refrigerator. Sterile storage containers should be readily available.

A mother should be encouraged to rent a pump for home use and around-the-clock pumping. These are available from medical supply stores, pharmacies, home care services, hospitals, and some lactation consultants. Insurance companies reimburse for the cost of rental when the milk is prescribed for a high-risk infant. The neonatologist can provide an appropriate letter of support. The hospital support staff who are coordinating the mother's care or the NICU staff should be sure that the mother understands how to use the equipment effectively. Ideally, NICUs have at least one staff member experienced in lactation counseling who will coordinate this effort under the direction of the obstetrician, pediatrician, and neonatologist. As more equipment and technology become available, the physician should be alert to avoid subjecting the mother to pressures of pump equipment entrepreneurs and unsolicited advice. The best remedy is for the NICU to provide on-staff, up-to-date experience and support to the mother in her efforts to provide milk and breastfeed her high-risk infant. Box 14-4 outlines key strategies for successful pumping when the infant is unable to suckle the breast. Many level three and four hospitals have at least one licensed International Board–certified lactation consultant (IBCLC) among their neonatal nursing staff who can see and assist all mothers who wish to provide their milk for their infant. All neonatal nurses should be familiar

---

BOX 14-4   Guidelines for initiating milk supply without infant suckling

1. Begin as soon after delivery as maternal condition permits.
2. Initiate use of electric pump while in hospital.
3. Begin slowly, increasing time over first week.
4. Pump on more regular basis as soon as engorgement is evident.
5. Pump at least five times in 24 hours.
6. Allow a rest period for uninterrupted sleep of at least 6 hours.
7. Pump a total of at least 100 minutes/day.
8. Use "double" pump to pump both breasts simultaneously; can cut total time proportionately.
9. Prepare breast with warm soaks, gentle stroking, and light massage to maximize production of milk.
10. Encourage skin-to-skin care (kangaroo care).

with the available pumps and their use and be supportive of mothers who are pumping.

Milk production for low-birth-weight or small-for-gestational-age infants

Maternal choice to breastfeed or provide milk for an LBW infant is influenced by many factors beyond those that interplay in most feeding decisions of normal full-term infants.[92] Lucas and associates[86,87] sought to answer two major questions in a study of 925 mother-infant pairs in five hospitals from 1982 to 1985: Do health care professionals in neonatal units exert a major influence on a mother's feeding preference and availability of her milk for her infant, and are there population differences between mothers who do and do not provide their milk?

Mothers in a study had delivered at a mean of 31 weeks' gestation infants weighing less than 1850 g with a mean of 1370 g. More educated mothers provided their milk (98%) than uneducated (40%). Higher socioeconomic class, lower parity or fewer living children, being married, and being over 20 years of age were associated with providing milk. Boys were more apt to receive mother's milk, as shown in other studies. Birth weight and extreme immaturity were not a determinant, nor was transfer of the infant to another center. In this study a mother who had cesarean delivery was more likely to breastfeed than one who had delivered vaginally.[130] In this study among five centers, the demographic characteristics of the mother were important, not the staff. This study did not look at success rates, however. Another study of breastfeeding LBW infants showed an inverse relationship between maturity and size; the smaller and less mature infants were not breastfed, nor were those with respiratory distress syndrome (RDS).[130]

Feeding premature infants at the breast

Large premature infants of 36 weeks' gestation or older may be nursed at the breast if otherwise stable. Particular care should be given to assist the mother in getting the infant to suckle, especially if the breast and nipples are large or engorged.[98,102]

Weight should be followed closely to prevent excessive weight loss. Infants who receive sugar water and formula supplements lose more weight than those who are nursed frequently at the breast without supplementation. If breastfeeding is going well, the infant could be discharged with the mother from the hospital as soon as the infant begins to gain substantially, with close follow-up at home.

Feeding at the breast when the infant is under 1500 g is considered too strenuous by many neonatologists. When the feeding of infants of less than 1500 g was examined, however, the growth of those fed at the breast was comparable with that of matched control infants fed expressed human milk by bottle.[71] Breastfeeding was started when sucking movements were observed. Initially, they all received supplementary human milk by tube plus 800 units vitamin D and 60 mg vitamin C daily. Unrestricted visiting of parents to the neonatal unit, an optimistic and knowledgeable attitude of the nursing staff toward breastfeeding, and the avoidance of a bottle for the infants are important to success. The authors also encourage the expression of milk by the mothers early in the postpartum period. The main deterrent to successful breastfeeding was lack of maternal interest and commitment.

Blaymore Bier and associates[12] undertook a clinical study of breastfeeding and bottle feedings in *extremely low birth weight* (ELBW) *infants* (birth weight 800 g or less) when they were considered ready to bottle feed. This was at a mean age since conception of 35 weeks (corrected gestational age). One breastfeeding and one bottle feeding were monitored each day for 10 days. Prefeeding and postfeeding weights, oxygen saturation, respiratory and heart rates, and axillary temperature were recorded. Higher oxygen saturation and higher temperatures during breastfeeding and less likelihood of desaturation below 90% were noted in the breastfed infants. The weights reflecting intake were higher in the bottle fed infants. The authors concluded that it was physiologically safe and less stressful for infants to breastfeed. The lower intake requires monitoring, however.[12]

The ontogenic and temporal organization of nonnutritive sucking during active sleep were studied by Hack and associates[54] in preterm infants.

One infant of the six studied had recognizable rhythmic sucking bursts at 28 weeks, and all had bursts by 31 to 32 weeks. The number of bursts increased and the interval between bursts decreased as the infants matured, with the earliest indications of intrinsic rhythm beginning at 30 weeks.

Nonnutritive sucking has become a subject of controversy in NICUs. Allowing premature infants to suck on a pacifier during gavage feedings was initially reported to be associated with increased weight gain and shorter hospitalizations.[52] When nutrient intake and other parameters were controlled, however, there were no advantages to nonnutritive sucking in somatic growth, serum proteins, energy absorption, or feeding tolerance, nor was there any increase in tropic hormones or growth promoters.[29,35] Infants have been observed to have transcutaneous oxygen saturation measurements increase by 3% to 4% during nonnutritive sucking.[28] Nonnutritive sucking does not appear to carry risk for infants destined for further bottle feeding but should be avoided for infants destined to breastfeed in order to avoid interference with normal sucking.

Of greater significance is the value of having these infants placed at the "emptied" breast during gavage tube feedings. When Narayanan and associates[100] studied this practice, they found no change in weight gain or length of hospital stay. It did, however, result in more successful and longer duration of breastfeeding after discharge. This technique was originally designed in our nursery to improve mother's milk production and encourage mothers who were becoming discouraged. As the infant matures and begins swallowing with sucking, it becomes unnecessary to pump the breast "empty" before presenting to the infant because any milk provided could be suckled and swallowed. Suckling at the breast initiates a peristaltic action that also triggers swallowing, and the physiologic response of the entire gastrointestinal tract (see Chapter 8). Suckling the breast also improves mother's success when pumping.

Kangaroo care

Kangaroo care is the term applied to skin-to-skin contact first introduced in 1979 in a hospital in Bogota, Colombia, because of a shortage of incubators, high death rate from infection, and abandonment of premature infants by their mothers. Since that time, many investigators have carefully evaluated kangaroo care and found it to be beneficial to mother and infant.

Dressed only in a diaper, the infant is held skin to skin against the mother's chest between her breasts, snug inside the mother's clothing, often for hours. The father can do the same. Many advantages have been noted, including more stable respirations, heart rates, and temperatures. The infants spend less time crying and more time in a quiet, alert state and deep sleep. Some studies suggest better weight gain and earlier discharge. Hurst and associates[63] also reported an increase in milk volume during pumping.

Mothers who give kangaroo care breastfeed longer and more frequently. They also report greater confidence in caring for their fragile infant than those who experience traditional care.[6] Many NICU nurseries encourage kangaroo care, and all parents are assisted in providing it whenever they are in the nursery to the benefit of both the mother and the infant.

Small-for-gestational-age infants

Infants who are below the 10th percentile (or 2 SD) in weight for their gestational age are termed *small for gestational age* (SGA). These infants may also be shorter in length and have smaller heads, depending on when in gestational life the insult to their growth occurred. The more general the growth failure, the earlier the intrauterine effect appears. For example, rubella in the first trimester causes total growth retardation, whereas hypertension in the mother in the third trimester predominantly affects weight. The more profound the growth retardation, the more difficult are the nutritional problems.

SGA infants are prone to be hypocalcemic; however, if they can be provided with adequate breast milk early, this complication may be avoided because the calcium/phosphorus ratio is more physiologic than formula. Other problems, including hypothermia and hypoglycemia, which lead to a vicious circle of acidosis and associated problems, can be triggered by unmonitored exposure of the infant to thermal stress in the first hours of life and failure to identify the hypoglycemia early. Hypoglycemia in an SGA infant cannot be ignored because the potential exists for significant stress to the nervous system, which can result in seizures requiring aggressive therapy and a detailed diagnostic workup. The SGA infant lacks glycogen stores.

Using human α-lactalbumin as a marker protein, Boehm and associates[17] demonstrated that SGA infants with intrauterine growth retardation have delayed postnatal decrease in macromolecular absorption and delayed intestinal maturation, even compared with premature infants of the same weight. Their management demands special care. The enzymes in human milk can facilitate catch-up maturation of the intestinal tract.

Thus, the perinatal nursery staff may appear to be obstructive to breastfeeding when they hover over this infant or even insist on transfer to the nursery. Initial breastfeeding at delivery is permissible; however, adequate external heat must be provided. Testing the blood sugar should be performed in the delivery room recovery area and the infant sent to the nursery if hypoglycemia or hypothermia cannot be controlled. Frequent breastfeeding can be initiated unless the blood sugar level is too low (below 30 mg/dL) or unresponsive to oral treatment. It may not be possible for even an actively lactating multipara to sustain an SGA infant initially, but the infant should be put to breast at least every 3 hours and given intravenous (IV) glucose as well.

SGA infants often have a poor suck and poor coordination with the swallow reflex. There may be considerable mucus with gagging and spitting. A simple lavage of the stomach with a No. 8 feeding tube (or No. 5, if the infant weighs less than 2600 g) and warmed glucose water usually relieves the gagging. Once this SGA infant begins to eat, he will do well and will require sufficient kilocalories to meet the needs of an AGA infant. The mother may need to use a breast pump to stimulate lactation initially and increase the volume she produces.

Children born small for gestational age are at neurodevelopmental disadvantage. When these infants receive enriched formula, it does improve their growth, but the breastfed SGA infant grew best in a series of children followed by Morley and associates.[95] Three groups fed regular formula, enriched formula, or breast milk were followed: 147 were randomized to regular formula, 152 received enriched formula, and there were 175 in the reference group of breastfeeders. The developmental scores using the Bayley Mental Development Index (MDI) or the Psychomotor Development Index (PDI) at 18 months were measured. There was no difference between formula groups. The breastfeeding infants had significantly higher PDI scores and a 6-point advantage in the BMI. The authors suggested that SGA infants clearly benefited by being breastfed.[95]

The transition from hospital to home for all families is a stressful time, but when the infant is premature and has been in the NICU for days, weeks, or months, transition can be extremely difficult. The stress can be reduced by discharge planning. Mother should spend as much time as possible with the infant, providing breastfeeding while she is present. A lactation consultant or trained staff member should observe these interactions. The presence of sucking and swallowing should be documented. Positioning and latch should be perfected by discharge if mother has received adequate assistance in the days and weeks before discharge.

Hospitals who have facilities to accommodate care-by-parent overnight are very helpful in the transition. At a minimum, the parent should have given all the medications and treatments prior to discharge as well as breastfeeding. If mother's supply is not adequate yet, she should be instructed in the use of the lactation supplementer prior to discharge along with a plan for amount and substance to be placed in the supplementer. If she has stored milk available, it can be used. If not, the neonatologist will have to order special care formula or special human milk supplementer, which is designed to be used separately from mixing with mother's milk as a feed. Mother should be instructed to continue pumping until the infant is exclusively breastfed and gaining weight adequately. Pumping three to four times a day to completely empty the breasts at home is critical. Preterm infants usually do not completely empty the breasts at first. They lack the suction strength and effective organization of sucking until they approach 40 weeks' corrected gestational age according to Meier.[94] These preterm infants need scheduling to ensure feeding every 3 hours to guarantee adequate production and intake.

Not all premature infants will need supplementation at home. Before and after weighings (Chapter 8) can be done while the infant is still in the hospital to measure the infant's intake at each feeding. Digital scales accurate to 2 g are available in all hospitals, and home models can be rented. When the infant is first discharged, it is helpful to both the physician and the parents to know what intake actually is. Some mothers produce large volumes of milk but the infant does not gain weight. Pumping first to remove the foremilk (and freeze it) and having the infant suckle the hind milk can help this problem. The pediatrician plays a critical role in the success of feeding after discharge. Monitoring of progress and knowledge of the unique concerns in breastfeeding the premature infant are key.

IMPROVING MILK PRODUCTION

1. Begin pumping as soon post partum as possible.
2. Use hospital grade double (two breast) pumps.
3. Pump 10 to 15 minutes every 3 hours until more than a few drops are produced (72 hours).
4. When amount increases, continue to pump for 2 minutes after the last drop is produced (total 20 to 30 minutes).
5. Keep a record of times pumped and volumes produced.
6. Pump at babies' bedside when possible.
7. Start with kangaroo care.
8. Stroke and massage breast during pumping.
9. As soon as infant is able, place at emptied breast to suckle or during gavage feedings.
10. Chapter 8 discusses pharmacologic stimulation of milk volume.

CONCLUDING RECOMMENDATIONS

Infants who weigh less than 1800 g at birth and have to be gavage fed and infants of any weight who are acutely ill present a complex problem. The mother should be instructed to express her milk initially and contribute any colostrum she produces. This can be given by gastric tube. A hospital grade electric pump is effective in helping a mother increase the volume produced. When the infant is born at 1000 g, requires ventilator support for days, and is not discharged for 8 weeks (Fig. 14-6), it is difficult to maintain a large volume of milk by pumping, but it can be done with supportive counseling by staff. Milk volumes usually increase when the infant begins actually to breastfeed, not unlike relactation (see Chapter 19) or increasing milk volume in other situations (Chapter 8).

When nipple feeding is possible, the infant can be put to the breast. It requires less energy to suckle at the breast than to feed from a bottle. The peristaltic motion of the tongue, which is the normal innate suckling mode, initiates the peristaltic motion of the gastrointestinal tract and triggers the swallow. If no pacifiers or rubber nipples have been given, the infant may be able to suckle at the breast before he reaches 1500 g. Figure 19-3 illustrates an infant who first nursed at 1100 g. If little or no breastfeeding has been done in the hospital and the mother has been unable to pump enough to sustain the daily needs, the infant may be frustrated at the breast when sent home from the hospital unless intervention is provided.

One can see that the reserves of the premature infant are limited if one studies the absolute and relative body compositions of infants at birth (Fig. 14-7). If one considers how little time it takes to starve a premature infant compared with a full-term infant, the risks of starving a premature infant while the infant adapts to nursing at the breast are real (Fig. 14-8). The solution to the problem is to provide nourishment while the infant stimulates maternal milk production by suckling at the breast. Equipment called a *nursing supplementer* will

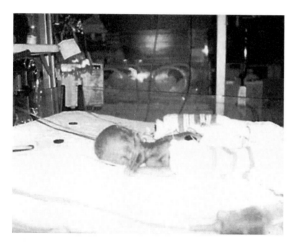

Figure 14-6. This 1100-g infant is shown at 4 hours of life in a busy neonatal intensive care unit. Infants in these situations require early intervention to ensure successful breastfeeding.

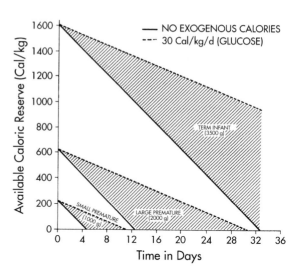

Figure 14-8. Estimated survival of starved and semistarved infants weighing 1000, 2000, and 3500 g at birth. (From Heird WC, Anderson TL: Nutritional requirements and methods of feeding low birth weight infants. In Gluck L et al (eds): Current Problems in Pediatrics, Vol. 7, No. 8. Chicago, Year Book, 1977.)

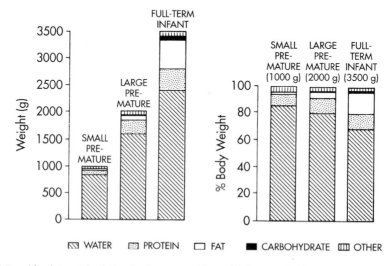

Figure 14-7. Absolute and relative body composition of infants weighing 1000, 2000, and 3500 g at birth. (From Heird WC, Anderson TL: Nutritional requirements and methods of feeding low birth weight infants. In Gluck L et al (eds): Current Problems in Pediatrics, Vol. 7, No. 8. Chicago, Year Book, 1977.)

provide this setup very effectively (see Fig. 19-4). It was developed to provide nourishment for the adopted infant who is being nursed by a mother who has not been pregnant or has never lactated and sustains the infant while the mother's milk supply develops (see Chapter 19). The same effect can be provided for the premature or sick infant who has not nursed at the breast since birth and needs nourishment while the mother's supply develops, even though she has been pumping.

The infant can continue to gain weight while stimulating the breast if a supplementer is used. The volume required from the nursing supplementer drops continually in a week or so. Occasional infants require the supplementer for a month. Mother should continue to pump after breastfeedings until her volume increases.

The nursing supplementer provides a simple means of ensuring adequate nourishment while adapting to the breast. It is preferable to using supplemental bottles because the infant is not confused by the rubber nipple, which requires a different mechanism of sucking than the human nipple. Furthermore, the suckling of the breast provides the continued stimulus necessary for increasing milk production. Cup feeding is an alternative to the bottle if the infant needs additional nourishment.

The parameters that are to be met before discharge home from the hospital include[56] sustained weight gain, growth in length and head circumference, and stable biochemical parameters (Table 14-14). Following discharge from the hospital, these same parameters should be met. If there is persistent faltering, fortifying breastfeeding may be indicated. This can be accomplished without interfering with the breastfeeding process again by using a lactation supplementer containing enriched breast milk that had been previously pumped or enriched formula.

Posthospitalization breastfeeding patterns of moderately preterm infants (30 to 35 weeks) were studied by Wooldridge and Hall[132] using daily feeding diaries in 55 women for the first month after discharge. Those women who were able to exclusively breastfeed before the end of the first week at home were able to maintain their supply. In general, those women who did not have an adequate supply the first week were unlikely to achieve it by week 4. The proportion of breastfeeds increased over the 4 weeks of observation, but only 56% achieved exclusive breastfeeds by 4 weeks.

TABLE 14-14   Postdischarge nutritional screening assessment

	Action values
Growth	
Weight gain	< 20 g/day
Length growth	< 0.5 cm/wk
Head circumference	< 0.5 cm/wk
Biochemical Test	
Phosphorus	< 4.5 mg/dL
Alkaline phosphatase	> 450 IU/L
Urea nitrogen	< 5 mg/dL

Modified from Hall, RT: Nutritional follow-up of the breastfeeding premature infant after hospital discharge. Pediatr Clin North Am 48: 435, 2001.

REFERENCES

1. Abrahms SA, Schanler RJ, Garza C: Bone mineralization in former very low birth weight infants fed either human milk or commercial formula. J Pediatr 112:956, 1988.
2. Adamkin DH: Enteral and total parenteral nutrition in the very low birth weight infant. I. Enteral nutrition. Neonatal Intensive Care 10:19, 1997.
3. American Academy of Pediatrics, Kleinman R (ed): Pediatric Nutrition Handbook, 5th ed. American Academy of Pediatrics, Elk Grove, Ill, 2004.
4. American Academy of Pediatrics, Section on Breastfeeding: The AAP and the use of human milk. Pediatrics 2004 (in press).
5. Anderson DM, William FH, Merkatz RB, et al: Length of gestation and nutritional composition of human milk. Am J Clin Nutr 37:810, 1983.
6. Anderson GC: Touch and the kangaroo care method. In Field TM (ed): Touch in Early Development. Mahwah, NJ, Erlbaum Associates, 1995.

7. Atkinson SA, Anderson GH, Bryan MH: Human milk: Comparison of the nitrogen composition in milk from mothers of premature and full-term infants. Am J Clin Nutr 33:811, 1980.

8. Atkinson SA, Radde IC, Chance GW, et al: Macromineral content of milk obtained during early lactation from mothers of premature infants. Early Hum Dev 4:5, 1980.

9. Beijers RJW, Graaf FVD, Schaafsma A, et al: Composition of premature breast milk during lactation: Constant digestible protein content (as in full term milk). Early Hum Dev 29:351, 1992.

10. Berseth CL: Effect of early feeding on maturation of the preterm infant's small intestine. J Pediatr 120:947, 1992.

11. Berseth CL: Gastrointestinal motility in the neonate. Clin Perinatol 23:179, 1996.

12. Blaymore Bier JA, Oliver T, Ferguson AE, et al: Human milk improves cognitive and motor development of premature infants during infancy. J Hum Lact 18:361, 2002.

13. Billeaud C, Senterre J, Rigo J: Osmolality of the gastric and duodenal contents in low birth weight infants fed human milk or various formulae. Acta Paediatr Scand 71:799, 1982.

14. Birch DG, Birch EE, Hoffman DR, et al: Retinal development in very-low-birth-weight infants fed diets differing in omega-3 fatty acids. Invest Ophthalmol Vis Sci 33:2365, 1992.

15. Bishop NJ, Dahlenburg SL, Fewtrell MS, et al: Early diet of preterm infants and bone mineralization at age five years. Acta Paediatr 85:230, 1996.

16. Bitman J, Wood L, Hamosh M, et al: Comparison of the lipid composition of breast milk from mothers of term and preterm infants. Am J Clin Nutr 38:300, 1983.

17. Boehm G, Jakobsson I, Mansson M, et al: Macromolecular absorption in small-for-gestational age infants. Acta Paediatr 81:864, 1992.

18. Brumberg H, LaGamma EF: Perspectives on nutrition: Enhance outcomes for premature infants. Pediatr Ann 32(9): 617, 2003.

19. Carey DE, Rowe JC, Goetz CA, et al: Growth and phosphorus metabolism in premature infants fed human milk, fortified human milk, or special premature formula. Am J Dis Child 141:511, 1987.

20. Cavell B: Gastric emptying in preterm infants. Acta Paediatr Scand 68:725, 1979.

21. Chan GM: Effects of powdered human milk fortifiers on the antibacterial actions of human milk. J Perinatol 23:620, 2003.

22. Chandra RK: Immunoglobulin and protein levels in breast milk produced by mothers of preterm infants. Nutr Res 2:27, 1982.

23. Chappell JE, Clandinin MT, Kerney-Volpe C, et al: Fatty acid balance studies in premature infants fed human milk or formula: Effect of calcium supplementation. J Pediatr 108:439, 1986.

24. Committee on Nutrition, American Academy of Pediatrics: Nutritional needs of the preterm infant. In Pediatric Nutrition Handbook, 5th ed. American Academy of Pediatrics, Elk Grove, Ill 2004.

25. Committee on Nutrition, European Society of Paediatric Gastroenterology and Nutrition: Nutrition and feeding of preterm infants. Acta Paediatr Scand Suppl 336:3, 1987.

26. Committee on Obstetric Practice, American College of Obstetricians and Gynecologists; Committee on the Fetus and Newborn, American Academy of Pediatrics: Guidelines for Perinatal Care, 4th ed. Elk Grove, Ill, American Academy of Pediatrics, 1997.

27. Davey AM, Wagner CL, Phelps DL, et al: Do premature infants with umbilical artery catheters tolerate oral feeds? Pediatr Res 31:199A, 1992.

28. de Carvalho M, Anderson DM, Giangreco A, et al: Frequency of milk expression and milk production by mothers of non-nursing premature neonates. Am J Dis Child 139:483, 1985.

29. DeCurtis M, McIntosh N, Ventura V, et al: Effect of nonnutritive suckling on nutrient retention in preterm infants. J Pediatr 109:888, 1986.

30. Dowling (deMonterice) D: Physiologic responses of breastfeeding and bottle feeding. Nurs Res 48:78, 1999.

31. Dunn L, Hulman S, Weiner J, et al: Beneficial effects of early hypocaloric enteral feeding on neonatal gastrointestinal function: Preliminary report of a randomized trial. J Pediatr 112:622, 1988.

32. Eibl MM, Wolf HM, Furnkranz H, et al: Prevention of necrotizing enterocolitis in low-birth-weight infants by IgA-IgG feeding. N Engl J Med 319:1, 1988.

33. Eidelmann AI, Hoffman NW, Kaitz M: Cognitive deficits in women after childbirth. Obstet Gynecol 81:764, 1993.

34. El-Mohaneles AE, Picard MB, Simmens SJ, et al: Use of human milk in the intensive care nursery decreases the incidence of nosocomial sepsis. J Perinatol 17:130, 1997.

35. Ernst JA, Rickard KA, Neal PR, et al: Lack of improved growth outcome related to non-nutritive sucking in very low birth weight premature infants fed a controlled nutrient. Pediatrics 83:706, 1989.

36. Feldman R, Eidelman AI: Direct and indirect effects of breast milk on the neurobehavioral and cognitive development of premature infants. Dev Psychobiol 43:109, 2003.

37. Forbes GB: Nutritional adequacy of human breast milk for premature infants. In Lebenthal E (ed): Textbook of Gastroenterology and Nutrition. New York, Raven, 1981.

38. Forbes GB: Human milk and the small baby. Am J Dis Child 136:577, 1982.

39. Forbes GB: Fetal growth and body composition: Implications for the premature infant. J Pediatr Gastroenterol Nutr 2(suppl):552, 1983.

40. Ford JE, Zechalko A, Murphy J, et al: Comparison of the B vitamin composition of milk from mothers of preterm and term babies. Arch Dis Child 58:367, 1983.

41. Garza C, Hopkinson J, Schanler RJ: Human milk banking. In Howell RR, Morriss FH, Pickering LK (eds): Human Milk in Infant Nutrition and Health. Springfield, IL, Thomas, 1986.

42. Goldman AS, Chheda S, Keeney SE, et al: Immunologic protection of the premature newborn by human milk. Semin Perinatol 18:495, 1994.

43. Goldman AS, Garza C, Nichols B, et al: Effects of prematurity on the immunologic system in human milk. J Pediatr 101:901, 1982.

44. Greer FR, McCormick A: Improved bone mineralization and growth in premature infants fed fortified own mother's milk. J Pediatr 112:961, 1988.

45. Greer FR, McCormick A, Kashyap ML, et al: Late hypertriglyceridemia in very low birth weight infants fed human milk exclusively. J Pediatr 111:466, 1987.

46. Greer FR, Tsang RC: Calcium, phosphorus, magnesium, and vitamin D requirements for preterm infants. In Tsang RC (ed): Vitamin and Mineral Requirements for Preterm Infants. New York, Marcel Dekker, 1985.

47. Groh-Wargo S, Toth A, Mahoney K: The utility of a bilateral breast pumping system for mothers of premature infants. Neonatal Network 14:31, 1995.

48. Gross SJ: Growth and biochemical response of preterm infants fed human milk or modified infant formula. N Engl J Med 308:237, 1983.

49. Gross SJ: Bone mineralization in preterm infants fed human milk with and without mineral supplementation. J Pediatr 111:450, 1987.

50. Gross SJ, Buckley RH, Wakil SS, et al: Elevated IgA concentration in milk produced by mothers delivered of preterm infants. J Pediatr 99:389, 1981.

51. Gross SJ, Gabriel E: Vitamin E status in preterm infants fed human milk or infant formula. J Pediatr 106:635, 1985.

52. Gross SJ, Slagle TA: Feeding the low birth weight infant. Clin Perinatol 20:193, 1993.

53. Guerrini P, Bosi G, Chierici R, et al: Human milk: Relationship of fat content with gestational age. Early Hum Dev 5:187, 1981.

54. Hack M, Estabrook MM, Robertson SS: Development of sucking rhythm in preterm infants. Early Hum Dev 11:133, 1985.

55. Hagelberg S, Lindblad BS, Lundsjo A, et al: The protein tolerance of very low birth weight infants fed human milk protein enriched mother's milk. Acta Paediatr Scand 71:597, 1982.

56. Hall RT: Nutritional follow-up of the breastfeeding premature infant after hospital discharge. Pediatr Clin North Am 48:453, 2001.

57. Hanlon MB, Tripp JH, Ellis RE, et al: Deglutition apnoea as indicator of maturation of suckle feeding in bottle-fed preterm infants. Dev Med Child Neurol 39:534, 1997.

58. Haug M, Laubach C, Burke M, et al: Vitamin E in human milk from mothers of preterm and term infants. J Pediatr Gastroenterol Nutr 6:605, 1987.

59. Heine W: Is mother's milk the most suitable food for low birth weight infants? Early Hum Dev 29:345, 1992.

60. Hibbard CM, Brooke OG, Carter ND, et al: Variations in the composition of breast milk during the first 5 weeks of lactation: Implications for the feeding of preterm infants. Arch Dis Child 57:658, 1982.

61. Hopkinson JM, Schanler RJ, Garza C: Milk production by mothers of premature infants. Pediatrics 81:815, 1988.

62. Hughes CA, Dowling RH: Speed of onset of adaptive mucosal hypoplasia and hypofunction in the intestine of parenterally fed rats. Clin Sci 59:317, 1980.

63. Hurst NM, Valentine CJ, Renfro L, et al: Skin-to-skin holding in the neonatal intensive care unit influences maternal milk volume. J Perinatol 17:213, 1997.

64. Hylander MA, Strobino DM, Dhanireddy R: Association of race, Apgar scores at five minutes and formula feeding with retinopathy of prematurity (ROP) among very low birth weight (VLBW) infants. Pediatr Res 41:199A, 1997.

65. Hylander MA, Strobino DM, Dhanireddy R: Human milk feedings and infection among very low birth weight infants. Pediatrics 102e:38, 1998.

66. Itabashi K, Hayashi T, Tsugoshi T, et al: Fortified preterm human milk for very low birth weight infants. Early Hum Dev 29:339, 1992.

67. Iwai Y, Takanashi T, Nakao Y, et al: Iron status in low birth weight infants on breast and formula feeding. Eur J Pediatr 145:63, 1986.

68. Jävenpää AL: Feeding the low-birth-weight infant, IV. Fat absorption as a function of diet and duodenal bile acids. Pediatrics 72:684, 1983.

69. Jävenpää AL, Raiha NCR, Rassin DK, et al: Preterm infants fed human milk attain intrauterine weight gain. Acta Paediatr Scand 72:239, 1983.

70. Jocson MAL, Mason EO, Schanler RJ: The effects of nutrient fortification and varying storage conditions on host defense properties of human milk. Pediatrics 100:240, 1997.

71. Jones E, Dimmock PW, Spencer SA: A randomised controlled trial to compare methods of milk expression after preterm delivery. Arch Dis Child Fetal Neonatal Ed 85:F91, 2001.

72. Kelly EJ, Newell SJ: Gastric ontogeny: Clinical implications. Arch Dis Child 71:F136, 1994.

73. Kuschel CA, Harding JE: Multicomponent fortified human milk for promoting growth in preterm infants (Cochrane Review). In The Cochrane Library, Issue 4. Chichester, UK, John Wiley & Sons, 2004.

74. LaGamma EF, Ostertag SG, Birenbaum H: Failure of delayed oral feedings to prevent necrotizing enterocolitis: Results of studying very low birthweight neonates. Am J Dis Child 139:385, 1985.

75. Lawrence RA: Infant nutrition. Pediatr Rev 5:133, 1983.

76. Lebenthal E, Leung Y-K: The impact of development of the gut on infant nutrition. Pediatr Ann 16:211, 1987.

77. Letarte J, Guyda H, Dussault JH, et al: Lack of protective effect of breastfeeding in congenital hypothyroidism: Report of 12 cases. Pediatrics 65:703, 1980.

78. Lewis-Jones DI, Reynolds GI: A suggested role for precolostrum in preterm and sick newborn infants. Acta Paediatr Scand 72:13, 1983.

79. Lubetsky R, Mandel D, Mimouni FB, Dollberg S: Diurnal variations in creamatocrits from expressed breast milk of preterm infants. Neonatal Fetal Nutr Metab abstract no. 644. Pediatr Res 55:644, 2003.

80. Lubit EC: Cleft palate orthodontics: Why, when, how? Am J Orthod 69:562, 1976.

81. Lucas A: Enteral nutrition. In Tsang RC, Lucas A, Uauy R, et al (eds): Nutritional Needs of the Preterm Infant. Baltimore, William & Wilkins, 1993.

82. Lucas A, Bishop NJ, King FL, et al: Randomized trial of nutrition for preterm infants after discharge. Arch Dis Child 67:324. 1992.

83. Lucas A, Bloom SR, Aynsley-Green A: Gut hormones and "minimal enteral feeding." Acta Paediatr Scand 75:719, 1986.

84. Lucas A, Cole TJ: Breast milk and neonatal necrotising enterocolitis. Lancet 336:1519, 1990.

85. Lucas A, Fewtrell MS, Morley R, et al: Randomized outcome trial of human milk fortification and developmental outcome in preterm infants. Am J Clin Nutr 64:142, 1996.

86. Lucas A, Morley R, Cole TJ, et al: Early diet in preterm babies and developmental status in infancy. Arch Dis Child 64:1570, 1989.

87. Lucas A, Morley R, Cole TJ, et al: Early diet in preterm babies and developmental status at 18 months. Lancet 335:1477, 1990.

88. Lucas A, Morley R, Cole TJ, et al: Breast milk and subsequent intelligence quotient in children born premature. Lancet 339:261, 1992.

89. Mathew OP: Science of bottle feeding. J Pediatr 119:511, 1991.

90. Mathew OP, Bhatia J: Sucking and breathing patterns during breast- and bottle-feeding in term neonates: Effects of nutrient delivery and composition. Am J Dis Child 143:588, 1989.

91. Mathur NB, Dwarkadas AM, Sharma VK, et al: Anti-infective factors in preterm human colostrums. Acta Paediatr Scand 79:1039, 1990.

92. Meberg A, Willgraff S, Sande HA: High potential for breastfeeding among mothers giving birth to pre-term infants. Acta Paediatr Scand 71:661, 1982.

93. Meetze WH, Valentine C, McGuigan JE, et al: Gastrointestinal priming prior to full enteral nutrition in very low birth weight infants. J Pediatr Gastroenterol Nutr 15:163, 1992.

94. Meier PP, Brown LP, Hurst NM: Breastfeeding the preterm infants. In Riordan J, Auerbach K (eds): Breastfeeding and Human Lactation, 2nd ed. Boston, Jones & Bartlett, 1998, p 449.

95. Morley R, Fewtrell MS, Abbott RA, et al: Neurodevelopment in children born small for gestational age: A randomized trial of nutrient-enriched versus standard formula and comparison with a reference breastfed group. Pediatrics 113:515, 2004.

96. Moro GE, Minoli I, Ostrom M, et al: Fortification of human milk: Evaluation of a novel fortification scheme and of a new fortifier. J Pediatr Gastroenterol Nutr 20:162, 1995.

97. Mortensen EL, Michaelsen KF, Sanders SA, et al: The association between duration of breastfeeding and adult intelligence. JAMA 287:2365, 2002.

98. Morton JA: The role of the pediatrician in extended breastfeeding of the preterm infant. Pediatr Ann 32:308, 2003.

99. Murphy JF, Neale ML, Matthews N: Antimicrobial properties of preterm breast milk cells. Arch Dis Child 58:198, 1983.

100. Narayanan I, Mehta R, Choudhury DK, et al: Sucking on the "emptied" breast: Non-nutritive sucking with a difference. Arch Dis Child 66:241, 1991.

101. Naayanan I, Prakash K, Prabhakar AK, et al: A planned prospective evaluation of the anti-infective property of varying quantities of expressed human milk. Acta Paediatr Scand 71:441, 1982.

102. Neifert MR, Seacat JM: Practical aspects of breastfeeding the premature infant. Perinatol Neonatol 12:24, 1988.

103. Newell SJ: Enteral feeding of the micro premie. Clin Perinatol 27:221, 2000.

104. Oski FA: Iron requirements of the premature infant. In Tsang RC (ed): Vitamin and Mineral Requirements in Preterm Infants. New York, Marcel Dekker, 1985.

105. Picciano MF: Nutrient composition of human milk. Pediatr Clin North Am 48:53, 2001.

106. Putet G, Rigo J, Salle B, et al: Supplementation of pooled human milk with casein hydrolysate: Energy and nitrogen balance and weight gain composition in very low birth weight infants. Pediatr Res 21:458, 1987.

107. Rönnholm KAR, Perheentupa J, Siimes MA: Supplementation with human milk protein improves growth of small premature infants fed human milk. Pediatrics 77:649, 1986.

108. Rönnholm KAR, Sipilä I, Siimes MA: Human milk protein supplementation for the prevention of hypoproteinemia without metabolic imbalance in breast milk-fed very low-birth-weight infants. J Pediatr 101:243,1982.

109. Savilahti E, Järvenpää A-L, Räihä NCR: Serum immunoglobulins in preterm infants: Comparison of human milk and formula feeding. Pediatrics 72:312, 1983.

110. Schanler RJ: Quality of growth in preterm infants: Use of fortified human milk. In Battaglia FC, Pedraz C, Sawatzki G, et al (eds): Maternal and Extrauterine Nutritional Factors: Their Influence on Fetal and Infant Growth. Madrid, Ediciones Ergon, 1996.

111. Schanler RJ: Suitability of human milk for the low birth-weight infant. Clin Perinatol 22:207, 1995.

112. Schanler RJ, Abrams SA: Postnatal attainment of intrauterine macromineral accretion rates in low birth weight infants fed fortified human milk. J Pediatr 126:441, 1995.

113. Schanler RJ, Garza C: Plasma amino acid differences in very low birth weight infants fed either human milk or

whey-dominant cow milk formula. Pediatr Res 21:301, 1987.

114. Schanler RJ, Garza C, Nichols BL: Fortified mother's milk for very-low-birth-weight infants: Results of growth and nutrient balance studies. J Pediatr 107:437, 1985.

115. Schanler RJ, Garza C, Smith EO: Fortified mother's milk for very-low-birth-weight infants: Results of macromineral studies. J Pediatr 107:767, 1985.

116. Schanler RJ, Hurst NM: Human milk for the hospitalized preterm infant. Semin Perinatol 18:476, 1994.

117. Senterre J, Patel G, Salle B, et al: Effects of vitamin D and phosphorus supplementation on calcium retention in preterm infants fed banked human milk. J Pediatr 103:305, 1983.

118. Slagle TA, Gross SJ: Effect of early low-volume enteral substrate on subsequent feeding tolerance in very low birth weight infants. J Pediatr 113:526, 1988.

119. Steichen JJ, Krug-Wispe SK, Tsang RC: Breastfeeding the low birth weight preterm infant. Clin Perinatol 14:131, 1987.

120. Stein H, Cohen D, Herman AAB, et al: Pooled pasteurized breast milk and untreated own mother's milk in the feeding of very low birth weight babies: A randomized controlled trial. J Pediatr Gastroenterol Nutr 5:242, 1986.

121. Stevenson DK, Yang C, Kerner JA, et al: Intestinal flora in the second week of life in hospitalized preterm infants fed stored frozen breast milk or a proprietary formula. Clin Pediatr 24:338, 1985.

122. Sturman JA, Rassin DK, Gaull GE: A mini review: Taurine in development. Life Sci 21:1, 1977.

123. Subcommittee on Nutrition during Lactation, Institute of Medicine. Washington, DC, National Academy Press, 1991.

124. Tikanoja T, Simell O, Järvenpää AL: Plasma amino acids in preterm infants after a feed of human milk or formula. J Pediatr 101:248, 1982.

125. Tsang RC, Lucas A, Uauy R, et al: Nutritional Needs of the Preterm Infant. Baltimore, Williams & Wilkins, 1993.

126. Tudehope D, Bayley G, Townsend M, et al: Breastfeeding practices and severe hyperbilirubinemia. J Pediatr Child Health 27:240, 1991.

127. Tyson JE, Lasky RE, Mize CE, et al: Growth, metabolic response, and development in very-low-birth-weight infants fed banked human milk or enriched formula. I. Neonatal findings. J Pediatr 103:95, 1983.

128. Uauy RD, Birch DG, Birch EE: Effect of dietary omega-3 fatty acids on retinal function of very low birth weight neonates. Pediatr Res 28:245, 1990.

129. Usowicz AG, Dab SB, Emery JR, et al: Liver disease in α-1-antitrypsin deficiency. JAMA 253:2679, 1985.

130. Verronen P: Breastfeeding of low birth weight infants. Acta Paediatr Scand 74:495, 1985.

131. Weaver LT, Ewing G, Taylor LC: The bowel habits of milk-fed infants. J Pediatr Gastroenterol Nutr 7:568, 1988.

132. Wooldridge J, Hall WA: Posthospitalization breastfeeding patterns of moderately preterm infants. J Perinat Neonat Nurs 17:50, 2003.

15

Breastfeeding the infant with a problem

Breastfeeding is a natural behavior for infants and provides the ideal nourishment, but some infants with complicating issues may need special assistance or adjustments. Prematurity is discussed in Chapter 14. Infants with structural abnormalities, metabolic challenges, and neurologic difficulties as well as stressed infants and twins and triplets will be discussed in this chapter.

PERINATAL ISSUES: POSTMATURE INFANTS

Postmature infants are full-grown, mature infants who have stayed in utero beyond the full vigor of the placenta and have begun to lose weight in utero. They are usually "older looking" and have a wide-eyed countenance. Their skin is dry and peeling, and subcutaneous tissue is diminished; thus, the skin appears too large. These infants have lost subcutaneous fat and lack glycogen stores. Initially, they may be hypoglycemic and require early feedings to maintain blood glucose levels of 40 mg/dL or higher. If breastfed, the infant should go to the breast early, taking special care to maintain body temperature, which is quite labile in postmature infants who lack the insulating fat layer. Blood sugar levels should be followed. These infants may feed poorly initially and require considerable prodding to suckle. If the infant becomes hypoglycemic despite careful management, consideration should be given to a feeding of 10% glucose in water. In extreme cases of hypoglycemia, an intravenous (IV) infusion may be necessary, and management should follow guidelines for any infant who has hypoglycemia that is resistant to routine early feedings. Because they lack glycogen stores, hypoglycemia may persist.

Calcium problems, on the other hand, although common in these infants, generally are rare if the infant is adequately breastfed early because of the physiologic calcium/phosphorus ratio in breast milk. Once postmature infants begin to feed well, they tend to catch up quickly and continue to adapt very well. Problems with hyperbilirubinemia seldom occur because their livers are mature.

Fetal distress and hypoxia

Infants who have been compromised in utero or during delivery because of insufficient placental reserve, cord accidents, or other causes of intrauterine hypoxia have very low Apgar scores at birth and need special treatment. An asphyxiated infant cannot be fed for at least 48 hours, and depending on associated findings, it may be 96 hours or more before it is safe to put food in the gastrointestinal tract, which has been poorly perfused during the hypoxia. The infant must be maintained on IV fluids. If the mother is to breastfeed,

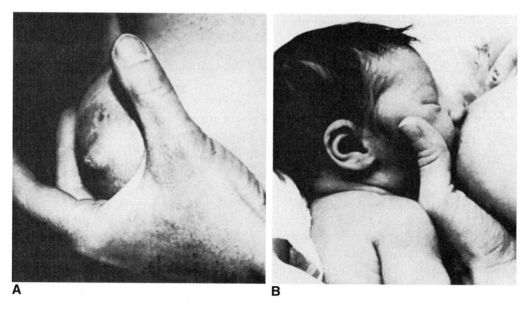

Figure 15-1.   Dancer hold. **A,** Hand position of mother. **B,** Infant in position at breast with support. (From McBride MC, Danner SC: Sucking disorders in neurologically impaired infants: Assessment and facilitation of breastfeeding. Clin Perinatol 14:109, 1987.)

her colostrum will be valuable to the infant and will be better tolerated by the infant's intestinal tract, which has usually suffered hypotoxic damage in these circumstances. *Hypoxia* decreases the motility of the gut and decreases stimulating hormones.

The mother will need help initiating lactation and understanding the pathophysiology of the infant's disease. These infants often have a poor suck and do not coordinate with the swallow, making nursing at the breast difficult. The mother may need to hold her breast in place and hold the infant's chin as well. These infants are especially susceptible to "nipple confusion," so means of sustaining nourishment other than a bottle should be sought. Weaning slowly from the IV hyperalimentation fluids while introducing breastfeeding is helpful. Using a dropper and employing the nursing supplementer are options if the milk supply from the breast is low. These infants may continue to feed poorly for neurologic reasons. They do not do better with a bottle. If the mother is taught to cope with the problem, nursing should progress satisfactorily. She may always need to hold her breast in place.

The infant can be held in positions that may help an individual baby adapt better. The "football hold" is a popular but poorly named position in which the infant is held to the mother's body with the feet to her side. The head and face are squarely in front of the breast and steadied by the mother's arm and hand on that side. Cupping the breast and the jaw in one hand facilitates the infant's seal around the breast with the mouth (Fig. 15-1). This position has been called the "dancer hold" by Sarah Coulter Danner, who has prepared a pamphlet for mothers feeding a neurologically impaired infant.* It is well illustrated and is directed toward the mother and her specific problem. One of the most valuable suggestions is the use of a sling or pleat seat to hold the infant's body in a flexed position, thus giving the mother both hands free to hold the head and the breast in position for feeding (Fig. 15-2).

---

*Danner SC, Cerutti ER: Nursing Your Neurologically Impaired Baby. Childbirth Graphics, Ltd, Division of WRS Group, Inc., PO Box 21207, Waco, TX 76702-1207.

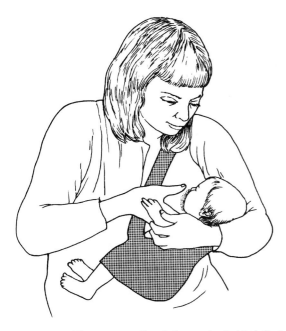

Figure 15-2. Pleat-seat or sling baby carrier holds infant in a flexed position that facilitates infant suckling, leaving mother's hands free to support her breast and the infant. (Redrawn from McBride MC, Danner SC: Sucking disorders in neurologically impaired infants: Assessment and facilitation of breastfeeding. Clin Perinatol 14:109, 1987.)

Pacing the feedings and pumping after feedings will increase mother's milk supply when the infant is unable to suck vigorously enough. Giving the pumped milk by lactation supplementer, small cup, or dropper ensures proper weight gain in the early weeks.[102] Holding the infant in a flexed position mimicking the fetal position relaxes an infant who is often hypertonic or arching away from the breast.

In a study of energetics and mechanics of nutritive sucking in preterm and term neonates, Jain and associates[75] compared 38-week infants with 35-week infants and noted that preterm infants use less energy to suck the same volume of milk. The preterm infant took up to 0.5 mL per suck and generated lower pressures and a lower frequency.

Exploring the hypothesis that milk flow achieved during feeding contributes to ventilatory depression during rubber-nipple feeding, Mathew[100] compared nipples with different flow rates. Decreases in minute ventilation and breathing frequency were significantly greater with high-flow nipples, thus confirming that milk flow influences breathing in the premature infant who is unable to self-regulate the flow.

The work of feeding, and especially the physical work of feeding at the breast, has been the argument against allowing an immature infant in the Western world to breastfeed at under 1800 g. Survival of low-birth-weight (LBW) infants in Third World countries has been dependent on early breastfeeding. Nonnutritive sucking using a pacifier was evaluated measuring transcutaneous oxygen tension, heart rate, and respiratory rate while sleeping. Infants were 32 to 35 weeks' postconceptual age.[21] The oxygen tension decreased 2.3 mm Hg during suckling the pacifier at 32 to 33 weeks and 4.0 mm Hg at 34 to 35 weeks but not at 36 to 39 weeks. Respiratory rates remained stable, and heart rate rose slightly. Transcutaneous oxygen pressure (to Po_2) and body temperature were monitored during feedings in five very low birth weight (VLBW) infants during bottle feeding and breastfeeding.[105,106] Tracings were made from the first oral feeding to time of discharge. Serial Po_2 values showed small undulations across baseline (above and below) while breastfeeding and substantial dips while bottle feeding with recovery, but not above baseline. The quality and quantity of variation were very different in the two modes, with large drops occurring during actual sucking of the bottle but only during burping or repositioning while breastfeeding. Meier[105] concludes that the findings do not support the widely held view that breastfeeding is more stressful. The comparative data suggest that both pacifier and bottle feeding are more stressful than suckling at the breast. If the infant has significant motor tone disabilities or lacks the usual oral reflexes in response to stimulus of the rooting and sucking reflexes, a neonatal neurologist should assess the infant before any routine exercises are initiated.

It has been suggested that perioral stimulation enhances an immature or neurologically impaired infant's ability to suck and to coordinate suck and swallow.[84] Perioral stimulation, consisting of stimulating the skin overlying the masseter and buccinator muscles by manually applying a quick-touch pressure stimulus lasting 1 second, was studied. This is accomplished by simultaneously squeezing (the buccal fat) both cheeks. Suck-monitoring equipment revealed that perioral stimulation increased the sucking rate, suggesting that this may facilitate sucking.[102] Exercising the mouths of infants who already have excessive mouth stimulation may not be appropriate.[84] Many infants in the neonatal intensive care unit (NICU) are being suctioned, tube fed and orally stimulated for other reasons.

When the infant is ready for nonnutritive sucking in the NICU, it is possible to allow sucking at the empty breast (prepumped) instead of a pacifier. Although it is not clear that digestion and gastrointestinal motility are enhanced by sucking,[115] enteral tube feedings are usually given while using a pacifier in most NICUs. Mothers who have been using an electric pump to produce milk for their VLBW infant find "nonnutritive" suckling at the breast by their infant very helpful. Premature infants with a postconceptual age of 35 weeks can discriminate between sweet and nonsweet tastes.[144] They respond with greater sucking when given glucose water rather than plain water, so that the popular vanilla-flavored pacifiers may be significantly preferred over the human nipple. These pacifiers should not be used in infants who breastfeed. Studies of nonnutritive suckling at the breast have been associated with more successful breastfeeding of longer duration. Whitelaw and associates[156] found skin-to-skin contact or kangaroo care to be associated with increased success and duration of breastfeeding. In a randomized trial of stable infants weighing 700 to 1500 g, half the mothers used skin-to-skin contact and half only fondled their infants. Skin-to-skin contact was deemed not only safe but enjoyable for the mother. We observed that the kangaroo care given in the NICU at the Providence Hospital in Anchorage, Alaska, which was surrounded by snow drifts and snow-covered mountains, was most successful in raising the body temperature and enhancing the maturation of their premature infants.

GALACTOGOGES: MEDICATION-INDUCED MILK PRODUCTION

Stimulating milk production pharmacologically in mothers of LBW infants who are pumping to provide milk for their infants has been recommended by several authors, as reported by Ehrenkranz and Ackerman.[41] They used 10 mg metoclopramide orally every 8 hours for 7 days, tapering over 2 more days. Milk production increased within 2 days, but after therapy decreased, milk production decreased. Prolactin levels also increased during the treatment.

Improved lactation occurred in 67% of mothers with no breast milk at onset and in 100% of mothers with poor supply given metoclopramide (10 mg three times a day for 10 days) by Gupta and Gupta.[61] They reported that the improvement persisted when the drug was discontinued. None of the 32 women had any symptoms or side effects. This drug is a substituted benzamide, which has selective dopamine-antagonist activity.

Although growth hormone (GH) has been observed to enhance milk supply, no recommended protocol exists for its clinical use. A study of 20 healthy mothers with insufficient milk who delivered between 26 and 34 weeks were given GH, 0.2 IU/kg/day subcutaneously for 7 days. A group of 10 received a placebo. Milk volume increased in the treated mothers. No change was noted in plasma GH levels, but an increase was seen in insulin-like growth factor (IGF). No other changes were noted during this short-term therapy.[60]

Other drugs have been noted to enhance milk production. Domperidome (Motilium) is currently unavailable in the United States unless a pharmacist is willing to fill a prescription. It is widely available in Canada, Europe, and Australia. It is fully discussed in Chapter 11. A dosage of 10 mg three times a day is reported to increase milk supply in some women. The drug is not without side effects, however. Other compounds are discussed in Chapter 11.

BREASTFEEDING TWINS AND TRIPLETS

Many case reports support that a mother can nurse twins and triplets. It has been documented for centuries that an individual mother can provide adequate nourishment for more than one infant. In 17th-century France, wet nurses were allowed to nurse up to six infants at one time. Foundling homes provided wet nurses for every three to six infants.

The key deterrent to nursing twins is not usually the milk supply but time. If the mother can nurse both infants simultaneously, the time factor is minimized (Fig. 15-3). Many tricks have been suggested to achieve this feat. As the infants become larger and more active, it may be difficult to keep them simultaneously nursing with only two hands to cope. However, twins trained from birth to nurse simultaneously will often continue to nurse in a position that allows both to nurse when they are older, even if the other is not nursing at the moment. If the mother has help at home to assist with feedings, breastfeeding can be accomplished. The first year of life for the mother of a set of twins is an extremely busy one and really requires additional help, particularly if the mother is going to breastfeed. She will need time for adequate rest and nourishment. She often benefits from suggestions from other mothers of twins. The incidence of prematurity with twins is 3 in 10, with triplets 9 out of 10, and with singletons just 1 in 10.

The challenge of breastfeeding twins was investigated by Addy,[2] who reviewed 173 questionnaires returned by mothers who were members of the Mothers of Twins Clubs of Southern California. This is a national organization that offers help and advice to mothers of twins. No other socioeconomic information was available. Forty-one mothers (23.7%) breastfed from birth, although 30% of the infants were premature. Of those who did not breastfeed, 9% were told not to do so by their physician, 11% did not think it was possible, and 11% did not think they would have enough milk for two. Of multiparas who had breastfed their first child, an equal number breastfed and bottle fed. Of those mothers who breastfed, 39 breastfed over 1 month and 12 over 6 months.

Eight healthy women breastfeeding twins and one breastfeeding triplets participated in a study by Saint and associates[127] to determine the yield and nutrient content of their milk at 2, 3, 6, 9, and 12 months post partum. At 6 months, they fed on the average 15 feeds per day. Fully breastfeeding women produced 0.84 to 2.16 kg of milk in 24 hours. Those partially

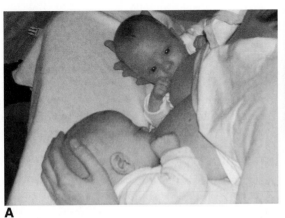 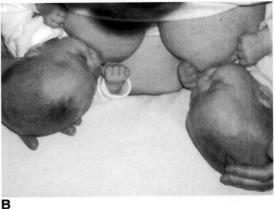

A **B**

Figure 15-3. Premature twins nursing simultaneously, resting on a nursing pillow.

breastfeeding produced 0.420 to 1.392 kg in 24 hours. The mother feeding triplets at 2½ months produced 3.08 kg/day, and the three infants were fed a total of 27 times per day. At 6 months the twins received 64% to 100% of total energy from breastfeeding and at 12 months received 6% to 13%. This demonstrates that the breast is capable of responding to nutritional demands on it, contrary to previous suggestions that milk production had a finite limit that was much less than a liter.

Guidelines for success in breastfeeding twins reported by Hattori admit there are many obstacles but suggest that the health care professional should provide extended support to mothers of multiples to promote successful breastfeeding.[66] An extra pair of helpful hands provide significant assistance and relieve some of the fatigue. The initiation and duration of breast milk feedings by mothers of multiples compared to mothers of singletons was studied by a mailed questionnaire with 358 responses (and 197 no responses). The mothers with multiples who answered were older, had higher incomes, were married, and were less likely to return to work by 6 months post partum. Initiation of breastfeeding was comparable between mothers of multiples and singletons, but mothers of multiples provided milk for a shorter period of time and mothers of preterm multiples breastfed the shortest period of time. At 6 months, 33% of mothers of term singletons were breastfeeding partially compared with 37% mothers of term multiples. For preterm singletons, 31% were breastfed compared with 16% of preterm multiples.[55]

FULL-TERM INFANTS WITH MEDICAL PROBLEMS

Infants who have self-limited acute illnesses, such as fever, upper respiratory infection, colds, diarrhea, or contagious diseases such as chickenpox, do best if breastfeeding is maintained. Because of breast milk's low solute load, an infant can be kept well hydrated despite fever or other increased fluid losses. If respiratory symptoms are significant, an infant seems to nurse well at the breast and poorly with a bottle. This observation has been documented many times when nursing mothers have roomed-in with their sick infants in the hospital. The studies of Johnson and Salisbury[76] on the synchrony of respirations in breastfeeding in contrast to the periodic breathing or gasping apnea pattern of the normal bottle fed infant may well provide the underlying explanation for the phenomenon of an acutely ill infant continuing to nurse at the breast.

In addition to the appropriateness of the human milk for a sick infant, there is the added comfort of nursing because of the closeness with the mother. If the infant is suddenly weaned, psychological trauma is added to the stress of the illness.

It may become difficult to distinguish the effect of the trauma of acute weaning from the symptoms of the primary illness, such as poor feeding or lethargy, if the acutely weaned infant fails to respond to adequate treatment. Going back to breastfeeding may be the answer because the stress of acute weaning will be removed.

It is not appropriate to give the mother medicine intended to treat the infant, especially antibiotics. This has been tried, to the detriment of the child, because variable amounts of the drug reach the infant, depending on the dose, dosage schedule, and amount of milk consumed. Maternal drugs can produce symptoms in the infant in some cases,[73] and thus maternal history of ingestants is important in assessing symptoms in the breastfed infant (Appendix D).

Guidelines for *buccal smear collection* in breastfed infants should be followed when genetic review is indicated. Buccal smear is a noninvasive, fast, and relatively inexpensive diagnostic method. It is used for gender determination as well as aneusomy, microdeletion syndromes, and a variety of polymerase chain reaction (PCR)-based molecular genetic tests. Maternal cells can contaminate smears taken from breastfed infants. The recommendation is to wait at least 1 hour after a feeding. Buccal mucosa should be cleansed thoroughly with a cotton swab applicator. These procedures apply to both neonates and older nursing children.[16]

Gastrointestinal disease

Bouts of diarrhea and intestinal tract disease are much less common in breastfed infants than in bottle fed infants, but when they occur, the infant should be maintained on the breast if possible.[128] Human milk is a physiologic solution that normally causes neither dehydration nor hypernatremia. Occasionally, an infant will have diarrhea or an intestinal upset because of something in the mother's diet. It is usually self-limited, and the best treatment is to continue to nurse at the breast. If the mother has been taking a laxative that is absorbed or has been eating laxative foods such as fruits in excess, she should adjust her diet. Intractable diarrhea should be evaluated as it would be in any infant. Allergy to mother's milk is extremely rare and would require substantial evidence to support the diagnosis. Allergy to a foreign protein passed into the milk such as bovine β-globulin can cause severe allergic symptoms in the infant.

Colitis while breastfeeding

Severe colitis in a totally breastfed infant, usually with onset in the neonatal period, suggests an intrinsic metabolic disorder in the infant or an exquisite intolerance to something in mother's milk, such as cow milk protein.[82] Six infants with protein-induced enterocolitis presenting in the first month of life with severe bloody diarrhea responded to weaning and use of hydrolyzed protein formula. Other cases have been reported requiring long periods of hyperalimentation and utilization of special formulas such as Nutramigen.

Induced colitis in infants is usually caused by some dietary insult, such as exposure to cow milk.[82,134] It has been reported in breastfed infants, most of whom responded to removal of cow milk from the maternal diet. Several had been given formula at birth. The symptoms included bloody diarrhea, and sigmoidoscopy revealed focal ulcerations, edema, and increased friability of the intestinal mucosa. On relief of symptoms by dietary change, the intestinal tract biopsy returns to normal. Removal of all bovine protein from mother's diet usually results in recovery while returning to breastfeeding.

A prospective study examined 35 consecutive infants who had fresh blood mixed with stools at approximately 4 weeks of age.[94] All infants were otherwise asymptomatic and had no infection, bleeding diathesis, or necrotizing enterocolitis (NEC). Thirty-one had histopathologic evidence of colitis characterized by marked eosinophilic infiltrate (more than 20 eosinophils per high-power field) compared with control subjects and low mean serum albumin. Ten of these 31 were exclusively breastfed, nine were fed cow milk formula, nine soy formula, two mixed breast milk and formula, and one Nutramigen. The low serum albumin and high peripheral eosinophil count suggested the diagnosis of allergic colitis. All cases cleared with dietary change. The breastfed infants were weaned, unfortunately, and not managed by dietary adjustment in the mother in this series.

Protein-induced colitis can follow a benign course with proper treatment. Israel and associates[72] studied 13 infants with blood from the rectum, negative stool cultures, and colonoscopic and histologic evidence of colitis. The infants were all less than 3½ months of age, and six were breastfed and five had been supplemented. All were gaining weight well. The mothers of the breastfed infants restricted cow milk in their diet, and the infants returned to exclusively breastfeeding. All recovered.

Dietary protein-induced proctocolitis in exclusively breastfed infants should be taken into consideration as a cause of rectal bleeding or blood-streaked stool in the neonatal period and early infancy (hematochezia). Benign eosinophilic proctocolitis by colonoscopy is best treated by the exclusion of the allergen from mother's diet. Resolution has taken place within 72 to 96 hours of elimination of the offending protein so temporarily stopping breastfeeding may not be necessary.[121]

An 8-week-old infant boy presented with irritability and projectile vomiting for an ultrasound to rule out pyloric stenosis. The ultrasound revealed colitis and further history revealed bloody stools. He responded to removing bovine protein from mother's diet and continuing to breastfeed.[115]

Harmon and associates[65] described a case of perforated pseudomembranous colitis in a breastfed infant. Other cases have been associated with giving antibiotics to the infant. The infant's stool was *Clostridium difficile* toxin positive, and the child required bowel resection for abscess and perforation. The mother had taken ciprofloxacin without consulting a physician for days before the infant's admission.

The Lactation Study Center has been notified of other cases of bloody diarrhea with a diagnosis of colitis that did appear to respond to maternal dietary restrictions. One infant showed brief improvement when all cow milk products were removed from the mother's diet and then had a relapse. Removing all bovine (both meat and milk) products from the maternal diet resulted in recovery without relapse with exclusive breastfeeding. In retrospect the mother recalled switching from a vegetarian diet to high meat, especially beef, intake throughout pregnancy.

A case of fucose intolerance is reported in a breastfed infant who was not intolerant of lactose but of the by-product of the oligosaccharides in human milk, passing large amounts of fucose in the stool.[17] The infant tolerated Pregestemil and then was weaned to regular formula.

It has been recommended by Haight[63] that the severe cases of allergic colitis and also severe gastrointestinal colic can be alleviated by treating the mother with pancreatic enzymes, 25 mg three times a day. It is safe for the mother and often dramatic for the infant. This is especially effective when eliminating cow protein has not solved the problem.

The management of protracted diarrhea in infants never breastfed is reported by many human milk banks on a case-by-case basis. Eleven of 24 children managed by MacFarlane and Miller[93] in a hyperalimentation referral unit recovered when fed banked human milk orally without protracted IV therapy. All the infants had been tried on all the available special formulas first. A study of oral rehydration in 26 children under the age of 2 years showed that the children who continued to breastfeed while receiving rehydration fluid had fewer stools and recovered more rapidly than those receiving only rehydration fluid.[78] The PIMA Infant Feeding Study clearly showed that in less

developed and more disadvantaged communities in the United States, exclusive breastfeeding protected against severe diarrhea and other gastrointestinal disorders.[47]

Lactose intolerance

Suckling milk is the defining characteristic of mammals. *Lactose,* the major carbohydrate in milk, is hydrolyzed by lactase-phlorhizin hydrolase, an enzyme of the small intestine. *Lactase* plays a critical role in the nutrition of mammalian neonates. Congenital lactase deficiency, present from birth, is extremely rare and is inherited as an autosomal recessive gene.[109] Most humans (except Northern Europeans) and other adult mammals do not drink milk beyond infancy; it causes indigestion and mild to severe gastrointestinal symptoms because of an adult's inability to digest lactose. Low lactase levels result from injury or genetic expression of lactase. The enzyme hydrolyzes lactose, phlorhizin, and glycosyl ceramides. A decline in lactase-specific activity occurs at the time of weaning in most mammalian species. In humans it may occur as early as 3 to 5 years of age; in other species the elevated juvenile levels of lactase-specific activity persist. The developmental patterns of lactase expression are regulated at the level of gene transcription.[109]

Premature infants and those recovering from severe diarrhea have transient lactose intolerance. The only treatment is a temporary lactose-free diet. Reports of lactose-hydrolyzed human milk suggest that banked human milk can be treated with lactase (Kerulac), which will hydrolyze the lactose (900 enzyme activity units to 200 mL breast milk degraded 82% of the lactose).[135] In one case the reason for using human milk was that the infant became infection prone when he was weaned from the breast at the time the initial diagnosis was made. He showed marked improvement with treated human milk. In the breastfed infant, lactase deficiency may be manifest by chronic diarrhea and marked failure to thrive.

An additional clinical syndrome related to slow gaining or failure to thrive is excessive lactose, resulting when the fat level in the milk is low and an excessive amount of milk is consumed because of the low calorie content. The first documented case was reported by Woolridge and Fisher.[160] Lactose production drives the milk-making capacity. When a feeding at one breast does not last long enough for the fat to let down, the result is low-calorie high-lactose milk. The authors recommend in such cases that an entire feeding be taken at one breast. (For further discussion of this phenomenon, see Chapter 8.)

Celiac disease, Crohn's disease, and inflammatory bowel disease

Some chronic diseases are better controlled with the infant kept on breast milk, and symptoms become more severe with weaning. Should an infant be weaned and do poorly on formula, relactation of the mother might be considered. With the availability of the nursing supplementer, this possibility is no longer remote (see Chapter 19).

Celiac disease or permanent gluten-sensitive enteropathy is an immunologic disease dependent on the exposure to wheat gluten or related proteins in rye and barley.[74]

Childhood *celiac disease* is disappearing, according to Littlewood and associates,[88] a trend they attribute to the increasing incidence of breastfeeding and the decreased use of untreated cow milk. They have seen a reduction in gastroenteritis. The delayed use of *gluten* in the diet may also be secondarily important. Infants who have been breastfed and had introduction of solids after 4 months have not been seen to have celiac disease.

In a retrospective study of 146 children with celiac disease, Greco and associates[58] initially confirmed that children breastfed 3 months or more showed a marked delay in onset of the disease unrelated to when gluten was introduced. In a case control study of 216 children in Italy with celiac disease and their siblings, Auricchio and associates[14] reported that infants formula fed from birth or infants breastfed less than 1 month have four times greater risk of celiac disease than infants breastfed over 1 month. The time of introduction of gluten into the diet was not a factor. The incidence in Ireland of celiac disease is also decreasing and was related by Stevens and associates[139] to the protective effect of breastfeeding. Troncone and associates[149] measured the passage of *gliadin* into breast milk after the ingestion of 20 g of wheat gluten. Fifty-four of 80 samples showed 5 to 95 ng/mL of gliadin, which peaked in the milk 2 to 4 hours after ingestion but did not appear in serum. The authors suggest that the transfer of gliadin from mother to infant might be critical for the development of an appropriate specific immune response. The epidemiologic data suggest that breastfeeding would be especially appropriate in celiac disease–positive families. The authors conclude that the presence of gliadin in the milk may be responsible for a protective effect and the development later of specific immune responses to gliadin. It need not be removed from mother's diet if the diagnosis is made while the infant is being breastfed.

A case-control study was done of the effect of infant feeding on celiac disease to investigate the association between duration of breastfeeding and age at first gluten introduction into the infant diet and the incidence and age of onset of celiac disease. A significant protective effect on the incidence of celiac disease was related to the duration of breastfeeding past 2 months. It was not related to the age of first gluten in diet, although the age of first exposure did affect the age of onset of symptoms.[118]

The risk of celiac disease was reduced in children aged less than 2 years in a study of 2000 Swedish children if they were still being breastfed when dietary gluten was introduced. The effect was more pronounced if breastfeeding continued after gluten was introduced. The authors conclude that gradual introduction of gluten-containing foods into the diet while breastfeeding reduces the risk of ever getting celiac disease.[74] The declining incidence of celiac disease and transient gluten intolerance (TGI) has been associated with changing feeding practices, which include later introduction of dietary gluten, the use of gluten-free foods for weaning (rice), and the increased initiation and duration of breastfeeding.[26]

The development of *Crohn's disease* later in life has increased in recent decades. Because it has been suggested that breast milk is essential for the development of the normal immunologic competence of the intestinal mucosa, investigators have studied the association between breastfeeding and later Crohn's disease. Bergstrand and Hellers[19] studied 826 patients who developed Crohn's disease between 1955 and 1974 and their matched control subjects. Mean length of breastfeeding was 4.59 months among patients and 5.76 among control subjects ($p < 0.01$). Patients with Crohn's disease were overrepresented among those with no or very short periods of breastfeeding. The role of infant feeding practices in the development of Crohn's disease in childhood was reported by Koletzko and associates[79] in a study of 145 families with similar results. Although Crohn's disease may develop in genetically susceptible people as a result of an immunologic response to unidentified antigen in the mucosa, early feeding practices are significant.

Early determinants of inflammatory bowel disease have pointed toward infectious diseases in childhood, especially measles, and even in utero infections as possible causative factors. It has become a major disease of adults in Europe with 5.12 cases per 1000 individuals over age 43 in the National Survey of Health and Development of 1946 (NSHD) and 2.02 to 2.54 cases per 1000 by age 33 years in the 1958 National Child Development Study (NCDS). In examining early determinants, these cohorts did not show a protective effect of breastfeeding. The authors comment, however, it recorded "ever breastfed" with no distinction for length of breastfeeding.[146]

Respiratory illness and otitis media

Infants who develop respiratory illnesses should be maintained at the breast. The added advantages of antibodies and antiinfective properties are valuable to the infant. Sick infants can nurse more easily than they can cope with a bottle. Furthermore, the comfort of having the mother nearby is important whenever the infant has a crisis; weaning during illness may be devastating to the infant.

Otitis media in infants occurs less frequently in breastfed infants. Recurrent otitis media is associated with bottle feeding in a study of 237 children, in contrast to prolonged breastfeeding, which had a long-term protective effect up to 3 years of age.[125]

A regional birth cohort of 5356 children was followed prospectively regarding the occurrence of infectious disease in the first year of life.[77] One third developed otitis media. Median age of onset was 8 months, and 10% had had three episodes by 1 year of age. Breastfeeding for 9 months or longer had a significant impact on otitis, as did the number of siblings and daycare. Otitis media in 3- to 8-year-old children in Greenland was studied as a national concern for the incidence and associated deafness. Children who were breastfed were spared, especially if nursed a long time.[117]

Young infants who have older siblings may well be exposed to some virulent viruses and bacteria. Developing croup or chickenpox, for instance, may make the infant seriously ill. Hydration can be maintained by frequent, short breastfeedings. Studies have shown that respirations are maintained more easily when feeding on human milk than on cow milk, even from a bottle. Nursing at the breast permits regular respirations, whereas bottle feeding is associated with a more gasping pattern. Thus, breastfed infants should continue to nurse when they are ill. If the infant is hospitalized, every effort should be made to maintain the breastfeeding to provide expressed breast milk if the infant can be fed at all. Staff should provide rooming-in for the mother if a care-by-parent ward is not available.

Colostrum and milk contain large amounts of IgA antibody, some of which is respiratory syncytial virus (RSV) specific. Breastfed but not bottle fed infants have IgA in their nasal secretions. Neutralizing inhibitors to RSV have been demonstrated in the whey of most samples of human milk tested.[148] IgG anti-RSV antibodies are present in milk and in reactive T lymphocytes. Breastfeeding-induced resistance to RSV was associated with the presence of interferon as well as virus-specific lymphocyte transformation activity, suggesting that breastfeeding has unique mechanisms for modulating the immune response of infants to RSV infection.[27] Clinical studies indicating a relative protection from RSV in breastfed infants were clouded by other factors.[147] The populations were unequal because of socioeconomic factors and smoking (i.e., bottle feeding mothers were in lower socioeconomic groups and smoked more). In general, if breastfed infants become ill, they have less severe illness.[147,148] Although breastfeeding protects, parental smoking and daycare are important negative factors as well in the incidence of respiratory infection. Respiratory illness in either the infant or the mother should be treated symptomatically and breastfeeding continued. If there is nasal congestion in the infant, nasal aspiration and saline nose drops before a feed are helpful.

Galactosemia

Galactosemia, caused by deficiency of galactose-1-phosphate uridyltransferase, is a rare circumstance in which the infant is unable to metabolize galactose and must be placed on a galactose-free diet. The disease can be rapidly fatal in the severe form. The infant may have severe and persistent jaundice, vomiting, diarrhea, electrolyte imbalances, cerebral signs, and weight loss. This does necessitate weaning from the breast to a special formula because human milk contains high levels of lactose, which is a disaccharide that splits into glucose and galactose. The diagnosis is suspected when reducing substances are found in the urine in the newborn, and it is confirmed by measuring the enzyme uridyltransferase in the red and white blood cells. The several forms can be distinguished by genetic testing, but except for the very mild form, the infant must be weaned to a lactose-free diet. An infection with *Escherichia coli* in the newborn period can be associated with this or other metabolic disorders. Galactosemia is screened for in most states along with phenylketonuria (PKU).

Inborn errors of metabolism

Other metabolic deficiency syndromes are usually only apparent as mild failure-to-thrive syndrome until the infant is weaned from the breast and the symptoms become severe. This particularly applies to inborn errors of metabolism caused by an inability to handle one or more of the essential amino acids. Infection is often a complication early in the lives of these infants with inborn errors most commonly due to *Escherichia coli* bacteria. While the acute infection is being treated, the infant may be weaned, and the metabolic disorder then becomes apparent precipitously.

Certain amino acids, including phenylalanine, methionine, leucine, isoleucine, and others associated with metabolic disorders, have significantly lower levels in human milk than in cow milk. Management of an amino acid metabolic disorder while breastfeeding depends on careful monitoring of blood and urine levels of the specific amino acids involved. Because these are essential amino acids, a certain amount is necessary in the diet of all infants, including those with disease. An appropriate combination of breastfeeding and a milk free of the offending amino acid should be developed. The care of such infants should be in consultation with a pediatric endocrinologist. Transient neonatal *tyrosinemia,* which has been reported to occur in a high percentage (up to 80%) of neonates fed cow milk, is associated with blood tyrosine levels 10 times those of adults. Wong and coworkers[159] have associated severe cases with learning disabilities in later years.

Screening programs that test all newborns have identified many victims early. Almost all programs test for PKU, galactosemia, and hypothyroidism, and increasingly maple syrup urine disease, homocystinuria, biotinidase deficiency, tyrosinemia, and now cystic fibrosis are included. Most cases (except galactosemia) can be managed with continued breastfeeding and diet modification. Congenital adrenal hyperplasia requires corticosteroids but the feeding can be breast milk. If it is the salt wasting variety, infant must have added salt.

Phenylketonuria

The most common of the amino acid metabolic disorders is phenylketonuria (PKU), in which the amino acid accumulates for lack of an enzyme. The treatment has been phenylalanine-free formula, available from Abbott Laboratories and Bristol-Myers, combined with added formula or breast milk to provide a little phenylalanine because every infant needs a small amount. If the infant is breastfed, the mother is usually willing to continue on an adjusted schedule. An infant may supplement the Lofenalac or Analog XP with breast milk. With careful monitoring of the blood levels and control of the amount of breastfeeding, a balance can be struck that permits optimal phenylalanine levels and breastfeeding. The infant will require some phenylalanine-free formula to provide enough calories and nutrients. A detailed outline of management called *Guide to Breast Feeding the Infant with PKU,* prepared by Ernest and associates,[44] is available from the Superintendent of Documents, U.S. Government Printing Office, Washington, DC 20402.

Literature values for phenylalanine range from 29 to 64 mg/dL in human milk. The amount for Lofenalac or Analog XP and human milk for a given baby are calculated by weight, age, blood levels, and needs for growth. As an example, a 3-week-old weighing 3.7 kg whose blood level was 52.5 mg/dL when he was ingesting an estimated 570 mL of breast milk would receive 240 mL Lofenalac and 360 mL breast milk (four breastfeedings a day with before and after weighing). The details of every step of management are available in the guide to assist the physician in planning treatment.[44] Test weighing, which is now a simple home procedure, greatly facilitates the accuracy of this management.

A simpler approach is described by Clark,[29] who suggests that as soon as the diagnosis is made, the infant be placed on the low-phenylalanine formula to reduce the levels in the plasma promptly. The mother should pump her breasts to maintain her milk supply. Human milk has less phenylalanine than formula, but it exceeds the tolerance of most infants with PKU. The breastfed infant is offered a small volume of special formula (10 to 30 mL) first and then completes the feeding at the breast. As long as the blood phenylalanine levels can be maintained between 120 and 300 μmol/L, exact intake need not be measured. Initially, weight

checks to ensure adequate growth are essential because poor intake leading to a catabolic state will interfere with control. Because human milk is low in phenylalanine, the offending amino acid, more than half the diet can be breast milk.

The weaning of this special infant should be similar to that of other infants. Adding solid foods can be initiated at 6 months.[29] The liquid part of the diet continues as before, that is, two feeding components of low-phenylalanine formula and breastfeeding plus solids with little or no phenylalanine (fruits, vegetables, low-protein foods). Rice and wheat contain too much phenylalanine. When the decision is made to wean from the breast, solid foods can be used to replace the phenylalanine in the breast milk as needed. Growth should be followed closely. When weaning is complete, the infant should be given other less bulky sources of protein free of phenylalanine. This stage will be carefully orchestrated by the endocrinologist and nutritionist. Because infants with PKU are more prone to thrush infection, the mother should be alerted to watch for symptoms in the infant and the onset of sore nipples that could be caused by *Candida albicans.* Treatment is nystatin for mother and baby initially. (See discussion in Chapter 16.)

The other benefits of human milk make the effort to breastfeed valuable for the infant and for the mother, who usually wants to continue to contribute to her infant's nurturing and nourishment. The prognosis for intellectual development is excellent if treatment is initiated early and the blood levels maintained at less than 10 mg/dL phenylalanine (120 to 300 μmol/L).

A retrospective study of 26 school-age children who had been breastfed or formula fed for 20 to 40 days before dietary intervention was conducted by Riva and associates.[122] The children who had been breastfed had a 14-point IQ advantage, which persisted at 12.9 points when corrected for maternal social and educational status. The age of treatment onset for PKU was not related to IQ scores. This study strongly supports the belief that breastfeeding in the prediagnostic stage has an impact on the long-range neurodevelopmental performance of PKU patients.

Nutrition management of infants with *organic acidemias* involves limiting the intake of the offending amino acid(s) to the minimum necessary for normal growth and development and suppressing amino acid degradation during catabolic periods by providing alternative fuels such as glucose. In some disorders, including isovaleric acidemia, specific treatment is included to increase the excretion of toxic metabolites by enhancing the body's capacity to make isovalerylglycine, a diisovalerylcarnitine. As more specific amino acid–free formulas are made available, a recipe for combining breastfeeding with the special formula can be engineered to specific infants' needs. The endocrinologist and nutritionist can provide such a recipe. Dietary precautions for the mother of a breastfeeding PKU child are to avoid the artificial sweetner, aspartame (Nutrasweet), which metabolizes to phenylalanine.

OTHER METABOLIC DISORDERS

Tyrosinemia type I is an inherited autosomal recessive trait. Symptoms are caused by accumulation of tyrosine and its metabolites in the liver. It is treated by dietary control consisting of low protein with limited phenylalanine and tyrosine. Some breastfeeding is possible combined with protein-free supplements. 2-(2-nitro-4-trifluoromethylbenzyl)-1-3-cyclohexanedione (NTBC) reduces the production of toxic metabolites. Liver failure is common. Dietary restrictions are lifelong.

Pompe disease (acid maltase deficiency or glycogen storage disease type II) is an inborn error of metabolism caused by a complete or partial deficiency of the enzyme acid alpha-gluconsidase that normally breaks down lysomal glycogen into glucose. Glycogen accumulates in the tissues, especially muscles. The disease takes various forms. Infantile onset has a poor prognosis and treatment is supportive. Because of the frequency of respiratory infection and difficulty feeding, breastfeeding would be palliative as liver disease is rapidly progressive.

Ornithine transcar amylase deficiency is a rare life-threatening genetic disorder. It is one of six urea cycle disorders named for the specific enzyme deficiency present.

A lack of enzyme results in excessive and symptomatic accumulation of ammonia in the blood (hyperammonemia). Symptoms vary but can occur within 72 hours of birth and include poor suck, irritability, vomiting, and progressive lethargy followed, if untreated, by hyptonia, seizures, respiratory distress, and coma. Infant onset disease is more common in males. Treatment involves limiting nitrogen intake and assisting nitrogen excretion with phenylbutrate (Buphenyl). Infants can be breastfed and receive nonprotein caloric supplement. The advantage of human milk is not only dietary but the infection protection and immune protective qualities. There is an essential amino acid formula available for those not breastfeeding.

There are many other variations of these enzyme deficiency diseases. Without treatment, they all lead to deterioration, mental retardation, and often organ failure especially liver failure.[158] The National Organization for Rare Disorders Inc. (NORD) provides information for professionals and the lay public as well as support groups. It lobbies for development of specific treatments (orphan drugs). Specific treatment information is available at their Web site, www.rarediseases.org, or by writing to Box 1968, Danbury, CT, 06813-1968.

Cystic fibrosis

Screening tests for cystic fibrosis have been initiated in many state-mandated metabolic screening programs for newborns so a greater number will be identified early. Meconium plug, especially large plugs and full-blown meconium ileus have a high correlation with pancreatic enzyme deficiency and cystic fibrosis. As clinicians are alerted to meconium plugs, early tests for cystic fibrosis can be carried out and management adjusted. Breastfeeding is optimal not only for the nutrition but the presence of enzymes to facilitate digestion and absorption of nutrients. Because infection is a critical morbidity in these children, the infection protection properties of human milk make a critical impact.

The first symptom in infants with cystic fibrosis (CF) is often failure to thrive. If the infant is breast-fed, the mother may be forced to wean, yet the infant feeds even less well and has no weight gain on formula. Infants do better if placed back on the breast. Pumping to increase mother's milk supply will help the child's hunger. In a study of CF centers, 77% recommended breastfeeding either alone on with pancreatic enzyme supplements.[91] The recommended breastfeeding duration was 3 to 6 months by 43% of the centers (Tables 15-1, 15-2, and 15-3). If supplementation is required, hydrolyzed formula is recommended. Generic and name-brand enzymes are not biologically equal, and some formulas were more frequently associated with greasy stools and abdominal cramping. Use of enzymes may be a way to improve tolerance and weight gain in these special breastfed infants rather than weaning to formula.[25] Prescribing pancreatic enzymes for the mother while breastfeeding is also a consideration.[63]

TABLE 15-1 Recommendations about breastfeeding by cystic fibrosis center directors for CFIM

Recommendations	Response,* no. (%)	
Breastfeeding		
Only	3	(2.6)
Plus pancreatic enzymes	39	(34.2)
Plus hydrolyzed formula	7	(6.1)
Plus pancreatic enzymes and hydrolyzed formula	39	(34.2)
Hydrolyzed formula with pancreatic enzymes	18	(15.8)
Hydrolyzed formula only	2	(1.8)
Not applicable and/or others category	6	(5.3)
Total	114	(100)

CFIM, Mothers of infants with cystic fibrosis.
*Many centers chose more than one answer; therefore, response rate for each answer is calculated as a percentage of total responses.
Modified from Luder E, Kattan M, Tanzer-Torres G, et al: Current recommendations for breast feeding in cystic fibrosis centers. Am J Dis Child 144:1153, 1990.

TABLE 15-2 Factors for discontinuation of breastfeeding according to cystic fibrosis center directors for CFIM

Factors for discontinuation	Response,* no. (%)	
Protein-energy malnutrition	69	(51.1)
Marked steatorrhea	29	(21.5)
Meconium ileus	16	(11.9)
Chronic bacterial pathogen(s) carrier	8	(5.9)
Not applicable and/or others category	13	(9.6)
Total	135	(100)

CFIM, Mothers of infants with cystic fibrosis.
*Many centers chose more than one answer; therefore, response rate for each answer is calculated as a percentage of total responses.
Modified from Luder E, Kattan M, Tanzer-Torres G, et al: Current recommendations for breastfeeding in cystic fibrosis centers. Am J Dis Child 144:1153, 1990.

α_1-Antitrypsin deficiency

Alpha$_1$-Antitrypsin (α_1AT) is a serum protease inhibitor that inactivates a number of proteases. More than 24 genetic variants of this disease are designated B through Z, with the M variant being most common. Children with α_1AT deficiency are at increased risk for liver disease, which occurs

TABLE 15-3 Duration of breastfeeding as reported by cystic fibrosis center directors for CFIM

Duration (months)	Centers,* no. (%)	
<3	34	(40)
3–6	37	(43)
>6	5	(5.8)
Not applicable and/or others category	10	(12)
Total	86	(100)

CFIM, Mothers of infants with cystic fibrosis.
*Many centers chose more than one answer; therefore, response rate for each answer is calculated as a percentage of total responses.
Modified from Luder E, Kattan M, Tanzer-Torres G, et al: Current recommendations for breastfeeding in cystic fibrosis centers. Am J Dis Child 144:1153, 1990.

most often during infancy and often progresses to cirrhosis and death. Udall and associates[151] investigated the relationship between early feedings and the onset of liver disease. Severe liver disease was present in eight (40%) of the bottle fed and one (8%) of the breastfed infants (breastfed for only 5 weeks). Of the 32 infants, 24 were still alive at the end of the study; 12 had been breastfed and 12 bottle fed during their first month of life. All eight of the deceased children had been bottle fed; SGA (small for gestational age) and preterm infants had been excluded from the study so that all infants were equally stable at birth and capable of breastfeeding. A bottle fed infant was seven times more likely to develop liver disease.

With the increasing early diagnosis of $\alpha_1 AT$ deficiency, encouraging a mother to breastfeed if her infant is affected would appear to have a significant impact on reducing the chance of long-range liver disease in her infant.

Acrodermatitis enteropathica (Danbolt-Closs syndrome)

Acrodermatitis enteropathica is a rare and unique disease in which feeding the infant with human milk may be lifesaving. It is an autosomal recessive disorder with an onset as early as 3 weeks old.[131] It is inherited as an autosomal recessive trait and is characterized by a symmetric rash around the mouth, genitalia, and periphery of the extremities. The rash is an acute vesicobullous and eczematous eruption often secondarily infected with *C. albicans*. It may be seen by the third week of life or not until late in infancy and has been associated with weaning from the breast. Failure to thrive, hair loss, irritability, and chronic severe intractable diarrhea are often life threatening. The disease has been associated with extremely low plasma zinc levels. Oral zinc sulfate has produced remission of the syndrome. Zinc deficiency was seen frequently in premature infants on peripheral alimentation until zinc was added to the solution.

Human milk contains less zinc than does bovine milk, with zinc concentrations of both decreasing throughout lactation. Eckert and associates[40] studied the zinc binding in human and cow milk and noted that the low-molecular-weight (LMW) binding ligand isolated from human milk may enhance absorption of zinc in these patients. Gel chromatography indicated that most of the zinc in cow milk was associated with high-molecular-weight fractions, whereas zinc in human milk was associated with LMW fractions. The copper/zinc ratio may also be of significance, because the ratio is lower in cow milk.

The zinc-binding ligand from human milk was further identified as prostaglandin E by chromatography, ultrafiltration, and infrared spectroscopy by Evans and Johnson.[45] Patients also have low arachidonic acid levels. Arachidonic acid is a precursor of prostaglandin. The efficacy of human milk in the treatment of acrodermatitis enteropathica results from the presence of the zinc-prostaglandin complex. The primary deficiency in the infant is an inability to absorb zinc except in this complex form.

The clinical significance of the relationship of human milk to onset of the disease and its treatment is in developing lactation in the mother of such an infant, rare as the disease may be. Delayed lactation or relactation is possible and should be offered as an option to the mother of such an infant (see Chapter 19).

Several reports of isolated cases of zinc deficiency during breastfeeding have appeared in the literature.[3,4,12] In some cases, zinc levels in the milk were low; in others, they were not measured.[161] One child had a classic "zinc-deficient" rash that responded to oral zinc therapy. One should keep in mind that any deficiency is possible and consider intake deficiency when symptoms occur in the breastfed infant. The basic defect is presumed to be related to gastrointestinal malabsorption of zinc.

The treatment of choice is oral administration of zinc in the sulfate or gluconate form. It is usually well tolerated, safe, inexpensive, effective, and expedient. When zinc deficiency occurs in a breastfed infant, the possibility of zinc deficiency in the milk, although a rare disorder, should be considered.[131]

Down syndrome

Infants with Down syndrome or other trisomies may be difficult to feed. When they are breastfed, the mother needs patience to teach the infant to suck with sufficient vigor to initiate the let-down reflex and to stimulate adequate production of milk. Using manual expression to start flow and holding the breast firmly for the infant so that the nipple does not drop out of the mouth when the infant stops suckling will assist the process.

Initially, an infant with Down syndrome may have surprisingly good tone and may even suck well at the breast, only to develop problems once the mother and infant have been discharged home. Providing support for the head, the jaw, and the general body hypotonia will require considerable coordination by the mother. Propping the baby firmly with a pillow in mother's lap or supporting the infant in a sling frees up a much-needed hand for steadying the jaw and breast (see Fig. 15-2).[102]

A nurse clinician knowledgeable and experienced in dealing with neurologically impaired infants should be available to the parents. The initial goals for the mother-infant pair are developing confidence in handling the infant, adjusting to the infant's problem, and dealing with the parental grief and sense of loss—loss of the normal infant that was expected. If the mother has breastfed other children, the emphasis on breastfeeding modifications are more successful, and milk supply usually responds to manual expression and pumping. Initiating sufficient stimulus to the breast to increase milk production is critical in the first few days to induce good prolactin response, especially in primiparas. Renting an electric breast pump is a good investment, justifiable for reimbursement from health insurance by physician prescription.

In developing a discharge plan for this infant, the pediatrician will need to coordinate the team to avoid the fragmented care that develops with a multiproblem situation, which may require the consultation of a geneticist, genetic counselor, cardiologist, and other medical experts to deal with the problems. Ideally, the pediatrician and the office nurse practitioner can provide the additional support and counsel necessary. Many families prefer to leave the hospital early to retreat to the comfort and privacy of their home and the health care provider they selected. Home visits by the pediatrician's staff can provide the necessary monitoring of weight gain and nutrition, as well as counseling by someone capable of handling all the problems that arise, including the breastfeeding. No referrals should be made without the pediatrician's knowledge and agreement. The pediatrician or family physician has the advantage of knowing both the family and the child.

In a study of 59 breastfed infants with Down syndrome, Aumonier and Cunningham[13] reported that 31 had no sucking difficulty, 12 were successfully nursing within a week, and 16 required tube feeding initially, which was associated with other medical problems, including LBW, cardiac lesions, and jaundice. Hyperbilirubinemia is common in trisomy and was seen in 49% of these study infants. Eighteen babies had multiple medical conditions, and 11 of them sucked poorly. The authors point out that the initial sucking ability of the infants did not appear to be a major cause for nonmaintenance of breastfeeding. Ten of the 13 mothers who discontinued breastfeeding cited insufficient milk as a contributing cause, which might have been prevented by early pumping of the breasts between feedings. With amniocentesis, genetic testing and screening in older mothers (over 35), many are diagnosed prenatally. Parents are then partly prepared before birth.

The birth of an infant with a major genetic abnormality is a shock, even to the strongest parents. If the mother wants to breastfeed, she should be offered all the encouragement and support necessary. Usually she needs to talk with someone just to express her anguish about the infant, not the feeding per se. A sympathetic nurse practitioner can be invaluable in providing the support as well as the expertise necessary to help with the various management problems. If the mother chooses not to breastfeed, appropriate support can also be provided without disrupting treatment continuity.

It is especially important that these infants be breastfed if possible because they are particularly prone to infection. Before the advent of antibiotics, they often died of overwhelming infection and rarely survived past 20 years of age. These infants and most other infants with developmental disorders do better with stimulation and affection, so the body contact and communication while at the breast are especially important. Those who have associated cardiac lesions not only can suckle, swallow, and breathe with less effort at the breast, but also can receive a fluid more physiologic for their needs. Breastfed or bottle fed, these infants gain poorly; thus, switching to a bottle does not solve the problem. The recommendation that the Down syndrome child receive extra vitamins was tested in a controlled study in children 5 to 13 years of age, and there was no sustained improvement in the children's appearance, growth, behavior, or development with added vitamins.[18]

Down syndrome is a lifelong condition. Developing a support system is important for the family. Support groups of other families in the community serve as vital peer support.

Hypothyroidism

Bode and associates[22] reported that an infant with congenital cretinism was spared the severe effects of the disease because he was breastfed. This was attributed to significant quantities of thyroid hormone in the milk. In a prospective study of 12 cases of hypothyroidism in breastfed infants, Letarte and associates[85] found no protective effect against the disease, nor was the onset of the disease delayed. Anthropometric measurements, biochemical values, and psychologic testing at 1 year of age did not differ from those in the 33 bottle fed hypothyroid infants. Abbassi and Steinour[1] also reported successful diagnosis of congenital hypothyroidism in four breastfed neonates.

Sack and associates[126] measured thyroxine (T_4) concentrations in human milk and found it to be present in significant amounts. Varma and associates[152] studied T_4, triiodothyronine (T_3), and reverse T_3 (rT_3) concentrations in human milk in 77 healthy euthyroid mothers from the day of delivery to 148 days post partum. They calculated from their data that if infants received 900 to 1200 mL of milk per day, they would receive 2.1 to 2.6 µg of T_4 per day, based on 238.1 ng/dL of milk after the first week. This amount of T_4 is much less than the recommended dose for the treatment of hypothyroidism (18.8 to 25 µg/day of levo-T_3). T_4 was essentially unmeasurable in the milk sampled. In another study, however, comparing 22 breastfed and 25 formula fed infants who were 2 to 3 weeks old, the levels of T_3 and T_4 were significantly higher in the breastfed infants.[62] No definite relationship between the levels of T_3 and rT_3 could be found.

A 6-week-old female was diagnosed to have congenital hypothyroidism by routine neonatal screening when T_4 was reported at 3 µg/dL (normal above 7 µg/dL).[33] The mother gave a history of multiple applications of povidone-iodine during pregnancy and continuing during lactation. Further testing revealed thyroid-stimulating hormone (TSH) levels of 0.9 µU/mL (normal 0.8 to 5 µU/mL). Iodine treatment was stopped and breastfeeding continued while treatment of thyroid replacement was begun. At 1 year, growth and development were normal. It is therefore suggested that neonatal screening for thyroid disease may be even more urgent if the clinical symptoms are apt to be masked in a breastfed infant. No contraindication exists to breastfeeding when the infant is hypothyroid, and it would be beneficial. Appropriate therapy should also be instituted promptly. Mandatory screening for hypothyroidism is available to newborns in developed countries. Many cases that screen positive do not have the characteristic signs and symptoms at birth. Breastfeeding is ideal for these infants.

Adrenal hyperplasia

In an analysis of 32 infants with salt-losing congenital adrenal hyperplasia who were in adrenal crisis, 8 had been breastfed, 5 had been breastfed with formula supplements, and 19 had been formula fed.[32] Infants who were breastfed were admitted to the hospital later than the formula fed infants, although the breastfed infants had lower serum sodium levels on admission. The breastfed infants did not vomit and remained stable longer, although they all had severe failure to thrive. Weaning initiated vomiting and precipitated crises in the breastfed infants. The authors suggest that congenital adrenal hyperplasia should be considered in a breastfed infant with failure to thrive. Electrolytes should be obtained before weaning to make the diagnosis and avoid precipitating a crisis by weaning. Then breastfeeding can continue as treatment is initiated.

Neonatal breasts and nipple discharge

The newborn may have swelling of the breasts for the first few days of life, whether male or female; this is unrelated to being breastfed. If the breast is squeezed, milk can be obtained. This has been called *witch's milk.* The constituents of neonatal milk were studied in the milks of 18 normal newborns and infants with sepsis, adrenal hyperplasia, CF, and meconium ileus.[20] Electrolyte values were similar to those in adult women in all the infants except one with a mastitis, in whom the sodium level was elevated and the potassium decreased. Total protein and lactose were also similar to those in adult women. The fat was different, increasing with postnatal age and being higher in short-chain fatty acids. It was indeed true milk.

Two infants, one female and one male, were reported to have bilateral bloody discharge from the nipples at 6 weeks of age. Cultures and smears were unrevealing.[20] No biopsy was done. The female infant's swelling and discharge cleared up after 5 months; the male's was still present at 10 weeks, when he was lost to follow-up. Galactorrhea or persistent neonatal milk has been reported in association with neonatal hyperthyroidism. In another report, a 21-day-old infant female was seen because of a goiter and galactorrhea. The infant had 50% 24-hour iodine-131 uptake and elevated prolactin levels, which slowly responded to Lugol's solution treatment for hyperthyroidism.[92]

Neonatal mastitis

Neonatal mastitis occurs infrequently, although it was a common event in the 1940s and 1950s, when staphylococcal disease was rampant in nurseries. It occurs in full-term infants 1 to 5 weeks of age and in as many females as males, usually unilaterally.[153] It is unrelated to maternal mastitis and usually occurs in bottle fed infants. Before IV antibiotic therapy, surgical incision and drainage were common. Prognosis for cure is excellent. In recent years the rare cases that occur are seen in conjunction with manipulation of the neonatal breast to express the natural secretion when the newborn breast is engorged (witch's milk).

Hyperbilirubinemia and jaundice

Jaundice in the newborn has become a source of considerable misinformation, confusion, and anxiety in recent years. There is a higher incidence of jaundice in full-term infants than a decade ago. More physicians are paying attention to the development of hyperbilirubinemia in newborns. These two factors serve to increase the frequency of the question of the role of breastfeeding in the development of hyperbilirubinemia. Some of the confusion and inconsistencies associated with the management can be attributed to the indecisive terminology. This discussion attempts to clarify the issues and outlines the causes and effects of hyperbilirubinemia.

Why the concern about jaundice?

Bilirubin is a cell toxin, as can be demonstrated dramatically by adding a little bilirubin to a tissue culture, which will be quickly destroyed. Excessive bilirubin causes concern because when there is free, unbound, unconjugated bilirubin in the system, it can be deposited in various tissues, ultimately causing necrosis of the cells. The brain and brain cells, if destroyed by bilirubin deposits, do not regenerate.[64] The full-blown end result is bilirubin encephalopathy, or *kernicterus,* which is essentially a pathologic diagnosis that depends on identifying the yellow pigmentation and necrosis in the brain, especially in the basal ganglion, hippocampal cortex, and subthalamic nuclei. About 50% of the infants with kernicterus at autopsy also have other lesions caused by bilirubin toxicity. There may be necrosis of the renal tubular cells, intestinal mucosa, or pancreatic cells or associated gastrointestinal (GI) hemorrhage.

The classic clinical manifestations of bilirubin encephalopathy are characterized by progressive lethargy, rigidity, opisthotonos, high-pitched cry, fever, and convulsions. The mortality rate is 50%. Survivors usually have choreoathetoid cerebral palsy, asymmetric spasticity, paresis of upward gaze, high-frequency deafness, and mental retardation.[37] Premature infants are particularly susceptible to bilirubin-related brain damage and may have kernicterus at autopsy without the typical clinical syndrome. A significant correlation exists between level of bilirubin and hearing impairment in newborns when other risk factors are present. Classic full-blown kernicterus rarely occurs today, but mild effects on the brain may be manifested clinically in later life as incoordination, hypertonicity, and mental retardation or perhaps learning disabilities, symptoms sometimes collectively called *minimal brain damage.*[64] *Bilirubin encephalopathy* is the appropriate term for conditions in which bilirubin is thought to be the cause of brain toxicity.

In response to the continued concern about hyperbilirubinemia, several collaborative long-range studies have been done.[59,95,96,129] Each one confirms the observation that in normal full-term infants who do not have an incompatibility, the neurodevelopmental outcome is normal, as is hearing acuity.[103,129] In a study of 60 breastfed infants in whom the maximum bilirubin was 18.3 mg% and the duration was 12 weeks or more, there were no late neurodevelopmental or hearing defects. The authors describe a peak level at 4 to 5 days and a second peak at the 14th to 15th day. All 60 infants had blood typing, direct and indirect Coombs' (antiglobulin) tests, blood count, glucose-6-phosphate dehydrogenase (G6PD) activity, urinalysis, urine culture, T_4 and TSH, total reducing substances in the urine, and spot tests for galactose and aminotransferase to rule out other causes of hyperbilirubinemia. The authors also reported a 14% incidence of familial jaundice, that is, a previous infant with jaundice (6 of 43 breastfeeders who had siblings).[157]

Mechanism of bilirubin production in the neonate

The normal full-term infant has a hematocrit in utero of 50% to 65%. Because of the low oxygen tension delivered to the fetus via the placenta, the fetus requires more hemoglobin (Hb) to carry the oxygen. As soon as the infant is born and begins to breathe room air, the need is gone. The infant bone marrow does not make more cells, and excess cells are destroyed and not replaced. The life span of a fetal red blood cell (RBC) is 70 to 90 days instead of the adult's 120 days. Normally when RBCs are destroyed, the released Hb is broken down to heme in the reticuloendothelial system (RES). The RES cells contain a microsomal enzyme, heme oxygenase, which is capable of oxidizing the α-methene bridge carbon of the heme molecule after the loss of the iron and the globin to form biliverdin, a green pigment.[49,53] *Biliverdin* is water soluble and is rapidly degraded to bilirubin. A gram of hemoglobulin will produce 34 mg of bilirubin.

The reticuloendothelial cell releases the bilirubin into the circulation, where it is rapidly bound to albumin. Indirect bilirubin is essentially insoluble (less than 0.01 mg% soluble) and is a yellow pigment. Adult albumin can bind two molecules of bilirubin, the first more tightly than the second. Newborn albumin has reduced molar binding capacities that vary with maturity and other factors,[124] such as pH, infection, and hypoglycemia.

Unconjugated bilirubin is removed from the circulation by the hepatocyte, which converts it by conjugation of each molecule of bilirubin with two molecules of glucuronic acid into direct bilirubin. *Direct bilirubin* is water soluble and is excreted via the bile to the stools. The balance between hepatic cell uptake of bilirubin and the rate of bilirubin production determines the serum unconjugated bilirubin concentration. Laboratory measurements include both bound and unbound indirect bilirubin.

Evaluation and management

Normal full-term newborns have serial bilirubin tests to determine the range of values. The cord bilirubin level may be as high as 2 mg% and rise over the first 72 hours to 5 to 6 mg%, which is barely in the visible range, and gradually tapers off, assuming adult levels of 1 mg% after 10 days. Fewer than 50% of normal infants are visibly jaundiced in the first week of life. Why any normal infant is visibly jaundiced is not known, although Gartner and Lee[53] suggest that it results from insufficient enzyme synthesis, inhibition of enzymatic activity by naturally occurring substances, deficient synthesis of the glucuronide donor uridine diphosphoglucoronic acid (UDPGA), or a combination of factors. This would suggest the jaundice is *idiopathic,* not physiologic. The level of bilirubin that is acceptable depends on a number of factors. In some premature infants, even bilirubin levels under 10 mg/dL may be of concern.

Factors that influence significance. For a given level of bilirubin, several associated factors may need to be considered. If the infant has acidosis, anoxia, asphyxia, hypothermia, hypoglycemia, or infection, even lower levels of bilirubin may have a significant risk of causing deposition of bilirubin in the brain cells. The most important factor is prematurity, which affects both liver and brain metabolism as well as albumin binding sites. An increased incidence of elevated bilirubin levels occurs in certain races and populations. Asian populations, including Chinese, Japanese, and Korean, and Native Americans may have bilirubin levels averaging 10 to 14 mg%. A higher incidence of autopsy-identified kernicterus also is seen in these populations. It does not seem to be related to G6PD deficiency, however, which is also common in these groups.

Determination of cause of jaundice. Following the chain of events from the RBC and its destruction in the newborn through the final excretion of conjugated bilirubin in the stools simplifies understanding the cause of a specific case of jaundice.[86] Causes include (1) increased destruction of RBCs, (2) decreased conjugation in the glucuronidase system, (3) decreased albumin binding, and (4) increased reabsorption from the GI tract.

When albumin binding is altered, the visibility of the jaundice is not affected. The bilirubin level may not be very high, but the substance is not bound to albumin and is available at lower levels to pass into the brain cells.[123] Premature infants have much lower albumin levels and thus have fewer binding sites. Drugs that also bind to albumin (e.g., aspirin, sulfadiazine) compete for binding sites. A lower level of bilirubin puts infants who have these medications in their system at risk because the bilirubin is unbound and available to enter tissue cells, including brain cells.

Reabsorption of bilirubin from stool in the GI tract can increase the bilirubin level. This occurs when the conjugated bilirubin that was excreted into the colon is unconjugated by the action of intestinal bacteria and reabsorbed, which happens when stools are decreased or slowed in passage. Poor feedings, pyloric stenosis, and other forms of intestinal obstruction are common causes of this type of jaundice. Some bacteria are more likely than others to unconjugate conjugated bilirubin.

Sepsis, on the other hand, was not found in more than 300 infants readmitted for hyperbilirubinemia while healthy and breastfeeding. Lower total bilirubin and direct bilirubin levels greater than 2.0 mg% in a sick baby have a high correlation with sepsis.[56]

Safe levels of bilirubin. Safe levels of bilirubin depend on a number of factors, including acidosis, hypoxia or anoxia, and sepsis. A handy rule of thumb is the correlation of birth weight in the premature infant and the indirect bilirubin level, using a value 2 to 3 mg lower when the infant has multiple problems. The risk of elevated bilirubin is related to the availability of albumin to bind the indirect bilirubin and prevent it from entering the brain cells. The amount of albumin is related to the degree of prematurity, and thus the rule of thumb is based on birth weight. When the infant is sick, fewer albumin-binding sites are available, and the bilirubin level of concern is even lower.

In a well infant weighing under 2000 g, the peak tolerated bilirubin level, above which an exchange transfusion might be done, corresponds roughly to weight as follows: 1800 g, 18 mg/dL; 1500 g, 15 mg/dL; 1200 g, 12 mg/dL; and 1000 g, 10 mg/dL. Phototherapy is usually initiated when the bilirubin is about 5 mg/dL lower than the exchange level. Because of stripping of bilirubin from the binding sites in the brain capillaries in some situations, such as prematurity, or presence of a competing drug in the serum, more bilirubin is available to be deposited than is measured to be "free" in the plasma.[124]

Any value of 20 mg/dL or greater warrants consideration of treatment. Jaundice visible under 24 hours of age is of special concern because it is usually associated with an incompatibility or infection. Rapidly rising bilirubin levels are also of concern, and a 0.5 mg/dL rise per hour is an indication for treatment.

The American Academy of Pediatrics (AAP) has published a practice parameter for the management of hyperbilirubinemia in the healthy term newborn (Table 15-4).[119] Term infants who are visibly jaundiced at or before 24 hours of life are not considered healthy and require a diagnostic workup regardless of feeding method. The AAP also addresses jaundice associated with breastfeeding in a healthy term infant as follows:

The AAP discourages the interruption of breastfeeding in healthy term newborns and encourages continued and frequent breastfeeding (at least 8 to 10 times every 24 hours). Supplementing nursing with water or dextrose water does not lower the bilirubin level in jaundiced, healthy, breastfeeding infants. Depending on the mother's preference and the physician's judgment, however, a variety of options are presented in Table 15-4 for possible implementation beyond observation, including supplementation of breastfeeding with formula or the temporary interruption of breastfeeding and substitution with formula if inadequate calories are contributing to the hyperbilirubinemia, either of which can be accompanied by phototherapy.[119]

Hyperbilirubinemia and breastfeeding. Two major clinical conditions exist (one common, one rare) that associate the breastfed infant with hyperbilirubinemia. Table 15-5 outlines the major clinical features of these two conditions. The more common condition has been called *early breast milk jaundice* by Gartner[49] and associates[51-53] but might be called *jaundice while breastfeeding,* because the failure to produce stool and the decreased intake of calories, probably not the breastfeeding, are at fault. Some bottle fed infants also are jaundiced, so the appropriate term would be *bottle feeding jaundice* for this group.

Early jaundice while breastfeeding. Many studies of bilirubin levels in normal newborn nurseries have been conducted looking at method of

---

TABLE 15-4   Management of hyperbilirubinemia in healthy term newborns

Age (hours)	Total serum bilirubin (TSB) level (mg/dL, μmol/L)			
	Consider phototherapy[*]	Phototherapy	Exchange transfusion if intensive phototherapy fails[†]	Exchange transfusion and intensive phototherapy
≤24[‡]	—	—	—	—
25–48	≥12 (170)	≥15 (260)	≥20 (340)	≥25 (430)
49–72	≥15 (260)	≥18 (310)	≥25 (430)	≥30 (510)
>72	≥17 (290)	≥20 (340)	≥25 (430)	≥30 (510)

[*]Phototherapy at these TSB levels is a clinical option, meaning that the intervention is available and may be used *on the basis of individual clinical judgment.*

[†]Intensive phototherapy should produce a decline of TSB of 1 to 2 mg/dL within 4 to 6 hours, and the TSB level should continue to fall and remain below the threshold level for exchange transfusion. If this does not occur, it is considered a failure of phototherapy.

[‡]Term infants who are clinically jaundiced at ≤24 hours old are not considered healthy and require further evaluation.

From Provisional Committee for Quality Improvement, Subcommittee on Hyperbilirubinemia, American Academy of Pediatrics: Practice parameters: Management of hyperbilirubinemia in the healthy term newborn. Pediatrics 94:558, 1994.

TABLE 15-5 Comparison of early and late jaundice associated with hyperbilirubinemia while breastfeeding

Early jaundice	Late jaundice
Occurs 2–5 days of age	Occurs 5–10 days of age
Transient: 10 days	Persists >1 month
More common in primiparas	All children of a given mother
Infrequent feeds	Milk volume not a problem
	May have abundant milk
Stools delayed and infrequent	Normal stooling
Receiving water or dextrose water	No supplements
Bilirubin peaks ≤15 mg/dL	Bilirubin may be >20 mg/dL
Treatment: none or phototherapy	Treatment: phototherapy
	Discontinue breast feeding temporarily
	Rarely, exchange transfusion
Associations: low Apgar scores, water or dextrose water supplement, prematurity	Associations: none identified

feeding. Unfortunately, very few have detailed frequency of feeds, supplementation, and stool pattern.[35,95,136] A review summarizing results in 13 studies covering more than 20,000 infants was reported by Schneider[130] to show a relationship between breastfeeding and jaundice. A pooled analysis of 12 studies showed 514 of 3997 breastfed infants to have total serum bilirubin levels of 12 mg/dL or higher versus 172 of 4255 bottle fed infants. In a smaller group of studies, 54 of 2655 breastfed infants had bilirubin levels of 15 mg/dL or greater versus 10 of 3002 bottle fed infants. Eleven of 13 studies reported that breastfed infants had higher mean bilirubin levels. In a series of more than 12,000 infants, the risk of a breastfed infant becoming jaundiced was 1:8. The risk of

becoming jaundiced for a premature infant was 3:6; for an Asian race, 3:56; and with prolonged rupture of membranes, 1:91. Jaundice is more common in normal newborns now compared with those in the 1950s, when bilirubin was rarely measured because it was a complicated test in normal babies, although hospital stays averaged 5 to 7 days.

Rates of significant jaundice in Australia rose from 0.9% to 3.5% from 1975 to 1987. The associated factors most likely to be present in jaundiced infants were infrequent breastfeeding, less frequent stooling, and excessive weight loss.[150] It is clear from many studies that more breastfed than bottle fed infants are jaundiced, and the cause requires further study.[132]

Relationship of bilirubin level to passage of stools. There are 450 mg of bilirubin in the intestinal tract meconium of the average newborn infant. Passing this meconium is critical to avoid the deconjugation and reabsorption of bilirubin from the gut into the serum. Failure to pass meconium is correlated with elevated serum bilirubin. Time of first stool is also correlated with level of serum bilirubin. Bottle fed infants were reported by de Carvalho and associates[36] to excrete more stool (82 g) and more bilirubin (23.8 mg) in the first 3 days than breastfed infants, who excreted 58 g of stool and 15.7 mg bilirubin. The serum bilirubin levels were 6.8 mg/dL in bottle fed and 9.5 mg/dL in breastfed infants. Furthermore, when the breastfed infants excreted more stools and more bilirubin, they had lower bilirubin levels. This relationship has been confirmed in other studies from days 3 to 21.[56]

Feeding practices and early hyperbilirubinemia. A retrospective study of over 200 infants in our nursery looked at weight loss, number of feedings, amount of supplementation with water or dextrose water, body temperature, number of stools, and third-day serum bilirubin. The infants who received water or dextrose water passed fewer stools, had higher bilirubin levels, and had more problems nursing beyond 4 days of life. Full-term breastfed infants who were receiving water or dextrose supplements had higher serum bilirubin levels on the sixth day of life than bottle fed babies in a study by Nicoll and associates.[113] Supplementation with water or dextrose did not reduce hyperbilirubinemia that had already developed. This is not surprising because bilirubin is excreted in the stool rather than the urine, and these jaundiced infants usually show no signs of dehydration.

When the number of feedings at the breast in the first 3 days of life was related to bilirubin levels, de Carvalho and associates[36] were able to display a significant relationship. The greater the number of breastfeedings, the lower was the bilirubin. Those infants with more than eight feedings per day were not significantly jaundiced. These authors also found that water and dextrose supplements were associated with higher bilirubin levels. When they studied feeding practices in breastfed infants, Kuhr and Paneth[80] noted that sugar-water intake in the first 3 days negatively affected the volume of breast milk available on the fourth day. The infants with high glucose intake had higher bilirubin levels. These studies do not appear to show a correlation between weight loss and bilirubin level, although breastfed infants may lose more weight than bottle fed infants.

When Stevenson[140] measured bilirubin production by calculating pulmonary carbon monoxide excretion in both breastfed and bottle fed infants, he found no difference in the amount of bilirubin produced in the two groups, suggesting the problem was excretion in the stool.

Caloric deprivation and starvation. Elevated bilirubin did not impede sucking ability in a study by Alexander and Roberts.[5] Reduced caloric intake or starvation has been associated with hyperbilirubinemia in adult humans and in many animals. Gartner[49] has described the association between starvation and early neonatal jaundice. Gartner and Lee[53] have postulated that starvation may increase bilirubin production, shift bilirubin pools, reduce hepatic bilirubin uptake, diminish hepatic bilirubin conjugation, or increase enteric bilirubin reabsorption. Adequate caloric intake may simply diminish intestinal bilirubin absorption. Infants with intestinal obstruction (pyloric stenosis) at birth or in the early weeks of life are often jaundiced.

Treatment of early hyperbilirubinemia. When Maisels and Gifford[95] measured serum bilirubin levels in the newborn and the relationship to breastfeeding, they reported 8 of 10 infants with serum bilirubin greater than 12.9 mg/dL were breastfed. They suggested that rather than use phototherapy to treat the jaundice, the cause (i.e., breastfeeding) should be treated by temporary cessation of breastfeeding. This approach implies a substance in the milk causes the problem, whereas it is the process of altered nourishment. The amount of stress for the mother generated by separation from her infant for phototherapy was measured by urine cortisol levels and compared with levels in mothers who roomed-in with their jaundiced infants during phototherapy. The separated mothers were more stressed and were more likely to discontinue breastfeeding than those who remained with their infant.[43]

In a controlled trial of four interventions,[111] 125 of the 1685 infants in the birth cohort whose bilirubin levels reached 17 mg/dL (291 μmol/L) were randomly assigned to treatment. The four interventions were (1) continue breastfeeding and observe; (2) discontinue breastfeeding and substitute formula; (3) discontinue breastfeeding, substitute formula, and use phototherapy; and (4) continue breastfeeding and use phototherapy. The bilirubin reached 20 mg/dL (342 μmol/L) in 24% of group 1, 19% of group 2, 3% of group 3, and 14% of group 4. Phototherapy clearly adds to the decline in bilirubin, and the authors suggest that the parents can be offered the management of their choice. Newman and Maisels[112] recommend that because jaundiced infants are rarely sick, the only laboratory work necessary is a blood type and Coombs' test; only when jaundice is excessive should bilirubin levels be followed closely. Infants with incompatibilities should be treated aggressively. In an attempt to apply logic to a very conflicting picture, a provocative report by Newman and Maisels[112] recommended a kinder, gentler approach to the evaluation and treatment of jaundice in the healthy term infant, with less interference with feeding.

The cumulative evidence from various studies published over the last 10 years, according to Gartner,[50] is that breastfeeding jaundice is the exaggeration of the first phase of physiologic jaundice of the newborn in the breastfed infant. It results from unphysiologic management of breastfeeding, expressed largely through insufficient frequency of breastfeeding. To treat the actual cause, that is, failed breastfeeding or inadequate stooling or underfeeding, the breastfeeding should be reviewed for frequency, length of suckling, and apparent supply of milk, adjusting the breastfeeding to improve any deficits. If stooling is the problem, the infant should be stimulated to stool. If starvation is the problem, the infant should receive additional calories (formula) while the milk supply is being increased by better breastfeeding techniques. The same would apply to bottle feeding jaundice (i.e., any infant with *idiopathic* jaundice who is being bottle fed and has a bilirubin level over 12.9 mg/dL). Stooling, frequency of feeds, and kilocalories would be improved. Box 15-1 provides a management schema for preventing or treating jaundice

in the breastfed infant. All infants must have the appropriate laboratory studies performed.

Breast milk jaundice. Apart from the frequent but low-level (usually under 12 mg/dL) hyperbilirubinemia, breastfeeding rarely is associated with delayed but prolonged hyperbilirubinemia, which, if unchecked, may exceed 20 mg/dL. This syndrome has been called variously *breast milk jaundice, late-onset jaundice,* or *breast milk jaundice syndrome.*[51] It occurs in less than 1 in 200 births; the numbers are imprecise because not all mothers breastfeed. This syndrome is associated with the milk of a particular mother and will occur with each pregnancy in varying degrees, depending on each infant's ability to conjugate bilirubin (i.e., a premature sibling might be more severely affected).[51] Early-onset jaundice is related to the process of breastfeeding, not the milk itself. It is essential to rule out other causes of prolonged or excessive jaundice, especially hemolytic disease, hypothyroidism, G6PD deficiency, inherited hepatic glucuronyl transferase deficiency (Gilbert syndrome, etc.), and intestinal obstruction.

The pattern of this jaundice is distinctly different. Normally, idiopathic jaundice peaks on the third day and then begins to drop. Breast milk jaundice, however, becomes apparent or continues to rise after the third day, and bilirubin levels may peak any time from the seventh to the tenth day, with untreated cases being reported to peak as late as the 15th day. Values have ranged from 10 to 27 mg/dL during this time. No correlation exists with weight loss or gain, and stools are normal.

The syndrome of breast milk jaundice was attributed by Arias and associates[11] to a substance in the milk of some mothers that inhibits the hepatic enzyme glucuronyl transferase, preventing the conjugation of bilirubin. The substance has been identified as 5β-pregnane-3α, 20α-diol, a breakdown product of progesterone and an isomer of pregnanediol that is not usually found in milk but occurs normally in about 10% of the lactating population. Although this substance had also been isolated from the milk and serum of mothers whose infants were not jaundiced, this work has not been duplicated.

BOX 15-1   Management outline for early jaundice while breastfeeding

1. Monitor all infants for initial stooling. Stimulate stool if no stool in 24 hours.
2. Initiate breastfeeding early and frequently. Frequent short feeding is more effective than infrequent prolonged feeding, although total time may be the same.
3. Discourage water, dextrose water, or formula supplements.
4. Monitor weight, voidings, and stooling in association with breastfeeding pattern.
5. When bilirubin level approaches 15 mg/dL stimulate stooling, augment feeds, stimulate breast milk production with pumping, and use phototherapy if this aggressive approach fails and bilirubin exceeds 20 mg/dL.
6. Be aware that no evidence suggests early jaundice is associated with "an abnormality" of the breast milk, so withdrawing breast milk as a trial is only indicated if jaundice persists longer than 6 days or rises above 20 mg/dL or the mother has a history of a previously affected infant.

In a definitive study of breast milk β-glucuronidase, Wilson and associates[157] examined 55 mother-infant pairs. No correlation was found between serum bilirubin levels and breast milk β-glucuronidase between days 3 and 6 post partum.

The role of lipoprotein lipase and bile salt–stimulated lipase in breast milk jaundice continues under investigation. The role of free fatty acids and the possibility of abnormal lipases are unresolved. The undisputed cause of breast milk jaundice continues to elude investigators.

As in early jaundice associated with breastfeeding, jaundiced infants at 3 weeks do not produce more bilirubin than their unjaundiced breastfed peers or bottle fed infants.

Gartner and Auerbach[52] have suggested that bilirubin reabsorption from the gut may be enhanced by the milk of mothers whose infants are jaundiced. The studies relate 60% reabsorption of bilirubin in the presence of this milk when reabsorption is usually close to zero. This abnormal milk also inhibited hepatic glucuronyl transferase and contained 10 times the free fatty acids in normal milk. The authors speculate that these three abnormal properties may enhance enterohepatic circulation of bilirubin, with this increased load of bilirubin exceeding the capacity of the liver.[49]

Diagnosis depends on circumstantial evidence, because no easy, rapid laboratory test exists. All other causes, including infection, should be ruled out in the usual manner and a thorough history taken, including medications and family history. If the mother has nursed other infants, were they jaundiced? Usually 70% of the previous children of a given mother whose infant has breast milk jaundice have been jaundiced. The difference may be related to the greater maturity of the liver of a given infant who then is able to handle the increased demands on the glucuronyl transferase system. To establish the diagnosis firmly, and this is necessary when the bilirubin level is above 16 mg/dL for more than 24 hours, a bilirubin reading should be obtained 2 hours after a breastfeeding and then breastfeeding discontinued for at least 12 hours.[112] The infant must be fed fluids and calories. The infant's mother should be assisted in pumping her breasts to main-tain her supply. Even more urgent is providing the mother with a sympathetic explanation of the problem and the process. After at least 12 hours without mother's milk, the bilirubin level should be measured. If a significant drop of more than 2 mg/dL occurs, it is diagnostic. When the level is below 15 mg/dL, the infant can be put to the breast. Bilirubin levels should be obtained to determine if the bilirubin rises again and, if so, how much. In most cases, in the time not breastfeeding the infant's body equilibrates the levels sufficiently, so there is only a slight increase in bilirubin on return to breastfeeding followed by a slow but steady drop. If that is the case, breastfeeding can continue. The bilirubin level should be checked at 10 to 14 days to be certain the bilirubin is truly clearing.

If the bilirubin has not dropped significantly after 12 hours off the breast, the time off the breast should be extended to 18 to 24 hours, measuring bilirubin levels every 6 hours. If the bilirubin rises while the infant is off the breast, the cause of jaundice is clearly not the breast milk; breastfeeding should be resumed and other causes for the jaundice reevaluated.

Phototherapy and breast milk jaundice. If the bilirubin is substantially over 20 mg/dL in a full-term infant (or proportionately lower in a preterm infant), it is important to lower the bilirubin promptly; thus, phototherapy should be initiated as soon as the blood work is drawn (Fig. 15-4). The relationship to breastfeeding can be established later. Often, IV fluids are also necessary.

If one is attempting to establish the diagnosis of breast milk jaundice, phototherapy should not be used while breast milk is being discontinued. If establishing the diagnosis is not necessary (perhaps because of the same diagnosis in older siblings), phototherapy can be used to bring the values to a more acceptable range (i.e., under 12 mg/dL). When phototherapy is discontinued, it is most important to establish that no rebound hyperbilirubinemia occurs. In addition, it is important to follow the infant at home after discharge through at least 14 days of life or longer if the values are not below 12 mg/dL. It should not be assumed that the diagnosis is breast milk jaundice when breastfeeding has been stopped and phototherapy initiated simultaneously.

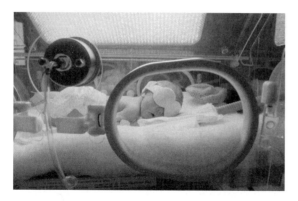

Figure 15-4. Phototherapy for a premature infant with two overhead banks of lights while lying on a fiberoptic blanket.

Late diagnosis of breast milk jaundice. With the frequency of early discharge from the hospital, especially for families enjoying the birthing center concept, breastfed infants are often discharged before jaundice for any reason has developed. Because breast milk jaundice is likely to be delayed to the fourth or fifth day, peaking at 10 to 14 days of age, most normal infants are already home. Occasionally, an infant is observed in the pediatrician's office at 10 days of age or older with a bilirubin level over 20 mg/dL, often 23 to 25 mg/dL. This necessitates the admission of the infant to the hospital for a complete bilirubin workup. It is important to recognize that other causes of hyperbilirubinemia must be ruled out, including blood-type incompatibilities. At this age it is also necessary to rule out biliary obstruction and hepatitis, which might have a high direct or conjugated bilirubin level.

Phototherapy is used for 4 to 6 hours to establish whether this therapy will be effective in dropping the level sufficiently. It is necessary to stop breastfeeding temporarily and start phototherapy immediately on admission while the diagnostic workup is being performed when the bilirubin is substantially over 20 mg/dL if a possible association with breast milk exists. Otherwise, breastfeeding may continue even though IV fluids may also be necessary.

The Agency for Health Care Research and Quality (AHCRQ) through its Evidence-based

Practice Centers (EPCs) published a report on the Management of Neonatal Hyperbilirubinemia in 2003 following an extensive review of over 4560 abstracts from which 241 articles were examined and 138 included in the report.[71] A summary of 28 reports spanning 30 years including 123 cases of kernicterus in term and near term infants affirmed the relationship of elevated bilirubin to kernicterus. They calculated that 6 to 10 jaundiced healthy infants with a total serum bilirubin (TSB) at or above 15 mg/dL would need to be treated with phototherapy to prevent TSB from rising above 20 mg/dL in one infant. They concluded that phototherapy combined with the cessation of breastfeeding and substitution with formula was the most efficient protocol. Recommendation was made that more research is needed as this approach was not tested.

In contrast, Chou and associates proposed a management of hyperbilirubinemia using a bench marking model in a 3-year prospective cohort study. They found association of high bilirubin with lower gestational age, older mother, exclusive or partial breastfeeding. The authors recommend assessing the breastfeeding and promoting breastfeeding, supplement if necessary but never with water, in combination with phototherapy as most efficacious.[28]

Suckling problems related to anatomy and neural disorders

Most problems with latch-on during breastfeeding can be solved with adjustment of position and approach, but a few cannot because the infant has an anatomic variation of the mouth or a neurodevelopmental problem. A thorough examination is required to evaluate the mouth and cheek for potential associated lesions and syndromes. Premature infants are more often identified with suckling problems because they not only are immature but also have been suctioned, intubated, and perhaps ventilated. Much has been put in their mouths. They may also have a high arched or grooved palate from the endotracheal tube.

When the mouth is carefully examined, an infant may have cysts on the dental ridge or under the tongue, the tongue may have limited range of motion, or the palate may be abnormal. A number of new observations are being reported in the literature, such as "bubble palate" or variation in infant palatal structure (VIPS). Snyder[137] recommends alternative positioning and repatterning oral behavior to increase the transfer of milk and reduce the trauma to the maternal nipple. Breastfeeding in the supine position with the infant prone encourages the infant's tongue to fall down and forward and keeps the nipple from being abraded by "the bubble." Marmet and Shell[97] describe a bubble palate as a concavity in the hard palate, usually about ⅜ to ¾ inch (1 to 2 cm) in diameter and ¼ inch (0.5 cm) deep. Similar adjustments to positioning would be appropriate for high arched palates.

Macroglossia presents a problem of too much tongue for the oral cavity. These infants do better at the breast than with a bottle. The main problem is to have the infant bring the tongue forward to avoid gagging.

Abnormal oral motor patterns are more common in premature infants and those who have been asphyxiated at birth. These movements include exaggerated tongue thrust (often from bottle feeding and nipple confusion), tonic bite, jaw thrust, jaw clenching, and lip pursing. Some of these behaviors are associated with postural muscle tone abnormalities.[154] Normal muscle tone and strength throughout breastfeeding, especially alignment of the head and neck, are required to form a stable base to anchor the oral and pharyngeal musculature.[114] Hypertonic and hypotonic infants may pose problems. Hypertonic infants are usually overflexed or overextended and have hypertonic mouths with tonic bite, jaw thrusting, and clenching. Inducing relaxation, minimizing handling, and using gentle strokes to calm the infant can be effective. If the infant is extended, flexion may be achieved with a pleat-seat carrier (see Fig. 15-2) or pillows. Flexed position in these infants relaxes the jaw and mouth and allows latching to take place. Finger feeding may help train these infants. If done just before a feed, the infant can be transferred to the breast smoothly.

Oral tactile hypersensitivity is often seen in infants who have had oral tubes, especially feeding tubes. Touching around the mouth causes feeding rejection. Decreased oral awareness may result in drooling and poor suckling. These infants may respond to stroking the oral area gently. Most infants have a very strong arching reflex, which is elicited by touching or applying pressure on the back of the head, causing the infant to arch back away from the breast. Positions that require the mother to hold the head (e.g., "football hold") may trigger this reflex. Infants prefer to be swaddled but always respond better to a firm supportive hold of the body, slightly flexing the arms, legs, and trunk. Pillows can be used for support of the baby or the mother's arms.

The development of an infant's oral motor and feeding skills parallels general physical development, especially gross and fine motor skills. When an infant is having persistent feeding problems, the infant needs total neuromotor assessment.[114] Minor problems may be solved by the firm supportive hold of a swaddled infant who is gently handled and encouraged.

Illingworth and Lister[70] first put forth the concept of a critical or sensitive period for the development of a skill. *Conditioned dysphagia* is a learned disorder, acquired and maintained through a behavioral conditioning process that occurs when a noxious stimulus is paired with the act of swallowing.[39] This is noted with suctioning of the mouth or nasopharynx and nasogastric feeding tubes in the neonatal intensive care unit (NICU).

An infant with a true feeding disorder requires an assessment with a neonatal oral-motor review by a trained physical therapist.[114] Training the infant to suckle will be required. These infants ultimately do best if sucking is limited to the breast. Cup feedings are more effective than bottle feeding.

INFANTS WITH PROBLEMS REQUIRING SURGERY

Immediate neonatal period
First-arch disorders

Feeding of any sort may be greatly hindered by abnormalities of the jaw, nose, and mouth. A receding chin may seem to be a minor problem and require only positioning the jaw forward. It is essential to establish that the jaw is not dislocated (Fig. 15-5). A mother can hook the angle of the jaw with her finger and draw it forward. If the tongue is too large for the jaw, the infant will actually nurse better at the breast than at the bottle because the human nipple fits into the mouth with less bulk. Infants with first-arch abnormalities usually require considerable help in feeding. A cleft palate may also be present. If choanal atresia is present, it may be necessary to insert semipermanent nasal tubes so that the infant can be fed orally until older; definitive surgery may be necessary later. Once the nasal tubes are in place, the infant can manage at the breast. Feeding by any technique, however, is never easy.

Cleft lip

A solitary cleft lip is usually repaired in the first few weeks of life. Before surgery the infant will need some help, but the infant can nurse at the breast if a seal around the areola can be developed. Actually the breast may fill the defect, and suckling will go well. The mother may be able to put her thumb in the cleft to create a seal as she holds the breast to the infant's mouth. It is important to encourage the infant to suck to strengthen the tongue and jaw muscles. If all else fails, a breast

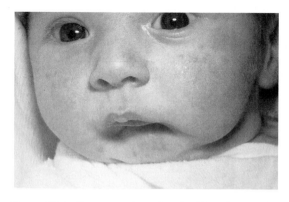

Figure 15-5. Demonstration of a significantly receding chin. (From Biancuzzo M: Breastfeeding the Newborn, Clinical Strategies for Nurses, 2nd ed. St. Louis, Mosby, 2003.)

shield can be tried, affixing a special cleft lip nipple to the shield. The mother will need to pump after feedings to increase milk supply. In some cases, the mother may have to express or pump milk and offer it by dropper or other means if sucking is ineffective. The pediatrician, plastic surgeon, and parents should work together as a team from the time of birth to determine a coordinated plan of treatment. Some surgeons have special protocols before and after surgery to ensure optimal healing. It is important to make all plans for feeding around the surgical plan. The literature reports individual mothers' experiences nursing infants with lip defects. The major caution in sharing these experiences is to consider that the supportive surgical approach may differ from those reported in the literature.[68] In these cases, the plastic surgeon is the captain of the team working with the pediatrician and support staff. As breastfeeding has increased lactation consultants have joined the team.

Cleft palate

The prognosis for successful feeding of an infant with a cleft palate depends on the size and position of the defect (soft palate, hard palate) as well as the associated lesions. Lubit[89] recommends the application of an orthopedic appliance to the neonatal maxilla to close the gap, thus aiding nursing, stimulating orofacial development, developing the palatal shelves, preventing tongue distortions, preventing nasal septum irritation, and decreasing the number of ear infections. This will make it easier for the plastic surgeon and help the mother psychologically as well. Lubit further relates that a cleft involving the secondary palate can interfere with normal nursing. For the infant to suckle, the nose must be sealed off from the mouth, creating a negative pressure in the oral cavity. The milk may also run out the nose. The absence of palatal tissue can prevent expulsion of milk from the nipple. The orthodontic appliance prosthetically restores the anatomy of the palate, permitting normal suckling.

Because the purpose of the negative pressure in the mouth is to hold the nipple and areola in place and not to extract milk from the breast, a seal is needed to keep the pressure. A mother may be able to perform the positioning task by holding the breast to her infant's mouth firmly between two fingers, as shown in Figures 8-13, 15-1, 15-2, and 15-6. The infant is then able to milk the areola and nipple with the tongue pressing it against the roof of the mouth, even with the cleft. The breast must be held in position just as a bottle must be held throughout the feeding.[57]

In assessing 143 infants with cleft lip and palate over a 5-year period, Clarren and associates[30] found that by assessing the infant's ability to generate negative intraoral pressure and to move the tongue against the nipple, they could identify effective feeding techniques. They summarized these findings in relation to the possibility of breastfeeding (Table 15-6). They point out that normal children with a cleft can swallow normally. A defect in the bony structure of the palate, however, creates a hole that is difficult to plug; thus, these children are more difficult to feed by any method.

The authors[30] point out that problems with intraoral muscular movements are associated with bilateral cleft lip, which causes severe anterior projection of the premaxilla that precludes stabilizing the nipple, and with wide palatal clefts, which

offer no back guard for tongue movements, and retroplaced tongues that cannot compress the nipple effectively. When there are neurologic problems causing dysrhythmic tongue movements or a weak tongue or grinding of the gum on the nipple, it is more than a simple anatomic problem and is usually part of a syndrome (e.g., first-arch syndrome). These children usually have swallowing problems as well (e.g., Pierre Robin syndrome).

Feeding procedures for each infant vary. Early assessment of the infant and the mother can usually lead to successful feeding within 1 to 2 days. The infant should not go hungry, and the mother should not spend hours struggling with a system that is not successful for her child. The Lact-Aid or the lactation supplementer can be very helpful, because the mother can control the flow by squeezing the reservoir, and the infant can have some suckling experience, which will strengthen the oral structure and avoid the trauma of invasive devices. The mother will need to pump to increase her milk supply.

Weatherley-White and associates[155] report a program of early repair in breastfeeding infants with cleft lip. Repair has been initiated earlier and

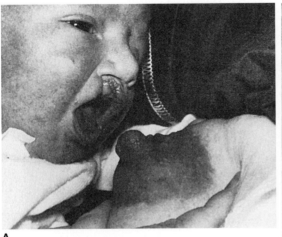 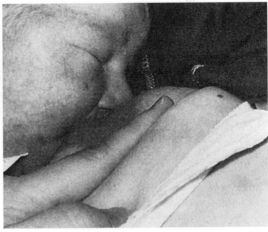

A   B

Figure 15-6. **A,** Infant with cleft lip and palate opening wide to latch on for a feeding. **B,** Same infant suckling at breast. Defect in lip and palate is comfortably filled by breast tissue. (Photos obtained with assistance of Marie Biancuzzo, RN, MSN.)

TABLE 15-6 **Assessment of sucking and feeding techniques for infants with clefts of lip and palate**

	Assessment		
	Generation of negative pressure	Ability to make mechanical movements	
Condition			Feeding techniques
Cleft lip and palate	−	+/−	Breastfeeding is unlikely. Deliver milk into infant's mouth.
Cleft palate only	+/−	+	Breastfeeding sometimes succeeds. Soft artificial nipples with large openings are effective. Infant may need delivery of milk into the mouth.
Cleft of soft palate	+/−	+	Breastfeeding or normal bottle feeding usually works well.
Pierre Robin malformation sequence	+/−	−	Breastfeeding is unlikely. Nipple position is critical. Many infants need delivery of milk into mouth.
Cleft lip only	+/−	+	Breastfeeding works well. Artificial nipple with large base works well.

+, Present; −, absent; +/−, partial.
From Clarren SK, Anderson B, Wolf LS: Feeding infants with cleft lip, cleft palate, or cleft lip and palate. Cleft Palate J 24:244, 1987.

earlier, but these authors present 100 consecutive repairs: 51 infants were older than 3 weeks, and 49 were younger, of whom 26 underwent surgery at age 1 week or less. There was no increase in complication rate and no increase in need for revision of repair. Sixty mothers were offered the opportunity to breastfeed immediately postoperatively; 38 began within hours. Of these, 16 infants breastfed more than 6 weeks, 22 converted by 6 weeks, and 22 were fed by cup or syringe. Breastfed infants gained more weight, and hospital stay was a day shorter. A prospective randomized trial of 40 infants showed that early postoperative breastfeeding after cleft lip repair is safe and results in more weight gain by 6 weeks after surgery when compared with infants randomized to be spoon-fed postoperatively.[34]

A position that is particularly effective is to have the infant straddle the mother's leg so he is directly facing the breast. If mother leans back slightly and the infant has to lean forward, structures fall in place to facilitate suckling. The breast needs to be held throughout the feeding.

Similar experience with early surgery and breastfeeding is confirmed by Fisher,[46] who reports performing reconstructive surgery in the Third World, where breastfeeding is undisputed and is very successful. He also reports greater success rate with breastfeeding but notes it requires the conviction not only of the surgeon and pediatrician but also of the nurse, nutritionist, mother, and grandmother. It takes the presence of all these elements for success but the absence of only one for failure.

As noted earlier, breastfed infants have fewer bouts with otitis media, which has been attributed to the position of the infant while feeding at the breast as well as the antiinfective properties of the milk. This is an important consideration in infants with cleft palates, who have been identified as having more ear infections in general than other infants.[39]

Children with cleft palates may also fail to thrive, not only as a function of their feeding difficulty but also because they may have an underlying increased metabolic need. In a study of 37 children with cleft palates and no other anomalies, the median birth weight was at the 30th percentile.[15] By 1 to 2 months, weights had dropped to the 20th percentile and did not recover to the 30th until 6 months of age.

It is important to have the plastic surgeon involved promptly after birth so management plans can be developed with the family immediately. This also avoids conflicting information from others.

Oral defects: feeding recommendations

Feeding infants with oral defects requires extra effort. Each infant is slightly different. Usually mothers learn to feed their own infants more effectively, even when bottle feeding, than the skilled professional can advise them. This amplifies that it requires a special patience and knack. Breastfeeding can be successful. Infants with cleft lip or palate should be managed as normal infants. Cupping of the infant's jaw and filling the defect with the mother's thumb while supporting the breast in place for suckling will allow effective breastfeeding in the infant with cleft lip. This has been referred to as the "dancer hold" (see Fig. 15-1).[102] The infant should be brought to the mother to feed and for rooming-in, as with any infant. Reinforcing that the infant is normal and merely needs some reconstructive surgery is important in helping the parents adjust. Parent-to-parent programs are most helpful. The primary care physician coordinates care with the specialist and the rest of the health care team.

Pediatric reconstructive surgeons usually have a team of professionals, including otolaryngologists, audiologists and affiliated therapists, social workers, and nurses, familiar and experienced with these first-arch problems. Parent support groups have often been developed through these sources. Most reconstructive surgeons will see the infant in the first 24 to 48 hours and reassure the parents while designing the plan of action. Usually a member of the nursing staff of the surgeon's practice will also

visit and provide the practical advice about feeding, especially if the mother chooses to breastfeed.[39]

Other syndromes may be associated with feeding difficulties because of an anatomic variation that interferes. *High arched palate* is seen in trisomies, in Turner syndrome, and in small premature infants who have been intubated, which causes a characteristic groove in the palate. In one study, 10 infants under 29 months of age with Turner syndrome had difficulty feeding from birth when compared with normal children.[101] Breastfeeding was less successful and terminated early. The infants were noted to have marked hypertonia of the cheeks and lips, dysfunctional tongue movements, and poor chewing skills later. The infants had difficulty latching on and had a slow, weak suck. The study infants did not demand food and had not developed a diurnal cycle of hunger and satiety. No efforts were reported to remedy these problems. Referral to a physiotherapist skilled in feeding disorders is the best place to start. A specially trained lactation consultant can provide the breastfeeding adaptations.

Intestinal tract disorders

Infants with anomalies of the GI tract that cause obstruction develop symptoms that are a function of the location of the problem in the GI tract.

Tracheoesophageal fistula. Tracheoesophageal (TE) fistula is apparent early and, depending on the exact anatomy of the lesions, results in respiratory symptoms and signs of intestinal obstruction. This is a surgical emergency. If no feedings have been given or no milk has been aspirated, surgery can be done as soon as possible. If pneumonia develops, the course is protracted and the infant may have to be maintained on peripheral venous alimentation until healing takes place and surgery can be done.

A mother who wants to breastfeed an infant with a TE fistula can manually express milk or pump, saving all samples in the freezer until the infant can take oral milk feedings. If the infant has a gastrostomy tube in place, small feedings may be started fairly early postoperatively, and human milk is ideal if available because of its easy digestibility and anti-infective properties. If there is initially a need to supplement the milk partially with IV fluids, the fluids can be calculated to make up the difference between needs and nutrients supplied by breast milk taken by tube. As nutrition progresses, if supply does not keep up with requirements, feedings can be supplemented with other nutrients. When ready for oral feedings, a full-term or large premature infant can nurse at the breast. Unless the mother is able to spend most of the day and night at the hospital, the infant will have to receive bottle or cup feedings as well (Fig. 15-7). If the mother has been able to store up enough milk, the infant may be able to fulfill needs from breast milk. Once the infant is discharged and begins to nurse at the breast every feeding for a few days, the supply will increase immediately. If concern exists about nutritional lag between needs and production, the Lact-Aid or lactation supplementer device can be used briefly to stimulate the breast without starving and exhausting the infant (see Chapter 19).

Gastroesophageal reflux. Gastroesophageal (GE) reflux—persistent nonprojectile, postpran-

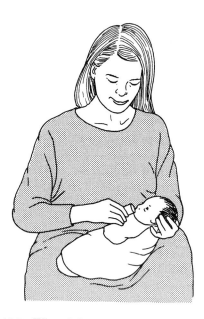

Figure 15-7. When infant must be fed but cannot be breastfed (e.g., when mother is ill), infant can be fed using a small, soft medicine cup. Infant is swaddled and held semiupright, and liquid is given inside lower lip.

dial vomiting or regurgitation—is being diagnosed with increasing frequency. Part of this increase is occurring in graduates of NICUs who have been tube fed or perhaps intubated. Previously compromised infants are more frequently bottle fed, thus the increase in bottle feeding associated with this diagnosis is to be expected. Little is written about GE reflux in breastfed infants because it usually does not occur or is asymptomatic. The position for feeding is more upright than for bottle feeding, and the suckling motion of the tongue, which triggers peristaltic waves from tongue to GI tract and an automatic swallow, provides some protection for breastfed infants.

The effect of milk type on physiologic GE reflux was evaluated in 37 breastfed and 37 bottle fed healthy term infants at 2 to 8 days of life by Heacock and associates.[67] The GE reflux episodes in breastfed infants were less frequent (83) and shorter than those in bottle fed infants (144). Breastfed infants had more quiet sleep than active sleep. There was no apparent difference in volume consumed. The pH of breast milk was initially slightly higher than formula; a significantly lower pH was found for refluxes in the breastfed infants. The researchers did not test whether the differences were caused by the variations in human milk and formula or the differences in suckling at the breast, a physiologic process, or sucking a bottle. If reflux is symptomatic in a breastfed infant, breastfeeding should be done with infant semiupright and he should be placed in an inclined seat after a feed. In rare cases, medication is necessary.

Pyloric stenosis. Pyloric stenosis occurs in about 2 to 5 of 1000 live births. A family tendency exists, but the disease is more common in first-born males. Usually it occurs between the second and sixth weeks of life, although it can occur any time after birth. Vomiting is characteristic, is intermittent at first and progresses to include every feeding, and is often projectile. These infants are eager feeders and go back for more milk until the weight loss and dehydration make them anxious and irritable.

Large epidemiologic studies have failed to show a relationship between pyloric stenosis and breastfeeding. Although pyloric stenosis and breastfeeding have both increased in the last decades, a relationship does not appear to exist. The study in western Australia links LBW, short gestational age, and paternal family history.[69] In Atlanta the rates were unchanged, but the infants were white male, had greater birth weight, were from upper-class families, and were most likely to be breastfed in this generation but not in 1970.[83]

In an analysis of 91 infants with pyloric stenosis born in Saskatchewan from 1970 to 1985, matched with control infants who did not have the disease and were born at the same time and place, the ratio of males to females was 4:1, and 39 of the 91 were firstborns. Bottle feeding was more prevalent in the disease group than in the control group.

In the investigation of vomiting, it is important to keep in mind that overfeeding can cause spitting and vomiting, even projectile vomiting, but it is not associated with weight loss, decreased urine and stools, and dehydration. Therapy consists of pyloromyotomy following correction of the dehydration and associated electrolyte abnormalities. If the procedure is uncomplicated (i.e., intestinal lumen was not entered), the infant can go back to the breast in 6 to 8 hours after a trial of water at 4 hours shows the infant is alert and sucking well. Mother should pump every 3 hours until infant can be fed. The breastfed infant may be discharged in 24 hours if nursing has gone well. If the duodenum is entered at the time of surgery, gastric decompression and IV fluids will be necessary and oral feeding delayed several days until signs of healing occur. A breastfed infant may resume nursing earlier than a bottle fed infant returns to formula because of the rapid emptying time of the stomach and the zero curd tension of the breast milk.

Disorders of the small intestine. Disorders such as duodenal obstruction, malrotation, jejunal obstruction, and duplications require surgery. Depending on the extent of the lesion, whether the bowel wall is opened, whether bowel segments are removed, and whether there are associated lesions such as annular pancreas, the infant will need postoperative maintenance on IV fluids and possibly alimentation. In a study of early postoperative feeding in infants with duodenal atresia ($n = 10$),

malrotation ($n = 6$) and jejunal atresia ($n = 1$), enteral feeding was started by postoperative day 2 in 14 cases. Breast milk was the most common nutrient (numbers and amounts not given). Thirteen infants were discharged (one died of sepsis).[142] The mother who chooses to breastfeed may or may not have ever nursed the infant prior to surgery, depending on the time of onset of symptoms and their severity. The mother should be counseled about the prognosis and encouraged to express milk manually and pump to provide her milk for her infant postoperatively. The decision should be made among the parents, surgeon, neonatologist, and pediatrician. Frequently, infants with atresias are also small or premature and have protracted recovery periods. If the infant will be breastfed, breast milk can be introduced earlier than formula.

Disorders of the colon. Disorders of the colon occur more often in full-term infants. *Hirschsprung's disease,* or *congenital aganglionic megacolon,* is the most common lesion. Passage of meconium is usually delayed; however, only 10% to 15% of all children with delayed passage of meconium have Hirschsprung's disease. Constipation and abdominal distention are the most frequent initial symptoms. They may begin during the first few days of life and gradually progress to include bilious vomiting. The clinical picture may be indistinguishable from meconium ileus, ileal atresia, or large bowel obstruction. In any infant with perforation of the colon, ileum, or appendix, Hirschsprung's disease should be considered. The breastfed infant may have milder symptoms and delayed onset of real stress because the breast milk stools are normally loose and seedy and easily passed. The pH and flora of the intestinal tract are also different, leading to less distention. Enterocolitis may occur at any age and is the major cause of death.

No data have been found to distinguish the incidence of this complication in breastfed and bottle fed infants, although an argument could be mounted regarding the projected value of secretory IgA (sIgA) and intestinal flora of the breastfed infant. The treatment depends on the symptoms, x-ray findings, and biopsy results for the identification of the aganglionic segment. Colostomy is usually done at the time of diagnosis, with definitive surgery later in the first year of life. Feedings can be resumed as soon as the infant is stable, after the colostomy has healed sufficiently to permit bowel activity. Human milk has the same advantages for early postoperative feeding in this disease as well because of its antiinfective properties and easy digestibility.

Meconium plug syndrome and meconium ileus. Meconium plug syndrome and meconium ileus are less common and less severe in breastfed infants who have received a full measure of colostrum, which has a cathartic effect and stimulates the passage of meconium. If either disorder is diagnosed, the infant should continue to nurse in addition to any other treatment, which should include an assessment for cystic fibrosis (CF) and pancreatic insufficiency.

Congenital chylothorax. Congenital chylothorax, although uncommon, is the most common cause of pleural effusion in the newborn period. It impacts the respiratory, nutritional, and immunologic systems and is potentially life-threatening. Most cases are single abnormalities, which may be associated with other anomalies, lymphangiectasia, or neuroblastoma. Management is controversial. Parenteral nutrition and mechanical ventilation have improved the outcome. If diagnosed prenatally, transabdominal thoracocentesis can be done and delivery initiated after 32 weeks. The chest can be tapped or put to continuous drainage.

Nutrition starts with total parenteral nutrition (TPN). Enteral feedings are started as soon as possible (about 5 to 7 days) using breast milk or regular formula. If the chylothorax worsened, oral feeds were stopped for another 3 to 7 days and then restarted special MCT (medium chain triglyceride)-rich formula (Pregestamil) and then in 2 to 4 weeks breast milk or regular formula. In a retrospective study by Al-Tawil and colleagues[6] 19 infants were reviewed, 18 were followed for 7 years and were successfully managed after about 7 weeks with breastfeeding or regular formula. In another study, the infants managed with TPN ($n = 9$) recovered more rapidly (mean 10 days) than those treated with medium chain triglycerides ($n = 8$) (mean 23 days). TPN treatment permitted progression to earlier oral feeds and earlier breastfeeding.[7] Iatrogenic chylothorax management is not as simple and may take weeks of TPN and then the use of defatted breast milk.

Necrotizing enterocolitis. Although necrotizing enterocolitis (NEC) has been known for 100 years, only since 1960 has it been identified with any frequency, which suggests an iatrogenic component. It is most common in premature infants and infants compromised by asphyxia. It has been associated with umbilical catheters, exchange transfusions, polycythemia, hyperosmolar feedings, and infection. Its cause is not clear. Work with animals has suggested that human breast milk, specifically colostrum, provides protection against the disease. A good control study to evaluate this in human infants has not been reported. A "dose or two" of human milk may not be enough. Reported cases of NEC have occurred so early in life that no feedings had been given. Present regimens of treatment call for cessation of all oral feedings and use of oral and systemic antibiotics, gastric decompression, plasma or blood transfusions, and rigorous monitoring for progression or perforation with serial x-ray studies as well as a septic workup. Further study is necessary to determine cause and possible prevention and the role colostrum or breast milk might play, as discussed earlier.

The organisms generally associated with NEC are gram-negative organisms such as *Bacteroides, Escherichia coli,* and especially *Klebsiella.* Brown and associates[24] reported that 89% of the infants with NEC had received cow milk formulas and that gram-negative bacteria and endotoxins were present in the stool. Colonization of breastfed infants with *Klebsiella* does not occur, and *Lactobacillus bifidus* predominates, according to Mata and Urrutia.[98] The unusual occurrence of NEC in Helsinki, at the University of Helsinki Children's Hospital intensive care nursery, is remarkable. All the premature infants are routinely fed colostrum and breast milk in Helsinki.

The role of bacterial colonization in NEC was further explored by Dal and Walker, who suggest that the beneficial effects of suppression of colonization of harmful bacteria and the stimulation of bifidobacterial growth is a valuable approach to the prevention and treatment of NEC. When standardized feeding protocols were studied by Kamisuka and colleagues, it was concluded that the protocols decreased the incidence of NEC independent of birth weight, prenatal steroid exposure, breast milk, and feeding timing. In a systemic review of the question of the value of donor milk versus formula for preventing NEC involving four studies from 1983 to 1990, the authors suggest that donor milk reduces the incidence of NEC in preterm or LBW infants.[104] NEC was three times less likely, confirmed NEC was four times less likely, actually barely statistically significant because of the small numbers of cases. It would take 900 infants from about 30 centers to confirm these findings because the incidence of NEC is low. Meanwhile, women who can contribute their colostrum and milk to their fragile infants should be encouraged to do so. Donor milk studies did not include colostrums which may account for less dramatic results.

Imperforate anus. Defects in the rectum and anal sphincter are usually diagnosed in the first few hours on physical examination. When the blind pouch is more generous, diagnosis may depend on the evaluation of failure to pass stool. Depending on associated lesions and fistulas to bladder or vagina, surgical decompression can be performed. Until this time, oral feedings are withheld. High lesions require an immediate colostomy with later final repair, whereas low lesions may be repaired at the primary procedure through a perineal approach. Infants may be breastfed as soon as any bowel activity can be permitted, often 2 to 3 days postoperatively.

Gastrointestinal bleeding. The most common cause of vomiting blood or passing blood via the rectum in a breastfed infant is a bleeding nipple in the mother, which may or may not be painful. Any time fresh blood is found in the vomitus or stool of any newborn, the blood should be tested for adult or fetal hemoglobin (Hb). If adult Hb, it indicates the source is maternal. This is done by a qualitative test, the Apt test: Mix red blood with 2 to 3 mL normal saline solution, and add this mixture to 3 mL of 10% NaOH (0.25 M). Mix gently. Observe for color change. Fetal Hb is stable in alkali and will remain pink, whereas adult Hb turns brown. Use a known adult sample as a color control. If the blood is adult Hb in a breastfed infant, the possibility of a cracked and bleeding nipple should be ruled out by examining the sample of expressed milk for color and guaiac, and inspection of the maternal breast (see Chapter 8).

If the blood is fetal Hb, the differential diagnosis for bleeding in any neonate should be followed. Breastfeeding can be maintained, unless a lesion requiring surgery is identified. More than 50% of cases of GI bleeding in the neonate go undiagnosed. Anorectal fissure is an uncommon cause in breastfed infants. Allergy to human milk itself has not been reported as a cause of intestinal bleeding. The distribution of causes of intestinal bleeding in the neonate, without selection for type of feeding, follows: idiopathic, 50%; hemorrhagic disorders, 20%; swallowed maternal blood, 10%; anorectal fissures, 10%; intestinal ischemia, 5%; and colitis, 5%. When the bleeding occurs beyond the newborn period, colitis (see earlier discussion) becomes a more frequent cause, as does Meckel diverticulum. Sullivan has reviewed the subject of cow milk–induced intestinal bleeding in infancy.[141]

Otitis media

Acute otitis media is a very common affliction among young children that has increased in incidence paralleling the increasing attendance at daycare. Population density and air pollution have also been identified as factors. In a Finnish study of 471 2- to 3-year-old children, 188 had three or more attacks of otitis media, 76 had one to two attacks, and 207 had none.[120] Incidence was increased in those who attended daycare or had several siblings. Prolonged breastfeeding (longer than 6 months) was associated with a decreased risk. A prospective study of 1011 children in Boston evaluated the duration of middle ear effusion, and it was significantly diminished by breastfeeding.[145]

Breastfeeding is protective against otitis media. With daycare exposure and other environmental risk factors, it does have a measurable minimizing effect. Breastfeeding is also more comfortable for the infant with a painful otitis when suckling at the breast than bottle feeding because of the physiologic suck/swallow mechanism. If the infant is having difficulty feeding, providing a dose of acetaminophen or ibuprofen before the feeding can be helpful.

Congenital dislocation of hip

When procedures or treatments need to be initiated for an infant previously thought to be normal, breastfeeding may not go smoothly. Using congenital dislocation of the hip as a prototype, Elander[42] looked at overall breastfeeding success. Compared with a randomly chosen control group of 113 infants, the 30 study infants who required the von Rosen splint were less successfully fed. However, a higher incidence of cesarean birth was seen in the study group (30% vs. 4%). There were equal numbers of primiparas (50% vs. 48%). Once breastfeeding was established, the long-range success rate was no different. Mothers were pleased to be able to do something special for their splinted children (i.e., breastfeed). This would suggest that special support and guidance regarding breastfeeding issues may be needed along with details on how to apply the splint and how to cope with the splint while positioning for breastfeeding.

Malformations of central nervous system

Malformations of the central nervous system (CNS) diagnosed at birth include the clinical spectrum from anencephaly and complete craniorachischisis to dermal sinuses. Defects of the spinal column range from complete spinal rachischisis to spina bifida occulta. Those that are incompatible with life or are inoperable present the additional problem to the mother who had planned to breastfeed of coping with her desire to nurse her infant. If the infant is to be given normal newborn care and the mother desires to nurse this infant, breastfeeding should be discussed by the pediatrician and parents together. It has been well demonstrated that parents grieve more physiologically if they have contact with their abnormal infants, but their imaginations are more vicious than some abnormalities of development. The professional's personal bias as to how to deal with this infant

should not overshadow the discussion with the parents. If the mother wants to nurse the infant who has no life expectancy and the infant is to be fed at all by mouth, she should have that choice.

Infants with CNS abnormalities requiring surgery can be breastfed until the procedure and postoperatively as soon as oral intake is permitted. In these cases, when the GI tract is not involved, breastfeeding can be initiated 6 to 8 hours postoperatively, at the surgeon's discretion. The risk of lung irritation from breast milk is minimal. The rapid emptying time of the stomach and presence of antiinfective factors serve as advantages in the postoperative course. The placing of a shunt for hydrocephalus is a common procedure and breastfeeding is an ideal feeding mode for this infant.

Surgery or rehospitalization beyond neonatal period

Anesthesia is a main concern when any patient is scheduled for surgery. Traditionally, the patient has been ordered "nothing by mouth" after midnight or 6 to 8 hours preoperatively. Young infants used to feeding every 4 hours are frantic when ready for the operating room.

Recommendations for fasting intervals preoperatively have changed with the belief that clear liquids are safe up to within 2 hours of anesthesia, with similar gastric volumes and pH at 2 hours and 8 hours.[132,138] Children under 1 year had not been studied until the report by Litman and associates,[87] who evaluated 77 infants between 2 weeks and 1 year of age. Bottle fed infants had no solids within 6 hours and only clear liquids up to 8 oz within 2 hours of surgery. Breastfed infants had no solids but were permitted to breastfeed up to within 2 hours of surgery. After 0.02 mg/kg oral atropine 30 to 45 minutes before surgery, induction anesthesia, and tracheal intubation, gastric fluid was aspirated by a blinded researcher who measured volume and pH. The study was discontinued when an unacceptable number of infants in the breastfed group had gastric volumes greater than 1 mL/kg (7 of 24 breastfed and 2 of 46 bottle fed). The pH of the gastric contents of bottle fed infants was less than 2.5 in 9 of 10 (90%)

infants with measurable fluid, whereas pH greater than 2.5 in breastfed infants was 3 of 8 (38%). Low pH is probably a greater risk than volume, but the residual in breastfed infants is much greater than with clear fluids.[87] Instructions to breastfeeding mothers should limit the amount of breastfeeding after 4 hours and permit feeding on a prepumped breast, predominantly for comfort up to 2 hours prior to surgery. According to the American Society of Anesthesiologists, adhering to these guidelines is essential for safety of the anesthesia.[10]

The infant who requires surgery or rehospitalization can and should be breastfed postoperatively in most cases. The gravity of the surgery and the length of the recovery phase will determine the time necessary for the mother to pump and manually express her milk to keep her supply available. The infant who is hospitalized is already traumatized by the separation, the strange surroundings and people, and the underlying discomfort of the disease process itself. If the infant is to be fed orally, feeding should be at the breast as often as possible. If the mother can room-in or the hospital has a care-by-parent ward, this works well. If obligations to other family members make it impossible for the mother to stay, she can pump her milk and bring it in fresh day by day or frozen if the time interval between visits is longer than a day. Freezing will destroy the cellular content, but this is not a major problem beyond the immediate neonatal period. The infant should not be subjected to the added trauma of being weaned from the breast when the infant needs the security and intimacy of nursing most, unless weaning is absolutely unavoidable.

The medical profession needs to be aware of this infant and mother and their special needs for support. An opportunity to discuss the breastfeeding aspect of the infant's management should be offered by the physician. The pediatrician should assume the advocacy role. The parents should not have to fight for the right to maintain breastfeeding. Plans for pumping and saving milk should be discussed and provided for. If the infant is recovering in an open ward or even a room with other infants and their parents without adequate privacy, a separate room should be provided for the mother to nurse or pump her milk. This room should be clean, neat, adequately illuminated, and equipped with a sink for washing hands. Storerooms, broom closets, and staff dressing rooms are inappropriate. If a mechanical pump is to be used, it should be kept clean and operable with disposable tubing and attachments that come in contact with the milk or the breast. If a breast pump is not provided on the pediatric floor, it should be available from the newborn or NICU service.

Arrangements for providing sterile containers for collecting milk and storing it are discussed (see Chapter 21). Occasionally a mother may become so concerned about the adequacy of her milk for her infant that she may nurse much too frequently. Actually her child will need much more nonnutritive cuddling and holding than usual. The physician may need to reassure the mother when pointing this out. The father should also be encouraged to understand all the tubes, bandages, and appliances the infant may have attached. He is an important member of the parenting team and should provide some of the soothing and especially the nonnutritive cuddling.

Congenital heart disease

When an infant who is diagnosed with congenital heart disease is already feeding at the breast, it is usually not a medical indication to interrupt the process unless surgery is imminent. Even infants with cyanotic heart disease, if they can be fed orally, can be breastfed. The "work" required to breastfeed is less than the "work" required to bottle feed. Heart and respiratory rates remain stable during feeding at the breast. If the infant is unable to generate enough sucking stimulus to the breast to increase the milk supply, an electric pump can be used between feedings to increase the mother's supply.

Not all infants with congenital heart disease are diagnosed at birth. When an infant is failing to thrive in spite of good breastfeeding, it is time to consider workup for cardiac or renal disease. Clinicians focus on the breastfeeding and may miss the "elephant in the room."

Cardiac surgeons frequently plan surgery for a certain weight or age. The mother can be assisted in helping the infant reach the goal. Human milk is low in sodium and easily digested, thus permitting frequent feedings. The nurse practitioner or lactation consultant should assist the mother in increasing her production and increasing fat content at each feeding. Feeding at one breast usually increases fat. In the case of a cardiac-compromised infant, using one breast also diminishes the stress of switching to the other side. The mother may need extra support and encouragement. Providing one's milk for one's sick infant may be extremely important. The breastfeeding relationship may be important for the infant as well. Research has shown that infants have important cardiovascular responses to nutrient intake.[110] These responses are regulated by changes in autonomic activity to the heart and vasculature. These early life-shaping interactions that occur when the offspring is fed by the mother have been demonstrated in the animal model. Interactions between mothers and their young serve as hidden regulators of physiologic function.

If oral intake must be restricted preoperatively or immediately postoperatively, "nonnutritive" suckling at the previously pumped breast can be very calming and comforting for the infant.

SUDDEN INFANT DEATH SYNDROME

Sudden infant death syndrome (SIDS) is the leading cause of death in infants after 1 month of age, accounting for one third of all deaths in the first year. Healthy, full-term infants account for 85% of the deaths.[48]

In a 3-year, multicenter, controlled study of SIDS in New Zealand reported in 1993,[133] The National COT Death Prevention Programme[107] sought to reduce the rising incidence of infant death by determining associated factors. Sleeping prone, maternal smoking, lack of breastfeeding, and the infant sharing a bed were the four modifiable risk factors. New Zealand launched a major prevention program to educate the public about these risk factors.[108] The American Academy of Pediatrics has launched a similar program focusing only on sleeping prone. Although breastfeeding offers protection,

there are cases of SIDS among breastfed infants; the incidence is much lower, however, than with bottle feeding. A case-control study in the United States by Frederickson and associates[48] analyzed births of infants weighing more than 2000 g between 1988 and 1989. There were 7102 control infants and 499 SIDS and 584 non-SIDS deaths. Breastfeeding offered dose-response protection against SIDS across races and socioeconomic levels. For white infants, the risk of SIDS increased 19% for every month of not breastfeeding and 100% for every month of nonexclusive breastfeeding. For black infants, the risk was 19% and 113%, respectively.

Numerous studies have been conducted to define further the associations with SIDS. Prone sleeping position continues to be the most important correlation, and the AAP continues the "back to sleep" campaign. The protective influence of breastfeeding is actually strongest among infants of smoking mothers. SIDS rates are higher among infants of mothers who smoke, but breastfeeding by a smoking mother lowers that to a rate equal to that of bottle fed infants. An association has also been suggested with pacifier use in bottle fed infants. Pacifiers are not known to lower SIDS rates among breastfed infants beyond normal breastfeeding rates. Should pacifiers be recommended to prevent SIDS, use should be limited to bottle feeders as pacifiers are associated with decreased duration of breastfeeding. Although some studies show a protective effect of bed sharing, the AAP has not endorsed bed sharing because of the reported risk of roll-over deaths and the need for additional studies.[143] Frederickson and associates[48] suggest that breastfeeding promotion, especially among low-income women where rates of breastfeeding are lowest and SIDS are higher, would reduce the national SIDS rates.

NURSING BOTTLE CARIES IN BREASTFED INFANTS

The development of rampant dental caries can occur in breastfed infants.[23] Usually the children have been nursed for 2 or 3 years, spending long stretches at the breast. One infant had early signs at 9 months, and by 18 months she required full mouth reconstruction.

The physician should be alert to the potential for dental decay when infants nurse frequently, especially through the night. Family history of dental enamel problems is worth investigating. Certainly these children are candidates for fluoride treatment.

The levels of mutant streptococci in saliva and plaque are higher in children with rampant cavities than in control subjects.[99] All breastfed infants have mutant streptococci and lactobacilli on their teeth. Tooth susceptibility is genetically programmed. Children with a strong family history of caries may need fluoride supplements while breastfeeding.[38] They are at special risk if they suckle all night after age 1 year. The most cariogenic solutions are soda, fruit juice, sweetened cow milk, chocolate milk, and sugar water.

REFERENCES

1. Abbassi V, Steinour TA: Successful diagnosis of congenital hypothyroidism in four breast-fed neonates. J Pediatr 97:259, 1980.
2. Addy HA: The breastfeeding of twins. J Trop Pediatr Environ Child Health 21:231, 1975.
3. Aggett PJ, Atherton DJ, More J, et al: Symptomatic zinc deficiency in a breast-fed preterm infant. Arch Dis Child 55:547, 1980.
4. Ahmed S, Blair AW: Symptomatic zinc deficiency in a breast-fed infant. Arch Dis Child 56:315, 1981.
5. Alexander GS, Roberts SA: Sucking behavior and milk intake in jaundiced neonates. Early Hum Dev 16:73, 1988.
6. Al-Tawil K, Ahmed G, Al-Hathal M: Congenital chylothorax. Am J Perinatol 17:121, 2000.
7. Alvarez JRF, Kalache KD, Grauel EL: Management of spontaneous congenital chylothorax: Oral medium-chain triglycerides versus total parenteral nutrition. Am J Perinatol 16:415, 1999.
8. American Academy of Pediatrics, Ronald E. Kleinman (ed): Pediatric Nutrition Handbook, 5th ed. Elk Grove, IL, American Academy of Pediatrics, 2004.
9. American Academy of Pediatrics, Section on Breastfeeding: The AAP and the use of human milk. Pediatrics 2005 (in press.
10. American Society of Anesthesiology Task Force on Preoperative Fasting: Practice Guidelines for Pre-operative Fasting in Elective Surgery. Park Ridge, IL, ASA, 2000.
11. Arias IM, Gartner LM, Seifter S, et al: Prolonged neonatal unconjugated hyperbilirubinemia associated with breast feeding and steroid pregnane-3α,20β-diol in maternal milk that inhibits glucuronide formation in vitro. J Clin Invest 43:2037, 1964.
12. Atinmo T, Omololu A: Trace element content of breast milk from mothers of preterm infants in Nigeria. Early Hum Dev 6:309, 1982.
13. Aumonier ME, Cunningham CC: Breastfeeding in infants with Down's syndrome. Child Care Health Dev 9:247, 1983.
14. Auricchio S, Follo D, de Ritis G, et al: Does breast feeding protect against the development of clinical symptoms of celiac disease in children? J Pediatr Gastroenterol Nutr 2:428, 1983.
15. Avedian LV, Ruberg RL: Impaired weight gain in cleft palate infants. Cleft Palate J 17:24, 1980.
16. Babovic-Vuksanovic D, Michels VV, Law ME, et al: Guidelines for buccal smear collection in breast-fed infants. Am J Med Genet 84:357, 1999.
17. Barfoot RA, McEnery G, Ersser RS, et al: Diarrhoea due to breast milk: A case of fucose intolerance? Arch Dis Child 63:311, 1988.
18. Bennett FC, McClelland S, Kriegsmann EA, et al: Vitamin and mineral supplementation in Down's syndrome. Pediatrics 72:707, 1983.
19. Bergstrand O, Hellers G: Breastfeeding during infancy in patients who later develop Crohn's disease. Scand J Gastroenterol 18:903, 1983.
20. Berkowitz CD, Inkelis SH: Bloody nipple discharge in infancy. J Pediatr 103:755, 1983.
21. Bernbaum JC, Pereira GR, Watkins JB, et al: Nonnutritive sucking during gavage feeding enhances growth and maturation in premature infants. Pediatrics 71:41, 1983.
22. Bode HH, Vanjonack WJ, Crawford JD: Mitigation of cretinism by breastfeeding. Pediatrics 62:13, 1978.
23. Brams M, Maloney J: "Nursing bottle caries" in breast-fed children. J Pediatr 103:415, 1983.
24. Brown EG, Ainbender E, Sweet AY: Effect of feeding stool endotoxins: Possible relationship to necrotizing enterocolitis. Pediatr Res 10:352, 1976.
25. Cannella PC, Bowser EK, Guyer LK, et al: Feeding practices and nutrition recommendations for infants with cystic fibrosis. J Am Diet Assoc 93:297, 1993.
26. Challacombe DN, Mecrow IK, Elliott K, et al: Changing infant feeding practices and declining incidence of celiac disease in West Somerset. Arch Dis Child 77:206, 1997.
27. Chiba Y, Minagawa T, Mito K, et al: Effect of breastfeeding on responses of systemic interferon and virus-specific lymphocyte transformation in infants with respiratory syncytial virus infection. J Med Virol 21:7, 1987.

28. Chou S-C, Palmer RH, Ezhuthachan S, et al: Management of hyperbilirubinemia in newborns: Measuring performance by using a benchmarking model. Pediatrics 112:1264, 2003.

29. Clark BJ: After a positive Guthrie—What next? Dietary management for the child with phenylketonuria. Eur J Clin Nutr 46(suppl I):S33, 1992.

30. Clarren SK, Anderson B, Wolf LS: Feeding infants with cleft lip, cleft palate, or cleft lip and palate. Cleft Palate J 24:244, 1987.

31. Committee on Obstetric Practice, American College of Obstetricians and Gynecologists, Committee on the Fetus and Newborn, American Academy of Pediatrics: Guidelines for Perinatal Care, 5th ed. Elk Grove, Ill, American Academy of Pediatrics, 2002.

32. Curtis JA, Bailey JD: Influence of breastfeeding on the clinical features of salt-losing congenital adrenal hyperplasia. Arch Dis Child 58:71, 1983.

33. Danziger Y, Pertzelan A, Mimouni M: Transient congenital hypothyroidism after topical iodine in pregnancy and lactation. Arch Dis Child 62:295, 1987.

34. Darzi MA, Chowdri NA, Bhat AN: Breast feeding or spoon feeding after cleft lip repair: A prospective, randomised study. Br J Plast Surg 49:24, 1996.

35. de Carvalho M, Klaus M, Merkatz RB: Frequency of breast-feeding and serum bilirubin concentration. Am J Dis Child 136:737, 1982.

36. de Carvalho M, Robertson S, Klaus M: Fecal bilirubin excretion and serum bilirubin concentrations in breastfed and bottle-fed infants. J Pediatr 107:786, 1985.

37. DeVries LS, Lary S, Whitelaw AG, et al: Relationship of serum bilirubin levels and hearing impairment in newborn infants. Early Hum Dev 15:269, 1987.

38. Deyano MP, Degana RA: Breastfeeding and oral health. NY State Dent J 59:30, 1993.

39. DiScippio W, Kaslon KR: Conditioned dysphagia in cleft palate children after pharyngeal flap surgery. Psychol Med 44:247, 1982.

40. Eckert CD, Sloan MV, Duncan JR, et al: Zinc binding: A difference between human and bovine milk. Science 195:789, 1977.

41. Ehrenkranz RA, Ackerman BA: Metoclopramide effect on faltering milk production by mothers of premature infants. Pediatrics 78:614, 1986.

42. Elander G: Breastfeeding of infants diagnosed as having congenital hip joint dislocation and treated in the von Rosen splint. Midwifery 2:147, 1986.

43. Elander G, Lindberg T: Hospital routines in infants with hyperbilirubinemia influence the duration of breastfeeding. Acta Paediatr Scand 75:708, 1986.

44. Ernest AE, McCabe ERB, Neifert MR, et al: Guide to breast feeding the infant with PKU. Washington, DC, U.S. Government Printing Office, 1980.

45. Evans GW, Johnson PE: Defective prostaglandin synthesis in acrodermatitis enteropathica. Lancet 1:52, 1977.

46. Fisher JC: Early repair and breastfeeding for infants with cleft lip. Plast Reconstr Surg 79:886, 1987.

47. Forman MR, Graubard BI, Hoffman HJ, et al: The PIMA infant study: Breastfeeding and gastroenteritis in the first year of life. Am J Epidemiol 119:335, 1984.

48. Frederickson DD, Sorenson JR, Biddle AK, et al: Relationship of sudden infant death syndrome to breast-feeding duration and intensity. Am J Dis Child 147:460, 1993.

49. Gartner LM: Disorders of bilirubin metabolism. In Nathan DG, Oski FA (eds): Hematology of Infancy and Childhood, 3rd ed. Philadelphia, WB Saunders, 1987.

50. Gartner LM: On the question of the relationship between breastfeeding and jaundice in the first 5 days of life. Semin Perinatol 18:502, 1994.

51. Gartner LM, Arias IM: Temporary discontinuation of breast feeding in infants with jaundice. JAMA 225:532, 1973.

52. Gartner LM, Auerbach KG: Breast milk and breastfeeding jaundice. Acta Pediatr 34:249, 1987.

53. Gartner LM, Lee KS: Effect of starvation and milk feeding on intestinal bilirubin absorption. Pediatr Res 14:498, 1980.

54. Garza C, Hopkinson J, Schanler RJ: Human milk banking. In Howell RR, Morriss FH, Pickering LK (eds): Human Milk in Infant Nutrition and Health. Springfield, IL, Thomas, 1986.

55. Geraghty SR, Kalkwarf HJ, Pinney SM, et al: The initiation and duration of breast milk feedings by mothers of multiples compared to mothers of singletons. ABM News Views 9:21, 2003.

56. Gourley GR, Kreamer B, Arend R: The effect of diet on feces and jaundice during the first three weeks of life. Gastroenterology 103:660, 1992.

57. Grady E: Breastfeeding the baby with a cleft of the soft palate: success and its benefits. Clin Pediatr 16:978, 1977.

58. Greco L, Mayer M, Grimaldi M, et al: The effect of early feeding on the onset of symptoms in celiac disease. J Pediatr Gastroenterol Nutr 4:52, 1985.

59. Grunebaum E, Amir J, Merlop P, et al: Breast milk jaundice: Natural history, familial incidence and late neurodevelopmental outcome of the infant. Eur J Pediatr 150:267, 1991.

60. Gunn AJ, Gunn TR, Rabone DL, et al: Growth hormone increases breast milk volumes in mothers of preterm infants. Pediatrics 98:279, 1996.

61. Gupta AP, Gupta PK: Metoclopramide as a lactagogue. Clin Pediatr 24:269, 1985.

62. Hahn HB, Spiekerman AM, Otto WR, et al: Thyroid function tests in neonates fed human milk. Am J Dis Child 137:220, 1983.

63. Haight M, personal correspondence.

64. Hansen TWR, Bratlid D: Bilirubin and brain toxicity. Acta Paediatr Scand 75:513, 1986.

65. Harmon T, Burkhart G, Applebaum H: Perforated pseudomembranous colitis in the breastfed infant. J Pediatr Surg 27:744, 1992.

66. Hattori R, Hattori H: Breastfeeding twins: Guidelines for success. Birth 26:37, 1999.

67. Heacock HJ, Jeffery HE, Baker JL, et al: Influence of breast versus formula milk on physiological gastroesophageal reflux in healthy, newborn infants. J Pediatr Gastroenterol Nutr 14:41, 1992.

68. Hemingway L: Breastfeeding a cleft-palate baby. Med J Aust 2:626, 1972.

69. Hitchcock NE, Gilmour AI, Gracey M, et al: Pyloric stenosis in western Australia, 1971-1984. Arch Dis Child 62:512, 1987.

70. Illingworth RS, Lister J: The critical or sensitive period, with special reference to certain feeding problems in infants and children. J Pediatr 65:839, 1964.

71. Ip S, Glicken S, Kulig J, et al: Management of neonatal hyperbilirubinemia, evidence report/technology assessment. No. 65, AHRQ Pub. No. 03-E011. Rockville, MD, U.S. Department of Health and Human Services, Agency for Health Care Research and Quality, January 2003.

72. Israel D, Levine J, Pettel M, et al: Protein induced allergic colitis (PAC) in infants. Pediatr Res 25:116A, 1989.

73. Ito S, Blajchman A, Stephenson M, et al: Prospective follow-up of adverse reactions in breast-fed infants exposed to maternal medication. Am J Obstet Gynecol 168:1393, 1993.

74. Ivarsson A, Hernell O, Stenlund H, et al: Breast-feeding protects against celiac disease. Am J Clin Nutr 75:914, 2002.

75. Jain L, Sivieri E, Abbasi S, et al: Energetics and mechanics of nutritive sucking in the preterm and term neonate. J Pediatr 111:894, 1987.

76. Johnson P, Salisbury DM: Breathing and sucking during feeding in the newborn. In Hofer MA (ed): Ciba Foundation Symposium No. 33. Parent-Infant Interaction. Amsterdam, Elsevier Scientific, 1975.

77. Kero P, Piekkala P: Factors affecting the occurrence of acute otitis media during the first year of life. Acta Paediatr Scand 76:618, 1987.

78. Khin-Maung-U, Nyant-Nyant-Wai, Myo-Khin, et al: Effect on clinical outcome of breastfeeding during acute diarrhoea. Br Med J 290:587, 1985.

79. Koletzko S, Sherman P, Corey M, et al: Role of infant feeding practices in development of Crohn's disease in childhood. Br Med J 298:1617, 1989.

80. Kuhr M, Paneth N: Feeding practices and early neonatal jaundice. J Pediatr Gastroenterol Nutr 1:485, 1982.

81. LaGamma EF, Ostertag SG, Birenbaum H: Failure of delayed oral feedings to prevent necrotizing enterocolitis: Results of studying very low birth weight neonates. Am J Dis Child 139:385, 1985.

82. Lake AM, Whitington PF, Hamilton SR: Dietary protein-induced colitis in breast-fed infants. J Pediatr 101:906, 1982.

83. Lammer EJ, Edmonds LD: Trends in pyloric stenosis incidence, Atlanta, 1968 to 1982. J Med Genet 24:482, 1987.

84. Leonard EL, Trykowski LE, Kirkpatrick BV: Nutritive sucking in high-risk neonates after perioral stimulation. Phys Ther 60:299, 1980.

85. Letarte J, Guyda H, Dussault JH, et al: Lack of protective effect of breastfeeding in congenital hypothyroidism: Report of 12 cases. Pediatrics 65:703, 1980.

86. Linn S, Schoenbaum SC, Monson RP, et al: Epidemiology of neonatal hyperbilirubinemia. Pediatrics 75:770, 1985.

87. Litman RS, Wu CL, Quinlivan JK: Gastric volume and pH in infants fed clear liquids and breast milk prior to surgery. Abstract for presentation to The American Society of Anesthesiology, Washington, DC, October, 1993.

88. Littlewood JM, Crollick AJ, Richards IDG: Childhood coeliac disease is disappearing. Lancet 2:1359, 1980.

89. Lubit EC: Cleft palate orthodontics: Why, when, how. Am J Orthodont 69:562, 1976.

90. Lucas A, Cole TJ: Breast milk and neonatal necrotising enterocolitis. Lancet 336:1519, 1990.

91. Luder E, Kattan M, Tanzer-Torres G, et al: Current recommendations for breastfeeding in cystic fibrosis centers. Am J Dis Child 144:1153, 1990.

92. Macaron C: Galactorrhea and neonatal hypothyroidism. J Pediatr 101:576, 1982.

93. MacFarlane PI, Miller V: Human milk in the management of protracted diarrhea of infancy. Arch Dis Child 59:260, 1984.

94. Machida HM, Smith AGC, Gall DG, et al: Allergic colitis in infancy: Clinical and pathologic aspects. J Pediatr Gastroenterol Nutr 19:22, 1994.

95. Maisels MJ, Gifford K: Normal serum bilirubin levels in the newborn and the effect of breastfeeding. Pediatrics 78:837, 1986.

96. Maisels MJ, Kring E: Risk of sepsis in newborns with severe hyperbilirubinemia. Pediatrics 90:741, 1992.

97. Marmet C, Shell E: Lactation forms: A guide to lactation consultant charting. Encino, CA, Lactation Institute and Breastfeeding Clinic, 1993.

98. Mata LJ, Urrutia JJ: Intestinal colonization of breast fed children in a rural area of low socioeconomic level. Ann NY Acad Sci 176:93, 1971.

99. Matee MIN, Mikx FHM, Maselle SYM, et al: Mutant streptococci and lactobacilli in breastfed children with rampant caries. Caries Res 26:183, 1992.

100. Mathew OP: Breathing patterns of preterm infants during bottle feeding: Role of milk flow. J Pediatr 119:960, 1991.

101. Mathisen B, Reilly S, Skuse D: Oral-motor dysfunction and feeding disorders of infants with Turner syndrome. Dev Med Child Neurol 34:141, 1992.

102. McBride MC, Danner SC: Sucking disorders in neurologically impaired infants: Assessment and facilitation of breastfeeding. Clin Perinatol 14:109, 1987.

103. McDonagh AF: Is bilirubin good for you? Clin Perinatol 17:359, 1990.

104. McGuire W, Anthony MY: Donor human milk versus formula for preventing necrotising enterocolitis in preterm infants: Systematic review. Arch Dis Child Fetal Neonatal Ed 88:F11, 2003.

105. Meier P: Bottle- and breast-feeding: Effects on transcutaneous oxygen pressure and temperature in preterm infants. Nurs Res 37:36, 1988.

106. Meier P, Anderson GC: Responses of small preterm infants to bottle- and breast-feeding. Matern Child Nurs J 12:97, 1987.

107. Mitchell EA, Aley P, Eastwood J: The National COT Death Prevention Programme in New Zealand. Aust J Publ Health 16:158, 1992.

108. Mitchell EA, Taylor BJ, Ford RPK, et al: Four modifiable and other major risk factors for cot death: The New Zealand study. J Paediatr Child Health 28(suppl 1):53, 1992.

109. Montgomery RK, Buller HA, Rings EHHM, et al: Lactose intolerance and the genetic regulation of intestinal lactase-phlorizin hydrolase. FASEB J 5:2824, 1991.

110. Myers MM, Shair HN, Hofer MA: Feeding in infancy: Short- and long-term effects on cardiovascular function. Experientia 48:322, 1992.

111. Newman TB, Maisels MJ: Does hyperbilirubinemia damage the brain of healthy full-term infants? Clin Perinatol 17:331, 1990.

112. Newman TB, Maisels MJ: Evaluation and treatment of jaundice in the term newborn: A kinder, gentler approach. Pediatrics 89:809, 1992.

113. Nicoll A, Ginsburg R, Tripp JH: Supplementary feeding and jaundiced newborns. Acta Paediatr Scand 71:759, 1982.

114. Palmer MM, Crawley K, Blanco IA: Neonatal oral-motor assessment scale: A reliability study. J Perinatol 13:28, 1993.

115. Paludetto R, Robertson SS, Hack M, et al: Transcutaneous oxygen tension during nonnutritive sucking in preterm infants. Pediatrics 74:539, 1984.

116. Patenaude Y, Bernard C, Schreiber R, et al: Cow's milk-induced allergic colitis in an exclusively breast-fed infant: Diagnosed with ultrasound. Pediatr Radiol 30:379, 2000.

117. Pedersen CB, Zachau-Christiansen B: Otitis media in Greenland children: Acute, chronic and secretory otitis media in three to eight year olds. J Otolaryngol 15:332, 1986.

118. Peters U, Schneeweiss S, Trautwein EA, et al: A case-control study of the effect of infant feeding on celiac disease. Ann Nutr Metab 45:135, 2001.

119. Provisional Committee for Quality Improvement, Subcommittee on Hyperbilirubinemia, American Academy of Pediatrics: Practice parameters: Management of hyperbilirubinemia in the healthy term newborn. Pediatrics 94:558, 1994.

120. Pukander J, Luotonen J, Timonen M: Risk factors affecting the occurrence of acute otitis media among 2- to 3-year-old urban children. Acta Otolaryngol Stockh 100:260, 1985.

121. Pumberger W, Pomberger G, Geissler W: Proctocolitis in breast fed infants: A contribution to differential diagnosis of haematochezia in early childhood. Postgrad Med J 77:252, 2001.

122. Riva E, Agostoni C, Biasucci G, et al: Early breastfeeding is linked to higher intelligence quotient scores in dietary treated phenylketonuric children. Acta Paediatr 85:56, 1996.

123. Robinson PJ, Rapoport SI: Binding effect of albumin on uptake of bilirubin by brain. Pediatrics 79:553, 1987.

124. Rowe JC, Wood DH, Rowe DW, et al: Nutritional hypophosphatemic rickets in a premature infant fed breast milk. N Engl J Med 300:293, 1979.

125. Saarinen UM: Prolonged breast feeding as prophylaxis for recurrent otitis media. Acta Paediatr Scand 71:567, 1982.

126. Sack J, Amado O, Lunenfeld B: Thyroxine concentration in human milk. J Clin Endocrinol Metab 45:171, 1977.

127. Saint L, Maggiore P, Hartman PE: Yield and nutrient content of milk in eight women breastfeeding twins and one woman breastfeeding triplets. Br J Nutr 56:49, 1986.

128. Sazawal S, Bhan MK, Bhandari N: Type of milk feeding during acute diarrhoea and the risk of persistent diarrhea: A case control study. Acta Paediatr Suppl 381:93, 1992.

129. Scheidt PC, Graubard BI, Nelson KB, et al: Intelligence at six years in relation to neonatal bilirubin level: Follow-up of the National Institute of Child Health and Human Development clinical trial of phototherapy. Pediatrics 87:797, 1991.

130. Schneider AP: Breast milk jaundice in the newborn. JAMA 255:3270, 1986.

131. Schneider JR, Fischer H, Feingold M: Acrodermatitis enteropathica. Am J Dis Child 145:212, 1991.

132. Schreiner MS, Triebwasser A, Keon TP: Ingestion of liquids compared with preoperative fasting in pediatric outpatients. Anesthesiology 75:593, 1990.

133. Scragg LK, Mitchell EA, Tonkin SL, et al: Evaluation of the cot death prevention programme in South Auckland. NZ Med J 106:8, 1993.

134. Shmerling DH: Dietary protein-induced colitis in breast-fed infants. J Pediatr 103:500, 1983.

135. Similä S, Kokkonen J, Kouvalainen K: Use of lactose-hydrolyzed human milk in congenital lactase deficiency. J Pediatr 101:584, 1982.

136. Sirota L, Nussinovirtch M, Landman J, et al: Breast milk jaundice in preterm infants. Clin Pediatr 27:195, 1988.

137. Snyder JB: Bubble palate and failure to thrive: A case report. J Hum Lact 13:139, 1997.

138. Splinter WM, Stewart JA, Muir JG: Large volumes of apple juice preoperatively do not affect gastric PH and volume in children. Can J Anaesth 37:36, 1990.

139. Stevens FM, Egan-Mitchell B, Cryan E, et al: Decreasing incidence of coeliac disease. Arch Dis Child 62:465, 1987.

140. Stevenson DK: Pulmonary excretion of carbon monoxide in human infants as an index of bilirubin production. In Maisels MJ (ed): Hyperbilirubinemia in the newborn: Report of the 85th Ross Conference on Pediatric Research. Columbus, Ohio, Ross Laboratories, 1983.

141. Sullivan PB: Cows' milk induced intestinal bleeding in infancy. Arch Dis Child 68:240, 1993.

142. Suri S, Eradi B, Chowdhary SK, et al: Early postoperative feeding and outcome in neonates. Nutrition 18:380, 2002.

143. Task Force on Infant Positioning and SIDS, American Academy of Pediatrics: Positioning and sudden infant death syndrome (SIDS): Update. Pediatrics 98:1216, 1996.

144. Tatzer E, Schubert MT, Timischl W, et al: Discrimination of taste and preference for sweet in premature babies. Early Hum Dev 12:23, 1985.

145. Teele DW, Klein JO, Rosner B, et al: Beneficial effects of breastfeeding on duration of middle ear effusion (MEE) after first episode of acute otitis media (AOM). Pediatr Res 14:494, 1980.

146. Thompson NP, Montgomery SM, Wadsworth ME, et al: Early determinants of inflammatory bowel disease: Use of two national longitudinal birth cohorts. Eur J Gastroenterol Hepatol 12:25, 2000.

147. Toms GL, Gardner PS, Pullan CR, et al: Secretion of respiratory syncytial virus inhibitors and antibody in human milk through lactation. J Med Virol 5:351, 1980.

148. Toms GL, Scott R: Respiratory syncytial virus and the infant immune response. Arch Dis Child 62:544, 1987.

149. Troncone R, Scarcella A, Donatiello A, et al: Passage of gliadin into human breast milk. Acta Paediatr Scand 76:453, 1987.

150. Tudehope D, Bayley G, Townsend M, et al: Breastfeeding practices and severe hyperbilirubinemia. J Pediatr Child Health 27:240, 1991.

151. Udall JN, Dixon M, Newman AP, et al: Liver disease in α-1-antitrypsin deficiency. JAMA 253:2679, 1985.

152. Varma SK, Collins M, Row A, et al: Thyroxine, tri-iodothyronine, and reverse tri-iodothyronine concentrations in human milk. J Pediatr 93:803, 1978.

153. Walsh M, McIntosh K: Neonatal mastitis. Clin Pediatr 25:395, 1986.

154. Walter RS: Issues surrounding the development of feeding and swallowing. In Tuchman DN, Walter RS (eds): Disorders of Feeding and Swallowing in Infants and Children: Pathophysiology, Diagnosis, and Treatment. San Diego, Singular, 1994.

155. Weatherley-White RCA, Kuehn DP, Kuehn DP, Mirrett P, et al: Early repair and breastfeeding for infants with cleft lip. Plast Reconstr Surg 79:879, 1987.

156. Whitelaw A, Heisterkamp G, Sleath K, et al: Skin-to-skin contact for very low birth weight infants and their mothers. Arch Dis Child 63:1377, 1988.

157. Wilson DC, Afrasiabi M, Reid MM: Breast milk beta-glucuronidase and exaggerated jaundice in the early neonatal period. Biol Neonate 61:232, 1992.

158. Winter S, Buist N: Clinical guide to inborn errors of metabolism. J Rare Dis. IV:18, 1998.

159. Wong PWK, Lambert AM, Komrowe GM: Tyrosinaemia and tyrosinuria in infancy. Dev Med Child Neurol 9:551, 1967.

160. Woolridge MW, Fisher C: Colic, "overfeeding" and symptoms of lactose malabsorption in the breastfed baby: A possible artifact of feed management. Lancet 2:382, 1988.

161. Zimmerman AW, Hambridge KM, Lepow ML, et al: Acrodermatitis in breastfed premature infants: Evidence for a defect of mammary gland zinc secretion. Pediatrics 69:176, 1982

16

$\mathscr{M}$edical complications of the mother

OBSTETRIC COMPLICATIONS

Cesarean delivery

When birth takes place by cesarean delivery, the mother becomes a surgical patient with all the inherent risks and problems. If the procedure is anticipated because of a previous cesarean birth, cephalopelvic disproportion, or some other identifiable reason, a mother can prepare herself psychologically for the event and usually tolerates the process better. When the procedure is unplanned and done during the process of labor, it is psychologically more traumatic, and the mother tends to feel as if she has failed in her female role. In addition to this unexpected disappointment, medical emergencies may also have an impact on the mother's well-being, such as a long, difficult labor; abruptio placentae; blood loss; toxemia; or infection.

The mother who plans to breastfeed after a cesarean birth should be able to do so if the infant is well enough. The method of delivery makes no significant difference to the timing of the milk coming in or the changes in the concentration of the major milk constituents in the first 7 days post partum.[138] Depending on the type of anesthesia and the associated circumstances, the mother may feel alert enough to put the infant to breast within the first 12 hours. Mothers frequently nurse in the first

hour after surgery. The obstetrician, surgeon, and the operating room nurses are key in making it happen.

Bupivacaine is being used as an epidural block for cesarean or vaginal delivery because it does not result in the decrease in muscle tone and strength reported in neonates whose mothers have received lidocaine or mepivacaine.[156,209] Bupivacaine and tetracaine are highly protein bound and appear in milk in very low concentrations, in contrast to lidocaine and mepivacaine, which are nonionized and unbound in serum. Because most local or regional anesthetics are used with epinephrine, which causes local vasoconstriction, thus slowing the rate of absorption, the anesthetic effects are prolonged and the amount secreted into the milk is minimal.

Epidural morphine is used for more prolonged analgesia and is used in cesarean delivery because it can then be continued post partum for the relief of postoperative pain. Bernstein and associates[19] showed that epidurally administered morphine enters the breast milk in very low levels compared with the levels in maternal urine, which were several thousand times higher. Most of the morphine in colostrum is in the conjugated form and thus pharmacologically inactive. Other studies report a milk/plasma ratio of 2:45; the amount received via the milk is calculated to be less than 50 μg/dL of milk, causing no untoward symptoms in any of the cases reported. At birth infants may have morphine in their system from transplacental transfer of intrapartum maternal dosing. Transplacental medication has depressed some infants and may interfere with early attempts to suckle.

In a cesarean delivery under controlled circumstances, the procedure is initiated using local anesthesia to the skin and fascial layers. Systemic anesthesia is given as soon as the cord is clamped, sparing the transfer of anesthetics to the newborn.

Regional anesthesia permits the mother to remain awake, and she may be ready to nurse as soon as the intravenous (IV) lines and urinary catheter are stabilized. The mother will need considerable help from the nursing staff. She should remain flat if she has had a spinal anesthetic to prevent developing a spinal headache. She can turn to one side and offer the breast by placing the infant on its side and stroking the infant's perioral area with the nipple. The normal full-term infant who has not been depressed by maternal medication should do well. If the mother can be turned to the other side, the infant may nurse on both sides. In this first encounter, the emphasis is on some suckling, not switching. The bedside rails will help the mother turn as well as provide safety for her.

Maternal fluids and medications in the first 48 hours postoperatively should not affect the infant adversely. Pain medication is required usually for about 72 hours. It is best given immediately after breastfeeding to permit the level to peak before the next feeding. The medication used should be limited to short-acting drugs that the adult eliminates quickly (i.e., within 4 hours) and that the newborn is able to excrete. Ibuprofen and acetaminophen are in that category; codeine is also acceptable (see Chapter 11). Low-grade fever may occur and should not interrupt lactation.

Some very positive factors are associated with breastfeeding for the mother who has had a cesarean delivery. Lactation is advantageous to the postoperative uterus in that the oxytocin production stimulated by suckling will assist in its involution. In addition, the traumatized psyche of a mother whose delivery did not occur naturally as planned is more quickly healed when she can demonstrate her maternal capabilities by breastfeeding.

Whether breastfeeding can be introduced early or must await stabilization of medical problems in the mother or infant, it is a reasonable goal for the mother to seek in most cases. Supportive nursing care is critical to establishing successful lactation. None of this can take place, however, unless the physician has carefully assessed the condition of the mother and the infant in light of the advantages and disadvantages of breastfeeding to both.

The management should include the following:
1. A postoperative care plan that includes sufficient rest. Most postpartum wards are not scheduled to include adequate rest for postoperative patients.
2. The family must be instructed on the needs for rest at home and assistance with the household chores. With shorter hospital stays, this is even more critical.
3. The impact on the infant should be considered when writing medication orders.
4. If the infant cannot be put to breast, arrangements should be made to pump the mother's breasts on a regular basis with a quality electric pump at least every 3 hours during waking hours, even if separation will last only a day or two.
5. If the mother is in intensive care, pumping can still be done by the skilled bedside nurse or lactation consultant.

Toxemia

Toxemia presents a problem in management any time it occurs. The clinical onset is insidious and may be accompanied by a variety of subtle symptoms, but the diagnosis depends on the presence of hypertension and proteinuria.[34] Toxemia usually begins after the 32nd week of gestation but has been observed to occur 24 to 48 hours or later post partum. Convulsions, renal disease, and cerebral hemorrhage in the mother are complications that can be prevented by careful management. Because serious toxicity in the mother may necessitate delivery of a premature infant or an infant compromised by a poorly perfused placenta or maternal medications, a number of contraindications to breastfeeding exist in the immediate postpartum period.

Initial treatment of the preeclamptic patient includes bed rest, preferably lying on her side in a quiet room that is darkened to prevent photic and auditory stimuli. Blood pressure and proteinuria should be carefully monitored. Sedation with phenobarbital or diazepam (Valium), salt restriction, and possibly diuretics such as thiazide or furosemide are used. Hydralazine (Apresoline) and methyldopa (Aldomet) or other antihypertensives may be indicated as well to bring down the blood pressure. Magnesium sulfate may also be used and is safest for the breastfeeding infant. Many patients recover quickly once the infant and placenta are delivered, requiring only 24 to 48 hours of postpartum sedation.

Often the infant is small for gestational age or premature and may require special or intensive care; therefore, the decision when to initiate breastfeeding depends on the infant's condition. If the infant is full term and well, breastfeeding is initiated when toxemia precautions are discontinued and when the mother's phenobarbital intake has been tapered off to about 180 mg/day or less, calculating that initially the amount of milk obtained is not so great as to provide a large dose of drug to the infant. Careful observation should ensure the infant is not depressed by the accumulation of phenobarbital. Phenobarbital is given to newborns for several indications and therefore is low risk. It is preferable to wait until the other medications can be discontinued, especially the diuretics, hydralazine, and methyldopa.

Once the risk of convulsions is past, some attention can be given to manual expression or pumping, even if the infant cannot be nursed yet. If medications are a problem temporarily, the milk may have to be discarded, but the expression of milk will serve to stimulate the breast and initiate lactation.

Diminution of stress is a critical factor in toxemia therapy, so maternal anxiety about being able to nurse must be managed with open discussion of the overall plan and nursing's role. On the other hand, the stress of early feedings that do not go well because the infant has been confused by initial bottle feedings may also present a hazard in the course of toxemia management. This can be minimized by cup feedings. The most important element in every case is *communication* with the patient about her expectations or needs regarding breastfeeding. The physician's therapeutic management design can put this in appropriate perspective. Because of the effects of oxytocin and prolactin, it may be therapeutic to breastfeed.

Retention of placenta and lactation failure

Three cases of failed onset of lactation were reported by Neifert and associates.[179] Although the original association of the placenta with delayed lactation was made a century ago, most reports of retained placenta merely discuss persistent hemorrhage as a recognized symptom. In each of three cases the failure of breast engorgement and leakage of milk was evident from delivery, but the hemorrhage and emergency curettage occurred at 1 week, 3 weeks, and 4 weeks post partum, respectively. In each case, spontaneous milk flow began immediately postoperatively, after the removal of placental fragments. The authors suggest that failure of lactogenesis may be an early sign of retained placenta that should not be ignored.[179]

Venous thrombosis and pulmonary embolism

Venous thrombosis and pulmonary embolism are the most common serious vascular diseases associated with pregnancy and the postpartum period.[34] Pulmonary embolism has assumed relatively greater importance because of the decline in morbidity and mortality rates from sepsis and eclampsia. *Varicose veins* also present more problems during pregnancy than at any other time. These diseases all represent common features in vein physiology as associated with the perinatal period.

The major concerns during lactation, in addition to the well-being of the mother, include the procedures that might be necessary to establish the diagnosis and the systemic medications necessary for treatment that could have an impact on the nursing infant via the milk. Accurate diagnosis is urgent and is far more complex than therapy. Besides the health of the mother in this life-threatening state, any program of contraception after childbirth is fundamentally affected by the established diagnosis of thromboembolism. Thus, the diagnosis must be accurate.

Diagnosis

Laboratory procedures such as evaluation of arterial blood gases, liver function studies, and fibrin/fibrinogen derivatives are not a problem to breastfeeding. The absence of fibrin split products in plasma and serum virtually excludes the diagnosis of embolism, although their presence does not confirm it. The most definitive diagnosis is made with radioactive scanning procedures and angiography.

Contrast venography is the most definitive method available for diagnosing deep vein thrombosis. The perfusion lung scan is the pivotal test for the investigation of patients with suspected pulmonary embolism. The radiopharmaceuticals used are technetium-99m-microaggregated albumin or microspheres (usual dose 3 mCi), which clear the milk promptly, thus requiring pumping and discarding the milk for 8 hours.[81] Pulmonary angiography, the most definitive test for pulmonary embolism, requires fluoroscopy, which is not a risk to the breastfeeding infant. The total dose is approximately 400 mrad and thus should not interfere with lactation. In deep vein thrombosis of the leg, fibrinogen leg scanning uses iodine-125 (^{125}I) fibrinogen, which requires 2 weeks of pumping and discarding the milk. Radioactive materials vary in their half-lives and disappearance time from breast milk. They all appear in breast milk (see Chapter 11).

Another diagnostic technique is duplex ultrasonography. It consistently visualizes the iliac veins. Impedance plethysmography (IPG) is noninvasive but not reliable for calf thromboses and is contraindicated in the lactating mother.[75] At present, computed tomography (CT) and ultrasound are effective in diagnosing major arterial aneurysms only.

Treatment

Anticoagulant therapy is the treatment of choice for established venous thrombosis with or without embolism. *Heparin* can be given parenterally, because this large molecule does not cross the placenta or appear in breast milk. This therapy is adequate for the hospitalized patient, in whom constant monitoring of coagulation is possible. *Warfarin* has been considered the best replacement for heparin, but it is secreted in the breast milk (see Chapter 11 and Appendix D). The amount transmitted is minuscule, and it is considered safe to breastfeed while taking warfarin. In long-term therapy the prothrombin time should be monitored at least monthly in the infant and vitamin K given if necessary.

The low-molecular-weight heparins are still large molecules and do not pass into the milk and are orally poorly absorbed.[88]

MEDICAL PROBLEMS

Mastitis

Mastitis is an infectious process in the breast that produces localized tenderness, redness, and heat, together with systemic reactions of fever, malaise, and sometimes nausea and vomiting. It no longer occurs in epidemics, as once seen in hospitals before the common use of antibiotics and when hospital stays were prolonged for normal childbirth. The infection, however, may be hospital acquired if the mother or infant is colonized with virulent bacteria before leaving the hospital.

Little appears in the medical literature about mastitis because women are rarely hospitalized for the problem and are treated at home and, in some cases, over the telephone. When staphylococcal disease was a major problem on postpartum wards, lactating and nonlactating women alike developed mastitis; thus the differentiation of two types: acute puerperal mammary *cellulitis,* a nonepidemic mastitis involving interlobular connective tissue, and acute puerperal mammary *adenitis,* which was epidemic and associated with an outbreak of skin infections in infants.

The current definition of *mastitis* includes fever of 38.5° C (101° F) or more, chills, flulike aching, systemic illness, and a pink, tender, hot, swollen, wedge-shaped area of the breast (Fig. 16-1).[182] Table 16-1 lists the significant differential points among mastitis, engorgement, and plugged duct.

The portal of entry of the disease is through the lactiferous ducts to a secreting lobule, through a nipple fissure to periductal lymphatics, or through hematogenous spread. The common organisms involved include *Staphylococcus aureus, Escherichia coli,* and (rarely) *Streptococcus.* Tuberculous mastitis does occur, and the infant often develops tuberculosis of the tonsils. In populations in which tuberculosis is endemic, it occurs in about 1% of cases of mastitis.[86]

Factors predisposing the woman to mastitis include poor drainage of a duct and then of an alveolus, presence of an organism, and lowered maternal defenses such as those associated with stress and fatigue (Figs. 16-1 and 16-2). Insufficient emptying and obstruction of ducts by tight clothing can cause plugged ducts, which can be prevented from becoming mastitis if identified early and treated vigorously with local massage, moist heat, and rest. Missing a feeding or having the infant suddenly sleep through the night may cause engorgement, plugging, and then mastitis.[202] Cracked or painful nipples may herald a problem, more because the mother avoids complete emptying on the painful side than because bacteria suddenly gain access. If

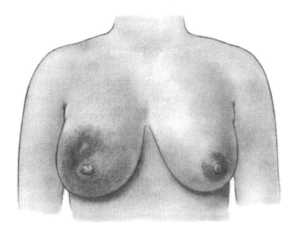

Figure 16-1. Mastitis of right breast, upper outer quadrant.

the mother has cracked, fissured, sore nipples, the breast pain and redness is more than likely mastitis.

Devereux[56] described 20 years of experience with 53 lactating patients who experienced 71 acute attacks of mastitis. The highest incidence was in the second and third weeks post partum. No infant was weaned because of the mastitis. No infants were sick in association with the mastitis. All but five mothers nursed subsequent infants. Six patients had mastitis with other pregnancies. Eight of 71 patients (11.1%) developed abscesses, six of which required incision and drainage. The bacterial cause was not stated. When antibiotic treatment was delayed beyond 24 hours, the abscess rate increased.

TABLE 16-1   Comparison of findings of engorgement, plugged duct, and mastitis

Characteristics	Engorgement	Plugged duct	Mastitis
Onset	Gradual, immediately post partum	Gradual, after feedings	Sudden, after 10 days
Site	Bilateral	Unilateral	Usually unilateral
Swelling and heat	Generalized	May shift; little or no heat	Localized, red, hot, swollen
Pain	Generalized	Mild but localized	Intense but localized
Body temperature	<38.4° C (101° F)	<38.4° C	>38.4° C
Systemic symptoms	Feels well	Feels well	Flulike symptoms

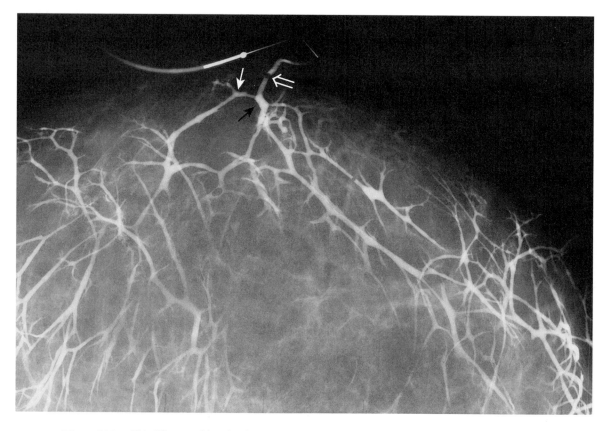

Figure 16-2.   This 38-year-old patient's craniocaudal view shows segmental duct draining a lobe in medial aspect of right breast. Ductal patterns differ among women. (From Logan-Young W, Hoffman NY: Breast Cancer: A Practical Guide to Diagnosis. Vol. 1, Procedures. Rochester, NY, Mt. Hope, 1994.)

Another series of 65 cases of mastitis, reported by Marshall and associates,[158] showed a 2.5% incidence of the disease among a population of 2534 lactating women. *S. aureus* was the offending organism in 23 of the 48 infected breasts that were cultured. In 19 normal (no mastitis) lactating women, only one grew this organism. Of the 65 women, 41 continued to nurse without difficulty for an average of 13 weeks longer. Three breast abscesses for a rate of 4.6% occurred in women who had chosen to wean. Onset was 5½ weeks post partum (range 5 days to 1 year). Of the 65, nine had missed feedings or acutely weaned, eight women had noticed a fissured nipple before the infection,

and the others were unanticipated. Treatment included 41 with penicillin V, 12 with ampicillin, and 8 with other antibiotics. Mastitis recurred in four of the women who continued to nurse.

Half the patients with mastitis in a series reported by Niebyl and associates[177] were infected with *S. aureus*, as determined by culture. They were treated with antibiotics, continued nursing on both sides, and observed no abscesses or problems in the infant. Investigators in The Gambia[200] observed mastitis in 2.6% of women, with recurrence common. They noted the milk was deficient in immunoglobulin A, complement C3, and lactoferrin when compared with that of other lactating mothers. The authors suggested these mothers were predisposed to mastitis. Coagulase-negative staphylococci isolated from the milk of mothers with mastitis has been shown to cause experimental acute mastitis when injected into mice and should be considered a possible etiologic agent in nursing women.[231]

Although breastfed infants usually remain well during bouts of acute mastitis in their mothers, Katzman and Wald[121] reported a case of scalded skin syndrome in an infant fed by a mother with mastitis that did not respond to ampicillin for 14 days. The child responded to intravenous (IV) nafcillin. The mother had a lesion on her areola on the infected breast, and she was told to use breast shields, although she was to continue nursing. Breast shields have been shown to decrease breast emptying by half. This case points out the urgency of evaluating both the mother and the infant when mastitis or any breastfeeding problem occurs.

Using leukocyte counts and microbiologic counts, Thomsen and associates[230] have separated breast inflammations into three clinical states: milk stasis (counts $<10^6$ leukocytes and $<10^3$ bacteria per milliliter of milk), noninfectious inflammation (counts of $>10^6$ leukocytes and $<10^3$ bacteria), and infectious mastitis (counts $>10^6$ leukocytes and $>10^3$ bacteria) (Tables 16-2 and 16-3). The authors concluded that no treatment was needed in stasis, but lack of treatment led to recurrence and lactation failure in noninfectious inflammation and abscess in mastitis. Emptying the breast (frequent feedings and pumping or hand-expressing three times a day after a feed) was sufficient in noninfectious inflammation and ameliorated the course in most cases of mastitis. However, recurrence was then inappropriately high. Mastitis requires antibiotics in addition to emptying the breast.[230]

Because cultures require time, when the bacteria count is finally available and the clinical course is clear, the noninfectious variety should already be cleared. Laboratory results are confirmatory; however, the skilled clinician can avoid the relapses and progression to abscess by close monitoring and selective aggressive treatment before the cultures are reported (see Tables 16-2 and 16-3).

TABLE 16-2 Categories of patients with inflammatory breast symptoms

Symptom	Leukocytes per milliliter of milk	Bacteria per milliliter of milk
Milk stasis	$<10^6$	$<10^3$
Noninfectious inflammation	$>10^6$	$<10^3$
Infectious mastitis	$>10^6$	$>10^3$

From Thomsen AC, Espersen T, Maigaard S: Course and treatment of milk stasis, noninfectious inflammation of the breast, and infectious mastitis in nursing women. Am J Obstet Gynecol 149:492, 1984.

TABLE 16-3 Course of infectious mastitis with and without treatment

Treatment	Number of cases	Duration of symptoms (days, mean)	Result (number of cases)	
			Normal lactation	Poor*
None	55	6.7	8	47
Emptying of breast	55	4.2	28	27
Antibiotics and emptying of breast	55	2.1	53	2

*Breast abscess, 6 cases; symptoms of sepsis, 12 cases; recurrence of symptoms, 21 cases; duration of >14 days, 10 cases; impaired lactation only, 27 cases.
From Thomsen AC, Espersen T, Maigaard S: Course and treatment of milk stasis, noninfectious inflammation of the breast, and infectious mastitis in nursing women. Am J Obstet Gynecol 149:492, 1984.

In lactating Gambian women, unilateral breast dysfunction is not an unusual finding.[199] It has been attributed to episodes of low-grade mastitis with the production of high-sodium milk, which the infant rejects. The unused breast involutes, and the functioning breast increases production. In subsequent pregnancies, function returns to the involved breast.

The clinician must inform patients of the need to contact the office if any unusual symptoms occur so that proper management can be initiated early, because prevention is the most effective treatment. Inappropriately or inadequately treated cases of mastitis predispose the patient to recurrent and ultimately chronic mastitis, which may last for months and require more antibiotics than would have been required initially. A mother should be instructed to contact her physician if she has local pain, heat, redness, or a fever while lactating. Red streaking on the breast may be inflammation of the lymphatics.

A study of 946 breastfeeding women from two sites (Michigan and Nebraska) was conducted by Foxman and colleagues.[73] The women were recruited prenatally and followed prospectively through 3 months post partum or until they stopped breastfeeding. Telephone interviews were done at 3, 6, 9, and 12 weeks. The diagnosis of mastitis was made by self-reported symptoms to their health care provider usually by telephone. The incidence of mastitis was 9.5%.

The strongest risk factor was a history of mastitis with a previous infant. Nipple cracks and sores prior to the mastitis, the use of antifungal cream, and feeding the infant more frequently than usual were key associated phenomena. For women with no prior history of breast infection, the use of a manual breast pump during the same week was a significant risk factor. As in other studies, the first time the infants slept through the night or mother leaves the baby for many hours and does not pump was a prominent feature. Quite apart from mastitis, one third of mothers reported nipple cracks and sores in the first week post partum, 64% of cases were diagnosed by telephone (physicians 59%, nurses 23%, and others 18%). The most common symptoms were breast tenderness (98%), fever (82%), malaise (87%), chills (78%), redness (98%), and hot spot (62%). The most frequent treatment was cephalexin (46%), amoxicillin (7%), ampicillin (7%), and Augmentin (7%).

Most series of acute mastitis clearly demonstrate that the cases that result in unfavorable outcome, including abscess and recurrent disease, had significant delay between onset of symptoms and request for medical advice.[161] When proper treatment is initiated promptly, the course of the disease is usually brief; if treatment is delayed, prolonged antibiotics become necessary. Treatment with less than 10 days of antibiotics is also associated with recurrence. (Refer to Chapter 14 for discussion of neonatal mastitis.)

Recommended management regimen

1. Continue to nurse on both breasts, but start the infant on the unaffected side while the affected side "lets down." Be sure to empty the affected side by feeding or pumping.
2. Insist on bed rest (mandatory). The mother can take the infant to bed and obtain assistance for the care of other family members.
3. Choose an antibiotic that can be tolerated by the infant as well as the mother (avoid sulfa drugs when the infant is under 1 month). The decision should be based on local sensitivities and length of time since delivery or exposure to resistant flora.

Empiric therapy without cultures should consider the common organisms causing mastitis: *S. aureus* (50%), *E. coli* or other gram-negative organisms, group A streptococci, *streptococcus pneumoniae* species, and *Bacteroides* species (especially with abscesses). Less common organisms include *Candida albicans* and *Mycobacterium tuberculosis*. First-line antibiotics that are safe for the mother and infant include first-generation cephalosporins or dicloxacillin/oxacillin. Treatment of suspected gram-negative organisms includes first-generation cephalosporins or amoxicillin/clavulanate (Augmentin). Treatment of abscesses should include some anaerobic coverage with Augmentin or clindamycin. Therapy for women with penicillin or cephalosporin allergy can include erythromycin or clindamycin. Suspected methicillin-resistant

S. aureus (MRSA) can be treated with vancomycin, clindamycin, or rifampin considering organism sensitivity.

An unusual case of *Streptococcus pneumoniae* mastitis was reported in a 38-year-old woman who was partially breastfeeding her 9-month-old infant. Cultures of breast milk had more than 10^6 *S. pneumoniae* bacteria/mL milk. Cultures of the infant's nose and throat also grew *S. pneumoniae,* although he was asymptomatic. Treatment was flucloxacillin. C-reactive protein was 177 mg/L at onset and 18.6 mg/L on day 6. The infant was presumed to have infected the mother.[246]

Regardless of the disease course, the antibiotic should be given for at least 10 to 14 days. Shorter courses are associated with a high incidence of relapse. Once relapsed, it can become chronic until the infant is weaned.

4. Apply ice packs or warm packs to the breast, whichever provides the most comfort. Experience indicates that heat provides drainage and pain relief.
5. Provide plenty of fluids for the mother.[187]
6. Give an analgesic such as acetaminophen or ibuprofen.
7. The mother should wear a supporting brassiere that does not cause painful pressure.

See Appendix P, Protocol 7 for information on management of mastitis.

Recurrent or chronic mastitis and candidal infection

Recurrent mastitis is usually caused by delayed or inadequate treatment of the initial disease. If antibiotics are started, they should be continued for a minimum of 10 to 14 days. Often, because the mother feels better, she discontinues them on her own. At the first recurrence, cultures should be sent of the midstream clean-catch specimen of breast milk and the infant's nasopharynx and oropharynx. The patient should be seen and the circumstances completely reviewed. An aggressive course of rest, nourishment, stress management, and complete drainage of the breast by suckling or pumping should be initiated. The antibiotics should be carefully selected and maintained for 2 weeks. Fluids should be increased. Failure of the second treatment is usually caused by failure to complete the entire treatment, which may also mean failure to get adequate rest and build up maternal resistance.

When the mastitis continues to recur, several possible reasons exist: chronic bacterial infection, secondary fungal infection, or underlying breast disease such as a cyst or tumor. If it is chronic bacterial disease, low-dose antibiotics can be instituted for the duration of lactation (erythromycin, 500 mg daily). Fungal infection is usually diagnosed by the nature of the pain, which is described as fiery throbbing pain along the duct system. Both mother and infant need treatment. If the infection is always in the same breast, examination of the breast for a unilateral unchanging lump or mass may indicate cyst, galactocele, or tumor. (The lactating breast is "lumpy," but the lumps are ever changing.) Needle aspiration or biopsy may be indicated. Ultrasound is a good diagnostic tool.

A secondary complication of recurrent mastitis is invasion of the breast by a yeast infection or a fungus such as *Candida albicans* (see Chapter 17), as is frequently seen after antibiotic treatment. Mothers describe the incredible pain when the infant nurses as feeling like hot cords burning in their chest wall. Between feedings, the surface of the breast may itch. This is usually fungal infection of the ducts. The best treatment is to massage nystatin cream (Mycostatin) or Mycolog, which also contains cortisone, into the nipple and areola after each feeding. The infant should also be given oral nystatin simultaneously, or the mother will be reinfected, even if the infant has no lesions. If the mother is known to have a recurrent vulvovaginitis, initiation of nystatin prophylactically should be considered when the antibiotics are begun. Although the infant may or may not have oral thrush or a diaper rash, he or she should be treated as well. The nipple may not look unusual despite exquisite pain. Overuse of nystatin may make it ineffective, and fluconazole has been used even in premature infants.

The incidence of fungal infections has increased dramatically in the past decade, probably because of the widespread use of antibiotics, which obliterate the normal flora credited with keeping fungal growth under control.[61] Young women often have vaginal yeast infections, which serve as a reservoir of infection. Milk is an excellent culture medium for the fungi, which thrive on carbohydrates. An infant may acquire the fungus during vaginal birth, becoming colonized and inoculating the breast during breastfeeding. The disease state flares up after a course of antibiotics.

Although the problem of fungal mastitis has been well recognized in dairy cattle, reports have only recently been creeping into the medical literature. A single case of cryptococcal mastitis in a 31-year-old (para 6), formerly breastfeeding woman with a long past lactation history of painful mass in the breast has been reported.[237] Subsequent removal revealed a granuloma that showed cryptococci. She had a recurrence 4 months later in the opposite breast. She then was treated with a systemic ketoconazole after removal of the granuloma and confirmation of continuing infection.

In a review of breast infections[188] from 1969 to 1982 in 17,000 cases seen at a mammary gland disease clinic, four cases of candidal mastitis were seen, all in lactating multiparas, 14 to 24 days post partum. Two were diabetics. Severe pruritus was described but no fever or general malaise. Cytologic and culture confirmation was made of *C. albicans*. The author treated the patients with local and oral antimycotics. Lactation was stopped with bromocriptine in these cases. Past antibiotic thrush infection has been associated with initial pruritus that degenerates to pain. Newer antifungal preparations are evolving from the azole family of antifungals. They are safer than amphotericin. Ketoconazole and miconazole have been replaced by fluconazole.[78] Fluconazole is effective against cryptococcosis, *Candida,* coccidioidomycosis, and other fungi. On the horizon are other triazoles as interest and effort in treating fungal infections have increased because of the risk in human immunodeficiency virus (HIV) infections (see Chapter 17).

Miconazole oral gel can be used for treating both the breast and the infant's mouth for at least 2 weeks. Gentian violet liquid (0.25% to 0.5%) can be used in resistant recurrent cases. It is applied to the nipple and areola and to the infant's mouth by swab three times a day and no longer than eight applications (3 days). It colors everything purple and masks the lesions. Clotrimazole can also be used. The prescription is for a 10-mg lozenge crushed and suspended in 5 g petrolatum or in 5 mL glycerine to make a topical ointment to be applied three times a day to the nipple and areola and orally to the infant's mouth (glycerine preparation only).[168]

Instructions to the mother should also include recommendations to treat any vaginal yeast infection with local therapy, decrease concentrated ingestion of sweets, and add yogurt or acidophilus to the diet. All clothing in contact with breasts and infant must be changed daily, washed, and dried in hot temperatures.

When the microbiology of 61 lactating women with burning nipple pain was compared with that of 64 lactating women without pain and 31 nonlactators, growth of *C. albicans* in the nipple and milk was identified in 19% of those with pain and in 3% of those without pain and not among the nonlactators. *S. aureus* was associated with nipple pain and nipple fissures. The authors note the difficulty in actually culturing the fungus.[5]

For recurrent fungal infection of the breast when nystatin is no longer effective, a course of fluconazole (Diflucan) can be given orally, 200 mg loading dose with 100 mg/day for 14 days. Side effects (e.g., nausea, vomiting, diarrhea) in the mother are minimal. Although fluconazole does pass into the milk, it is approved for use under 6 months and has a safety profile for newborns. It is currently used in neonatal intensive care units. A single dose peaks in the milk at 2 hours, and the milk/plasma (M/P) ratio is less than 1. The infant should be maintained on nystatin to avoid relapse. Freezing pumped breast milk infected with *Candida* does not kill the fungus. The milk must be pasteurized or discarded.

All burning breast pain is not thrush. History should include a presence of tendency for fungal infections, recent antibiotic therapy, or other supporting evidence in order to assume it is thrush. Diagnosis should be confirmed by culture. The most common cause of failure of treatment is incorrect diagnosis. Burning pain may be caused by staphylococcal disease and treated with appropriate antibiotics. Therapies that include antifungals, antibiotics, and antiinflammatories in one preparation serve to sensitize the flora and diminish effectiveness and encourage the clinician to prescribe over the telephone without a diagnosis.

Abscess formation

Abscess can also be a complication of mastitis and is usually the result of delayed or inadequate treatment. A true abscess will require surgical drainage but should be treated with antibiotics, rest, warm soaks, and complete emptying of the breast at least every few hours.

The drainage should be cultured and sensitivities determined so that antibiotics can be adjusted accordingly. The increasing number of oxacillin-resistant *S. aureus* (ORSA) cases occurring in hospitals places women recently delivered or hospitalized within 28 days at risk. An infection with ORSA may require vancomycin therapy, the only antibiotic effective against it. ORSA may start as an inflammation of the lymphatics (Fig. 16-3).

The milk will remain clean unless the abscess ruptures into the ductal system. Usually it drains externally. Nursing can be maintained when the breast is surgically drained as long as the incision and drainage tube are sufficiently far from the areola so that they are not involved in feeding. In any event, the breast should be manually drained of milk frequently to maintain the milk supply until feeding can resume (sufficient healing usually occurs in 4 days). The infant can continue to feed on the unaffected side. The infant should always be monitored for infection, and simultaneous therapy should be initiated, especially with staphylococcal or streptococcal disease.

Isolated cases of abscesses, which have been drained surgically but also drain milk during a feeding or pumping, have been reported to the

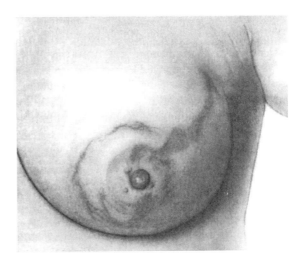

Figure 16-3. Infammation of lymphatics of breast demonstrating drainage of breast. Generalized infection of breast, especially staphylococcal, occasionally presents as lymph duct infection.

Lactation Study Center. With adequate systemic antibiotics and careful but thorough draining of the breast by suckling or pumping, healing gradually takes place even while the mother continues to lactate. When the drain is removed, the incision can be closed and breastfeeding resumed on that breast. The mother should be instructed to press firmly over the incision with sterile gauze to keep milk from flowing from the wound during feedings. The cause of this milk drainage is a severed milk duct, an unavoidable complication of draining a deep abscess. It will heal completely within 3 to 4 weeks. Rarely is weaning from the involved breast necessary. Continued lactation usually facilitates the healing and abrupt weaning and subsequent engorgement, which interfere with healing.

Laboratory findings

Cultures of the breast milk, when indicated, should be done after the breast has been cleaned with water and the mother's hands have been thoroughly washed. The milk stream should be initiated by manual expression and the first 3 mL discarded to obtain a midstream clean-catch specimen. One should check for antibody coating in the bacteria found in the milk to confirm its relationship to the disease.[229] It is important to remember that the normal cell count of uninfected human milk is 1000 to 4000/mm³. The presence of cells should not be automatically construed as infection.

A leukocyte count greater than 10⁶/mL of milk is considered diagnostic, plus a bacterial count greater than 10³ bacteria/mL of milk (see Table 16-1).

The levels of sodium and chloride in milk from mastitic breasts have been reported in the literature to be extremely elevated (Na $\geq$ 100 mEq/L, Cl $\geq$ 80 mEq/L, potassium $\leq$ 8 mEq/dL).[42] Usually, electrolyte abnormalities are associated with recurrent mastitis or chronic subclinical mastitis. The quickest screen for the problem is for the mother to compare the tastes of milk from each side. Elevated sodium will be salty.

Bilateral mastitis

Bilateral non-Hodgkin's lymphoma of the breast presented as mastitis in a 37-year-old woman with fever, chills, and pain, swelling, and redness of both breasts.[32] She was treated with antibiotics. She had a history of non-Hodgkin's lymphona (NHL) 7 years earlier. Biopsy of the red indurated skin revealed recurrent lymphoblastic lymphoma, which responded to chemotherapy. The breast can be involved as a primary site or a site of recurrence of NHL, although it is rare.

Streptococcal mastitis also presents as a bilateral infection and bilateral mastitis should always be treated as streptococcus unless cultures disprove it. The infant needs to be treated as well.

Granulomatous mastitis is a benign inflammatory breast disease of unknown etiology. It is rare and frequently presents similar to a carcinoma. It occurs in premenopausal women shortly after child birth and has been correlated with breastfeeding and the use of oral contraceptives. An autoimmune component has been suggested. It presents with galactorrhea, inflammation, breast mass, tumorous indurations and ulcerations of the skin. On mammography and sonography, there are nodular opacities. The diagnosis is made histologically with signs of chronic granulomatous inflammation. Treatment is surgical excision and steroid therapy.[57]

Pituitary and prolactinemic disorders
Galactorrhea

After an infant stops breastfeeding, it is not unusual for the mother to be able to express milk from the breasts for many weeks, although spontaneous flow ceases in 14 to 21 days. Postlactation milk is partially a function of the length of established lactation. When spontaneous lactation persists for more than 3 months after the infant has stopped nursing, the cause should be sought. The physician should evaluate the mother to make a specific diagnosis.

Galactorrhea is characterized by spontaneous milky, multiduct, bilateral nipple discharge. It is thought to result from increased prolactin production, either by the pituitary or by removal of hypothalamic inhibition.[236] Pituitary adenomas may be the cause. Galactorrhea can occur with normal ovulatory function for 1 or more years post partum if everything else appears normal. Galactorrhea has been reported to occur in thyrotoxicosis with such frequency (80%) that it should be part of the differential diagnosis for galactorrhea. Amenorrhea and galactorrhea are also associated with hypothyroidism, which is not surprising because thyrotropin-releasing hormone (TRH) is known to be a prolactin-stimulating hormone. More complex disorders are rare and are usually named for the physician who first described them.

During pregnancy a risk of pituitary tumor expansion exists, especially with large tumors. In a series of cases of microprolactinomas, Ikegami and associates[102] noted no symptom of tumor enlargement in pregnancy. The serum prolactin levels were at or below pregnancy levels post partum. The authors thought these breastfeeding patients diagnosed as having Chiari-Frommel syndrome could actually have occult microadenomas that might become radiologically evident later.[74]

Prolactin levels are elevated in about half the patients with galactorrhea, and the prolactin levels show little correlation with the copiousness of milk flow in the patients. Prolactin levels in milk and plasma in women with inappropriate lactation were compared with those of normally lactating women by Adamopoulos and Kapolla.[2] Women with galactorrhea had milk prolactin concentrations similar to nursing mothers, but plasma levels were significantly lower than in lactating women except for pituitary adenoma-related galactorrheas. Levels in milk remain relatively constant, whereas plasma levels vary by time of day and various stimuli.

Some drugs, including phenothiazines, tricyclic antidepressants, rauwolfia alkaloids, theophylline, amphetamines, methyldopa, and even some contraceptives, can cause galactorrhea. A copper intrauterine device (IUD) was associated with normoprolactinemic galactorrhea in a fertile woman. When the IUD was removed, the secretion stopped, and when it was reinserted, the flow began again.[79]

The major causes of galactorrhea associated with amenorrhea are (1) medications (e.g., tranquilizers, antidepressants, reserpine, methyldopa, narcotics, oral contraceptives), (2) local stimulation of the nipples and breast, (3) hypothalamic dysfunction, (4) Forbes-Albright syndrome, (5) hypothyroidism, (6) chest lesion, (7) renal disease, and (8) a nonpituitary prolactin-producing tumor (lungs or kidney). A patient has *idiopathic galactorrhea* if prolactin levels, menses, and fertility are normal. Idiopathic galactorrhea has five possible explanations[17]:

1. The abnormality may be in the breast itself, which is unusually sensitive to circulating prolactin.
2. The breast may have an increased number of prolactin receptors.
3. Prolactin levels may be intermittently high.
4. Excessive sleep-induced increases may occur in prolactin, which normally rises during sleep.
5. Biologically active prolactin may be elevated and is not immunoreactive (i.e., is not detected by immunoassay).

Prolactin exists in three sizes: small (molecular weight 25,000 daltons), large (50,000 daltons), and very large (100,000 daltons). Most of the biologic activity occurs in the small form. The large forms are immunoreactive but weakly biologically active. Thus, in patients with persistent galactorrhea with normal prolactin levels by immunoassay, magnetic resonance imaging (MRI) is necessary to rule out a tumor producing the large prolactin molecules.[17]

Hyperprolactinemia

Hyperprolactinemia with and without galactorrhea has been identified in patients with multiple sclerosis,[128] especially in relapse, suggesting hypothalamic dysfunction and not a pituitary prolactinoma.[93] Hyperprolactinemia is also seen in some connective tissue disorders[120] (see later discussion).

Since 1971, when human prolactin was identified as a distinct lactogenic hormone and was isolated and measurable by a specific radioimmunoassay, previously unrecognized clinical entities associated with hyperprolactinemia have been identified. *Physiologic hyperprolactinemia* occurs with excessive breast manipulation and is the reason induced lactation and relactation are physiologically possible. In susceptible women, a visit to the doctor, stress, a pelvic examination, venipuncture, or surgical procedures can produce elevated serum prolactin. The half-life of prolactin in these circumstances is 50 to 60 minutes. Placing a heparin lock and drawing a second sample an hour later that is lower may explain this.

Table 16-4 lists causes of hyperprolactinemia. Pathologic conditions associated with hyperprolactinemia include hypothyroid and hyperthyroid disease, chronic renal failure, and chest wall lesions such as thoracotomy scars and herpes zoster. Galactorrhea, or the secretion of a lactose/fat-containing fluid independent of pregnancy, can occur in any of these hyperprolactinemic states. In general, pharmacologic hyperprolactinemia does not exceed 100 ng/mL. If a woman has achieved pregnancy with hyperprolactinemia, postpartum lactation is possible.

Chiari-Frommel syndrome

Patients with persistent postpartum or postlactation lactation extending over months or years should be evaluated for Chiari-Frommel syndrome, especially if abnormal menses exist.[74] Often, irregular

TABLE 16-4   Causes of chronic hyperprolactinemia in the female

Type	Causes
Physiologic	Excessive breast manipulation
	Stress, surgery, venipuncture, etc.
Pharmacologic	Depletion of tuberoinfundibular dopamine stores (by extrusion from intracellular granule to cytosol)
	Reserpine
	Blockade of dopamine receptor binding
	Phenothiazines (chlorpromazine, thioridazine, prochlorperazine, perphenazine, trifluoperazine)
	Thioxanthenes (chlorprothixene)
	Butyrophenones (haloperidol)
	Benzamines (metoclopramide, sulpiride)
	Dibenzoxapine antidepressants (amoxapine)
	Inhibition of dopamine release
	Chronic opiate use (methadone, morphine)
	Blockade of histamine (H_2) receptor binding
	Cimetidine
	Estrogen-containing oral contraceptives
	Interference with dopamine synthesis
	α-Methyldopa
	Calcium channel blockers
	Verapamil
	Mechanism unknown
	Tricyclic antidepressants (imipramine, amitriptyline)
	Papaverine derivatives
Pathologic	Primary hypothyroidism
	Hypothalamic disorders
	Neoplastic, infectious, vascular, degenerative, or granulomatous hypothalamic lesions
	Pituitary stalk section
	Pituitary disorders
	Prolactin-secreting adenoma
	Acromegaly, Cushing's disease, Nelson syndrome
	Ectopic production of prolactin
	Bronchogenic carcinoma, hypernephroma
	Chronic renal failure
	Chest wall lesions
	Surgical scars, herpes zoster
Functional	Idiopathic (no demonstrable tumor)

Modified from Katz E, Adashi EY: Hyperprolactinemic disorders. Clin Obstet Gynecol 33:623, 1990.

menses will have occurred before the pregnancy as well. The galactorrhea will occur whether the mother breastfeeds or does not breastfeed. The clinical manifestations of Chiari-Frommel syndrome are not only persistent lactation with possible breast engorgement, but also oligomenorrhea or amenorrhea, obesity, uterine and ovarian failure, and in some cases hypothyroidism (Table 16-5). Spontaneous remission within 5 years occurs in 40% of patients.

TABLE 16-5 **Comparison of characteristics of various hyperprolactinemic disorders**

Syndrome	Amenorrhea	Galactorrhea	Postpartum	Pituitary tumor
Del Castillo	+	+	0	0
Chiari-Frommel	+	+	+	0
Forbes-Albright	+	+	±	+

From Gould BK, Randall RV, Kempers RD, et al: Galactorrhea. Springfield, IL, Thomas, 1974.

Other possible causes of the galactorrhea include other hypothalamoadenohypophyseal disorders, including infection and trauma, ectopic production or lactogenic hormone as in hypernephroma, or end-organ hypersensitivity to prolactin.

Hyperprolactinemic women do not respond to breast stimulation with a rise in prolactin as breast-feeding women do, which can be demonstrated with two levels drawn before and after pumping. The hyperprolactinemic patient has no acute response to suckling in her growth hormone levels either, indicating that the central dopaminergic tonus was not altered but shows regulatory dysfunction.[74]

Del Castillo's syndrome

Del Castillo's syndrome was first described in 1932.[83] All patients have had galactorrhea and amenorrhea without evidence of pituitary tumor and with negative urinary gonadotropins and a small uterus but normal secondary sex characteristics and normal breasts, nipples, and areolae. Remission is rare, as is pregnancy. Clomiphene citrate (Clomid) has been reported to be useful in decreasing the galactorrhea and achieving pregnancy (see Table 16-5).

Forbes-Albright syndrome

Forbes-Albright syndrome was first described in 1954 by Forbes, who reported 15 cases of nonacromegalic women who had persistent lactation and amenorrhea or irregular menses, low urinary follicle-stimulating hormone (FSH), and pituitary tumor on x-ray films.[71] Both medical and surgical treatments have been used. Pregnancy may cause a recurrence of the galactorrhea (see Table 16-5).

Sheehan's syndrome and hypopituitarism

Sheehan's syndrome is caused by postpartum hemorrhage of such severe degree that it leads to pituitary thrombotic infarction and necrosis or other vascular injury to the pituitary, including hypoperfusion. It is the only commonly recognized endocrine disorder associated with lactation failure.[2] It occurs in 0.01% to 0.02% of postpartum women. A highly vascular organ, the pituitary gland is particularly vulnerable to decreased blood flow at the end of gestation because of its increased size. It is thus more sensitive to hypoperfusion and necrosis. The degree of hypopituitarism is variable; hypoprolactinemia generally results following necrosis of the pituitary stalk, causing mammary involution and failure of lactation.[74]

Other signs of pituitary failure are diabetes insipidus, amenorrhea, hypothyroidism, loss of axillary hair, or sparse regrowth of pubic hair post partum. Spontaneous recovery can occur, depending on the degree of infarction and regeneration.

Secretion of pituitary hormones including prolactin is usually deficient, and thus the patient may fail to lactate post partum; this is considered a key clinical sign of the syndrome. Studies have reported women with Sheehan's syndrome who do lactate; the diagnosis had to be established by other means. This is believed to result from the pituitary *lactotropes,* which have compensatory activity of hypothalamoadenohypophyseal function.[235] Patients usually manifest hyposecretion of all pituitary hormones, with decreased thyroid and adrenal function. They may experience oligomenorrhea or amenorrhea and uteroovarian atrophy. Often the obstetric crisis that caused the hemorrhage has also required hysterectomy, however, and these findings are obscured.

Prolactin-stimulating drugs such as sulpiride to augment milk yields require investigation, although they have been successful in women delivering prematurely and unable to breastfeed immediately.[11] In a case of presumed Sheehan's syndrome in our service, use of nasal oxytocin spray (see Chapter 8) with each feeding for about 2 weeks resulted in a gradual increase in milk production. The mother weaned herself from the drug and the infant from the lactation supplementer over the next 2 weeks, achieving full lactation for 6 months.

Diabetes insipidus in a patient with Sheehan's syndrome requiring vasopressin injection therapy was described by Isbister.[103] The woman had been diagnosed and treated for 2 years before becoming pregnant and experiencing a normal labor and delivery. For 10 days post partum, she required no replacement therapy. She breastfed without difficulty for 2 months until she was hospitalized with pneumonia. Lactation was temporarily interrupted until the infant was brought to the hospital. Lactation was reestablished by suckling at the breast and supplementing the infant with formula. The vasopressin injection did not cause a let-down or influence the feeding patterns. It was concluded that the patient produced adequate oxytocin but lacked antidiuretic hormone (ADH).

Treatment

In a review of normal lactation and galactorrhea, Benjamin[17] outlines four treatments for pituitary adenomas: (1) identify nonpituitary causes and eliminate (e.g., medications), (2) do nothing, (3) perform surgery, or (4) administer bromocriptine. Also, a significant cause of galactorrhea or hyperprolactinemia can be breast stimulation. Stimulation of breast and nipple can cause prolactin to rise 60 to 120 ng/mL (normal levels 15 to 25 ng/mL).

Acute lactation failure

Acute lactation failure (when women abruptly lose their milk) has been noted historically in times of great crises, fright, or accident. Two such cases have been reported in the literature by Ruvalcaba[206] after the Mexico City earthquake in 1985. Stress-induced lactation failure is described in a gravida 3 woman, 24 years old, who had been exclusively breastfeeding for 3 months and had fed two previous children for 14 and 18 months. The day of the quake, the building she was in collapsed. She ran home to her children past demolished buildings and could not produce a drop of milk when her infant suckled then or subsequently. Multiple attempts over the next weeks failed to produce a drop. The second woman was 39 weeks pregnant and had been dripping colostrum for several weeks, as she had with her previous three pregnancies. The day of the quake, her house collapsed, her husband and two children were missing for several hours, and her sister was killed. She never leaked another drop of colostrum and was never able to breastfeed.[206]

Alactogenesis

Familial puerperal alactogenesis is described as probably a genetically transmitted, isolated prolactin deficiency. It is a rare disorder with only a few cases reported. Zargar and associates[249] describe a mother and her daughter with eight pregnancies between them with no evidence of lactation at any time. Their only abnormal laboratory value was their prolactin levels, which were undetectable.

Hypergalactia

Hypergalactia is excessive milk production. It is often heralded by the initiation of milk production beginning in pregnancy, often as early as 25 weeks' gestation, and is characterized by persistent leaking that soaks the clothing and is independent of breast stimulation. Some women will note a drop or two on stimulation or while showering during pregnancy. This is considered to be within normal limits. Hypergalactia then persists after delivery with constant leaking between feedings. Mothers can pump or express several ounces after each feeding with no effort. This does not appear to minimize the leaking. Many women find early in lactation that they have a strong let-down reflex with a soaking spray of milk initially. This is not hypergalactia and usually diminishes over 1 or 2 weeks.

If this phenomenon persists for more than 1 or 2 weeks, an evaluation for prolactinoma is in order. A baseline level and a stimulus-associated level of prolactin after 10 minutes of suckling or pumping with a breast pump should be obtained. If the patient has associated symptoms of headache or visual disturbances, further workup for pituitary adenoma would be appropriate. The phenomenon, however, may not be associated with any identifiable pathology. Idiopathic hypergalactia may diminish over months of breastfeeding. It occurs more often with first pregnancies and may not recur with subsequent pregnancies.

Treatment is palliative, including a tight, well-fitting brassiere that is well padded between feedings. A trial of low-dose estrogen, as available in oral contraceptives, may be effective. A careful history to identify any medications or herbs that are galactagogues or any form of stimulus other than breastfeeding is essential to management. Although bromocriptine would theoretically be effective, it would only be indicated in patients with hyperprolactinemia associated with pituitary adenoma. In such a patient the diagnosis should be established first. Bromocriptine has potentially serious side effects and should not be used casually.

Excessive milk production has also been associated with hyperthyroidism and postpartum thyroiditis.

Hyperactive let-down reflex

Hyperactive let-down reflex may occur especially among primiparas. It is characterized by a spray of milk on initiation of a feeding. If the other breast is checked, it also is flowing. The infant is often overwhelmed by the rate of flow and begins to choke or is gulping frantically to keep up. Milk runs out the corners of the mouth. When the milk is high volume but low fat, it may be accompanied by increased gas formation and colic.[247]

Treatment involves controlling the flow. Initially, expressing a little milk (and saving it in the freezer) until the flow slows and then putting the infant to the breast usually solves the problem.

If the fat of hindmilk is slow to come, additional milk can be expressed until the fat begins to be secreted. The high-fat milk or hindmilk will decrease the relative volume of lactose and the relative amount of gas produced, reducing the colic, thrashing about during feedings, and green stools.

The mother may reduce the flow during feedings by folding the nipple down and wearing a firm brassiere. Pressing her arm across the breast can also diminish flow.

Diabetes mellitus

Interest in lactation among diabetic women is high, and clinical research on the topic is gradually increasing.[13,31,36,107] The laboratory has been the site of considerable study of the disease in the animal model and of the role of insulin.[13] The breast is known to be a target organ for insulin, and there are insulin receptors in the mammary gland acini. The mammary gland is an insulin-sensitive tissue where acute changes in insulin concentration result in a rapid alteration in the rate of lipogenesis and the utilization of glucose. Cultures of mammalian breast tissue serve as ideal laboratory models for the exploration of insulin activity.[152]

Pregnancy has become a more common event in the well-controlled diabetic woman, and fertility rates compare with those of nondiabetic women. Much has been said about labor and delivery in the diabetic mother and almost nothing about lactation in these mothers. Textbooks on diabetes often do not mention lactation, except those written before 1960, perhaps reflecting the national trends away from breastfeeding. A mother, although diabetic, should be offered the same opportunity to breastfeed that is offered to all patients unless her disease has so incapacitated her that any metabolic stress is contraindicated. When the progress of the infant of a diabetic mother is uneventful and the infant can be treated normally, no contraindication exists to breastfeeding. Lactation may be more difficult in diabetic mothers, perhaps as a result of cesarean delivery or the need to keep the infant in a special care unit for the first few days of life.[183]

Congenital malformations in infants of diabetic mothers are more common (two to six times the normal rate) or about 8% to 10% of insulin-dependent diabetes mellitus (IDDM) births. They cover all organ systems. Congenital cardiac disease continues to be most common. At birth, the major problems are macrosomia complicating delivery, hypoglycemia, respiratory distress syndrome (RDS), hypocalcium, and hypomagnesemia, polycythemia, and hyperbilirubinemia. Thus, close monitoring is mandatory while providing as "normal" an experience as possible.

Cordero and colleagues[46] reported 530 infants born to 332 women with diabetes and 177 women with IDDM; 191 (36%) were large for gestational age, 76 (14%) were under 34 weeks' gestation, 115 (22%) were 34 to 37 weeks' gestation, and 339 (64%) at term. Almost half (47%) were admitted to the neonatal intensive care unit (NICU) due to RDS prematurity, hypoglycemia, or congenital malformation. Hypoglycemia occurred in 137 (27%) and more commonly among mothers with severe types of diabetes; 182 (34%) had RDS. Although 244 infants were admitted to normal newborn care, 43 had to be transferred for hypoglycemia. Routine care failures were less frequent among breastfed infants. The authors recognize the improvements in care of the mother; however, they caution about hypoglycemia and RDS in infants who are overstressed. They recommend observation of the infant in a special care nursery, especially when the mother's disease is advanced. They further say breastfeeding should be encouraged in these mothers.

In a retrospective study of 25 mothers who were insulin dependent before pregnancy, there were both successful (13) and unsuccessful (12) breastfeeders.[69] The successful ones were slightly older and better educated and had had diabetes longer (13.7 years versus 8.2 years). The infants were half a week more mature and spent less time in the intensive care nursery (ICN) (1.8 days versus 7.2 days). Delay to first breastfeeding and introduction of a bottle in the ICN were no different, and both groups of mothers experienced an adjustment period. Observations about diet, insulin, and control of diabetes were similar in the two groups and paralleled the observations made in the study by Ferris and associates.[69]

During the last stages of pregnancy in normal women, a more or less constant excretion of lactose occurs in the urine, with the peak reached on the day of delivery. After delivery the lactose excretion immediately drops to a low level, where it remains for from 2 to 5 days, followed by a sudden large excretion of lactose.[214] *Lactosuria* in the diabetic mother may lead to diagnostic confusion. It normally occurs late in pregnancy and in the postpartum period before the infant takes much milk, if the mother does not nurse, or if the supply of milk exceeds the infant's requirement. Lactose reabsorbed from the breasts is excreted in the urine. Urine sugar tests are not reliable during lactation.

The sparing effect of lactation on the insulin requirement has been observed by many, beginning with Joselin and associates.[111] The depression of the level of the blood sugar in normal nursing diabetic women may lead to hypoglycemic symptoms. The simultaneous lactosuria may be misdiagnosed as glucosuria and excessive insulin taken. The improved tolerance has been explained by the transference of sugar from the blood to the breast for conversion to galactose and lactose. Joselin and associates[111] reported that the majority of patients at the Joselin Clinic, as well as those at Johns Hopkins Hospital, breastfed in whole or in part. They recommended the increased administration of the B vitamins for the diabetic mother during lactation.

Milk composition in diabetes has been studied by Butte and associates[35] in a group of moderately well controlled insulin-dependent women (type I) at 3 months post partum. Diabetic women in pregnancy and post partum have been observed to have low levels of prolactin, placental lactogen, and parathyroid hormone. Whether the observed decreased placental blood flow is associated with diminished mammary blood flow in lactation has not been established.

In this small sample size, no significant difference was seen in the values for total nitrogen, lactose, fat, and calories given the normally wide variations found among control subjects as well. Mineral content was not different except for sodium, which averaged 140 µg/g compared with reference milk's 100 µg/g. The glucose concentrations were significantly higher in the milk of diabetic women, and this varied greatly without any pattern throughout the 24-hour collections, although lactose fluctuated little. The mean glucose value was 0.70 ± 0.11 mg/g in diabetic women and 0.32 ± 0.08 mg/g in the reference women. During the collections the diabetic women were noted to have periods of hyperglycemia. Total milk volumes were not measured in Butte's study, but the infants were noted to gain weight appropriately.[35] Measurements of glycosylated hemoglobin within a month of the milk collections were noted to be $8.1\% \pm 0.6\%$, that is, above the normal range of 4.0% to 7.6%. It is appropriate for the clinician to be aware of the slightly elevated sodium levels, especially if mastitis develops. The glucose elevations probably have little clinical significance to the infant because glucose makes up only about 0.4% of the total energy content.

When milk volume and composition were measured serially on days 3 to 7 post partum in a diabetic woman by Bitman and associates,[21] sodium, potassium, chloride, lactose, protein, calcium, magnesium, and citrate were within the limits of a nondiabetic reference population. Unlike Butte and associates,[35] Bitman and coworkers[21] found that fat content was lower, with free fatty acids 2% of total lipid on day 3 but 23% on days 4 through 7. Lipoprotein lipase was increased on days 4 and 5. Other changes suggested impaired fatty acid synthesis and high concentrations of polyunsaturated fatty acids. Jensen and associates[108] studied serum levels at 3, 14, and 42 days post partum from a large group of women. Serum cholesterol levels decreased significantly from days 3 and 14 to day 42 in both diabetic women and control subjects. Because lipids are a major source of calories, the lipid content of milks of diabetic women will require further study.

Diet for lactating diabetic mothers

Although it is clearly demonstrated that all lactating mothers have an increased energy requirement, it is critical to the diabetic woman to identify this need and provide for it in dietary adjustments (Fig. 16-4). The 300 kcal required by the infant initially means at least 500 to 800 additional kilocalories in the mother's diet. Because the milk is synthesized from maternal stores and substrates, the plasma glucose levels in the lactating diabetic mother will be lower. The daily maternal insulin requirement is usually much less. The balance is

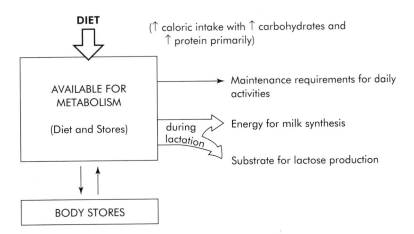

Figure 16-4.   Glucose utilization in lactation. (From Asselin BL, Lawrence RA: Maternal disease as a consideration in lactation management. Clin Perinatol 14:17, 1987.)

significant between the needs of the infant and the energy and nutrition production in the mother. Most postpartum women, including the diabetic mother, have fat stores developed during pregnancy in preparation by the body for lactation. The diabetic woman, when balancing diet and insulin, needs to consider that the course of lactation mobilizes these fat stores as substrate for the mammary gland. It has been recommended that the diet include no less than 100 g of carbohydrate and 20 g of protein. This balance will permit the continued mobilization of fat stores to produce the glucose needed for mother and milk. When a diabetic mother increases fat metabolism, there is always the risk of ketonemia and ketonuria. Ketonemia and ketonuria indicate a need for increased kilocalories in both the diabetic and the nondiabetic mother. With some careful observations of blood sugar levels and anticipatory guidance, lactation can be managed without hypoglycemia or hyperglycemia. With the availability of newer glucometers, this measurement is more easily accomplished.

A critical analysis of dietary intake and outcome of lactation in a group of women with insulin-dependent diabetes mellitus (IDDM) was undertaken by Ferris and associates[69] in three major obstetric services in Connecticut. Sixteen of the 30 women with IDDM chose to breastfeed and 14 to bottle feed (53%), compared with the 57% of the general maternity population at that time. The authors found that the women with IDDM who sustained lactation received average diet prescriptions of 31 kcal/kg/day (based on maternal weight at 3 days post partum) or 35 kcal/kg/day (based on preconceptual weight). The mothers who stopped nursing had received only 25 kcal/kg/day (based on maternal weight at 3 days post partum) or 31 kcal/kg/day (based on preconceptual weight). The latter was the same as that for bottle feeding diabetic women. When compared with general recommendations, the recommended dietary allowance (RDA) for lactation is 2000 kcal plus 500 kcal extra. Only one mother who continued to nurse and none who had stopped nursing met this requirement. Mothers who lactated successfully actually consumed more than they thought, and those who "failed" consumed less than they thought when it was calculated, which supports the recommendation that breastfeeding mothers with IDDM need a knowledgeable dietary counselor as well as other support systems. The weight loss patterns of these women reinforced this observation. Those women who stopped lactating lost considerably more weight than the successful breastfeeders, the bottle feeders, or the normal control subjects. Fasting blood sugar levels were lower (60 mg/dL) in the successful lactators without an increased insulin dosage.

Adjustments to lactation for diabetic mothers

The mildly, or class A, diabetic woman whose condition can be controlled by diet alone must modify her diet to include the increased caloric needs, especially ensuring adequate protein intake. Class A diabetic women who have been taught to control the problem in pregnancy by diet often continue this dietary awareness after delivery, and thus appropriate counseling for lactation should continue. The IDDM mother usually is able to increase her diet and maintain her insulin level, although some may find insulin requirements are also reduced. Monitoring blood sugar levels and acetone is necessary at first to achieve the correct balance.

Although hypoglycemia does not cause a reduction in lactose in the milk, the phenomenon of hypoglycemia itself causes increased secretion of epinephrine in insulin shock. The epinephrine inhibits milk production and the ejection reflex. Acetone signals a need for increased calories and carbohydrate. In addition, elevated acetone can cause increased acetone in the milk itself, which is a stress to the newborn's liver. If one merely increases insulin to clear the acetone, it may predispose the patient to hypoglycemia. Each mother will identify the point below which she cannot reduce her insulin dosage without producing acetonuria. While the infant is nursing exclusively at the breast, adjustment is usually smooth. Weaning may present some need for day-to-day adjustment, because the amount of milk taken by the infant varies. Many infants take more one day and less the next, and the amount is less predictable. If blood sugar levels cannot be controlled by diet during this time, insulin must be decreased. If the weaning is gradual and continuous, the adjustment is similar.

Social support, including help and encouragement with baby care and family responsibilities, was a significant difference between successful and unsuccessful breastfeeding among diabetic women in the report by Gagne and associates.[77] The management problems, on the other hand, were not related to breastfeeding per se but to management of the diabetes. Physicians managing the maternal diabetes and the infant must work in concert to help the mother adjust her diabetes management to lactation and must understand the issues of diet and insulin.

Problems among mothers with IDDM in first days after delivery

Fewer infants of mothers with diabetes are put to the breast in the first few days, as noted by Ferris and associates.[69] Most infants of diabetic mothers are admitted to the neonatal intensive care unit (NICU) for 8 hours or more of observation. Not only does this delay breastfeeding, but it also increases the amount of formula and number of bottle feedings. The breastfeeding women with IDDM fed for the first time at 35 ± 5 hours, whereas the bottle feeding mothers did so for the first time in 43 ± 24 hours! In this study, only two diabetic mothers and no control mothers were offered a pump. All the mothers who stopped breastfeeding had infants who received a total of 9 oz or more of formula while in the NICU.

Weaning was precipitated in these mothers by problems they saw with the baby, such as crying, fussing, and problems suckling, not because of insufficient milk. No woman with IDDM was told by her physician to stop. Control mothers all cited insufficient milk as the cause of weaning. Severity of the disease correlated with the decision to bottle feed and to wean early.

Supportive hospital management is critical to successful lactation in diabetic mothers as well.[13] When 42 mothers with IDDM who breastfed were followed by Whichelow and Doddridge,[243] they found the most important factor in success was the lapsed time to the first breastfeeding. This is usually a function of the infant's medical stability. They were able to initiate a change in hospital policy that minimized separation of infant and mother. Duration of lactation was inversely related to the delay in the first suckling.[13]

The insulin requirement at 3 months in Whichelow and Doddridge's study[243] was an average 43 U daily, compared with 50 U prepregnancy in bottle feeders, and 40 U at 3 months, compared with 45 U prepregnancy in the breastfeeders. Ferris and associates[69] reported that insulin dosages were no different among breastfeeders and bottle feeders, but the numbers were not provided. The subjects in Butte and associates's study[35] received less insulin while lactating (35 ± 10 U/day compared with 63 ± 14 U/day during pregnancy).

Special features of lactation for diabetic mothers

Some diabetic mothers enjoy a postpartum remission of their diabetes that may be minimal or complete. The remission may last through lactation, or for several years. This remission has been attributed to the hormone interactions that affect the hypothalamus and pituitary gland during pregnancy, labor, delivery, and lactation. Many diabetic women report a feeling of well-being during lactation.

Diabetic women are prone to infection,[31] and therefore *mastitis* presents a particular problem. With careful anticipatory care, avoidance of fatigue, and antibiotics for at least 10 days when indicated, mastitis should not pose a threat. Candidal infections are more common because of the glucose-rich vaginal secretions, and most diabetic women are alert to the early signs of a fungal vaginitis. When the infant is delivered by cesarean section, there is no exposure in the birth canal. Infection of the nipples can also occur from *Candida albicans,* even though the infant does not have obvious thrush. Early specific treatment with nystatin ointment to the breast and nystatin suspension for the infant whenever sore nipples do not respond to the usual nonspecific treatment is recommended. Treatment of both mother and infant simultaneously is necessary or they will reseed each other. (See discussion of candidiasis later in this chapter.)

Infants of diabetic women present a special problem in breastfeeding because they are often premature, frequently have respiratory distress syndrome and hyperbilirubinemia, and may be poor feeders at first. Hypoglycemia is the immediate problem, and its management may initially preclude dependency on breast milk as the sole source of nourishment. Because less than half do develop problems, many need not be separated from their mothers. For those that require special or intensive care, lactation may have to be postponed briefly, depending on the infant's status.

Providing an electric breast pump and assistance in pumping is essential if the infant is too ill to be fed. Attention to this detail is important regardless of the reason for separation of the mother and infant.[13]

The hypoglycemia of the infant of a diabetic woman occurs early and is proportional to the level of hyperglycemia in the mother at delivery. Cord blood sugar and microsugar levels at ½ and 1 hour of age provide the curve of glucose disappearance and potential for hypoglycemia. If lactation can be established, the glucose can be managed by breastfeeding, but it must be closely monitored so that intervention can be initiated when necessary. There is also a high incidence of hypocalcemia in infants of diabetic mothers, which is believed to result from functional hypoparathyroidism because phosphorus and calcitonin levels are normal.[165] The role of magnesium in this balance has not been clearly defined but needs to be monitored.

Hyperbilirubinemia occurs more frequently in infants of diabetic mothers. Beta-glucuronidase and bilirubin measurements were made on 10 breastfed infants of diabetic women and 10 normal breastfed control infants by Sirota and associates.[217] The concentrations of β-glucuronidase were higher in the serum of the milk of diabetic mothers, and the bilirubin levels were higher in their infants. None of the control infants required phototherapy, whereas 50% of the infants of the women with IDDM did. Other investigators compared β-glucuronidase and bilirubin levels in a group of normal breastfed infants on the third and fifth days of life and found no correlation between the values. Although infants of diabetic women clearly are more prone to hyperbilirubinemia, the central cause remains elusive.

Breastfeeding and onset of diabetes

Epidemiologic reports[25,72] continue to accumulate suggesting that breastfeeding has a protective effect on the onset of diabetes in childhood. Children in western Australia who were studied to the age of 14 years revealed an incidence of 0.59 diabetic children per 1000.[82] No significant trends or associations with illness were made, except that breastfeeding beyond 1 week of age was less frequent in diabetic than nondiabetic cohorts. In a study of 95 children of women with diabetes and their nondiabetic siblings and peers, the incidence of breastfeeding was only 18% but was comparable in all three groups. Twice as many diabetic children had received soy formula as the other children. In a study of IDDM in Scandinavian populations, fewer children with childhood-onset diabetes were breastfed, and those who were breastfed were breastfed for shorter periods.[25] The authors suggest that insufficient breastfeeding of genetically susceptible newborn infants may lead to β-cell infection and IDDM in later life. The prevalence of diabetes in black populations throughout Africa, where breastfeeding is common, is usually considerably lower than in Western countries among those of African descent.[136]

The Colorado IDDM Registry was studied retrospectively to determine the possible relationship between breastfeeding and development of childhood diabetes in comparison with randomly selected control subjects.[163] There was less IDDM among breastfed infants, and the longer the breastfeeding, the greater the effect. The population percentage with attributable risk ranged from 2% to 26%. Because of the increasing incidence of childhood diabetes throughout Scandinavia, a prospective study was conducted following children for 7 years. Results demonstrate a clear relationship between lack of breastfeeding and IDDM in the first 7 years of life, or conversely a protective effect of breastfeeding, which is strongest with at least 4 months of exclusive breastfeeding.[25]

Other investigators have been exploring the possible relationship of early exposure to cow milk and the onset of diabetes. It is suggested there is both a genetic and an environmental component to the etiology of the disease. Karjalainen and associates[119] report the identification of a bovine albumin peptide as a possible trigger of IDDM. The antibodies to this peptide are said to react with P69, a β-cell surface protein that may represent the target antigen for milk-induced β-cell-specific immunity. The antibodies decline over 1 to 2 years to normal values. Much lower values were found in all the control children.

Utilizing the Colorado IDDM Registry, Kostraba and associates[135] compared children with high and low genetic risk for IDDM by an HLA-DQB1 molecular marker and a group of matched normal control subjects. Early exposure to cow milk and solid foods was strongly associated with IDDM in genetically high-risk individuals. The authors suggest that the inclusion of the HLA-encoded risk in the analyses demonstrates the combined effect of genetic and environmental factors.

The association of serum immunoglobulin A (IgA) antibodies with milk antigens in patients with severe arteriosclerosis is under review. The presence of antibodies against dietary antigens is well documented. Its relevance is under study by Muscari and associates[174] and others.

Rennie[201] showed a relationship between the consumption of cow milk and the incidence of diabetes between the ages of 0 to 14 years in countries around the world (Fig. 16-5). The association between IDDM and early exposure to cow milk may be explained by the generation of a specific immune response to β-casein. A cellular and humoral anti-β-casein immune response is triggered by exposure to cow milk and may cross-react with β-cell antigen. Sequential homologies exist between β-casein and several β-cell molecules.[38] The introduction of cereal under 6 months of age was shown to increase the incidence of diabetes in at-risk children. Much work remains to be done. In the meantime, this may

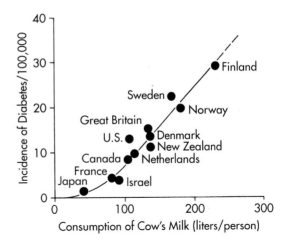

Figure 16-5. Annual comsumption of cow milk and incidence of diabetes (ages 0 to 14). (Modified from Rennie J: Formula for diabetes? Sci Am 267:24, 1992.)

be one more reason for mothers to consider breastfeeding, especially in families at high risk for diabetes, and delaying the introduction of solid food until 6 months of age as recommended by WHO/UNICEF for all children.[54,59]

Thyroid disease

The thyroid gland is intimately involved with hormone activity of pregnancy. The metabolic and hormonal demands of pregnancy alter the thyroid gland. Conversely, the outcome of pregnancy may be altered by changes in the thyroid gland. Thyroxine-binding globulin increases secondary to the increased estrogens. The normal pregnant woman may be euthyroid, but changes occur in the basal metabolic rate, radioactive iodine uptake, and thyroid size.

Thyroid disease is four times more common in women than men, and thyroid abnormality is common in pregnancy. The diagnosis is more difficult to make during pregnancy because of problems with the interpretation of thyroid function tests. Treatment must take into account the presence of the fetus once the management decision is made.

Thyroid disease is increasingly common post partum and often presents as depression. No postpartum woman should be started on antidepressive drugs without a thyroid screen, especially if she has not been symptomatic before pregnancy.

Maternal hypothyroidism

It has long been held that hypothyroidism is associated with infertility. There is a low incidence of hypothyroidism during pregnancy. Because of the difficulty in maintaining pregnancy in hypothyroid individuals, the number of women who are truly hypothyroid at delivery is also low. Some women who are maintained on thyroid treatment for one reason or another do bear children. If hypothyroidism is diagnosed, it should be treated with full replacement therapy equivalent to 3 grains of desiccated thyroid daily. The medication should be continued after delivery. The mother should be permitted to breastfeed without question. Data from Bode and associates[24] indicate there is measurable thyroid hormone in the milk of normal women. Breastfeeding is not contraindicated.

In experimental animals when the thyroid is removed before onset of lactation, lactation cannot be initiated. In hypothyroid states in the animal model, there may be associated hypoprolactinemia. This would suggest that a woman with hypothyroidism should be well controlled by thyroid replacement therapy to ensure full lactation. If the mother is truly hypothyroid, particular care should be used to rule out hypothyroidism in the infant, using neonatal screening with thyroxine (T_4) and thyroid-stimulating hormone (TSH) if necessary. Diagnosis can be performed by evaluating maternal blood values and is not a hazard to the nursling.[234] Because of the small amount of thyroid hormone in breast milk, a breastfed hypothyroid child may be undiagnosed unless laboratory values are carefully reviewed.

An increase in hypothyroidism is being identified post partum, especially when normal women have prolonged "baby blues" and fatigue or appear to have new-onset depression. Screening for thyroid disease is appropriate before prescribing antidepressants. Self-medication has led women to initiate treatment with St. John's wort, thus masking the thyroid disease. A thorough history is always important, including self-medication with other drugs and herbs. Herbals are being recommended by paraprofessionals during lactation and therefore the physician should be especially vigilant when taking a history and should include specific questions about herbal use.

Maternal hyperthyroidism

The diagnostic procedures and therapeutic management of the mother with possible hyperthyroidism present some hazards to the breastfed infant. The diagnosis can be made without radioactive material. The combination of an elevated serum T_4 level and a normal resin triiodothyronine (T_3) uptake is helpful. These two determinations can be combined to obtain a free-T_4 index, which reflects these determinations in a single value. Whether the patient eventually has a thyroidectomy or not, her thyrotoxicosis must first be medically stabilized.

In the experimental hyperthyroid model, rats given chronic doses of thyroid hormone, beginning before mating, were able to carry the pregnancy and delivery without difficulty but were unable to lactate. The mammary gland made milk, but the dams were unable to allow suckling and could not experience milk let-down.[203]

Postpartum thyroiditis has also increased in frequency to about 1 in 20 women. It is characterized by symptoms of hyperthyroidism with pounding tachycardia, rapid weight loss, insatiable appetite, and excessive milk production.[118] One case reported to the lactation center was notable for the stimulating reaction to prenatal vitamins (possible iodine effect), caffeine, and high-protein beverages.

A distinction between postpartum thyroiditis and Graves disease should be made (Box 16-1). Those with postpartum thyroiditis initially appear to suffer from hyperthyroidism but become hypothyroid at about 6 weeks and usually require thyroid replacement indefinitely.

The treatment for hyperthyroidism includes antithyroid medication with thiourea compounds, which inhibit the synthesis of thyroid hormone by blocking iodination of the tyrosine molecule. Propylthiouracil (PTU) and methimazole (Tapazole)

BOX 16-1   Characteristics of postpartum thyroiditis and Graves disease

	Post partum thyroiditis	Graves disease
Blood levels	Modest elevations	Significant elevation
Microsomal antibody	+	++
TSI (thyroid stimulating immunoglobulin)	Normal	High
Gland size	Sli enlargement	Significant enlargement
Diagnostic tests	Irradiating tests not indicated	Diagnostic tests with I_{131} should be avoided while lactating
Symptoms	Moderate sx	Marked sx
Thyroid levels over time	Return to normal 4–6 weeks	Unchanged
Treatment	Symptomatic: Propranolol Watch and wait (PTU no effect) May need thyroid therapy when becomes hypothyroid	Start with propranolol, add propylthiouracil (PTU)
Safety while lactating	No contraindications	Medications—all OK I_{131} treatment contraindicated— may need surgery

are the drugs of choice for the mother. The major difficulty in their use in pregnancy is that PTU may cause fetal goiter and possibly hypothyroidism. The goiter is thought to be the result of inhibition of fetal thyroid hormone production by PTU with resulting increase in fetal TSH and thyroid gland enlargement. In 41 pregnancies in 30 patients receiving antithyroid medication, five infants developed goiters. Goiter development was not dose related. It has been recommended that the maternal therapy also include desiccated thyroid on the basis that the various components of thyroid metabolism cross the placenta at different rates.[34] An infant may show withdrawal symptoms at birth and present as hyperthyroid and hypermetabolic.

The lactating mother presents a somewhat similar problem. Thiouracil appears in the milk in significant levels and is contraindicated. Methimazole appears in the milk with a milk/plasma (M/P) ratio of 1. A 40-mg dose of methimazole would yield 70 µg for the infant. Lamberg and associates[142] treated 12 lactating women with a methimazole derivative, carbimazole, in doses ranging from 5 to 15 mg daily, which is comparable with 3.3 to 10 mg methimazole. All the infants maintained normal thyroid function studies at 4, 14, and 21 days. Two

infants were followed to 3 and 4 months and remained normal.

Levels of PTU in milk were reported by Kampmann and associates,[116] who calculated that minimal amounts reach the milk because the drug is ionized and protein bound. They found no evidence of effect in the infants with careful follow-up with T_4 and TSH measurements. It has been suggested that the infant can be breastfed and monitored biochemically. Microtechniques are available for determining T_3, T_4, and TSH levels, and monitoring should not be a technical problem.[233] Physical examination would reveal bradycardia or other signs of hypothyroidism and goiter. It has also been suggested that the infant may be given 0.125 and 0.25 grain of thyroid daily.

This situation requires close medical surveillance and continual monitoring by microanalysis. The clinical judgment rests with the physician as to whether sufficient medication is reaching the infant. The older infant (over 6 months of age) who is receiving other dietary intake such as solids would be at less risk than the newborn, who depends solely on breast milk. Lamberg and associates[142] recommend PTU doses of up to 150 mg/day.

When PTU is not an effective drug for the mother, Cooper[44] suggests methimazole or carbimazole in doses up to 10 mg with close monitoring of the breastfeeding infant and thyroid function tests biweekly. Lamberg and associates[142] recommend methimazole doses up to 15 mg/day.

Because iodine appears in milk and the M/P ratio is greater than 1.0, a lactating mother with thyroid disease should not be given iodine for any reason.

Polycystic ovarian syndrome (PCOS)

Polycystic ovarian syndrome (PCOS) is one of the disorders of androgen excess that begins at puberty and progresses slowly. Mild androgen expression in women is characterized by body hair growth, acne, and seborrhea. Prepubertal acne is not part of normal puberty and should be evaluated for androgen excess. A synonyn for PCOS is hyperandrogenic anovulation. Excess androgens result in abnormal release of the pituitary hormones that normally control menstruation and ovulation; thus, women with PCOS have irregular menses and erratic or no ovulation. Other symptoms besides infertility and hirsutism are amenorrhea, obesity, functional bleeding, dysmenorrhea, virilization, and biphasic body temperature. Obesity may be associated with abnormal fat distribution (upper body android). This fat distribution is associated with risk of diabetes, hypertension, arteriosclerosis, and gallbladder disease. It is strongly associated with insulin resistance. Insulin resistance appears to be due to receptor abnormalities with too few receptor cells and corresponding circulating hyperinsulinemia. Drug therapy for the hyperandrogenism does not change the insulin resistance. In contrast, lowering the insulin with drug therapy does improve the hyperandrogenism.

Acathosis nigricans is also seen with the insulin resistance (especially in axilla, neck folds, and anticubital creases). The disease has been renamed by some hyperandrogenic chronic anovulation.

Pregnancy can be accomplished with clomiphene citrate or naturally if there is some ovulation.

Maternal excessive androgens do not appear to affect the fetus because the placenta converts androgens to estrogens. The initiation of lactation may be a challenge.

Insufficient milk supply has been observed in PCOS women who classically do everything right: breast changes in pregnancy, early frequent feeds, good latch, and pumping. Metoclopramide does minimally increase supply while the drug is taken. Supplementation is usually required.

The cause of the lack of milk production may be that estrogen and prolactin receptors have been "down regulated" by the androgen. Perhaps high estrogen post partum suppresses prolactin. Is insulin resistance at the core of the problem? In some cases, the mammary tissue is inadequate.

With this constellation of symptoms, the clinician would be wise to refer the mother back to her obstetrician for evaluation if she has not been worked up.

The traditional efforts to increase milk supply should be tried: pumping, domperidone, other galactogogues.

Because insulin plays an important role in lactogenesis and in the insulin-resistant components of PCOS, metformin (Wellbutrin) has been tried with minimal success. These women also pumped and used various galactogogues. The metformin did produce engorgement and increase in milk production. Because it was not initiated until lactation failure was apparent, the authors suggested it should be initiated when lactation begins in women with a history compatible with PCOS.[76]

Cystic fibrosis

Patients with cystic fibrosis (CF) are living longer and enjoying more stable lives as diagnostic and therapeutic advances in the disease continue. Reports have appeared indicating that a number of women with CF have become pregnant and have delivered normal infants. A case was reported of such a mother who had high sodium levels (132 and 280 mEq/L) in her milk. This mother had not been breastfeeding and expressed her milk for the studies only. As pointed out by Alpert and Cormier,[3] milk from involuting breasts is different, and sodium may be closer to serum levels. Sodium levels are always elevated when measured in nonlactators. Since that time, Welch and associates[242] reported one case and Alpert and Cormier[3] reported two cases of successful breastfeeding with maternal CF. Sodium and chloride levels in the milks were normal, as the women were fully lactating.

Hamosh and associates[89] have investigated the fat content of the milk of mothers with CF and report lowered levels of fatty acids.

Another case of successful breastfeeding by a woman with CF is reported by Smith and associates.[218] The infant grew along the 50th percentile for height, weight, and head circumference. Milk samples (fore and hind) at 11 weeks post partum had sodium levels of 11 mmol/L (normal 2 to 19 mmol/L).

Michael and Mueller[166] reviewed five women with CF and their infants. Evaluations indicating their need for enzyme therapy and their pulmonary disease status classified these women as mild cases. The infants averaged 37.4 ± 1.5 weeks' gestation with birth weights of 3.0 ± 0.5 kg. Sweat tests were negative for all the infants. Duration of breastfeeding ranged from 3 to 30 weeks. Four of the five infants maintained good growth during breastfeeding. Four of the five mothers were at or above their standard body weight throughout lactation. The authors conclude that women with mild CF can not only sustain a pregnancy but also support the growth of a healthy infant through breastfeeding while maintaining their own weight.[166]

Current recommendations for breastfeeding by mothers with CF have been published by Luder and associates[154] following a survey of CF centers (Tables 16-6 and 16-7). For mothers with CF, 11% of centers recommend breastfeeding, 8% do not recommend it, 42% tailor their recommendations to the mother's health, and 32% make recommendations on the basis of the mother's wishes. Of the centers, 41% report breastfeeding duration of less than 3 months. Table 16-7 lists factors that preclude breastfeeding and factors contributing to discontinuation, as reported by directors of CF centers.

TABLE 16-6   Recommendations about breastfeeding by cystic fibrosis (CF) center directors for mothers with CF*

Recommendation	Response, no. (%)
Recommend breastfeeding	14 (11.2)
Do not recommend breastfeeding	10 (8.0)
Recommendation made according to each patient's health status	52 (41.6)
Recommendation made according to each patient's personal wishes	40 (32.0)
Not applicable and/or others category	9 (7.2)
Total	125 (100)

*Many centers chose more than one answer; therefore, the response rate for each answer is calculated as a percentage of total responses.
Modified from Luder E. Kaltan M. Tanzer-Torres G, et al: Current recommendations for breastfeeding in cystic fibrosis centers. Am J Dis Child 144:1153, 1990.

Eighty-one centers (94%) have support services available throughout the course of lactation.

As the survival of patients with CF continues to improve and more women reach the childbearing years, an increasing number will choose to breastfeed.[154] Additional research is necessary to help mothers with CF maintain their health while lactating and to monitor growth in infants with CF and their general health status while breastfeeding. Breastfeeding usually enhances the health of

TABLE 16-7   Duration of breastfeeding as reported by cystic fibrosis (CF) center directors for mothers with CF

Duration (months)	Centers, no. (%)
<3	35 (41)
3–6	9 (10)
>6	1 (1.2)
Not applicable and/or others category	41 (48)
Total	86 (100)

Modified from Luder E. Kaltan M, Tanzer-Torres G, et al: Current recommendations for breastfeeding in cystic fibrosis centers. Am J Dis Child 144:1153, 1990.

an infant with CF because it helps to protect against infection and provide active enzymes (see Chapter 15).

Studies demonstrate that mothers with pulmonary and pancreatic disease of CF can breastfeed and that their infants do well. It is appropriate, however, to test milk samples occasionally for sodium, chloride, and total fat and to follow the infant's growth pattern critically.

Hyperlipoproteinemia

The study of a mother with type I hyperlipoproteinemia nursing her second child is reported by Steiner and associates.[222] The milk and plasma were carefully analyzed, and it appeared that the deficit of lipoprotein lipase extended to the mammary gland. The milk had low total lipids and a bizarre composition of fatty acids. Her milk differed greatly from her plasma triglycerides in comparison to normal mothers, whose fatty acid profile in the milk matched the plasma. Low concentrations of essential linoleic ($C_{18:2, 20.4}$) and arachidonic ($C_{20:4}$) acids in her milk made it inadequate for her infant. Other women in the literature have been reported to develop pancreatitis during pregnancy.

Galactosemia

The case of a 25-year-old woman, who had been diagnosed herself at the age of 3 weeks to have galactosemia, was reported by Forbes and associates[71] at the time of her first baby, whom she breastfed. The woman had blood transferase activity that hovered from zero to 1.9 U (normal 18 to 25 U/g hemoglobin). Despite irregular menses, she conceived and delivered a normal female who thrived on breastfeeding exclusively. Solid foods were added at 5 months. The analysis of her milk at 4½ weeks post partum revealed protein 1.42 g/dL, lactose 7.5 g/dL, fat 4.25 g/dL, and calculated energy content 74 kcal/dL. Fatty acid profile was normal except for 18:3, which was low. Macrominerals were all within normal range. Glucose was 26 mg/dL and galactose less than 15 mg/dL. The authors point out that because "lactose can be

found from uridine diphosphogalactose (by means of epimerase) and glucose (a reaction stimulated by lactalbumin) in the absence of transferase enzyme, one could have predicted that lactose would be present in her milk.[71]

Phenylketonuria

The success of newborn screening and early treatment has resulted in a population of adolescents with phenylketonuria (PKU) moving into the childbearing years with normal intelligence. Matalon and associates[160] reported a pregnancy and lactation experience in a woman who had stopped her diet and did not seek medical care until 16 weeks' gestation. They also reported their experience with 32 young adults who had discontinued their diets. The authors make the following recommendations:

1. Diet restrictions for PKU should not be discontinued at any age, especially in women.
2. Strict control should begin before conception to bring blood phenylalanine levels to 4 mg/dL or lower.
3. Breastfeeding is permitted.

Matalon and associates[160] report that the milk of mothers with PKU controlled by diet is normal (Table 16-8).

Radiation exposure

The diagnosis and treatment of a lactating woman with malignancy may well necessitate the use of radioactive compounds or antimetabolites. Because the breast is a minor route of excretion

TABLE 16-8 Amino acid levels (mmol/dL) in milk of mothers with phenylketonuria (PKU)

Amino acid	PKU milk	Reference values
Phenylalanine	0.5	0.62
Tyrosine	0.5	1–2
Taurine	36.7	41–45

Iron, zinc, copper, magnesium, and selenium were also within normal range.

for most of these compounds, it is probably inappropriate to continue nursing during such exposure. Although the dose of the material in a single aliquot of milk may be small, the effects are cumulative (see Appendix D). No long-range studies indicate the outcome of offspring exposed in utero. In addition, a mother with malignancy should be encouraged to spare all her resources to overcome the disease. Lactation is as draining in such a situation as pregnancy.

Diagnostic or therapeutic measures using radioactive materials are contraindicated in pregnancy and lactation because they tend to accumulate in the fetal and neonatal thyroid gland and the maternal breast. If radioactive testing is deemed essential before treatment can be carried out, a test dose of iodine-123 (^{123}I) can be given and breastfeeding discontinued for 66 hours. (The half-life of ^{123}I is 13.2 hours; $5 \times 13.2 = 66$ hours.) The validity of the test during lactation has been questioned because the mammary gland may divert a disproportionate amount of ^{123}I to the milk. The milk should be expressed during the 66-hour period and discarded.[28]

Breast cancer

In the young cancer patient, another concern is what risk lactation adds to the mother's long-range prognosis.[204] The automatic response tends to be not to become pregnant and, in any event, not to breastfeed. This question was examined by Hornstein and associates,[100] who indicate that "the current data suggest that pregnant women with early breast carcinoma may be treated in the same way as nonpregnant women without affecting the pregnancy." Disease that is detected toward the end of pregnancy may be treated with surgery immediately, and then the patient may receive adjuvant therapy if indicated after delivery. Advanced disease should be treated aggressively, and the infant delivered and not breastfed. During lactation, the diagnosis of breast carcinoma requires the immediate suppression of lactation by medications other than estrogens. The carcinoma is then treated by standard methods. When a woman has already had

a radical mastectomy for breast cancer, she can have subsequent pregnancies, but they should be delayed until the period of greatest risk is over (i.e., at least 3 to 5 years). She may also breastfeed.

Kalache and associates[113] report that 7% of fertile women have one or more pregnancies after mastectomy. Seventy percent of these pregnancies have occurred within 5 years after treatment. Women who have pregnancies after potentially curative mastectomy have survival rates of 5 to 10 years—as good or better than those who do not become pregnant. The patients with the best prognosis, however, may be a function of selection because they are healthier and thus able to become pregnant. Uneventful pregnancy does not guarantee cure, although the highest rate of recurrence is in the first 3 years and gradually declines. It is never zero. Metastases to the axilla increase the risk. Recurrence in the chest wall during pregnancy can be treated with local shielded radiation, but anything more extensive requires aggressive intervention.

The importance of careful monitoring during pregnancy is obvious. One of the major contributors to a more grave prognosis of the original disease that appears during pregnancy and lactation is not the underlying disease, but the difficulty detecting the lesion during pregnancy and lactation and the reluctance of patient and physician to make a diagnosis and initiate treatment. The greatest risk of neoplastic growth occurs in the first 20 weeks of pregnancy, when the immune system is suppressed and growth of the mammary tissues is at its peak under the stimulus from estrogen, progesterone, and prolactin levels.[148,205] No data were provided on the influence of postmastectomy lactation on long-range survival. Some women have wanted to nurse on the remaining breast. The decision would necessitate consideration of the individual situation. It represents a different risk/benefit ratio than pregnancy itself. Extensive epidemiologic studies of large populations of women do not indicate that breastfeeding has any relationship to the overall risk of breast cancer. Epidemiologic data about breastfeeding on the remaining breast are not available.[148]

The incidence of cancer in the remaining breast has fueled the question of prophylactic contralateral mastectomy. The women who are at greatest risk for cancer in the second breast are those who have a family history of breast cancer in their mother or sister, who have had onset in childbearing years, or whose original cancer involved multiple lesions in the primary breast. In their discussion of the other breast, Leis and Urban[148] state that if a postmastectomy patient were to become pregnant and deliver, "it would be rare indeed that the patient would allow or the attending physician would condone the use of the remaining breast for nursing." Although some women cherish the remaining breast, most in the experience of Leis and Urban[148] are ashamed of it and keep it hidden.

Lactation after primary radiation therapy for carcinoma of the breast was reported in a major literature search by Burns[33] to have occurred successfully in one patient whose primary lesion was in the tail of Spence. One year after radiation, she became pregnant and successfully breastfed. She had less milk on the treated side. Her malignancy had not recurred. Another patient received radiotherapy after biopsy for an invasive duct carcinoma known to be present for a year. She had a week of boost therapy 8 weeks later. She became pregnant a year later, delivering a full-term infant 22 months after the original radiation. She successfully established lactation on the uninvolved side but was unable to obtain any response from the irradiated breast. No comment was made about the radiated breast's response to pregnancy. She weaned her infant at 6 weeks.[52] Two years after treatment the patient had no evidence of recurrence.

The incidence of breast cancer diagnosed during pregnancy in a large series was 3 per 10,000 pregnancies, or 1% to 2% of breast cancer cases. Delay in diagnosis is the primary reason for the seemingly worse prognosis overall for breast cancer diagnosed during pregnancy and lactation, with the duration of symptoms averaging 5 to 15 months. The incidence of spread to the axilla is 70% to 80% in the perinatal period compared with a 40% to 50% node-positive rate in nonpregnant women.[98]

Any dominant mass during pregnancy or lactation should be evaluated promptly. Mammography may be difficult to interpret, however, because of the increased water density of the breast. Radiation exposure is minimal if the abdomen is properly shielded. A fine-needle biopsy will distinguish cystic from solid lesions. A solid mass can be biopsied during pregnancy or lactation.[208] The risk of milk fistulas is very low. Suppression of lactation is not necessary. Once the diagnosis of cancer is made, staging is essential before treatment is begun. Staging during pregnancy is more difficult because of the need for ionizing radiation.[92]

Further surgery, including mastectomy, can be done during pregnancy and lactation. Because radiation and chemotherapy will also be necessary, breastfeeding is not recommended. When breast cancer is diagnosed during lactation, treatment should be initiated promptly and the infant weaned when chemotherapy is begun.

When young patients are treated with breast-conserving therapy and radiation for early-stage breast cancer, they may experience full-term pregnancies subsequently. Successful breastfeeding on the untreated breast as well as the treated breast is possible after conservative lumpectomy and radiation in some patients. The volume and the duration of lactation are less on the treated side. When the incision is circumareolar, successful lactation is less likely. Usually the function of the untreated breast is unaffected.[95]

Treatment with chemotherapy is changing as new protocols are developed. When a woman who is breastfeeding is diagnosed with a malignancy requiring chemotherapy, it is possible that the compounds used have a very short half-life and therefore clear the system in 48 to 72 hours (half-life $\times$ 5 = clearance time). Mothers determined to breastfeed can indeed pump and discard the required time and resume breastfeeding. It takes a flexible infant for this schedule as well. Each chemotherapeutic agent would have to be evaluated for half-life and clearance time.

Autoimmune thrombocytopenic purpura

Reports are conflicting regarding the passage of antibodies to platelets via the breast milk in mothers with autoimmune thrombocytopenic purpura.[90,122,164] Laboratory efforts to demonstrate absorption of these antibodies from the breast milk failed. One case report detailed the successful breastfeeding of a severely affected premature infant who had required exchange transfusion and multiple platelet transfusions at birth.[159] No relapses occurred with introduction of maternal milk at 5 days of age. Steroids were discontinued at 2 weeks, and the infant thrived at the breast.

Rheumatoid arthritis and other connective tissue disorders

The influence of lactation on the development and progression of rheumatoid arthritis (RA) has been the subject of several epidemiologic studies. Previous observations noted an increased risk of RA developing post partum, particularly after the first pregnancy. A national cohort of 187 women who developed RA within 12 months of pregnancy were studied. Of the 88 women who developed the disease after their first pregnancy, 71 breastfed (81%) compared with only half of control mothers. A smaller risk was noted after the second pregnancy. No added risk with the third pregnancy was associated with breastfeeding. The increase in risk was highest in those women whose disease was erosive and rheumatoid factor positive. The authors suggest that this may be a hormonal influence, especially by the proinflammatory hormone prolactin.[27]

Other investigators reviewed a cohort of 176 women with RA who had at least one child and a mean age of 46 years at diagnosis.[109] They concluded that parity and to a lesser degree breastfeeding before RA onset worsened the prognosis for severe disease. Oral contraceptive use had a protective effect.[110]

The evidence regarding reproductive events as risk factors for RA is conflicting. A population-based study of 63,090 women followed from 1961 to 1989 examined reproductive factors and mortality rates. The role of parity, age at first and last birth, or age at menarche and menopause showed no relationship to RA. A protective effect of lactation was noted, however, with total time of lactation associated with decreased mortality rate from RA with a dose-response relationship.[30,*]

Rheumatic disease may necessitate treatment of pregnant and lactating patients with disease-modifying active rheumatic disease (D-MARD) drugs or immunosuppressive drugs. For lack of information, breastfeeding is not recommended by Ostensen[190] in patients requiring antimalarials, penicillamine, cyclosporine, or cytotactic drugs. Intramuscular gold and sulfasalazine impose no risk to the breastfed infant, however. Information about milk levels and general recommendations appear in Appendix D. Levels in milk of aurothioglucose, aurothiomalate, chloroquine, hydroxychloroquine, and sulfasalazine have less than 10% of maternal dose in milk, and in the few cases studied, the infants had no side effects.[190] Cyclosporine is not recommended as a therapy during breastfeeding.

Prolactin levels are greatly elevated during pregnancy in women with systemic lupus erythematosus (SLE).[106] Most patients with SLE have elevated prolactin levels, as do patients with RA, osteoarthritis, fibromyalgia, and polymyalgia. A dysregulation of pituitary response has been suggested as the etiology in RA. The role of prolactin in other autoimmune disorders is not understood but supports the concept that a close relationship exists between neuroendocrine and immune systems.

If symptoms can be controlled with nonsteroidal antiinflammatory drugs (NSAIDs), such as acetaminophen, ibuprofen, hydroxychloroquine (Plaquenil), Keterolac, and Piroxicam, which are all acceptable according to the AAP list, then treatment is not a problem during lactation. The use of corticosteroids (prednisone 120 mg/day) is considered safe. Injections into the joint of steroids, even the more potent triamci-

---

*Karlson and colleagues reported that women who breastfeed more than a total of 24 months reduce their risk of rheumatoid arthritis by 50%. This finding was part of a study of more than 120,000 women. (Karlson EW, Mandl LA, Hankinson SE, Grodstein F: Do breast-feeding and other reproductive factors influence future risk of rheumatoid arthritis?: Results from the Nurses' Health Study. Arthritis Rheum 50:3458, 2004.)

nolone, provide low doses in the serum and can be tolerated for brief courses. The D-MARD drugs, which include methotrexate, gold salts, and azathioprine, are critical to management and cannot be delayed in a patient with a confirmed diagnosis and joint pain with an elevated sedimentation rate. They are toxic and breastfeeding is contraindicated. Gold salts have been found in milk and in a nursing infant.[241]

Postpartum flare of inflammatory polyarthritis may be induced by breastfeeding according to a prospective study of over 100 women with RA.[15] The first-time breastfeeders had increased disease activity 6 months post partum based on symptoms, joint counts, and C-reactive protein levels. Not all women had flares, and long-term implications were not investigated. It was less frequent and less severe in those who had breastfed previously. The authors relate it to prolonged elevated levels of prolactin.[15]

Primary *Sjögren's syndrome* is known to be associated with hyperprolactinemia, but because of the characteristic abnormalities of secreting glands, lactation may not be successful.[10] Sjögren's syndrome has also been seen in association with Raynaud's phenomenon[104] (see later discussion). Breastfeeding is not contraindicated.

Hypertension

The published literature on the excretion of antihypertensive agents into human milk has been reviewed by White[244] because successful management of hypertension is pharmacologic. Before one considers the drugs involved, it is appropriate to consider that lactation may present some therapeutic advantages. The high levels of prolactin may be physiologically soothing to the mother, and it has been shown in animals that females given high levels of prolactin respond with nesting and mothering behavior. The breast is also an organ of secretion, and a liter or so of fluid is produced a day. In dehydrated women, lactation continues while urine production diminishes. The appropriate use of low-dose diuretics may control hypertension, whereas high-dose thiazides can cause suppression of lactation. Chlorothiazide, hydrochlorothiazides, and chlorthalidone are mini-

mally excreted in milk (see Chapter 11 and Appendix D), as are spironolactone and its metabolite canrenone, according to single-dose kinetics.

Propranolol has been widely studied and is probably the safest of the beta blockers during lactation because of its low level in milk compared with other beta blockers, which are weak bases with an average pK_a of 9.2 to 9.5, predisposing them to appear in slightly acidic human milk. *Methyldopa* appears in low amounts in milk, but its direct action on the pituitary to suppress prolactin release presents a theoretic risk of suppressing milk production. The obstetrician should be aware of this potential if lactation is going poorly. *Reserpine* poses a recognized risk to the infant during delivery and post partum. Other drugs appropriate to hypertension management are discussed in Chapter 11.

Cardiac, liver, and renal transplantation

The number and survival times of patients receiving heart transplants are increasing, as is their quality of life. In young recipients, childbearing becomes important. Teratogenicity has not been reported with traditional immunosuppressive agents such as prednisone and azathioprine or with cyclosporine. Osteoporosis prophylaxis is important in pregnancy and lactation associated with chronic use of prednisone. A successful pregnancy after cardiac transplantation is reported with the birth of a normal infant who had normal growth and development for the 3 years of follow-up. The infant was not breastfed.[126]

Successful pregnancy after liver transplant has been reported in at least six patients.[216] Immunosuppression was maintained throughout pregnancy, and the infants were normal. Breastfeeding was not recommended because of the cyclosporine therapy.

Of infants born to mothers with renal transplants, 60% to 70% have uncomplicated neonatal courses. Thymic atrophy, leukopenia, anemia, thrombocytopenia, chromosome aberrations in lymphocytes, and certain abnormalities of the immune system have been seen.[126]

Breastfed infants of mothers with renal transplants have normal blood counts and show no increase in infection and above-average growth rates.[134] The immunosuppressants azathioprine, 6-mercaptopurine, and 6-methylprednisolone have been found in milk in very low levels. Cyclosporine, however, has been detected in breast milk at levels approximating maternal concentrations. The advice when cyclosporine is the drug has been not to breastfeed, with varying decisions about 6-mercaptopurine and azathioprine.

Pregnancy following renal transplant is relatively safe when renal function is adequate before conception and when maintenance immunosuppressive therapy is instituted. Most patients receive azathioprine and prednisone or methylprednisolone. When the actual levels of these compounds were studied in two patients, one of whom breastfed her infant,[47] measurements of IgA were also done because of the concept that immunosuppressed women might produce immunoincompetent milk.

The levels of 6-mercaptopurine in the milk averaged 3.4 ng/mL in one patient and 18 ng/mL in the other. The therapeutic level is 50 ng/mL with the use of the normal daily dose. The levels of methylprednisolone in the milk (daily dose 6 mg) were at or below the levels measured in normal drug-free control subjects. The IgA determination in the milk was similar in both transplant and control mothers. The breastfed infant whose mother had a transplant had normal blood cell counts, no increase in infections, and an above-average growth rate.[47]

Breastfeeding and maternal donor renal allografts

With the advent of renal transplants, a new mode of investigation with the role of human milk in the host-graft relationship has developed.[13] Large numbers of living maternal lymphocytes are present in human milk. Campbell and associates[37] investigated the question of whether exposure of an infant to maternal lymphocytes during breastfeeding would affect the subsequent reactivity of a patient to a maternal donor-related renal transplant. They studied the posttransplant course of 55 patients with a primary maternal donor transplant, 27 of whom were breastfed and 28 of whom were not. The 1-year graft function rate was 82% for those breastfed and 57% for the bottle fed ($p \leq 0.05$) infants. Five-year follow-up did not sustain the statistically significant difference. Paternal donor relationship in a small group of patients did not reveal significant difference.

The same group of investigators (Kois and associates[133]) reported that a history of breastfeeding was associated with improved results in a different patient population (HLA-semiidentical sibling donors). Breastfed patients in whom both donor and recipient were breastfed by the same mother showed dramatic improvements in graft-function rates compared with nonbreastfed counterparts at all intervals studied up to 9 years ($p \leq 0.001$). The authors[133] concluded that the breastfeeding effect is not entirely specific for maternal antigens, because both sibling donor and maternal donor transplantation was improved. They consider a history of being breastfed an important variable in clinically related renal transplantation.

Because these studies used retrospective questionnaires, they did not take into account the length of time breastfeeding took place, which included all cases "ever breastfed." Although this is potentially important, studies of graft recipients' donors are another means of understanding more about the role of breast milk for the human species.

In a study of renal transplants, 45 breastfed subjects with maternal donor transplants were compared with 43 bottle fed subjects with maternal donor transplants and 62 subjects with paternal donor transplants.[70] No statistically significant differences were seen in graft survival between the groups. Length of breastfeeding was not stated.

Glomerular disease and lactation

A high percentage of pregnant patients show their first evidence of renal disease probably not because pregnancy precipitates the disease but because it is the first time these young women have had urinalysis and blood pressure studies. The series of glomerular disease in pregnancy published by

Surian and associates[224] reported that in most cases the disease is not made worse by pregnancy. A disease with a poor prognosis such as membranoproliferative glomerulonephritis is neither worsened nor bettered by pregnancy. When the nonpregnant serum creatine and urea nitrogen levels exceed 3 mg/dL and 300 mg/dL, respectively, normal pregnancy is uncommon. Lupus nephropathy, however, has a very poor prognosis in pregnancy with considerable fetal loss and morbidity.[53]

Hypertension as a complication influences the obstetric complication rate and the fetal outcome. The infant may be premature, small for gestational age (SGA), or both. The option to breastfeed is a matter of the risk/benefit ratio.[13] It involves not only the medical status of the mother but also that of the infant and the drugs that must be used to keep the mother stable. The obstetrician, nephrologist, and neonatologist must determine the appropriateness of breastfeeding on a case-by-case basis.

Osteoporosis

Tremendous attention has been focused on osteoporosis in women, particularly following childbirth and lactation. Clearly the demands for calcium and phosphorus during the perinatal period are great, but they can be met by diet with any degree of attention. In addition to dairy products and other supplemented foods such as orange juice, there are other sources of calcium (Table 16-9). Modern advertising in the wave of the calcium hysteria has suggested women take various medicinal forms of calcium. The incidence of calcium-containing renal calculi has increased as a result.

A syndrome of severe osteoporosis is associated with pregnancy and lactation. Three cases are reported by Gruber and associates.[85] These young women had vertebral fractures and skeletal complications, but most of their studies were normal except for their bony structure. They had no osteo-

TABLE 16-9   Calcium content of foods (mg per serving)

100±	150±	200±	250±
10 Brazil nuts	1 cup ice cream	1 cup beet greens	1 cup almonds
1 med stalk broccoli	1 cup oysters	1 oz cheddar or Muenster cheese	1 oz Swiss or Parmesan cheese
1 cup instant Farina	1 cup cooked rhubarb		1 cup cooked collard greens
3 oz canned herring	3 oz canned salmon with bones		
1 cup cooked kale			
1 T blackstrap molasses	1 cup cooked spinach		1 cup cooked dandelion greens
3 T light (reg) molasses	1 oz feta or mozzarella cheese		
1 cup cooked navy beans			4 oz self-rising flour
3.5 oz soybean curd (tofu)	½ cup cooked chopped collard greens		1 cup milk
			3 oz sardines
3.5 oz sunflower seeds			½ cup cooked ricotta cheese
5 T maple syrup			
1 cup cottage cheese, regular or lowfat			

From Kleinman RE (ed): Pediatric Nutrition Handbook, 5th ed. Elk Grove, Ill, American Academy of Pediatrics, 2004.

malacia, however. They apparently recovered after lactation ceased and had no residual high-turnover osteoporosis. The authors suggest an association with low calcium in the diet.[85]

Bone density changes during pregnancy and lactation in active women were followed in a longitudinal study by Drinkwater and Chesnut.[60] The variations at the femoral neck, radial shaft, tibia, and lumbar spine were attributed to mechanical stress of weight gain and changes in posture in pregnancy and lactation. Further studies have confirmed that lactation-associated bone-mineral mobilization does not require parathyroid hormone (PTH) or parathyroid tissue.[96]

Extended lactation (≥70% of infant energy intake provided for ≥6 months) is associated with bone loss; however, there is evidence of return to baseline by 12 months.[220] Those who breastfed a month or less lost no bone mass. Age, diet, body size, and physical activity were not correlated in these healthy white women. Six months after weaning there was a return to normal bone densities.

Hypomagnesemia caused by lactational losses

A case of hypomagnesemic tetany caused by excessive lactation was reported in 1963 by Greenwald and associates.[84] The 20-year-old patient had been fully nursing her own 3-month-old infant and contributing 50 oz a day to the local milk bank. She was hospitalized with painful muscle spasms of her hands and feet that improved slightly but did not clear with calcium (serum level 9.6 mg/dL). Serum magnesium levels were low (0.4 mEq/L).

Kamble and Ookalka[114] reported on a 24-year-old woman who was breastfeeding a 15-day-old full-term infant. She presented with the sudden onset of rapidly progressive weakness of all her limbs. She had successfully breastfed two previous children. Her electrocardiogram (ECG) showed "hypokalemia" and multiple ventricular premature beats. Serum magnesium was 0.5 mmol/L (normal 0.8 to 1.7 mmol/L); milk magnesium was 4.9 mmol/L (normal 1.6 mmol/L). Serum calcium was

2.8 mmol/L, phosphate 1.1 mmol/L, and PTH normal. Urinary potassium was 36 mmol/L. After treatment with potassium and magnesium, the ECG and muscle tone returned to normal. This woman continued to breastfeed. She had three times the normal level of magnesium in her milk.

Lactational hypomagnesia is well described in the bovine model.

Crohn's disease and ulcerative colitis

Ulcerative colitis and Crohn's disease (and recently RA) are treated with salazosulfapyridine (SASP). Because of the concern about exposing the fetus to sulfisoxazole at the end of pregnancy or during lactation owing to the suggestion that sulfa drugs, even at low levels, predispose to kernicterus, this therapy has been discontinued in the third trimester. Recently, it was noted that sulfapyridine (SP), the main split product of SASP, has a low affinity for albumin-binding sites.

Esbjorner and associates[66] studied the binding capacities in both mothers and babies and found them low. They measured cord blood levels in the mothers of 11.5 µmol/L and in the infants of 20 µmol/L. Follow-up infant blood levels showed a clearance in 70 to 90 hours. Infants who were being breastfed did not increase their levels of SASP or SP. The milk/serum levels for SP were 0.4 to 0.6, and those for SASP were undetectable. Infant serum samples were 10% of maternal SP levels, and only one infant had detectable SASP. No children had complications of hyperbilirubinemia or kernicterus. All the infants were term infants without major complications. The authors[66] concluded that it is safe to continue the SASP throughout pregnancy and lactation in full-term infants. The effect on premature infants is under study. Prednisone therapy is usually safe because levels in milk are low.[4]

Epilepsy

A history of epilepsy in a mother is of concern for the obstetrician during pregnancy, and much has been written on the topic. Seizures in pregnancy are more dangerous to the fetus than is the medication. Antiepileptic drugs (AEDs) include phenobarbital, primidone, phenytoin, carbamazepine, ethosuximide, valproic acid, diazepam, and topiramate (Topamax). The concern regarding lactation includes the effect of the disease on the fetus in terms of major and minor malformations, the level of drugs in the infant's serum at birth, and the state of the mother post partum. Breastfeeding may provide a means of gradually withdrawing the infant from maternal medication and avoiding the syndrome of withdrawal[26] (i.e., hyperirritability, tremor, vomiting, poor sucking, hyperventilation, sleep disturbances). A good mother-infant relationship is important for a mother with epilepsy. Brodie[29] recommends alternating the breast with an occasional bottle (once a day or more) if the infant is sedated by maternal medication to reduce the effect.

Table 16-10 lists the half-lives of various AEDs. These compounds have a sedating effect and may prevent the infant from suckling adequately in the first few days. Attention must be paid to the infant's behavior to avoid not only undernutrition but also failure to provide sufficient stimulus to the breast. The infant may need some supplementation and the mother some stimulus with an electric pump, carefully coordinated with support.

Whether the infant is breastfed or bottle fed, it is necessary to establish that the mother will remain seizure free and be able to care for the infant. Forty-two infants of 32 epileptic mothers were studied by Kaneko and associates[117] for harmful side affects of AEDs while breastfeeding. The duration of poor sucking was correlated with the drug and the levels. The poor weight gain of the mixed-fed infants (breast/bottle) was associated with vomiting and infant drowsiness during feeding. These authors recommend mixing feedings (breastfeeding and formula) early post partum to reduce the medication to the infant until levels in infant serum taper a little and the infant's metabolism increases to promote drug clearance. Full breastfeeding can then proceed if care has been taken to establish a good milk supply with supplementary pumping.

Neuropathies associated with breastfeeding

A number of neurologic symptoms have been described in association with lactation. During periods of engorgement, pressure on nerves in the axilla, especially from an engorged tail of Spence (see Chapter 2), has caused numbness and tingling down the arms on the flexor surface to the ulnar distribution of the hands similar to crutch palsy. The numbness and tingling usually abate as soon as the infant nurses and then gradually return as the breast fills again. Symptoms gradually disappear after several weeks as engorgement disappears.

Symptoms similar to those associated with tennis elbow—pain and tingling with flexion of the forearm—have developed in nursing women who

TABLE 16-10	Pharmacokinetic data on antiepileptic drugs (AEDs) in newborns		
AED	Free fraction (% unbound)	Volume distribution (L/kg)	Half-life (hr)
Phenobarbital	57–72	0.6–1.5	40–500
Primidone	?	?	7–60
Phenytoin	15–30	0.7–2.0	15–105
Carbamazepine	?	1.1–2.6	8–28
Ethosuximide	?	?	40
Valproic acid	~15	0.2–0.4	14–88
Diazepam	~14	1.8–2.1	40–400
Topiramate	85	0.7	18–24

are pumping milk with a Kaneson-style hand pump.[245] Similar symptoms have been experienced by mothers just holding a newborn over time, especially primiparas and especially heavy infants.

Carpal tunnel syndrome has been described in pregnancy, causing paresthesia of the hands. Two cases were reported by Yagnik[248] in which symptoms developed 1 month post partum in breastfeeding women. The diagnosis was confirmed by electromyography (EMG) and nerve conduction studies. The second case was bilateral. Symptoms disappeared after the infants were weaned. Five other cases are described in the literature: all the women were breastfeeding, all showed improvement with temporary suspension of breastfeeding, and all recovered completely within a month of complete weaning.[219]

In a retrospective study by mail[239,240] of 27 women who had developed carpal tunnel syndrome post partum, the women affected were older (mean age 31.5 years) and were primiparous, and 24 of 27 were breastfeeding. The three bottle feeders had less severe symptoms that cleared in less than 1 month. Symptoms (predominantly paresthesias, clumsiness, and pain) began at a mean of 3.5 weeks post partum and lasted 6.5 months. Resolution began after 2 weeks of beginning to wean. Two women required surgical intervention. All were symptom free within a year.[239] The recommended treatment for carpal tunnel syndrome is conservative, with rest, diuretics, hand splint, and local corticosteroid injection, because it is usually reversible. No women had residual signs or symptoms, so perseverance with lactation and symptomatic treatment is appropriate.

Raynaud's phenomenon

Raynaud's phenomenon was first described by Maurice Raynaud in 1862 as episodic digital ischemia provoked by cold and emotion. The true cause remains obscure despite elaborate efforts to identify it.[64] It is widely thought to be a cutaneous manifestation of a generalized vascular disorder often associated in complex cases with scleroderma and vasoconstriction of the kidneys, heart, and lungs. Patients with Raynaud's phenomenon have significantly more migraine headaches.[112] The basic research on the subject does not mention vasospasm of the nipples.[64] The digital vessels of patients are more sensitive to the cold. Not all vasospasm is Raynaud's phenomenon.

Five cases of Raynaud's phenomenon of the nipple are described in the literature as severe blanching and debilitating pain.[144] Several women had white, blue, and red color changes but only of the nipple. All were treated with nifedipine (10 mg three times a day or 30 mg by slow-release tablet). Nifedipine (Adalat, Procardia) is an antihypertensive calcium-channel blocker. It does pass into the milk and is estimated to provide about 7.0 µg/kg/day (5%) of the pediatric dose. The American Academy of Pediatrics (AAP) rates nifedipine a 6, which suggests it is safe during lactation. All the women responded with a decrease or obliteration of the painful blanching. Oral bioavailability is only 50%, which reduces the risk to the breastfeeding infant.

The clinical parameters used to diagnose this disease are not universal.[62] Some history or other evidence of Raynaud's phenomenon is essential when associating it with nipple blanching.[22] Before prescribing a medication, the other therapeutic first options should be initiated.[143] Discontinuing smoking or avoiding secondhand smoke is imperative. Steady ambient temperature and warm clothing are important. Adding fish oil to the diet has helped some victims, as has evening primrose oil, which is a rich source of essential polyunsaturated fatty acid, especially γ-linoleic acid. Evening primrose oil has been used effectively in patients with mastalgia of unknown origin.

Peripheral tissue ischemia in neonates has been treated with topical nitroglycerin ointment, which is well absorbed through intact skin. Effects are usually seen within 30 to 60 minutes and last 6 to 8 hours.[22] Because of the risk of hypotension, constant observation is necessary. Although this is theoretically an effective therapy for blanched nipples, no studies report on its safety, and no data are available on its secondary effect on the infant, who would receive it through the milk or directly from the nipple. When mothers ingest nitrates, little is found in the milk and it is rapidly cleared from serum. Other medications that have been used for Raynaud's phenomenon include angiotensin-converting enzyme (ACE) inhibitors (e.g., captopril, enalapril) and prostaglandins for severe prolonged attacks.

Smoking

The number of women who breastfeed and smoke varies from 5% to 20% of breastfeeding women. Mothers who smoke choose bottle feeding more frequently than women who do not smoke. Of those smokers who are breastfeeding on discharge from the hospital, more have discontinued breastfeeding by 6 weeks than those who do not smoke.[155]

Smoking behavior patterns prenatally, during pregnancy, and post partum, as studied by O'Campo and associates,[185] show that 41% of women quit during pregnancy, with the highest rate of quitters being older, better educated, and white. Among black women, only the intention to breastfeed affected behavior. Early postpartum relapse rates differed by ethnicity, with formula feeding being the strongest predictor. Clinicians may be able to assist women in their resolve to quit as well as to breastfeed by providing strong support at the critical time in the early postpartum period.

The pharmacologic effects of nicotine have been studied in the fetuses of experimental animals. The active components of cigarette smoke, nicotine and carbon monoxide, have been implicated in the birth weight reduction seen in infants of mothers who are heavy smokers. Nicotine has acetylcholine-like actions on the central nervous system (CNS), skeletal muscle, and upper sympathetic and parasympathetic ganglia. Nicotine initially stimulates and then depresses. Nicotine has been shown to interfere with the let-down reflex, but it does not appear to disrupt lactation once it has been initiated. Smoking has been associated with a poor milk supply. It has been reported that women who smoke 10 to 20 cigarettes a day have 0.4 to 0.5 mg of nicotine/L in their milk. Calculations indicate this is equivalent to a dose of 6 to 7.5 mg of nicotine in an adult. In an adult, 4 mg

of nicotine has produced symptoms, and the lethal dosage is in the range of 40 to 60 mg for adults. On the basis of gradual intake over a day's time, the neonate would metabolize it in the liver and excrete the chemical through the kidney.

Multiple studies of nicotine and cotinine concentrations in the nursing mother and her infant have confirmed that although bottle fed infants born to smoking mothers and raised in a smoking environment have significant levels of nicotine and metabolites in their urine, breastfed infants have higher levels.[51,140,153] A direct correlation exists between the mother's plasma level and the amount in the milk, but not with the amount in the infant's urine in a study of smokers.[140,211] When the infant was removed from the environment and secondhand smoke, the correlation between milk and infant urine levels was high. The half-life of nicotine in the milk of smokers was reported by Steldinger and Luck[223] to be 95 minutes. Nicotine levels were higher in milk than in maternal serum because maternal serum is basic and milk is acidic. The total amount of nicotine and metabolites depends on the number of cigarettes per day and the time between the last cigarette and breastfeeding.[153]

When lactating women who smoked more than 15 cigarettes a day were compared with lactating women who did not smoke at all, the basal prolactin levels were significantly lower in smokers, but suckling-induced acute increments in serum prolactin and oxytocin-linked neurophysin were not influenced.[7] These experiments showed no influence on oxytocin when two cigarettes were smoked before a feeding. Serum nicotine and plasma epinephrine, but not dopamine or norepinephrine, were significantly increased in the mothers during smoking.

Somatostatin levels in plasma in smoking breastfeeding women were significantly higher at onset of lactation on day 4 post partum and throughout lactation. *Somatostatin* is a widely distributed peptide with multiple hormonal and neurogenic actions. It inhibits the release of prolactin; it inhibits gastrointestinal functions; and its presence in milk suggests it may be produced by the mammary gland. That milk yield is significantly decreased in smoking women was demonstrated by deuterium-dilution methods by Vio and associates.[234] Similar results were reported in the mothers of premature infants initiating lactation by pump in a carefully controlled study by Hopkinson and associates.[99] The smokers weaned their babies more quickly than nonsmokers.[155] The heavy smokers had the lowest prolactin levels and weaned earliest.

Newborn infants nursed by smoking mothers and kept in the newborn nursery to avoid passive smoke showed serum concentration of nicotine 0.2 ng/mL and cotinine, the main metabolite, 5 to 30 ng/mL.[48] Newborns excrete measurable amounts in their urine as well. Infants exposed to passive smoking but not breastfed also had nicotine in their urine. Thus breastfeeding by smoking women contributes to the nicotine in infants.

The effect of maternal smoking on the infant includes decreased growth (Fig. 16-6). Weight increase of infants of smokers was 340 ± 170 g compared with 550 g ± 130 g in control subjects over 14 days, as reported by Vio and associates.[234] In another comparison group of breastfeeders, Schulte-Hobein and associates[211] reported no significant weight difference when the infants were 1 year old. Gross motor and mental development

also were no different. A group of infants followed from the sixth month of pregnancy through 1 year of age included breastfed infants of 74 smokers, breastfed infants of 195 nonsmokers, and bottle fed infants of 64 smokers. Every 10 cigarettes smoked while breastfeeding was related to an additional 3% infant body mass at 1 year of age. This group of infants whose mothers smoked paradoxically had significantly higher body mass and were heavier than those of nonsmokers.[151]

Children of smokers had more respiratory illnesses in the first year and had been weaned sooner.[87] In a matched-pair group of 28 smokers and 28 nonsmokers, the smokers weaned at 4.5 months and the nonsmokers at 6.7 months. The infants of smokers required treatment for respiratory infection with antibiotics 38 times and the infants of nonsmokers 19 times. The relationship to colic in infants breastfed by a smoker is significant.[207] Forty percent of infants breastfed by smokers (≥5 cigarettes/day) had infantile colic, defined as 2 to 3 hours a day of excessive crying, compared with 26% of those breastfed by nonsmokers, according to Matheson and Rivrud[162] ($p < 0.005$). This observation has been made for bottle fed infants with one or more smokers in the home. A case of presumed nicotine poisoning was reported by Bisdom[20] in 1937 in a 6-week-old nursling whose mother smoked 20 cigarettes a day. The infant was restless and insomniac, with "spastic vomiting," diarrhea, rapid pulse, and "circulatory disturbances." The milk contained nicotine, and discontinuing breastfeeding caused "withdrawal," which was treated symptomatically. In a report of hair analysis as a marker for fetal exposure to nicotine and cotinine from maternal smoking by Klein and associates,[129] there was a direct correlation of hair levels to maternal levels. Measurable levels were found in mothers and infants exposed to passive smoke. Hair analysis may be an estimate of long-term systemic exposure.

Sudden infant death syndrome (SIDS) is more common in infants of smokers. Breastfed infants of smokers have a SIDS rate equal to that of bottle fed infants of nonsmokers. Infants of smokers have more respiratory disease, as do infants exposed to

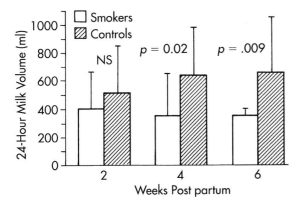

Figure 16-6. Milk production of smokers. (From Hopkinson JM, Schanler RJ, Fraley JK, et al: Milk production by mothers of premature infants: Influence of cigarette smoking. Pediatrics 90:934, 1992.)

passive smoke. This effect is improved if the infant is breastfed.

Many women who want to stop smoking have tried *nicotine gum*.[150] Its safety in lactation has not been determined. Levels of nicotine in mothers and the physiologic effect on their fetuses have been measured by Doppler effect in Sweden. Nicotine gum exposes the child only to nicotine and its metabolites and not to the other effects of smoking, including thiocyanate and carbon monoxide. The Swedish Nicorette chewing gum containing 4 mg nicotine was compared with one cigarette (high dose provides 1.6 mg). The gum did not appear to affect the fetus. Maternal plasma levels after a high-dose cigarette are double the levels after the gum or a low-dose cigarette. Nicorette gum in the United States contains 2 mg nicotine, which produces a plasma level of 11.8 ng/mL (Table 16-11).

The *nicotine patch* provides nicotine transdermally continuously while worn (it is recommended that it be removed while sleeping). The estimated rate of release of nicotine depends on the total dose in the patch, the number of layers, and the size of the patch (skin contact area). Up to 114 mg nicotine may be in a patch with a delivery rate of 21 to 22 mg/hour. Lower doses (7 mg/24 hour) can be prescribed. The serum level will vary accordingly.

In counseling the nursing mother who smokes, consideration should be given to the data, which suggest that mothers should not smoke while nursing or in the infant's presence. If it is not possible to stop, they should cut down and also consider

---

TABLE 16-11   Available nicotine in tobacco products and nicotine therapies

Tobacco products	Nicotine treatments
Smoking tobacco	***Nicotine gum***
1-g cigarette contains about 1.5% nicotine, or 13–19 mg/cigarette	Nicotine polyacrolex, Nicorette
Cigar 15–40 mg	Contains 2 mg nicotine/piece in United States or 4 mg/piece in Canada and Europe
Cigarette butt 5–7 mg/butt	Buffered to pH of 8.5 for enhanced absorption
	Nicotine rapidly and completely absorbed through oral mucosa
	About 30 minutes of chewing releases 90% of nicotine
Snuff	1 hour of chewing 2-mg piece produces 11.8 ng/mL and 4-mg piece 23.2 ng/mL nicotine plasma concentrations
1.5% nicotine	Gum must be chewed to release nicotine
Snuff contains about 30 g, of which 1.5% is nicotine, or total of 45 mg	
Dry snuff inhaled	
Wet snuff more alkaline and absorbed more readily, reaching plasma levels of cigarette smoking in 10 minutes	***Nicotine transdermal systems***
	Usually in three doses
	Provide 21, 14, and 7 mg of nicotine over 16–24 hours
Chewing tobacco	Provide average plasma nicotine concentrations of 17, 12, and 6 ng/mL, respectively (smoking provides 20–50 ng/mL)
2.5%–8% nicotine	21 mg/24 hr equivalent to smoking for 15 hours
Sweeter in taste than smoking tobacco	Elimination half-life of transdermally absorbed nicotine 3–6 hours
"Chaw" 7.8 mg nicotine/g of tobacco	
8–10 "chaws" equivalent to smoking 30–40 cigarettes	

low-nicotine cigarettes. Feedings should be delayed as long as possible after smoking.

Bupropion (Wellbutrin) has been used in smoking cessation programs. A trade name product, Zyban, is marketed for this purpose. Bupropion is an antidepressant drug unrelated to the tricyclics. It has a large volume of distribution and is highly protein bound, which may explain why it is not detected in the breastfed infant even though the milk/plasma ratio 2.5 to 8.5. The AAP considers its effect unknown but of some concern (Category 4).

Because some vegetables contain measurable amounts of nicotine (but not cotinine), they should be avoided as well. Highest levels are found in eggplant, green and pureed tomatoes, and cauliflower. Ten grams of eggplant provides 1 μg of nicotine, the same amount obtained in 3 hours in a room with minimal tobacco smoke.[58]

Clove cigarettes

Clove cigarettes contain 60% to 70% tobacco and 30% to 40% clove. Exposure to tar, nicotine, and carbon monoxide is twice that from regular cigarettes. *Eugenol,* the major active ingredient, is used as a topical dental anesthetic. It is more toxic in smoke than by ingestion.

Marijuana

If the mother smokes marijuana, an entirely different risk is created. Animal studies have shown that structural changes occur in the brain cells of newborn animals nursed by mothers whose milk contained cannabis. Nahas and associates[175,176] describe impairment of deoxyribonucleic acid (DNA) and ribonucleic acid (RNA) formation and of proteins essential for proper growth and development. Results seen in some humans suggest that serious and long-lasting effects can occur. Impairment of judgment and behavioral changes may interfere with an individual's ability to care for the infant or adequately breastfeed. If the mother smokes while nursing, the infant not only ingests the drug in her milk but also inhales the effect of the smoke from the environment. Because brain cell development is still taking place in the first months of life, any remote chance that DNA and RNA metabolism is altered should be viewed with concern.

The mother who requires hospitalization
Emergency admission

The mother who suddenly develops an emergency condition that requires hospitalization presents a unique problem in management. The emergency condition must be dealt with appropriately, whether medically, surgically, or psychiatrically. It is equally important in all three situations to deal with the patient as a lactating mother. Failure to do so may have an impact on the successful outcome of the primary condition.

Medical admission. Medical problems such as acute infection or metabolic disturbances should be analyzed in relationship to lactation, to the infant, and to any other children at home. Is it contagious? In the case of lactation, will the drugs pass into the breast milk? If so, are there alternative treatments? What is the prognosis for recovery? Is the recovery phase more or less than 2 weeks, and is maintaining lactation realistic? This decision should not be made without an understanding of the mother's commitment to further breastfeeding. If the prognosis is poor for recovery or the drugs involved are contraindicated for the infant but necessary for the mother, provision should be made for the mother's adjustment. Abrupt cessation of lactation can cause a fever and a flulike syndrome, which will confuse the management picture. It may be advisable to include the mother's obstetrician or pediatrician in the discussion to provide the mother with the necessary support to accept alternatives (see Chapter 11).

For instance, the management of asthma during pregnancy or lactation must consider the risk of drugs to the infant. Inhaled β_2-agonist medication (metaproterenol, terbutaline, albuterol) by metered dose delivers the least drug to the infant. Steroid therapy may be dramatic in the acute disease, and the breast milk levels are minimal and will drop slowly, providing a weaning mechanism from the drug. Theophylline, as with caffeine, can cause irritability and wakefulness in the infant and is no longer considered the primary treatment. The approach is initially focused to decrease the inflammation and not the spasm.

Surgical admission. As with any surgical procedure, communication must occur among the surgeon(s), anesthesiologist, other consultants, and the primary care physician to establish the process for breastfeeding when a lactating woman is the patient. Surgical emergencies such as trauma, appendicitis, or chylocystitis[16] require immediate attention, including anesthesia and surgery.

Breast biopsy during pregnancy and lactation represents special challenges to the surgeon and pathologist. The risk of milk fistula and infection is increased, although no published data are available. The risk is low in peripheral biopsies and high in central biopsies involving the areola. In 105 benign biopsies, 71% of patients had conditions similar to nonpregnant, nonlactating women. Those lesions peculiar to pregnancy and lactation in decreasing order of frequency are fibroadenoma, lipoma, papilloma, fibrocystic disease, galactocele, and inflammation. Localized breast infarcts also occur either from overgrowth of preexisting fibroadenoma or spontaneously. The risk of cancer diagnosis in one series was 22% of breastfeeding women compared with 19% of nonpregnant, nonlactating women overall. Most lumps were preexisting, but growth rate was accelerated by pregnancy.[194]

Thiopental sodium (thiopentone) as an induction agent was studied in lactating women, a group who had cesarean births and a group who had been fully lactating for at least 2 weeks and were to have elective surgery.[9] The dosage was 5.0 mg/kg for the first group and 5.4 mg/kg for the second. The maximum concentrations in colostrum were 1.3 ± 0.5 μmol/L and 3.4 ± 0.68 μmol/L in the mature milk, which were lower levels than those in the maternal serum (2.21 ± 0.31 and 7.09 ± 1.4, respectively). The maximum dose of drug in 100-mL mature milk was calculated to be 0.090 mg and in colostrum 0.034 mg. No effect was anticipated or seen in the fully breastfeeding infants.

Alfentanil has been measured in colostrum of nonlactating women having tubal ligations post partum. When the women were in the operating room before medication, both breasts were pumped with an electric pump for 10 minutes.[9] The women received diazepam, d-turbocurarine, succinylcholine, and thiopental sodium. Mothers were maintained on mechanical ventilation for the procedure. Then 50 μg/kg alfentanil was given intravenously with additional 10-μg/kg doses as needed for control. Four hours after the last injection of alfentanil, colostrum was collected from the right breast and at 28 hours from the left breast. The mean level at 4 hours was 0.88 ng/mL and 0.05 ng/mL at 28 hours. The drug cleared the colostrum rapidly.[80]

In the immediate postpartum period, tubal ligation may be performed on a multiparous woman. This type of procedure requires anesthesia and a brief interruption of mother-infant contact. The choice of anesthetic is important. Specific information is slowly accumulating regarding actual milk levels and infant responses. The highest morphine levels were reached about 30 minutes after the intravenous, intramuscular, or epidural doses and were slightly higher than the maternal plasma levels at all points. Some specimens were pumped from lactating patients having tubal ligations in the immediate postpartum period.[67] The peak dose was estimated at 500 ng/mL in the milk. Because of the low oral bioavailability of morphine in the breastfed infant, the drug is of minimal risk.[19,67]

Interpleural bupivacaine in the seventh right interspace 10 cm from the spinous process was given for operative and postoperative pain to a woman for biliary surgery who was breastfeeding a 10-month-old infant four times a day.[14] The dosage of bupivacaine was 0.13 mL/kg/hour. Peak maternal serum level was 1.6 μg/mL at 47 hours. The drug was undetectable in the infant's blood; maximum milk levels occurred immediately postoperatively. Despite numbness of the right nipple, breastfeeding continued uninterrupted except for time in the operating room. The numbness would suggest that the pain fibers are from the thoracic spinal nerves and the suckling sensory nerve fibers from the median branches of the intracostal nerves.

Major surgical trauma has a rapid, profound, and long-lasting effect on gonadal activity and less effect on adrenal activity. Prolactin levels rise significantly and return to baseline slowly. Initiating lactation postoperatively may be influenced by hormonal changes and the effects of pain.

With self-limited trauma or disease with a short postoperative course, as in appendicitis, the mother can go back to breastfeeding on her return home. If the hospitalization will be more prolonged, as in trauma with immobilizing fractures, different considerations are important. The infant can be brought to the hospital several times a day for nursing. Unless the mother is mobile enough to provide some of the infant's bedside care, rooming-in is too taxing to the recovering patient. It is also stressful to other patients and staff who are not equipped for neonates. The mother would require a single room. If she has provision for her own nursing care or if the nursing staff is agreeable, an arrangement could be worked out. The only contraindication would be whether it would interfere with recovery.

When bone healing is important, attention should be given to the dietary demands of bone healing and lactation, especially in calcium, phosphorus, and vitamin intakes. If the mother is to be cared for but immobilized at home, nursing is easier, but provision for ample assistance is mandatory. The need for assistance does not differ for the breastfed or bottle fed infant of the same age. Home care services are available in most communities.

Psychiatric admission. The onset of a psychiatric crisis in a lactating mother rarely occurs unless the mother has already been identified as having a psychiatric problem. Childbirth has an established etiologic role in postpartum psychosis. A report in the literature, however, details a case of mania precipitated in a mother each time she weaned her children from the breast but at no other time. We had treated a patient with a known psychiatric disorder who decompensated during pregnancy, did well during lactation, and had difficulty after weaning. With her fourth child, she weaned abruptly at 3 months and committed suicide 2 weeks later.

Breastfeeding of itself does not cause psychosis. Women with a postpartum psychosis have acutely decompensated when they wean abruptly. Thus, the management of weaning is a very important part of the mother's treatment, and the process should be orchestrated by the psychiatrist and not the pediatrician or obstetrician.

As the number of women who breastfeed increases, there will be increased understanding of the relationship of these physiologic events to psychiatric disease.[145] The role of the mother in lactation will be a part of her psychiatric care, and the decision to breastfeed or not should be worked out with her psychiatrist. Most psychiatric wards can accommodate young infants whether they are breastfed or bottle fed, so it is less of a novelty than on medical or surgical wards. The management of postpartum psychosis includes the concerns of the mother caring for the infant as part of recovery. The drugs used when the mother is nursing should be appropriate for both mother and nursing infant.

Elective admission

At times a lactating mother may have to plan for hospitalization. The urgency will be determined by the underlying disease. If the admission date can be made for over a month away, there is time for gradual weaning of the infant, if necessary. If weaning is appropriate or necessary, the impact will largely be determined by the age of the infant. A very young infant who would profit greatly by continued breastfeeding is one type of problem. If the infant is a year old, it may be less traumatic for the child to be weaned when the separation is going to be greater than 48 to 72 hours. A child who is also receiving solids and some other liquids from a cup can be sustained during the separation without much more than sadness. If the caregiver and the surroundings are familiar, the support of this infant is easier. For the mother of the older child, the impact of forced separation during hospitalization is also easier and less likely to produce "milk fever."

The young infant can be sustained by cup feedings, bottle feedings, or "cross-nursing" by another lactating mother until the infant can be breastfed by the mother again. The mother in the first few months of lactation will have more problems with engorgement, discomfort, and even malaise.

Provision should be made to express or pump milk to maintain the supply if the mother will be nursing again or pumping minimally for comfort if lactation is to be discontinued. Milk can be collected in sterile bottles and sent home for the infant. When the admission is elective, plans can be made in advance to have a pump available, renting one if the hospital is not equipped. Methods for collecting, refrigerating, and transporting milk home to the infant can be planned along with her other needs, such as a babysitter.

During an elective admission for a self-limited disease, rooming-in for the infant may be possible if the circumstances of the illness permit. The prime purpose of the hospitalization is to treat an illness. If surgery is involved, rooming-in should not be a stress to the mother when she is in the operating room, in the recovery room, or heavily medicated. Day-of-surgery, same-day surgery, and ambulatory surgery units have minimized hospital stays and the need for alternative nourishment for the infant.

The purpose of this section is to point out that it is possible to maintain lactation when hospitalization is necessary for the mother. It is also possible to have the infant accompany the mother, or vice versa, in a rooming-in arrangement. The theoretic threat of infection in the hospital setting is outweighed by the advantages of human milk in most cases. On the other hand, the decision rests with the physician in charge of the case, who will have the responsibility of looking at the total picture, including the medical problem in question, the necessary treatment, and the short-range prognosis for resuming normal breastfeeding. The expertise of the mother's obstetrician and the infant's pediatrician may be invaluable. They can also assist in coping with family and friends who have confused the mother with their personal experiences or opinions.

Evaluation of nipple discharge

Reports of nipple discharge usually exclude problems during lactation. In a consecutive series of 8703 breast surgeries, Leis and Urban[148] noted that 7.4% of patients had a discharge. To be significant, they point out, a discharge should be true, sponta-

neous, persistent, and nonlactational. Discharges can be milky, multicolored and sticky, purulent, clear (watery), yellow (serous), pink (serosanguineous), and bloody (sanguineous). The latter four are the surgically significant ones except in lactation.

Most nipple discharges are caused by benign lesions, and many do not require surgical intervention.[147] They could, however, represent a malignant condition and deserve careful investigation. Nipple discharges associated with lactation have a different etiologic incidence profile, but they are no less significant. In general, discharge is more common in older women. Most texts discussing discharge from the nipple are written by surgeons, and the distinction regarding the relationship to breastfeeding is not made.

A *discharge* from the nipple is defined as fluid that escapes spontaneously. A *secretion,* on the other hand, is fluid present in the ducts that must be collected by nipple aspiration or by other means, such as a conventional breast pump or gentle massage and expression from the ducts (*nonspontaneous secretion*).[127]

Nipple secretion is usually not observed in nonlactating women because the lactiferous sinuses are plugged with dense keratotic material. The secretions are seen on histologic sections. If the keratotic plugs are removed, fluid can be aspirated by use of a simple device in most women.[127] Various solutions have been injected into the duct system, and their absorption into tissue, lymphatics, and blood have been traced. The presence of fluid among nonlactating women depends on age, race, and menstrual, menopausal, and breast disease status.[6] The latter being the most important, lactation is still the ultimate secretory product.

Needle aspiration *biopsy* and aspiration biopsy cytology have made it possible to achieve a diagnosis without open biopsy and are standard clinical procedures for the evaluation of many palpable breast masses.[130] They are also used for nonpalpable lesions and can be used for multiple nodules, in mastitis, for evaluating vague masses and painful areas, and for assay of hormonal receptors. Biopsy is a prompt, cost-effective, safe procedure and can be done without interrupting lactation, often in the office setting.

Breast cytologic examination is an important part of an evaluation during pregnancy and lactation and any other time. During pregnancy the ductal lobular system undergoes marked hyperplasia with rapid proliferation of the epithelial linings as they form new ductules.[189] Lymphocytes, plasma cells, and eosinophils infiltrate during the proliferation process. After 16 weeks, colostrum-like fluid is present in the ducts. Cytologic appearance of the breast during pregnancy is very cellular; the cell types are the same as in the resting breast, although the proportions differ.[97] Epithelial cells are numerous and suggest a papillary structure. Neutrophils are abundant as well. The most common cell types are foam cells, leukocytes, histiocytes, and gland epithelial cells consisting of single cells and cell clusters.[97] The foam cells in pregnant patients exhibit nuclear enlargement, binucleation, multinucleation, and increased cytoplasmic vacuolization compared with those of nonpregnant women. Unexpectedly large numbers of ductal epithelial cells are present in pregnancy and lactation. Groups of cells are papillary in structure and similar to the papillary fronds of an intraductal papilloma. In the immediate postpartum period, the lactating woman's secretions are virtually acellular at the end of the first week; nonlactators exhibited cellularity characteristics of pregnancy, according to work by Holmquist and Papanicolaou.[97]

Biopsies during the third trimester of pregnancy, as described by Kline and Lash,[131] had "tufts of cells forming spurs or invaginations into duct and alveolar lumens and similar structures that were desquamated into lumens and groups of cells found in the breast secretions." The investigators also commented that the "spurs" were closely associated with the formation of new alveoli, suggesting their origin. Delicate capillary networks within these tufts of cells might easily be traumatized and result in the bloody secretion described in pregnancy and early lactation. Kline and Lash[132] reported the persistence of the antepartum cellular findings in 31 of 72 postpartum women. The correlation to lactation or its suppression was not made. Biopsies, however, demonstrated findings similar to those in pregnancy; these changes lasted up to 2 months.

Conclusions drawn from multiple studies by King and Goodson[127] are that breast-fluid cytologic examination during pregnancy and lactation reveals the following:

1. Increased cellularity is seen and is most marked in late pregnancy.
2. Cellularity is variable post partum.
3. Increased numbers of duct epithelial cells in groups are similar to intraductal papilloma or papillary hyperplasia.
4. Blood may be found in pregnancy and lactation in the absence of clinical lesion.
5. Interpretation of secretions in pregnancy and lactation justifies caution.

Cytologic findings referred to as "hyperplasia" in lactation have no apparent association with increased risk of breast cancer.[55] Lesions usually not associated with increased risk of cancer are apocrine metaplasia, cyst, duct ectasia, fibroadenoma, fibrosis, mastitis, periductal mastitis, squamous metaplasia, and milk hyperplasmia.

Milky discharge

Persistent bilateral lactation is the presentation following breastfeeding and, as noted, may represent pituitary disease. If no surgical disease (e.g., adenoma) exists, medical treatment to suppress prolactin (e.g., estrogens, bromocriptine) is no longer employed and involution is left to take place naturally. In the nonlactating woman, this finding is called *galactorrhea* and is a spontaneous, milky, multiduct, bilateral discharge (see earlier discussion).[196]

Multicolored and sticky discharge

Multicolored, sticky, spontaneous bilateral discharges from multiple ducts usually show only normal skin flora when cultured.[148] It is usually green but may be yellow, brown, red brown, or gray; it is Hemostix or guaiac negative. The discharge can occur from puberty to the postmenopausal years and is most common in parous women. It is often associated with nipple manipulation, especially when seen in the third trimester or early lactation. Simple cases can be treated with good hygiene and discontinuing nipple manipulation. If it occurs at delivery, lactation can be initiated after cleansing and removal and discarding of early secretion. Normal colostrum usually follows.

Duct ectasia, or *comedomastitis,* is the most common cause of multicolored sticky discharge.[196] It begins as a dilatation of the terminal ducts and may occur during pregnancy, although it is most common between the ages of 35 and 40. It is rare in virgins and most common in women who have lactated. An irritating lipid forms in the ducts, producing an inflammatory reaction and nipple discharge. Cytologic examination shows debris and epithelial cells. Duct ectasia may be associated with burning pain, itching, and swelling of the nipple and areola. Palpation reveals a wormlike tube once called *varicocele tumor of the breast.* As the disease progresses, a mass may develop that mimics cancer, and chronic inflammation leads to fibrosis. Surgery is not indicated unless the discharge becomes bloody. The disease is usually treated with thorough cleansing with pHisoHex or povidone-iodine (Betadine) daily and avoidance of nipple manipulation. Lactation would aggravate preexisting diseases but would not be an absolute contraindication. When the nipple becomes inflamed and clogged with a thick sticky gray-green discharge with no apparent cause especially nearing menopause, treatment is warm compresses, antibiotics, and if necessary, surgical removal of the duct.

Purulent discharge

Purulent discharge is caused by acute puerperal mastitis, chronic lactation mastitis, central breast abscess, or plasma cell mastitis. It is usually unilateral, involving one or two ducts. Once diagnosed, the treatment is antibiotics. When an abscess does not clear after withholding of lactation and adequate treatment, a biopsy should be done to rule out secondary necrosis and infection of an underlying lesion. Ultrasound or other imaging may assist in the diagnosis.

Watery, serous, serosanguineous, and bloody discharges

A volunteer survey among members of the Nursing Mothers Association of Australia resulted in a report of 37 cases in 32 women who had bloody or serosanguineous secretion in either pregnancy or lactation. The condition usually occurred in the first pregnancy (27 of 37) or was a recurrence in a second pregnancy (five cases), with one case occurring in the third pregnancy. It was usually bilateral, although onset might be unilateral. The earliest case started in the fourth month of pregnancy, although most began at birth and in early lactation. More than 50% of the women had practiced prenatal nipple "exercising." Most cases cleared within 3 to 7 days of onset of lactation. These cases were distinct from trauma, cracked nipple, or mastitis.

The Lactation Study Center frequently receives calls regarding pink (guaiac positive) or frankly bloody milk, referred to by some as "rusty-pipe syndrome." It is painless and may go unnoticed unless the mother is pumping her milk or her infant vomits blood that is positive for adult hemoglobin (Apt test), eliminating cases of bleeding of the newborn gastrointestinal tract, which is positive for fetal blood by Apt test. If the infant tolerates the milk, breastfeeding can continue and the blood usually disappears in 3 to 7 days.

The explanation for this phenomenon is probably the increased vascularization of the breast coupled with the rapid development of the alveolae.[132] If the blood persists or is recurrent, the breast should be evaluated by mammography.

The cytology of breast secretions obtained during the third trimester from 50 pregnant women aged 16 to 39 years was reported by Kline and Lash.[132] There was increased cellularity with epithelial cell clusters and capillary groupings forming "spurs" or invaginations into duct and alveolar lumina. The authors noted that the spurs were closely associated with the formation of new alveoli; the delicate capillary networks within these tufts could be easily traumatized and result in blood escaping into the breast secretions.

The other cells found in secretions during pregnancy and lactation when breast secretions were aspirated were foam cells, leukocytes, histiocytes, and gland epithelial cells.[65] Foam cells are also referred to as *colostrum bodies* and have large nucleae or are binuclear or multinucleated. When lactation is suppressed post partum, the secretion is almost acellular by the seventh day.[132]

Nipple discharges are primarily of surgical significance. They are the second most common indication for breast surgery. Watery or colorless, serous or yellow, serosanguineous or pink and sanguineous discharges are more common over the age of 50, but younger women do not escape them.[196] Bloody discharge in pregnancy and lactation is most often caused by vascular engorgement or breast trauma. The next most common causes in pregnancy and lactation are intraductal papilloma (50%) and fibrocystic disease (31%). Because the type of discharge does not identify the malignant or nonmalignant nature of the problem, all patients with unusual discharge should be seen by an appropriate surgeon for diagnosis.

Nipple discharges with blood visible or detected by cytologic examination are common during pregnancy and lactation. Lafreniere[141] estimated that 15% of asymptomatic lactating women have blood in their early secretions when they are examined cytologically. An intraductal papilloma is a small, usually noncancerous growth protruding into a duct near the nipple in women 35 to 45 years old. Discharge is bloody or sticky spontaneous from one duct only. Treatment is surgical removal of the duct with pathologic examination.

In intraductal papilloma the discharge is usually spontaneous, unilateral, and from a single duct. It is occasionally associated with a nontender lump in the subareolar area. Symptoms may include bleeding, which is usually painless during pregnancy. It is possible to excise the involved duct and wedge of tissue, leaving the rest intact to preserve mammary function, when surgery is required for intraductal papilloma. Painless bleeding during pregnancy may be bilateral or unilateral and may cease after delivery. After serious disease has been ruled out by physical examination and cytologic evaluation, lactation is possible.[141]

To be significant, a discharge should be true, persistent, spontaneous, and nonlactational. Single-duct unilateral discharges are more apt to be surgically significant. A true discharge comes from a duct to the surface of the nipple. Pseudodischarges occur on the surface and may be associated with inverted nipples, eczematoid lesions, trauma, herpes simplex, infections of the Montgomery glands, and mammary duct fistulas. Discharges are more common in women taking oral contraceptives, tranquilizers, or rauwolfia alkaloids and in those who are postmenopausal and menopausal. Cytologic examination should be part of any examination for an abnormal discharge from the breast, although a high percentage of false negative tests occur as well as some false positive results. Absence of a mass is reassuring but should not dissuade one from further diagnostic studies.

Paget's disease of the breast is an uncommon type of cancer that occurs in only 1% to 4% of all women with breast cancer. Signs and symptoms include itching, burning, redness or scaling of the surface of the nipple and areola. There may be a bloody discharge. The nipple may appear flattened against the breast. It has been mistaken for candidiasis during lactation, greatly delaying proper treatment. A biopsy of the areola is necessary. Mastectomy is usually recommended, although early lumpectomy may be adequate. Chemotherapy and radiation are recommended.

Lumps in the breast

The lactating breast is lumpy to palpation, and the lumps shift day by day. The most common cause of a persistent lump is a plugged duct (see Chapter 8); the second most common cause is a mass associated with mastitis. Lumps that persist beyond a few days and do not respond to palliative treatment deserve investigation.[192,193] In young pregnant or lactating women, ultrasound is the ideal method for evaluation of the breast. It visualizes the breast architecture dynamically and facilitates differentiation between benign cysts and solid lesions and further suggests if a solid mass is benign or malignant. It could be a benign shape with smooth edges. It also establishes a baseline for subsequent follow-up. The American College of Radiology (ACR) standard for the performance of a breast ultrasound examination states that breast sonography is the initial imaging technique to evaluate palpable masses in women under 30 or in pregnant and lactating women.[1]

Ultrasound is also useful to diagnose and guide drainage of breast collections and check for abscess when mastitis presents. A small abscess identified early can be treated with percutaneous drainage before surgical drainage is necessary. When a mass is to be evaluated, the mother should nurse immediately before the procedure. If there is a mass in a lactating breast that warrants biopsy, percutaneous core biopsy can be done.

Adenomas of the breast and ectopic breast under lactational influences were reviewed by O'Hara and Page.[186] They reported five ectopic lactating adenomas located in the axilla, chest wall, and vulva. Tubular adenomas have been associated with lactation and show lactational changes in a fibroadenoma, thus making diagnosis difficult by fine-needle aspiration. Fine-needle aspiration of the breast has been recommended as a safe, simple diagnostic tool to use in an ambulatory setting without interrupting lactation.[146]

Once a breast mass is palpated, prompt evaluation is indicated to rule out breast cancer. A palpable lump in pregnancy has been noted by investigators to delay the time to treatment as long as 8 months.[18]

Three percent of women diagnosed with breast cancer are pregnant or lactating.[194] Data suggest that pregnant or lactating women with breast cancer, stage for stage, have similar survival rates as nonpregnant women. Average delay during the perinatal period is 2.2 months compared with 0.59 month in the total population of breast cancer patients; thus, a higher proportion of pregnant women are in advanced stages when first seen.[212] Lumpectomy can be performed during pregnancy and lactation.

Fibrocystic disease

Fibrocystic disease is a diffuse parenchymal process in the breasts that has many synonyms, none of which is satisfactory. The process involves hormonally produced benign proliferations of the alveolar system of varying degrees that occur in response to the normal menstrual cycle. A patient with full-blown disease has pain, tenderness, palpable thickenings, and nodules of varying sizes that are most symptomatic with menses. Fibrocystic disease is prominent in the childbearing years and regresses during pregnancy. It is not a contraindication to breastfeeding. Some women have achieved relief by totally eliminating caffeine and related products from their diet.

Diagnostic procedures include mammography and aspiration biopsy. When no fluid is obtained and a smooth, freely movable mass is present, lumpectomy can be performed. Microscopic examination will clarify the diagnosis and the need for further treatment.

Galactography

Galactography is radiography of the mammary ducts after the injection of radiopaque contrast material (see Fig. 16-2). It is done to identify the cause of abnormal nipple discharge, especially when there is no palpable or radiologically detectable lesion. Cytologic examination of the discharge material should always be done first. Positive cytologic examination is helpful, but false negative results do occur. The procedure involves cannulation of the duct with a blunt needle under sterile precautions with the slow injection of 2.0 mL of sterile, water-soluble contrast material. Preexisting mastitis or abscess is a contraindication to the procedure (see Fig. 16-1).

The nipple discharge may be caused by ductal ectasia, fibrocystic changes, papilloma, papillomatosis, or intraductal carcinoma. Galactography is performed to localize the abnormality and not to make a histologic diagnosis, because the appearance of some benign and malignant lesions overlaps significantly. In lactating women, fewer than 10% with abnormal discharge are malignant (Fig. 16-7).

Breast cysts

Benign cysts of the breast are being identified in younger and younger women, probably because of the more careful self-examination of the breast now recommended. They should be removed and biop-

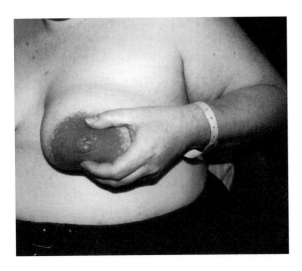

Figure 16-7.   Bi-fed nipple or double nipple. Note milk at both orifices and third on face or surface of areola. With gentle pressure all three orifices have major spray.

sied but do not interfere with lactation. Fibroadenomas that result from a disturbance in the normal menstrual cycle usually proliferate and regress before age 30. Pregnancy and lactation stimulate their growth. They are firm, smooth, lobulated masses and are freely movable without fixation. They can be diagnosed radiologically. They can be removed while the patient is under local anesthesia, if necessary, without causing cessation of breast-feeding.

Lipomas

Lipomas are very common in the breast, which has considerable fat in its stroma. They are usually solitary, asymptomatic, slowly growing, freely movable, soft, and well delineated. They can be easily identified radiologically or with ultrasound imagery in the lactating breast, which has less fat present.

Fat necrosis

Fat necrosis is usually associated with trauma and is caused by local destruction of fat cells with release of free lipid and variable hemorrhage. Organization with fibrosis may lead to fixation. Fat necrosis can be identified radiologically and appears as a fat density or oil cyst with a capsule.

Hematomas

Hematomas of the lactating breast may occur from trauma or in women receiving anticoagulant therapy. They generally regress without treatment. When they occur with minimal trauma, the presence of a tumor should be considered.

Breast hypertrophy with pregnancy (gigantomastia)

Massive hypertrophy of the breast with pregnancy is a rare condition of unknown etiology referred to as *gigantomastia of pregnancy*.[170] It is reported in all races during the childbearing years but is less common than juvenile or virginal hypertrophy,[23] which usually has its onset between ages 11 and 19. When associated with pregnancy, hypertrophy usually begins during the first trimester and progresses until delivery and may even lead to necrosis and incapacity. The first report was in 1948, and a total of 55 cases have been reported in the world literature.[170]

The typical case involves a previously healthy pregnant woman who observes excessive enlargement bilaterally early in pregnancy. The breasts may double or triple in size, becoming not only grotesque but incapacitating. They are firm, edematous, and tense, with a prominent venous pattern. The rapidity of the changes predisposes to necrosis, infection, and hemorrhage. According to the literature, after delivery, in the immediate postpartum period, in most cases the breasts recede to almost their previous size. With subsequent pregnancies, they almost always enlarge again and even more extensively.

A patient reported to our center who had moderate breast hypertrophy during pregnancy and massive enlargement during the immediate postpartum period. She had planned to breastfeed but was completely incapacitated. Her caregivers described her breasts as the size of basketballs. Some pain relief was achieved with a Velcro abdominal binder applied to support the breasts and provide some counterpressure. Pillows for support under the arms were also used. Ice packs did little for relief, and analgesics were mildly palliative. The mother was hospitalized for weeks, unable to get out of bed.

Gentle pumping helped establish milk flow, and breastfeeding was initiated. Breast size diminished sufficiently to allow discharge home. At about 3 months post partum, the excessive enlargement recurred, weaning was unpreventable, and surgical intervention was planned. Another patient with massive enlargement during pregnancy was assisted to breastfeed post partum and did well until 6 weeks when she developed mastitis requiring hospitalization and weaning to cure the overwhelming septicemia. There was a recurrence with the second pregnancy and she had reduction mammoplasty following delivery.

The cause of gigantomastia is unknown, but most authors agree it is hormonal in nature,[170] whether it is an overproduction or an overreaction of the target organ to the stimulus. Various hormonal therapies, including estrogen, testosterone, and hydrocortisone, have not been effective. Diuretics have been mildly helpful for some. Liver dysfunction has been postulated but essentially discarded when all studies of liver function were normal.

Pseudohyperparathyroidism has been associated with this condition, with improvement after therapy for the underlying disease. A case of gigantic mammary hypertrophy during pregnancy was associated with severe nonparathyroid hypercalcemia. Vigorous diuresis reduced the calcium level to 11.1 mg/dL. No galactorrhea was present, and the prolactin level was 26 ng/mL. No enlargement of parathyroids was detected. An emergency partial bilateral mastectomy was performed because of necrosis and bleeding. Intraoperatively, 16 U of blood were required. The breast tissue removed weighed 12.5 kg (left) and 11.3 kg (right). Pathologic examination showed virginal hypertrophy with no duct formation. Postoperatively, the serum calcium level returned to normal.[232]

If delivery is not imminent, surgical intervention to relieve severe pain, massive infections, ulceration, hemorrhage, or necrosis is an alternative. After delivery the patient should be counseled about the risk of recurrence and the option of reduction mammoplasty, preserving the nipple and duct system.[212] Surgery is sometimes life-saving.

Lactation after delivery has not been described in these patients.[170]

Surgical procedures

Surgical manipulation of the breast may result in residual loss of sensation for several months but only rarely permanently. The nerve involved is the anterior cutaneous branch of the fourth lateral cutaneous nerve, which passes deep into the breast tissue unaccompanied by arteries. Preoperative and postoperative evaluation of breast sensation was reported by Courtiss and Goldwyn.[49] Preoperatively, they found the areola to be the most sensitive. For 2 weeks following augmentation mammoplasty, sensation was decreased to the areola and nipple. Erectility did return in all patients. The return of significant sensitivity, however, usually took 6 months or longer, even 2 years, with the larger implants being associated with the greatest loss. Hyperesthesia and paresthesia were also reported.

Immediately after reduction mammoplasty (see next section), breasts were insensitive to testing, and it took about 6 months for sensation to return. The greater the resection, the greater was the loss of sensation. Nipple erectility returned before complete sensation in the skin in about 2 months, but complete recovery took about 1 year. With mastopexy for sagging breasts, normal sensation in the skin returned in about 2 months, but complete recovery could take up to a year.[49]

Augmentation mammoplasty

Augmentation mammoplasty has become a more acceptable procedure, and techniques have improved tremendously.[225] The implantation of inert material is the approach. Young women may request it and then choose to lactate. There should be no destruction of breast tissue or interruption of ducts, nerve supply, or blood supply to the gland or nipple so that breastfeeding is possible and successful (Fig. 16-8). The incision is inferior near the chest wall and not periaveolar. Injections of silicone are no longer used. The silicone caused fibrosis and duct destruction.[225]

Implants for augmentation present different problems and different risk/benefit ratios than implants done after mastectomy as prostheses. An

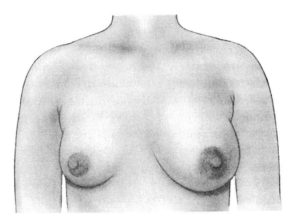

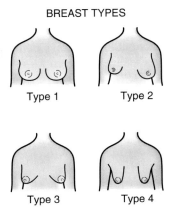

Figure 16-9. Asymmetric breasts, with right breast significantly smaller.

and Drug Administration (FDA) concluded after extensive study that it is not necessary to remove intact implants or to check milk for silicone when the prosthesis is intact and the woman chooses to breastfeed. Measurements of levels of silicone and degradation products in urine and milk are not readily available. Silicone and simethicone are present in many medications and toiletries, and silicon is the second most common element on the earth's surface. Nonaugmented cadavers have measurable amounts of silicone in tissues.

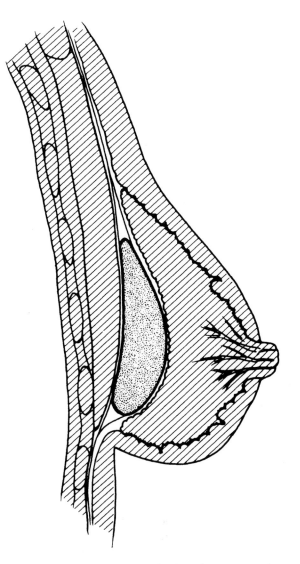

Figure 16-8. Placement of implant in augmentation mammoplasty, with no interruption of vital ducts, nerve supply, or blood supply.

BREAST TYPES

Type 1

Type 2

Type 3

Type 4

Figure 16-10. Breasts are asymmetric and often variably shaped. Tubular breasts (*Type 4*) usually have minimal functioning tissue.

indication that still remains is the unilateral use when one breast is significantly underdeveloped (Figs. 16-9 and 16-10). The underdeveloped breast may present a problem of underproduction during lactation. The flood of reports of rupture of the implants and the leakage of silicone into the breast tissue caused considerable alarm. The U.S. Food

The FDA's position is that breast implants filled with silicone gel will be available only through controlled clinical trials.[125] Women needing reconstruction will be assured of access. This is based on the lack of knowledge about the safety of silicone implants 35 years after their introduction. It has not been recommended that these implants be removed, except on a case-by-case basis for medical reasons.[125]

Silicon analysis of breast and periprosthetic capsular tissue from patients with saline or silicone gel breast implants demonstrated that silicon levels of breast tissue specimens from saline prostheses were in the same range as those of control subjects. The levels in the periprosthetic tissue with intact saline implants were significantly higher than those of control subjects but not as high as those of ruptured silicone gel implants.[210]

Polyurethane implants are no longer available. They had been associated with long-lasting complications, the most common being contractions. Polyurethane is a polymer formed by reaction of diisocyanates and polyols. The polymer sponge breaks down into its reactive monomers, toluene-2,4- and -2,6-diisocyanate. Diamine metabolites have been identified in the urine of patients implanted with the material.[39] The disfigurement of the breast from fibrosis and contractions has led to their removal from the market.

More than 700 articles are found in the literature relating to illness and silicone gel implants, many of them single-case reports. After a thorough study of the literature the Practice Committee of the American Academy of Neurology reports that studies to date (1) show no clear relationship between silicone breast implants and connective tissue disease and (2) do not support a causal relationship between silicone breast implants and neurologic disorders at present.[68] Renewed efforts to make silicone implants available should include data on infants born and those breastfed while implants are in place. No such data are currently available.

Breasts requiring augmentation mammoplasty may lack adequate functional breast tissue. A woman may want to have this evaluated by real-time ultrasound before the insertion of an implant if she plans to breastfeed later.

Postlactation involution

Postlactation involution of a severe degree occasionally occurs. After multiple pregnancies and lactation, some women note considerable regression and seeming atrophy after weaning, which alarms them. The fat deposition has not recurred when the ducts regress. In most of these women the breasts return to their normal contour in about 3 years if no further pregnancy or lactation has occurred. Loss of tissue turgor and fat padding occurs without pregnancy or lactation as well (Fig. 16-11). Augmentation is possible, if desired, once childbearing is completed. If subsequent pregnancy occurs, the breast regenerates and lactates well.

Reduction mammoplasty

Some women have breasts so large that they cause shoulder and back pain, deep grooves in the shoulders from brassiere straps, and negative self-image. These women sometimes want surgical correction. Reduction mammoplasty is more destructive than augmentation because of the necessity of replacing the nipple symmetrically, which requires interrupting the ducts.[225,226] Although reconstructive surgeons report that these women do not want to breastfeed, it is our experience that many of them do choose to breastfeed later when they bear a child and are suddenly aware of their maternal role. At surgery they are consumed with their perceived affliction. The surgeon should clearly discuss the options with the patient or provide a procedure that leaves the ducts intact. If the ducts are intact, breastfeeding can be successful postoperatively. The nerve must also be intact for tactile sensations to trigger let-down.

In general, surgery of the breast for nonmalignant lesions does not preclude breastfeeding unless the ductal structure has been interrupted. Surgeons need to consider mammary function in counseling young women about breast surgery.

A prospective study of 319 normal healthy women by Neifert and associates[178] identified 22 women with previous breast surgery, including 11 excisional biopsies, 5 augmentations, 4 reductions, and 2 chest surgeries involving breast tissue. Ten of the 22 had periareolar incisions (4 reductions, 1 augmentation, 5 excisional biopsies). In this series, previous breast surgery was significantly correlated with the final outcome of lactation, that is, a threefold risk of insufficiency compared to women without surgery. Those women with a periareolar incision had a fivefold risk of lactation insufficiency. Breast reduction was the condition most highly correlated with insufficiency.

It has been reported that large breasts are a major image issue for some young women who take extreme efforts to lose weight and decrease their breast size. In the management of several patients with bulimia, in spite of the fact surgery to change the body is not recommended, these patients had reduction mammoplasty by a skilled plastic surgeon. Postoperatively, they recovered from their underlying disease.[137]

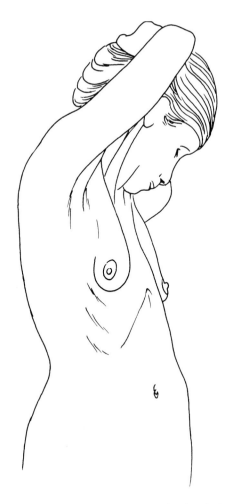

Figure 16-11.   Extreme postlactation involution.

A follow-up study by Harris and associates[92] of 73 patients, all in the childbearing years, was done by mailed questionnaire. In the series of 68 patients with reduction mammoplasty procedures who responded, 20 patients became pregnant. All 20 lactated; 7 (35%) breastfed successfully; and 13 (65%) decided not to breastfeed or discontinued breastfeeding for a variety of personal reasons. These patients had all undergone an inferiorly based pedicle reduction mammoplasty, which retains the ability to lactate because the nipple and areola are maintained on a ductal pedicle.[92]

Dermatitis that involves the breast
Bacterial dermatitis

Infections of the skin can also involve the breast. Impetigo is extremely contagious and spreads by contact. If it affects the breast, it should be vigorously treated locally and systemically. Breastfeeding should be interrupted until lesions are clear. Milk should be pumped and discarded until systemic treatment has been under way for at least 24 hours. The infant should be inspected daily for possible lesions and treated vigorously if under 3 months of age. Local treatment may be adequate early in older children.

Viral dermatitis

Herpes simplex and herpes zoster lesions on the breast are a contraindication for breastfeeding (see Chapter 17). Chickenpox lesions similarly are a contraindication for breastfeeding until the lesions clear unless the infant has already contracted the disease. When lesions of herpes are unilateral, breastfeeding can take place on the other breast. Herpes simplex in a neonate can be life threatening, so the source of the lesion should be determined to measure the risk of a lesion occurring on the other breast.

Contact dermatitis

Lesions from contact with irritating material usually do not affect the infant, so breastfeeding is not contraindicated unless the process interferes with maternal healing or puts the mother at risk for infection. Latex allergic dermatitis can usually be treated with cortisone ointment (by prescription to achieve adequate dosing), and breastfeeding can continue. The offending material should be eliminated. Latex may be in moisture-proof padding for nursing brassieres. Some nipple shields are latex and have no purpose in lactation management. Silicone nipple shields can be used if indicated.

Herpes gestationis is a noncontagious, noninfectious bullous disease of the skin that occurs during pregnancy and the puerperium.[75] It occurs only when there is placental tissue and so can occur with choriocarcinomas and hydatidiform moles. There is a genetic predisposition and increased frequency of HLA antigens as in autoimmune diseases. It begins with itching followed by erythema and edema of subcutaneous tissue. Within days or weeks, papules and plaques form that are somewhat urticarial. Lesions can be anywhere including palms and soles but not face, scalp, or mucosa. Diagnosis is confirmed by biopsy. Onset is most commonly midpregnancy but it can be immediately post partum. It lasts for weeks. Neonatal gestationis occurs in 10% of cases and is transient and milder. It is believed to be related to placental exposure.

Breastfeeding is not contraindicated. Treatment is symptomatic, usually with corticosteroids. The itching is intense. It usually abates after delivery.

PUPP syndrome (pruritic urticarial papules and plaques of pregnancy) is the most common dermatosis of pregnancy (1 in 200 patients). Cause is unknown but no hormonal or autoimmune abnormalities have been found.[75] It is more common in primigravidas with prominent striae and uterine distention (twins, hydramnios). Lesions typically begin on abdomen as erythematous papules surrounded by a narrow pale halo that coalesce into urtical plaques. It spreads to thighs and arms in 2 to 3 days. Diagnosis is confirmed by biopsy to distinguish from gestationis. Treatment is symptomatic. It is not contagious or infectious. Breastfeeding is appropriate. Lesions on the breast will have to be evaluated, but the disease does fade post partum.

Mastocytosis is a local mast cell density and overactivity resulting in a hive-like histamine-mediated reaction to any one of a variety of irritants from simple physical contact to chemical contacts to drug reactions. The lesions are benign, often solitary, and tend to fade over time. It flares when it is mechanically stimulated. It presents as a recurrent hive and may have hyperpigmented papule or plaque. Biopsy (which is rarely necessary) shows eosinophiles and mast cells. Mastocytosis does not interfere with breastfeeding.

Poison ivy (*Rhus* infection) anywhere on the body except the breast poses no problem to the suckling infant. The toxin from the plant is dissipated from the involved skin within 6 hours after contact. Toxic oils may remain on shoes or clothing until they are washed. The contents of the vesicles do not cause disease in others. The risk involved with continuing to breastfeed if the lesions are on the nipple or areola results from the possibility of secondary infection from infant to mother, which will cause skin breakdown and delayed healing. Treatment with hydrocortisone ointment 1% will hasten healing. Milk should be pumped and may be fed to the infant. Breastfeeding can resume as soon as lesions have healed, usually 4 to 5 days, and the risk of secondary infection is gone.

Anaphylaxis and breastfeeding

Anaphylaxis can be associated with breastfeeding. Urticaria and angioedema can be triggered by a number of factors, including physical stimuli, bites, stings, hormones, collagen vascular disease, and cyclooxygenase inhibitors.

The patient reported by Mullins and associates[171] had symptoms when achieving a let-down with breastfeeding. The first episode occurred at first feeding with the first infant. The events were restricted to the early postpartum period. The role of progesterone is not clear, although in other cases unrelated to lactation, suppressing ovulation cleared the symptoms. Although the patient did not react to a skin test with oxytocin, manual expression of the breast precipitated laryngeal edema and hypotension, as did every attempt to breastfeed. Lactation was suppressed by bromocriptine and there were no recurrences. The patient remained symptom free for 5 years until the birth of her fourth child. At 48 hours post partum, urticaria, upper airway angioedema, and hypotension occurred within minutes of each breastfeeding. She was again given bromocriptine, lactation ceased, and she was symptom free.

Less dramatic urticaria reported during lactation usually occurs at onset of let-down. The itching may be intense. Some relief has been achieved by medicating the mother about 15 minutes before breastfeeding with antihistamines. An alternative is a low-dose, sustained-release antihistamine preparation such as loratadine (Claritin), which does pass into milk but at levels less than 0.03% of the maternal dose. Because it dries mucous membranes and decreases secretions, such a preparation could decrease milk supply over time. Low-dose corticosteroids taken prior to symptoms or daily is an alternative treatment.

Cephalgia and lactational headache

The association of headache with lactation has been described in the literature and reported to our Lactation Study Center. Migraine headaches differ from lactational headaches.[215] *Migraine* is a unilateral hormonally sensitive, episodic headache disorder that may worsen during pregnancy and lactation.[238] Women are reported to have frequent headaches between the third and the sixth day post partum. Research on periparietal migraines fails to mention the mode of infant feeding. The relationship to prolactin is of interest to neurogenic theorists because prolactin levels are high during migraine headaches. Hyperprolactinemic infertility is associated with increased headaches. The theory is that although hyperprolactinemia does not cause headaches per se, headaches and hyperprolactinemia reflect a derangement of neurotransmission.[115,221]

A detailed description of the onset of headache is provided by Askmark and Lundberg[12] in a 26-year-old woman who was gravida 4, para 2, Ab 2. At her previous term pregnancy, she had intense headaches the weeks before delivery. These increased in intensity, necessitating a complete diagnostic workup by 32 weeks. Because of the headache and facial edema, a cesarean delivery was done at 32⅔ weeks. The headache and edema cleared in 2 days and recurred at 1 month about 2 minutes into breastfeeding. Each event lasted for 2 to 7 minutes. On occasion the headache would briefly clear while the infant interrupted feeding to burp or change breasts. There was no change in blood pressure and no exertion. Measurements of serum vasopressin, which is a vasoconstrictor, did not show a rise, and oral propranolol given 1 hour before nursing did not prevent the headache. Prolactin levels rose gradually and persisted long after the headache stopped. Oxytocin was not measured. The patient weaned the infant, and the headaches stopped. Wall[238] reported five milder but similar cases.

Headaches are reported to occur during sexual intercourse, which is also associated with oxytocin, a vasoconstrictor. This condition is called *benign orgasmic cephalgia* There are reported causes of serious vascular problems (stroke) with such events.

Medical evaluation of such a complaint requires the usual evaluation for headache. When associated with lactation and after assessment of pulse and blood pressure, a trial of oxytocin can be given by nasal spray to test the association with oxytocin. A prolactin level at baseline and after 10 minutes of breast stimulation might provide some information. With a negative workup for causes of headache, lactational headache can be considered. It appears to be self-limited. When lactational headache is seen in conjunction with preeclampsia or hypertension and edema, a thorough review is essential to avoid an eclampic crisis.

Multiple sclerosis

Studies historically have reported an increased risk of exacerbation in multiple sclerosis (MS) during the postpartum period but have not considered the impact of breastfeeding. In a study of 435 women regarding their pregnancy and breastfeeding experience, Nelson and associates[180] report that 191 pregnancies occurred in a nonprogressive phase of MS. During the 9 months of pregnancy, the exacerbation risk was 10%. During the first 9 months post partum, the risk was more than three times higher, or 34%. The rate of exacerbation was highest in the first 3 months (44 of 65 women, or 68%) and tapered through 6 months post partum. In 96 of 191 pregnancies, breastfeeding was initiated, and the average duration was 6.3 months. The exacerbation rate was 37.5% for breastfeeders compared with 31.5% for nonbreastfeeders. The average time of onset was similar—3.0 and 3.1 months, respectively. The exacerbation pattern was similar in breastfeeding and bottle feeding women and was not correlated with duration of breastfeeding.*

Patients may wish to start or resume therapy to decrease risks of exacerbation post partum. The medication utilized is glatiramer (Copaxone). It is a mixture of polymers of four amino acids—L-alanine, L-glutaminic acid, L-lysine, and L-tyrosine—and is similar to myelin.[88] It has a large molecular weight, so it does not pass into the milk, and minimal oral bioavailability, so it would not be absorbed by the infant. It metabolizes into basic amino acids, which are already present in human milk. The mother receives the drug daily by injection because of its absent oral uptake. It is thus considered appropriate for use during lactation.

---

*A protective effect of vitamin D intake on risk of developing MS has been confirmed in the Nurses Health Studies I and II involving more than 238,000 women. It is further hypothesized that vitamin D supplementation will postpone or delay MS progression. Postpartum progression of MS may be related to vitamin D need in lactation and not lactation itself. Munger KL, Zhang SM, O'Reilly E, et al: Vitamin D intake and incidence of multiple sclerosis. Neurology 62:60, 2004.

The relationship between the mode of feeding in infancy and MS development in later life was examined by Pisacane and associates.[197] Patients with MS were less likely than healthy control subjects to have been breastfed for a prolonged period. Of the 93 MS patients and 93 control subjects, 76% of controls and 55% of MS patients breastfed for 7 months or longer (odds ratio 0.38).

Counseling a woman with MS regarding pregnancy should include discussion of the postpartum statistics. Breastfeeding is not contraindicated but unfortunately does not appear to protect against exacerbations. It does allow a mother the opportunity to provide her infant with a special gift.

PSYCHOLOGICAL PROBLEMS WHILE BREASTFEEDING

Early works, including those of Hippocrates in the *Third Book of Epidemics* from the fourth century BC, described the "mental derangements" of women who recently delivered and were breastfeeding.[213] These disorders were considered to be etiologically linked to childbirth and lactation as a discrete disease entity. The women were described as febrile and toxic. With the introduction and liberal use of antibiotics, these symptoms disappeared. An extensive review by Seager[213] notes that after the middle of the 20th century, the incidence of infection and delirious reactions dropped precipitously. Some investigators now believe that no unique pattern of illness exists in puerperal compared with nonpuerperal women. Whereas childbearing might render certain predisposed women more vulnerable to an acute psychiatric episode, the pattern of mental illness in women in the perinatal period does not differ from that seen in other women or in men. The terms *puerperal disorders* and *postpartum psychoses* have been removed from the nomenclature.

What has often been suspected has now been proved by Eidelman and associates[63]: Postpartum women have transient deficits in cognitive function, particularly in memory function. Test results on the Wechsler Logical Memory Test and the Wechsler Visual Reproduction Test were compared with results of similar but nonpregnant childless women, third trimester, high-risk pregnant women, and fathers of newborns. Intrapartum analgesics mitigated the cognitive deficit. These results should be considered in planning postpartum education.

Interest in the temporal relationship of the postpartum period to psychiatric disorders continues, however, especially because the incidence of mental illness is lower in pregnant women than in matched nonpregnant women for age, race, and socioeconomic status. The highest incidence of hospitalization for mental problems in women 15 to 44 years of age is 1 to 2 months post partum.[213] Although the risk of mental illness increases 15-fold post partum, most reviews never consider the distinction between mothers who breastfeed and those who do not. Elaborate discussions of the influence of fluctuating hormone levels ignore lactation and the possible protective nature of the high levels of prolactin and oxytocin during lactation (Table 16-12).

The major clinical issue when significant mental illness occurs during breastfeeding is the question of medications. The use of *lithium* for bipolar disorders during lactation has been of concern because lithium does enter the milk, and lithium in any dosage has been considered a risk in an infant under 1 year of age. Infants have been reported to be hypotonic, flaccid, and "depressed" when the nursing mother is taking lithium, whereas others have remained asymptomatic. The AAP currently has placed lithium on its acceptable in lactation list, but each case should be reviewed individually.

Lithium is a heavy metal and has pharmacologically unique properties. It is a small molecule, which crosses the placenta and into milk. It is not protein bound and has a low volume of distribution. Milk/plasma ratios are 0.24 to 0.66. Levels in the breastfed infant are one third of maternal levels and the infant receives about 0.1 mEq/kg/day.[88] Toxic levels in the serum are 1.5 to 2.0 mEq/L. Lithium is excreted in the urine, so hydration is critical for the breastfeeding infant because renal clearance may be reduced in the neonate.[241]

Monitoring the infant is essential. Watch for symptoms of overdose, lethargy, hyptonia, and electrocardiographic changes. Blood levels can be quickly measured. There have been no controlled studies looking at the breastfeeding infant of a mother taking lithium.

In a study of 147 postpartum women 6 to 8 weeks after delivery of a normal, healthy infant, the Edinburgh, Montgomery-Asberg, and Raskin psychological scales were completed. Fifteen percent of women were depressed on all three scales.[71] Significant correlations were seen between depression ratings and salivary progesterone and prolactin. Progesterone was positively associated with depression in bottle feeding women and negatively associated in breastfeeding women. Prolactin levels were inappropriately low in depressed breastfeeders. The authors suggest management should be different for breastfeeding and bottle feeding women.[91]

Chlorpromazine or phenothiazine used in psychotic disorders appears in the milk in small amounts. Even at doses of 1200 mg, it does not appear to accumulate. Doses of 100 mg/day do not appear to cause symptoms in the infants. *Fluoxetine* (Prozac) appears in breast milk at one fourth to one fifth the levels in maternal plasma.[105] (See Chapter 11.)

Clinical experience with significantly depressed patients has shown that abrupt weaning from the breast may precipitate severe depression or even suicidal behavior. Whenever weaning is initiated in a woman with a psychiatric disorder, it should be initiated gradually and take place over 2 to 4 weeks or longer.

The impact of mental illness on the lactation process has been evaluated. Depressed mothers had more difficulties during breastfeeding than other women, and their attitudes were more negative. Depressed mothers complained more of too little milk or too much, of too much crying, of too little sleep, and of not getting enough support and help. It is difficult to determine cause and effect. Tamminen and Salmelin[227] noted frequent difficulties when they studied psychosomatic interaction between mother and infant during breastfeeding. They found that "depressed mothers in particular did not

TABLE 16-12 Timing of onset, symptoms, and incidence of maternal psychological problems

Problem	Onset	Duration	Symptoms	Incidence
The "blues" ("baby blues")	3–5 days post partum typically	A few days	Lability of mood; tearfulness; cognitive confusion; forgetfulness; headaches; depersonalization; negative feelings toward baby; restlessness; irritability; nightmares	30%–84%; mean incidence across studies 55.75%
Postpartum depression	Within first post partum year	At least 2 weeks, but usually longer	Tearfulness; despondency; feelings of inadequacy; numbness; suicidal ideation; sadness; reduced appetite and interest; insomnia; oversensitivity; feelings of helplessness and hopelessness; excessive dependency; anxiety and despair; irrational fears about infant or mother's health	27% had depressive symptoms at 3–5 months post partum 20% mild and 8% severe depression at 6 weeks post partum; 40% mild and 17% severe depression at 12 months post partum 12% major and minor depression combined at 9 weeks post partum 10%–14% experienced depression of clinical severity at 3 days post partum 6.1% with major depression and 10.4% with minor depression at 8 weeks post partum
Postpartum psychosis	Typically within 2–4 weeks or as late as 8 weeks post partum	Depends on diagnosis and treatment prescribed	Heightened or reduced motor activity; hallucinations; marked deviation in mood; severe depression, mania, or both; confusion; delirium	1–2 per 1000 post partum women

Modified from Kendall-Tackett KA, Kantor GK: Postpartum depression. In Sage Series in Clinical Nursing Research. Newbury Park, CA, Sage, 1993.

seem to understand that problems in nursing may be due to somatic rather than psychic reasons. Depressed mothers lacked satisfaction in the mother-infant relationship, failing to create reciprocity with their infant."

In assessing the relationship between infant-feeding method and maternal role adjustment at 1 month, studies find that women who breastfeed their infants have less anxiety and more mutuality, the adaptation of appropriate maternal behavior to the infant's state and behavioral cues and the ability to adjust mothering activities to the infant's needs.[227]

It is not possible from present knowledge to state definitely the impact of breastfeeding on the potential for mental illness in the mother, but breastfeeding clearly enhances mothering and mother-infant interaction and mutuality.[181] Under most circumstances, it is better to continue breastfeeding than to terminate it unnecessarily or prematurely.

Postpartum depression

Much has been written in the lay press about the "baby blues," and many mothers, predominantly primiparas, will admit to a few hours or a day of incredible emotional seesawing some time in the first week after delivery. Episodes in which a mother dissolves in tears when she has "so much to be thankful for" is the usual description. This is a transient state that has been attributed to the tremendous change in hormonal levels after the delivery of the placenta, although no studies confirm this belief. It is usually successfully treated with reassurance and rest. True postpartum depression does occur, however, and contrary to popular fantasy, it occurs in women who are breastfeeding but usually only in women with a problem before pregnancy (see Table 16-12).

The incidence of psychiatric disorders during pregnancy is remarkably lower than age-adjusted rates in the general population. Rates in the postpartum period, however, increase dramatically to 1 to 2 per 1000, with 50% to 75% involving affective disorders, 10% to 20% schizophrenic illness, 2% to 12% organic psychiatric disorders, and 12% anxiety disorders.[41] Studies of clinically depressed postpartum women reveal that two out of three have a major depression. In an extensive review of postpartum mental illness, Seager[213] noted that with the introduction and use of antibiotics in the mid-1950s, many symptoms, described as puerperal fever or milk fever, resulting in toxic-confusional or delirious behavior no longer are reported.

A growing number of investigators have been unable to demonstrate significant evidence for a unique pattern of mental illness in puerperal compared with nonpuerperal psychiatric disorders. Although childbearing might make a woman more vulnerable to psychiatric stress, the patterns of illness symptomatology, course, and outcome are no different from those of nonpuerperal women or males. The relative risk of serious psychiatric illness when it is immediately preceded by the event of childbirth is 15-fold.[123] Causal mechanisms, however, remain uncertain. Prevailing views support a concept of multifactorial causes or the summation of stresses. Factors of ambivalence or negative attitude toward pregnancy, primary role conflict, lack of emotional and practical support, and increased numbers of life events are all part of the picture.

The relationship between breastfeeding and depression was studied by Kumar and Robson[139] in mothers who totally breastfed and in those who totally bottle fed. No relationship was found between depression and feeding method. A prospective study following 103 women post partum recorded a 13% incidence of marked postnatal depressive illness and an additional 16% of minor depressive illness of at least 4 weeks' duration. No correlation was made with method of feeding until the mothers were asked about their feeding methods and oral contraceptive use in an attempt to determine the influence of hormones on depression. The authors speculated that the prolactin, estrogen, and progesterone levels would vary with the amount of breastfeeding, amount of other foods consumed by the baby, and amount of hormones taken in the form of contraceptives.[139] In this study the bottle feeders received estrogen and progesterone as contraceptives, but breastfeeders received only progesterone. Total breastfeeders who were not taking contraceptives were somewhat more likely to report depressive symptoms. Feelings of fatigue may have influenced this. The mothers least likely to be depressed were those who were likely to have normal hormonal levels, that is, partial breastfeeders not taking contraceptives. Clearly, breastfeeding women are not immune to postpartum depression.[50]

The impact of the mother's depression on her breastfeeding and nursing attitudes was reported by Tamminen and Salmeun[227] in a study of 119 healthy primiparous women using the Beck Depression Inventory (BDI) attitude scales and other questionnaires. Eight percent of the participants were clinically depressed, but 25% did not return the questionnaire, which is possibly more common in depressed subjects. Depressed mothers had more difficulty with breastfeeding.

In a continuing study as part of a larger study, qualitative analysis of mother-infant interactions during breastfeeding showed depressed mothers to be less able to sense the infant's needs, cues, and problems.[184] Furthermore, they saw the problems in psychological terms; that is, the infant did not want their milk or did not like it.[227] They did not understand that difficulties in breastfeeding could be somatic in nature. Depressed mothers achieved less satisfaction and mutual pleasure in breastfeeding.

The impact of postpartum depression on the emotional and cognitive development of infants was found to be adverse in several studies, because depressed mothers are typically unresponsive to infant cues, which are manifest with flat affect or withdrawal.[172] Postnatally depressed mothers are likely to be socially isolated and emotionally unsupported. The relationship among family life events, maternal depression, and teacher and maternal ratings of child behavior up to age 6 was reported. Both maternal depression and family life events made significant contributions to negative child behavior.[169]

The prevalence of postpartum depression varied between 7% and 14% over 34 weeks of postpartum monitoring of a cohort of 293 women studied by Pop and associates.[198] Peak incidence (14%) was at 10 weeks post partum; in other studies the peak incidence has been as high as 40%. The symptoms of postpartum and other depressions are similar; however, the puerperium is a time of unique stress.[195] Table 16-12 lists major findings related to the "baby blues," postpartum depression, and psychosis.[124] The cause is uncertain, with hormonal change being a continuing theme. Other perinatal events have been noted to trigger true depression, especially negative birth experiences. At-risk infants, including premature infants, sick infants, and those with disabilities, are often triggers for maternal depressive episodes.[198]

Breastfeeding can be a source of distress for many new mothers who do not have a good support system at home, especially when no one knowledgeable about breastfeeding is available. The La Leche League International has made an enormous difference with their mother-to-mother program. Isolation often contributes to the depression, and having telephone contact with a league mother or resources such as a lactation consultant to assess the breastfeeding progress may be therapeutic.

The physician and other health care team members should be sensitive to the subtle signs and vague symptoms. When a woman says, "I am overwhelmed," "Nothing will ever be the same," or "I feel hopeless or out of control," the other person must listen to her. When she is anxious or nervous or has insomnia, especially waking in the early morning when she is exhausted, the person must consider depression.[124] Use of a depression scale may be helpful when the mother answers general questions such as "How are things going?" with "Fine." A referral for professional psychiatric help or to a support program or hotline is the minimal response.

Studies support the recommendation that the primary care physician should identify the mother with depression using a simple inventory such as the 10-item Edinburgh Postnatal Depression Scale (EPDS) (Box 16-2). The EPDS has been validated and specifically designed for use by the primary

BOX 16-2   Edinburgh Postnatal Depression Scale (EPDS)

The Edinburgh Postnatal Depression Scale (EPDS) has been developed to assist primary care health professionals to detect mothers suffering from postnatal depression, a distressing disorder more prolonged than the "blues" (which occur in the first week after delivery) but less severe than puerperal psychosis.

Previous studies have shown that postnatal depression affects at least 10% of women and that many depressed mothers remain untreated. These mothers may cope with their baby and with household tasks, but their enjoyment of life is seriously affected, and it is possible that there are long-term effects on the family.

The EPDS was developed at health centers in Livingston and Edinburgh. It consists of 10 short statements. The mother underlines which of the four possible responses is closest to how she has been feeling during the past week. Most mothers complete the scale without difficulty in less than 5 minutes.

The validation study showed that mothers who scored above a threshold 12/13 were likely to be suffering from a depressive illness of varying severity. Nevertheless, the EPDS score should *not* override clinical judgment. A careful clinical assessment should be carried out to confirm the diagnosis. The scale indicates how the mother has felt *during the previous week*, and in doubtful cases it may be usefully repeated after 2 weeks. The scale will not detect mothers with anxiety neuroses, phobias, or personality disorders.

Instruction for users

1. The mother is asked to underline the response which comes closest to how she has been feeling in the previous 7 days.
2. All 10 items must be completed.
3. Care should be taken to avoid the possibility of the mother discussing her answers with others.
4. The mother should complete the scale herself, unless she has limited English or has difficulty with reading.
5. The EPDS may be used at 6–8 weeks to screen postnatal women. The child health clinic, postnatal check-up, or a home visit may provide suitable opportunities for its completion.

EDINBURGH POSTNATAL DEPRESSION SCALE (EPDS)
J. L. Cox, J. M. Holden, R. Sagovsky
Department of Psychiatry, University of Edinburgh

Name:

Address:

Baby's age:

As you have recently had a baby, we would like to know how you are feeling. Please **UNDERLINE** the answer which comes closest to how you have felt **IN THE PAST 7 DAYS**, not just how you feel today.

Here is an example, already completed.
I have felt happy:
   Yes, all the time
   <u>Yes, most of the time</u>
   No, not very often
   No, not at all
This would mean: "I have felt happy most of the time" during the past week. Please complete the other questions in the same way.

In the past 7 days:

1. I have been able to laugh and see the funny side of things
   As much as I always could
   Not quite so much now
   Definitely not so much now
   Not at all

2. I have looked forward with enjoyment to things
   As much as I ever did
   Rather less than I used to
   Definitely less than I used to
   Hardly at all

*3. I have blamed myself unnecessarily when things went wrong
   Yes, most of the time
   Yes, some of the time
   Not very often
   No, never

4. I have been anxious or worried for no good reason
   No, not at all
   Hardly ever

Continued

BOX 16-1   Edinburgh Postnatal Depression Scale (EPDS)—cont'd

Yes, sometimes

Yes, very often

*5. I have felt scared or panicky for no very good
reason

Yes, quite a lot

Yes, sometimes

No, not much

No, not at all

*6. Things have been getting on top of me

Yes, most of the time I haven't been able to cope
at all

Yes, sometimes I haven't been coping as well as
usual

No, most of the time I have coped quite well

No, I have been coping as well as ever

*7. I have been so unhappy that I have had difficulty
sleeping

Yes, most of the time

Yes, sometimes

Not very often

No, not at all

*8. I have felt sad or miserable

Yes, most of the time

Yes, quite often

Not very often

No, not at all

*9. I have been so unhappy that I have been crying

Yes, most of the time

Yes, quite often

Only occasionally

No, never

*10. The thought of harming myself has occurred to
me

Yes, quite often

Sometimes

Hardly ever

Never

J. L. Cox, MA, DM, FRCP(Edin), FRCPsych, Professor of Psychiatry, Department of Postgraduate Medicine, University of Keele. Consultant
Psychiatrist. City General Hospital, Stoke-on-Trent, formerly Senior Lecturer. Department of Psychiatry, University of Edinburgh (Correspondence to:
University of Keele, Thormburrow Drive, Hartshill, Stoke-on-Trent. Staffs S177QB): J. M. Holden, BSc., SRN, HVCert, Research Psychologist.
R. Sagovsky, MB, ChB, MRCPsych, Research Psychiatrist, Department of Psychiatry, University of Edinburgh.
*Response categories are scored 0, 1, 2, and 3 according to increased severity of the symptom.
Items marked with an asterisk are reverse-scored (i.e., 3, 2, 1, and 0). The total score is calculated by adding together the scores for each of the 10 items.
Users may reproduce the scale without further permission, providing they respect copyright (which remains with the British Journal of Psychiatry) by
quoting the names of the authors, the title, and the source of the paper in all reproduced copies (Br J Psychiatry 150:782, 1987).
From Cox JL, Holden JM, Sagovsky R: Detection of postnatal depression. Development of the 10-item Edinburgh Postnatal Depression Scale. Br J
Psychiatry 150:78, 1987.

health care team during routine health care visits
and it relies on self-reporting.[172]

In a study conducted in the well baby clinic of a
large teaching hospital,[40] universal screening for
postpartum depressive symptoms during the first
year of infant's life using the Edinburgh Postnatal
Depression Scale was administered at each well
baby visit: 46% of visits had a filed completed
form, 21% of completed forms had scores $\geq$ 10,
and 27% of all mothers who completed forms during the year had at least one score $\geq$ 10 (highly
depressive symptoms). These clients were referred
to social services. The authors concluded that pediatricians can play an active role in early detection
and referral for postpartum depression.[40]

Appearing in the same journal was a report
exploring maternal beliefs and perceptions about discussing the stress of parenting and symptoms of
depression with their child's pediatrician. The population was from five community-based practices. The
mothers were aware of the impact of their emotional
health on their infants. Many were reluctant to discuss parenting stress and depressive symptoms with
their child's pediatrician because of mistrust and fear
of judgment. They like open communication with
their pediatrician and are receptive to written materials about parenting stresses and depression from their
pediatrician but do not want verbal counsel.[94]

The role of infant factors in postnatal depression and mother-infant interactions was evaluated

in a large group of infants born to 188 primiparous women at risk for postnatal depression and a smaller group born to 43 mothers at low risk. By 8 weeks post partum, poor motor scores and high irritability in the infant were strongly predictive of maternal depression. These factors also predicted less optimal infant behavior in face-to-face interactions with the mother at 8 weeks.[167]

When the crying behaviors of 3- and 6-month-old infants were compared, infants of depressed mothers cried significantly more per day than infants of nondepressed mothers at 3 months but not at 6 months of age.[167]

A significant association exists with depressive disorder preceding the early cessation of breast-feeding, according to the results of two large, independent samples of puerperal women.[45] This was confirmed in a study in several large teaching centers examining the causes of early weaning pointing out the effect of maternal depression and lack of clinical support.[228] Other factors associated with early weaning were low social class, low education, and young age of the mother. Depression is more common in winter in the Northern Hemisphere, when days are short and darkness is prolonged. The relationship of lower prolactin levels in the winter is not understood.[191]

REFERENCES

1. ACR Bulletin. Accessed at www.acr.org/, March 2002.
2. Adamopoulos DA, Kapolla N: Prolactin concentration in milk and plasma of puerperal women and patients with galactorrhea. J Endocrinol Invest 7:273, 1984.
3. Alpert SE, Cormier AD: Normal electrolyte and protein content in milk from mothers with cystic fibrosis: An explanation for the initial report of elevated milk sodium concentration. J Pediatr 102:77, 1983.
4. American Academy of Pediatrics, Committee on Drugs: The transfer of drugs and other chemicals into human milk. Pediatrics 108:776, 2001.
5. Amir LH, Garland SM, Dennerstein L, et al: Candida albicans: Is it associated with nipple pain in lactating women? Gynecol Obstet Invest 41:30, 1996.
6. Anbazhagan R, Bartek J, Monaghan P, et al: Growth and development of the human infant breast. Am J Anat 192:407, 1991.
7. Andersen AN, Lund-Andersen C, Larsen JF, et al: Suppressed prolactin but normal neurophysin levels in cigarette smoking breast-feeding women. Clin Endocrinol 17:363, 1982.
8. Andersen AN, Tabor A: Prl, TSH, GH and LH responses to metoclopramide and breast-feeding in normal and hyperprolactinaemic women. Acta Endocrinol 100:177, 1982.
9. Andersen LW, Qvist T, Hertz J, et al: Concentrations of thiopentone in mature breast milk and colostrum following an induction dose. Acta Anaesthesiol Scand 31:30, 1987.
10. Angya JM, Gutierrez MA, Scopelitis E, et al: Hyperprolactinemia in primary Sjögren's syndrome. Arthritis Rheum 37:10, 1994.
11. Aono T, Aki T, Koike K, et al: Effect of sulpiride on poor puerperal lactation. Am J Obstet Gynecol 143:927, 1982.
12. Askmark H, Lundberg PO: Lactation headache—A new form of headache? Cephalalgia 9:119, 1989.
13. Asselin BL, Lawrence RA: Maternal disease as a consideration in lactation management. Clin Perinatol 14:71, 1987.
14. Baker PA, Schroeder D: Interpleural bupivacaine for postoperative pain during lactation. Anesth Analg 69:400, 1989.
15. Barrett JH, Brennan P, Fiddler M, et al: Breast-feeding and postpartum relapse in women with rheumatoid and inflammatory arthritis. Arthritis Rheum 43:1010, 2000.
16. Basso L, McCollum PT, Darling MRN, et al: A study of cholelithiasis during pregnancy and its relationship with age, parity, menarche, breastfeeding, dysmenorrhea, oral contraception and a maternal history of cholelithiasis. Surg Gynecol Obstet 175:41, 1992.
17. Benjamin F: Normal lactation and galactorrhea. Clin Obstet Gynecol 37:887, 1994.
18. Berens P, Newton ER: Breast masses during lactation and the role of the obstetrician in breastfeeding. ABM News Views 3(2):4, 1997.
19. Bernstein J, Patel N, Moszczynski Z, et al: Colostrum morphine concentrations following epidural administration. Anesth Analg 68:S23, 1989.
20. Bisdom CJW: Alcohol and nicotine poisoning in nurslings. Maandschrift Kindergenees Kunde Leyden 6:332, 1937.
21. Bitman J, Hamosh M, Hamosh P, et al: Milk composition and volume during the onset of lactation in a diabetic mother. Am J Clin Nutr 50:1364, 1989.
22. Black C: Update on Raynaud's phenomenon. Br J Hosp Med 52:555, 1994.
23. Bland KI, Romnell LJ: Congenital and acquired disturbances of breast development and growth. In Bland KI, Copeland EM III (eds): The Breast: Comprehensive

Management of Benign and Malignant Diseases. Philadelphia, WB Saunders, 1991.

24. Bode HH, Vanjonack K, Crawford JD: Mitigation of cretinism by breast feeding. Pediatrics 62:13, 1978.

25. Borch-Johnsen K, Joner G, Mandrup-Poulsen T, et al: Relation between breastfeeding and incidence rates of insulin-dependent diabetes mellitus. Lancet 2:1083, 1984.

26. Bossi L: Neonatal period including drug disposition in newborns: review of the literature. In Janz D, Dam M, Richens A, et al (eds): Epilepsy, Pregnancy, and the Child. New York, Raven, 1982.

27. Brennan P, Silman A: Breast-feeding and the onset of rheumatoid arthritis. Arthritis Rheum 37:808, 1994.

28. Briggs GG, Freeman RK, Yaffe S: Drugs in Pregnancy and Lactation, 3rd ed. Baltimore, Williams & Wilkins, 1990.

29. Brodie MJ: Management of epilepsy during pregnancy and lactation. Lancet 336:426, 1990.

30. Brun JG, Nilssen S, Kvale G: Breastfeeding, other reproductive factors and rheumatoid arthritis: A prospective study. Br J Rheumatol 34:542, 1995.

31. Buchanon TA, Unterman TG, Metzger BE: Medical management of diabetes in pregnancy. Clin Perinatol 12:625, 1985.

32. Buddhadeb D, Perry MC: Bilateral non-Hodgkin's lymphoma of the breast mimicking mastitis. South Med J 90:328, 1997.

33. Burns PE: Absence of lactation in a previously radiated breast. Int J Radiat Oncol Biol Phys 13:1603, 1987 (letter).

34. Burrow GN, Ferris TF: Medical Complications during Pregnancy. Philadelphia, WB Saunders, 1975.

35. Butte NF, Garza C, Burr R, et al: Milk composition of insulin-dependent diabetic women. J Pediatr Gastroenterol Nutr 6:936, 1987.

36. Bybee DE, Metzger BE, Freinkel N, et al: Amniotic fluid prolactin in the third trimester of pregnancies complicated by gestational or pregestational diabetes mellitus. Metabolism 39:714, 1990.

37. Campbell DA, Lorber MI, Sweeton JC, et al: Breastfeeding and maternal-donor renal allografts. Transplantation 37:340, 1984.

38. Cavallo MG, Fava D, Monetini L, et al: Cell-mediated immune response to β-casein in recent-onset insulin-dependent diabetes: Implications for disease pathogenesis. Lancet 348:926, 1996.

39. Chan SC, Birdsell DC, Gradeen CY: Detection of toluenediamines in the urine of a patient with polyurethane-covered breast implants. Clin Chem 37:756, 1991.

40. Chaudron LH, Szilagyi PG, Kitzman HJ, et al: Detection of postpartum depressive symptoms by screening at well-child visits. Pediatrics 113:551, 2004.

41. Coble PA, Day NL: The epidemiology of mental and emotional disorders during pregnancy and the postpartum period. In Cohen RL (ed): Psychiatric Consultation in Childbirth Setting. New York, Plenum, 1988.

42. Conner AE: Elevated levels of sodium and chloride in milk from mastitic breast. Pediatrics 63:910, 1979.

43. Consensus Meeting: Is "fibrocystic disease" of the breast precancerous? Arch Pathol Lab Med 110:171, 1986.

44. Cooper DS: Antithyroid drugs: to breastfeed or not to breastfeed. Am J Obstet Gynecol 157:234, 1987.

45. Cooper PJ, Murray L, Stein A: Psychological factors associated with the early termination of breastfeeding. J Psychosom Res 37:171, 1993.

46. Cordero L, Treuer SH, Landon MB, et al: Management of infants of diabetic mothers. Arch Pediatr Adolesc Med 152:249, 1998.

47. Coulam CB, Moyer TP, Jiang NS, et al: Breastfeeding after renal transplantation. Transplant Proc 14:605, 1982.

48. Counsilman JJ, Mackay EV: Cigarette smoking by pregnant women with particular reference to their past and subsequent breastfeeding behaviour. Aust NZ Obstet Gynecol 25:101, 1985.

49. Courtiss EH, Goldwyn RM: Breast sensation before and after plastic surgery. Plastic Reconstruct Surg 58:1, 1976.

50. Cox JL, Connor Y, Kendall RE: Prospective study of the psychiatric disorders of childbirth. Br J Psychiatry 140:111, 1982.

51. Dahlström A, Lundell B, Curvall M, et al: Nicotine and cotinine concentrations in the nursing mother and her infant. Acta Paediatr Scand 79:142, 1990.

52. David FC: Lactation following primary radiation therapy for carcinoma of the breast. Int J Radiat Oncol Biol Phys 11:1425, 1985.

53. Davidson JM, Katz AI, Lindheimer MD: Kidney disease and pregnancy: Obstetric outcome and long term renal prognosis. Clin Perinatol 12:497, 1985.

54. Davis MK: Breastfeeding and chronic disease in childhood and adolescence. Pediatr Clin North Am 48:125, 2001.

55. Dawson EK: A histological study of the normal mamma in relation to tumor growth. II. The mammary gland in pregnancy and lactation. Edinburgh Med J 42:569, 633, 1935.

56. Devereux WP: Acute puerperal mastitis. Am J Obstet Gynecol 108:78, 1970.

57. Diesing D, Axt-Fliedner R, Hornung D, et al: Granulomatous mastitis. Arch Gynecol Obstet 269:233, 2003.

58. Domino EF, Hornbach E, Demana T: The nicotine content of common vegetables. N Engl J Med 329:437, 1993.

59. Dosch HM, Becker DJ: Infant feeding and autoimmune diabetes. Adv Exp Med Biol 503:133, 2002.

60. Drinkwater BL, Chesnut CH: Bone density changes during pregnancy and lactation in active women: a longitudinal study. Bone Mineral 14:153, 1991.

61. Edwards JE Jr: Should all patients with candidemia be treated with antifungal agents? Clin Infect Dis 15:422, 1992 (editorial).

62. Eglash A: Vasospasm of the nipples. ABM News Views 2(1):1, 1996.

63. Eidelman AI, Hoffmann NW, Kaitz M: Cognitive deficits in women after childbirth. Obstet Gynecol 81:764, 1993.

64. Engelhart M: Clinical and physiological studies of Raynaud's phenomenon. Danish Med Bull 38:458, 1991.

65. Engels S: An investigation of the origin of the colostrum cells. J Anat 87:362, 1953.

66. Esbjorner E, Jarnerot G, Wranne L: Sulphasalazine and sulphapyridine serum levels in children of mothers treated with sulphasalazine during pregnancy and lactation. Acta Paediatr Scand 76:137, 1987.

67. Feilberg VL, Rosenborg D, Christensen CB, et al: Excretion of morphine in human breast milk. Acta Anaesthesiol Scand 33:426, 1989.

68. Ferguson JH: Silicone breast implants and neurologic disorders. Neurology 48:1504, 1997.

69. Ferris AM, Dalidowitz CK, Ingardia CM, et al: Lactation outcome in insulin-dependent diabetic women. J Am Diet Assoc 88:317, 1988.

70. Flores HC, Cromwell JW, Leventhal JR, et al: Does previous breastfeeding affect maternal donor renal allograft outcome? A single-institution experience. Transplant Proc 25:212, 1993.

71. Forbes GB, Barton LD, Nicholas DL, et al: Composition of milk produced by a mother with galactosemia. J Pediatr 113:90, 1988.

72. Fort P, Lanes R, Dahlem S, et al: Breastfeeding and insulin-dependent diabetes mellitus in children. J Am Coll Nutr 5:439, 1986.

73. Foxman B, D'Arcy H, Gillespie B, et al: Lactation mastitis: Occurrence and medical management among 946 breastfeeding women in the United States. Am J Epidemiol 155:103, 2002.

74. Frantz AG, Wilson JD: Endocrine disorders of the breast. In Wilson JD, Foster DW (eds): Textbook of Endocrinology, 7th ed. Philadelphia, WB Saunders, 1985.

75. Gabbe SG, Niebyl JR, Simpson JL (eds): Obstetrics: Normal Problem Pregnancies, 3rd ed. New York, Churchill Livingstone, 1996.

76. Gabby M, Kelly H: Use of metformin to incrase breast milk production in women with insulin resistance: Case series. ABM News Views 9:20, 2003.

77. Gagne MP, Leff EW, Jefferis SC: The breastfeeding experience of women with type I diabetes. Health Care Women Int 13:249, 1992.

78. Galgiani JN: Fluconazole, a new antifungal agent. Ann Intern Med 113:177, 1990.

79. Giampietro O, Ramacciotti C, Moggi G: Normoprolactinemic galactorrhea in a fertile woman with a copper intrauterine device (copper IUD). Acta Obstet Gynecol Scand 63:23, 1984.

80. Giesecke AH Jr, Rice LJ, Lipton JM: Alfentanil in colostrum. Anesthesiology 63:A284, 1985.

81. Ginsberg JS, Hirsh J: Thromboembolic disorders of pregnancy. In Reese EA, Hobbins JC, Mahoney MJ, et al (eds): Medicine of the Fetus and Mother. Philadelphia, JB Lippincott, 1992.

82. Glatthaar D, Whittall DE, Welborn TA, et al: Diabetes in western Australian children: Descriptive epidemiology. Med J Aust 148:117, 1988.

83. Gould BK, Randall RV, Kempers RD, et al: Galactorrhea. Springfield, IL, Thomas, 1974.

84. Greenwald JH, Dubin A, Cardon L: Hypomagnesemic tetany due to excessive lactation. Am J Med 35:854, 1963.

85. Gruber HE, Gutteridge DH, Baylink DJ: Osteoporosis associated with pregnancy and lactation: bone biopsy and skeletal features in three patients. Metab Bone Dis Rel Res 5:159, 1984.

86. Gupta R, Gupta AS, Duggal N: Tubercular mastitis. Int Surg 67:422, 1982.

87. Häkansson A, Cars H: Maternal cigarette smoking, breast-feeding and respiratory tract infections in infancy. Scand J Prim Health Care 9:115, 1991.

88. Hale TW: Medications and Mother's Milk, 10th ed. Amarillo, TX, Pharmasoft Publishing, 2002.

89. Hamosh M, Bitman J, Wood DL, et al: Human milk in cystic fibrosis: Composition and enzyme content. Pediatr Res 16:164A, 1982.

90. Hanson LA: The mammary gland as an immunological organ. Immunol Today 3:168, 1982.

91. Harris B, Johns S, Fung H, et al: The hormonal environment of postnatal depression. Br J Psychol 154:660, 1989.

92. Harris L, Morris SF, Freiberg A: Is breastfeeding possible after reduction mammoplasty? Plast Reconstr Surg 89:836, 1992.

93. Hattori N, Ishihara T, Ikekubo K, et al: Autoantibody to human prolactin in patients with idiopathic hyperprolactinemia. J Clin Endocrinol Metab 75:1226, 1992.

94. Heneghan AM, Mercer MB, DeLeone NL: Will mothers discuss parenting stress and depressive symptoms with their child's pediatrician? Pediatrics 113:460, 2004.

95. Higgins S, Haffty BG: Pregnancy and lactation after breast-conserving therapy for early stage breast cancer. Cancer 73:2175, 1994.

96. Hodnett DW, DeLuca HF, Jorgensen NA: Bone mineral loss during lactation occurs in absence of parathyroid tissue. Am J Physiol 262:E230, 1992.

97. Holmquist DG, Papanicolaou GN: The exfoliative cytology of the mammary gland during pregnancy and lactation. Ann NY Acad Sci 63:1422, 1956.

98. Hoover HC: Breast cancer during pregnancy and lactation. Surg Clin North Am 70:1151, 1990.

99. Hopkinson JM, Schanler RJ, Fraley JK, et al: Milk production by mothers of premature infants: Influence of cigarette smoking. Pediatrics 90:934, 1992.

100. Hornstein E, Skornick Y, Rozin R: The management of breast carcinoma in pregnancy and lactation. J Surg Oncol 21:179, 1982.

101. Humenick SS, Hill PD, Anderson MA: Breast engorgement: Patterns and selected outcomes. J Hum Lact 10:87, 1994.

102. Ikegami H, Aono T, Koizumi K, et al: Relationship between the methods of treatment for prolactinomas and the puerperal lactation. Fertil Steril 47:867, 1987.

103. Isbister C: Diabetes insipidus with a normal draught reflex. Med J Aust 43:234, 1956.

104. Isenberg DA, Black C: Raynaud's phenomenon, scleroderma, and overlap syndromes. Br Med J 310:795, 1995.

105. Isenberg KE: Excretion of fluoxetine in human breast milk. J Clin Psychiatry 51:169, 1990.

106. Jara LJ, Lavelle C, Espinoza LR: Does prolactin have a role in the pathogenesis of systemic lupus erythematosus? J Rheumatol 19:1333, 1992.

107. Jarrett RJ: Breastfeeding and diabetes. Lancet 2:1283, 1984 (letter).

108. Jensen RG, Ferris AM, Lammi-Keefe CJ: Cholesterol levels and the breastfeeding mom. JAMA 262:2092, 1989.

109. Jorgensen C, Maziad H, Bologna C, et al: Kinetics of prolactin release in rheumatoid arthritis. Clin Exp Rheumatol 13:705, 1995.

110. Jorgensen C, Picot MC, Bologna C, et al: Oral contraception, parity, breastfeeding, and severity of rheumatoid arthritis. Ann Rheum Dis 55:94, 1996.

111. Joselin EP, Root HF, White P, et al: The Treatment of Diabetes Mellitus. Philadelphia, Lea & Febiger, 1959.

112. Kahaleh B, Matucci-Cerinic M: Raynaud's phenomenon and scleroderma. Arthritis Rheum 38:1, 1995.

113. Kalache A, Vessey MP, McPherson K: Lactation and breast cancer. Br Med J 280:223, 1980.

114. Kamble TK, Ookalka DS: Lactation hypomagnesemia. Lancet 2:155, 1989.

115. Kamman E, Jones J: Hyperprolactinemia and headache. Am J Obstet Gynecol 145:668, 1983.

116. Kampmann J, Johansen K, Hansen JN, et al: Propylthiouracil in human milk. Lancet 1:736, 1980.

117. Kaneko S, Suzuki K, Sato T, et al: The problems of antiepileptic medication in the neonatal period: Is breastfeeding advisable? In Janz D, Dam M, Richens A, et al (eds): Epilepsy, Pregnancy, and the Child. New York, Raven, 1982.

118. Kapcala LP: Galactorrhea and thyrotoxicosis. Arch Intern Med 144:2349, 1984.

119. Karjalainen J, Martin JM, Knip M, et al: A bovine albumin peptide as a possible trigger of insulin-dependent diabetes mellitus. N Engl J Med 327:302, 1992.

120. Katz E, Adashi EY: Hyperprolactinemic disorders. Clin Obstet Gynecol 33:622, 1990.

121. Katzman DK, Wald ER: Staphylococcal scalded skin syndrome in a breastfed infant. Pediatr Infect Dis J 6:295, 1987.

122. Kelemen E, Szalay F, Peterfy M: Autoimmune (idiopathic) thrombocytopenic purpura in pregnancy and the newborn. Br J Obstet Gynecol 85:239, 1978 (letter).

123. Kendall RE, Wainwright S, Hailey A, et al: The influence of childbirth on psychiatric morbidity. Psychol Med 6:297, 1976.

124. Kendall-Tackett KA, Kantor GK: Postpartum Depression. Sage Series in Clinical Nursing Research. Newbury Park, CA, Sage, 1993.

125. Kessler DA: The basis of the FDA's decision on breast implants. N Engl J Med 326:1713, 1992.

126. Key TC, Resnik R, Dittrich HC, et al: Successful pregnancy after cardiac transplantation. Am J Obstet Gynecol 160:367, 1989.

127. King EB, Goodson WH III: Discharges and secretions of the nipple. In Bland KI, Copeland EM III (eds): The Breast: Comprehensive Management of Benign and Malignant Diseases. Philadelphia, WB Saunders, 1991.

128. Kira J-I, Harada M, Yamaguchi Y, et al: Hyperprolactinemia in multiple sclerosis. J Neurol Sci 102:61, 1991.

129. Klein J, Chitayat D, Koren G: Hair analysis as a market for fetal exposure to maternal smoking. N Engl J Med 328:66, 1993.

130. Kline TS, Kline IK: Breast: Guides to Clinical Aspiration Biopsy. New York/Tokyo, Igaku-Shoin Medical Publishers, 1989.

131. Kline TS, Lash SR: Nipple secretion in pregnancy: A cytologic and histologic study. Am J Clin Pathol 37:626, 1962.

132. Kline TS, Lash SR: The bleeding nipple of pregnancy and postpartum period: A cytologic and histologic study. Acta Cytol 8:336, 1964.

133. Kois WE, Campbell DA, Lorber MI, et al: Influence of breastfeeding on subsequent reactivity to a related renal allograft. J Surg Res 37:89, 1984.

134. Kossoy LR, Herbert CM, Wentz AC: Management of heart transplant recipients: Guidelines for the obstetrician-gynecologist. Am J Obstet Gynecol 159:490, 1988.

135. Kostraba JN, Cruickshanks KJ, Lawler-Heavner J, et al: Early exposure to cow's milk and solid foods in infancy, genetic predisposition, and risk of IDDM. Diabetes 42:288, 1993.

136. Kostraba JN, Steenkiste AR, Dorman JS, et al: Early infant diet and risk of IDDM in blacks and whites. Diabetes Care 15:626, 1992.

137. Kreipe RE, Lewand AG, Dukarm CP, et al: Outcome for patients with bulimia and breast hypertrophy after reduction mammaplasty. Arch Pediatr Adolesc Med 151:176, 1997.

138. Kulski JK, Smith M, Hartmann PE: Normal and caesarean section delivery and the initiation of lactation in women. Aust J Exp Biol Med Sci 59:405, 1981.

139. Kumar R, Robson K: Neurotic disorders during pregnancy and the puerperium: preliminary report of a prospective study of 119 primigravidae. In Sandler MJ (ed): Mental Illness in Pregnancy and the Puerperium. London, Oxford University Press, 1978.

140. Labrecque M, Marcoux S, Weber J-P, et al: Feeding and urine cotinine values in babies whose mothers smoke. Pediatrics 83:93, 1989.

141. Lafreniere R: Bloody nipple discharge during pregnancy: A rationale for conservative treatment. J Surg Oncol 43:228, 1990.

142. Lamberg BA, Ikonen E, Osterlund K, et al: Antithyroid treatment of maternal hyperthyroidism during lactation. Clin Endocrinol 21:81, 1984.

143. Lawlor-Smith LS, Lawlor-Smith CL: Raynaud's phenomenon of the nipple: A preventable cause of breastfeeding failure. Med J Aust 166:448, 1996.

144. Lawlor-Smith LS, Lawlor-Smith CL: Vasospasm of the nipple: A manifestation of Raynaud's phenomenon; case reports. Br Med J 314:644, 1997.

145. Lawrence R: Lactation, breastfeeding, infant care and mental illness. In Kuczmerczy AR, Reading AE (eds): Handbook of Behavioral Obstetrics and Gynecology. New York, Plenum, 1994.

146. Lee GF: Fine-needle aspiration of the breast: The outpatient management of breast lesions. Am J Obstet Gynecol 156:1532, 1987.

147. Leis HP: Management of nipple discharge. World J Surg 13:736, 1989.

148. Leis HP, Urban JA: The other breast. In Gallager HS (ed): The Breast. St Louis, Mosby, 1978.

149. Leppert PC, Howard FM: Primary Care for Women. Philadelphia, Lippincott-Raven, 1997.

150. Lindblad A, Mar Ahsál K: Influence of nicotine chewing gum on fetal blood flow. J Perinat Med 15:13, 1987.

151. Little RE, Lambert MD III, Worthington RB, et al: Maternal smoking during lactation: Relation to infant size at one year of age. Am J Epidemiol 140:544, 1994.

152. Lobato MF, Careche M, Ros M, et al: Effect of prolactin and glucocorticoids on P-enolpyruvate carboxykinase activity in liver and mammary gland from diabetic and lactating rats. Mol Cell Biochem 67:19, 1985.

153. Luck W, Nau H: Nicotine and cotinine concentrations in serum and urine of infants exposed via passive smoking or milk from smoking mothers. J Pediatr 107:816, 1985.

154. Luder E, Kaltan M, Tanzer-Torres G, et al: Current recommendations for breastfeeding in cystic fibrosis centers. Am J Dis Child 144:1153, 1990.

155. Lyon AJ: Effects of smoking on breast feeding. Arch Dis Child 58:378, 1983.

156. Magno R, Berlin A, Karlsson K, et al: Anesthesia for cesarean section. IV. Placental transfer and neonatal elimination of bupivacaine following epidural analgesia for elective cesarean section. Acta Anaesthesiol Scand 20:141, 1976.

157. Marasco L, Marmet C, Shell E: Polycystic ovary syndrome: A connection to insufficient milk supply? J Hum Lact 16:143, 2000.

158. Marshall BR, Hepper JK, Zirbel CC: Sporadic puerperal mastitis. JAMA 233:1377, 1975.

159. Martin JN, Morrison JC, Files YC: Autoimmune thrombocytopenic purpura: Current concepts and recommended practices. Am J Obstet Gynecol 150:86, 1984.

160. Matalon R, Michals K, Gleason L: Maternal PKU: Strategies for dietary treatment and monitoring compliance. Ann NY Acad Sci 477:223, 1986.

161. Matheson I, Aursnes I, Horgen M, et al: Bacteriological findings and clinical symptoms in relation to clinical outcome in puerperal mastitis. Acta Obstet Gynecol Scand 67:723, 1988.

162. Matheson I, Rivrud GN: The effect of smoking on lactation and infantile colic. JAMA 261:42, 1989.

163. Mayer EJ, Hamman RF, Gay EC, et al: Reduced risk of IDDM among breastfed children: The Colorado IDDM Registry. Diabetes 37:1625, 1988.

164. Meschengieser S, Lazzari MA: Breastfeeding in thrombocytopenic neonates secondary to maternal autoimmune thrombocytopenic purpura. Am J Obstet Gynecol 154:1166, 1986.

165. Metcalfe MA, Baum JD: Family characteristics and insulin dependent diabetes. Arch Dis Child 67:731, 1992.

166. Michael SH, Mueller DH: Impact of lactation on women with cystic fibrosis and their infants: A review of five cases. J Am Diet Assoc 94:159, 1994.

167. Milgrom J, Westley DJ, McCloud PI: Do infants of depressed mothers cry more than other infants? J Paediatr Child Health 31:218, 1995.

168. Montello JM, Darby MH, Faubel K, et al: Clotrimazole by thumb. N Engl J Med 301:1005, 1979.

169. Morrow-Tlucak M, Haude RH, Ernhart CB: Breastfeeding and cognitive development in the first two years of life. Soc Sci Med 26:635, 1988.

170. Moss TW: Gigantomastia with pregnancy. Arch Surg 96:27, 1968.

171. Mullins RJ, Russell A, McGrath GJ, et al: Breastfeeding anaphylaxis. Lancet 338:1279, 1991.

172. Murray L, Cooper PJ, Stein A: Postnatal depression and infant development: Emotional and cognitive development of infants may be adversely affected. Br Med J 302:978, 1991.

173. Murray L, Stanley C, Hooper R: The role of infant factors in postnatal depression and mother-infant interactions. Dev Med Child Neurol 38:109, 1996.

174. Muscari A, Volta U, Bonazzi C, et al: Association of serum IgA antibodies to milk antigens with severe atherosclerosis. Atherosclerosis 77:251, 1989.

175. Nahas GG: Marijuana. JAMA 233:79, 1975.

176. Nahas GG, Suciu-Foca N, Armand J-P, et al: Inhibition of cellular mediated immunity in marijuana smokers. Science 183:419, 1974.

177. Niebyl JR, Spence MR, Parmley TH: Sporadic (nonepidemic) puerperal mastitis. J Reprod Med 20:97, 1978.

178. Neifert M, DeMarzo S, Seacat J, et al: The influence of breast surgery, breast appearance and pregnancy-induced breast changes on lactation sufficiency as measured by infant weight gain. Birth 17:31, 1990.

179. Neifert MR, McDonough SL, Neville MC: Failure of lactogenesis associated with placental retention. Am J Obstet Gynecol 140:477, 1981.

180. Nelson LM, Franklin GM, Jones MC, et al: Risk of multiple sclerosis exacerbation during pregnancy and breastfeeding. JAMA 259:3441, 1988.

181. Newton N, Newton M: Psychologic aspects of lactation. N Engl J Med 277:1179, 1967.

182. Newton NR, Newton M: Relationship of ability to breast-feed and maternal attitudes toward breast feeding. Pediatrics 5:869, 1950.

183. Nigro G, Campea L, DeNovellis A, et al: Breastfeeding and insulin-dependent diabetes mellitus. Lancet 1:467, 1985.

184. Nordstrom UL, Dallas JH, Morton HG, et al: Mothering problems and child morbidity amongst "mothers with emotional disturbances." Acta Obstet Gynecol Scand 67:155, 1988.

185. O'Campo P, Brown H, Faden RR, et al: The impact of pregnancy on women's prenatal and postpartum smoking behavior. Am J Prev Med 8:8, 1992.

186. O'Hara MF, Page DL: Adenomas of the breast and ectopic breast under lactational influences. Hum Pathol 16:707, 1985.

187. Olsen A: Nursing under conditions of thirst or excessive ingestion of fluids. Acta Obstet Gynecol 20:313, 1940.

188. Opri F: Mammary mycoses. Chemotherapy 28(suppl): 561, 1982.

189. Osborne MP: Breast development and anatomy. In Harris JR, Hellman S, Henderson IC, et al (eds): Breast Diseases. Philadelphia, JB Lippincott, 1987.

190. Ostensen M: Treatment with immunosuppressive and disease modifying drugs during pregnancy and lactation. Am J Reprod Immunol 28:148, 1992.

191. Partonen T: Prolactin in winter depression. Med Hypotheses 43:163, 1994.

192. Paulus DD: Benign diseases of the breast. Radiol Clin North Am 21:27, 1983.

193. Pellegrini JR, Wagner RF Jr: Polythelia and associated conditions. Am Fam Physician 28:129, 1983.

194. Petrek JA: Abnormalities of the breast in pregnancy and lactation. In Harris JR, Lippman ME, Morrow M, et al (eds): Diseases of the Breast. Philadelphia, Lippincott-Raven, 1996.

195. Picazo O, Fernandez-Guasti A: Changes in experimental anxiety during pregnancy and lactation. Physiol Behav 54:295, 1993.

196. Pilnik S, Leis HP: Nipple discharge. In Gallager HS (ed): The Breast. St. Louis, Mosby, 1978.

197. Pisacane A, Impagliazzo N, Russo M, et al: Breastfeeding and multiple sclerosis. Br Med J 308:1411, 1994.

198. Pop VJM, Essed GGM, deGeus CA, et al: Prevalence of postpartum depression. Acta Obstet Gynecol Scand 72:354, 1993.

199. Prentice A, Prentice AM: Unilateral breast dysfunction in lactating Gambian women. Ann Trop Pediatr 4:19, 1984.

200. Prentice A, Prentice AM, Lamb WH: Mastitis in rural Gambian mothers and the protection of the breast by milk antimicrobial factors. Trans R Soc Trop Med Hyg 79:90, 1985.

201. Rennie J: Formula for diabetes? Sci Am 267:24, 1992.

202. Riordan J, Auerbach KG: Breastfeeding and Human Lactation, 2nd ed. Boston, Jones and Bartlett, 1998.

203. Rosato RR, Gimenez MS, Jahn GA: Effect of chronic thyroid hormone administration on pregnancy, lactogenesis and lactation in the rat. Acta Endocrinol (Copenh) 127:547, 1992.

204. Rudland PS: Histochemical organization and cellular composition of ductal buds in developing human breast: Evidence of cytochemical intermediate between epithelial and myoepithelial cells. J Histochem Cytochem 39:1471, 1991.

205. Russo IH, Russo J: Progestagens and mammary gland development: Differentiation versus carcinogenesis. Acta Endocrinol (Copenh) 125:7, 1991.

206. Ruvalcaba RHA: Stress-induced cessation of lactation. West J Med 146:228, 1987.

207. Said G, Patois E, Lellouch J: Infantile colic and parenteral smoking. Br Med J 289:660, 1984.

208. Sakakura T: New aspects of stroma-parenchyma relations in mammary gland differentiation. Int Rev Cytol 125:165, 1991.

209. Scanlon JW, Ostheimer GW, Lurie AO, et al: Neurobehavioral responses and drug concentrations in newborns after maternal epidural anesthesia with bupivacaine. Anesthesiology 45:400, 1976.

210. Schnur PL, Weinzweig J, Harris JB, et al: Silicon analysis of breast and periprosthetic capsular tissue from patients with saline or silicone gel breast implants. Plast Reconstr Surg 98:798, 1996.

211. Schulte-Hobein B, Schwartz-Bickenbach D, Abt S, et al: Cigarette smoke exposure and development of infants throughout the first year of life: Influence of passive smoking and nursing on nicotine levels in breastmilk and infant's urine. Acta Paediatr Scand 81:550, 1992.

212. Scott-Conner CEH, Schorr SJ: The diagnosis and management of breast problems during pregnancy and lactation. Am J Surg 170:401, 1995.

213. Seager CP: A controlled survey of postpartum mental illness. J Ment Sci 106:214, 1960.

214. Siemiatycki J, Colle E, Campbell S, et al: Case-control study of IDDM. Diabetes Care 12:209, 1989.

215. Silberstein SD: Headaches and women: treatment of the pregnant and lactating migraineur. Headache 33:533, 1993.

216. Sims CJ, Porter KB, Knuppel RA: Successful pregnancy after a liver transplant. Am J Obstet Gynecol 161:532, 1989.

217. Sirota L, Ferrera M, Lerer N, et al: Beta glucuronidase and hyperbilirubinemia in breastfed infants of diabetic mothers. Arch Dis Child 67:120, 1992.

218. Smith PK, Tamlin N, Robertson E: Breastmilk and cystic fibrosis. Med J Aust 157:283, 1992.

219. Snell NJC, Coysh HL, Snell BJ: Carpal tunnel syndrome presenting in the puerperium. Practitioner 224:191, 1980.

220. Sowers MF, Corton G, Shapiro B, et al: Changes in bone density with lactation. JAMA 269:3130, 1993.

221. Stein G: Headaches in the first postpartum week and their relationship to migraine. Headache 21:201, 1981.

222. Steiner G, Myher JJ, Kuksis A: Milk and plasma lipid composition in a lactating patient with type I hyperlipoproteinemia. Am J Clin Nutr 41:121, 1985.

223. Steldinger R, Luck W: Half lives of nicotine in milk of smoking mothers: Implications for nursing. J Perinat Med 16:261, 1988.

224. Surian M, Imbasciati E, Cosci P, et al: Glomerular disease and pregnancy. Nephron 36:101, 1984.

225. Synderman RK: Augmentation mammoplasty. In Gallager HS (ed): The Breast. St. Louis, Mosby, 1978.

226. Synderman RK: Reduction mammoplasty. In Gallager HS (ed): The Breast. St. Louis, Mosby, 1978.

227. Tamminen TM, Salmelin RK: Psychosomatic interaction between mother and infant during breastfeeding. Psychother Psychosom 56:78, 1991.

228. Taveras EM, Capra AM, Braveman PA, et al: Clinician support and psychosocial risk factors associated with breastfeeding discontinuation. Pediatrics 112:108, 2003.

229. Thomsen AC: Infectious mastitis and occurrence of antibody-coated bacteria in milk. Am J Obstet Gynecol 144:350, 1982.

230. Thomsen AC, Espersen T, Maigaard S: Course and treatment of milk stasis, noninfectious inflammation of the breast, and infectious mastitis in nursing women. Am J Obstet Gynecol 149:492, 1984.

231. Thomsen AC, Mogensen SC, Jepsen FL: Experimental mastitis in mice induced by coagulase-negative staphylococci isolated from cases of mastitis in nursing women. Acta Obstet Gynecol Scand 64:163, 1985.

232. VanHeerden JA, Gharib H, Jackson IT: Pseudohyperparathyroidism secondary to gigantic mammary hypertrophy. Arch Surg 123:80, 1988.

233. Varma SK, Collins M, Row A, et al: Thyroxine, tri-iodothyronine, and reverse tri-iodothyronine concentrations in human milk. J Pediatr 93:803, 1978.

234. Vio F, Salazar G, Infante C: Smoking during pregnancy and lactation and its effects on breastmilk volume. Am J Clin Nutr 54:1011, 1991.

235. Voegeli DR: Galactography. In Peters ME, Voegeli DR, Scanlon KA (eds): Breast Imaging. New York, Churchill Livingstone, 1989.

236. Vorherr H: The Breast: Morphology, Physiology, and Lactation. New York, Academic Press, 1974.

237. Walia HS, Abraham TK, Shaikh H: Fungal mastitis. Acta Chir Scand 153:133, 1987.

238. Wall VR: Breastfeeding and migraine headaches. J Hum Lact 8:209, 1992.

239. Wand JS: The natural history of carpal tunnel syndrome in lactation. J R Soc Med 82:349, 1989.

240. Wand JS: Carpal tunnel syndrome in pregnancy and lactation. J Hand Surg 15B:93, 1990.

241. Weiner CP, Buhimschi C: Drugs for pregnant and lactating women. Philadelphia, Churchill Livingstone, 2004.

242. Welch MJ, Phelps DL, Osher AB: Breastfeeding by a mother with cystic fibrosis. Pediatrics 67:664, 1981.

243. Whichelow MJ, Doddridge MC: Lactation in diabetic women. Br Med J 287:649, 1983.

244. White WB: Management of hypertension during lactation. Hypertension 6:297, 1984.

245. Williams JM, Auerbach KG, Jacobi A: Lateral epicondylitis (tennis elbow) in breastfeeding mothers. Clin Pediatr 28:42, 1989.

246. Wüst J: Streptococcus pneumoniae as an agent of mastitis. Eur J Clin Microbiol Infect Dis 14:156, 1995 (letter).

247. Woolridge MW: The "anatomy" of infant sucking. Midwifery 2:164, 1986.

248. Yagnik PM: Carpal tunnel syndrome in nursing mothers. South Med J 80:1468, 1987.

249. Zargar AH, Masoodi SR, Laway BA, et al: Familial puerperal alactogenesis: Possibility of a genetically transmitted isolated prolactin deficiency. Br J Obstet Gynecol 104:629, 1997.

17

Transmission of infectious diseases through breast milk and breastfeeding

ROBERT M. LAWRENCE

A large body of evidence clearly demonstrates the protective effects of breastfeeding and documents the transmission of specific infections to the infant through breast milk. The fear and anxiety that arise with the occurrence of any infectious disease are even greater in the situation of the breastfeeding mother-infant dyad. Uncertainty and lack of knowledge often lead to proscribing against breastfeeding out of fear, which then deprives the infant of the potential protective, nutritional, and emotional benefits of breastfeeding exactly at the time when they are most needed (see the dynamic nature of immunologic benefit, Chapter 5). Decisions concerning breastfeeding in the mother with an infectious illness should balance the potential benefits of breastfeeding versus the known or estimated risk of the infant acquiring a clinically significant infection via breastfeeding and the potential severity of the infection.

Documenting transmission of infection from mother to infant by breastfeeding requires not only the exclusion of other possible mechanisms of transmission but also the demonstration of the infectious agent in the breast milk and a subsequent clinically significant infection in the infant caused by a plausible infectious process. The first step is to establish the occurrence of a specific infection (clinically or immunologically evident) in the mother and demonstrate the persistence of the infectious agent in the mother such that it could still be transmitted to the infant. Isolation or identification of the infectious agent from the colostrum, breast milk, or an infectious lesion of the breast is important but not necessarily proof of transmission to the infant. Epidemiologic evidence of transmission must be considered, including identifying characteristics of the organism that relate an isolate from the infant to the maternal isolate. Infectious organisms can reach the breast milk either by secretion in the fluid or cellular components of breast milk or by contamination of the milk at the time of or after expression. A reasonable mechanism of infection via breast milk should be evident and proved through either animal or human studies. Demonstration of a subclinical or clinically evident infection in the infant should follow these outlined steps.

Exclusion of other possible mechanisms of transmission (exposure to the mother or other persons/animals via airborne, droplet, arthropod, or vector modes of transmission or through direct contact with other infectious fluids) would complete the confirmation of transmission of infection via breastfeeding. It is essential to exclude prenatal or perinatal transmission of infection to the fetus/infant, but doing this can often be difficult.

Clinical case reports or studies confirming the isolation of an infectious agent from the milk are important. To determine a reasonable estimate of the risk of infection via breast milk, larger epidemiologic studies are needed, comparing infection rates in breastfed infants versus formula fed infants, addressing the issues just identified. Timing of breastfeeding is important relative to the timing of maternal infection and to the presence of a pathogen in colostrum or breast milk. The duration of breastfeeding is another important variable to consider in the estimate of risk, because shedding of a pathogen in breast milk may be intermittent.

These considerations are only some of the variables to be taken into account, in general, to assess the risk of transmission of an infectious agent from mother to infant via breast milk or breastfeeding. Efforts to prove transmission of infection in a particular maternal-infant dyad can be just as difficult and must consider many of the same factors.

This chapter focuses on a discussion of specific, clinically relevant, infectious agents and diseases, with reasonable estimates of the risk of infection to the infant from breastfeeding. The basic tenet concerning breastfeeding and infection is that *breastfeeding is rarely contraindicated in maternal infection.* The few exceptions relate to specific infectious agents with strong evidence of transmission and to the association of the infant's illness with significant morbidity and mortality.

The risk or benefit of breastfeeding relative to immunization of the mother or infant is discussed for certain microorganisms. Chapter 11 addresses use of antimicrobial agents in the breastfeeding mother, and Chapter 5 reviews how breastfeeding may protect against infection. Chapter 21 addresses specific concerns relating to banked breast milk and includes standards developed by the Human Milk Banking Association of North America to guide the appropriate handling of banked human milk relative to possible infectious agents.

INFECTION CONTROL CONSIDERATIONS

Isolation precautions have undergone some revisions in terminology and conceptualization.[99] Understanding that the transmission of microorganisms can occur with a known infection and with unrecognized sources of infection, recommendations have been made for standard precautions to be applied to all patients to protect health care workers from potentially infectious body fluids. Additionally, precautions based on the predominant modes of transmission have been recommended to protect against infection through the airborne route, direct contact, or contact with droplets. Although these precautions are intended to be used in clinical situations to protect health care workers, they may be applied in certain situations to the mother-infant dyad to prevent transmission of infectious agents from one to the other or to other hospitalized mothers and infants. These precautions are useful most often when the mother and infant are still hospitalized. The use of such precautions within the home is not meant to limit breastfeeding. They are intended to allow breastfeeding in the majority of cases and to facilitate the continuation of breastfeeding with some additional safeguards in certain situations, after short temporary periods of stopping breastfeeding and when to safely use expressed breast milk (see Appendix E).

Standard precautions

Standard precautions include preventing contact with blood, all body fluids, secretions and excretions, nonintact skin, and mucous membranes by

(1) careful handwashing before and after every patient contact; (2) use of gloves when touching body fluids, nonintact skin, or mucous membranes or any items contaminated with body fluids (linens, equipment, devices, etc.); (3) use of nonsterile gowns to prevent contact of clothing with body fluids; (4) use of masks, eye protection, or face shields when splashing with body fluids is possible; and (5) appropriate disposal of these materials. Standard precautions should be applied to all patients regardless of actual or perceived risks. *The CDC (Centers for Disease Control and Prevention) does not consider breast milk a body fluid with infectious risks for such policies.*

In considering the breastfeeding infant-mother dyad and standard precautions, body fluids other than breast milk should be avoided, and only in specified situations should breast milk also be avoided. In general, clothing or a gown for the mother and bandages, if necessary, should prevent direct contact with nonintact skin or secretions. Avoiding infant contact with maternal mucous membranes requires mothers to be aware of and understand the risks and to make a conscious effort to avoid this type of contact. The use of gloves, gowns, and masks by the infant for protection is neither practical nor appropriate. The recommendations concerning the appropriateness of breastfeeding and breast milk are addressed for specific infectious agents throughout this chapter. Human immunodeficiency virus (HIV) infection is an example of one infection that can be prevented by the use of standard precautions, including avoiding breast milk and breastfeeding. The recommendations concerning breastfeeding and HIV and the various variables and considerations involved are discussed later.

Airborne Precautions

Airborne precautions are intended to prevent transmission via droplet nuclei (dried respiratory particles smaller than 5 μm that contain microorganisms and can remain suspended in the air for long periods) or dust particles containing microorganisms. Airborne precautions include the use of a private room with negative-air-pressure ventilation and masks at all times. In the case of pulmonary tuberculosis (TB), respiratory protective devices (requiring personal fitting and seal testing before use) should be worn. Airborne precautions are recommended with measles, varicella or disseminated zoster, and TB. Breastfeeding in the situation of these maternal infections is prohibited for the infectious period. This is to protect against airborne contact with the mother and to allow the infant to be fed the mother's expressed breast milk by another individual. The exception to allowing breast milk would be local involvement of the breast by varicella-zoster lesions or *Mycobacterium tuberculosis*, such that the milk becomes contaminated by the infectious agent.

Transmission via droplets occurs when an individual produces droplets that travel only a short distance in the air and then contact a new host's eyes, nose, mouth, or skin. The common mechanisms for producing droplets include coughing, sneezing, talking (singing or yelling), suctioning, intubation, nasogastric tube placement, and bronchoscopy. Droplet precautions include the use of a private room (preferred) and a mask if within 3 feet (0.9 m) of the patient, in addition to standard precautions applied to all patients. Droplet precautions are recommended for adenovirus, diphtheria, respiratory infections, *Haemophilus influenzae, Neisseria meningitidis* or invasive infection, influenza, mumps, mycoplasma, parvovirus, pertussis, plague (pneumonic), rubella, and streptococcal pharyngitis, pneumonia, or scarlet fever. The institution of droplet precautions with a breastfeeding mother who has these infections should be specified for each particular infection. This may require some period of separation for the infant and mother (for duration of the illness, for short-term or complete treatment of the mother, for the infectious period) with use of expressed breast milk for nutrition in the interim. Prophylactic treatment of the infant, maternal use of a mask during breastfeeding or close contact combined with meticulous handwashing, and the mother's avoidance of touching her mucous membranes may be adequate and reasonable with regard to certain infections.

Contact Precautions

Contact precautions are meant to prevent transmission of infection via direct contact (contact between the body surfaces of one individual with another) and indirect contact (contact of a susceptible host with an object contaminated with microorganisms from another individual). Contact precautions include cohorting or a private room, gloves and gowns at all times, and handwashing after removal of gown and gloves. Contact precautions are recommended for a long list of infections, such as diarrhea in diapered or incontinent patients with *Clostridium difficile* infection, *Escherichia coli* O157:H7, shigella, rotavirus, hepatitis A, respiratory illness with parainfluenza virus or respiratory syncytial virus, multidrug-resistant bacteria (e.g., enterococci, staphylococci, gram-negative organisms), enteroviral infections, cutaneous diphtheria, impetigo, herpes simplex virus infection, herpes zoster (disseminated or in immunocompromised individuals), pediculosis, scabies, *Staphylococcus aureus* skin infection, viral hemorrhagic fevers (e.g., Ebola, Lassa), conjunctivitis and abscesses, cellulitis, or decubiti that cannot be contained by dressings.[61] With regard to the breastfeeding infant-mother dyad, implementation of precautions for each of these infections in the mother requires meticulous attention to gowning and handwashing by the mother, as well as a specialized plan for each situation.

Each of these transmission-based precautions can be used together for organisms or illnesses that can be transmitted by more than one route. They should always be used in conjunction with standard precautions, which are recommended for all patients. The *Red Book: Report of the Committee on Infectious Diseases* by the American Academy of Pediatrics (AAP)[62] remains an excellent resource for infection control guidelines and recommendations to prevent transmission in specific situations and infections.

CLINICAL SYNDROMES AND CONDITIONS

Microorganisms produce a whole spectrum of clinical illnesses affecting the mother and infant. Many situations carry the risk of transmission of the involved organism from the mother to the infant, or vice versa; in general, however, the infant is at greater risk because of such factors as inoculum size and immature immune response. As always, the infection must be accurately diagnosed in a timely manner. Empiric therapy and initial infection control precautions should begin promptly, based on the clinical syndrome and the most likely etiologic agents. When dealing with a maternal infection, clarifying the possible modes of transmission and estimating the relative risk of transmission to the infant are essential first steps to decision making concerning the issues of isolating the mother from the infant and the appropriateness of continuing breastfeeding or providing expressed breast milk. Breastfeeding infrequently is contraindicated in specific maternal infections. Often the question of isolation and interruption of breastfeeding arises when symptoms of fever, pain, inflammation, or other manifestations of illness first develop in the mother and the diagnosis is still in doubt. A clinical judgment must be made as to the site of infection, probable organisms involved, possible or actual mechanisms of transmission of these organisms to the infant, estimated virulence of the organism, and likely susceptibility of the infant. Additionally, by the time the illness is clearly recognized or diagnosed in the mother, the infant has already been exposed. Given the dynamic nature of the immunologic benefits of breast milk, continuation of breastfeeding at the time of diagnosis or illness in the mother can provide the infant protection rather than continued exposure in most illnesses. Rarely is stopping breastfeeding necessary. Many situations associated with maternal fever do not require separation of the mother and infant, such as engorgement of the breasts, atelectasis, localized nonsuppurative phlebitis, or urinary tract infection (UTI).

Appendix E lists a number of clinical syndromes, conditions, and organisms that require infection control precautions in the hospital. This appendix also includes short lists of possible etiologic agents for these conditions and appropriate precautions and recommendations concerning breastfeeding for different scenarios or organisms. This chapter considers specific infectious agents that are very common, clinically significant, or of particular interest.

BACTERIAL INFECTIONS

Anthrax

Bacillus anthracis, a gram-positive, spore-forming rod, causes zoonotic disease world wide. Human infection typically occurs due to contact with animals or their products. Three forms of human disease occur: cutaneous anthrax (the most common), inhalation anthrax, and gastrointestinal disease (rare). Person-to-person transmission can occur as a result of discharge from cutaneous lesions, but there is no evidence of human-to-human transmission of inhalational anthrax. There is no evidence of transmission of anthrax via breast milk. Standard contact isolation is appropriate for hospitalized patients or patients with draining skin lesions.

The issue of anthrax as a biologic weapon has exaggerated its relative importance as a cause of human disease. The primary concerns regarding anthrax and breastfeeding are antimicrobial therapy or prophylaxis in breastfeeding mothers and the possibility that the infant and mother were exposed by intentional aerosolization of anthrax spores. The Centers for Disease Control and Prevention have published recommendations for treatment and prophylaxis in infants, children, and breastfeeding mothers.[47] Those recommendations include the use of ciprofloxacin, doxycycline, and amoxicillin as well as several other agents without discontinuing breastfeeding. There is little available information on ciprofloxacin and doxycycline in breast milk for the prolonged periods of therapy or prophylaxis (60 days) and their

possible effect on infant's teeth and bone/cartilage growth over that time period. Depending on the clinical situation and sensitivity testing of the identified anthrax strain, other agents can be substituted to complete the 60-day course. The AAP has approved the use of ciprofloxacin and doxycycline for breastfeeding women for short courses of therapy (less than several weeks).

Simultaneous exposure of the infant and mother could occur from primary aerosolization or from spores "contaminating" the local environment. In either case decontamination of the mother-infant dyad's environment should be considered.

Breastfeeding can continue during the mother's therapy for anthrax, as long as she is physically well. Open cutaneous lesions should be carefully covered and depending on the situation, simultaneous prophylaxis for the infant may be appropriate.

Botulism

Considerable justifiable concern has been expressed because of the reports of sudden infant death from botulism. Infant botulism is distinguished from food-borne botulism from improperly preserved food containing the toxin and from wound botulism from spores entering the wound. Infant botulism occurs when the spores of *Clostridium botulinum* germinate and multiply in the gut and produce the botulinal toxin in the gastrointestinal tract.[14] The toxin binds presynaptically at the neuromuscular junction, preventing acetylcholine release. The clinical picture is a descending, symmetric flaccid paralysis. Not every individual who has *C. botulinum* identified in the stool experiences a clinical illness. The age of the infant seems to relate to their susceptibility to illness. The illness is mainly in children younger than 12 months of age; the youngest patient described in the literature was 6 days old. Most children become ill between 6 weeks and 6 months of age. The onset of illness seems to occur earlier in formula fed infants compared with breastfed infants. When a previously healthy infant under 6 months of age develops constipation, then weakness and difficulty sucking, swallowing, crying, or breathing, botulism is a likely diagnosis. The organisms should be looked for in the stools, and electromyography (EMG) may or may not be helpful.

In a group reviewed by Arnon and associates,[16] 33 of 50 patients hospitalized in California were still being nursed at onset of the illness. A beneficial effect of human milk was observed in the difference in the mean age at onset, with breastfed infants being twice as old as formula fed infants with the disease. The breastfed infants' symptoms were milder. Breastfed infants receiving iron supplements developed the disease earlier than those who were breastfed but unsupplemented. Of the cases of sudden infant death from botulism, no infants were breastfed within 10 weeks of death. All were receiving iron-fortified formulas. In most cases, no specific food course of *C. botulinum* can be identified, but honey is the food most often implicated and corn syrup has been implicated in infants older than 2 months of age. Honey may contain botulism spores, which can germinate in the infant gut. However, botulin toxin has not been identified in honey. It has been recommended that honey not be given to infants under 12 months of age. This includes putting honey on a mother's nipples to initiate an infant's interest in suckling.

Arnon[15] reviewed the first 10 years of infant botulism monitoring worldwide. The disease has been reported from 41 of the 50 states and from eight countries on four continents. The relationship to breastfeeding and human milk is unclear. In general, the acid stools (pH 5.1 to 5.4) of human milk fed infants encourage *Bifidobacterium* species. Few facultative anaerobic bacteria, or clostridia, existing as spores, are present in breastfed infants. In contrast, formula fed infants have stool pHs ranging from 5.9 to 8.0, with few *bifidobacteria*, primarily gram-negative bacteria, especially coliforms and *Bacteroides* species. *C. botulinum* and toxin production declines with pH and usually stops below 4.6. Breast milk also contains the protective immunologic components.

The relationship between the introduction of solid foods or weaning in both formula fed and breastfed infants and the onset of botulism remains unclear. For the breastfed infant, the introduction of solid food may cause a major change in the gut with a rapid rise in the growth of enterobacteria and enterococci followed by progressive colonization by *Bacteroides* species, clostridia, and anaerobic streptococci. Feeding solids to formula fed infants minimally changes the gut flora as these organisms already predominate. Although more hospitalized infants have been breastfed, sudden-death victims are younger and have been formula fed, which supports the concept of immunologic protection in the gut of the breastfed infant.

Much work remains to understand this disease. Clinically, constipation, weakness, and hypotonicity in a previously healthy child constitute botulism until ruled out especially with recent dietary changes. At this time, no reason exists to suspect breastfeeding as a risk for infant botulism, and some evidence suggests a possible protective effect from breastfeeding. Breastfeeding should continue if botulism is suspected in the mother or infant.

Brucellosis

Brucella melitensis has been isolated in the milk of animals. Foods and animals represent the primary sources of infection in humans. Brucellosis demonstrates a broad spectrum of illness in humans, from subclinical to subacute to chronic illness with nonspecific signs of weakness, fever, malaise, body aches, fatigue, sweats, arthralgia, and lymphadenitis. In areas where the disease is enzootic, childhood illness has been described more frequently. The clinical manifestations in children are similar to those in adults.[167] Infection can occur during pregnancy, leading to abortion (infrequently), and can produce transplacental spread, causing neonatal infection (rarely). The transmission of *B. melitensis* through breast milk has been implicated in neonatal infection, although not proved.[167,168] Interruption of breastfeeding with breast pumping and discarding the milk to continue stimulation of milk production is appropriate; breastfeeding should then continue after an initial period of 48 to 72 hours of therapy in the mother. Acceptable medications for treating the mother while continuing breastfeeding include streptomycin, tetracycline, trimethoprim-sulfamethoxazole (TMP-SMX), and rifampin (see Appendix E).

Chlamydial infections

Chlamydial infection is the most frequent sexually transmitted disease (STD) in the United States and is a frequent cause of conjunctivitis and pneumonitis in the infant from perinatal infection. The major determinant of whether chlamydial infection occurs in the newborn is the prevalence rate of chlamydial infection of the cervix.[228] Specific chlamydial immunoglobulin A (IgA) has been found in colostrum and breast milk in a small number of postpartum women who were seropositive for *Chlamydia*. No information is available on the role of milk antibodies in protection against infection in the infant.[243] It is not believed that *Chlamydia* is transmitted via breast milk. Use of erythromycin or tetracycline to treat the mother and oral erythromycin and ophthalmic preparations of tetracyclines, erythromycin, or sulfonamides to treat suspected infection in the infant are appropriate during continued breastfeeding. Separating the infant from a mother with chlamydial infection or stopping breastfeeding is not indicated.

Diphtheria

Corynebacterium diphtheriae causes several forms of clinical disease, including membranous nasopharyngitis, obstructive laryngotracheitis, and cutaneous infection. Complications can include airway obstruction from membrane formation and toxin-mediated central nervous system (CNS) disease or myocarditis. The overall incidence of diphtheria has declined even though immunization does not prevent infection but does prevent severe disease from toxin production. Fewer than five cases are reported annually in the United States.

Transmission occurs via droplets or direct contact with contaminated secretions from the nose, throat, eye, or skin. Infection occurs in individuals whether they have been immunized or not, but infection in those not immunized is more severe and prolonged. As long as the skin of the breast is not involved, no risk of transmission exists via breast milk. No toxin-mediated disease from toxin transmitted through breast milk has been reported in an infant.

Breastfeeding, along with chemoprophylaxis and immunization of the infant, is appropriate in the absence of cutaneous breast involvement (see Appendix E).

Haemophilus influenzae

Haemophilus influenzae type B can cause severe invasive disease such as meningitis, sinusitis, pneumonia, epiglottitis, septic arthritis, pericarditis, and bacteremia. Shock can also occur. Since the increased utilization of the *H. influenzae* type B conjugate vaccines, invasive disease caused by *Haemophilus* has decreased dramatically, more than 95%, in the United States. Most invasive disease occurs in children 3 months to 3 years of age. Older children and adults rarely experience severe disease but do serve as sources of infection for young children. Children younger than 3 months of age seem to be protected because of passively acquired antibodies from the mother, and some additional benefit may be received from breast milk.

Transmission occurs through contact with respiratory secretions, and droplet precautions are protective. No evidence suggests transmission through breast milk or breastfeeding. There is evidence that breast milk limits the colonization of *H. influenzae* in the throat.[126]

In the rare case of maternal infection, an inadequately immunized infant in the household is an indication to provide rifampin prophylaxis and close observation for all household contacts, including the breastfeeding infant. Expressed breast milk can be given to the infant during the 24-hour separation after the mother's initiation of antimicrobial therapy, or if the mother's illness prevents breastfeeding, it can be reinitiated when the mother is able (see Appendix E).

Leprosy

Although uncommon in the United States, leprosy occurs throughout the world. This chronic disease presents with a spectrum of symptoms depending on the tissues involved (typically the skin, peripheral nerves, and mucous membranes of the upper respiratory tract) and the cellular immune response to the causative organism, *Mycobacterium leprae*. Transmission occurs through long-term contact with individuals with untreated or multibacillary (large numbers of organisms in the tissues) disease.

Leprosy is not a contraindication to breastfeeding, according to Jeliffe and Jeliffe.[138] The importance of breastfeeding and urgency of treatment are recognized by experts who treat the infant and mother early and simultaneously. No mother-infant contact is permitted except to breastfeed. Dapsone, rifampin, and clofazimine are typically and safely used for the infant and mother regardless of the method of feeding (see Appendix D).

Listeriosis

Listeriosis is a relatively uncommon infection that can have a broad range of manifestations. In immunocompetent individuals, including pregnant women, the infection can vary from being asymptomatic to presenting as an influenza-like illness, occasionally with gastrointestinal (GI) symptoms or back pain. Severe disease occurs more frequently in immunodeficient individuals or infants infected in the perinatal period (pneumonia, sepsis, meningitis, granulomatosis infantisepticum).

Although listeriosis during pregnancy may manifest as mild disease in the mother and is often difficult to recognize and diagnose, it is typically associated with stillbirth, abortion, and premature delivery. It is believed that transmission occurs through the transplacental hematogenous route, infecting the amniotic fluid, although ascending infection from the genital tract may occur.[83] Early and effective treatment of the mother can prevent fetal infection and sequelae.[140,165] Neonatal infection occurs as either early- or late-onset infection from transplacental spread late in pregnancy,

ascending infection during labor and delivery, infection during passage through the birth canal, or, rarely, during postnatal exposure.

No evidence in the literature suggests transmission of *Listeria* through breast milk. Treatment of the mother with ampicillin, penicillin, or TMP-SMX is not a contraindication to breastfeeding as long as the mother is well enough. Expressed colostrum or breast milk also can be given as long as the infant is able to feed orally. The management of lactation and feeding in neonatal listeriosis is conducted supportively, as it is in any situation in which the infant is extremely ill, beginning feeding with expressed milk or directly breastfeeding as soon as reasonable.

Meningococcal infections

Neisseria meningitidis most often causes severe invasive infections, including meningococcemia or meningitis often associated with fever and a rash and progressing to purpura, disseminated intravascular coagulation (DIC), shock, coma, and death.

Transmission occurs via respiratory droplets. Spread can occur from an infected, ill individual or from an asymptomatic carrier. Droplet precautions are recommended until 24 hours after initiation of effective therapy. Despite the frequent occurrence of bacteremia, no evidence indicates breast involvement or transmission through breast milk.

The risk of maternal infection to the infant after birth is from droplet exposure and exists whether the infant is breastfeeding or bottle feeding. In either case the exposed infant should receive chemoprophylaxis with rifampin, 10 mg/kg/dose every 12 hours for 2 days (5 mg/kg/dose for infants less than 1 month of age), or ceftriaxone, 125 mg intramuscularly (IM) once, for children less than 12 years of age. Close observation of the infant should continue for 7 days, and breastfeeding during and after prophylaxis is appropriate. The severity of maternal illness may prevent breastfeeding, but it can continue if the mother is able, once the mother and infant have begun receiving antibiotics for 24 hours. A period of separation from the index case for the first 24 hours of effective therapy is recommended; expressed breast milk can be given during this period.

Pertussis

Respiratory illness caused by *Bordetella pertussis* evolves in three stages: *catarrhal* (nasal discharge, congestion, increasing cough), *paroxysmal* (severe paroxysms of cough sometimes ending in an inspiratory whoop, i.e., whooping cough), and *convalescent* (gradual improvement in symptoms).

Transmission is via respiratory droplets. The greatest risk of transmission occurs in the catarrhal phase, often before the diagnosis of pertussis. The nasopharyngeal culture usually becomes negative after 5 days of antibiotic therapy. Chemoprophylaxis for all household contacts is routinely recommended. No evidence indicates transmission through breast milk, with similar risk to breastfed and bottle fed infants.

In the case of maternal infection with pertussis, chemoprophylaxis for all household contacts, regardless of age or immunization status, is indicated. In addition to chemoprophylaxis of the infant, close observation and subsequent immunization (in infants older than 6 weeks of age) are appropriate. Despite chemoprophylaxis, droplet precautions and separation of the mother and infant during the first 5 days of effective maternal antibiotic therapy are recommended. Expressed breast milk can be provided to the infant during this period.

Tuberculosis

The face of TB is changing throughout the world. In the United States the incidence of TB rose during 1986 through 1993 and has been declining since then.[40] Increased rates of TB were noted in adults between 25 and 45 years of age, and because these are the primary childbearing years, the risk of transmission to children increased.

Tuberculosis during pregnancy has always been a significant concern for patient and physician alike.[213] It is now clear that the course and prognosis of TB in pregnancy are less affected by the pregnancy and more determined by the location and extent of disease, as defined primarily by the chest radiograph, and by the susceptibility of the individual patient. Untreated TB in pregnancy is associated with maternal and infant mortality rates of 30% to 40%.[229] Effective therapy is crucial to the clinical outcome in both pregnant and nonpregnant women. TB during pregnancy rarely results in congenital TB.

Any individual in a high-risk group for TB should be screened with a tuberculin skin test (TST). No contraindication or altered responsiveness to the TST exists during pregnancy or breastfeeding. Interpretation of the TST should follow the most recent guidelines, using different sizes of induration in different-risk populations as cutoffs for a positive test, as proposed by the CDC.[43] Figure 17-1 outlines the evaluation and treatment of a pregnant woman with a positive TST.[249]

Treatment of active TB should begin as soon as the diagnosis is made, regardless of the fetus' gestational age, because the risk of disease to the mother and fetus clearly outweighs the risks of treatment. Isoniazid, rifampin, and ethambutol have been used safely in all three trimesters. Isoniazid and pyridoxine therapy during breastfeeding is safe, although the risk of hepatotoxicity in the mother may be a concern during the first 2 months post partum.[245]

Congenital TB is extremely rare if one considers that 7 to 8 million cases of TB occur each year worldwide and that less than 300 cases of congenital TB have been reported in the literature. As with other infectious diseases presenting in the perinatal period, distinguishing congenital infection from perinatal or postnatal TB in the infant can be difficult.

Postnatal TB infection in infancy typically presents with severe disease and extrapulmonary extension (meningitis, lymphadenopathy, and bone, liver, spleen involvement). Airborne transmission of TB to infants is the major mode of postnatal infection because of close and prolonged exposure in enclosed spaces, especially in their own household, to any adult with infectious pulmonary TB. Potential infectious sources could be the mother or any adult caregiver, such as babysitters, daycare workers, relatives, friends, neighbors, and even health care workers.

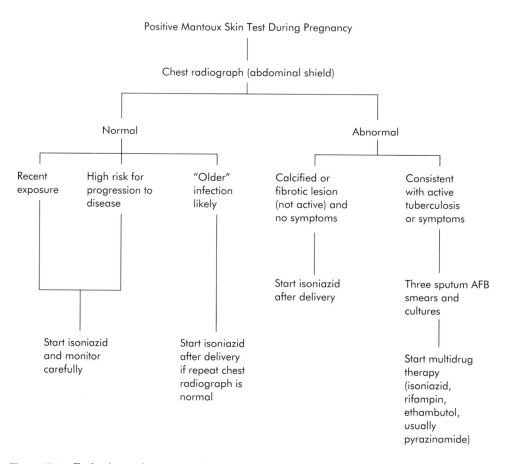

Figure 17-1. Evaluation and treatment of pregnant woman with positive tuberculin skin test. (From Starke JR: Tuberculosis, an old disease but a new threat to mother, fetus, and neonate. Clin Perinatol 24:107, 1997.)

The suspicion of TB infection or disease in a household with possible exposure of an infant is a highly anxiety-provoking situation (Fig. 17-2). Although protection of the infant from infection is foremost in everyone's mind, separation of the infant from the mother should be avoided when reasonable. Every situation is unique, and the best approach will vary according to the specifics of the case and accepted principles of TB management. The first step in caring for the potentially exposed infant is to determine accurately the true TB status of the suspected case (mother or household contact). This prompt evaluation should include a complete history (previous TB infection or disease, previous or ongoing TB treatment, TST status, symptoms suggestive of active TB, results of most recent chest radiograph, sputum smears, or cultures), physical examination, a TST if indicated, a new chest radiograph, and mycobacterial cultures and smears of any suspected sites of infection. All household contacts should be evaluated promptly, including history and TST with further evaluation as indicated.[43] Continued risk to the infant can occur from infectious household contacts who have not been effectively evaluated and treated.

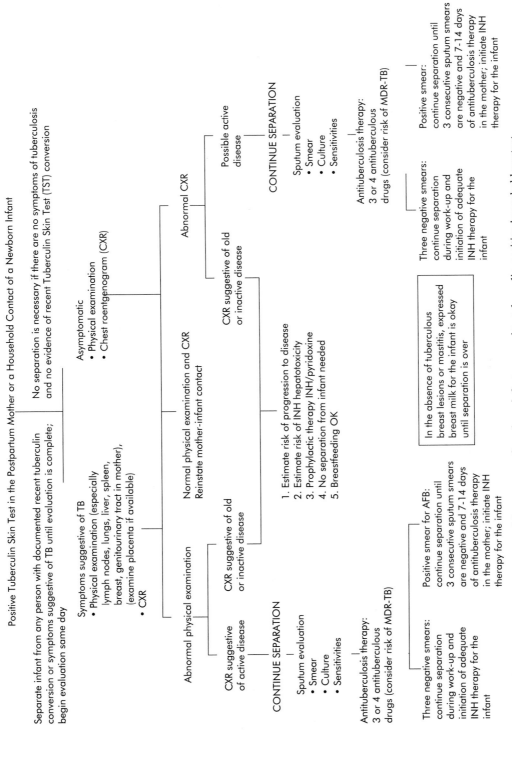

Figure 17-2. Management of newborn infant exposed to tuberculin-positive household contact.

The infant should be separated temporarily from the suspected source if symptoms suggest active disease or a recent TST documents conversion, and separation should continue until the results of the chest radiograph. Because of considerable variability in the course of illness and the concomitant infectious period, debate continues without adequate data about the appropriate period of separation.[178] This should be individualized given the specific situation. HIV testing and assessment of the risk of multidrug-resistant TB (MDR-TB) should be done in every case of active TB. Sensitivity testing should be done on every *Mycobacterium tuberculosis* isolate. Table 17-1 summarizes the management of the newborn infant whose mother (or other household contact) has TB.

Initiation of prophylactic isoniazid therapy in the infant has been demonstrated to be effective in preventing TB infection and disease in the infant. Therefore, continued separation of the infant and mother is unnecessary once therapy in both mother and child has begun.[75] The real risk to the infant requiring separation is from airborne transmission. Separation of the infant from a mother with active pulmonary TB is appropriate, regardless of the method of feeding. However, in many parts of the world, once therapy in the mother and prophylaxis with isoniazid in the infant has begun, the infant and mother are not separated. With or without separation, the mother and infant should continue to be closely observed throughout the course of maternal therapy to ensure good compliance with medication by both the mother and infant and to identify, early on, any symptoms in the infant suggestive of tuberculosis.

Tuberculous mastitis occurs very rarely in the United States but does occur occasionally in other parts of the world[110] and can lead to infection in the infant, frequently involving the tonsils. The mother usually has a single breast mass and associated axillary lymph node swelling and infrequently develops a draining sinus. TB of the breast can also present as a painless mass or edema. Involvement of the breast can occur with or without evidence of disease at other sites. Evaluation of extent of disease is appropriate, including lesion cultures by

needle aspiration, biopsy, or wedge resection and milk cultures. Therapy should be with multiple antituberculosis medications, but surgery should supplement this, as needed, to remove extensive necrotic tissue or a persistently draining sinus.[13] Neither breastfeeding nor breast milk feeding should be done until the lesion is healed, usually 2 weeks or more. Continued antituberculosis therapy for 6 months in the mother and isoniazid for the infant for 3 to 6 months is indicated.

In the absence of tuberculous breast infection in the mother, transmission of TB through breast milk has not been documented. Thus, even though temporary separation of the infant and mother may occur pending complete evaluation and initiation of adequate therapy in the mother and prophylactic isoniazid therapy (10 mg/kg/day as a single dose) in the infant, breast milk can be expressed and given to the infant during the short separation. Breastfeeding can safely continue whether the mother, infant, or both are receiving antituberculosis therapy. Antituberculosis medications (isoniazid, rifampin, pyrazinamide, aminoglycosides, ethambutol, ethionamide, *p*-aminosalicylic acid) have been safely used in infancy, and therefore the presence of these medications in smaller amounts in breast milk is not a contraindication to breastfeeding.

Although conflicting, reports indicate that breastfeeding by TST-positive mothers does influence the infant's response to bacille Calmette-Guérin (BCG) vaccine, the TST, and perhaps the *M. tuberculosis* bacillus. Despite efforts to identify either a soluble substance or specific cell fractions (gamma/delta T cells) in colostrum and breast milk that affect the infant's immune responsiveness, no unified theory explains the various reported changes and no evidence has identified a consistent, clinically significant effect.[27,146,202,231]

Staphylococcal infections

Staphylococcal infection in the neonate can be caused by either *Staphylococcus aureus* or coagulase-negative staphylococci (most often *Staphylococcus epidermidis*) and can manifest in a wide

TABLE 17-1 Management of newborn whose mother (or other household contact) has tuberculosis (TB)

Mother/infant status	Additional workup recommended[1]	Therapy for mother/contact	Therapy for infant	Separation[2]	Breast milk[3]	Breast-feeding[3]
1. TB infection, no disease[4]	None for mother/contact	Prophylactic[5]	None	No	Yes	Yes
2. TB infection: abnormal CXR not suggestive of active disease		Decide active vs. inactive disease				
a. Symptoms or physical findings suggestive of active TB	Aerosolized sputums (culture, smears)[6]	Active disease: empiric[5] Inactive disease: prophylactic[5]	Isoniazid[7] None	Yes No	Yes Yes	No[8] Yes
b. No symptoms or physical findings suggestive of active TB	Aerosolized sputums in select cases	Prophylactic[5]	None	No	Yes	Yes
3. TB infection: abnormal CXR suggestive of active disease	Aerosolized sputums (culture, smears)[6]	Empiric therapy[5]	Isoniazid[7]	Yes	Yes	No[8]
4. Active pulmonary TB: suspected multi/drug-resistant (MDR) TB	Aerosolized sputums (culture, smears)[6]	Consult TB specialist for best regimen[9]	Consult pediatric TB specialist[9] Consider bacille Calmette-Guérin (BCG) vaccine	Yes	Yes	No
5. TB disease: suspected mastitis[10]	Aerosolized sputums (culture, smears)[6]	Empiric[5]	Isoniazid[7]	Yes	No[11]	No

(Continued)

TABLE 17-1 Management of newborn whose mother (or other household contact) has tuberculosis (TB)—cont'd

	Perform/interpret CXR within 24 hours	Yes, until CXR interpreted (see a and b)	Yes	No
6. TB infection: status undetermined[12]				
a. Abnormal CXR not suggestive of active disease	Proceed as in 2	As in 2	As in 2	
b. Abnormal CXR suggestive of active disease	Proceed as in 3	As in 3	As in 3	

Notes:

1. Further workup should always include evaluation of TB status of all other household (or close) contacts by tuberculin skin testing (TST), review of symptoms, physical examination, and chest x-ray film (CXR). Sputum smears and cultures should be done as indicated.

2. Separation should occur until interpretation of CXR confirms absence of active disease, or with active disease, separation should continue until individual is no longer considered infectious: three negative consecutive sputum smears, adequate ongoing empiric therapy, and decreased fever, cough, and sputum production. *Separation* means in a different house or location, not simply separate rooms in a household. Duration of separation should be individualized for each case in consultation with TB specialist.

3. This assumes no evidence of breast involvement, suspected TB mastitis, or lesion (except in status 5, when breast involvement is considered). Risk to infant is via aerosolized bacteria in sputum from the lung. Expressed breast milk can be given even if separation of mother and infant is advised.

4. TST positive, no symptoms or physical findings suggestive of TB, negative CXR.

5. *Prophylactic therapy:* isoniazid 10 mg/kg/day, maximum 300 mg for 6 months; pyridoxine 25 to 50 mg/day for 6 months. *Empiric therapy:* standard 3- or 4-drug regimens for 2 months, and treatment should continue for total of 6 months with isoniazid and rifampin when organism is shown to be sensitive. Suspected MDR-TB requires consultation with TB specialist to select optimum empiric regimen and for ongoing monitoring of therapy and clinical response.

6. Sensitivity testing should be done on any positive culture.

7. Isoniazid 10 mg/kg/day for 3 to 9 months depending on mother's or contact's status; repeat TST at 3 months and obtain normal CXR in infant before stopping isoniazid. Before beginning therapy, workup of infant for congenital or active TB may be appropriate. This workup should be determined by clinical status of infant and suspected, potential risk. TST after 4 weeks of age, with CXR, complete blood count, and erythrocyte sedimentation rate. Liver function tests, cerebrospinal fluid analysis, gastric aspirates, sonography/computed tomography of liver/spleen, and chest if congenital TB is suspected.

8. Breastfeeding is proscribed when separation of mother and infant is indicated because of risk of aerosolized transmission of bacteria. Expressed breast milk given to infant via bottle is acceptable in absence of mastitis or breast lesions.

9. Consult with TB specialist about MDR-TB. Empiric therapy will be chosen based on the most recent culture sensitivities of index patient or perhaps suspected source case, if known, as well as medication toxicities and other factors.

10. TB mastitis usually involves a single breast with associated axillary lymph node swelling and, infrequently, a draining sinus tract. It can also present as a painless mass or edema of breast.

11. With suspected mastitis or breast lesion caused by TB, even breast milk is contraindicated, until lesion or mastitis heals, usually 2 weeks or more.

12. Patient has a documented, recent TST conversion but has not been completely evaluated. Evaluation should begin and be evaluated in less than 24 hours to minimize separation of this person from infant. Further workup should proceed as indicated by symptoms, physical findings, and CXR results.

Data from Committee on Infectious Diseases, American Academy of Pediatrics: *Red Book: Report of the Committee on Infectious Diseases*, 26th ed. Elk Grove Village, IL. The Academy, 2003.

range of illnesses. Localized infection can be impetigo, cellulitis, or wound infection, and invasive or suppurative disease includes sepsis, pneumonia, osteomyelitis, arthritis, and endocarditis. *S. aureus* requires only a small inoculum (10 to 250 organisms) to produce colonization in the newborn, most often of the nasal mucosa and umbilicus.[132] By the fifth day of life, 40% to 90% of the infants in the nursery will be colonized with *S. aureus*.[87] The organism is easily transmitted to others from mother, infant, family, or health care personnel through direct contact. Outbreaks in the nursery were common in the past. Mothers, infants, health care workers, and even contaminated, unpasteurized, banked breast milk were sources of infection.[205] Careful use of antibiotics, changes in nursery layout and procedures, standard precautions, and cohorting as needed have decreased the spread of *S. aureus* in nurseries. Now the occurrence of methicillin-resistant *S. aureus* (MRSA) is a more common problem, requiring cohorting and occasionally epidemiologic investigation and careful infection control intervention. Breastfeeding can continue during diagnosis and treatment of closed, minor staphylococcal infection in the mother along with standard precautions.

S. aureus is the most common cause of mastitis in lactating women. One case of *staphylococcal scalded skin syndrome* (SSS) was reported by Katzman and Wald[142] in an infant breastfed by a mother with a lesion on her areola that did not respond to ampicillin therapy for 14 days. Subsequently the infant developed conjunctivitis with *S. aureus*, which produced an exfoliative toxin, and a confluent erythematous rash without mucous membrane involvement or Nikolsky's sign. No attempt to identify the exfoliative toxin in the breast milk was made, and the breast milk was not cultured for *S. aureus*. The child responded to intravenous (IV) therapy with nafcillin. This emphasizes the importance of evaluating the mother and infant at the time of a suspected infection and the need for continued observation of the infant for evidence of a pyogenic infection or toxin-mediated disease, especially with breast lesions.

This case also raises the issue of when and how infants and mothers become colonized with *S. aureus* and what factors lead to illness and infection in each. Empiric therapy may be indicated depending on the infant's clinical status. For patients with major open lesions caused by *S. aureus* that cannot be fully contained, with MRSA, or with SSS, the CDC recommends contact precautions in addition to standard precautions for the duration of the illness. The concern is that staphylococci can be easily transmitted, colonization occurs, and potentially serious infection can occur later. With SSS the primary site of infection can be minimal (e.g., conjunctivitis, infection of a circumcision site), but a clinically significant amount of toxin can be produced and lead to severe disease in the infant. However, it seems reasonable that after initiating appropriate antistaphylococcal therapy for the mother for 24 hours, standard precautions and breastfeeding can be continued whether or not mastitis is present. Some individuals recommend bathing the mother and infant once with hexachlorophene to change the skin flora, but this does not address nasal carriage of *S. aureus*. With the current increasing prevalence of community-acquired MRSA various regimens for eradicating colonization with *Staphylococcus* have been proposed, although none have been proved highly efficacious in controlled trials. Usually these regimens include systemic therapy with one or two antimicrobial agents to which the organism is sensitive, topical antibiotics to both nares at least twice daily, and intermittent bathing with hexachlorophene or a similar agent. Often simultaneous treatment of all family members is recommended to eradicate colonization in the household. It is uncertain what role pets play in colonization of family members with *Staphylococcus aureus*. Evaluation of the infant's status at the time of decision making, continued close observation of the infant, and timely empiric therapy as needed in the infant are also appropriate. The mother and infant can room-in together, without contact with other mothers or infants until discharge.

Toxic shock syndrome (TSS) can result from *S. aureus* or *Streptococcus pyogenes* infection and probably from a variety of antigens produced by other organisms. TSS-1 has been identified as a "superantigen" affecting the T lymphocytes and other components of the immune response, producing an unregulated and excessive immune response and resulting in an overwhelming systemic clinical response. TSS has been reported in association with vaginal delivery, cesarean birth, mastitis, and other local infections in the mother. Mortality rate in the mother may be as high as 5%.

The case definition of staphylococcal TSS includes meeting all four major criteria: fever greater than 38.9° C, rash (diffuse macular erythroderma), hypotension, and desquamation (associated with subepidermal separation seen on skin biopsy). The definition also includes involvement of three or more organ systems (gastrointestinal, muscular, mucous membrane, renal, hepatic, hematologic, or central nervous system); negative titers for Rocky Mountain spotted fever, leptospirosis, and rubeola; and lack of isolation of *S. pyogenes* from any source or *S. aureus* from the cerebrospinal fluid (CSF).[232] A similar case definition has been proposed for streptococcal TSS.[281] Aggressive empiric antibiotic therapy against staphylococci and streptococci and careful supportive therapy are essential to decreasing illness and death. Oxacillin, nafcillin, first-generation cephalosporins, clindamycin, erythromycin, and vancomycin are all acceptable antibiotics, even for the breastfeeding mother. The severity of illness in the mother may preclude breastfeeding, but it can be reinitiated when the mother is improving and wants to restart. Standard precautions, but allowing breastfeeding, are recommended.

Staphylococcal enterotoxin F (SEF) has been identified in breast milk specimens collected on days 5, 8, and 11 from a mother who developed TSS at 22 hours post partum.[269] *S. aureus* that produced SEF was isolated from the mother's vagina but not from breast milk. The infant and mother lacked significant antibody against SEF in their sera. The infant remained healthy beyond 60 days of follow-up. SEF is pepsin inactivated at pH 4.5 and therefore is probably destroyed in the stomach environment and presents little or no risk to the breastfeeding infant.[25] Breastfeeding can continue if the mother is able.

Coagulase-negative staphylococcal infection (S. epidermidis is the predominant isolate) produces minimal disease in healthy, full-term infants but is a significant problem in hospitalized or premature infants. Factors associated with increased risk of this infection include prematurity, high colonization rates in specific nurseries, invasive therapies (e.g., IV lines, chest tubes, intubation), and antibiotic use. Illness produced by coagulase-negative staphylococci can be invasive and severe in high-risk neonates, but rarely in mothers. At 2 weeks of age, for infants still in the nursery, *S. epidermidis* is a frequent colonizing organism at multiple sites, with colonization rates as high as 75% to 100%. Serious infections with coagulase-negative staphylococci (e.g., abscesses, IV line infection, bacteremia/sepsis, endocarditis, osteomyelitis) require IV therapy. Many strains are resistant to penicillin and the semisynthetic penicillins, so sensitivity testing is essential. Empiric or definitive therapy may require treatment with vancomycin, gentamicin, rifampin, teicoplanin, linezolid, or combinations of these for synergistic activity. Transmission of infection in association with breastfeeding appears to be no more common than with bottle feeding. Infection control includes contact and standard precautions, as with *S. aureus*. Occasionally, during presumed outbreaks, careful epidemiologic surveillance may be required, including cohorting, limiting overcrowding and understaffing, surveillance cultures of infants and nursery personnel, reemphasis of meticulous infection control techniques for all individuals entering the nursery, and rarely, removal of colonized personnel from direct infant contact.

Streptococcal infections
Group A

Streptococcus pyogenes (β-hemolytic group A *Streptococcus* [GAS]) is a common cause of skin and throat infections in children, producing pharyngitis, cellulitis, and impetigo. Illnesses produced by GAS can be classified in three categories: (1) impetigo, cellulitis, or pharyngitis without invasion or complication; (2) severe invasive infection with bacteremia, necrotizing fasciitis, myositis, or systemic illness (e.g., streptococcal TSS); and (3) autoimmune-mediated phenomena, including acute rheumatic fever and acute glomerulonephritis. GAS can also cause puerperal sepsis, endometritis, and neonatal omphalitis. Significant morbidity and mortality rates are associated with invasive GAS infection; mortality rate is approximately 20% to 50%, with almost half the survivors requiring extensive tissue débridement or amputation.[218] Infants are not at risk for the autoimmune sequelae of GAS (rheumatic fever or poststreptococcal glomerulonephritis). Transmission is through direct contact (rarely indirect contact) and droplet spread. Outbreaks of GAS in the nursery are rare, unlike with staphylococcal infections. Either mother or infant can be initially colonized with GAS and transmit it to the other.

In the situation of maternal illness (extensive cellulitis, necrotizing fasciitis, myositis, pneumonia, TSS, mastitis), it is appropriate to separate the mother and infant until effective therapy (penicillin, ampicillin, cephalosporins, erythromycin) has been given for 24 hours. Breastfeeding should also be suspended and may resume after 24 hours of therapy.

Group B

Group B Streptococcus (GBS, *S. agalactiae*) is a significant cause of perinatal bacterial infection. In parturient women, infection can lead to asymptomatic bacteriuria, UTI (often associated with premature birth), endometritis, or amnionitis. In infants, infection usually occurs between birth and 3 months of age (1 to 4 cases per 1000 live births). It is routinely classified by the time of onset of illness in the infant: early onset (0 to 7 days, majority less than 24 hours) and late onset (7 to 90 days, generally less than 4 weeks). Infants may develop sepsis, pneumonia, meningitis, osteomyelitis, arthritis, or cellulitis. Early-onset GBS disease is often fulminant, presenting as sepsis or pneumonia with respiratory failure. Almost three quarters of neonatal disease is early onset. Type III is the most common serotype causing disease.

Transmission is believed to occur in utero and during delivery. Colonization rates of mothers and infants have varied between 5% and 35%. Postpartum transmission is thought to be uncommon, although it has been documented. Risk factors for early-onset GBS disease include delivery before 37 weeks' gestation, rupture of membranes for longer than 18 hours before delivery, intrapartum fever, heavy maternal colonization with GBS, or low concentrations of anti-GBS capsular antibody in maternal sera.[62,63] The common occurrence of severe GBS disease before 24 hours of age in the neonate has lead to prevention strategies. Revised guidelines developed by the AAP Committees on Infectious Diseases and on the Fetus and Newborn[63] have tried to combine various variables for increased risk of GBS infection (prenatal colonization with GBS, obstetric and neonatal risk factors for early-onset disease) and provide intrapartum prophylaxis to those at high risk (Fig. 17-3).

Late-onset GBS disease is thought to be the result of transmission during delivery or in the postnatal period from maternal, hospital, or community sources. Dillon and associates[73] demonstrated that 10 of 21 infants with late-onset disease were colonized at birth, but the source of colonization was unidentified in the others. Gardner and associates[97] showed that only 4.3% of 46 children who were culture negative for GBS at discharge from the hospital had acquired GBS by 2 months of age. Anthony and associates[12] noted that many infants are colonized with GBS, but the actual attack rate for GBS disease is low and difficult to predict.

Acquisition of GBS through breast milk or breastfeeding is rare. Three cases of late-onset GBS disease associated with GBS in the maternal milk have been reported.[146,230] Two of the three mothers had bilateral mastitis, and the third was asymptomatic. It was not clear when colonization of the infants occurred or when infection or disease began. The authors discussed the possibility that the infants were originally colonized during delivery, subsequently colonized the mothers' breasts during breastfeeding, and then became reinfected at a later time. Butter and DeMoor[38] showed that infants initially colonized on their heads at birth

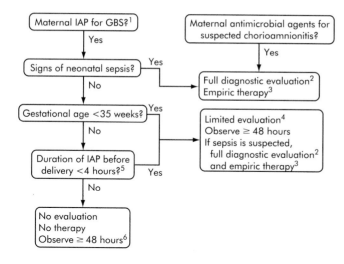

¹ If no maternal IAP for GBS was administered despite an indication being present, data are insufficient on which to recommend a single management strategy.

² Includes complete blood cell (CBC) count with differential, blood culture, and chest radiograph if respiratory abnormalities are present. When signs of sepsis are present, a lumbar puncture, if feasible, should be performed.

³ Duration of therapy varies depending on results of blood culture, cerebrospinal fluid findings (if obtained), and the clinical course of the infant. If laboratory results and clinical course do not indicate bacterial infection, duration may be as short as 48 hours.

⁴ CBC including WBC count with differential and blood culture.

⁵ Applies only to penicillin, ampicillin, or cefazolin and assumes recommended dosing regimens.

⁶ A healthy-appearing infant who was ≥38 weeks' gestation at delivery and whose mother received ≥4 hours of IAP before delivery may be discharged home after 24 hours if other discharge criteria have been met and a person able to comply fully with instructions for home observation will be present. If any one of these conditions is not met, the infant should be observed in the hospital for at least 48 hours and until criteria for discharge are achieved.

Figure 17-3. Empiric management of neonate born to mother who received intrapartum antimicrobial prophylaxis (IAP) for prevention of early-onset group B streptococcal (GBS) disease. CBC, complete blood count; CSF, cerebrospinal fluid. This algorithm is not an exclusive course of management. Variations that incorporate individual circumstances or institutional preferences may be appropriate. (From Committee on Infectious Diseases, American Academy of Pediatrics: Red Book Report of the Committee on Infectious Disease, 26th ed. Elk Grove, Ill, American Academy of Pediatrics, 2003, p 590.

had GBS cultured from their throat, nose, or umbilicus 8 days later. Whenever they cultured GBS from the nipples of mothers, the authors also found it in the nose or throat of the infants.

When a breastfed infant develops late-onset GBS disease, it is appropriate to culture the milk and treat the mother to prevent reinfection if the milk is culture positive for GBS, with or without clinical evidence of mastitis. There are rare reports of reinfection of the infant. Eradication of GBS colonization in the infant or the mother may be difficult with amoxicillin or rifampin. Breastfeeding can continue depending on the infant's ability to feed during GBS disease. Routine culturing of infants or breast milk to detect colonization is not recommended or useful. (See Chapter 16 for management of mastitis in the mother.) A mother or infant colo-

nized or infected with GBS should be managed with standard precautions[62] while in the hospital. GBS endometritis in the mother necessitates separation of mother and infant for the first 24 hours of the mother's therapy, but expressed breast milk can be given to the infant during the separation. Timely evaluation of the infant for infection or illness and empiric therapy for GBS in the infant are appropriate until the child has remained well and cultures are subsequently negative at 72 hours. Occasionally, epidemiologic investigation in hospital will utilize culturing to detect a source of late-onset GBS disease in the nursery. This can be useful when more than one case of late-onset disease is detected with the same serotype. Cohorting in such a situation may be appropriate, but prophylactic therapy to eradicate colonization is impractical. Unlike GAS infection, GBS infection in nurseries has not been reported to cause outbreaks.

Gonococcal infections

Maternal infection with *Neisseria gonorrhoeae* can produce a large spectrum of illness ranging from uncomplicated vulvovaginitis, proctitis, pharyngitis, conjunctivitis, or more severe and invasive disease, including pelvic inflammatory disease (PID), meningitis, endocarditis, or disseminated gonococcal infection. The risk of transmission from the mother to the infant occurs mainly during delivery in the passage through the infected birth canal and occasionally from postpartum contact with the mother (or her partner). There is negligible risk of transmission from breast milk, and *N. gonorrhoeae* does not seem to cause local infection of the breast. Infection in the neonate is most often ophthalmia neonatorum and less often a scalp abscess or disseminated infection. Mothers with presumed or documented gonorrhea should be reevaluated for other STDs, especially *Chlamydia trachomatis* and syphilis, because some therapies for gonorrhea are not adequate for either of these infections.

With the definitive identification of gonorrhea in the mother, empiric therapy should begin immediately, and the mother should be separated from the infant until completion of 24 hours of adequate therapy. Treatment of the mother with ceftriaxone, cefixime, penicillin, or erythromycin is without significant risk to the infant. Single-dose treatment with spectinomycin, ciprofloxacin, ofloxacin, or azithromycin has not been adequately studied but would presumably be safe for the infant given the 24-hour separation and a delay in breastfeeding without giving the infant the expressed breast milk (pump and discard). Doxycycline use in the nursing mother is not recommended.

Careful preventive therapy for ophthalmia neonatorum should be provided, and close observation of the infant should continue for 2 to 7 days, the usual incubation period. Empiric or definitive therapy against *N. gonorrhoeae* may be necessary depending on the infant's clinical status and should be chosen on the basis of the maternal isolate's sensitivity pattern. The mother should not handle other infants until 24 hours of adequate therapy, and the infant should be separated from the rest of the nursery population, with or without breastfeeding.

VIRAL INFECTIONS

Arboviruses

Arboviruses were originally a large collection of viruses grouped together because of the common mode of transmission through arthropods. They have now been reclassified into several different families: Bunyaviridae, Togaviridae, Flaviviridae, Reoviridae, and others. They include more than 30 human pathogens.

These organisms primarily produce either CNS infections (encephalitis, meningoencephalitis) or undifferentiated illnesses associated with fever and rash, severe hemorrhagic manifestations, and involvement of other organs (hepatitis, myalgia, polyarthritis). Infection with this array of viruses may also be asymptomatic and subclinical, although how often this occurs is uncertain. Some of the notable human pathogens include Bunyaviridae (California serogroup viruses), Hantavirus, Hantaan virus, Phlebovirus (Rift Valley fever), Nairovirus (Crimean-Congo hemorrhagic fever [CCHF]), Alphavirus (western, eastern, and Venezuelan equine encephalomyelitis viruses), Flavivirus (St. Louis encephalitis virus, Japanese encephalitis virus, dengue viruses, yellow fever virus, tick-borne encephalitis viruses), and Orbivirus (Colorado tick fever). Other than for CCHF and for reported cases of Colorado tick fever associated with transfusion, direct person-to-person spread does not seem to occur.

No evidence indicates that these organisms can be transmitted through breast milk. Standard precautions are sufficient. With any of these infections in a breastfeeding mother, the severity of the illness may determine the mother's ability to continue breastfeeding. Providing the infant with expressed breast milk is acceptable.

In general, treatment for these illnesses is supportive. However, ribavirin appears to decrease the severity of and mortality from Hantavirus pulmonary syndrome, hemorrhagic fever with renal failure, and CCHF. Ribavirin has been described as teratogenic in various animal species and is contraindicated in pregnant women. No information is available concerning ribavirin in breast milk, with little information available on the use of IV or oral ribavirin in infants.

Arenaviruses

Arenaviruses are single-stranded ribonucleic acid (RNA) viruses that infect rodents and are acquired by humans through the rodents. The six major human pathogens in this group are (1) lymphocytic choriomeningitis virus (LCMV), (2) Lassa fever virus, (3) Junin virus (Argentine hemorrhagic fever), (4) Machupo virus (Bolivian hemorrhagic fever), (5) Guanarito virus (Venezuelan hemorrhagic fever), and (6) Sabia virus. The geographic distribution of these viruses and the illness they cause are determined by the living range of the host rodent (reservoir). The exact mechanism of transmission to humans is unknown and hotly debated.[19,44,91] Direct contact and aerosolization of rodent excretions and secretions are probable mechanisms.

LCMV is well recognized in Europe, the Americas, and other areas. Perinatal maternal infection can lead to severe disease in the newborn, but no evidence suggests transmission through breast milk.[21,150] Standard precautions with breastfeeding are appropriate.

Lassa fever (West Africa) and Argentine hemorrhagic fever (Argentine pampas) are usually more severe illnesses with dramatic bleeding and involvement of other organs, including the brain. These fevers more frequently lead to shock and death than do the forms of hemorrhagic fever caused by the other viruses in this group. Person-to-person spread of Lassa fever is believed to be common, and transmission within households does occur.[144] This may relate to prolonged viremia and excretion of the virus in the urine of humans for up to 30 days.[207] The possibility of persistent virus in human urine, semen, and blood after infection exists for each of the arenaviruses. The possibility of airborne transmission is undecided. Current recommendations by the CDC[44] are to use contact precautions for the duration of the illness in situations of suspected viral hemorrhagic fever. No substantial information describes the infectivity of various body fluids, including breast milk, for these different viral hemorrhagic fevers. Considering the severity of the illness in the mother and the risk to the infant, it is reasonable to avoid breastfeeding in these situations if alternative forms of infant nutrition can be provided.

As more information becomes available, reassessment of these recommendations is advisable. There is a vaccine in clinical trials in endemic areas for Junin virus and Argentine hemorrhagic fever. Preliminary studies suggest it is very effective, but data are still being accumulated concerning the vaccine's use in children and pregnant or breastfeeding women.

Cytomegalovirus

Cytomegalovirus (CMV) is one of the human herpesviruses. Congenital infection of infants, postnatal infection of premature infants, and infection of immunodeficient individuals represent the most serious forms of this infection in children. The time at which the virus infects the fetus or infant and the presence or absence of antibodies against CMV from the mother are important determinants of the severity of infection and the likelihood of significant sequelae (congenital infection syndrome, deafness, chorioretinitis, abnormal neurodevelopment, learning disabilities).[151] About 1% of all infants are born excreting CMV at birth, and approximately 5% of these congenitally infected infants will demonstrate evidence of infection at birth (approximately 5 symptomatic cases per 10,000 live births). Approximately 15% of infants born after primary infection in the pregnant woman will manifest at least one sequela of prenatal infection.[62]

Various studies have detected that 3% to 28% of pregnant women have CMV in cervical cultures and that 4% to 5% of pregnant women have CMV in their urine.[81,115] Perinatal infection certainly occurs through contact with virus in these fluids but usually is not associated with clinical illness in full-term infants. The lack of illness is believed to result from transplacental passive transfer of protective antibodies from the mother.

Postnatal infection later in infancy occurs via breastfeeding or contact with infected fluids (e.g., saliva, urine) but, again, rarely causes clinical illness in full-term infants. Seroepidemiologic studies have documented transmission of infection in infancy, with higher rates of transmission occurring in daycare centers, especially when the prevalence of CMV in the urine and saliva is high. CMV has been identified in the milk of CMV-seropositive women at varying rates (10% to 85%) using viral cultures or CMV deoxyribonucleic acid polymerase chain reaction (DNA-PCR).[115,192,248,271] CMV is more often identified in the breast milk of seropositive mothers than in vaginal fluids, urine, and saliva. The CMV isolation rate from colostrum is lower than that from mature milk.[115,247] The reason for the large degree of variability in identification of CMV in breast milk in these studies probably relates to the intermittent nature of reactivation and excretion of the virus, in addition to the variability, frequency, and duration of sampling of breast milk in the different studies. Some authors have hypothesized that the difference in isolation rates between breast milk and other fluids is caused by viral reactivation in cells (leukocytes or monocytes) in the breast leading to "selective" excretion in breast milk.[192] Vochem and associates[271] reported that the rate of virolactia was greatest at 3 to 4 weeks post partum, and Yeager and associates[285] reported significant virolactia between 2 and 12 weeks post partum. Antibodies (e.g., secretory IgA) to CMV are present in breast milk, along with various cytokines and other proteins (e.g., lactoferrin). These may influence virus binding to cells, but they do not prevent transmission of infection.[3,4,151,181,192,206,282]

Several studies have documented increased rates of postnatal CMV infection in breastfed infants (50% to 69%) compared with bottle fed infants (12% to 27%) observed through the first year of life.[81,181,248,271] In these same studies, full-term infants who acquired CMV infection postnatally were only rarely mildly symptomatic at the time of seroconversion or documented viral excretion. Also, no evidence of late sequelae from CMV was found in these infants.

Postnatal exposure of susceptible infants to CMV, including premature infants without passively acquired maternal antibodies against CMV, infants born to CMV-seronegative mothers, and immunodeficient infants, can cause significant clinical illness (pneumonitis, hepatitis, thrombocytopenia).[113,173] In one study of premature infants followed up to 12 months, Vochem and associates[271] found CMV transmission in 17 of 29 infants (59%) exposed to CMV virolactia and breastfed compared with no infants infected of 27 exposed to breast milk without CMV. No infant was given CMV-seropositive donor milk or blood. Five of the 12 infants who developed CMV infection after 2 months of age had mild signs of illness, including transient neutropenia, and only one infant had a short increase in episodes of apnea and a period of thrombocytopenia. Five other premature infants with CMV infection before 2 months of age had acute illness, including sepsis-like symptoms, apnea with bradycardia, hepatitis, leukopenia, and prolonged thrombocytopenia.[271]

Exposure of CMV-seronegative or premature infants to CMV-positive milk (donor or natural mother's) should be avoided.[239] Various methods of inactivating CMV in breast milk have been reported, including Holder pasteurization, freezing ($-20°$ C for 3 days), and brief high temperature ($72°$ C for 10 seconds).[81,92,107,246,285] One small, prospective study suggests that freezing breast milk at $-20°$ C for 72 hours protects premature infants from CMV infection via breast milk. Sharland and associates reported on 18 premature infants (<32 weeks) who were uninfected at birth and exposed to breast milk from their CMV seropositive mothers.[239] Only one of 18 (5%) infants became positive for CMV at 62 days of life, and this infant was clinically asymptomatic. This transmission rate is considerably lower than others reported in the literature. CMV seronegative and leukocyte–depleted blood products were used routinely. Banked breast milk was pasteurized and stored at $-20°$ C for various time periods and maternal expressed breast milk was frozen at $-20°$ before use whenever possible. The infants received breast milk for a median of 34 days (range, 11 to 74 days) and they were observed for a median of 67 days (range, 30 to 192 days). Breast milk samples pre- or postfreezing were not analyzed by PCR or culture for the presence of cytomegalovirus.[239] Yasuda and associates reported on 43 preterm infants (median gestational age 31 weeks) demonstrating a peak in CMV DNA copies, detected by a real-time PCR assay, in breast milk at 4 to 6 weeks post partum. Thirty of the 43 infants received CMV DNA-positive breast milk. Three of the 30 had CMV DNA detected in their sera, but none of the three had symptoms suggestive of CMV infection. Much of the breast milk had been stored at $-20°$ C before feeding, which the authors propose is the probable reason for less transmission in this cohort.[284] The efficacy of such treatments to prevent CMV infection in premature infants has not been studied prospectively in a randomized control trial.

CMV-seropositive mothers can safely breastfeed their full-term infants because, despite a higher rate of CMV infection than in formula fed infants observed through the first year of life, infection in this situation is not associated with significant clinical illness or sequelae.

Dengue disease

Dengue viruses (serotypes dengue 1 to 4) are Flaviviruses associated primarily with febrile illnesses and rash; dengue fever (DF), dengue hemorrhagic fever (DHF,) and dengue shock syndrome (DSS). Although DHF and DSS occur frequently in children under 1 year of age, they are infrequently described in infants younger than 3 months of age.[112] Boussemart and associates[33] reported on two cases of perinatal/prenatal transmission of dengue and discussed eight additional cases in neonates from the literature. Prenatal or intrapartum transmission of the same type of dengue as the mother was confirmed by serology, culture, or PCR.

It has been postulated that more severe disease associated with dengue disease occurs when the individual has specific IgG against the same serotype as the infecting strain in a set concentration, leading to antibody-dependent enhancement (ADE) of infection. The presence of preexisting dengue serotype specific IgG in an infant implies either previous primary infection with the same serotype, passive acquisition of IgG from the mother (who had a previous primary infection with the same serotype), or perhaps acquisition of specific IgG from breast milk. There is no evidence in the literature for more severe disease in breastfed infants compared with formula fed infants.

There has been no interhuman transmission of dengue virus in the absence of the mosquito vector and no evidence of transmission via breast milk. Breastfeeding during maternal or infant dengue disease should continue as determined by the mother's or infant's severity of illness.

Epstein-Barr virus

Epstein-Barr virus (EBV) is a common infection in children, adolescents, and young adults. It is usually asymptomatic but most notably causes infectious mononucleosis and has been associated with chronic fatigue syndrome (CFS), Burkitt's lymphoma, and nasopharyngeal carcinoma. Because EBV is one of the human herpesviruses, concern has been raised about lifelong latent infection and the potential risk of infection to the fetus and neonate from the mother. Primary EBV infection during pregnancy is unusual because few pregnant women are susceptible.[102,130] Although abortion, premature birth, and congenital infection from EBV are suspected, no distinct group of anomalies is linked to EBV infection in the fetus or neonate. Also, no virologic evidence of EBV as the cause of abnormalities has been found in association with suspected EBV infection.

Culturing of EBV from various fluids or sites is difficult. The virus is detected by its capacity to transform B lymphocytes into persistent lymphoblastoid cell lines. PCR and DNA hybridization studies have detected EBV in the cervix and in breast milk. One study, which identified EBV-DNA in breast milk cells in more than 40% of women donating milk to a breast milk bank, demonstrated that only 17% had antibody to EBV (only IgG, no IgM).[139]

The question of the timing of EBV infection and the subsequent immune response and clinical disease produced requires continued study. Differences exist among the clinical syndromes manifest at different ages. Infants and young children are asymptomatic, have illness not recognized as related to EBV, or have mild episodes of illness, including fever, lymphadenopathy, rhinitis and cough, hepatosplenomegaly, or rash. Adolescents or young adults who experience primary EBV infection more often demonstrate infectious mononucleosis syndrome or are asymptomatic. CFS is more common in adolescents and young adults. Burkitt's lymphoma, observed primarily in Africa, and nasopharyngeal carcinoma, seen in southeast Asia, where primary EBV infection usually occurs in young children, are tumors associated with early EBV infection.[256] These tumors are related to "chronic" EBV infection and tend to occur in individuals with persistently high antibody titers to EBV viral capsid antigen and early antigen. The questions of why these tumors occur with much greater frequency in these geographic areas and what cofactors (including altered immune response to infection) may contribute to their development remain unanswered.[17]

It also remains unknown to what degree breast milk could be a source of early EBV infection compared with other sources of EBV infection in the infant's environment. Similar to the situation of postnatal transmission of CMV in immunocompetent infants, clinically significant illness rarely is associated with primary EBV infection in infants. More data concerning the pathogenesis of EBV-associated tumors should be obtained before proscribing against breastfeeding is warranted, especially in areas where these tumors are common but the protective benefits of breastfeeding are high. In areas where Burkitt's lymphoma and nasopharyngeal carcinoma are uncommon, EBV infection in the mother or infant is not a contraindication to breastfeeding.

Filoviridae

Marburg and Ebola viruses cause severe and highly fatal hemorrhagic fevers. The illness often presents with nonspecific symptoms (conjunctivitis, frontal headache, malaise, myalgia, bradycardia) and progresses with worsening hemorrhage to shock and subsequent death in 50% to 90% of patients. Person-to-person transmission through direct contact, droplet spread, or airborne spread is the common mode of transmission. However, the animal reservoir or source of these viruses in nature for human infection has not been identified. Attack rates in families are 5% to 16%.[207] No postexposure interventions have proved useful in preventing spread, and no treatment other than supportive is currently available.

No information is available concerning these viruses in breast milk or additional risks or benefits from breastfeeding. Contact precautions are recommended for Marburg virus infections and contact and airborne precautions for Ebola virus infection. Given the high attack and mortality rates, these precautions should be carefully instituted and breastfeeding not allowed. If any other suitable source of nutrition can be found for the infant, expressed breast milk should also be proscribed for the infant of a mother with either of these infections.

Human herpesvirus 6

Human herpesvirus 6 (HHV-6) is a cause of exanthema subitum (roseola, roseola infantum) and is associated with febrile seizures. HHV-6 appears to be most similar to CMV based on genetic analysis. No obvious congenital syndrome of HHV-6 infection has been identified, although prenatal infection has been reported.[79] Seroepidemiologic studies show that most adults have already been infected by HHV-6. Therefore, primary infection during pregnancy is unlikely, but reactivation of latent HHV-6 infection may be more common. No case of symptomatic HHV-6 prenatal infection has been reported. The significance of reactivation of HHV-6 in the pregnant woman and the production of infection and disease in the fetus and infant remains to be determined. Primary infection in children occurs most often between 6 and 12 months of age, when maternally acquired passive antibodies against HHV-6 are waning. Febrile illnesses in infants younger than 3 months of age have been described with HHV-6 infection, but infection before 3 months or after 3 years is uncommon.

Various studies involving serology and restriction enzyme analysis of HHV-6 isolates from mother/infant pairs support the idea that postnatal transmission and perhaps perinatal transmission from the mother are common sources of infection. At least one study was unable to detect HHV-6 in breast milk by PCR analysis in 120 samples, although positive control samples seeded with HHV-6-infected cells did test positive.[80]

Given the limited occurrence of clinically significant disease and the absence of sequelae of HHV-6 infection in infants and children, the almost universal acquisition of infection in early childhood (with or without breastfeeding) and the absence of evidence that breast milk is a source of HHV-6 infection, breastfeeding can continue in women known to be seropositive for HHV-6.

Herpes simplex virus

Herpes simplex virus types 1 and 2 (HSV-1, HSV-2) can cause prenatal, perinatal, and postnatal infection in the fetus and infant. Prenatal infection can lead to abortion, prematurity, or a recognized congenital syndrome. Perinatal infection is the most common (1 in 2000 to 5000 live births, 700 to 1500 cases per year in the United States) and is often fatal or severely debilitating. The factors that facilitate intrapartum infection and predict the severity of disease have been extensively investigated. Postnatal infection is uncommon but can occur from a variety of sources, including oral or genital lesions and secretions in mothers or fathers, hospital or home caregivers, and breast lesions in breastfeeding mothers.

A number of case reports have documented severe HSV-1 or HSV-2 infections in infants in association with HSV-positive breast lesions in the mother.[77,212,255] Cases of infants inoculating the mother's breast have also been reported.

Breastfeeding, in the absence of breast lesions, in HSV-seropositive or culture-positive women is reasonable when accompanied by careful handwashing, covering other lesions, and avoiding fondling or kissing with oral lesions until all lesions are crusted. Breastfeeding during maternal therapy with oral or IV acyclovir can continue safely. Inadequate information exists concerning valacyclovir, famiciclovir, ganciclovir, and foscarnet in breast milk to make a recommendation at this time. Breastfeeding in women with active herpetic lesions on their breasts should be proscribed until the lesions are dried. Treatment of the mother's breast lesion with topical, oral, or even IV antiviral preparations may hasten recovery and decrease the length of viral shedding.

Rotaviruses

Rotavirus infections usually result in diarrhea accompanied by emesis and low-grade fever. In severe infections the clinical course can include dehydration, electrolyte abnormalities, and acidosis and can contribute to malnutrition in developing countries. In developed countries, rotavirus is often associated with diarrhea requiring hospitalization in children less than 2 years of age. Fecal-oral transmission is the most common route, but fomites and respiratory spread may also occur. Spread of infection occurs most often in homes with young children or in daycare centers and institutions. In hospitalized infants or mothers with rotavirus infection, contact precautions are indicated for the duration of the illness. No evidence indicates prenatal infection from rotavirus, but perinatal or postnatal infection from contact with the mother or others can occur.

There are no documented cases of transmission of rotavirus via breast milk. Breast milk does contain antibodies to rotavirus for up to 2 years. Although breastfeeding does not prevent infection with rotavirus, it seems to decrease the severity of rotavirus-induced illness in children less than 2 years old.[60,84,125] At least one study suggested that this may represent simply the postponement of severe rotavirus infection until an older age.[60] This delay in rotavirus infection until the child is older may be beneficial in that the older child may be able to tolerate the infection or illness with a lower likelihood of becoming dehydrated or malnourished. Continuing breastfeeding during an episode of rotavirus illness with or without vomiting is appropriate and often helpful.

Several types of rotavirus vaccines are undergoing study in a variety of situations. Evidence indicates that maternal immunization with rotavirus vaccine can increase both transplacental acquisition of antibodies and secretory IgA (sIgA) in breast milk.[209] Additionally, oral rotavirus vaccines have been able to stimulate a good serologic response in both formula fed and breastfed infants, although the antigen titers may need to be modified to create an optimal response in all infants.[56] The actual protective effect of these vaccines in different situations and strategies will require measurement in prospective studies.

Rubella virus

Congenital rubella infection has been well described, and the contributing variables to infection and severe disease have been elucidated. The primary intervention to prevent congenital rubella has been to establish the existence of maternal immunity to rubella before conception, including immunization with rubella vaccine and reimmunization if indicated. Perinatal infection is not clinically significant. Postnatal infection occurs infrequently in children younger than 1 year of age because of passively acquired maternal antibodies. The predominant age of infection is 5 to 14 years old, and more than half of those with infections are asymptomatic. Postnatal rubella is a self-limited, mild viral infection associated with an evanescent rash, shotty adenopathy, and low-grade transient fever. It most often occurs in the late winter and spring. Infants with

congenital infection shed the virus for prolonged periods from various sites and may serve as a source of infection throughout the year. Contact isolation is appropriate for suspected and proved congenital infection for at least 1 year, including exclusion from day care and avoidance of pregnant women, whereas postnatal rubella infection requires droplet precautions for 7 days after the onset of rash.

Rubella virus has been isolated from breast milk after natural infection (congenital or postnatal) and after immunization with live attenuated vaccine virus. Both IgA antibodies and immunoreactive cells against rubella have been identified in breast milk. Breastfed infants can acquire vaccine virus infection via milk but are asymptomatic. Because postpartum infection with this virus (natural or vaccine) is not associated with clinically significant illness, no reason exists to prevent breastfeeding after congenital infection, postpartum infection, or maternal immunization with this virus.

Varicella-zoster virus

Varicella-zoster virus (VZV) infection (varicella/chickenpox, zoster/shingles) is one of the most communicable diseases of humans, in a class with measles and smallpox. Transmission is believed to occur via respiratory droplets and virus from vesicles. Varicella in pregnancy is a rare event, although disease can be more severe with varicella pneumonia, and can be fatal.

Congenital VZV infection occurs infrequently, causing abortion, prematurity, and congenital malformations. A syndrome of malformations has been carefully described with congenital VZV infection, typically involving limb deformity, skin scarring, and nerve damage, including to the eye and brain.[101]

Perinatal infection can lead to severe infection in the infant if maternal rash develops 5 days or less before delivery and within 2 days after delivery. Illness in the infant usually develops before 10 days of age and is believed to be more severe because of the lack of adequate transfer of antibody from the mother during this period and transplacental spread of virus to the fetus and infant during viremia in the mother. Varicella in the mother occurring prior to 5 days before delivery allows sufficient formation and transplacental transfer of antibodies to the infant to ameliorate disease even if the infant is infected with VZV. Mothers who develop varicella rash more than 2 days after delivery are less likely to transfer virus to the infant transplacentally; they pose a risk to the infant from postnatal exposure, which can be diminished by the administration of varicella-zoster immune globulin (VZIG) to the infant. Postnatal transmission is believed to occur through aerosolized virus from skin lesions or the respiratory tract entering the susceptible infant's respiratory tract. Airborne precautions are therefore appropriate in the hospital setting. Infants infected with VZV in utero or in the perinatal period (less than 1 month of age) are more likely to develop zoster (reactivation of latent VZV) during childhood or as young adults. Table 17-2 summarizes management of varicella in the hospitalized mother or infant.[101]

Postnatal varicella from nonmaternal exposure can occur but is generally mild when it develops after 3 weeks of age or when the mother has passed on antibodies against VZV via the placenta. Severe postnatal varicella does occur in premature infants or infants of varicella-susceptible mothers. When the mother's immune status relative to VZV is uncertain and measurement of antibodies to VZV in the mother or infant cannot be performed promptly (less than 72 hours), administration of VZIG to the infant exposed to varicella or zoster in the postnatal period is indicated. Ideally the mother's varicella status should be known before pregnancy, when varicella virus vaccine could be given if indicated.

VZV virus has not been cultured from milk, but VZV-DNA has been identified in breast milk.[288] Antibody against VZV has also been found in breast milk.[174] One case of suspected transfer of VZV to an infant via breastfeeding has been reported, but virus may have been transmitted by respiratory droplet or exposure to rash before the mother began antiviral therapy.[288] Isolation of the infant from the mother and interruption of breast-feeding should occur only while the mother remains clinically infectious, regardless of the method of feeding. Expressed breast milk can be given to the infant if no skin lesions involve the breasts, as soon as the infant has received VZIG. Persons with varicella rash are considered noninfectious when no new vesicles have appeared for 72 hours and all lesions have crusted, usually in 6 to 10 days. Immunocompetent mothers who develop zoster can continue to breastfeed if the lesions do not involve the breast and can be covered, because antibodies against VZV are provided to the infant via the placenta and breast milk and will diminish the severity of disease even if not preventing it. Conservative management in this scenario would include giving the infant VZIG as well (see Table 17-2).

Measles

Measles is another highly communicable childhood illness that can be more severe in neonates and adults. Measles is an exanthematous febrile illness following a prodrome of malaise, coryza, conjunctivitis, and cough and often Koplik's spots in the mouth. The rash usually appears 10 to 14 days after exposure. Complications can include pneumonitis, encephalitis, and bacterial superinfection. With the availability of vaccination, measles in pregnancy is rare (0.4 in 10,000 pregnancies),[101] although respiratory complications (primary viral pneumonitis, secondary bacterial pneumonia), hepatitis, or other secondary bacterial infections often lead to more severe disease in these situations.

Prenatal infection with measles may cause premature delivery without disrupting normal uterine development. No specific group of congenital malformations have been described in association with in utero measles infection, although teratogenic effects of measles infection in the pregnant woman may rarely manifest in the infant.

Perinatal measles includes transplacental infection when measles occurs in the infant in the first 10 days of life. Infection from extrauterine exposure usually develops after 14 days of life. The severity of illness after suspected transplacental

TABLE 17-2	**Guidelines for preventive measures after exposure to chickenpox in the nursery or maternity ward**		

| | Chickenpox lesions present | | |
Type of exposure or disease	Mother	Neonate	Disposition
A. Siblings at home have active chickenpox when neonate and mother are ready for discharge from hospital.	No	No	1. Mother: if she has a history of chickenpox, she may return home. Without a history, she should be tested for varicella-zoster virus (VZV) antibody titer.[*] If test is positive, she may return home. If test is positive, she may return home. If test is negative, varicella-zoster immune globulin (VZIG)[†] is administered and she is discharged home. 2. Neonate: may be discharged home with mother if mother has history of varicella or is VZV antibody positive. If mother is susceptible, administer VZIG to infant and discharge home or place in protective isolation.
B. Mother has no history of chickenpox; exposed during period 6-20 days antepartum.[‡]	No	No	1. Exposed mother and infant: send home at earliest date unless siblings at home have communicable chickenpox.[§] If so, may administer VZIG and discharge home, as above. 2. Other mothers and infants: no special management indicated. 3. Hospital personnel: no precautions indicated if there is a history of previous chickenpox or zoster. In absence of history, immediate serologic testing is indicated to determine immune status.[*] Nonimmune personnel should be excluded from patient contact until 21 days after an exposure. 4. If mother develops varicella 1 to 2 days post partum, infant should be given VZIG.

[*]Send serum to virus diagnostic laboratory for determination of antibodies to VZV by a sensitive technique (e.g., FAMA, LA, ELISA). Personnel may continue to work for 8 days after exposure pending serologic results because they are not potentially infectious during this period. Antibodies to VZV >1:4 probably are indicative of immunity.

[†]VZIG is available through the American Red Cross. The dose for a newborn is 1.25 mL (1 vial). The dose for a pregnant woman is conventionally 6.25 mL (5 vials).

[‡]If exposure occurred less than 6 days antepartum, mother would not be potentially infectious until at least 72 hours post partum.

[§]Considered noninfectious when no new vesicles have appeared for 72 hours and all lesions have crusted.

(Continued)

spread of virus to the infant varies from mild to severe and does not seem to vary with the antepartum or postpartum onset of rash in the mother. It is uncertain what role maternal antibodies play in the severity of the infant's disease. More severe disease seems to be associated with severe respiratory illness and bacterial infection. Postnatal exposure leading to measles after 14 days of life is generally mild, probably because of passively acquired antibodies from the mother. Severe measles in children younger than 1 year of age may occur because of declining passively acquired antibodies and complications of respiratory illness and rare cases of encephalitis.

TABLE 17-2 Guidelines for preventive measures after exposure to chickenpox in the nursery or maternity ward—cont'd

| Type of exposure or disease | Chickenpox lesions present | | Disposition |
	Mother	Neonate	
C. Onset of maternal chickenpox occurs antepartum‡ or post partum.	Yes	No	1. Infected mother: isolate until no longer clinically infectious. If seriously ill, treat with acyclovir.‖ 2. Infected mother's infant: administer VZIG† to neonates born to mothers with onset of chickenpox less than 5 days before delivery and isolate separately from mother. Send home with mother if no lesions develop by the time mother is noninfectious. 3. Other mothers and infants: send home at earliest date. VZIG may be given to exposed neonates. 4. Hospital personnel: same as B-3.
D. Onset of maternal chickenpox occurs antepartum.§			1. Mother: isolation unnecessary. 2. Infant: isolate from other infants but not from mother. 3. Other mothers and infants: same as C-3 (if exposed). 4. Hospital personnel: same as B-3 (if exposed).
E. Congenital chickenpox	No	Yes	1. Infected infant and mother: same as D-1 and D-2. 2. Other mothers and infants: same as C-3. 3. Hospital personnel: same as B-3.

‖Dosage of acyclovir for pregnant woman is 30 mg/kg/day; for seriously ill infant with varicella, 750 to 1500 mg/m²/day.
From Gershon AA: Chickenpox, measles and mumps. In Remington JS, Klein JO (ed): Infectious Diseases of the Fetus and Newborn Infant. 4th ed. Philadelphia. WB Saunders, 1995.

Measles virus has not been identified in breast milk, whereas measles-specific antibodies have been documented.[1] Infants exposed to mothers with documented measles while breastfeeding should be given immune globulin and isolated from the mother until 72 hours after the onset of rash, which is often only a very short period after diagnosis of measles in the mother. The breast milk can be pumped and given to the infant because sIgA begins to be secreted in breast milk within 48 hours of onset of the exanthem in the mother. Table 17-3 summarizes management of the hospitalized mother and infant with measles exposure or infection.[101]

Mumps

Mumps is an acute transient benign illness with inflammation of the parotid gland and other salivary glands and often involving the pancreas, testicles, and meninges. Mumps occurs infrequently in pregnant women (1 to 10 cases in 10,000 pregnancies) and is generally benign. Mumps virus has been isolated from saliva, respiratory secretions, blood, testicular tissue, urine, CSF in cases of meningeal involvement, and breast milk. The period of infectivity is believed to be between 7 days before and 9 days after the onset of parotitis, with the usual incubation period being 14 to 18 days.

TABLE 17-3   Guidelines for preventive measures after exposure to measles in the nursery or maternity ward

Type of exposure or disease	Measles (prodrome or rash) present[*]		Disposition
	Mother	**Neonate**	
A. Siblings at home have measles[*] when neonate and mother are ready for discharge from hospital.	No	No	1. Neonate: protective isolation and immune globulin (IG) indicated unless mother has unequivocal history of previous measles or measles vaccination.[†] 2. Mother: with history of previous measles or measles vaccination, she may either remain with neonates or return to older children. Without previous history, she may remain with neonate until older siblings are no longer infectious, or she may receive IG prophylactically and return to older children.
B. Mother has no history of measles or measles vaccination exposure 6 to 15 days antepartum.[‡]	No	No	1. Exposed mother and infant: administer IG to each and send home at earliest date unless siblings at home have communicable measles. Test mothers for susceptibility if possible. If susceptible, administer live measles vaccine 8 weeks after IG. 2. Other mothers and infants: same unless clear history of previous measles or measles vaccination in the mother. 3. Hospital personnel: unless clear history of previous measles or measles vaccination, administer IG within 72 hours of exposure. Vaccinate 8 weeks or more later.
C. Onset of maternal measles occurs antepartum or post partum.[§]	Yes	Yes	1. Infected mother and infant: isolate together until clinically stable, then send home. 2. Other mothers and infants: same as B-3 except infants should be vaccinated at 15 months of age. 3. Hospital personnel: same as B-3.
D. Onset of maternal measles occurs antepartum or post partum.[§]	Yes	No	1. Infected mother: isolate until no longer infectious.[§] 2. Infected mother's infant: isolate separately from mother. Administer IG immediately. Send home when mother is no longer infectious. Alternatively, observe in isolation for 18 days for modified measles,[‖] especially if IG administration was delayed more than 4 days. 3. Other mothers and infants: same as C-2. 4. Hospital personnel: same as B-3.

[*]Catarrhal stage or less than 72 hours after onset of exanthem.
[†]Vaccination with live attenuated measles virus.
[‡]With exposure less than 6 days antepartum, mother would not be potentially infectious until at least 72 hours post partum.
[§]Considered infectious from onset of prodrome until 72 hours after onset of exanthem.
[‖]Incubation period for modified measles may be prolonged beyond the usual 10 to 14 days.
From Gershon AA: Chickenpox, measles and mumps. In Remington JS, Klein JO (ed): Infectious Diseases of the Fetus and Newborn Infant, 4th ed. Philadelphia, WB Saunders, 1995.

Prenatal infection with the mumps virus causes an increase in the number of abortions when infection occurs in the first trimester. A small increase in the number of premature births was noted in one prospective study of maternal mumps infection.[101] No conclusive evidence suggests congenital malformations associated with prenatal infection, not even with endocardial fibroelastosis, as originally reported in the 1960s.

Perinatal mumps (transplacentally or postnatally acquired) has rarely if ever been documented. Natural mumps virus has been demonstrated to infect the placenta and infect the fetus, and live attenuated vaccine virus has been isolated from the placenta but not from fetal tissue in women vaccinated 10 days before induced abortion. Antibodies to mumps do cross the placenta.

Postnatal mumps in the first year of life is typically very benign. No epidemiologic data suggest that mumps infection is more or less common or severe in breastfed infants compared with formula fed infants. Although mumps virus has been identified in breast milk and mastitis is a rare complication of mumps in the mature female, no evidence indicates that breast involvement occurs more frequently in lactating women. If mumps occurs in the mother, breastfeeding can continue because exposure has already occurred throughout the 7 days before the development of the parotitis, and sIgA in the milk may help to mitigate the symptoms in the infant.

Polioviruses

Poliovirus infections (types 1, 2, and 3) cause a range of illness, with 90% to 95% subclinical, 4% to 8% abortive, and 1% to 2% manifest as paralytic poliomyelitis. A review by Bates[22] from 1955 of 58 cases of poliomyelitis in infants younger than 1 month of age demonstrated paralysis or death in more than 70% and only one child without evidence of even transient paralysis. More than half the cases were ascribed to transmission from the mothers, although no mention was made of breastfeeding. Breastfeeding rates at the time were about 25%.

Prenatal infection with polioviruses does cause an increased incidence of abortion. Prematurity and stillbirth apparently occur more frequently in mothers who developed paralytic disease versus inapparent infection.[129] Although individual reports of congenital malformations in association with maternal poliomyelitis exist, no epidemiologic data suggest that polioviruses are teratogenic. Also, no evidence indicates that live attenuated vaccine poliovirus given during pregnancy is associated with congenital malformations.[58,114]

Perinatal infection has been noted in several case reports of infants infected in utero several days before birth who had severe disease manifesting with neurologic manifestations (paralysis) but without fever, irritability, or vomiting. Additional case reports of infection acquired postnatally demonstrate illness more consistent with poliomyelitis of childhood. These cases were more severe and involved paralysis, which may represent reporting bias.[58]

No data are available concerning the presence of poliovirus in breast milk, although antibodies to poliovirus types 1, 2, and 3 have been documented.[174] In this era of increasing worldwide poliovirus vaccination, the likelihood of prenatal or perinatal poliovirus infection is decreasing. Maternal susceptibility to poliovirus should be determined before conception and poliovirus vaccine offered to susceptible women. An analysis of the last great epidemic in Italy in 1958 was done using a population-based case-control study.[211] In 114,000 births, 942 infants were reported with paralytic poliomyelitis. A group of matched control subjects was selected from infants admitted to the hospital at the same time. Using the dichotomous variable of never breastfed and partially breastfed, 75 never-breastfed infants were among the cases and 88 among the control group. The authors determined an odds ratio of 4:2, with 95% confidence interval of 1.4 to 14, demonstrating that the risk of paralytic poliomyelitis was higher in infants never breastfed and lowest among those exclusively breastfed. Because by the time the diagnosis of poliomyelitis is made in a breastfeeding mother, the exposure of the infant to poliovirus from maternal secretions has already occurred, and because the breast milk already contains antibodies that may be protective, no reason exists to interrupt breastfeeding. Breastfeeding also does not interfere with successful immunization against poliomyelitis with oral or inactivated poliovirus vaccine.[46]

Tumor virus in breast milk

No documented evidence indicates that women with breast cancer have RNA of tumor virus in their milk. No correlation between RNA-directed DNA polymerase activity has been found in women with a family history of breast cancer. RNA-directed DNA polymerase activity, a reserve transcriptase, is a normal feature of the lactating breast.[59,89,222]

Epidemiologic studies

Epidemiologic data conflict with the suggestion that the tumor agent is transmitted through the breast milk. The incidence of breast cancer is low among groups who had nursed their infants, including lower economic groups, foreign-born groups, and those in sparsely populated areas.[169] The frequency of breast cancer in mothers and sisters of a woman with breast cancer is two to three times that expected by chance. This could be genetic or environmental. Cancer actually is equally common on both sides of the family of an affected woman. If breast milk were the cause, it should be transmitted from mother to daughter. When mother-daughter incidence of cancer was studied, no relationship was found to breastfeeding.

Sarkar and associates[226] reported that human milk, when incubated with mouse mammary tumor virus, caused degradation of the particular morphology and decreased infectivity and reverse transcriptase activity of the virions. They suggest that the significance of this destructive effect of human milk on mouse mammary tumor virus may account for the difficulty in isolating the putative human mammary tumor agent. Sanner[225] showed that the inhibitory enzymes in milk can be removed by special sedimentation technique. He ascribes the discrepancies in isolating virus particles in human milk to these factors, which inhibit RNA-directed DNA polymerase.

Current position

The fear of cancer in the breastfed female offspring of a woman with breast cancer does not justify avoiding breastfeeding. Breastfed women have the same breast cancer experience as nonbreastfed women, and no increase is seen in benign tumors. Daughters of breast cancer patients have an increased risk of developing benign and malignant tumors because of their heredity, not because of their breastfeeding history.[180,184]

Unilateral breastfeeding (limited to the right breast) is a custom of Tanka women of the fishing villages of Hong Kong. Ing and associates[133] investigated the question, "Does the unsuckled breast have an altered risk of cancer?" They studied breast cancer data from 1958 to 1975. Breast cancer occurred equally in the left and the right breasts. Comparison of patients who had nursed unilaterally with nulliparous patients and with patients who had borne children but not breastfed indicated a highly significantly increased risk of cancer in the unsuckled breast. The authors conclude that in postmenopausal women who have breastfed unilaterally, the risk of cancer is significantly higher in the unsuckled breast. They believed that breastfeeding may help protect the suckled breast against cancer.[133]

Others[176] have suggested that Tanka women are ethnically a separate people and that left-sided breast cancer may be related to their genetic pool and not to their breastfeeding habits. No mention has been made of other possible influences, such as the impact of their role as "fishermen" or any inherent trauma to the left breast.[207]

In 1926, Lane-Claypon[204] stated that the breast that had never lactated was more liable to become cancerous. Nulliparity and absence of breastfeeding had been considered important risk factors for breast cancer. MacMahon and associates[169] reported in 1970 that age at first full-term pregnancy was the compelling factor, and the younger the mother, the less the risk.

In a collective review of the etiologic factors in cancer of the breast in humans, Papaioannou concludes, "Genetic factors, viruses, hormones, psychogenic stress, diet and other possible factors, probably in that order of importance, contribute to some extent to the development of cancer of the breast."[204]

Wing[279] concluded in her 1977 review on human milk and health that "in view of the complete absence of any studies showing a relationship between breast-feeding and increased risk of breast cancer, the presence of virus-like particles in breast milk should not be a contraindication to breastfeeding." Henderson and associates[116] made a similar statement in 1974, whereas Vorherr[272] concluded in 1979 that the roles of pregnancy and lactation in the development and prognosis of breast cancer had not been determined.

Gradually, studies have appeared challenging the dogma. Brinton and associates,[35] McTiernan and Thomas,[177] and Layde and associates[158] showed the clearly protective effects of breastfeeding. Another example is a study conducted to clarify whether lactation has a protective role against breast cancer in an Asian people, regardless of confounding effects of age at first pregnancy, parity, and closely related factors.[287] In a hospital-based case-control study of 521 women without breast cancer, statistical adjustment for potential confounders and a likelihood ratio test for linear trend were done by unconditional logistic regression. Total months of lactation regardless of parity was the discriminator. Regardless of age of first pregnancy and parity, lactation had an independent protective effect against breast cancer in Japanese women.[287] Although breast cancer incidence is influenced by genetics, stress, hormones, and pregnancy, breastfeeding clearly has a protective effect. "There is a reduction in the risk of breast cancer among premenopausal women who have lactated. No reduction in the risk of breast cancer occurred among postmenopausal women with a history of lactation," according to Newcombe and associates,[191] reporting a multicenter study in 1993.

Hepatitis in the mother

The diagnosis of hepatitis in the pregnant woman or nursing mother causes significant anxiety. The first issue is determining the etiology of the hepa-titis, which then allows an informed discussion of the risk to the fetus/infant. The differential diagnosis of acute hepatitis includes (1) common causes of hepatitis, such as hepatitis A, B, C, and D; (2) uncommon causes of hepatitis, such as hepatitis E and G, CMV, echoviruses, enteroviruses, EBV, HSV, rubella, VZV, yellow fever virus; (3) rare causes of hepatitis, such as Ebola virus, Junin virus and Machupo virus (cause hemorrhagic fever), Lassa virus, and Marburg virus; and (4) nonviral causes, such as hepatotoxic drugs, alcoholic hepatitis, toxoplasmosis, autoimmune hepatitis, bile duct obstruction, ischemic liver damage, Wilson's disease, α_1-antitrypsin deficiency, and metastatic liver disease. The following sections focus on hepatitis viruses A to G. Other infectious agents that can cause hepatitis are considered individually in other sections. Box 17-1 provides hepatitis terminology.

Martin and associates[172] outline a succinct diagnostic approach to the patient with acute viral hepatitis and chronic viral hepatitis (Figs. 17-4 and 17-5). The approach involves using the four serologic markers (IgM anti-HAV, HBsAg, IgM anti-HBcAg, anti-HCV) as the initial diagnostic tests. Simultaneous consideration of other etiologies of acute liver dysfunction is appropriate depending on the patient's history. If the initial diagnostic tests are all negative, subsequent additional testing for anti-HDV, HCV-RNA, HGV-RNA, anti-HEV, or HEV-RNA may be necessary. If initial testing reveals positive HBsAg, testing for anti-HDV, HBeAg, and HBV-DNA is appropriate. These additional tests are useful in defining the prognosis for the mother and the risk of infection to the infant. During the diagnostic evaluation, it is appropriate to discuss with the mother or parents the theoretic risk of transmitting infectious agents that cause hepatitis via breastfeeding. The discussion should include an evaluation of the positive and negative effects of suspending or continuing breastfeeding until the exact etiologic diagnosis is determined. The relative risk of transmission of infection to the infant can be estimated and specific preventive measures provided for the infant (Table 17-4).

BOX 17-1   Terminology for hepatitis

Hepatitis A Virus (HAV)

IgM anti-HAV	Immunoglobulin M antibody against HAV
HAV-RNA	HAV ribonucleic acid

Hepatitis B Virus

HBsAg	Hepatitis B surface antigen
HBeAg	Hepatitis Be antigen
HBcAg	Hepatitis B core antigen
Anti-HBe	Antibody against hepatitis Be antigen
IgM anti-HBcAg	IgM antibody against hepatitis B core antigen
HBV-DNA	HBV deoxyribonucleic acid
HBIG	Hepatitis B immune globulin

Hepatitis C Virus (HCV)

Anti-HCV	Antibody against HCV
HCV-RNA	HCV ribonucleic acid

Hepatitis D Virus (HDV)

Anti-HDV	Antibody against HDV

Hepatitis E Virus (HEV)

HEV-RNA	HEV ribonucleic acid

Hepatitis G Virus (HGV)

HGV-RNA	HGV ribonucleic acid
TT Virus (TTV)	
TTV-DNA	TT virus deoxyribonucleic acid

Other

NANBH	Non-A, non-B hepatitis
ISG	Immune serum globulin

Hepatitis A

Hepatitis A virus (HAV) is usually an acute self-limited infection. The illness is typically mild, and generally subclinical in infants. Occasionally, HAV infection is prolonged or relapsing, extending over 3 to 6 months, rarely is fulminant, but does not lead to chronic infection. The incidence of prematurity after maternal HAV infection is increased, but no evidence to date indicates obvi-ous birth defects or a congenital syndrome.[235,292] HAV infection in premature infants may lead to prolonged viral shedding.[219] Transmission is most often person to person (fecal-oral), and transmission in food-borne or water-borne epidemics has been described. Transmission via blood products and vertical transmission (mother to infant) are rare.[273] Transmission in daycare settings has been clearly described.

Infection with HAV in the newborn is uncommon and does not seem to be a significant problem. The usual period of viral shedding and presumed contagiousness lasts 1 to 3 weeks. Acute maternal HAV infection in the last trimester or in the postpartum period could lead to infection in the infant. Symptomatic infection can be prevented by immune globulin (IG) administration, and 80% to 90% of disease can be prevented by IG administration within 2 weeks of exposure. HAV vaccine can be administered simultaneously with IG without affecting the seroconversion rate to produce rapid and prolonged HAV serum antibody levels.

Transmission of HAV via breast milk has been implicated in one case report, but no data exist on the frequency of isolating HAV from breast milk.[273] Because HAV infection in infancy is rare and usually subclinical without chronic disease, and because exposure has already occurred by the time the etiologic diagnosis of hepatitis in the mother is made, no reason exists to interrupt breastfeeding with maternal HAV infection. The infant should receive IG and HAV vaccine, administered simultaneously.

Hepatitis B

Hepatitis B virus (HBV) infection leads to a broad spectrum of illness, including asymptomatic seroconversion, nonspecific symptoms (fever, malaise, fatigue), clinical hepatitis with or without jaundice, extrahepatic manifestations (arthritis, rash, renal involvement), fulminant hepatitis, and chronic HBV infection. Chronic HBV infection occurs in up to 90% of infants infected via perinatal and vertical transmission and in 30% of children infected between 1 to 5 years of age. Given the increased

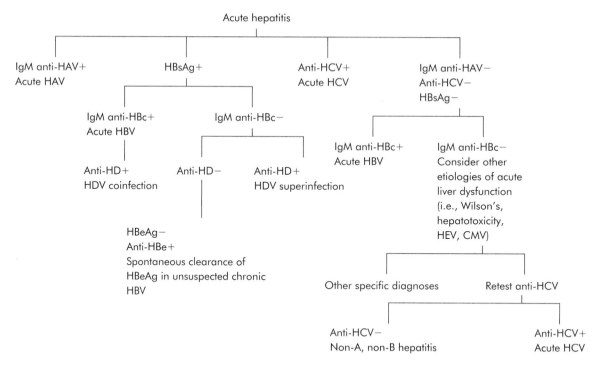

Figure 17-4.   Diagnostic approach to patient with acute viral hepatitis. See Box 17-1 for definitions of abbreviations. (From Martin P, Friedman L, Dienstag J: Diagnostic approach. In Zuckerman A, Thomas H (eds): Viral Hepatitis: Scientific Basis and Clinical Management. Edinburgh, Churchill Livingstone, 1993.)

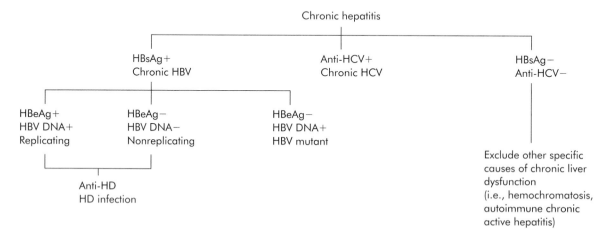

Figure 17-5.   Diagnostic approach to patient with chronic viral hepatitis. See Box 17-1 for definitions of abbreviations. (From Martin P, Friedman L, Dienstag J: Diagnostic approach. In Zuckerman A, Thomas H (eds): Viral Hepatitis: Scientific Basis and Clinical Management. Edinburgh, Churchill Livingstone, 1993.)

TABLE 17-4 Viral hepatitis in association with breastfeeding*

Hepatitis	Virus	Identified in breast milk	Factors for peri/postnatal transmission	Prevention	Breastfeeding†
A	Picornaviridae (RNA)	?	Vertical transmission uncertain or rare HAV in pregnancy associated with premature birth	ISG HAV vaccine	Limited evidence of transmission via breastfeeding or of serious disease in infants Breastfeeding OK after ISG and vaccine
B	Hepadnaviridae (DNA)	HBsAg HBV-DNA	Increased risk of vertical transmission with HBeAg+, in countries where HBV is endemic or early in maternal infection, before Ab production	HBIG HBV vaccine	Low theoretic risk Virtually no risk after HBIG and HBV vaccine Breastfeeding OK after HBIG and vaccine
C	Flavivirus (RNA)	HCV-RNA detected	Increased risk when mother HIV+ and HCV+ or with increased HCV-RNA titers Vertical transmission uncommon	None	Positive theoretic risk Inadequate data on relative risk Breastfeeding OK after informed discussion with parents
D	Deltaviridae (RNA negative strand, circular)	?	Requires coinfection/superinfection with HBV Vertical transmission rare	None (except to prevent HBV infection, give HBIG/HBV vaccine)	Prevent HBV infection with HBIG and vaccine Breastfeeding OK after HBIG and vaccine
E	Caliciviridae (RNA)	+	Severe disease in pregnant women (20% mortality)	ISG and subunit vaccine being tested	Usually subclinical infection in children Breastfeeding OK
G	Related to calicivirus and flaviviruses (RNA)	?	Vertical transmission occurs	None	Inadequate data
TT	TT virus (DNA, circular, single stranded)	TIV-DNA detected	Vertical transmission occurs	None	Inadequate data

*See Box 17-1 for abbreviations. Ab, Antibody; HIV, human immunodeficiency virus.

†With any type of infectious hepatitis, discussion of what is known and not known concerning transmission should be related to the mother/parents, and together an informed decision can be made concerning breastfeeding.

Data from Committee on Infectious Diseases, American Academy of Pediatrics: Red Book: Report of the Committee on Infectious Diseases, 26th ed. Elk Grove, IL, The Academy, 2003.

risk of significant sequelae from chronic infection (chronic active hepatitis, chronic persistent hepatitis, cirrhosis, primary hepatocellular carcinoma), prevention of HBV infection in infancy is crucial. Transmission of HBV is usually through blood or body fluids (stool, semen, saliva, urine, cervical secretions).[62]

Vertical transmission either transplacentally or perinatally during delivery has been well described throughout the world. Vertical transmission rates in areas where HBV is endemic (Taiwan and Japan) are very high, whereas transmission to infants from HBV carrier mothers in other areas where HBV carrier rates are low is uncommon.[250] Transmission of HBV to infants occurs in up to 50% of infants when the mother is acutely infected immediately before, during, or soon after pregnancy.[291]

Hepatitis B surface antigen (HBsAg) is found in breast milk, but transmission by this route is not well documented. Beasley and associates[23,24] demonstrated that although breast milk transmission is possible, seroconversion rates are no different between breastfed and nonbreastfed infants in a long-term follow-up study of 147 HBsAg-positive mothers. Transmission, when it does happen, probably occurs during labor and delivery. The AAP Committee on Infectious Diseases stated in 2003 that "studies from Taiwan and England have indicated that breastfeeding by HBsAg-positive women does not increase significantly the risk of infection among their infants."[62]

Screening of all pregnant women for HBV infection is an essential first step to preventing vertical transmission. Universal HBV vaccination at birth and during infancy, along with administration of hepatitis B immune globulin (HBIG) immediately after birth to infants of HBsAg-positive mothers, prevents HBV transmission in more than 95% of cases. Breastfeeding by HBsAg-positive women is not contraindicated, but immediate administration of HBIG and HBV vaccine should occur. Two subsequent doses of vaccine should be given at the appropriate intervals and dosages for the specific HBV vaccine product. This decreases the small theoretic risk of HBV transmission from breastfeeding to almost zero.

When acute peripartum or postpartum hepatitis occurs in the mother and HBV infection is a possibility, with its associated increased risk of transmission to the infant, a discussion with the mother or parents should identify the potential risks and benefits of continuing breastfeeding until the etiology of the hepatitis can be determined. If an appropriate alternative source of nutrition is available for the infant, breast milk should be withheld until the etiology of the hepatitis is identified. HBIG and HBV vaccine can be administered to the infant who has not already been immunized or has no documented immunity against HBV.[251] If acute HBV infection is documented in the mother, breastfeeding can continue once immunization has begun.

Hepatitis C

Acute infection with hepatitis C virus (HCV) can be indistinguishable from hepatitis A or B infection; however, it is typically asymptomatic or mild. HCV infection is the major cause of blood-borne non-A, non-B hepatitis (NANBH). Chronic HCV infection is reported to occur 70% to 85% of the time regardless of age at time of infection. Sequelae of chronic HCV infection are similar to those associated with chronic HBV infection. Bortolotti and associates[32] described two groups of children with HCV infection whom they observed for 12 to 48 months. The first group of 14 children, who acquired HCV infection early in life, presumably from their mothers, all demonstrated biochemical evidence of liver disease in the first 12 months of life. Two of these children subsequently cleared the viremia and had normal liver function, an additional three children developed normal liver function despite persistent HCV viremia, and the remaining children had persistent viremia and abnormal liver function. The second group of 16 children, with chronic HCV infection, remained free of clinical symptoms of hepatitis, but 10 (62%) of them had mild alanine aminotransferase (ALT) elevations, and 7 (44%) of the 16 who had liver biopsies had histologic evidence of mild to moderate hepatitis.

The two commonly identified mechanisms of transmission of HCV are transfusions of blood or blood products and IV drug use. However, other routes of transmission exist, because HCV infection occurs even in the absence of obvious direct contact with significant amounts of blood. Other body fluids contaminated with blood probably serve as sources of infection. Transmission through sexual contact occurs infrequently and probably requires additional contributing factors, such as coinfection with other sexually transmitted agents or high viral loads in serum and other body fluids. Studies of transmission in households without other risk factors has demonstrated either very low rates of transmission or no transmission.

The reported rates of vertical transmission vary widely. In mothers with unknown HIV status or known HIV infection, the rates of vertical transmission were 4% to 100%, whereas the rates varied between 0% and 42% in known HIV-negative mothers.[74] These same studies suggest that maternal coinfection with HIV, HCV genotype, active maternal liver disease, and the serum titer of maternal HCV-RNA may be associated with increased rates of vertical transmission.[170,195,290] The correlation between HCV viremia, the HCV viral load in the mother and vertical transmission of HCV is well documented.[185,224,257,286] The clinical significance and risk of liver disease after vertical transmission of HCV are still unknown. The timing of HCV infection in vertical transmission is also unknown. In utero transmission has been suggested by some studies,[86] whereas intrapartum or postpartum transmission was proposed by Ohto and associates[196] when they documented the absence of HCV-RNA in the cord blood of neonates who later became HCV-RNA positive at 1 to 2 months of age. More recently, Gibb and associates reported two pieces of data supporting the likelihood of intrapartum transmission as the predominant time of vertical transmission: (a) low sensitivity of PCR for HCV RNA testing in the first month of life with a marked increase in sensitivity after that for diagnosing HCV infection in infants and (b) a lower transmission risk for elective cesarean section (without prolonged rupture of membranes) compared with vaginal or emergency cesarean section delivery.[103]

The risk of HCV transmission via breast milk is uncertain. Anti-HCV antibody and HCV-RNA has been demonstrated in colostrum and breast milk, although the levels of HCV-RNA in milk did not correlate with the titers of HCV-RNA in serum.[111,164] Nevertheless, transmission of HCV via breastfeeding (and not in utero, intrapartum, or from other postpartum sources) has not been proved in the small number infants studied. Transmission rates in breastfed and nonbreastfed infants appear to be similar, but various important factors have not been controlled, such as HCV-RNA titers in the mothers, examination of the milk for HCV-RNA, exclusive breastfeeding versus exclusive formula feeding versus partial breastfeeding, and duration of breastfeeding.[103,164,170,183,185,197,290] Zanetti and associates[290] documented the absence of HCV transmission in 94 mother-infant pairs when the mother had only HCV (no HIV) infection and no transmission in 71 mother-infant pairs who breastfed, including 23 infants whose mothers were seropositive for HCV-RNA. Eight infants in that study were infected with HCV, their mothers had both HIV and HCV, and three of these eight infants were infected with both HIV and HCV. The HCV-RNA levels were significantly higher in the mothers coinfected with HIV compared with those mothers with HCV alone.

Overall, (1) the risk of HCV infection via breastfeeding is very low, (2) the risk of HCV infection appears to be more frequent in association with HIV infection and higher levels of HCV-RNA in maternal serum, (3) no effective preventive therapies (IG or vaccine) exist, and (4) the risk of chronic HCV infection and subsequent sequelae with any infection is high. It is, therefore, appropriate to discuss the theoretic risk of breastfeeding in HCV-positive mothers with the mother or parents and to consider proscribing breast milk when appropriate alternative sources of nutrition are available for the infant. HIV infection is a separate contraindication to breastfeeding. Additional study is necessary to determine the exact role of breastfeeding in the transmission of HCV, including the quantitative measurement of HCV-RNA in colostrum and breast milk, the relative risk of HCV transmission in exclusively or partially breastfed infants versus the risk in formula fed infants, and the effect of duration of breastfeeding on transmission.

The current position of the CDC is that no data indicate that HCV virus is transmitted through breast milk. Therefore, breastfeeding by a HIV-negative mother is not contraindicated.[20]

Infants born to HCV-RNA-positive mothers require follow-up through 18 to 24 months of age to determine the infant's HCV status, regardless of the mode of infant feeding. Infants should be tested for alanine aminotransferase and hepatitis C virus RNA at 3 months and 12 to 15 months of age. Alanine aminotransferase and anti-hepatitis C virus antibody should be tested at 18 to 24 months of age in order to confirm the infant's status: uninfected, ongoing hepatitis C infection, or past hepatitis C virus infection.

Hepatitis D

Hepatitis delta virus (HDV) is a defective RNA virus that causes hepatitis only in persons also infected with HBV. The infection occurs as either an acute coinfection of HBV and HDV or a super-infection of HBV carriers. This "double" infection results in more frequent fulminant hepatitis and chronic hepatitis, which can progress to cirrhosis. The virus uses its own HBV-RNA (circular, negative-strand RNA) with an antigen, HDAg, surrounded by the surface antigen of HBV, HBsAg. HDV is transmitted in the same way as HBV, especially through the exchange of blood and body fluids. HDV infection is uncommon where the prevalence of HBV is low. In areas where HBV is endemic, the prevalence of HDV is highly variable. HDV is very common in tropical Africa and South America as well as in Greece and Italy but is uncommon in the Far East and in Alaskan Eskimos, despite the endemic occurrence of HBV in these areas.[244]

Transmission of HDV has been reported to occur from household contacts and, rarely, through vertical transmission. No data are available on transmission of HDV by breastfeeding. HDV infection can be prevented by blocking infection with HBV; therefore, HBIG and HBV vaccine are the best protection. In addition to HBIG and HBV vaccine administration to the infant of a mother infected with both HBV and HDV, discussion with the mother or parents should include the theoretic risk of HBV and HDV transmission through breastfeeding. As with HBV, once HBIG and HBV vaccine have been given to the infant, the risk of HBV or HDV infection from breastfeeding is negligible. Therefore, breastfeeding after an informed discussion with the parents is acceptable.

Hepatitis E

Hepatitis E virus (HEV) is a cause of sporadic and epidemic, enterically transmitted NANBH, which is typically self-limited and without chronic sequelae. HEV is notable for causing high mortality rate in pregnant women. Transmission is primarily via the fecal-oral route, commonly contaminated water or food. High infection rates have been reported in adolescents and young adults (ages 15 to 40 years). Tomar reported that 70% of cases of HEV infections in the pediatric population in India manifest as acute hepatitis. Maternal-neonatal transmission was documented when the mother developed hepatitis E infection in the third trimester. Although HEV was demonstrated in breast milk, no transmission via breast milk was confirmed in the report. Five cases of transfusion associated hepatitis E were reported.[262] Epidemics are usually related to contamination of water. Person-to-person spread is minimal, even in households and daycare settings. Although IG may be protective, no controlled trials have been done. Animal studies suggest that a recombinant subunit vaccine may be feasible.[216]

HEV infection in infancy is rare, and no data exist on transmission of HEV by breastfeeding. There is no evidence of clinically significant postnatal HEV infection in infants or of chronic sequelae in association with HEV infection and no documented HEV transmission through breast milk. Currently no contraindication exists to breastfeeding with maternal HEV infection. IG has not been shown to be effective in preventing infection, and no vaccine is available for HEV.

Hepatitis G

Hepatitis G virus (HGV) has recently been confirmed as a cause of NANBH distinct from hepatitis viruses A through E. Several closely related genomes of HGV, currently named GBV-A, -B, and -C, appear to be related to HCV, the Pestiviruses, and the Flaviviruses. Epidemiologically, HGV is most often associated with transfusion of blood, although studies have identified nontransfusion-related cases. HGV genomic RNA has been detected in some patients with acute and chronic hepatitis and a small number of patients with fulminant hepatits. GBV-C/HGV has also been found in some patients with inflammatory bile duct lesions, but the pathogenicity of this virus is unconfirmed. HGV-RNA has been detected in 1% to 3% of healthy blood donors in the United States.[6] Feucht and associates[88] described maternal-to-infant transmission of HGV in three of nine children. Two of the three mothers were coinfected with HIV and the third with HCV. None of these infants developed signs of liver disease. Neither the timing nor the mode of transmission was clarified. Lin and associates[163] reported no HGV transmission in three mother-infant pairs after cesarean delivery and discussed transplacental spread via blood as the most likely mode of HGV infection in vertical transmission. Wejstal and associates reported on perinatal transmission of HGV to 12 of 16 infants born to HGV viremic mothers, identified by PCR. HGV did not appear to cause hepatitis in the children.[274]

Fischler and associates[90] followed eight children born to HGV-positive mothers and found only one to be infected with HGV. That child remained clinically well, while his twin, also born by cesarean delivery and breastfed, remained HGV negative over 3 years of observation. Five of the other six children breastfed for variable periods without evidence of HGV infection. Ohto and associates examined HGV mother-to-infant transmission. Of 2979 pregnant Japanese women who were screened, 32 were identified as positive for GBV-C/HGV RNA by PCR; 26 of 34 infants born to the 32 HGV positive women were shown to be HGV RNA positive. Reportedly, none of the infants demonstrated a clinical picture of hepatitis, although two infants had persistent mild elevations (less than two times normal) of alanine aminotransferase. The viral load in mothers, who transmitted HGV to their infants, was significantly higher than in nontransmitting mothers. Infants delivered by elective cesarean section had a lower rate of infection (3 in 7) compared with infants born by emergency cesarean section (2 of 2) or born vaginally (21 of 25). In this study, HGV infection in breastfed infants was four times more common than in formula fed infants, but this difference was not statistically significant because only four infants were formula fed. The authors report there was no correlation between infection rate and duration of breastfeeding. Testing of the infants was not done frequently and early enough routinely through the first year of life to determine the timing of infection in these infants.[197] Schröter and associates reported transmission of HGV to 3 of 15 infants born to HGV RNA positive mothers at 1 week of age. None of 15 breast milk samples were positive for GBV-C/HGV RNA, and all of the children who were initially negative for HGV RNA in serum remained negative at follow-up between 1 to 28 months of age.[234]

The foregoing data suggest that transmission is more likely to be vertical, prior to, or at delivery rather than via breast feeding. The pathogenicity and the possibility of chronic disease due to HGV infection remain uncertain at this time. Insufficient data are available to make a recommendation concerning breastfeeding by the HGV-infected mother.

TT Virus

TT virus is a recently identified virus found in a patient (TT) with posttransfusion hepatitis not associated with the other hepatitis related viruses A through G. TTV has been described as an unenveloped, circular, single-stranded DNA virus.[199]

This virus is prevalent in healthy individuals, including healthy blood donors, as well as having been identified in patients with hepatitis. TTV DNA has been detected in infants of TTV-positive and TTV-negative mothers. Ohto and associates reported no TTV DNA was detected in cord blood from 38 infants, and it was detected in only 1 of 14 samples taken at 1 month of age. They noted an increasing prevalence, from 6 months (22%) to 2 years (33%), which they ascribed to acquisition via nonparenteral routes. In comparisons of the TTV DNA in TTV-positive mothers and their positive infants; 6 of 13 showed high level nucleotide sequence similarity, and 7 of 13 differed by greater than 10%.[198]

Schröter and associates reported on TTV DNA in breast milk examined retrospectively. Notably, TTV DNA was detected in 22 of 23 serum samples of infants at 1 week of age, who were born to 22 women viremic for TTV DNA. Twenty-four women who were negative for TTV DNA gave birth to 24 children who were initially negative for TTV DNA and remained negative throughout the observation period (mean 7.5 months, range 1 to 28 months). TTV DNA was detected in 77% of breast milk samples from TTV viremic women and in none of the breast milk samples from TTV-negative women. There was no clinical or laboratory evidence of hepatitis found in the 22 children who were observed to be TTV DNA positive during the period of this study.[234] Other authors have reported TTV in breast milk detected by PCR. They describe the absence of TTV DNA in infants at 5 days and 3 months of age, and 4 of 10 infants were positive for TTV DNA at 6 months of age, suggesting the late acquisition of infection via breastfeeding.[135]

TT virus is transmitted in utero and is found in breast milk. There is no evidence of clinical hepatitis in infants related to TTV infection, nor is there evidence for a late chronic hepatitis. Given the current available information there is no reason to proscribe breastfeeding by TTV-positive mothers. There is certainly more to be understood concerning the chronic nature of this infection and the possible pathogenesis of liver disease.

Human papillomavirus

Human papillomavirus (HPV) is a DNA virus with at least 70 different types. These viruses cause warts, genital dysplasia, cervical carcinoma (types 6 and 11), and laryngeal papillomatosis. Transmission occurs through direct contact and sexual contact. Laryngeal papillomas are believed to result from acquiring the virus in passage through the birth canal. Infection in pregnant women or during pregnancy does not lead to an increase in abortions or the risk of prematurity, and no evidence indicates intrauterine infection.

Diagnosis is usually by histologic examination or DNA detection. Spontaneous resolution does occur, but therapy for persistent lesions or growths in anatomically problematic locations is appropriate. Therapy can be with podophyllum preparations, trichloroacetic acid, cryotherapy, electrocautery, and laser surgery. Interferon is being tested in the treatment of laryngeal papillomas, with mixed results.[71] Prevention against transmission means limiting direct or sexual contact, but this may not be sufficient because lesions may not be evident, and transmission may still occur.

The breast is a rare site of involvement. Without breast lesions, there is no apparent risk from breast milk, and breastfeeding is acceptable.

Parvovirus

Human parvovirus B19 causes a broad range of clinical manifestations, including asymptomatic infection (most frequent manifestation in all ages), erythema infectiosum (fifth disease), arthralgia and arthritis, red blood cell (RBC) aplasia (less often decreased white blood cells or platelets), chronic infection in immunodeficient individuals, and rarely myocarditis, vasculitis, or hemophagocytic syndrome.

Vertical transmission can lead to severe anemia and immune-mediated hydrops fetalis, which can be treated, if accurately diagnosed, by intrauterine transfusion. Inflammation of the liver or CNS can be seen in the infant, along with vasculitis. If the child is clinically well at birth, hidden or persistent abnormalities are rarely identified. No evidence indicates that parvovirus B19 causes an identified pattern of birth defects.

Postnatal transmission usually occurs person to person via contact with respiratory secretions, saliva, and rarely blood or urine. Seroprevalence in children at 5 years of age is less than 5%, with the peak age of infection occurring during the school-age years (5% to 40% of children infected). The majority of infections are asymptomatic or undiagnosed seroconversions.[263] Severe disease, such as prolonged aplastic anemia, occurs in individuals with hemoglobinopathies or abnormal RBC maturation. Attack rates have been estimated to be 17% to 30% in casual contacts but up to 50% among household contacts. In one study of 235 susceptible pregnant women, the annual seroconversion rate was 1.4%.[149]

There are no reports of transmission to an infant through breastfeeding. Excretion in breast milk has not been studied because of limitations in culturing techniques. Rat parvovirus has been demonstrated in rat milk. The very low seroconversion rate in young children and the absence of chronic or frequent severe disease suggest that the risk of parvovirus infection via breast milk is not significant. The possibility of antibodies against parvovirus or other protective constituents in breast milk has not been studied. Breastfeeding by a mother with parvovirus infection is acceptable.

RETROVIRUSES

Human T-cell leukemia virus type I

The occurrence of human T-cell leukemia virus type I (HTLV-I) is endemic in parts of southwestern Japan,[55,68,121,141,281] the Carribean, South America,[108] and sub-Saharan Africa. HTLV-I is associated with adult T cell leukemia/lymphoma (ATL) and a chronic condition with progressive neuropathy. The progressive neuropathy is called HTLV-I associated myelopathy or tropical spastic paraparesis (HAM/TSP).[93] Other illnesses have been reported in association with HTLV-I infection including dermatitis, uveitis, arthritis, Sjögren's syndrome in adults, and infective dermatitis and persistent lymphadenitis in children. Transmission of HTLV-I occurs most often through sexual contact, via blood or blood products, and via breast milk. Infrequent transmission does occur in utero or at delivery and with casual or household contact.[187]

Seroprevalence generally increases with age and varies widely in different regions and in populations of different backgrounds. In some areas of Japan, seropsitivity can be as high as 12% to 16%, but in South America, Africa, and some Caribbean countries the rates are 2% to 6%. In Latin America seropostive rates can be as high as 10% to 25% among female sex workers or attendees to STD clinics.[108] In blood donors in Europe, the seroprevalence of HTLV-I has been reported at 0.001% to 0.03%. The seroprevalence in pregnant women in endemic areas of Japan is as high as 4% to 5% and in nonendemic areas as low as 0.1% to 1.0%. HTLV-1 is not a major disease in the United States.[25] In studies from Europe the seroprevalence in pregnant women has been noted to be up to 0.6%. These pregnant women were primarily of African or Caribbean descent.[94]

HTLV-I antigen has been identified in breast milk of HTLV-I positive mothers.[147] Another report shows that basal mammary epithelial cells can be infected with HTLV-I and can transfer infection to peripheral blood monocytes.[162] Human milk from HTLV-I positive mothers caused infection in marmosets.[148,283] HTLV-I infection clearly occurs via breastfeeding and a number of reports document an increased rate of transmission of HTLV-I to breast-fed infants compared with formula fed infants.[7,8,10,11,119,120,258] Ando and associates in two separate reports demonstrated a parallel decline in antibodies against HTLV-I in both formula fed and breastfed infants to a nadir at about 1 year of age and a subsequent increase in antibodies from 1 to 2 years of age. The percentage of children seropositive at 1 year of age was 3.0% and 0.6%, at 1.5 years of age it was 15.2% and 3.9%, and at 2 years of age it was 41.9% and 4.6% in the breastfed and formula fed groups, respectively. A smaller group of children followed out through 11 to 12 years of age demonstrated no newly infected children after

2 years of age and no loss of antibody in any child who was seropositive at 2 years of age.[10,11]

Transmission of HTLV-I infection via breastfeeding is also clearly associated with the duration of breastfeeding.[258,259,276,277] It has been postulated that the persistence of passively acquired antibodies against HTLV-I offers some protection through 6 months of life (Table 17-5).

Other factors relating to HTLV-I transmission via breast milk have been proposed. Yoshinaga and associates presented data on the HTLV-I antigen producing capacity of peripheral blood and breast milk cells and showed an increased mother-to-child transmission rate when the mother's blood and breast milk produced large numbers of antigen-producing cells in culture.[289] Hisada and associates reported on 150 mothers and infants in Jamaica, demonstrating that a higher maternal provirus level and a higher HTLV-I antibody titer were independently associated with HTLV-I transmission to the infant.[124] Ureta-Vidal and associates reported an increased seropositivity rate in children of mothers with a high proviral load and elevated maternal HTLV-I antibody titers.[265]

Various interventions have been proposed to decrease HTLV-I transmission via breastfeeding. Complete avoidance of breastfeeding was shown to be an effective intervention by Hino and associates in large population of Japanese in Nagasaki.[122] There was an 80% decrease in transmission by avoiding breastfeeding. Breastfeeding for a shorter duration is another effective alternative. Ando and

associates showed that freezing and thawing breast milk decreased the infectivity of HTLV-I.[9] Sawada and associates demonstrated in a rabbit model that HTLV-I immune globulin protected against HTLV-I transmission via milk.[227] It is reasonable to postulate that any measure that would decrease the maternal provirus load or increase the anti-HTLV-I antibodies available to the infant might decrease the risk of transmission. The overall prevalence of HTLV-I infection during childhood is unknown because the majority of individuals do not manifest illness until much later in life. The timing of HTLV-I infection in a breastfeeding population has been difficult to assess because of passively acquired antibodies from the mother and issues related to testing. Furnia and associates estimated the time of infection for a cohort of 16 breastfed infants in Jamaica.[95] The estimated median time of infection was 11.9 months as determined by PCR as compared with the estimated time of infection, based on whole virus Western blot, of 12.4 months.

In areas where the prevalence of HTLV-I infection (in the United States, Canada, or Europe) is rare, the likelihood that a single test for antibody against HTLV-I would be a false positive test is high compared with the number of true positive tests. Repeat testing is warranted in many situations.[55] Quantification of the antibody titer and the proviral load is appropriate in a situation when mother-to-child transmission is a concern. A greater risk of progression to disease in later life

---

TABLE 17-5   HTLV-I Transmission Related to the Duration of Breastfeeding

Author (reference)	Duration	Seroconversion Rate	Number of Children*
Takahashi[258]	≤6 months	4.4%	4/90
	≥7 months	14.4%	20/139
	(bottle-fed)	5.7%	9/158
Takezaki[259]	≤6 months	3.9%	2/51
	>6 months	20.3%	13/64
Wiktor[277]	< 12 months	9%	8/86
	≥ 12 months	32%	19/60

* Number of children positive for HTLV-I over the number of children examined.

has not been shown for HTLV-I infection through breast milk, but early-life infections are associated with the greatest risk of adult T-cell leukemia.[254]

The mother and family should be informed about all these issues. If the risk of lack of breast milk is not too great and formula is readily available and culturally acceptable, then the proscription of breastfeeding or at least a recommendation to limit the duration of breastfeeding to 6 months or less is appropriate to limit the risk of HTLV-I transmission to the infant. Freezing and thawing breast milk before giving it to the infant might be another reasonable intervention to decrease the risk of transmission. Neither immune globulin nor antiviral agents against HTLV-I are available at this time.

Human T-cell leukemia virus type II

Human T-cell leukemia virus type II (HTLV-II) is endemic in specific geographic locations, including Africa, the Americas, the Caribbean, and Japan. Transmission is primarily through IVDU, contaminated blood products, and breastfeeding. Sexual transmission occurs but its overall contribution to the prevalence of HTLV-II in different populations remains uncertain. Many studies have examined the presence of HTLV-I and II in blood products. PCR testing and selective antibody tests suggest that about one half of the HTLV seropositivity in blood donors is caused by HTLV-II.

HTLV-II has been associated with two chronic neurologic disorders similar to those caused by HTLV-I, tropical or spastic ataxia.[166] A connection between HTLV-II and glomerulonephritis, myelopathy, arthritis, T-hairy cell leukemia, and large granulocytic leukemia has been reported.

Mother-to-child transmission has been demonstrated in both breastfed and formula fed infants. It appears that the rate of transmission is greater in breastfed infants.[94,117,134,152,153,193,268,270] HTLV-II has been detected in breast milk.[117] Nyambi and associates reported that HTLV-II transmission did correlate with the duration of breastfeeding. The estimated rate of transmission was 20%. The time to serconversion (after the initial loss of passively acquired maternal antibodies) for infected infants seemed to range between 1 and 3 years of age.[193] Avoidance of breastfeeding and limiting the duration of breastfeeding are the only two possible interventions with evidence of effectiveness for preventing HTLV-II mother-to-child transmission.

With the current understanding of retroviruses, it is appropriate in cases of documented HTLV-II maternal infection to recommend avoiding or limiting the duration of breastfeeding and provide alternative nutrition when financially practical and culturally acceptable. The mother should have confirmatory testing for HTLV-II and measurement of the proviral load. The infant should be serially tested for antibodies to HTLV-II and have confirmatory testing if still seropositive after 12 to 18 months of age. Further investigation into the mechanisms of transmission via breast milk and possible interventions to prevent transmission should occur as it is for HIV-1 and HTLV-I.

Human immunodeficiency virus type 1

Human immunodeficiency virus type 1 (HIV-1) is transmitted through human milk. Refraining from breastfeeding is a crucial aspect of preventing perinatal HIV infection in the United States and many other countries. The dilemma is the use of replacement feeding in countries where breastfeeding provides infants with significant protection from illness and death due to other infections. The question of the contribution of breastfeeding in mother-to-child HIV-1 transmission is not a trivial one; when one considers the following:

1. The World Health Oganization (WHO) has estimated that there were 40 million people living with HIV-1 in 2003.
2. Over 90% of the children younger than 13 years old infected with HIV-1 have been infected by mother-to-child transmission.
3. WHO estimates that 5 million people were newly infected with HIV-1 in 2003, with children younger than 15 years old making up 700,000 of that 5 million.

4. Breastfeeding contributes an estimated 10% to 20% increase in the overall mother-to-child transmission rates, over and above intrauterine and intrapartum transmission.

The evidence of HIV transmission via breastfeeding is irrefutable. Two recent publications summarize the current evidence for HIV transmission via breastfeeding in the literature.[214,264] Since 1985, case reports have documented HIV transmission via breast milk to children around the world.[123,136,160,293] Primary HIV infection in breastfeeding mothers, with the concomitant high viral load, is associated with a particularly high rate of HIV transmission via breast milk. Palasanthiran and associates estimated that risk at 27%.[203] Large observational studies have demonstrated higher rates of HIV transmission in breastfed infants of mothers with chronic HIV infection compared with formula fed infants.[30,69,85] A systematic analysis of published reports estimated the additional risk of perinatal HIV transmission due to breastfeeding to be 14% (95% CI: 7% to 22%).[78] More recently published cohort studies similarly attributed additional risk of HIV transmission due to breastfeeding at 4% to 22% over and above the risk from prenatal and intrapartum transmission.[26,67,82] Laboratory reports demonstrate the presence of cell-free virus and cell-associated virus in breast milk as well as various immunologic factors that could block or limit infection.[37,109,188,190,200,233,261,266] A dose response has been observed, correlating the HIV viral load in human milk as well as the mother's plasma viral load with an increased transmission risk for the breastfed infant.[210,217,221,236]

Many of the potential risk factors associated with human milk transmission of HIV have been described. The cumulative risk of HIV transmission is higher the longer the duration of breastfeeding.[69,161,182,186,267] Maternal characteristics related to transmission of HIV via human milk include younger maternal age, higher parity, lower CD4+ counts, higher plasma viral loads, and breast abnormalities (mastitis, abscess, or nipple lesions). Characteristics of human milk that relate to a higher risk of transmission include higher viral load in the milk, lower concentrations of antiviral substances

(lactoferrin, lysozyme), and lower concentrations of virus-specific cytotoxic T-lymphocytes, secretory IgA, and IgM. Mixed breastfeeding is also associated with a higher risk of HIV transmission compared with exclusive breastfeeding.[64,65,260] The measurable benefits of breast milk versus the relative risk of HIV transmission to the infant due to exclusive breastfeeding (with optimization of other factors to decrease HIV transmission) has not yet been studied in a prospective fashion.[159]

There are a number of potential interventions to prevent breastfeeding transmission of HIV-1 that can be utilized (Box 17-2). The simplest and most effective is the compete avoidance of human milk. This is a practical solution in places like the United States and other countries where replacement feeding as well as other strictly medical interventions are feasible and reasonable, and the risk of not providing breast milk to the infant is negligible. In resource-poor situations, where the risk of other infections is high without the benefits of breast milk, then breastfeeding is appropriate along with any reasonable interventions to decrease HIV transmission via breast milk.

The complete avoidance of breastfeeding in certain situations may lead to increased risk of death due to other reasons besides HIV transmission. One study from Kenya showed improved HIV-1-free survival rates in a formula fed group of children born to HIV-positive mothers, but the breastfed and formula groups had similar mortality rates (24.4% versus 20.0%, respectively) as well as similar incidences of diarrhea and pneumonia over the first 2 years of life.[175] There was no difference in the two groups in terms of the prevalence of malnutrition, but the breastfed infants had better nutritional status in the first 6 months of life.

Potentially effective interventions include exclusive breastfeeding, early weaning, education, and support to decrease the likelihood of mastitis or nipple lesions. Other possible interventions include treating the mother with antiretroviral therapy to decrease the human milk viral load, treating the milk itself to decrease the viral load (by pasteurization or other methods),[200,201] treating acute conditions in the mother and the infant (e.g., mastitis,

BOX 17-2   Recommendations on breastfeeding and transmission of human immunodeficiency virus (HIV)

- Women and their health care providers need to be aware of the potential risk of transmission of HIV infection to infants during pregnancy and in the peripartum period, as well as through breast milk.
- Documented, routine HIV education and routine testing with consent of all women seeking prenatal care are strongly recommended so that each woman knows her HIV status and the methods available both to prevent the acquisition and transmission of HIV and to determine whether breastfeeding is appropriate.
- At delivery, education about HIV and testing with consent of all women whose HIV status during pregnancy is unknown are strongly recommended. Knowledge of the woman's HIV status assists in counseling on breastfeeding and helps each woman understand the benefits to herself and her infant of knowing her serostatus and the behaviors that would decrease the likelihood of acquisition and transmission of HIV.
- Women who are known to be HIV infected must be counseled not to breastfeed or provide their milk for the nutrition of their own or other infants.
- In general, women who are known to be HIV seronegative should be encouraged to breastfeed. However, women who are HIV seronegative but at particularly high risk of seroconversion (e.g., injection drug users and sexual partners of known HIV-positive persons or active drug users) should be educated about

HIV with an individualized recommendation concerning the appropriateness of breastfeeding. In addition, during the perinatal period, information should be provided on the potential risk of transmitting HIV through breast milk and about methods to reduce the risk of acquiring HIV infection.
- Each woman whose HIV status is unknown should be informed of the potential for HIV-infected women to transmit HIV during the peripartum period and through breast milk and the potential benefits to her and her infant of knowing her HIV status and how HIV is acquired and transmitted. The health care provider needs to make an individualized recommendation to assist the woman in deciding whether to breastfeed.
- Neonatal intensive care units should develop policies that are consistent with these recommendations for the use of expressed breast milk for neonates. Current standards of the U.S. Occupational Safety and Health Administration (OSHA) do not require gloves for the routine handling of expressed human milk. However, health care workers should wear gloves in situations in which exposure to breast milk might be frequent or prolonged, such as in milk banking.
- Human milk banks should follow the guidelines developed by the U.S. Public Health Service, which include screening all donors for HIV infection and assessing risk factors that predispose to infection, as well as pasteurization of all milk specimens.

From Lawrence RA: A review of the medical benefits and contraindications to breastfeeding in the United States. In Maternal and Child Health Technical Information Bulletin, Washington, DC, US Health Resources and Services Administration, 1997.

breast lesions, infant candidiasis), and enhancing the infant's own defenses via immunization or antiretroviral therapy. There is limited information of the practicality and effectiveness of many of these interventions in clinical trials. Some of these may not be feasible in certain settings such as pasteurization or maternal antiretroviral therapy. Others may not be culturally acceptable such as treating expressed breast milk prior to giving it to the infant

or even exclusive breastfeeding. Any method of treating the breast milk, to decrease viral load, will need to be clinically assessed as to its effect on the nutritional and protective benefits for the infant, including nutritional status, growth, development, and overall survival. It is unlikely that any single intervention or a combination of them will effectively decrease the risk of HIV-1 mother-to-child transmission to zero.[70]

The potential effect of breastfeeding on the HIV-positive mother needs to be assessed in relation to the mother's health status. Two studies have examined this and reported conflicting results. The first study from Kenya demonstrated a significantly higher mortality rate in breastfeeding mothers compared with a formula feeding group in the 2 years after delivery. The hypothesized explanation offered by the authors for this difference was increased metabolic demands, greater weight loss, and nutritional depletion.[189] A second study from South Africa showed an overall lower mortality rate in the two groups with no significant difference in mortality rate over 10 months of observation.[66]

In summary, breastfeeding of infants by HIV-positive mothers does lead to an increased risk of HIV infection in the infant. There is much still to be understood about the mechanisms of HIV transmission via breast milk and the action and efficacy of interventions to prevent such transmission. The complete avoidance of breastfeeding remains a crucial component for the prevention of perinatal HIV infection in the United States and many other countries. In resource-poor settings, where breastfeeding is the norm and where it provides vital nutritional and infection protective benefits, the WHO, UNICEF, and UNAIDS recommend education, counseling, and support for HIV-infected mothers so they can make an informed choice concerning infant feeding. Mothers choosing to breastfeed should receive additional education, support, and medical care to minimize the risk of HIV transmission and to optimize their own health status during and after breastfeeding. Mothers choosing to use replacement feedings should receive parallel education, support, and medical care for themselves and their infants to minimize the effect of the lack of breastfeeding. The decision about infant feeding for the HIV-positive mother remains a true dilemma—a choice between two equally unsatisfactory alternatives. It is only through continued research and education concerning the potential interventions to prevent HIV transmission via breast milk that we can minimize transmission and optimize infant nutrition and health.

Human immunodeficiency virus type 2

Human immunodeficiency virus type 2 (HIV-2) is an RNA virus in the nononcogenic, cytopathic lentivirus genus of retroviruses. It is genetically closer to *simian immunodeficiency virus* (SIV) than to HIV-1. The clinical disease associated with HIV-2 has similar symptoms to HIV-1 infection, but progresses at a slower rate to severe immunosuppression.

HIV-2 is endemic in west Africa and parts of the Caribbean and found infrequently in Europe and North and South America.[131,194] It is transmitted via sexual contact, blood, or blood products and from mother to child.

Routine testing for HIV-2 is recommended in blood banks. Antibody tests used for HIV-1 are only 50% to 90% sensitive for detecting HIV-2.[41] Specific testing for HIV-2 is appropriate whenever clinically or epidemiologically indicated.

Vertical transmission occurs infrequently. Ekpini and associates followed a large cohort of west African mothers and infants; 138 HIV-1 positive women, 132 HIV-2 positive women, 69 women seropositive for both HIV-1 and 2, and 274 HIV seronegative women. A few cases of perinatal HIV-2 transmission occurred, but no case of late postnatal transmission was observed.[82]

It is probable that HIV-2 transmission via breast milk is less common than with HIV-1, but there is insufficient data to say the risk of transmission is zero. Mothers who test positive for HIV-2 should be tested for HIV-1, and guidelines for breastfeeding should follow those for HIV-1 until additional information is available.

Rabies

Rabies virus produces a severe infection with progressive CNS symptoms (anxiety, seizures, altered mental status) that ultimately proceeds to death; few reports of survival exist. Rabies occurs worldwide except in Australia, Antarctica, and several island groups. In 1992 more than 36,000 cases of rabies were reported to WHO, a number that is probably a marked underestimate of the actual cases.[42] Between 1990 and 2003, there were 37 cases of human rabies in the United States.[45,52] Postexposure prophylaxis is given to thousands of patients each year.

Rabies virus is endemic in various animal populations, including raccoons, skunks, foxes, and bats. Because of aggressive immunization programs, rabies in domesticated dogs and cats in the United States is uncommon. The virus is found in the saliva and nervous tissue of infected animals. Transmission occurs by bites, licking, or simply contact of oral secretions with mucous membranes or nonintact skin. Many cases of rabies in humans now lack a history of some obvious contact with a rabid animal. This may be a result of the long incubation period (generally 4 to 6 weeks, but can be up to 1 year, with reports of incubation periods of several years), a lack of symptoms early in an infectious animal, or airborne transmission from bats in enclosed environments (caves, laboratories, houses). Person-to-person transmission via bites has not been documented, although it has occurred in corneal transplants.[31] No evidence indicates transmission through breast milk.

In the case of maternal infection with rabies, many scenarios can occur before the onset of progressive, severe CNS symptoms. The progression and severity of maternal illness can preclude breastfeeding, but separation of the infant from the mother is appropriate regardless of the mother's status and method of infant feeding. Breastfeeding should not continue when the mother has symptoms of rabies, and the infant should receive postexposure immunization and close observation. Depending on the scenario, the nature of the mother's illness, the possible exposure of the infant to the same source as the mother, and the exposure of the child to the mother, postexposure immunization of the infant may be appropriate. A more common scenario is the mother's apparent exposure to rabies (without exposure for the infant), necessitating postexposure immunization of the mother with rabies vaccine. In the majority of cases, in the absence of maternal illness, breastfeeding can reasonably continue during the mother's five-dose immunization series over 28 days. In a rare situation in which apparent exposure of the mother and infant to rabies occurs together, postexposure treatment of both mother and infant should be instituted, and breastfeeding can continue.

Respiratory syncytial virus

Respiratory syncytial virus (RSV) is a common cause of respiratory illness in children and is relatively common in adults, usually producing milder upper respiratory tract infection in adults. No evidence indicates that RSV causes intrauterine infection, adversely affects the fetus, or causes abortion or prematurity. RSV does produce infection in neonates, causing asymptomatic infection, afebrile upper respiratory tract infection, bronchiolitis, pneumonia, and apnea. Mortality rate can be high in neonates, especially in premature infants and ill full-term infants, particularly those with preexisting respiratory disease (hyaline membrane disease, bronchopulmonary dysplasia) or cardiac disease associated with pulmonary hypertension.

RSV is believed to be transmitted via droplets or direct contact of the conjunctiva, nasal mucosa, or oropharynx with infected respiratory secretions. Documentation of RSV infection is rarely made in adults, and spread from the mother or other household contacts probably occurs before a diagnosis can be made. Therefore, risk of RSV transmission from breast milk is probably insignificant compared with transmission via direct or droplet contact in families. In nurseries, however, it is appropriate to make a timely diagnosis of RSV infection in the neonate to gain the benefit of treatment with ribavirin and to isolate the infant from the others to prevent spread in the nursery. RSV infection should be suspected in any infant with rhinorrhea, nasal congestion, or unexplained apnea, especially in October through March in temperate climates. Prophylaxis against RSV with specific intravenous immune globulin (RSV-IGIV) during this season for infants at highest risk of severe disease may be appropriate.

Considerable debate surrounds the effect of passively acquired antibodies against RSV on the occurrence and severity of illness in the neonate and infant. It appears that a higher level of neutralizing antibody against RSV in the neonate decreases the risk of severe RSV disease.[105,154] However, some controversy remains concerning the measurable benefit of breastfeeding for preventing serious RSV disease.[2,36,76] Different studies have shown benefit and others no effect. Controlling for possible confounding factors (e.g., smoking, crowded living conditions) in these studies has been difficult. At this point, no reason exists to stop breastfeeding with maternal RSV infection, and infants with RSV infection should breastfeed unless their respiratory status precludes it.

Severe acute respiratory syndrome (SARS)

This term could be applied to any acute serious respiratory illness caused by or associated with a variety of infections agents; however, since 2003 it has been linked with SARS-associated coronavirus. In the global outbreak of 2002–2003 there were over 8400 probable cases of SARS and over 800 deaths. More than the actual number of affected individuals or its associated mortality rate (approximately 10% overall, but closer to 50% in persons over 65 years of age), it was what we did not know about this new unusual illness, and the tremendous publicity surrounding it, that made SARS such a sensation. We now know the cause of this illness, known as the SARS-associated coronavirus (SARS-CoV). SARS-CoV was shown to not be closely related to these previously characterized coronavirus groups.[171,220] Despite intense international collaboration to study the illness and the virus, there are still many things we do not know about it, such as the degree of infectiousness (Ro), the actual period of transmissibility, all the modes of transmission, how many people have an asymptomatic infection compared to those with symptoms or severe illness, how to make a rapid diagnosis of confirmed cases, and where it originated, just to name a few.

At least 21 cases of probable SARS in children have been described in the literature.[29,128,240,242] In general, the illness in children is a mild, nonspecific respiratory illness, but in adolescents it is more likely to progress to severe respiratory distress, as it does in adults. It has been reported that children are less likely to transmit SARS than adults.[128] The overall clinical course, the radiologic evolution, and the histologic findings of these illness are consistent with the host's immune response playing a significant role in disease production.

Five infants were born to mothers with confirmed SARS. The infants were born prematurely (26 to 37 weeks) presumably due to maternal illness. Although two of the five infants had serious abdominal illnesses (other coronaviruses have been associated with reported outbreaks of necrotizing enterocolitis), the presence of SARS-CoV could not be demonstrated in any of these infants.[240]

There was no mention of the mode of feeding for any of the reported cases of young children with SARS or the infants born to mothers with SARS. As with other respiratory viruses predominantly transmitted by droplets, transmission via breast milk is an insignificant mode of transmission, if it occurs at all. The benefits of breastfeeding being what they are, mothers with SARS should continue breastfeeding if they are able or expressed breast milk can be given to the infant, until the mother is able to breastfeed.

Smallpox

In this era of worry about biologic terrorism, smallpox is an important concern. The concern for the infant (breastfed or formula fed) is direct contact with the mother or a household member with smallpox. Smallpox is highly contagious in the household setting due to person-to-person spread via droplet nuclei or aerosolization from the oropharynx and direct contact with the rash. Additional potential exposures for the infant include the release of a smallpox aerosol into the environment by terrorists, contact with a smallpox-contaminated space or the clothes of household members exposed to an aerosol, and infection via contact with the mother's or a household member's smallpox vaccination site. These risks are the same for breastfed and formula fed infants. There is no evidence for transmission of the smallpox virus via breast milk.

Relative to smallpox, a contact is defined as a person who has been in the same household or had face-to-face contact with the patient (with smallpox) after the onset of fever. Patients do not transmit infection until after progression from the fever stage to the development of the rash. An exposed contact does not need to be isolated from others during the postcontact observation period (usually 17 days) until the person develops fever. Temperature should be monitored daily in the exposed contact. Personal contact and breastfeeding between mother and infant can continue until the onset of fever, when immediate isolation (at home) should begin. Providing expressed breast milk for the infant of a mother with smallpox should be avoided because of the extensive nature of the smallpox rash and the possibility of contamination (from the rash) of the milk during the expression process. There is no literature documenting transmission of the smallpox virus via expressed breast milk.

The other issue for the breastfeeding infant is the question of maternal vaccination with smallpox in a pre-event vaccination program. Children over 1 year of age can be safely and reasonably vaccinated with smallpox in the face of a probable smallpox exposure. Smallpox vaccination of infants younger than 1 year of age is contraindicated. Breastfeeding is listed as a contraindication to vaccination in the pre-event vaccination program. It is unknown whether vaccine virus or antibodies are present in breast milk. The risk of infection due to contact or aerosolization of virus from a mother's smallpox vaccination site is the same for the breastfed and formula fed infant. The Advisory Committee on Immunization Practices also does not recommend pre-event smallpox vaccination of children younger than 18 years old.[275]

A report documents tertiary contact vaccinia in a breastfeeding infant.[96] A U.S. military person received a primary smallpox vaccination and developed a local reaction at the inoculation site. Despite reportedly observing appropriate precautions, the individual's wife developed vesicles on both areolae (secondary contact vaccinia). Subsequently, the breastfeeding infant developed lesions on her philtrum, cheek, and tongue. Both the mother and infant remained well and the infections resolved without therapy. Culture and PCR testing confirmed vaccinia in both the mother's and the infant's lesions. The breast milk was not tested.[96]

Sepkowitz reported on 27 cases of secondary vaccinia in households in a review from 1931 to 1981.[239] The CDC reported 30 suspected cases of secondary/tertiary vaccinia with 18 of those cases confirmed by culture or PCR. The 30 cases were related to 578,286 vaccinated military personnel. This is an incidence of 5.2 cases per 100,000 vaccinees and 7.4 cases per 100,000 primary vaccinees.[53] In a separate report on the civilian pre-event smallpox vaccination program, 37,802 individuals were vaccinated between January and June 2003 and there were no reported cases of contact vaccinia.[51]

The risk of contact vaccinia is low. The risk is from close or intimate contact. In the above-mentioned case, the risk for the infant was contact with the mother's breasts, the inadvertent site of her contact vaccinia. Breastfed and formula fed infants are equally at risk from close contact in the household of a smallpox vaccinee or a case of secondary vaccinia, and separation from the individual is appropriate in both situations. If the breast of the nursing mother is not involved, then expressed breast milk can be given to the infant.

West Nile virus

West Nile virus disease in the United States is one of the best examples of an emerging infectious disease taking on new importance in public awareness about health issues. In 2003, there were 9136 human cases of West Nile infection reported to the CDC (through 2/11/2004). Cases were reported from 45 states, including 6256 (68%) cases of West Nile fever (milder cases), 2718 (30%) cases of West Nile meningoencephalitis, and 228 deaths related to West Nile disease.[54] West Nile virus is endemic in Israel and parts of Africa. Outbreaks have been reported from Romania (1996), Russia (1999), Israel (2000), and Canada (2002) as well as the United States (1999–2003).[208]

It is estimated that 150 to 300 asymptomatic cases of West Nile infection occur for every 20 febrile illnesses and for every one case of meningoencephalitis associated with West Nile virus. West Nile fever is usually a mild illness of 3 to 6 days' duration. The symptoms are relatively nonspecific, including malaise, nausea, vomiting, headache, myalgia, lymphadenopathy, and rash. West Nile disease is characterized by severe neurologic symptoms (e.g., meningitis, encephalitis, or acute flaccid paralysis, and occasionally optic neuritis, cranial nerve abnormalities, and seizures). Children are infrequently sick with West Nile virus infection and infants younger than 1 year of age have rarely been reported.[208] The case-fatality rate for 2003 in the United States was approximately 2.5%, but has been reported as high as 4% to 18% in hospitalized patients. The case-fatality rate for persons over 70 years of age is considered to be higher, 15% to 29% among hospitalized patients in outbreaks in Romania and Israel.[208]

The primary mechanism of transmission is via a mosquito bite. Mosquitoes from the genus *Culex* are primary vectors. The bird-mosquito-bird cycle serves to maintain and amplify the virus in the environment. Humans and horses are incidental hosts. The pathogenesis of the infection is believed to occur via replication of the virus in the skin and lymph nodes, leading to a primary viremia which seeds secondary sites before a second viremia causes the infection of the central nervous system and other affected organs.[39,72] Transmission has been reported in rare instances during pregnancy[5,48] via organ transplant[137] and percutaneously in laboratory workers.[50] West Nile virus transmission occurs via blood and blood product transfusion,[127] and the incidence has been estimated to be as high as 21 per 10,000 donations during epidemics in specific cities.[28] There is no evidence of direct person-to-person transmission without the mosquito vector.

There is one reported case of possible West Nile virus (WNV) transmission via breastfeeding.[49] The mother acquired the virus via packed red blood cell transfusions after delivery. The second unit of blood she received was associated with other blood products from the same donation causing West Nile infection in another transfusion recipient. Eight days later the mother had a severe headache and was hospitalized with fever and a CSF pleocytosis on day 12 after delivery. The mother's CSF was positive for WNV-specific IgM antibody. The infant had been breastfed from birth through the second day of hospitalization of the mother. Samples of breast milk were WNV-specific IgG and IgM positive on day 16 after delivery and WNV-specific IgM positive on day 24. The same milk was WNV-RNA positive by PCR testing on day 16, but not on day 24 after delivery. The infant tested positive for WNV-specific IgM in serum at day 25 of age, but remained well without fever. There was reportedly no clear-cut exposure to mosquitoes for the infant. The cord blood and placenta were not available to be tested. IgM antibodies can be found in low concentrations in breast milk, but this is not common or as efficient as the transfer of IgA, sIgA, or IgG into breast milk. This is the only case currently reported in the literature. Live virus has not been cultured from the samples of breast milk.

Based on the information from this single case in which the infant remained well, and considering the lack of significant disease due to West Nile virus infection in young children, there is no reason to proscribe breastfeeding in the case of maternal West Nile virus infection if the mother is well enough to breastfeed. As with many other maternal viral illnesses, by the time the diagnosis is made in the mother, the infant may have already been exposed during maternal viremia and possible virolactia. The infant can and should continue to receive breast milk for the potential specific immunologic benefit.

SPIROCHETES

Lyme disease

Lyme disease, as with the other human illnesses caused by spirochetes, especially syphilis, is characterized by a protean course and distinct phases (stages) of disease. Lyme borreliosis was described in Europe in the early 20th century. Since the 1970s, tremendous recognition, description, and investigation of Lyme disease have occurred in the United States and Europe. Public concern surrounding this illness is dramatic.

Lyme disease is a multisystem disease characterized by involvement of the skin, heart, joints, and nervous system (peripheral and central). Stages of disease are identified as *early localized* (erythema migrans [EM], often accompanied by arthralgia, neck stiffness, fever, malaise, and headache), *early disseminated* (multiple EM lesions, cranial nerve palsies, meningitis, conjunctivitis, arthralgia, myalgia, headache, fatigue, and, rarely, myocarditis), and *late disease* (recurrent arthritis, encephalopathy, and neuropathy). The varied manifestations of disease may relate to the degree of spirochetemia, the extent of dissemination to specific tissues, and the host's immunologic response.

The diagnosis of Lyme disease is often difficult in part because of the broad spectrum of presentations, inapparent exposure to the tick, and the lack of adequately standardized serologic tests. Culture of the spirochete, *Borrelia burgdorferi*, is not readily available. ELISA, immunofluorescent assay (IFA), and immunoblot assay are the usual tests. PCR detection of spirochetal DNA requires additional testing in clinical situations to clarify and standardize its utility.

Gardner[98] reviewed infection during pregnancy, summarizing a total of 46 adverse outcomes from 161 cases reported in the literature. The adverse outcomes included miscarriage and stillbirth (11% of cases), perinatal death (3%), congenital anomalies (15%), and both early- and late-onset progressive infection in the infant. Silver[241] reviewed 11 published reports and concluded that Lyme disease during pregnancy is uncommon, even in endemic areas. Although the spirochete can be transmitted transplacentally, a significant immune response in the fetus is often lacking, and the association of Lyme infection with congenital abnormalities is weak.[252,278]

Little published information exists on whether *B. burgdorferi* can be transmitted via breast milk.

One report showed the detection of *B. burgdorferi* DNA by PCR in the breast milk of two lactating women with untreated EM, but no evidence of Lyme disease or transmission of the spirochete in the one infant followed for 1 year.[233] No attempt to culture the spirochete was made, so it is not possible to determine if the detectable DNA was from viable spirochetes or noninfectious fragments. In that same study, of 56 women with untreated EM who had detectable *B. burgdorferi* DNA in the urine, 32 still had detectable DNA in the urine 15 to 30 days after starting treatment, but none had it 6 months after initiating therapy. Ziska and associates reported on the management of nine cases of Lyme disease in women associated with pregnancy; seven of the nine women were symptomatic at conception and six received antibiotics throughtout pregnancy. Follow-up of the infants, showed no transmission of Lyme disease, even in the seven infants who had been breastfed.[294]

The lack of adequate information on transmission of *B. burgdorferi* via breast milk cannot be taken as proof that it is not occurring. If one extrapolates from data on syphilis and the *Treponema pallidum* spirochete, it would be prudent to discuss the lack of information on the transmission of *B. burgdorferi* via breast milk with the mother or parents and to consider withholding breast milk at least until therapy for Lyme disease has begun or been completed. If the infection occurred during pregnancy and treatment has already been completed, the infant can breastfeed. If infection occurs post partum or the diagnosis is made post partum, infant exposure may have already occurred. Again, discussion with the mother or parents about withholding versus continuing breastfeeding is appropriate.

After prenatal or postnatal exposure, the infant should be closely observed and empiric therapy considered if the infant develops a rash or symptoms suggestive of Lyme borreliosis. Treatment of the mother and infant with ceftriaxone, penicillin, or amoxicillin is acceptable during breastfeeding relative to the infant's exposure to these medications. Doxycycline should not be administered for more than 14 days while continuing breastfeeding because of possible dental staining in the neonate. Continued surveillance for viable organisms in breast milk and evidence of transmission through breastfeeding is recommended.

A large body of information is available on various "Lyme vaccines" used in dogs, but these vaccines are only partially protective and must be repeated yearly. Preliminary information suggests that a vaccine for use in humans safely produces good serologic responses, but protective efficacy has not been demonstrated, and no information exists on its use during pregnancy or breastfeeding.

Syphilis

Syphilis is the classic example of a spirochetal infection that causes multisystem disease in various stages. Both acquired syphilis and congenital syphilis are well-described entities. *Acquired syphilis* is almost always transmitted through direct sexual contact with open lesions of the skin or mucous membranes of individuals infected with the spirochete, *Treponema pallidum. Congenital syphilis* occurs by infection across the placenta (placentitis) at any time during the pregnancy or by contact with the spirochete during passage through the birth canal. Any stage of disease (primary, secondary, tertiary) in the mother can lead to infection of the fetus, but transmission in association with secondary syphilis approaches 100%. Infection with primary syphilis during pregnancy, without treatment, leads to spontaneous abortion, stillbirth, or perinatal death in 40% of cases. Similar to acquired syphilis, congenital syphilis manifests with moist lesions or secretions from rhinitis (snuffles), condylomata lata, or bullous lesions. These lesions and secretions contain numerous spirochetes and are therefore highly infectious.

Postnatal infection of the infant can occur through contact with open, moist lesions of the skin or mucous membranes in the mother or other infected individuals. If the mother or infant has potentially infectious lesions, isolation from each other and from other infants and mothers is recommended. If lesions are on the breasts or nipples, breastfeeding or using expressed milk is contraindi-

cated until treatment is complete and the lesions have cleared. Spirochetes are rarely identified in open lesions after more than 24 hours of appropriate treatment. Penicillin remains the best therapy.

Evaluation of the infant with suspected syphilis should be based on the mother's clinical and serologic status, history of adequate therapy in the mother, and the infant's clinical status. Histologic examination of the placenta and umbilical cord, serologic testing of the infant's blood and CSF, complete analysis of the CSF, long bone and chest radiographs, liver function tests, and a complete blood cell count are all appropriate given the specific clinical situation. Treatment of the infant should follow recommended protocols for suspected, probable, or proven syphilitic infection.[62]

No evidence indicates transmission of syphilis via breast milk in the absence of a breast or nipple lesion. When the mother has no suspicious breast lesions, breastfeeding is acceptable as long as appropriate therapy for suspected or proven syphilis is begun in the mother and infant.

PARASITES

Toxoplasmosis

Toxoplasmosis is one of the most common infections of humans throughout the world. The infective organism, *Toxoplasma gondii*, is ubiquitous in nature. The prevalence of positive serologic test titers increases with age, indicating past exposure and infection. The cat is the definitive host, although infection occurs in most species of warm-blooded animals.

Postnatal infection with toxoplasmosis is usually asymptomatic. Symptomatic infection typically manifests with nonspecific symptoms, including fever, malaise, myalgia, sore throat, lymphadenopathy, rash, hepatosplenomegaly, and occasionally a mononucleosis-like illness. The illness usually resolves without treatment or significant complications.

Congenital infection or infection in an immunodeficient individual can be persistent and severe, causing significant morbidity and even death. Although most infants with congenital infection are asymptomatic at birth, visual abnormalities, learning disabilities, and mental retardation can occur months or years later. There is a clearly defined syndrome of *congenital toxoplasmosis*, with the most severe manifestations involving the CNS, including hydrocephalus, cerebral calcifications, microcephaly, chorioretinitis, sei-zures, or simply isolated ocular involvement. The risk of fetal infection is related to the timing of primary maternal infection, although transmission can occur with preexisting maternal toxoplasmosis. In the last months of pregnancy the protozoan is more readily transmitted to the fetus, but the infection is more likely to be subclinical. Early in pregnancy the transmission to the fetus occurs less frequently but does result in severe disease. Treatment of documented congenital infection is currently recommended, although the duration and optimal regimen have not been determined, and reversal of preexisting sequelae generally does not occur.[215]

Prevention of infection in susceptible pregnant women is possible by avoiding exposure to cat feces or the organism in the soil. Pregnant or lactating women should not change cat litter boxes, but if they must, it should be done daily and while wearing gloves. The oocyst is not infective for the first 24 to 48 hours after passage. Mothers can avoid ingestion of the organism by fully cooking meats and carefully washing fruits, vegetables, and food preparation surfaces.[62]

In various animal models, *T. gondii* has been transmitted through the milk to the suckling young. The organism has been isolated from colostrum as well. The newborn animals became asymptomatically infected when nursed by an infected mother whose colostrum contained *T. gondii*. Only one report has identified *T. gondii* in human milk, and some question surrounds the reliability of that report.[156] Transmission during breastfeeding in humans has not been demonstrated. Breast milk may contain appropriate antibodies against *T. gondii*. Given the benign nature of postnatal infection, the absence of documented transmission in human breast milk, and the poten-

tial antibodies in breast milk, no reason exists to proscribe breastfeeding by a mother known to be infected with toxoplasmosis.

Giardia lamblia

Giardiasis is a localized infection limited to the intestinal tract, causing diarrhea and malabsorption. Immunocompetent individuals show no evidence of invasive infection, and no evidence exists documenting fetal infection from maternal infection during pregnancy. Giardiasis is rare in children under 6 months of age, although neonatal infection from fecal contamination at birth has been described.[18] Human milk has an in vivo protective effect against *G. lamblia* infection, as documented by work from central Africa, where the end of breastfeeding heralds the onset of *Giardia* infection.[100] This has been reaffirmed in undeveloped countries around the world.

The protective effect of breast milk has been identified in the milk of noninfected donors.[104] The antiparasitic effect does not result from specific antibodies but rather from lipase enzymatic activity. The lipase acts in the presence of bile salts to destroy the trophozoites as they emerge from their cysts in the gastrointestinal tract. Hernell and associates[118] demonstrated that free fatty acids have a marked giardiacidal effect, which supports the conclusion that lipase activity releasing fatty acids is responsible for killing *G. lamblia*.

G. lamblia have also been reported to appear in the mother's milk, and the parasite has been transmitted to newborns via that route. The exact relationship of breastfeeding to transmission of *G. lamblia* and the effect on the infant continue to be studied, even though symptomatic infection in the breastfed infant is rare.[104] Breastfeeding by mothers with giardiasis is mainly problematic because of the medications used for therapy. Metronidazole's safety in infants has not been established, and little information is available on quinacrine hydrochloride and furazolidone in breast milk. Paramomycin, a nonabsorbable aminoglycoside, is a reasonable alternative recommended for treatment of pregnant women. Breastfeeding by the mother with symptomatic giardiasis is acceptable when consideration is given to the presence of the therapeutic agents in the breast milk.

Trichomonas vaginalis

Trichomonas vaginalis is a flagellated protozoan that can produce vaginitis (see Chapter 16) but frequently causes asymptomatic infection in both males and females. The parasite is found in 10% to 25% of women in the childbearing years. It is transmitted predominantly by sexual intercourse, but it can be transmitted to the neonate by passage through the birth canal. This parasite often coexists with other STDs, especially gonorrhea.

Infection during pregnancy or while taking oral contraceptives is more difficult to treat. Some evidence suggests that infection with and growth of the parasite are enhanced by estrogens or their effect on the vaginal epithelium. No evidence indicates adverse effects on the fetus in association with maternal infection during pregnancy. Occasionally the female newborn has a vaginal discharge during the first weeks of life caused by *T. vaginalis*. This is thought to be influenced by the effect of maternal estrogen on the infant's vaginal epithelium and acquisition of the organism during passage through the birth canal. The organism does not seem to cause significant disease in the healthy infant. No documentation exists on transmission of *T. vaginalis* via breast milk.

The difficulty encountered with maternal infection during lactation stems from metronidazole (Flagyl), the drug of choice, being contraindicated for infants. Case reports describe treatment of neonates with metronidazole without adverse effect. Although topical agents containing povidone-iodine (Betadine) or sodium lauryl sulfate (Trichotine) can be effective when given as douches, creams, or suppositories, metronidazole remains the treatment of choice. The AAP advises using metronidazole only with the physician's discretion and considers its effect on the nursing infant unknown but possibly a concern. The potential concerns are metronidazole's disulfiram-like effect in association with alcohol, tumorigenicity in animal studies, and the leukopenia and neurologic side effects described in adults. On the other hand, metronidazole is given to children beyond the neonatal period to treat serious infections with various other parasites, such as *Entamoeba histolytica*.

The current recommendation for lactating women is to try local treatment first, and if these fail, then to try metronidazole. A 2-g single-dose treatment produces peak levels after 1 hour, and discarding expressed breast milk for the next 12 to 24 hours is recommended. If this treatment also fails, a 1-g twice-daily regimen for 7 days or a 2-g single daily dose for 3 to 5 days is recommended, with discarding of some breast milk close to the dose and timing of feedings distant from the dose. Infants who exclusively breastfeed are presumed at greater risk from exposure to metronidazole than those who are only partially breastfed.

Malaria

Malaria is recognized as a major health problem in many countries. The effect of malaria infection on pregnant and lactating women and thus on the developing fetus, neonate, and growing infant can be significant. The four species of malaria, *Plasmodium vivax*, *P. ovale*, *P. malariae*, and *P. falciparum*, vary in the specific aspects of the disease they produce. *P. vivax* exists throughout the world, but *P. falciparum* predominates in the tropics and is most problematic in its chloroquine-resistant form. Malaria in the United States is most often seen in individuals traveling from areas where malaria is endemic. The parasite can exist in the blood for weeks, and infection with *P. vivax* and *P. malariae* can lead to relapses years later. Transmission occurs through the bite of the anopheline mosquito and can occur via transfusion of blood products and transplacentally.

Congenital malaria is rare but seems to occur more often with *P. vivax* and *P. falciparum*. It usually presents in the first 7 days of life (range 1 day to 2 months). It may resemble neonatal sepsis, with fever, anemia, and splenomegaly occurring in the most neonates and hyperbilirubinemia and hepatomegaly in less than half.

Malaria in infants younger than 3 months of age generally manifests with less severe disease and death than in older children. Possible explanations include the effect of less exposure to mosquitoes, passive antibody acquired from the mother, and the high level of fetal hemoglobin in the infant at this age.[18] The variations in the infection rates in children under 3 months of age during the wet and dry seasons support the idea that postnatal infection is more common than congenital infection. No evidence indicates that malaria is transmitted through breast milk. The greatest risk to the infant is exposure to the anopheline mosquito infected with malaria.

The main issues relative to malaria and breastfeeding are how to protect both the mother and the infant effectively from mosquitoes and what drugs for treating malaria in the mother are appropriate during lactation. Protection from mosquito bites includes screened-in living areas, mosquito nets while sleeping, protective clothing with or without repellents on the clothes, and community efforts to eradicate the mosquitoes. Chloroquine, quinine, and tetracycline are acceptable during breastfeeding. Sulfonamides should be avoided in the first month of the infant's life, but pyrimethamine-sulfadoxine (Fansidar) can be used later.

Mefloquine is not approved for infants or pregnant women. However, the milk/plasma ratio for mefloquine is less than 0.25, there is a large volume of distribution of the drug, high protein binding of the drug limits its presence in breast milk, and the relative importance of breastfeeding in areas where malaria is prevalent shifts the risk/benefit ratio in favor of treatment with mefloquine. The single dose recommended for treatment or the once-weekly dose for prevention allows for continued breastfeeding with discarding of the milk for short periods after a dose (1 to 6 hours). Maternal plasma levels of primaquine range from 53 to 107 ng/mL, but no information is available on levels in human milk. Primaquine is used in children, and once daily dosing in the mother would allow discarding milk with peak levels of drug. Therefore, breastfeeding during maternal malaria even with treatment is appropriate with specific medications.

CANDIDA INFECTIONS

Candida consists of multiple species. The most common species affecting humans include *C. albicans* as the dominant agent and *C. tropicalis, C. krusei,* and *C. parapsilosis,* as well as many other uncommon species. In general, *Candida* exists as a commensal organism colonizing the oropharynx, gastrointestinal tract, vagina, and skin without causing disease until some change disrupts the balance between the organism and the host. Mild mucocutaneous infection is the most common illness, which can lead to vulvovaginitis, mastitis or uncommonly oral mucositis in the mother, and thrush (oral candidiasis) and candidal diaper rash in the infant.

Invasive candidal infection occurs infrequently, usually when the individual has other illness, impaired resistance to infection (HIV, diabetes mellitus, neutropenia; decreased cell-mediated immunity in premature infants or low birth weight or very low birth weight infants), or disrupted normal mucosal and skin barriers and has received antibiotics or corticosteroids. Invasive disease can occur through local spread, as may occur more often in the genitourinary tract (urethra, bladder, ureters, kidneys), but usually develops in association with candidemia. The bladder and kidney are more frequently involved, but when dissemination occurs via candidemia, a careful search for other sites of infection should be made (e.g., retina, liver, spleen, lung, meninges).[179]

Transmission usually occurs from healthy individuals colonized with *Candida* through direct contact with them or through contact with their oral or vaginal secretions. Intrauterine infection can occur through ascending infection up through the birth canal but is rare. No distinct syndrome of congenital candidal infection exists. Most often the infant is infected in passing through the birth canal and remains colonized. Postnatal transmission can occur through direct contact with caregivers.

The mother and infant each serve as an immediate source of recolonization for one another, especially during the direct contact of breastfeeding. For this reason, the infant and breastfeeding mother should be treated simultaneously when treating thrush, vulvovaginitis, diaper candidiasis, or mastitis. Colonization with this organism usually occurs in the absence of any clinical evidence of infection. Simultaneous treatment should occur even in the absence of any clinical evidence of *Candida* infection or colonization in the apparently uninvolved individual of the breastfeeding dyad.

There are no well-controlled clinical trials defining the most appropriate or most effective method(s) of treatment for candidal infection in the breastfeeding mother-infant pair. The list of possible treatment products is extensive and includes many anecdotal and empirical regimens followed. In the face of this absence of data, Dr. Brent has conducted a survey of members of The Academy of Breastfeeding Medicine concerning the respondents' approach to diagnosis and treatment of thrush in the breastfeeding dyad.[34] Most of the respondents relied on the history and physical examination of the infant, but only a third rated the examination of the mother as very important in making a diagnosis. Only 7% reported using laboratory testing to make the diagnosis. Twenty-one percent of the respondents reported using only oral nystatin for the infant when the mother was asymptomatic. Almost half treated the infant and the mother with topical nystatin, and 13% used oral nystatin for the infant and oral fluconazole for the mother when the mother had breast pain. Less than 5% used oral fluconazole for both infant and mother and other therapies were used by about 15% of the respondents. For recurrence of persistence of the thrush, more respondents reported treating the mother or both the infant and mother with fluconazole, and almost a quarter reported using other therapies.

Treatment of mucocutaneous candidiasis should probably begin with a topical agent, such as nystatin, clotrimazole, miconazole, econazole, butaconazole, terconazole, or ciclopirox. Treatment should continue for at least 2 weeks, even with obvious improvement in 1 or 2 days. Failures most often result from inadequate therapy involving the frequency of application, careful washing and drying before application, or in the case of diaper candidiasis, decreasing the contact of the skin with moisture as well. There have been reports that nystatin oral suspension is less effective for the treatment of oral candidiasis in infants, now as compared to the past, supposedly due to increasing resistance.[106] Gentian violet (diluted to 0.25% to 1.0%) applied to the breast or painted onto the infant's mouth is being recommended more frequently. Other topical preparations have been recommended for the mother's breast including mupirocin, grapefruit-seed extract, or mixtures of mupirocin, betamethasone ointments, and miconazole powder. Again controlled clinical trails for efficacy and toxicity are not available.

When good adherence to the proposed regimen with topical agents fails, or when the infant or mother are severely affected by pain and decreased breastfeeding, systemic therapy is appropriate. Fluconazole and ketoconazole are the most commonly used systemic agents for oral or diaper candidiasis and vulvovaginitis or mastitis. Fluconazole has a better side effect profile than ketoconazole, and there is more available data concerning its safe use in children younger than 6 months of age and even neonates and premature infants.[57,106,143] Fluconazole is not currently approved for use in infants under 6 months of age. For severe invasive infections in the infant amphotericin B with or without oral flucytosine, intravenous fluconazole, or voriconazole are reasonable choices in different situations. Use of itraconazole or caspofungin in infants has not been adequately studied to date. Maternal use of fluconazole during breastfeeding is not contraindicated because only a small amount of medicine compared with the usual infant dose would reach the infant in breast milk. Amphotericin or caspofungin therapy in the mother is also not contraindicated because these are both poorly absorbed from the gastrointestinal tract. Whenever the mother is treated for candidal mastitis or vulvovaginitis, the infant should be treated simultaneously at least with nystatin oral suspension as the first choice of medication.

Any predisposing risk factors for candidal infection in the mother and infant should be reduced or eliminated to improve the chance of rapid, successful treatment and to decrease the likelihood of chronic or recurrent disease. For the mother, such interventions might include decreasing sugar consumption, stopping antibiotic use as soon as possible, and consuming some form of acidophilus (yogurt, milk, or pills) to establish a normal colonizing bacterial flora. For the infant, breastfeeding can help enhance the growth of specific colonizing bacterial flora such as lactobacillus, which can successfully limit fungal growth. Breastfeeding should continue with appropriate support and problem solving with a professional knowledgeable about breastfeeding.

SUMMARY

HIV-1, HIV-2, HTLV-I, and HTLV-II are the only infectious diseases that are considered absolute contraindications to breastfeeding in developed countries. When the primary route of transmission is via direct contact or respiratory droplets/particles, temporary separation of the mother and infant may be appropriate (whether the infant is breastfed or formula fed), but expressed breast milk should be given to the infant for the organism-specific immunologic benefits in the mother's milk. In most instances, by the time a specific diagnosis of an infection is made in the mother, the infant has already been exposed to the organism and providing expressed breast milk to the infant should continue. (Refer to Appendix E for specifc exceptions, such as Lassa fever.) Relative to antimicrobial therapy for the mother and continued breastfeeding, the majority of the medications commonly used in adults can be used to treat the same infection in the infant. The additional amount of medication received by the infant via the breast milk is usually insignificant. In almost all instances, an appropriate antimicrobial agent for treating the mother can be chosen which is also compatible with breastfeeding.

Unless there is a documented risk to the infant for transmission of an infectious agent via breast milk which leads to a clinically significant illness in the infant, breastfeeding should continue.

REFERENCES

1. Adu FD, Adeniji JA: Measles antibodies in the breast milk of nursing mothers. Afr J Med Med Sci 24:385, 1995.
2. Albargish KA, Hasony HJ: Respiratory syncytial virus infection among young children with acute respiratory tract infection in Iraq. East Medit Health J 5(5):941, 1999.
3. Alford C: Breast milk transmission of cytomegalovirus (CMV) infection. In Mestecky J, Blair C, Ogra PL (eds): Immunology of Milk and the Neonate. New York, Plenum, 1991.
4. Alford CA, Stagno S, Pass RF, et al: Congenital and perinatal cytomegalovirus infections. Rev Infect Dis 12:S745, 1990.
5. Alpert SG, Fergerson J, Noel LP: Intrauterine West Nile virus: Ocular and systemic findings. Am J Ophthalmol 136:733, 2003.
6. Alter HJ: The cloning and clinical implications of HGV and HGBV-C. N Engl J Med 334:1536, 1996.
7. Ando Y, Saito K, Nakano S, et al: Bottle feeding can prevent transmission of HTLV-I from mothers to their babies. J Infect 19:25, 1989.
8. Ando Y, Nakano S, Saito K, et al: Transmission of adult T-cell leukemia retrovirus (HTLV-I) from mother to child: Comparison of bottle- with breastfed babies. Jpn J Cancer Res 78:322, 1987.
9. Ando Y, Kakimoto K, Tanigawa T, et al: Effect of freeze-thawing breast milk on vertical HTLV-I transmission from seropositive mothers to children. Jpn J Cancer Res 80:405, 1989.
10. Ando Y, Matsumoto Y, Nakano S, et al: Long-term follow up study of vertical HTLV-I infection in children breastfed by seropositive mothers. J Infect 46(3):177, 2003.
11. Ando Y, Matsumoto Y, Nakano S, et al: Long-term follow-up study of HTLV-I infection in bottle-fed children born to seropositive mothers. J Infect 46:9, 2003.
12. Anthony BF, Okada DM, Hobel CJ: Epidemiology of group B streptococcus: maternal and nosocomial sources for acquisition. J Pediatr 95:431, 1979.
13. Armstrong L, Garay SM: Tuberculosis and pregnancy and tuberculous mastitis. In Rom WN, Garay SM (eds): Tuberculosis. Boston, Little, Brown, 1996.
14. Arnon SS: Infant botulism. Ann Rev Med 31:541, 1980.
15. Arnon SS: Infant botulism: Anticipating the second decade. J Infect Dis 154:201, 1986.

16. Arnon SS, Damus K, Thompson B, et al: Protective role of human milk against sudden death from infant botulism. J Pediatr 100:568, 1982.

17. Arvin AM, Maldonado YA: Other viral infections of the fetus and newborn. In Remington JS, Klein JO (eds): Infectious Diseases of the Fetus and Newborn Infant, 4th ed. Philadelphia, WB Saunders, 1995.

18. Arvin AM, Maldonado YA: Protozoan and helminth infections (including *Pneumocystis carinii*). In Remington JS, Klein JO (eds): Infectious Diseases of the Fetus and Newborn Infant, 4th ed. Philadelphia, WB Saunders 1995.

19. Bannister BA: Stringent precautions are advisable when caring for patients with viral hemorrhagic fevers. Rev Med Virol 3:3, 1993.

20. Barden LS: Personal communication. 1998.

21. Barton LL, Budd SC, Morfitt WS, et al: Congenital lymphocytic choriomeningitis virus infection in twins. Pediatr Infect Dis J 12:942, 1993.

22. Bates T: Poliomyelitis in pregnancy, fetus and newborn. Am J Dis Child 90:189, 1955.

23. Beasley RP: Transmission of hepatitis by breastfeeding. N Engl J Med 292:1354, 1975 (letter).

24. Beasley RP, Stevens CE, Shiao I, et al: Evidence against breast feeding as a mechanism for vertical transmission of hepatitis B. Lancet 2:740, 1975.

25. Bergdoll MS, Crass BA, Reisser, et al: A new staphylococcal enterotoxin, enterotoxin F, associated with TSS *Staphylococcus aureus* isolate. Lancet 1:1017, 1981.

26. Bertolli J, St Louis ME, Simonds RJ, et al: Estimating the timing of mother-to-child transmission of human immunodeficiency virus in a breast-feeding population in Kinshasa, Zaire. J Infect Dis 174(4):722, 1996.

27. Bertotto A, Gerli R, Castellucci G, et al: Mycobacteria-reactive T cells are present in human colostrum from tuberculin-positive, but not tuberculin-negative nursing mothers. Am J Reprod Immunol 29:131, 1993.

28. Biggerstaff BJ, Petersen LR: Estimated risk of transmission of the West Nile virus through blood transfusion in the US, 2002. Transfusion 43(8):1007, 2003.

29. Bitnun A, Allen U, Heurter H, et al: Children hospitalized with severe acute respiratory syndrome–related illness in Toronto. Pediatrics 112(4):e261, 2003.

30. Blanche S, Rouzioux C, Moscato ML, et al: A prospective study of infants born to women seropositive for human mmunodeficiency virus type 1. HIV Infection in Newborns French Collaborative Study Group. N Engl J Med. 320:1643, 1989.

31. Bleck TP, Rupprecht CE: Rhabdoviruses. In Richman DD, Whitley RJ, Hayden FG (eds): Clinical Virology. New York, Churchill Livingstone, 1997.

32. Bortolotti F, Resti M, Giacchino R, et al: Hepatitis C virus infection and related liver disease in children of mothers with antibodies to the virus. J Pediatr 130:990, 1997.

33. Boussemart T, Babe P, Sibille G, et al: Prenatal transmission of dengue: Two new cases. J Perinatol 21(4):255, 2001.

34. Brent NB: Thrush in the breastfeeding dyad: Results of a survey on diagnosis and treatment. Clin Pediatr 40:503, 2001.

35. Brinton LA, Hoover R, Fraumeni JF Jr: Reproductive factors in the aetiology of breast cancer. Br J Cancer 47:757, 1983.

36. Bulkow LR, Singleton RJ, Karron RA, Harrison LH: Alaska RSV Study Group: Risk factors for severe respiratory syncytial virus infection among Alaska native children. Pediatrics 109(2):210, 2002.

37. Buranasin P, Kunakorn M, Petchclai B, et al: Detection of human immunodeficiency virus type 1 (HIV-1) proviral DNA in breast milk and colostrum of seropositive mothers. J Med Assoc Thai 76(1):41, 1993.

38. Butter MNW, DeMoor CE: Streptococcus agalactiae as a cause of meningitis in the newborn and bacteraemia in adults. Antonie Van Leeuwenhoek 33:439, 1967.

39. Campbell GL, Marfin AA, Lanciotti RS, Gubler DJ: West Nile virus. Lancet Infect Dis 2:519, 2002.

40. Cantwell M, Snider DE Jr, Cauthen G, et al: Epidemiology of tuberculosis in the United States, 1985-1992. JAMA 272:535, 1994.

41. Centers for Disease Control and Prevention: Testing for antibodies to HIV-2 in the United States. MMWR 41:1, 1992.

42. Centers for Disease Control and Prevention: Compendium of animal rabies control, 1995. MMWR 44(RR-2):1, 1995.

43. Centers for Disease Control and Prevention: Screening for tuberculosis and tuberculosis infection in high-risk populations. MMWR 44(RR-11):19, 1995.

44. Centers for Disease Control and Prevention: Update: Management of patients with suspected viral hemorrhagic fever—United States. MMWR 44:475, 1995.

45. Centers for Disease Control and Prevention: Human rabies—Washington, 1995. MMWR 44:625, 1995.

46. Centers for Disease Control and Prevention, Advisory Committee on Immunization Practices: Poliomyelitis prevention in the United States: Introduction of a sequential vaccination schedule of inactivated poliovirus vaccine followed by oral poliovirus vaccine—United States. MMWR 46:1, 1997.

47. Centers for Disease Control and Prevention: Recommendations for antimicrobial prophylaxis for children and breastfeeding mothers and treatment of children with anthrax. MMWR 50:1014, 2001.

48. Centers for Disease Control and Prevention: Intrauterine West Nile virus infection—New York, 2002. MMWR 51:1135, 2002.

49. Centers for Disease Control and Prevention: Possible West Nile virus transmission to an infant through breastfeeding—Michigan, 2002. MMWR 51:877, 2002.

50. Centers for Disease Control and Prevention: Laboratory-acquired West Nile virus infections—United States, 2002. MMWR 51:1133, 2002.

51. Centers for Disease Control and Prevention: Update: Cardiac and other adverse events following civilian smallpox vaccination—United States, 2003. MMWR 52:639, 2003.

52. Centers for Disease Control and Prevention: First human death associated with raccoon rabies—Virginia, 2003. MMWR 52:1102, 2003.

53. Centers for Disease Control and Prevention: Secondary and tertiary transfer of vaccinia virus among U.S. military personnel—United States and worldwide, 2002-2004. MMWR 53(5):103, 2004.

54. Centers for Disease Control and Prevention: Division of vector-borne infectious diseases. Surveillance and control case count of West Nile virus, 2003. Available at http://www.cdc.gov/ncidod/dvbid/westnile/surv&control CaseCount03_detailed.htm. Accessed February 15, 2004.

55. Centers for Disease Control and Prevention, U.S. Public Health Service Working Group: Recommendations for counseling persons infected with human T-lymphotropic virus, types I and II. MMWR 42(RR-9):1, 1993.

56. Ceyhan M, Kaura G, Secmeer G, et al: Take of rhesus-human reassortment tetravalent rotavirus vaccine in breast-fed infants. Acta Pediatr 82:223, 1993.

57. Chapman RL: Candida infections in the neonate. Curr Opin Pediatr 15(1):97, 2003.

58. Cherry JD: Enteroviruses: Polioviruses (poliomyelitis), coxsackieviruses, and enteroviruses. In Feigin RD, Cherry JD (eds): Textbook of Pediatric Infectious Diseases, 3rd ed. Philadelphia, WB Saunders, 1992.

59. Chopra H, Ebert P, Woodside N, et al: Electron microscopic detection of simian-type virus particles in human milk. Nat Biol 243:159, 1973.

60. Clemens J, Rao M, Eng M, et al: Breastfeeding and the risk of life-threatening rotavirus diarrhea: Prevention or post-ponement? Pediatrics 92:680, 1993.

61. Committee on Infectious Diseases, American Academy of Pediatrics: Red Book Report of the Committee on Infectious Disease, 26th ed. Elk Grove Village, Ill, American Academy of Pediatrics, 2003, p. 150.

62. Committee on Infectious Disease, American Academy of Pediatrics: Red Book Report of the Committee on Infectious Disease, 26th ed. Elk Grove Village, Ill, American Academy of Pediatrics, 2003.

63. Committee on Infectious Diseases, American Academy of Pediatrics: Red Book Report of the Committee on Infectious Disease, 26th ed. Elk Grove, Ill, American Academy of Pediatrics, 2003, p. 590.

64. Coutsoudis A, Pillay K, Spooner E, et al: Influence of infant-feeding patterns on early mother-to-child transmission of HIV-1 in Durban, South Africa: A prospective cohort study. South African Vitamin A Study Group. Lancet 354:471, 1999.

65. Coutsoudis A, Pillay K, Kuhn L, et al: Method of feeding and transmission of HIV-1 from mothers to children by 15 months of age: prospective cohort study from Durban, South Africa. South African Vitamin A Study Group. AIDS 15:379, 2001.

66. Coutsoudis A, Coovadia H, Pillay K, Kuhn L: Are HIV-infected women who breastfeed at increased risk of mortality? AIDS 15:653, 2001.

67. Datta P, Embree JE, Kreiss JK, et al: Mother-to-child transmission of human immunodeficiency virus type: Report from the Nairobi Study. J Infect Dis 170:1134, 1994.

68. Davis MK: Human milk and HIV infection: Epidemiologic and laboratory data. In Mestecky J, Blair C, Ogra P (eds): Immunology of Milk and the Neonate. New York, Plenum, 1991.

69. De Martino M, Tovo PA, Tozzi, et al: HIV-1 transmission through breast-milk: Appraisal of risk according to duration of feeding. AIDS 6:991, 1992.

70. Del Fante P, Jenniskens F, Lush L, et al: HIV, breastfeeding and under 5 mortality: Modelling the impact of policy decisions for or against breastfeeding. J Trop Med Hyg 96:203, 1994.

71. Derkay CS: Task force on recurrent respiratory papillomatosis. Acta Otolaryngol Head Neck Surg 121:1386, 1995.

72. Deubel V, Fiette L, Gounon P, et al: Variations in biological features of West Nile viruses. Ann NY Acad Sci 951:195, 2001.

73. Dillon HC Jr, Khare S, Gray BM: Group B streptococcal carriage and disease: A 6 year prospective study. J Pediatr 110:31, 1987.

74. Dinsmoor MJ: Hepatitis in the obstetric patient. Infect Obstet 11:77, 1991.

75. Dormer BA, Swarit JA, Harrison I, et al: Prophylactic isoniazid protection of infants in a tuberculosis hospital. Lancet 2:902, 1959.

76. Downham M, Scott R, Sims DG, et al: Breast-feeding protects against respiratory syncytial virus infections. Br Med J 2:274, 1976.

77. Dunkle LM, Schmidt RR, O'Connor DM: Neonatal herpes simplex infection possibly acquired via maternal breast milk. Pediatrics 63:250, 1979.

78. Dunn DT, Newell ML, Ades AE, et al: Risk of human immunodeficiency virus type 1 transmission through breastfeeding. Lancet 340:585, 1992.

79. Dunne WM, Demmler GJ: Serologic evidence for congenital transmission of human herpesvirus 6. Lancet 340:121, 1992.

80. Dunne WM, Jevon M: Examination of human breastmilk for evidence of human herpesvirus 6 by PCR. J Infect Dis 168:250, 1993.

81. Dworsky M, Yow M, Stagno S, et al: Cytomegalovirus infection of breast milk and transmission in infancy. Pediatrics 72:295, 1983.

82. Ekpini ER, Wiktor SZ, Satten GA, et al: Late postnatal mother-to-child transmission of HIV-1 in Abidjan, Cote d'Ivoire. Lancet 349:1054, 1997.

83. Enocksson E, Wretlind B, Sterner G, et al: Listeriosis during pregnancy and in neonates. Scand J Infect Dis Suppl 71:89, 1990.

84. Espinosa F, Paniagua M, Hallander H, et al: Rotavirus infections in young Nicaraguan children. Pediatr Infect Dis J 16:564, 1997.

85. European Collaborative Study: Children born to women with HIV-1 infection: Natural history and risk of transmission. Lancet 337:253, 1991.

86. European Paediatric Hepatitis C Virus Network: Effects of mode of delivery and infant feeding on the risk of mother-to-child transmission of hepatitis C virus. Br J Obstet Gynaecol 108:371, 2001.

87. Fairchild JP, Graber CD, Vogel EH, et al: Flora of the umbilical stump: 2479 cultures. J Pediatr 53:538, 1958.

88. Feucht HH, Zollner B, Polywka S, et al: Vertical transmission of hepatitis G. Lancet 347:615, 1996.

89. Fieldsteel AH: Nonspecific antiviral substances in human milk against arbovirus and murine leukemia virus. Cancer Res 34:712, 1974.

90. Fischler B, Lara C, Chen M, et al: Genetic evidence for mother-to-infant transmission of hepatitis G virus. J Infect Dis 176:281, 1997.

91. Fisher-Hoch SP: Stringent precautions are not advisable when caring for patients with viral hemorrhagic fevers. Rev Med Virol 3:7, 1993.

92. Friis H, Andersen HK: Rate of inactivation of cytomegalovirus in raw banked milk during storage at −20 degrees C and pasteurisation. Br Med J Clin Res 285:1604, 1982.

93. Fujino T, Nagata Y: HTLV-I transmission from mother to child. J Reprod Immunol 47(2):197, 2000.

94. Fujiyama C, Fuyiyoshi T, Miura T, et al: A new endemic focue of human T-lymphotropic virus type II carriers among Orinoco natives in Colombia. J Infect Dis 168:1075, 1993.

95. Furnia A, Lal R, Maloney E, et al: Estimating the time of HTLV-I infection following mother-to-child transmission in a breast-feeding population in Jamaica. J Med Virol 59(4):541, 1999.

96. Garde V, Harper D, Fairchok MP: Tertiary contact vaccinia in a breastfeeding infant. JAMA 291(6):725, 2004.

97. Gardner SE, Mason EO Jr, Yow MD: Community acquisition of group B streptococcus by infants of colonized mothers. Pediatrics 66:873, 1980.

98. Gardner T: Lyme disease. In Remington JS, Klein JO (eds): Infectious Diseases of the Fetus and Newborn Infant, 4th ed. Philadelphia, WB Saunders, 1995.

99. Garner JS: Hospital Infection Control Practices Advisory Committee: Guidelines for isolation precautions in hospitals. Infect Control Hosp Epidemiol 17:53, 1996.

100. Gendrel D, Richard-Lenoble D, Kombila M, et al: Giardiasis and breastfeeding in urban Africa. Pediatr Infect Dis J 8:58, 1989.

101. Gershon AA: Chickenpox, measles and mumps. In Remington JS, Klein JO (eds): Infectious Diseases of the Fetus and Newborn Infant, 4th ed. Philadelphia, WB Saunders, 1995.

102. Gervais F, Joncas JH: Seroepidemiology in various population groups of the greater Montreal area. Comp Immunol Microbiol Infect Dis 2:207, 1979.

103. Gibb DM, Goodall RL, Dunn DT, et al: Mother-to-child transmission of hepatitis C virus: Evidence for preventable peripartum transmission. Lancet 356(9233):904, 2000.

104. Gillin FD, Reiner DS, Gault MJ: Cholate-dependent killing of *Giardia lamblia* by human milk. Infect Immunol 47:619, 1985.

105. Glezen WP, Paredes A, Allison JE, et al: Risk of respiratory syncytial virus infection for infants from low-income families in relationship to age, sex, ethnic group, and maternal antibody level. J Pediatr 98:708, 1981.

106. Goins RA, Ascher D, Waecker N, et al: Comparison of fluconazole and nystatin oral suspensions for treatment of oral candidiasis in infants. Pediatr Infect Dis J 21:1165, 2002.

107. Goldblum RM, Dill CW, Albrecht TB, et al: Rapid high temperature treatment of human milk. J Pediatr 104:380, 1984.

108. Gotuzzo E: HTLV-I: A new problem for latin America. ASM News 67:3 2001.

109. Guay LA, Hom DL, Mmiro F, et al: Detection of human immunodeficiency virus type 1 (HIV-1) DNA and p24 antigen in breast milk of HIV-1-infected Ugandan women and vertical transmission. Pediatrics 98(3 Pt 1):438, 1996.

110. Gupta R, Gupta AS, Duggal N: Tubercular mastitis. Int Surg 67:422, 1982.

111. Gurakan B, Oran O, Yigit S, et al: Vertical transmission of hepatitis C virus. N Engl J Med 331:399, 1994 (letter).

112. Halstead SB, Lan NT, Myint TT, et al: Dengue hemorrhagic fever in infants: Research opportunities ignored. Emerg Infect Dis 8(12):1474, 2002.

113. Hamprecht K, Maschmann J, Vochem M, et al: Epidemiology of transmission of cytomegalovirus from mother to preterm infant by breastfeeding. Lancet 357(9255):513, 2001

114. Harjulhto T, Aro T, Hovi T, et al: Congenital malformations and oral poliovirus vaccination during pregnancy. Lancet I:771, 1989.

115. Hayes K, Danks DM, Gibas H, et al: Cytomegalovirus in human milk. N Engl J Med 287:177, 1972.

116. Henderson BE, Powell D, Rosario I, et al: An epidemiologic study of breast cancer. J Natl Cancer Inst 53:609, 1974.

117. Heneine W, Woods T, Green D, et al: Detection of HTLV-II in breast milk of HTLV-II infected mothers. Lancet 340:1157, 1992.

118. Hernell O, Ward H, Blackberg L: Killing of *Giardia lamblia* by human milk lipases: An effect mediated by lipolysis of milk lipids. J Infect Dis 153:715, 1986.

119. Hino S: Milk-borne transmission of HTLV-I as a major route in the endemic cycle. Acta Pediatr Jpn 31:428, 1989.

120. Hino, S, Sugiyama H, Doi H, et al: Breaking the cycle of HTLV-I transmission via carrier mothers milk. Lancet 2:158, 1987.

121. Hino S, Katamine S, Miyata H, et al: Primary prevention of HTLV-I in Japan. J AIDS Hum Retrovirol 13S:515, 1996.

122. Hino S, Katamine S, Miyata H, et al: Primary prevention of HTLV-1 in Japan. Leukemia 11:S57, 1997.

123. Hira SK, Mangrola UG, Mwale C, et al: Apparent vertical transmission of human immunodeficiency virus type 1 by breast-feeding in Zambia. J Pediatr 117(3):421, 1990.

124. Hisada M, Maloney EM, Sawada T, et al: Virus markers associated with vertical transmission of human T lymphotropic virus type 1 in Jamaica. Clin Infect Dis 34:1551, 2002.

125. Hjelt K, Granbella PC, Haagen O, et al: Rotavirus antibodies in the mother and her breastfed infant. J Pediatr Gastroenterol Nutr 4:414, 1985.

126. Hokama T, Sakamoto R, Yara A, et al: Incidence of *Haemophilus influenzae* in the throats of healthy infants with different feeding methods. Pediatr Int 41(3):277, 1999.

127. Hollinger FB, Kleinman S: Transfusion transmission of West Nile virus: A merging of historical and contemporary perspectives. Transfusion 43:992, 2003.

128. Hon K, Leung CW, Cheng W, et al: Clinical presentations and outcomes of severe acute respiratory syndrome in children. Lancet 361:1701, 2003.

129. Horn P: Poliomyelitis in pregnancy: A twenty-year report from Los Angeles County, California. Obstet Gynecol 6:121, 1955.

130. Horowitz CA, Henle W, Henle G, et al: Long-term serologic follow-up of patients for Epstein-Barr virus after recovery from infectious mononucleosis. J Infect Dis 151:1150, 1985.

131. Horsburgh CR, Holmberg SC: The global distribution of human immunodeficiency virus type 2 (HIV-2) infection.Transfusion 28:192, 1988.

132. Hurst V: *Staphylococcus aureus* in the infant upper respiratory tract. I. Observations on hospital-born babies. J Hyg 55:299, 1957.

133. Ing R, Ho JHC, Petrakis NL: Unilateral breast feeding and breast cancer. Lancet 2:124, 1977.

134. Ishak R, Harrington WJ, Azeuedo VN, et al: Identification of human T-cell lymphotropic virus type IIa infection in the Kayapo, an indigenous population of Brazil. Aids Res Hum Retrovirol 11(7):813, 1995.

135. Iso K, Suzuki Y, Takayama M: Mother-to-infant transmission of TT virus in Japan. Int J Gynecol Obstet 75:11, 2001.

136. Italian Register for HIV Infection in Children: HIV-1 infection and breastmilk. Acta Paediatr Suppl 400:51, 1994.

137. Iwamoto W, Jernigan DB, Guasch A, et al: Transmission of West Nile virus from an organ donor to four transplant recipients. N Engl J Med 348:2196, 2003.

138. Jeliffe DB, Jeliffe EFP: Human milk in the modern world. Oxford, Oxford University Press, 1978.

139. Junker AK, Thomas EE, Radcliffe A, et al: Epstein-Barr virus shedding in breast milk. Am J Med Sci 302:220, 1991.

140. Kalstone C: Successful antepartum treatment of listeriosis. Am J Obstet Gynecol 164:57, 1991.

141. Kaplan JE, Abrams E, Shaffer N, et al: Low risk of mother-to-child transmission of human T lymphotropic virus type II in non-breastfed infants. J Infect Dis 166:892, 1992.

142. Katzman DK, Wald ER: Staphylococcal scalded skin syndrome in a breastfed infant. Pediatr Infect Dis J 6:295, 1987.

143. Kaufman D, Boyle R, Hazen KC, et al: Fluconazole prophylaxis against fungal colonization and infection in preterm infants. N Engl J Med 345:1660, 2001.

144. Keelyside RA, McCormick JB, Webb PA, et al: Case-control study of Mastomys natalensis and humans in Lassa virus-infected households in Sierra Leone. Am J Trop Med Hyg 32:829, 1983.

145. Keller MA, Rodriguez AI, Alvarez S, et al: Transfer of tuberculin immunity from mother to infant. Pediatr Res 22:277, 1987.

146. Kenny JF, Zedd AJ: Recurrent group B streptococcal disease in an infant associated with the ingestion of infected mother's milk. J Pediatr 91:158, 1977.

147. Kinoshita K , Hino S, Amagasaki T, et al: Demonstration of adult T-cell leukemia virus antigen in milk from three sero-positive mothers. Gann 75;103, 1984.

148. Kinoshita K, Yamanouchi K, Ikeda S, et al: Oral infection of a common marmoset with human T-cell leukemia virus type I (HTLV-I by fresh human milk of HTLV-I carrier mothers.) Jpn J Cancer Res 76:1147, 1985.

149. Koch WC, Adler SP: Human parvovirus B19 infection in women of childbearing age and within families. Pediatr Infect Dis J 8:83, 1989.

150. Komrower GM, Williams BL, Stones PB: Lymphocytic choriomeningitis in the newborn. Lancet 1:697, 1955.

151. Kumar ML, Nankervis GA, Jacobs IB, et al: Congenital and postnatally acquired cytomegalovirus infections: long-term follow-up. J Pediatr 104:674, 1984.

152. Lal RB, Renan A, Gongora-Biaanchi A, et al: Evidence for mother-to-child transmission of human T-lymphotropic virus type II. J Infect Dis 168:586, 1993.

153. Lal RB, Owen SM, Segurado AAC, Gongora-Bianchi RA: Mother-to-child transmission of human T-lymphotropic virus type II (HTLV-II). Ann Intern Med 120:300, 1994.

154. Lamprecht CL, Krause HE, Mufson MA: Role of maternal antibody in pneumonia and bronchiolitis due to respiratory syncytial virus. J Infect Dis 134:211, 1976.

155. Lane-Claypon JE: A further report on cancer of the breast, with special reference to its associated antecedent conditions. Report No. 32. London, Reports of the Ministry of Health, 1926.

156. Langer H: Repeated congenital infection with *Toxoplasma gondii*. Obstet Gynecol 21:318, 1963.

157. Lawrence RA: A review of the medical benefits and contraindications to breastfeeding in the United States. Maternal and Child Health Technical Information Bulletin, U.S. Health Resources and Services Administration, October 1997.

158. Layde PM, Webster LA, Braughman AL, et al: The independent associations of parity, age at first full term pregnancy, and duration of breastfeeding with risk of breast cancer. J Clin Epidemiol 42:963, 1989.

159. Lederman SA: Estimating infant mortality from HIV and other causes in breastfeeding and bottle-feeding populations. Pediatrics 89:290, 1992.

160. Lepage P, Van de Perre P, Carael M, et al: Postnatal transmission of HIV from mother to child [letter]. Lancet 2:400, 1987.

161. Leroy V, Newell ML, Dabis F, et al: International multicentre pooled analysis of late postnatal mother-to-child transmission of HIV-1 infection. Ghent International Working Group on Mother-to-Child Transmission of HIV. Lancet 352(9128):597, 1998.

162. LeVasseur RJ, Southern SO, Southern PJ: Mammary epithelial cells support and transfer productive human T cell lymphotropic virus infections. J Hum Virol 1:214, 1998.

163. Lin HH, Kao JH, Chen PJ, et al: Mechanism of vertical transmission of hepatitis G. Lancet 347:1116, 1996.

164. Lin HH, Kao JH, Hsu H, et al: Absence of infection in breast fed infants born to hepatitis C virus- infected mothers. J Pediatr 126:589, 1995.

165. Liner RI: Intrauterine listeria infection: prenatal diagnosis by biophysical assessment and amniocentesis. Am J Obstet Gynecol 163:1596, 1990.

166. Lowis GW, Sheremata WA, Minagar A: Ejpidemiologic features of HTLV-II: Serologic and molecular evidence. Ann Epidemiol 12:46, 2002.

167. Lubani MM, Dudin KI, Sharda DC, et al: Neonatal brucellosis. Eur J Pediatr 147:520, 1988.

168. Lubani MM, Dudin KI, Sharda DC, et al: A multicenter therapeutic study of 1100 children with brucellosis. Pediatr Infect Dis J 8:75, 1989.

169. MacMahon B, Lin TM, Lowe CR, et al: Lactation and cancer of the breast: A summary of an international study. Bull WHO 42:185, 1970.

170. Manzini P, Saracco G, Cerchier A, et al: Human immunodeficiency virus infection as risk factor for mother-to-child hepatitis C virus transmission: persistence of anti-hepatitis C virus in children is associated with the mother's anti-hepatitis C virus immunoblotting pattern. Hepatology 21:328, 1995.

171. Marra MA, Jones SJ, Astell CR, et al: The genome sequence of the SARS-associated coronavirus. Science 300:1399, 2003.

172. Martin P, Friedman L, Dienstag J: Diagnostic approach. In Zuckerman A, Thomas H (eds): Viral Hepatitis: Scientific Basis and Clinical Management. Edinburgh, Churchill Livingstone, 1993.

173. Maschmann J, Hamprecht K, Kietz K, et al: Cytometalovirus infection of extremely low-birth weight infants via breast milk. Clin Infect Dis 33:1998, 2001.

174. May JT: Antimicrobial factors and microbial contaminants in human milk: Recent studies. J Pediatr Child Health 30:470, 1994.

175. Mbori-Ngacha D, Nduati R, John G, et al: Morbidity and mortality in breastfed women: A randomized clinical trial. JAMA 286(19):2413, 2001.

176. McManus IC: Predominance of left-sided breast tumors. Lancet 2:297, 1977.

177. McTiernan A, Thomas DB: Evidence for a protective effect of lactation on risk of breast cancer in young women: Results from a case-control study. Am J Epidemiol 124:353, 1986.

178. Menzies D: Effect of treatment on the contagiousness of patients with active pulmonary tuberculosis. Infect Control Hosp Epidemiol 18:582, 1997.

179. Miller MJ: Fungal infections. In Remington JS, Klein JO (eds): Infectious Diseases of the Fetus and Newborn Infant, 4th ed. Philadelphia, WB Saunders, 1995.

180. Miller RN, Fraumeni JF: Does breast feeding increase the child's risk of breast cancer? Pediatrics 49:645, 1972.

181. Minamishima I, Ueda K, Minematsu T, et al: Role of breast milk in acquisition of cytomegalovirus infection. Microbiol Immunol 38:549, 1994.

182. Miotti PG, Taha TE, Kumwenda NI, et al: HIV transmission through breastfeeding: A study in Malawi. JAMA 282(8):781, 1999.

183. Molin GD, D'Aquaro P, Ansaldi F, et al: Mother-to-infant transmission of hepatitis C virus: Rate of infection and assessment of viral load and IgM anti-HCV as risk factors. J Med Virol 67(2):137, 2002.

184. Morgan RW, Vakil DV, Chipman ML: Breastfeeding family history and breast disease. Am J Epidemiol 99:117, 1974.

185. Moriya T, Sasaki F, Mizui M, et al: Transmission of hepatitis C virus from mothers to infants: Its frequency and risk factors revisited. Biomed Pharmacother 49:59, 1995.

186. Nagelkerke NJ, Moses S, Embree JE, et al: The duration of breastfeeding by HIV-1 infected mothers in developing countries: Balancing benefits and risks. J AIDS Hum Retrovirol 8:176, 1995.

187. Nakano S, Ando Y, Ichijo M, et al: Search for possible routes of vertical and horizontal transmission of adult T-cell leukemia virus. Gann 75:1044, 1984.

188. Nduati RW, John GC, Richardson BA, et al: Human immunodeficiency virus type 1-infected cells in breast milk: Association with immunosuppression and and vitamin A deficiency. J Infect Dis 172:1461, 1995.

189. Nduati R, Richardson BA, John G, et al: Effect of breastfeeding on mortality among HIV-1 infected women: A randomised trial. Lancet 357:1651, 2001.

190. Newburg DS, Linhardt RJ, Ampofo SA, et al: Human milk glycosaminoglycans inhibit HIV glycoprotein gp 120 binding to its host cell CD4 receptor. J Nutr 125:419, 1995.

191. Newcombe PA, Storer BE, Longnecker MP: Lactation and a reduced risk of premenopausal breast cancer. N Engl J Med 330:81, 1994.

192. Numazaki K: Human cytomegalovirus infection of breast milk. FEMS Immunol Med Micro 18:91, 1997.

193. Nyambi PN, Ville Y, Louwagie J, et al: Mother-to-child transmission of human T-cell lymphotoropic virus types I and II (HTLV-I/II) in Gabon: A prospective follow-up of 4 years. J AIDS Hum Retrovirol 12:187, 1996.

194. O'Brien TR, George JR, Holmberg SD: HIV-2 infection in the United States: Epidemiology, diagnosis and public health implications. JAMA 267:2775, 1992.

195. Ohto H, Okamoto H, Mishiro S: Vertical transmission of hepatitis C virus. N Engl J Med 331:400, 1994 (letter).

196. Ohto H, Terazawa S, Sasaki N, et al: Transmission of hepatitis C virus from mothers to infants. N Engl J Med 330:744, 1994.

197. Ohto H, Ujiie N, Sato A, et al, for the vertical transmission of hepatitis viruses collaborative Study Group: Mother-to-infant transmission of GB virus type C/HGV. Trasnsfusion 40:725, 2000.

198. Ohto H, Ujiie N, Takeuchi C, et al for the vertical transmission of hepatitis viruses Collaborative Study Group: TT virus infection during childhood. Transfusion 42:892, 2002.

199. Okamoto H, Mayumi M: TT Virus: Virological and genomic characteristics and disease associations. J Gastroenterol 36:519, 2001.

200. Orloff SL, Wallingford JC, McDougal JS: Inactivation of human immunodeficiency virus type I in human milk: effects of intrinsic factors in human milk and of pasteurization. J Hum Lact 9:13, 1993.

201. Oxtoby MJ: Human immunodeficiency virus and other viruses in human milk: Placing the issues in broader prospective. Pediatr Infect Dis J 7:825, 1988.

202. Pabst HF, Grace M, Godel J, et al: Effect of breast-feeding on immune response to BCG vaccination. Lancet I:295, 1989.

203. Palasanthiran P, Ziegler JB, Stewart GJ, et al: Breast-feeding during primary maternal human immunodeficiency virus infection and risk of transmission from mother to infant. J Infect Dis 167:441, 1993.

204. Papaioannou AN: Etiologic factors in cancer of the breast in humans: Collective review. Surg Gynecol Obstet 138:257, 1974.

205. Parks YA, Nuy MF, Aukett MA, et al: Methicillin-resistant Staphylococcus aureus in milk. Arch Dis Child 62:82, 1987.

206. Peckham CS, Johnson C, Ades A, et al: Early acquisition of cytomegalovirus infection. Arch Dis Child 62:780, 1987.

207. Peters CJ: Arenaviruses. In Richman DD, Whitley RJ, Hayden FG (eds): Clinical Virology. New York, Churchill Livingstone, 1997.

208. Petersen LR, Marfin AA: West Nile virus: A primer for the clinician. Ann Intern Med 137:173, 2002.

209. Pickering LK, Morrow AL, Herrera I, et al: Effect of maternal rotavirus immunization on milk and serum antibody titers. J Infect Dis 172:723, 1995.

210. Pillay K, Coutsoudis A, York D, et al: Cell-free virus in breast milk of HIV-1–seropositive women. 1. J AIDS 24(4):330, 2000.

211. Pisacane A, Grillo G, Cafiero M, et al: Role of breastfeeding in paralytic poliomyelitis. Br Med J 305:1367, 1992.

212. Quinn PT, Lofberg JV: Maternal herpetic breast infection: Another hazard of neonatal herpes simplex. Med J Aust 2:411, 1978.

213. Raucher HS, Grimbetz I: Care of the pregnant woman with tuberculosis and her newborn infant: A pediatrician's perspective. Mt Sinai J Med 53:70, 1986.

214. Read JS, and the Committee on Pediatric AIDS: Human milk, breastfeeding, and transmission of human immunodeficiency virus type 1 in the United States. Pediatrics 112:5, 2003.

215. Remington JS, McLeod R, Desmonts G: Toxoplasmosis. In Remington JS, Klein JO (eds): Infectious Diseases of the Fetus and Newborn Infant, 4th ed. Philadelphia, WB Saunders, 1995.

216. Reyes GR: Hepatitis E virus. In Richman DD, Whitley RJ, Hayden FG (eds): Clinical Virology. New York, Churchill Livingstone, 1997.

217. Richardson BA, John-Steward GC, Hughes JP, et al: Breast-milk infectivity in human immunodeficiency virus type 1-infected mothers. J Infect Dis 187:736, 2003.

218. Roggiani M, Schlievert PM: Streptococcal toxic shock syndrome, including necrotizing fasciitis and myositis. Curr Opin Infect Dis 7:423, 1994.

219. Rosenblum LS, Villarino ME, Nainan OV, et al: Hepatitis A outbreak in a neonatal intensive care unit: Risk factors for transmission and evidence of prolonged viral excretion among preterm infants. J Infect Dis 164:476, 1991.

220. Rota PA, Oberste MS, Monroe SS, et al: Characterization of a novel corona virus associated with severe acute respiratory syndrome. Science 300:1994, 2003.

221. Rousseau CM, Nduati RW, Richardson BA, et al: Longitudinal analysis of human immunodeficiency virus type 1 RNA in breast milk and of its relationship to infant infection and maternal disease. J Infect Dis 187(5):741, 2003.

222. Roy-Burman P, Rongey RW, Henderson BE, et al: Attempts to detect RNA tumour virus in human milk. Nat Biol 244:146, 1973.

223. Ruff AJ, Coberly J, Halsey NA, et al: Prevalence of HIV-1 DNA and p24 antigen in breastmilk and correlation with maternal factors. J AIDS 7:68, 1994.

224. Ruiz-Extremera A, Salmeron J, Torres C, et al: Follow-up of transmission of hepatitis C to babies of human immunodeficiency virus-negative women: The role of breast-feeding in transmission. Pediatr Infect Dis J 19(6):511, 2000.

225. Sanner T: Removal of inhibitors against RNA-directed DNA polymerase activity in human milk. Cancer Res 36:405, 1976.

226. Sarkar NH, Charney J, Doion AS, et al: Effect of human milk on mouse mammary tumor virus. Cancer Res 33:626, 1973.

227. Sawada T, Iwahara Y, Ishii K, et al: Immunoglobulin prophylaxis against milkborne transmission of human T cell leukemia virus type 1 in rabbits. J Infect Dis 164:1193, 1991.

228. Schachter J, Grossman M: Chlamydial infections. Ann Rev Med 32:45, 1981.

229. Schaefer G, Zervoudakis IA, Fuchs FF, et al: Pregnancy and pulmonary tuberculosis. Obstet Gynecol 46:706, 1975.

230. Scheiner RL, Coates T, Shackelford PG, et al: Possible breast milk transmission of group B streptococcal infection. J Pediatr 91:159, 1977.

231. Schlesinger JJ, Covelli HD: Evidence for transmission of lymphocyte responses to tuberculin by breast-feeding. Lancet I:529, 1977.

232. Schlievert PM: Toxic shock syndrome. Postgrad Med 94:108, 1993.

233. Schmidt B, Aberer E, Stockenhuber C, et al: Detection of *Borrelia burgdorferi* DNA by PCR in the urine and breast-milk of patients with Lyme borreliosis. Diagn Microbiol Infect Dis 21:121, 1995.

234. Schröter M, Polywka S, Zollner B, et al: Detection of TT virus DNA and GB virus type C/Hepatitis G virus RNA in serum and breast milk: Determination of mother-to-child transmission. J Clin Microbiol 38(2):745, 2000.

235. Schwer M, Moosa A: Effects of hepatitis A and B in pregnancy on the mother and fetus. S Afr Med J 54:1092, 1978.

236. Semba RD, Kumwenda N, Hoover DR, et al. Human immunodeficiency virus load in breast milk, mastitis and mother-to-child transmission of human immunodeficiency virus type 1. J Infect Dis 180:93, 1999.

237. Senturia, YD, Ades AE, Peckham CS, Giaquinto C: Breast-feeding and HIV infection. Lancet 2:400, 1987.

238. Sepkowitz KA: How contagious is vaccinia? N Engl J Med 348:439, 2003.

239. Sharland M, Khare M, Bedford-Russell A: Prevention of postnatal cytomegalovirus infection in preterm infants. Arch Dis Child Fetal Neonat Ed 86:F140, 2002.

240. Shek, CC, Ng PC, Genevieve PG, et al: Infants born to mothers with severe acute respiratory syndrome. Pediatrics 112:4; 2003.

241. Silver HM: Lyme disease during pregnancy. Infect Obstet 11:93, 1997.

242. Sit SC, Yau EKC, Lam YY, et al: A young infant with severe acute respiratory syndrome. Pediatrics 112(4):e257, 2003.

243. Skaug K, Otnaess Ab, Orstavik I, et al: Chlamydial secretory IgA antibodies in human milk. Acta Pathol Microbiol Immunol Scand 90:21, 1982.

244. Smedile A, Niro G, Rizzetto M: Hepatitis D virus. In Richman DD, Whitley RJ, Hayden FG (eds): Clinical Virology. New York, Churchill Livingstone, 1997.

245. Snider DE Jr, Powell KE: Should women taking antituberculous drugs breast feed? Arch Intern Med 144:589, 1984.

246. Speer CHP, Gahr M, Pabst MJ: Phagocytosis- associated oxidative metabolism in human milk macrophages. Acta Pediatr Scand 75:444, 1986.

247. Stagno S, Cloud GA: Working parents: The impact of day care and breast-feeding on cytomegalovirus infection in offspring. Proc Natl Acad Sci USA 91:2384, 1994.

248. Stagno S, Reynolds DW, Pass RF, et al: Breast milk and the risk of cytomegalovirus infection. N Engl J Med 302:1073, 1980.

249. Starke JR: Tuberculosis, an old disease but a new threat to mother, fetus, and neonate. Clin Perinatol 24:107, 1997.

250. Stevens CE, Beasley PR, Tsui J, et al: Vertical transmission of hepatitis B antigen in Taiwan. N Engl J Med 292:771, 1975.

251. Stevens CE, Taylor PE, Tong MJ, et al: Yeast-recombinant hepatitis B vaccine: Efficacy with hepatitis B immune globulin in prevention of perinatal hepatitis B virus transmission. JAMA 257:2612, 1987.

252. Strobino B, Abid S, Gerwitz M: Maternal lyme disease and congenital heart disease: A case-control study in an endemic area. Am J Obstet Gynecol. 180(3):711, 1999.

253. Subcommittee on Nutrition During Lactation, Food and Nutrition Board, Institute of Medicine, National Academy of Sciences: Nutrition during Lactation. Washington, DC, National Academy Press, 1991.

254. Sugiyama H, Doi H, Yamaguchi, et al: Significance of postnatal mother-to-child transmission of HTLV-I on the development of adult T-cell leukemia/lymphoma. J Med Virol 20:253, 1986.

255. Sullivan-Bolyai JZ, Fife KH, Jacobs RF, et al: Disseminated neonatal herpes simplex virus type I from a maternal breast lesion. Pediatrics 71:455, 1983.

256. Sumaya CV: Epstein-Barr virus. In Feigin RD, Cherry JD (eds): Textbook of Pediatric Infectious Diseases, 3rd ed. Philadelphia, WB Saunders, 1992.

257. Tajiri H, Miyoshi Y, Funada S, et al: Prospective study of mother-to-infant transmission of hepatitis C virus. Pediatr Infect Dis J 20(1):10, 2001.

258. Takahashi K, Takezaki T, Oki T, et al (the mother-to-child transmission study group, Osame M, Miyata K, Nagata Y, Sonoda S): Inhibitory effect of maternal antibody on mother-to-child transmission of human T-lymphotropic virus type I. Int J Cancer 49:673, 1991.

259. Takezaki T, Tajima K, Ito M, et al: Short-term breast-feeding may reduce the risk of vertical transmission of HTLV-I. The Tsushima ATL Study Group. Leukemia 11(suppl 3):60, 1997.

260. Tess BH, Rodrigues LC, Newell ML, et al: Infant feeding and risk of mother-to-child transmission of HIV-1 in Sao

Paulo State, Brazil. Sao Paulo Collaborative Study for Vertical Transmission of HIV-1. J AIDS Hum Retrovirol 19:189, 1998.

261. Thiry L, Sprecher-Goldbrecker S, Jonckheer T, et al: Isolation of the AIDS virus from cell-free breastmilk of three healthy virus carriers. Lancet 2:891, 1985.

262. Tomar BS. Hepatitis E in India. Zhonghua Min Guo Xiao Er Ke Yi Xue Hui Zhi 39(3):150, 1998.

263. Torok TJ: Human parvovirus B19. In Remington JS, Klein JO (eds): Infectious Diseases of the Fetus and Newborn Infant, 4th ed. Philadelphia, WB Saunders, 1995.

264. UNAIDS/UNICEF/WHO: HIV and infant feeding. A review of HIV transmission through breastfeeding. Geneva, Switzerland: WHO/UNAIDS, 1998. Available at http://www.unaids.org/publicatins/documents/mtct/hiv-mod3.doc. Accessed January 21, 2004

265. Ureta-Vidal A, Angelin-Duclos C, Tortevoye P, et al: Mother-to-child transmission of human T-cell leukemia/lymphoma virus type I: Implication of high antiviral antibody titer and high proviral load in carrier mothers. Int J Cancer 82(6):832, 1999.

266. Van de Perre P, Simonon A, Hitimana D, et al: Infective and antiinfective properties of breastmilk from HIV-1 infected women. Lancet 341:914, 1993.

267. Van de Peere P, Simonon A, Msellati P, et al: Postnatal transmission of the human immunodeficiency virus type 1 from mother to infant: A prospective cohort study in Kigali, Rwanda. N Engl J Med 3325:593, 1991.

268. Van Dyke RB, Heneine W, Perrin M, et al: Mother-to-child transmission of human T-lymphotropic virus type II. J Pediatr 127:927, 1995.

269. Vergeront JM, Everson ML, Crass BA, et al: Recovery of staphylococcal enterotoxin F from the breast milk of a woman with toxic-shock syndrome. J Infect Dis 146:456, 1982.

270. Vitek CR, Gracia FI, Giusti RA, et al: Evidence for sexual and mother-to-child transmission of human T lymphotrophic virus type II among Guaymi Indians, Panama. J Infect Dis 171:1022, 1995.

271. Vochem M, Hamprecht K, Jahn G, et al: Transmission of cytomegalovirus to preterm infants through breast milk. Pediatr Infect Dis J 17:53, 1998.

272. Vorherr H: Pregnancy and lactation in relation to breast cancer risk. Semin Perinatol 3:299, 1979.

273. Watson JC, Fleming DW, Borella AJ, et al: Vertical transmission of hepatitis A resulting in an outbreak in a neonatal intensive care unit. J Infect Dis 167:567, 1993.

274. Wejstal R, Manson AS, Widell A, Norkrans G: Perinatal transmission of hepatitis G virus (GB virus type C) and hepatitis C virus infections—A comparison. Clin Infect Dis 28(4):816, 1999.

275. Wharton M, Strikas RA, Harpaz R, et al; Advisory Committee on Immunization Practices; Healthcare Infection Control Practices Advisory Committee: Recommendations for using smallpox vaccine in a pre-event vaccination program. Supplemental recommendations of the Advisory Committee on Immunization Practices (ACIP) and the Healthcare Infection Control Practices. Advisory Committee (HICPAC). MMWR Recomm Rep 52(RR-7):1, 2003.

276. Wiktor SZ, Pate EJ, Barnett M, et al: Maternal-infant transmission of HTLV-I: Frequency and time course of seroconversion. Abstract W-53. Proceedings of the Fifth International Conference of Human Retrovirology, Tokyo, May 1992.

277. Wiktor SZ, Pate EJ, Rosenberg PS, et al: Mother-to-child transmission of human T-cell lymphotropic virus type I associated with prolonged breast- feeding. J Hum Virol 1:37, 1997.

278. Williams CL, Strobino B, Weinstein A, et al: Maternal Lyme disease and congenital malformations: A cord blood serosurvey in endemic and control areas. Paediatr Perinat Epidemiol 9(3):320, 1995.

279. Wing JP: Human versus cow's milk in infant nutrition and health. Curr Probl Pediatr 8(1):1, 1977 (entire issue).

280. Wong-Staal F, Gallo RC: Human T-lymphocyte retroviruses. Nature 312:395, 1985.

281. Working Group on Severe Streptococcal Infections: Defining GAS streptococcal toxic shock syndrome: Rationale and consensus definition. JAMA 269:390, 1993.

282. Wu J, Tang ZY, Wu YX, et al: Acquired cytomegalovirus infection of breast milk in infancy. Chin Med J 102:124, 1989.

283. Yamanouchi K, Kinochita K, Moriuchi R, et al: Oral transmission of human T-cell leukemia virus type 1 into a common marmoset as an experimental model for milk-borne transmission. Jpn J Cancer Res 76:481, 1985.

284. Yasuda A, Kimura H, Hayakawa M, et al: Evaluation of cytomegalovirus infections transmitted via breast milk in preterm infants with a real-time polymerase chain reaction assay. Pediatrics 111:1333, 2003.

285. Yeager AS, Palumbo PE, Malachowski N, et al: Sequelae of maternally derived cytomegalovirus infections in premature infants. J Pediatr 102:918, 1983.

286. Yeung LTF, King SM, Roberts EA: Mother-to-infant transmission of hepatitis C virus. Hepatology 34(2):223, 2001.

287. Yoo K-Y, Tajima K, Kuroishi T, et al: Independent protective effect of lactation against breast cancer: A case-control study in Japan. Am J Epidemiol 135:726, 1992.

288. Yoshida M, Yamagami N, Tezuka T, et al: Case report: Detection of varicella-zoster virus DNA in maternal breast milk. J Med Virol 38:108, 1992.

289. Yoshinaga M, Yashiki S, Fujiyoshi T, et al: A maternal factor for mother-to-child transmission: Viral antigen-producing capacities in culture of peripheral blood and breast milk cells. Jpn J Cancer Res 86:649, 1995.

290. Zanetti AR, Tanzi E, Paccagnini S, et al: Mother-to-infant transmission of hepatitis C virus. Lancet 345:289,1995.

291. Zeldis JB, Crumpacker CS: Hepatitis. In Remington JS, Klein JO (eds): Infectious Diseases of the Fetus and Newborn Infant, 4th ed. Philadelphia, WB Saunders, 1995.

292. Zhang RJ, Zeng JS, Zhang HZ: Survey of 34 pregnant women with hepatitis A and their neonates. Chin Med J 103:552, 1990.

293. Ziegler JB, Cooper DA, Johnson RO, et al: Postnatal transmission of AIDS-associated retrovirus from mother to infant. Lancet 1:896, 1985.

294. Ziska MH, Giovanello T, Johnson MJ, Baly J: Disseminated Lyme disease and pregnancy. 9th Annual International Scientific Conference on Lyme Disease and Other Tick-Borne Disorders, Boston, MA, April 19–20, 1996.

$\mathcal{H}$uman milk as a prophylaxis in allergy

THE NATURAL HISTORY OF ATOPIC DISEASE

The association of allergy with cow milk has been documented in the literature for decades.[20,52,72] The incidence of this allergy in the general population has been noted to increase progressively since the original comments on the subject by Rowe[74] in 1931. The incidence has reportedly increased 10 times in 20 years and has been attributed to increased recognition, increased incidence of exposure to known allergens, and a gradual decrease in infection as a source of morbidity because use of antibiotics and immunization revealed an underlying allergic component to chronic symptoms. Glaser[25] attributed this rapid increase in the development of allergic diseases to the abandonment of breast-feeding when safe pasteurized milk became available. It was noted that 20% of all children were allergic by 20 years of age.

Studies of office pediatrics have shown that one third of the visits are a result of allergy.[87] One third of all chronic conditions under age 17 result from allergy and one third of lost school days from asthma. In the evaluation of 2000 consecutive unselected newborns in pediatric practice, 50% had family histories of allergy. Grulee and associates[31] observed as early as 1934 that eczema was seven times more common in infants fed cow milk than in breastfed infants. McCombs and associates[65] reported in 1979 that asthma caused more than 2000 deaths and the loss of 94 million days of activity and initiated 183,000 hospital admissions and more than 1 million hospital days in 1 year in the United States alone.

Asthma is the most common chronic disease of childhood, affecting an estimated 6.3 million children, according to a Centers for Disease Control and Prevention (CDC) report in 2001.[69,92] These data indicate that in the United States people with asthma collectively have more than 100 million days of restricted activity and 470,000 hospitalizations annually, with more than 5000 deaths annually. Asthma hospitalization rates have been highest among blacks and children, with mortality rates consistently highest among blacks ages 15 to 24 years. Asthma costs the American public billions of dollars annually.

The question of heredity

Heredity undoubtedly plays a part in the development of allergic disease, an observation first recorded by Maimonides in his *Treatise on Asthma* in the 12th century. Most studies in the past 60 years have concurred with the concept of a recessive mode of inheritance.[42]

Kern[51] has noted that the outstanding etiologic factor in human hypersensitivity is heredity. He states that few diseases exist in which heredity is so clearly identified and so common.

Hamburger[34] reported that children with two atopic parents had a 47% chance of developing atopic disease. One atopic parent meant a 29% chance of developing atopy, and the risk dropped to 13% with no allergic parent.

Falliers and associates,[16] in a study of asthmatic monozygotic twins, observed similar serum immunoglobulin E (IgE), blood eosinophil counts, and positive skin tests to allergens in both twins but dissimilar responses to infection and methacholine. This finding suggests there is also an acquired component to bronchial hyperactivity. Apparently several mechanisms are involved in antigen processing.

To identify infants at high risk for developing atopy, several approaches have been suggested. Cord serum total IgE levels of greater than 100 U/mL are associated with five to ten times greater risk than lower levels. Eosinophilia and lymphocytes may prove to be markers, but at present only the family allergy history and the cord blood IgE have been significantly reliable predictors.[3]

Glaser speculated in the 1930s that if a child were at high risk for developing allergy, prophylaxis should be able to change the outcome. The original work on prophylaxis was done by Glaser and Johnstone[28] and reported in 1953. Only 15% of a group of children whose mothers controlled their own diet in pregnancy and controlled the infant's diet and environment at birth did develop eczema, whereas 65% of the sibling controls and 52% of nonrelated controls receiving cow milk developed similar allergic illnesses. Although as a retrospective study it was open to some criticism, it did begin to look at a very significant issue, that is, reducing the incidence of allergic manifestations in high-risk individuals by a new type of preventive measure.

A second study was designed in 1953 and carried out prospectively by Johnstone and Dutton[43] to investigate dietary prophylaxis of allergic disease. They observed a difference of more than 10 years

in the incidence of asthma and perennial allergic rhinitis in those fed soybean milk (18%) and those fed evaporated milk (50%). No infant in this study of 283 children was breastfed, however. Halpern and associates[33] reported the study of 1753 children fed breast milk, soy milk, and cow milk from birth to 6 months of age who were followed until they were 7 years or older. The children included those with high-risk, low-risk, and no-risk family histories for allergy. No difference in outcome was related to early diet, but a relationship to the family history was seen.

In a prospective study to identify the development of reaginic allergy, infants of allergic parents were placed in a study or control group. The study group followed an allergen-avoidance regimen, including breastfeeding. At 6 months and 1 year, the study infants had less eczema than the control infants, as well as lower serum total IgE levels.[52]

PROPHYLAXIS OF ATOPIC DISEASE

Efforts to alter the incidence of atopic illness have continued to challenge investigators, who now have access to increased methodologic sophistication. Prevention of IgE-mediated disorders can be directed at interfering with any of the major forces responsible for the phenotypic expression of atopy. Practically, however, it is not yet possible to mask IgE genes or manipulate cellular components of the response organ. Clinicians are limited to manipulating the effect of the environment by reducing the allergenic load.

Review of the plethora of studies directed at measuring the impact of dietary manipulations on the incidence of atopic disease demonstrates that retrospective studies show little or no difference in the incidence of asthma and eczema. Prospective studies, however, tend to demonstrate a significant reduction in atopic disease in the treated group (Table 18-1). In looking at these data, it is important to recognize that some studies did not consider the risk of the population developing atopic disease on

TABLE 18-1	Prevention of atopy: prospective studies				
Study	Year published	No. of years followed	No. of subjects[*]	Type of milk/feeding	Impact on atopy[†]
Johnstone and Dutton[43]	1966	10	235	Soy, cow	↓ Asthma, rhinitis
Matthew et al[63]	1977	1	53 (26)	Breast, soy	↓ Eczema
Chandra[9]	1979	>2	134	Breast	↓ Eczema, asthma
Saarinen et al[76]	1979	3	(256)	Breast	↓ Eczema, food allergy, asthma
Hamburger[35]	1981	1	(300)	Breast	↓ Eczema, asthma
Kaufman and Frick[49,50]	1976, 1981	2	(94)	Breast	↓ Asthma
Hide and Guyer[38]	1981	1	843 (266)	Breast <6 mo, soy, cow (maternal diet not controlled)	↓ Eczema slight, rhinitis
Gruskay[32]	1982	15	908 (328)	Breast 4 mo, soy, cow	↓ Breast symptoms; soy no effect
May et al[64]	1982	½	67 normal	Soy, cow, modern formula	↑ Antibodies with no disease symptoms
Businco et al[6]	1983	2	(101)	Breast <6 mo; soy, cow	↓ Asthma, eczema
Kajosaari and Saarinen[48]	1983	1	(135)	All breast milk <6 mo; half solid foods early	↑ Eczema/food intolerance in those fed solids
Moore et al[67]	1985	1	525	Study—breastfed 3 mo; control —SMA	Not clear: 74% failed to breastfeed or gave cow's milk in study group
Zeiger et al[98]	1989	4	288	Maternal avoidance diet last trimester Controls unrestricted; mothers diet; infants given Nutramigen	↓ Atopy 16% in restricted infants ↑ Atopy in control infants (to 27%) ↓ Urticaria/GI symptoms in restricted group
Sigurs et al[86]	1992	4	115	All breastfed; 65 mothers restricted diet for first 3 mo of lactation; 50 no restrictions	↓ Atopy/asthma among both groups ↓ Greater among restricted group

[*] Number in study; parentheses indicate number at risk for atopy.
[†]Arrows indicate decrease or increase compared with control group.
Modified from Businco L, Marchetti F, Pellegrini G, et al: Prevention of atopic disease in "at-risk newborns" by prolonged breastfeeding. Ann Allergy 51:296, 1983.

TABLE 18-2   Relationship of maternal total serum IgE level to cord and 4-month serum IgE level in prophylaxis group infants

Maternal IgE (U/mL)	Cord IgE (U/mL)		4-months IgE (U/mL)	
	<0.5 Number (%)	≥0.5 Number (%)	<5.0 Number (%)	≥5.0 Number (%)
≤100	35 (71)	14 (29)	41 (87)	6 (13)
>100	14 (42)	19 (58)	24 (73)	9 (27)
Total	49	33	65	15

$p < 0.01$ by chi square for maternal IgE <100 vs. >100 U/mL for cord IgE with a trend ($p < 0.08$) at 4-month IgE measurement.
From Hamburger RN, Heller S, Mellon MH, et al: Current status of the clinical and immunologic consequences of a prototype allergic disease prevention program. Ann Allergy 51:281, 1983.

a hereditary basis. In other studies, breastfeeding may have been carried out for only a few weeks or months. The evidence is clear that 6 months or longer of exclusive breastfeeding makes a difference. No study controlled for smoking in the household, and no data were reported on incidence of respiratory syncytial virus. In addition, some studies did not control the breastfeeding mother's diet, the weaning foods, or use of cow milk beverages.

Hamburger and associates[36] carried out prospective prophylactic studies to include measuring IgE and skin radioallergosorbent test (RAST) on mother, father, and infant. They found a significant correlation between maternal IgE and infant IgE and potential allergy in the infant (Tables 18-2 and 18-3). This study was done by controlling the environment and the diet. The process was initiated in pregnancy to begin by protecting the fetus and then was continued at birth. Therefore, considerable attention was directed toward breastfeeding in this and other studies.

Human milk consistently contains antibodies, especially secretory immunoglobulin A (sIgA) to major food proteins. The levels are influenced by the mother's own external antigen exposure.

In a study of 500 babies born to families at high risk for allergies, one group was deliberately not given cow milk and was fed soy milk by random assignment.[66] No benefit resulted from withholding cow milk, but breastfeeding even for a short period was clearly associated with a lower incidence of wheezing, prolonged colds, diarrhea, and vomiting. Smoking and environmental molds were also associated with wheezing. Merrett and associates[66] concluded from this that breastfeeding played a significant role in prophylaxis.

TABLE 18-3   Relationship of paternal total serum IgE level to cord and 4-month serum IgE level in prophylaxis group infants

Paternal IgE (U/mL)	Cord IgE (U/mL)		4-months IgE (U/mL)	
	<0.5 Number (%)	≥0.5 Number (%)	<5.0 Number (%)	≥5.0 Number (%)
≤100	29 (63)	17 (37)	40 (83)	8 (17)
>100	10 (56)	8 (44)	14 (82)	3 (18)
Total	39	25	54	11

From Hamburger RN, Heller S, Mellon MH, et al: Current status of the clinical and immunologic consequences of a prototype allergic disease prevention program. Ann Allergy 51:281, 1983.

The effect of breastfeeding on allergic sensitization is both *direct* through the elimination of nonhuman milk protein as an exposure to antigen and *indirect* by affecting the absorption of antigen through the intestinal tract.[52] Maternal antibody is transferred to the breastfed infant as part of what has been called the *enteromammary immune system* (Fig. 18-1).[53] The secretory IgA (sIgA) antibody present in the milk is the result of the mother's enteric immune response to antigens in her gut. sIgA in her milk provides protection against bacterial, viral, and toxic exposures. Prospective studies have shown that infants at high risk for atopic illness from a hereditary standpoint had significantly less disease when breastfed, especially if reared in a protected environment with delayed use of solid foods, compared with children of similar risk fed cow milk and regular solid foods. Serum IgE concentrations were also greatly reduced under 6 months and 12 months of age in the breastfed group.[89]

Infants with a low incidence of T lymphocytes are at greater risk to develop allergies if fed cow milk rather than breast milk, according to Juto[44] and Bjorksten.[45] Infants with reduced T cells fed cow milk also demonstrated higher serum IgE levels and peripheral eosinophil counts. Juto and Strannegard[46] also reported that with careful prophylaxis, greater than 50% of infants who had both parents with IgE levels above 100 µg/mL (100 µg = 1.0 mg) showed elevated cord and 4-month IgE levels. More than 80% of those infants whose parents had IgE levels below 100 µg/mL (100 µg = 1.0 mg), however, had both low cord blood and low 4-month IgE levels. Such data confirm the genetic effect of both maternal and paternal genes.

The predictive value of cord blood IgE in the development of atopic disease was tested by Chandra and associates[12] in a study of 226 infants, 120 of whom had a positive family history of atopic disease in first-degree relatives (parents and siblings) and 106 whose family history was

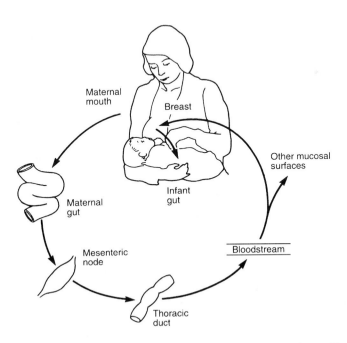

Figure 18-1.   Maternal serum antibodies affect passage of foreign antigens into milk and processing of antigen in infant's intestine. (Redrawn from Kleinman RE: The role of developmental immune mechanisms in intestinal allergy. Ann Allergy 51:222, 1983.)

negative for atopy. Using 0.7 U/mL or less of IgE, these authors found the level of cord blood IgE correlated significantly with the subsequent development of atopic disease. These investigators further tested the effect of feeding.[13] In the group with IgE levels less than 0.7 mg/dL who were breastfed, none developed atopy, and only one on formula did by 2 years of age. Of the 39 breastfed infants with elevated IgE, 12 developed atopy (30.7%), whereas in the 31 with elevated IgE who were formula fed, 26 (83.3%) developed eczema or wheezing in the first 2 years, a highly significant finding ($p = 0.001$). Of the entire study group, 12% of breastfed and 32% of formula fed infants developed atopy. The authors[13] consider cord blood IgE antibody levels a significant marker for development of atopy when the level of 0.7 or less µg/mL is used. The history of family atopy was a significant indicator of high IgE levels.

Investigating the influence of maternal food antigen avoidance during pregnancy and lactation on the incidence of atopic eczema in infants, Chandra and associates[13] reported the outcome of a randomly assigned prospective study of 120 women with a history of a previous child with atopic disease. The study group avoided all milk, dairy products, eggs, fish, beef, and peanuts throughout pregnancy and lactation. The control group had no restrictions. Maternal antigen avoidance was associated with less and milder eczema, particularly in those who were breastfed. Of 55 women who completed the avoidance regimen, 17 infants developed atopy, 5 from the 35 who were breastfed and 12 from the 20 who were formula fed. Of the 54 unrestricted mothers, 11 of 36 breastfed infants and 13 of 18 formula fed infants developed atopy. The researchers thus concluded that avoidance of common dietary allergens during pregnancy and lactation enhances the preventive beneficial effect of exclusive breastfeeding on the incidence of atopic eczema among high-risk infants.[13] Diets eliminating dairy products and eggs are deficient in calcium, however, and require special efforts to correct this by diet or supplementation.

In one study, 162 women with respiratory allergies to animal danders or pollens were randomly allocated to two groups: one on a diet of limited eggs and cow milk and the other on a diet of a daily egg and a liter of cow milk the last 3 months of pregnancy. Genetic factors rather than maternal diet during pregnancy were thought to have a greater effect on the incidence of atopic diseases in the first 18 months of life.[57] Almost all the infants in both groups were breastfed, a few received soy milk, and 13 received some cow milk formula. Mothers had no diet restrictions during lactation. Thus, as an isolated effort, diet restriction for the last trimester of pregnancy does not influence neonatal allergy in the first 18 months when it is associated with environmental allergens and not with diet.

Long-term effects of allergy prophylaxis

In an 18-month study of atopic outcome, atopic mothers were randomly allocated to an intervention group or an unrestricted-diet group, and both were compared to nonatopic mothers on unrestricted diets.[59] The intervention was a milk/dairy product-free diet during late pregnancy and lactation. After 7 weeks of the diet, serum β-lactoglobulin and immunoglobulin G (IgG) levels in the mother were collated to the levels in the cord blood. The infants were examined at 12 and 18 months by a single-blind allergy assessment by a pediatrician. The infants born to nonatopic parents had significantly less allergy than those born to atopic mothers with the unrestricted diets.[58] The "restricted-diet group" of infants had comparable levels to the atopy-free group and had significantly less allergy than the unrestricted-diet group. The nature of the parents' disease also played a role in the type of illness in both groups.

A prospective longitudinal study of 988 healthy infants from birth to 6 years of age recorded feeding-history episodes of lower respiratory tract infection in the first 3 years of life and recurrent episodes of wheezing.[97] Being breastfed was associated with lower rates of recurrent wheeze (3.1% vs. 9.7%, $p < 0.01$) for nonatopic children. The authors concluded that recurrent wheeze at age 6 is

TABLE 18-4   Odds ratios and confidence intervals for recurrent wheeze at age 6 years by logistic regression

Factor	Total group (n = 970)		Nonatopic children (n = 420)		Atopic children (n = 280)	
	Odds ratio (confidence interval)[*]					
Not breastfed	1.49	(0.80-2.77)	3.03[†]	(1.05-8.69)	1.36	(0.49-3.73)
Maternal education ≤12 yr	1.48	(0.87-2.53)	1.58	(0.56-4.43)	0.92	(0.36-2.38)
Hispanic	2.48[‡]	(1.39-4.40)	2.45	(0.82-7.27)	2.50[†]	(1.01-6.18)
Maternal hay fever	2.66[§]	(1.49-4.72)	2.64	(0.96-7.22)	2.35[†]	(1.07-5.16)
Wheezing lower respiratory tract illness in first 6 mo	1.68	(0.88-3.19)	1.86	(0.55-6.25)	2.01	(0.74-5.48)

[*]Excludes children who were missing information for one or more of these factors.
[†]$p < 0.05$.
[‡]$p < 0.005$.
[§]$p < 0.0005$.
From Wright AL, Holberg CJ, Taussig LM, et al: Relationship of infant feeding to recurrent wheezing at age 6 years. Arch Pediatr Adolesc Med 49:762, 1995.

less common among nonatopic children who were breastfed as infants. This effect was independent of whether or not the child had a wheezing lower respiratory tract illness in the first 6 months of life (Table 18-4). These authors recorded smoking history, but it did not alter the compelling influence of breastfeeding on the outcome.

Additional long-term studies have demonstrated that children who had ever been breastfed had a 50% lower incidence of wheezing than those who had not breastfed and that the effect persisted for the 7 years of the study in nonatopic children.[4] These authors attribute this in part to breastfeeding's protective effect against respiratory illness. They did not distinguish minimal from prolonged breastfeeding.

In a 17-year prospective study of 150 healthy children, researchers did consider length of breastfeeding.[75] The three groups had been breastfed less than 1 month or not at all, 1 to 6 months, or more than 6 months. Prolonged breastfeeding was associated with the least eczema at 1 to 3 years, as well as fewer food and respiratory allergies. At age 17 years the trends continued, leading the authors to conclude that breastfeeding is protective against atopic eczema, food allergy, and respiratory asthma throughout childhood and adolescence (Figs. 18-2 and 18-3).[75]

IMMUNOLOGIC ASPECTS OF ALLERGY

Interest in identifying the immunologic aspects of clinical allergy led to a number of additional studies on infant feeding.[35,36] Kletter and associates[54] reported that hemagglutinating antibodies to cow milk were

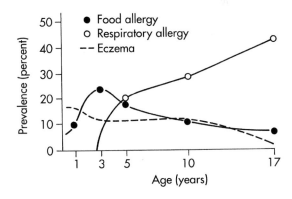

Figure 18-2.   Prevalence of atopic eczema, food allergy, and respiratory allergy in full cohort of initially 236 children during follow-up for 17 years. (Modified from Saarinen UM, Kajossari M: Breastfeeding as prophylaxis against disease: prospective follow-up study until 17 years old. Lancet 346:1065, 1995.)

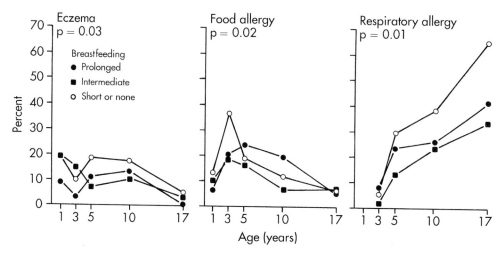

Figure 18-3. Prevalence of atopic eczema, food allergy, and respiratory allergy in infant feeding groups during follow-up for 17 years. Tests for differences during the appropriate age periods (eczema 1 to 3 years, food allergy 1 to 3 years, respiratory allergy at 5, 10, and 17 years) were done by analysis of variance and covariance with repeated measures. (Modified from Saarinen UM, Kajossari M: Breastfeeding as prophylaxis against disease: prospective follow-up study until 17 years old. Lancet 346:1065, 1995.)

present in the sera of some newborns but usually at levels lower than those of the mother. The earliest rise in titer was detected at 1 month, and a peak was seen at 3 months in infants given cow milk from birth. Antibodies belonged mainly to the IgG group, with their rise and fall paralleling hemagglutinating antibodies. IgA antibodies were in low titer, and IgM antibodies were rarely detected. The delayed exposure to cow milk in breastfed infants resulted in lower mean values of cow milk antibodies, and peak values were attained more slowly. An inverse relationship exists between duration of breastfeeding and levels of titers of humoral antibodies.

Freed and Green[18] investigated antibody-facilitated digestion and its implications for infant nutrition. They suggest a model of digestion in which oligopeptides in the small bowel are bound to secretory antibodies, which hold them in contact with proteases. This facilitates the breakdown and utilization of the oligopeptides. They consider immunity and digestion to be closely related. Breastfeeding with colostrum and then mature human milk provides the immature gut of the infant with both immunity and "digestivity."

The presence of periods of transient IgA deficiency in saliva in the first 12 months of life has been identified as a possible risk factor for the development of asthma, bronchial hyperactivity, and atopy.[29]

Eighteen patients with documented malabsorption of cow milk who were studied by Savilahti and associates[77-79] improved by feeding them human milk after challenge with powdered milk. Eight patients had clinical reactions; the number of IgA- and IgM-containing cells increased by almost 2.5 times in the intestinal mucosa. When breast milk feedings resumed, the findings returned to normal. Serum antibodies of both hemagglutination and IgA increased. No change was seen in IgE antibodies or serum complement. Many other findings, including villous atrophy and round cell infiltration, were noted. After age 2 years, all the infants became tolerant of milk, which may indicate that immunologic immaturity is part of the pathogenesis. Walker[95] presented similar arguments and conclusions in a symposium discussion.

When studying problems related to infant feeding, it is difficult to randomize groups to breastfeed or not, and many women are particularly adamant about breastfeeding with a strong family history of allergy. This was a factor in a study of 69 preterm infants and subsequent allergic symptoms in childhood, as well as the premature infant's intestine being more permeable to proteins and the immune system more immature. The long-term incidence of atopy, however, was no different between the feeding groups at age 11, although those receiving breast milk had a strong family history of atopy.[79]

Low IgA content of milk, especially low colostral IgA, has been correlated with cow milk allergy in a group of 198 infants, seven of whom became allergic to cow milk.[78] All other measurements (immunoglobulins G, A, M; cow milk–specific antibodies; β-lactoglobulin) were similar among all 198 infants. The authors[58] suggest that an infant is more likely to develop cow milk allergy if the mother has insufficient protective factors, namely, IgA.

Some discrepancies between studies may be explained by measuring the concentration of bovine IgG in human milk using different methods. When levels were tested on the same milk samples using competition radioimmunoassay (RIA), competition enzyme-linked immunosorbent assay (ELISA), and sandwich ELISA, IgG levels were significantly higher using RIA or ELISA.[61] Levels in the milk of mothers on a dairy product–free diet for a month still have measurable levels by RIA and ELISA but not by sandwich ELISA.

To resolve the question of the presence of specific secretory IgE (sIgE) for cow milk protein in the sera of breastfed infants who had never received cow milk, Cantisani and associates[8] measured sIgE in the sera of six breastfed infants with atopic dermatitis who were never in contact with cow milk. The sIgE to bovine β-lactoglobulin was not detected in any of the sera examined.

Studying the role of heredity in allergy, Kaufman and Frick[49] described unilateral family history as allergy in one parent and bilateral as involving both parents. They followed 94 infants from birth for 24 months. Significantly more infants developed allergy if they were from a bilaterally allergic family. In the first 3 months

there was less atopic dermatitis in the breastfed infants with unilateral history than with bilateral history. Businco and associates[6] present similar relationships to family history in a study of breastfed infants.

These data are augmented by findings by Murray[68] examining nasal-secretion eosinophilia in relationship to respiratory allergy, associated with a screening procedure for hearing loss. In a group of children with a history of allergy in the immediate family, an association between early introduction of solid food and the presence of a nasal-secretion eosinophilia was significantly positive.

Further follow-up on the Isle of Wight Infant Feeding Survey was conducted by Hide and Guyer[38,39] when the children were 2 and 4 years old, producing data on 486 of the original 843 children. The authors reported not only on eczema and asthma but also on recurrent croup. Both asthma and recurrent croup showed strong predictability with a positive family history. More atopy was seen in the breastfed group; however, more mothers with a family history of eczema choose to breastfeed. Breastfeeding had a protective effect against asthma at 1 year but not at 4 years. Recurrent croup did not have a clear relationship to feeding method, but any breastfeeding at all was considered breastfeeding. The authors found a male preponderance and a close association with other signs of allergy in children with recurrent croup.

Although modern processing of cow milk has diminished the problem, it has not eliminated it. Given high-risk factors or strong family history of allergy, an effort to avoid unnecessary exposure to known allergens is an easy way to avoid some medical problems (Table 18-5).

PATTERNS OF CLINICAL DISEASE ASSOCIATED WITH COW MILK ALLERGY IN CHILDHOOD

Cow milk allergy affects 2% to 7% of infants. Many poorly defined illnesses and pathologic lesions have been associated with the ingestion of

TABLE 18-5 Some diseases possibly preventable by protecting relatively immunodeficient infants from adverse antigen experience

Disease	Status
Eczema	Established
Asthma	Probable
Hay fever	Probable
Infantile gut and respiratory infection	Probable
Intestinal allergy	Probable
Septicemia and renal *E. coli* infection	Probable
Sudden death	Probable
Ulcerative colitis	Possible

From Soothill JF: Some intrinsic and extrinsic factors predisposing to allergy. Proc R Soc Med 69:439, 1976.

milk, making clear diagnosis difficult.[40] Definitions have been proposed by the American Academy of Allergy and Immunology and are described in a consensus paper,[40,94] as follows:

- *Food intolerance* is an adverse reaction to the ingestion of a food related to an enzyme deficiency.
- *Food adverse reaction with unknown mechanism* is an idiosyncrasy; there is no associated immunologic mechanism.
- *Food allergy* or *food hypersensitivity* is an adverse reaction to food caused by one or more immune hypersensitivity mechanisms and is not confined to IgE.
- *Food anaphylaxis* reactions are immediate hypersensitivity involving the immunologic activity of IgE homocytotropic antibody and release of chemical mediators.
- *Anaphylactoid reaction* to food is an anaphylaxis-like reaction to food as a result of non-immune release of chemical mediators.

Symptoms associated with food allergy include asthma, eczema, urticaria, and rhinitis, as well as colic and failure to thrive with chronic respiratory and gastrointestinal disease.[94] Well-defined but uncommon syndromes, including pulmonary hemo-

siderosis, bronchitis, protein- and iron-losing enteropathy, neonatal thrombocytopenia, and colitis, have been reported to result from cow milk allergy in both breastfed and formula fed infants.[10] Sleep disturbances have been reported in a series of children evaluated with a prospective double-blind crossover design.[47] Another symptom reported in two siblings was insatiability despite adequate weight gain.[15] This was confirmed by history and reproducible reaction to dietary elimination and subsequent oral challenges.

The *intestinal permeability test* is a noninvasive but rigorous technique for detecting the deleterious effect of food on the intestinal mucosa of allergic children. It requires overnight fasting of 6 hours, test feeding, and nothing but water for 5 additional hours to collect urine samples for analysis. A 1-month-old breastfed infant with a history of regurgitation, diarrhea, difficult feeding, and malaise did not respond clinically to the elimination of dairy products from the mother's diet.[14] When the intestinal permeability test was performed with the mother's milk before and after dietary elimination of milk, there was no change. When the mother eliminated pork and egg, however, clinical and test results improved.

ACUTE REACTIONS TO COW MILK IN BREASTFED INFANTS

Hippocrates and Gojen described classic cases of milk allergy.[74] External reaction to cow milk was first described in the literature in the 19th century by Schloss[83] in 1920 and Tisdale and Erb[90] in 1925. At that time the reaction was noted to occur at the first feeding of cow milk provided in an effort to wean from the breast at several months of age. The event included sudden crying as if in pain; swelling of the lips, tongue, and throat; stridor; and even generalized urticaria and wheezing lasting for up to an hour.

This type of cow milk allergy is the first of two types described by Gerrard and Shenassa[21] and others. The second type is the well-known reaction to large amounts of cow milk in a cow milk–fed infant and is manifested by vomiting, diarrhea, or colic and is not associated with cow milk–specific IgE antibodies. It usually subsides over time. The acute anaphylactic reactions, however, are associated with α-lactalbumin, β-lactoglobulin, and casein immunity.

Schwartz and associates[82] studied 29 breastfed or soy formula fed infants who had experienced acute urticarial reactions while being fed cow milk for the first time. One infant had the reaction in the newborn nursery, suggesting in utero sensitization. When charts were carefully reviewed, 16 infants were identified as having been given formula, often without an order, in the newborn nursery. Twelve could have been sensitized in utero or through the breast milk. The authors identified elevated serum IgE levels; positive RASTs for α-lactalbumin, β-lactoglobulin, and casein; and recurrent wheezing in 55% of infants (16 of 29).

In a follow-up study challenging this group of children with whey and casein hydrolysate products, Schwartz[80] and associates[81] found 69% with positive prick tests to whey hydrolysate and 38% positive to casein hydrolysate. Children with reactions to cow milk and both hydrolysates had very severe reactions, including urticaria, angioedema, and wheezing. Hydrolysates of cow milk protein are not therefore hypoallergic. Breastfeeding with occasional, small amounts of cow milk can be a major risk factor in the development of IgE-mediated cow milk allergy in the rare, susceptible infant. Early exposures may occur in utero, through the breast milk, or with inadvertent feeds. Schwartz suggests that isolated cow milk not be given to exclusively breastfed infants in the newborn period.[80,81]

The study confirms the importance of heredity in this acute reaction by its occurrence in twins and human leukocyte antigen (HLA)-identical siblings as well as in children of 28 (89%) parent pairs also sensitive to cow milk. Genetic homogeneity could not be demonstrated by HLA typing.

A case of anaphylactic shock from cow milk hypersensitivity in a breastfed infant has been reported by Lifschitz and associates.[56] They describe three episodes of shock from two separate feedings of formula and one while breastfeeding.

After a prolonged course and the diagnosis of colitis, associated with numerous eosinophils, the infant was able to breastfeed at 21 days of age without difficulty after his mother had been placed on a cow milk–free diet. When challenged, however, with breast milk that had been pumped and stored while the mother was still consuming dairy products, the infant went into profound shock. The child was finally stabilized on breast milk and meat-based formula. At 6 months, cereal was added to the diet. At 12 months, soy and cow milk were well tolerated.

Intrauterine sensitization and allergy in the newborn breastfed infant were described by Matsumura and associates[62] in Japan. Glaser[26] also identified that under certain conditions an infant with a predisposition for allergy may become actively sensitized in utero because of the mother's overindulgence in certain foods in pregnancy. For example, Shannon[85] demonstrated in 1922 the presence of egg antigen in human breast milk. The infant then responded to reexposure with allergic symptoms on first contact with that same food.[21,55] Kuroume and associates[55] showed that with intrauterine sensitization, hemagglutinating antibody titers against lactalbumin and soybean in the amniotic fluid are high. They suggest using measurement of amniotic fluid as an instrument to predict future allergy. Infant colic associated with maternal ingestion of cow milk is discussed in Chapter 14.

Multiple studies continue to confirm the value of elimination diets in pregnancy for women at high risk for having an allergic infant.[7,19,37] These studies not only report a significantly reduced incidence of symptoms in the infants, but also a significant reduction in β-lactoglobulin-specific IgA and α-casein-specific IgA levels in maternal serum and milk. Similar observations have been made with the elimination of egg. Consistently breastfeeding was associated with reduced incidence of atopy in the infant with, and to a lesser degree without, dietary restrictions in mothers.

When Giovannini and associates[23] studied growth and metabolic parameters of infants fed special formulas for atopy prevention, they noted differences compared with infants exclusively breastfed. Lower body mass index values and higher blood urea nitrogen levels were seen at 3 months.[24] Plasma aminoacidograms showed higher essential amino acids but lower branched-chain amino acids. Furthermore, the plasma taurine levels were lower in the formula fed infants even though the formulas had added taurine. These observations have been confirmed by other investigators, who are most concerned about the elevated threonine levels.[73]

The allergens of specific foods ingested by the mother have now been identified in the milk. β-Lactoglobulin was studied by Machtinger and Moss[60] and identified in milk. These same investigators measured IgA in milk and attempted to correlate these levels with symptoms in the infants. High IgA levels were seen in asymptomatic infants. Cant and associates[7] found 49 eczematous infants who were solely breastfed to be sensitized to cow milk and egg protein; these researchers also concluded that infants can be sensitized by foods eaten by the mother. They were able to demonstrate ovalbumin in the breast milk of 14 of 19 mothers tested 2 to 4 hours after eating raw egg, whether or not their infants had tested positive to egg albumin.

Troncone and associates[91] collected samples of breast milk at various times after the mothers were fed 20 g of gluten, following a period of deliberate gluten avoidance. Gliadin was found in 54 of 80 samples; levels peaked at 2 to 4 hours. Gliadin could not be detected in maternal serum. The transfer of gliadin to the infant through the milk could be one of the factors producing a protective effect, because breastfeeding is known to decrease the risk of celiac disease.[30]

The impact of early feeding

A multidisciplinary review of the literature (1966–2001) by a group of Scandinavian researchers was undertaken to access the impact of early feeding in infancy and its impact on later atopic manifestations. Early feeding mode was breast milk, cow milk, and/or formula. The search located 4323 articles of which 4191 were eliminated because they lacked information on both exposure and health effects. The remaining 132 articles were analyzed in the final analysis, and 56 were considered conclusive. The review group of 12 university scientists from Sweden, Norway, and Denmark concluded that breastfeeding seems to protect from the development of atopic disease. This effect was even stronger in children with atopic heredity. They further recommended that when breast milk is unavailable or insufficient, extensively hydrolyzed formulas are better than unhydrolyzed or partially hydrolyzed formulas to reduce the risk of some atopic manifestations.

Once again, the definition of breastfeeding was important. Many articles included as breastfeeding were any breastfeeding. Exclusive breastfeeding as defined by WHO, meaning that no other food or drink be given, was critical to the analysis by these authors.

In an addendum to this article, these authors comment on two publications published after this review that reported that long-term breastfeeding by an asthmatic mother may in a limited group of children increase the risk of developing asthma.[70,96]

In a large study from Germany,[1] each week of breastfeeding increased the risk of eczema in children with atopic parents. In contrast, a large study from Australia[71] reported a protective effect of breastfeeding unaffected by maternal asthma, atopy, or infection.

van Odijk[93] and associates explain this apparent incongruity by the fact that maternal diets were not accounted for and the fact that the mother's milk in Australia contains lower ratios of n5/n3 fatty acids. Considering reports by Jensen and associates[41] regarding fish oils as previously noted, this is plausible (see Chapter 4).

The authors comment in their review that financial aid for the studies by formula companies seemed to show a bias. The review was funded by grants from the National Institute of Public Health in Sweden and the Foundation for Research into Health Care and Allergy and the Swedish Council for Building Research. The reader is referred to the article by van Odijk[93] for extensive bibliography.

The authors provide the following consensus statement:

For all children:

1. Exclusive breastfeeding reduces the risk of asthma. (Note: The definition of asthma is referred to the author's definition.)
2. Any breastfeeding decreases the risk of recurrent wheezing. (Note: Recurrent wheezing is mainly caused by viral infection.)
3. These protective effects increase with the duration of breastfeeding up to at least 4 months.
4. The protective effects seem to persist at least during the first decade of life.
5. Breastfeeding protects against the development of atopic dermatitis.
6. Exposure to small doses of cow milk during the first days of life appears to increase the risk of cow milk allergy but does not affect the incidence of atopic diseases later on.

In children with atopic heredity:

1. The beneficial effects of breastfeeding seen in all children are particularly strong in infants with atopic heredity.
2. In addition, breastfeeding protects against cow milk allergy.
3. When breastfeeding is insufficient, extensively hydrolyzed cow milk formula, as opposed to nonhydrolyzed cow milk formula, reduces the risk of cow milk allergy.
4. Extensively hydrolyzed cow milk formulas also somewhat reduces the risk to develop atopic dermatitis and asthma or other wheezing.
5. Partially hydrolyzed cow formula also reduces this risk, but to a lesser degree.

RECOMMENDATIONS FOR MANAGEMENT

It has been suggested that for the first 6 weeks or so of life, the intestinal tract is immature anatomically and immunologically. The early absorption of protein macromolecules in young animals is well recognized.[84] The subepithelial plasma cells of the lamina propria mucosae and lymph nodes do not make IgA initially. Gradually, the levels increase until they reach adult values at 2 years of age. Children with a strong family history of allergy have a more prolonged deficiency of IgA, lasting 3 months or longer. The early introduction of foods other than human milk has been associated with a rise in antibodies in the blood and eosinophilia, as noted earlier. Providing infants with breast milk so that they will not become sensitized to it is the most direct way of dealing with the problem.[27]

The total approach to the potentially allergic infant involves exclusion of known common food allergens from the pregnant mother's diet and avoidance of products known to cause problems in members of that family (Table 18-6).[88] From birth until 6 months, the infant should receive no cow milk formula. In addition, the diet of the mother should be restricted as in pregnancy and the environment made as allergen free as possible. If not breastfed, the infant should receive cow milk–free formula. Even though this regimen will not totally prevent all the potentials for allergy, it will help to minimize the insults by foreign protein. Another compelling reason to consider prophylaxis is the costly medical care required for the affected individual (Fig. 18-4).[11]

The possible alleviation of atopic eczema in a breastfed infant by maternal supplementation with a fish oil concentrate has been reported by Jensen and associates.[41] A 6-week-old infant who had eczema from the first week of life despite treatment cleared when the mother, who was part of a study of effects of fish oil supplementation, began the supplementation. The eczema returned when the fish oil was stopped and cleared again when the mother added fish to her diet.

This clinical experience has been corroborated in the laboratory. Essential fatty acids are important in promoting the renewal of the protective hydrolipidic layer of the skin. Altered essential fatty acid metabolism has been associated with atopic dermatitis,[23] and reduced levels of γ-linolenic acid and dihomo-α-linolenic acid appear in the plasma of patients with atopic

TABLE 18-6   Idealized strategy and mechanisms for the prevention of allergic diseases in humans

Strategy	Mechanisms
Identify at-risk families	Document IgE reactivity in parents with history of allergic disorders or with existing atopic child
Prevent intrauterine sensitization	Reduce maternal dietary allergenic load during last trimester, when potential for sensitization increases
Prevent postnatal sensitization to:	
1. Food allergens	
a. Transmitted through breast milk	Continue maternal avoidance diet during lactation
b. Ingested by infant	Withhold *all* nonbreast-milk foods except casein hydrolysate formula for at least 6 months
2. Environmental allergens	Encourage, instruct, and document avoidance of animals, mites, dust, and molds, as well as unnecessary medications
Maximize immunologic competence	Encourage, instruct, and support breastfeeding for at least 6 months
Minimize nonspecific enhancing factors	Discourage parental smoking; encourage avoidance of viral illnesses (?); delay pertussis immunization (?)

From Hamburger RN, Heller S, Mellon MH, et al: Current status of the clinical and immunologic consequences of a prototype allergic disease prevention program. Ann Allergy 51:281, 1983.

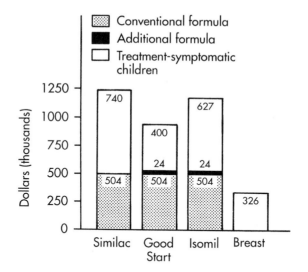

Figure 18-4.   Estimated cost of management of symptomatic children with atopy in Newfoundland. Costs include physician fees, laboratory tests, hospitalization, and medication. For those fed Similac, cost of management until age 5 is $740,000 per annum. Standard cow milk formula (e.g., Similac) during first 6 months of life for all infants with parental history of allergy would cost $504,000. In those fed hydrolyzed formula (e.g., Good Start), cost is about the same as for standard formula, but with savings of about 50% on management. An almost similar magnitude of reduction in allergic disease by feeding extensively hydrolyzed casein formula (e.g., Nutramigen) would cost three times more than in the cow milk group because of higher purchase value of such a formula. (Modified from Chandra RK: Five-year follow-up of high-risk infants with family history of allergy who were exclusively breast-fed or fed partial whey hydrolysate, soy, and conventional cow's milk formulas. J Pediatr Gastroenterol Nutr 24:388, 1997.)

dermatitis. The ratio of linoleic acid to the sum of its metabolites was found to be the relevant feature related to atopy. Increased marine fat consumption by the breastfeeding mother appears to improve the ratio of polyunsaturated fatty acids,[5] although this treatment has not been incorporated into routine care.

Human milk is a carrier of biochemical messages through its hormones, growth factors, cytokines, and whole cells. Nucleotides, glutamine, and lactoferrin have been shown to influence gastrointestinal development and host defenses. Basically, three separate processes are involved in the reaction of the immune system toward allergen challenge.[2] Deregulation in each of them may increase the susceptibility to developing gastrointestinal allergy. It is speculated that breast milk may help to shift the balance toward tolerance rather than sensitization when the infant is exposed to an allergen.[2]

Walker[95] summarizes his extensive research on the subject by stating that antigens have been shown to cross the intestinal barrier in physiologic and pathologic states. He further states that it is most important to prevent excessive penetration of antigens in patients who are susceptible to the disease by implementing the following steps:

1. Identify the population at risk.
2. Encourage breastfeeding in infancy.
3. Decrease antigen load with elemental formulas.
4. Continue to conduct direct research at identification and prevention.

SUMMARY

The role of prophylactic management in pregnancy and the initiation of breastfeeding at birth have a major impact on the long-term incidence of reactive airway disease. Beyond the medical risks, the high cost of medical management must be considered when an infant is not breastfed.

REFERENCES

1. Bergmann RL, Edenharter G, Bergmann KE, et al: Breastfeeding duration is a risk factor for atopic eczema. Clin Exp Allergy 32:205, 2002.
2. Bernt KM, Walker WA: Human milk as a carrier of biochemical messages. Acta Paediatr Suppl 930:27, 1999.
3. Bousquet J, Menardo J, Viala J, et al: Predictive value of cord serum IgE determination in the development of "early-onset" atopy. Ann Allergy 51:291, 1983.
4. Burr M, Limb ES, Maguire MJ, et al: Infant feeding, wheezing, and allergy: A prospective study. Arch Dis Child 68:724, 1993.
5. Businco L, Ioppi M, Morse NL, et al: Breast milk from mothers of children with newly developed atopic eczema has low levels of long chain polyunsaturated fatty acids. J Allergy Clin Immunol 91:1134, 1993.
6. Businco L, Marchetti F, Pellegrini G, et al: Prevention of atopic disease in "at-risk newborns" by prolonged breastfeeding. Ann Allergy 51:296, 1983.
7. Cant AJ, Bailes JA, Marsden RA, et al: Effect of maternal dietary exclusion on breast fed infants with eczema: Two controlled studies. Br Med J 293:231, 1986.
8. Cantisani A, Giuffrida MG, Fabris C, et al: Detection of specific IgE to human milk proteins in sera of atopic infants. Fed Eur Biochem Soc 412:515, 1997.
9. Chandra RK: Prospective studies on the effect of breast feeding on incidence of infection and allergy. Acta Pediatr Scand 68:691, 1979.
10. Chandra RK: Long-term health consequences of early infant feeding. In Atkinson SA, Hanson LA, Chandra RK (eds): Breastfeeding, Nutrition, Infection, and Infant Growth in Developed And Emerging Countries. St. Johns, Newfoundland, Canada, ARTS Biomedical, 1990.
11. Chandra RK: Five-year follow-up of high-risk infants with family history of allergy who were exclusively breast-fed or fed partial whey hydrolysate, soy, and conventional cow's milk formulas. J Pediatr Gastroenterol Nutr 24:380, 1997.
12. Chandra RK, Puri S, Cheema PS: Predictive value of cord blood IgE in the development of atopic disease and role of breastfeeding in its prevention. Clin Allergy 15:517, 1985.
13. Chandra RK, Puri S, Suraiya C, et al: Influence of maternal food antigen avoidance during pregnancy and lactation on incidence of atopic eczema in infants. Clin Allergy 16:563, 1986.
14. de Boussieu D, Dupont C, Badoval J: Allergy to non-dairy proteins in mother's milk as assessed by intestinal permeability tests. Allergy 49:882, 1994.
15. Ducharme FM, Rousseau E, Seidman EG, et al: Apparent insatiability: An unrecognized manifestation of food intolerance in breast-fed infants. Pediatrics 93:1006, 1994.
16. Falliers CJ, Cardoso RR de A, Bane HN, et al: Discordant allergic manifestations in monozygotic twins: Genetic

identity vs. clinical, physiologic, and biochemical differences. J Allergy 47:207, 1971.

17. Fidler N, Koletzko B: The fatty acid composition of human colostrums. Eur J Nutr 39:31, 2000.

18. Freed DLJ, Green FHY: Hypothesis: Antibody-facilitated digestion and its implications for infant nutrition. Early Hum Dev 1:107, 1977.

19. Fukushima Y, Kawata Y, Onda T, et al: Consumption of cow milk and egg by lactating women and the presence of β-lactoglobulin and ovalbumin in breast milk. Am J Clin Nutr 65:30, 1997.

20. Gerrard JW: Allergy in infancy. Pediatr Ann 3:9, 1974.

21. Gerrard JW, Shenassa M: Sensitization to substances in breast milk: Recognition, management and significance. Ann Allergy 51:300, 1983.

22. Gerrard JW, Shenassa M: Food allergy: Two common types as seen in breast and formula fed babies. Ann Allergy 50:375, 1983.

23. Giovannini M, Agostoni C, Fiocchi A, et al: Antigen-reduced infant formulas versus human milk: Growth and metabolic parameters in the first 6 months of life. J Am Coll Nutr 13:357, 1994.

24. Giovannini M, Fiocchi A, Agostoni C, et al: Nutrition in infancy and childhood. In Wüthrich B, Ortolani C (eds): Highlights In Food Allergy. Basel, Karger, 1996.

25. Glaser J: Prophylaxis of allergic disease in infancy and childhood. In Speer F, Dockhorn RJ (eds): Allergy and Immunology in Children. Springfield, IL, Thomas, 1973.

26. Glaser J: Intrauterine sensitization and allergy in the newborn breast fed infant. Ann Allergy 35:256, 1975 (editorial).

27. Glaser J, Dreyfuss EM, Logan J: Dietary prophylaxis of atopic disease. In Kelley VC (ed): Brennemann's Practice of Pediatrics, Vol. 2. Hagerstown, MD, Harper & Row, 1976.

28. Glaser J, Johnstone DE: Prophylaxis of allergic disease in newborn. JAMA 153:620, 1953.

29. Gleeson M, Cripps AW, Clancy RL, et al: The significance of transient mucosal IgA deficiency on the development of asthma and atopy in children. Adv Exp Med Biol 371B:861, 1995.

30. Greco L, Mayer M, Grimaldi M, et al: The effect of early feeding on the onset of symptoms in celiac disease. J Pediatr Gastroenterol Nutr 4:52, 1985.

31. Grulee GG, Sanford HN, Herron PH: Breast and artificial feeding. JAMA 103:735, 1934.

32. Gruskay FL: Comparison of breast, cow, and soy feedings in the prevention of onset of allergic disease. Clin Pediatr 21:486, 1982.

33. Halpern SR, Sellars WA, Johnson RB, et al: Development of childhood allergy in infants fed breast, soy, or cow milk. J Allergy Clin Immunol 51:139, 1973.

34. Hamburger RN: Allergy and the immune system. Am Sci 64:157, 1976.

35. Hamburger RN: Development of atopic allergy in children. In Johansson SGO (ed): International Symposium on Diagnosis and Treatment of IgE-Mediated Diseases. Amsterdam, Excerpta Medica, 1981.

36. Hamburger RN, Heller S, Mellon MH, et al: Current status of the clinical and immunologic consequences of a prototype allergic disease prevention program. Ann Allergy 51:281, 1983.

37. Herrmann ME, Danneman A, Grüters A, et al: Prospective study on the atopy preventive effect of maternal avoidance of milk and eggs during pregnancy and lactation. Eur J Pediatr 155:770, 1996.

38. Hide DW, Guyer BM: Clinical manifestations of allergy related to breast and cow's milk feeding. Arch Dis Child 56:172, 1981.

39. Hide DW, Guyer BM: Clinical manifestations of allergy related to breastfeeding and cow's milk-feeding. Pediatrics 76:973, 1985.

40. Hill DJ, Hosking CS: Patterns of clinical disease associated with cow milk allergy in childhood. Nutr Res 12:109, 1992.

41. Jensen RG, Ferris AM, Lammi-Keefe CJ, et al: Possible alleviation of atopic eczema in a breastfed infant by maternal supplementation with a fish oil concentrate. J Pediatr Gastroenterol Nutr 14:474, 1992 (letter).

42. Johnstone DE: The natural history of allergic disease in children. In Proceedings of Advances in Pediatric Allergy Workshop, Rome, 1982.

43. Johnstone DE, Dutton AM: Dietary prophylaxis of allergic disease in children. N Engl J Med 274:715, 1966.

44. Juto P: Elevated serum immunoglobulin E in T cell-deficient infants fed cow's milk. J Allergy Clin Immunol 66:402, 1980.

45. Juto P, Bjorksten B: Serum IgE in infants and influence of type of feeding. Clin Allergy 10:593, 1980.

46. Juto P, Strannegard O: T lymphocytes and blood eosinophils in early infancy in relation to heredity for allergy and type of feeding. J Allergy Clin Immunol 64:38, 1979.

47. Kahn A, Mozin MJ, Rebuffat E, et al: Milk intolerance in children with persistent sleeplessness: A prospective double-blind crossover evaluation. Pediatrics 84:595, 1989.

48. Kajosaari M, Saarinen UM: Prophylaxis of atopic disease by six months' total solid food elimination. Acta Paediatr Scand 72:411, 1983.

49. Kaufman HS, Frick OL: The development of allergy in infants of allergic parents: A prospective study concerning the role of heredity. Ann Allergy 37:410, 1976.

50. Kaufman HS, Frick OL: Prevention of asthma. Clin Allergy 11:549, 1981.

51. Kern RA: Prophylaxis in allergy. Ann Intern Med 12:1175, 1939.

52. Kleinman RE: The role of developmental immune mechanisms in intestinal allergy. Ann Allergy 51:222, 1983.

53. Kleinman RE, Walker WA: The enteromammary immune system: an important new concept in breast milk host defense. Dig Dis Sci 24:876, 1979.

54. Kletter B, Gery I, Freier S, et al: Immune response of normal infants to cow milk. I. Antibody type and kinetics of production. Int Arch Allergy 40:656, 1971.

55. Kuroume T, Oguri M, Matsumura T, et al: Milk sensitivity and soybean sensitivity in the production of eczematous manifestations in breast-fed infants with particular reference to intrauterine sensitization. Ann Allergy 37:41, 1976.

56. Lifschitz CH, Hawkins HK, Guerra C, et al: Anaphylactic shock due to cow's milk protein hypersensitivity in a breast-fed infant. J Pediatr Gastroenterol Nutr 7:141, 1988.

57. Lilja G, Dannaeus A, Foucard T, et al: Effects of maternal diet during late pregnancy and lactation on the development of atopic diseases in infants up to 18 months of age—In vivo results. Clin Exp Allergy 18:473, 1989.

58. Lovegrove JA, Hampton SM, Morgan JB: The immunological and long-term outcome of infants born to women following a milk-free diet during late pregnancy and lactation: A pilot study. Br J Nutr 71:223, 1994.

59. Lovegrove JA, Morgan JB, Hampton SM: Dietary factors influencing levels of food antibodies and antigens in breast milk. Acta Paediatr 85:778, 1996.

60. Machtinger S, Moss R: Cow's milk allergy in breastfed infants: The role of allergen and maternal secretory IgA antibody. J Allergy Clin Immunol 77:341, 1986.

61. Maeda S, Morikawa A, Tokuyama K, et al: The concentration of bovine IgG in human breast milk measured using different methods. Acta Paediatr 82:1012, 1993.

62. Matsumura T, Kurome T, Iwasaki I, et al: Congenital sensitization to food in humans. Jpn J Allergy 16:858, 1967.

63. Matthew DJ, Taylor B, Norman AP, et al: Prevention of eczema. Lancet 1:321, 1977.

64. May CD, Fomon SJ, Remigio L: Immunologic consequences of feeding infants with cow milk and soy products. Acta Paediatr Scand 71:43, 1982.

65. McCombs R, Lowell F, Ohman J: Myths, morbidity, and mortality in asthma. JAMA 242:1521, 1979.

66. Merrett TG, Burr ML, Butland BK, et al: Infant feeding and allergy: 12-month prospective study of 500 babies born into allergic families. Ann Allergy 61:13, 1988.

67. Moore WJ, Midwinter RE, Morris AF, et al: Infant feeding and subsequent risk of atopic eczema. Arch Dis Child 60:722, 1985.

68. Murray AB: Infant feeding and respiratory allergy. Lancet 1:497, 1971.

69. National Asthma Education Program: Expert Panel Report II. Atlanta, Centers for Disease Control and Prevention, 1996.

70. Oberle D, Von Kries R, Von Mutius E: Asthma and breast feeding. Thorax 56:896, 2001.

71. Oddy WH, DeKlerk NH, Sly PD, et al: The effects of respiratory infections, atopy, and breastfeeding on childhood asthma. Eur Respir J 19:899, 2002.

72. Ratner B: A possible causal factor of food allergy in certain infants. Am J Dis Child 36:277, 1928.

73. Rigo J, Salle BL, Cavero E, et al: Plasma amino acid and protein concentrations in infants fed human milk or a whey protein hydrolysate formula during the first month of life. Acta Paediatr 83:127, 1994.

74. Rowe AH: Food Allergy. Philadelphia, Lea & Febiger, 1931.

75. Saarinen UM, Kajossari M: Breastfeeding as prophylaxis against disease: prospective follow-up study until 17 years old. Lancet 346:1065, 1995.

76. Saarinen UM, Kajosaari M, Backman A, et al: Prolonged breast-feeding as prophylaxis for atopic disease. Lancet 1:163, 1979.

77. Savilahti E: Intestinal immunoglobulins in children with coeliac disease. Gut 13:958, 1972.

78. Savilahti E, Tainio V-M, Salmenpera L, et al: Low colostral IgA associated with cow's milk allergy. Acta Paediatr Scand 80:1207, 1991.

79. Savilahti E, Tuomikoski-Jaakkola P, Järvenpää A-L, et al: Early feeding of preterm infants and allergic symptoms during childhood. Acta Paediatr 82:340, 1993.

80. Schwartz RH: IgE-mediated allergic reactions to cow's milk. Immunol Allergy Clin North Am 11:717, 1991.

81. Schwartz RH, Keefe MW, Harris N, et al: The spectrum of IgE-mediated acute allergic reactions to cow's milk in children as determined by skin testing with cow's milk protein hydrolysate formulas. Pediatr Asthma Allergy Immunol 3:207, 1989.

82. Schwartz RH, Kubicka M, Dreyfuss EM, et al: Acute urticarial reactions to cow's milk in infants previously fed breast milk or soy milk. Pediatr Asthma Allergy Immunol 1:81, 1987.

83. Schloss OM: Allergy in infants and children. Am J Dis Child 19:433, 1920.

84. Shannon WR: Demonstration of food proteins in human breast milk by anaphylactic experiments in guinea pigs. Am J Dis Child 22:223, 1921.

85. Shannon WR: Eczema in breast-fed infants as a result of sensitization to foods in the mother's diet. Am J Dis Child 23:392, 1922.

86. Sigurs N, Hattevig G, Kjellman B: Maternal avoidance of eggs, cow's milk, and fish during lactation: Effect on allergic manifestations, skin-prick tests and specific IgE antibodies in children at age 4 years. Pediatrics 89:735, 1992.

87. Soothill JF: Some intrinsic and extrinsic factors predisposing to allergy. Proc R Soc Med 69:439, 1976.

88. Soothill JF: Prevention of atopic allergic disease. Ann Allergy 51:229, 1983.

89. Stevenson DD, Orgell HA, Hamburger RN, et al: Development of IgE in newborn human infants. J Allergy Clin Immunol 48:61, 1971.

90. Tisdale FF, Erb IH: Extreme sensitization in infants to cow's milk protein. J Can Med Assoc 15:497, 1925.

91. Troncone R, Scarcella A, Donatiello A, et al: Passage of gliadin into human breast milk. Acta Paediatr Scand 76:453, 1987.

92. U.S. Department of Health and Human Services, Centers for Disease Control and Prevention, National Center for Health Statistics: Vital and Health Statistics, Summary Health Statistics for U.S. Children: National Health Interview Survey, 2001. Series 10, Number 216, November 2003.

93. van Odijk J, Kull I, Borres MP, et al: Breastfeeding and allergic disease: A multidisciplinary review of the literature (1966-2001) on the mode of early feeding in infancy and its impact on later atopic manifestations. Allergy 58:883, 2003.

94. Vandenplas Y, Bahna SL, Bousquet J, et al: Extraintestinal manifestations of food allergy in infants and children. Nutr Res 12:161, 1992.

95. Walker WA: Antigen absorption from the small intestine and gastrointestinal disease. Pediatr Clin North Am 22:731, 1975.

96. Wright AL, Holberg CJ, Taussig LM, et al: Factors influencing the relation of infant feeding to asthma and recurrent wheeze in childhood. Thorax 56:192, 2001.

97. Wright AL, Holberg CJ, Taussig LM, et al: Relationship of infant feeding to recurrent wheezing at age 6 years. Arch Pediatr Adolesc Med 149:758, 1995.

98. Zeiger RS, Heller S, Mellon MH, et al: Effect of combined maternal and infant food-allergen avoidance on development of atopy in early infancy: a randomized study. J Allergy Clin Immunol 84:72, 1989.

19

Induced lactation and relactation (including nursing the adopted baby) and cross-nursing

I nduced lactation is the process by which a non-puerperal woman is stimulated to lactate—in other words, breastfeeding without pregnancy. Relactation is the process by which a woman who has given birth but did not initially breastfeed is stimulated to lactate. This may also apply to a mother who may have initially breastfed her infant, weaned the infant, and then chooses to reinstitute lactation. Relactation can also involve a woman who previously breastfed a biologic child and now is adopting a newborn.

HISTORICAL PERSPECTIVE

Induced lactation and relactation are not new concepts but rather are well known to history and to other cultures. The motivation historically has been to provide nourishment for an infant whose mother has died in childbirth or is unable to nurse for some reason. A friend or relative would take on the care of the child and with it the responsibility to nourish the infant at the breast, because no other alternatives were available.

Relactation has been used in times of disaster or epidemics to provide safe nutrition to weaned or motherless infants. Numerous accounts of induced lactation are recorded in medical literature and reviewed in the writings of Brown.[6] Mead[26] recorded the phenomenon in her writings about New Guinea in 1935. Other anthropologists have made similar observations in other preindustrialized societies of women who have not borne children and, after a few weeks of placing the suckling infant to the breast, produce milk adequate to nourish the infant.[37] Until recently, Western world literature reported the phenomenon as an anecdotal report as part of the discussion of aberrant lactation. In 1971 Cohen[11] reported a patient who had been nursing an adopted child very successfully for weeks when first seen in his pediatric office.

Today, the interest in induced lactation in the industrialized world stems from a desire on the part of some adopting mothers to nurture the adopted child at the breast even if they were unable to carry the infant in utero. The interest in relactation comes from mothers of sick or premature infants who want to breastfeed their infants after the days and weeks of neonatal intensive care are over. These mothers, although post partum, have not been lactating.

INDUCED VERSUS INAPPROPRIATE LACTATION

The process of induced lactation is separate from *galactorrhea,* or inappropriate lactation, which has been described in the medical literature for more than 100 years.[43] Abnormal lactation has been observed in a number of circumstances in nulliparous and parous women and even in males. There are many eponyms for these conditions, usually based on the name of the physician who first described the syndrome, such as Chiari-Frommel and Ahumada-del Castillo.

Normally in the absence of suckling, lactation ceases 14 to 21 days after delivery. Milk flow that continues beyond 3 to 6 months after abortion or any termination of pregnancy is termed *abnormal* or *inappropriate lactation,* or *galactorrhea. Galactorrhea* also refers to lactation in a woman 3 months after weaning or the secretion of milk in a nulliparous woman in association with hyperprolactinemia and amenorrhea. Although these cases are pathologic in nature and therefore different from the groups under discussion, it is noteworthy that some knowledge of the initiation and maintenance of lactation has been gained from the study of these syndromes.

ANIMAL STUDIES

Information on the incidence of nonoffspring nursing in 100 mammalian species has been assembled by Packer and associates.[31] The incidence of nonoffspring nursing is increased by captivity. It is more common in species with large litters (polytocous taxa) and differs from that which occurs with single young species (monotocous taxa). In the latter, it is more common for females to continue nursing after they have lost their own young. Among nondomesticated animals, spontaneous lactation has been observed repeatedly only in the dwarf mongoose *(Helogale parvula).*

Lactation has been induced for scientific and commercial purposes in nonpregnant and nonpar-

turient animals by the continual systematic application of a mechanical milking apparatus to the mammary gland of the animal.[23] The response is effected through the release of mammotropic hormone from the anterior pituitary gland. This effect is abolished if the pituitary stalk is transected. Ruminants respond to the addition of estrogen or estrogen-progesterone combinations, which facilitate mammary growth. Experiments in goats involved applying ointment containing estradiol benzoate to the udders of virgins, which resulted in development of the udder and milk yield almost comparable to normal postpartum animals.[12] It was subsequently shown, however, that a combination of estrogen-progesterone not only resulted in better milk yield, but histologically the lobuloalveolar growth was normal, whereas with estrogen alone growth was cystic and irregular. It was also demonstrated that ovariectomized goats could be stimulated to lactation with these two hormones, with resultant normal histology of the udder and good milk production. Initiation of regular milkings had a significant impact on production of milk.

Because lactation can be stimulated when the ovaries have been removed but not when the pituitary stalk has been severed, this has significance for understanding some of the postpartum lactation failures in women. Again in ruminants, growth hormone and thyroid hormone have been shown to increase milk yield, although prolactin does not. This suggests that prolactin is not deficient in ruminants. Selye and McKeown[36] showed in 1934 that suckling stimulus inhibits sexual cyclicity in rats. They further showed that when the main milk ducts to all the nipples are cut and the escape of milk has been rendered impossible, the mechanical stimulation of the nipples by nursing would also inhibit the sexual cyclicity of the normal estric, nonlactating adult rat. These studies demonstrate the significance of suckling in triggering the lactation cycle and suppressing ovulation.

Because the motivation, goals, and physiologic problems may be slightly different, induced lactation and relactation are discussed separately.

INDUCED LACTATION

When a mother chooses to nurse her adopted infant, the goal is usually to achieve a mother-infant relationship that may also have the benefit of some nutrition.[27] In that perspective, success can be evaluated on the basis of whether the infant will suckle the breast and achieve some comfort and security from this opportunity and close relationship with the new mother. As has been well described by Avery,[4] this is nurturing with the emphasis on *nurturing,* not on "breastfeeding" or nutrition. A mother who is interested in inducing lactation to nurse an adopted infant may need to understand that she may never be able to sustain the infant completely by her milk alone without supplementation. Neither the physician nor the mother should be disappointed. The nurturing goal is still achieved.

Preparation of the breast

Normally the breast is prepared by the proliferation of the ductal and alveolar system through pregnancy in anticipation of the time when lactation will begin.[26] Thus, it is appropriate to assume that a period of similar preparation should take place in induced lactation. It has been suggested that the woman should begin systematically to express the breasts manually and stimulate the nipples for up to 2 months before the arrival of the infant, if time permits. A hand pump or other pumping devices can be used, but manual expression may work as well or better. Sometimes some secretion can be produced in this manner if it is carried out systematically on a uniform schedule throughout the day. The schedule should be practical, that is, include times when a mother could take a moment for this activity, such as morning and night plus any times she uses the bathroom or can conveniently handle her breasts.

A more aggressive approach involves hormones and medications. During pregnancy, the breast is prepared by the hormones generated by the pregnancy, estrogen, progesterone, and human placental lactogen (see Fig. 3-2).

In order to mimic this environment, it has been suggested that starting a course of estrogen and progesterone would be appropriate, namely, prescribing oral contraceptive dosing that does suppress ovulation (such as Ortho-Novum). This dosing should be maintained without a pause as it would be during pregnancy.[29] Unfortunately, adopting women do not have 9 months to prepare, so priming the breast with hormones may not be possible as the hormones need to be discontinued a month before anticipated lactation.

Concomitant with hormone therapy should be breast stimulation with systematic pumping with a good electric double pump. Timing should begin gradually 5 minutes three times a day, then 10 minutes increasing to every 4 hours. Pumping about the same time every day is helpful. It usually takes about a month before drops of milk appear. This is a good time to start domperidone.* The schedule adopted by Newman[29] in Canada is 10 mg three times a day increasing over a month's time to 20 mg four times a day. Newman suggests using domperidone from the beginning.[29] Without a placenta, the adoptive mother does not have "prolactin inhibiting" hormone to block the breast from responding to the prolactin secreted because of the breast stimulation. When domperidone is initiated, milk should appear in increasing quantities. Many women have achieved success by pumping alone initially and then adding galactogues.

In other cultures in which lactation is induced as a survival tactic for the infant, no period of preparation is available. The infant is put to the adoptive mother's breast and allowed to suckle. Emphasis has been placed on herbal teas as galactogogues and good nourishment for the mother, while the infant is also given prechewed food, gruel, or animal milk. Mead[26] attributed much of the success of induced lactation to the ingestion of ample supplies of coconut milk by the new mother. Coconuts are well known in herbal medicine; the oil pressed from ripe fruit is used for wound healing and inflammation.[33]

Adoption is not an easy process, and in fact, it can be quite stressful to become an instant parent.

---

*Domperidone is not available in the United States.

In assisting such a mother, consideration should be given to the infant's age, previous feeding experience, and any medical problems that may exist. Provision for additional nourishment during the process of establishing some milk secretion is most important. Onset of lactation varies from 1 to 6 weeks, averaging about 4 weeks after initiation of stimulation with the appearance of the first drops of milk. When the infant is actually nursing at the breast and being nourished by supplements, milk may appear as early as 1 to 2 weeks.

Some infants are easily confused by switching back and forth between breast and bottle because the sucking technique is slightly different. Other nourishment can be offered by dropper, by small medicine cup, or as solid foods. A unique system is available, however, for providing nourishment for the infant while suckling at the breast. It involves the use of a device to provide a source of nourishment while the infant suckles at the breast, thus stimulating production. It is further described later in this chapter and in Appendix F and is called *Lact-Aid Nursing Trainer System* or *Supplemental Nursing System* (Medela's SNS).

Other drug schedules to induce lactation

As described in Chapter 3, estrogen and progesterone stimulate the proliferation of the alveolar and ductal systems. These hormones work in association with an increase in prolactin production. Although the prolactin level is high during pregnancy, milk secretion is inhibited by the presence of the estrogen, progesterone, and placental lactogen, the prolactin-inhibiting hormone. After delivery has occurred and the placenta is removed, there is a marked fall in these hormones, and prolactin initiates milk production.[41] Efforts to stimulate this hormonal response have had variable success and are not usually recommended because of the possible effect on the infant through the milk. Women taking oral contraceptives have been noted in some cases to have breast enlargement. In addition, although estrogen and progesterone may enhance proliferation, they may inhibit lactation per se, so they must be discontinued well before lactation is planned to begin.

The dosage of conjugated estrogens recommended by Waletzky and Herman[45] is 2.5 mg twice a day for 14 days beginning on the fourth day of a regular menstrual cycle. Giving 0.35 mg norethindrone once daily for the morning dose of estrogen prevents breakthrough bleeding. Medication is given for 2 weeks and is comparable in dosage to 2 weeks of oral contraceptives. This therapy may be accompanied by some side effects. The regimen should include direct efforts to stimulate lactation by pumping the breasts.

A report from Papua New Guinea, where inducing lactation is critical to adequate infant nutrition, recommends priming the breast tissue of nulliparous women or those who have not lactated with 50-μg ethinyl estradiol three times a day for a week.[20] Medroxyprogesterone (Depoprovera) has been used to initiate lactation in nonpuerperal women. A dose of 100 mg is given intramuscularly a week before stimulating the breast with massage and pumping. Galactogogues such as metoclopramide, domperidone, or herbals can be introduced. This approach was reported in Papua New Guinea, and claimed success in 24 of 27 women.[32] When relactation is the goal in women who have previously lactated, pumping and massaging alone are initiated.

Growth hormone (GH) and prolactin have considerable genetic similarity, as reflected in some overlap of function.[10] High concentrations of GH can cause lobuloalveolar development and casein expression. GH may play a role in optimization of milk production during lactation and even an accessory role in the induction of lactogenesis. Both natural and recombinant human growth hormones (hGHs) are potent inductors of milk synthesis in pregnant and lactating rats. This effect is attributed to their effect on the prolactin receptor.[10]

Oxytocin is a critical component in the milk ejection reflex and may be helpful in the early initiation of ejection. Physiologically, stimulation of the nipple in the lactating woman results in the release of oxytocin by the hypothalamus, which then triggers the release of milk by stimulating the contraction of myoepithelial cells and the ejection of milk (see Chapter 8). The effect of intranasal administration of oxytocin on the let-down reflex in lactating women was well described by Newton and Egli.[30] (Oral administration by tablet is not as effective, because oxytocin is destroyed in the stomach; therefore, oral administration must be sublingual.) Oxytocin nasal spray has been used in cases of nonpuerperal lactation with some success in enhancing let-down but not necessarily altering the volume produced. The original oxytocin product Syntocin is no longer available, but a pharmacist by prescription can place the intravenous preparation in a dropper bottle or a nasal spray container. The intravenous preparation is one quarter the strength of the old nasal spray (40 units/mL). Therefore, the dose needs to be increased fourfold: 4 to 6 drops per dose in one nares and feed the infant or pump immediately (Chapter 8). The dose can be repeated. Continued use of oxytocin over weeks has been associated with diminished effect or even suppression of lactation. The chief benefit of oxytocin is often to break the cycle of failure and instill a feeling of confidence once it has been demonstrated that some secretion can be produced.

Chlorpromazine has been observed to act as a galactogogue as well as a tranquilizer when given to patients in large doses (up to 1000 mg or more). The effect has been observed in both male and female patients in mental institutions. The drug has been reported to increase pituitary prolactin secretion severalfold. It acts via the hypothalamus, probably by reducing levels of prolactin inhibitory factor. Using this information, women well motivated to lactate who have attempted induced lactation by suckling a normal infant have had the process enhanced by small doses of chlorpromazine.[8]

In a program to induce lactation in refugee camps in India and in Vietnam, nonlactating women were given 25 to 100 mg of chlorpromazine three times a day for a week to 10 days while infants were initially put to breast. Brown[7] reports apparent enhancement of lactation with this treatment. Chlorpromazine has the added pharmacologic effect of acting as a tranquilizer. The program of management in these women was supportive in other ways and also included the usual herbal medicines associated with lactation

in these Eastern cultures. There was no control group. It is possible that the drug contributed to both the physiologic and the psychological well-being of the women wanting to lactate. It has been suggested that the desire to lactate is a strong component of success, because women whose breasts are frequently stimulated sexually do not begin to lactate.

Theophylline can also increase pituitary prolactin secretions.[44] Therefore, both tea and coffee should enhance prolactin secretion and thus lactation. Excessive amounts may inhibit milk let-down, however.

Because the role of prolactin is the initiation and maintenance of lactation, whereas oxytocin regulates the glandular emptying through the milk-ejection reflex, it is reasonable to speculate that enhancing prolactin release would be productive in inducing lactation. The exact activating mechanism of the neuronal reflex arc from breast to brain has not been deciphered. Secretion of prolactin appears to be influenced, if not controlled, by changes in hypothalamic dopamine turnover. Correspondingly, suckling has been observed to deplete dopamine stores.

Investigation of other drugs that are known to stimulate prolactin release has identified some possible therapeutic materials.[1] Kramer[20] and McNeilly and associates[25] have reported that *metoclopramide* induces prolactin release regardless of the route of administration. Prolactin levels are increased three to eight times normal levels within 5 minutes when a 10-mg dose is given either intravenously or intramuscularly. The effect is achieved within an hour when metoclopramide is given orally. The effect persists for 8 hours. The suggested regimen is 10 mg of metoclopramide, four times a day for a week.[14] This is then gradually tapered (see Chapter 11).

Metoclopramide also is used in neonates with esophageal reflux. The side effects are irritability and diarrhea. Rarely, susceptible infants experience dystonic reactions, which have been described in adults. Metoclopramide has also been used in combination with chlorpromazine, 25 mg four times a day, in Papua New Guinea.[20] Metoclopramide has been used to enhance lactation as well, especially among mothers of premature infants.[14]

The regulation of prolactin secretion in humans has been studied to further the understanding of abnormal lactation as well as to provide information on the regulation of pituitary function of the brain.[13] It has been shown experimentally that the hypothalamus secretes prolactin inhibitory factor (PIF), which acts on the mammotropin-releasing cells of the pituitary to inhibit release of the hormone prolactin. The hypothalamus can also regulate prolactin secretion by a stimulatory mechanism, the secretion of thyrotropin-releasing hormone (TRH). When human volunteers (nonpregnant, nonlactating) are given infusions of TRH, increases in thyrotropin and prolactin are observed within minutes of injection, with values peaking in 20 minutes. The level of thyroid hormone in the volunteers initially influences the results. Hypothyroid patients have been observed to secrete excessive amounts of

prolactin, whereas hyperthyroid patients are relatively insensitive to TRH. This may explain some of the variable results obtained with prolactin-stimulating drugs used to enhance lactation. Studies of relactation have been done using TRH but not of newly induced lactation. Thyroid activity has not been measured. Table 19-1 summarizes the influence of drugs on prolactin secretion.

Any pharmacologic regimen to stimulate milk production is most effective if it is initiated after the breast tissue has responded to mechanical stimulation because the hormones that act as the prolactin-stimulating compounds are thought by many to be ineffective in unprimed breast tissue. Jelliffe[18] points out that the most important factor for continued production of milk is not drugs or hormones but "mulging." He explains that *mulging* (stimulation) is a word created in 1975 by N. W. Pirie to mitigate the confusion between the words *sucking* and *suckling*. The word comes from the Latin *mulgere,* to milk. Suck, according to the dictionary,[16]

TABLE 19-1   Influence of drugs on prolactin secretion

Pharmacologic agents	Plasma prolactin concentration	Mechanism of drug action
L-Dopa	Decrease	Increase in hypothalamic dopamine-catecholamine levels, leading to enhanced activity of prolactin inhibitory factor (PIF)
Ergot alkaloids (ergocornine, ergocryptine)	Decrease	Direct inhibition of adenohypophyseal prolactin secretion; possible increase of hypothalamic PIF activity (continued PIF function)
Thyrotropin-releasing hormone (TRH; pyroglutamyl-histidyl-prolinamide)	Increase	Direct stimulation of adenohypophyseal lactotrophs for increased prolactin secretion
Theophylline		
Phenothiazines (chlorpromazine)	Increase	Decreases in hypothalamic dopamine-catecholamine levels, leading to diminution of PIF activity
Metoclopramide	Increase	Inhibition of hypothalamic PIF secretion through dopamine antagonism
Sulpiride	Increase	Increase in hypothalamic prolactin- releasing hormone
Growth hormone (GH)	Increase	Causes lobulo-alveolar development and casein expression
Recombinant human growth hormones (hGHs)	Increase	Affects prolactin receptors

Modified from Vorherr H: Human lactation and breast feeding. In Larson BL (ed): Lactation, New York, Academic Press, 1978.

means to draw into the mouth by means of a partial vacuum created by action of the lips and the tongue. Suckle, however, refers specifically to the breast and means "to give suck to," as at the breast, or to take nourishment from the breast; thus, by definition a bottle is not suckled.

Composition of milk

Concern has been expressed that the composition of the milk produced by stimulation of suckling rather than as a result of pregnancy might differ from "normal human milk."[39] Such induced milk is not different in other species that have been studied extensively, including bovine and rat. In developing countries, the fact that the infants showed normal growth and weight gain was taken as evidence that induced milk is adequate.

Vorherr[43,44] reported the analysis of the galactorrheal secretion produced by the breast after hyperstimulation; Table 19-2 shows the comparative analysis. The induced lactational milk did not differ from puerperal milk. Brown[6] reported

higher values of fat, protein, and lactose in galactorrheal milk, but the volume of secretion was small in these subjects.

The composition of the breast secretion produced by two women who induced lactation artificially by breast hyperstimulation was close to the composition obtained for women with normal lactation, according to Kulski and associates (see Table 19-2).[22] These investigators also examined the milk of a woman in whom lactation had occurred when medicated with a psychotropic drug (haloperidol). She had been pregnant 4 years previously. Her galactorrhea lasted 38 months. Her milk had composition like that of colostrum for a week but resembled mature milk at 1 month. A woman with hypothyroidism and elevated prolactin and TSH had colostrum-like milk for 53 days of sampling. Two women with galactorrhea and amenorrhea associated with pituitary tumor and hyperprolactinemia had transient colostrum-like secretion, which changed to mature appearing milk.

Protein values of milk samples from five mothers without biologic pregnancies were measured by

TABLE 19-2	Composition of normal breast milk and "galactorrhea milk"		
Milk components and properties	Normal breast milk	"Galactorrhea milk"	Induced lactation
Components			
Fat (g/dL)	3.7	3–8	
Lactose (g/dL)	7.0	3–5	5.4
Total protein (g/dL)	1.2	2–7	1.6
Sodium (mg/dL)	15	70	22.0
Potassium (mg/dL)	50	5	19.8
Calcium (mg/dL)	35	38	
Chlorine (mg/dL)	45	50	18.4
Phosphorus (mg/dL)	15	2	
Ash (mg/dL)	20	40–70	
Properties			
Specific gravity	1030–1033	1031	
Milk pH	6.8–7.3	7.3	
Daily volume	400–800 mL	1–120 mL	

From Vorherr H: The Breast: Morphology, Physiology and Lactation. New York, Academic Press, 1974; and Kulski JK, Hartmann PE, Saint WJ, et al: Changes in the milk composition of non-puerperal women. Am Obstet Gynecol 139:597, 1981. Reprinted with permission from the American College of Obstetricians and Gynecologists.

Kleinman and associates.[19] Two of the mothers had nursed previous babies, and three had never been pregnant and had never breastfed. These authors did not distinguish between them. The mean total protein concentration of milk samples from the "nonbiologic" mothers differs from the "biologic" mothers (Figs. 19-1 and 19-2). If the goal of induced lactation is nurturing, these differences are clinically less important. However, the clinician needs to keep these values in mind when counseling a mother-infant dyad about induced-lactation nutrition, especially if the infant was premature or small for gestational age. A creamatocrit test for fat and energy content is an appropriate first step (see Chapter 21).

In tandem nursing, when a mother continues to nurse an older child and puts an adopted newborn on the breast simultaneously, the composition of milk will not return to colostrum as it does with a biologic pregnancy.

Lactation has been induced in males usually when a father tries to replace the mother who has died suddenly. A young married male provided our

center with several liters he had collected and frozen over a year's time of taking estrogen and progesterone and using mechanical breast stimulation. The milk was sent to an analytic laboratory but was lost in transit. It appeared to be milk.

Management of the mother and infant

The collected experiences of counseling women in the Western world who want to induce lactation have reported on several thousand women. The request for information and advice is increasing and becoming widespread throughout the United States and other Western countries.[39]

Because there are simple means of supplementing the nutritional needs of the infant, the counseling should center on the relationship and the nurturing aspects. When the process is undertaken in preindustrialized nations, the antiinfective properties become important even though total nourishment may not be possible. Success is measured by having the infant content to nurse at the breast.

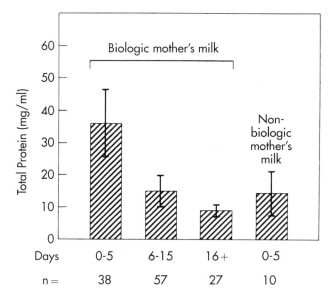

Figure 19-1. Total protein changes over time: biologic versus nonbiologic mother's milk, protein value ± standard deviation. (From Kleinman R, Jacobson L, Hormann E, et al: Protein values of milk samples from mothers without biologic pregnancies. J Pediatr 97:613, 1980.)

The woman should be encouraged to come to the physician's office for a counseling visit before the arrival of the adoptive infant to discuss the process of induced lactation. Actually, parents who are planning to adopt an infant should have at least one visit with their pediatrician so that some understanding of parenting can be discussed, just as any couple should do before the birth of their first child. At this visit, while discussing lactation with the couple, it is helpful to explore their motives and general concepts of what is involved. All authors on the subject have pointed out that the husband's interest in and support of lactation is critical to success. His participation in the preparation of the breasts may be a means by which the father can share intimately and con-structively in the process.

Instruction of the mother in preparation of the breast for suckling is critical in induced lactation, whereas with puerperal lactation it may not be necessary at all. Exercises to stimulate the nipple should be undertaken several times a day and will be most successful if they are scheduled for times when and situations in which it is easy, feasible, and readily remembered. A few minutes multiple times a day is more successful and less likely to *overemphasize* milk versus mothering than rigid excessive exercises once or twice a day. Manual manipulation with gentle traction or horizontal and vertical stretching can be suggested. Avery[4] suggests that the father be encouraged to assist in breast massage and other techniques. She notes that "many adoptive parents felt that this tech-nique (fondling and suckling of the breasts by the husband) added to the mutual sharing in prepara-tion for adoptive nursing similar to the closeness many couples experience in preparing for natural childbirth." Raphael[35] reports that among 40 adoptive nursing mothers, dozens of variations on the theme of preparation were used. A positive attitude seemed to be the only consistent factor.

The need for dietary counseling is obvious. Lip service in behalf of well-balanced nutritious meals is not enough. Discussion should center around the absolute needs in kilocalories, fluids, and nutrients to produce milk (see Chapter 9).

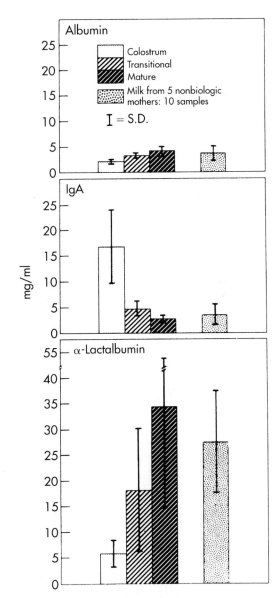

Figure 19-2. Concentrations of albumin, immunoglobu-lin A (IgA), and β-lactalbumins: biologic versus nonbio-logic mother's milk. S.D., Standard deviation. (From Kleinman R, Jacobson L, Hormann E, et al: Protein val-ues of milk samples from mothers without biologic preg-nancies. J Pediatr 97:614, 1980.)

The physician should point out that stimulation of the nipples may well cause amenorrhea. Although the variation in menses is not uniform, decreased flow, irregular cycles, and total cessation of menstrual flow are possible. Conversely, the menstrual cycle may be maintained and the flow of milk may seem to vary during menses. Changes in breast size, heaviness, and feeling of fullness may accompany the induced lactation. The woman may have an associated weight gain of 10 to 12 lb (4.5 to 5.4 kg), on the average,[4] attributed to the response of the body to developing stores for lactation, just as in pregnancy (i.e., increased fluid retention and appetite increase). The weight gain may be a simple phenomenon of excessive intake. There is no need to gain excessive weight, however, during this experience. Mothers (who may be nutritionally depleted) in non-Western countries who induce lactation are given added diet, nourishment, and herbal teas but do not usually gain weight. Failure to experience change in breast size, menstrual regularity, or weight should not be construed as a failed response as it might be in pregnancy.

Auerbach and Avery[3] reported a retrospective questionnaire study of 240 women: 83 had never been pregnant or lactated, 55 had been pregnant but never lactated, and 102 had breastfed one or more biologic children before the adoptive nursing (lactation). Most respondents used more than one technique to stimulate their nipples. These mothers stated that the most effective method of nipple stimulation was nipple exercises combined with infant suckling. Hand-operated pumps caused soreness and irritation. The nipple exercises included nipple stroking, massaging the breast, and rolling the nipple between thumb and finger.

In this study the infant's willingness to suckle improved over time and was related to the age at which the infant was first put to breast. Infants who were under 8 weeks of age had over a 75% success rate; those over 8 weeks of age had only 50% success. No infants failed to thrive, but nearly all needed some type of supplementation. Mothers who had nursed a biologic baby before were able to wean from supplementation partially or com-

pletely. This group was also more disappointed if they had to supplement.[3]

The following simple guidelines, developed as a result of experiences reported by several authors and many mothers, may be helpful to the physician in counseling the mother to induce lactation:

1. Before arrival of the baby, initiate frequent, brief manual stimulation of nipples and breasts, increasing time gradually to about 10 minutes per session. Initiate mechanical pumping stimulus after 2 weeks or so of manual stimulus, if time permits. Hand pumps usually cause more soreness. Modern electric pumps with milking action and pressure cycling are most effective. Pumps that can be controlled in cycle frequency and strength are best. Double-sided pumps maximize stimulus and save time.
2. On arrival of the baby, depending on the infant's age, limit sucking to breastfeeding, using a lactation supplementer if necessary.
3. Breastfeed before any other nourishment is provided for a given feeding.
4. Avoid stressing baby with hunger.
5. When supplementing, use donor human milk or prepared formula, not cow milk, with its long stomach-emptying time and potential for allergic response.
6. Avoid rubber nipples and pacifiers to encourage appropriate suckling at breast.
7. Provide other supplements by dropper, spoon, cup, or supplementer.
8. Create a positive atmosphere; "mother the mother."

A trial of oxytocin nasal spray once the infant is established at the breast may facilitate let-down and even encourage prolactin release.

Rigid conformity to a system of feeding may be a symptom of a more serious problem. Women who are rigid and compulsive may have trouble lactating because of the inability to have a good ejection reflex, which can be inhibited by stress and emotional conflict. Mothers who demonstrate an inordinate attention to volume of production of milk over and above the value of the relationship may feel as if they have failed.

Nutritional supplementation

The need to supplement the infant's intake while the milk supply is being developed should be discussed. The older infant who has already been receiving solid foods can be continued on solids by spoon with careful attention to nutritional content so that the diet includes a balance of protein and other nutrients. Supplements with milk or formula should be appropriate to the age of the infant. The infant under 12 months should receive infant formula rather than whole milk if donor breast milk is not available. The milk supplements should be full strength, 20 kcal/oz, and provided during the feeding by dropper or supplementer or after the nursing by dropper, spoon, or cup in preference to rubber nipple, which may confuse the infant during adaptation to nursing at the breast.

Postmenopausal lactation

Women have had postmenopausal infants thanks to modern fertility techniques and hormone therapy. The question "Can they breastfeed?" arises. They will require maintenance hormone therapy paralleling levels in postpartum lactating women. The oxytocin and prolactin should respond with removal of the placenta and suckling of the infant at the breast. Three cases have been reported to the lactation center who were successful in producing milk. No long-term follow-up was obtained.

A postmenopausal woman may wish to induce lactation. Some of these women are young and had surgical menopause; however, most of them had emergency hysterectomies and still retain their ovaries. The situations are different; the treatment is different.

In natural menopause, the woman may be on hormone replacement therapy, which should be modified to match pregnancy levels of estrogen and progesterone. A program of regular systematic dual pumping should be initiated with the addition of galactogogues such as domperidone once the breast has responded with enlargement and turgescence and the first drops of milk. The woman who has retained her ovaries can be managed in the same manner as a normal woman.

Support systems

The process of induced lactation requires considerable commitment and determination.[46] It is far more arduous a task than initiating postpartum lactation, but it is possible and worth the effort, according to the many mothers who have attempted it. The situation is better managed if a doula is available. It is appropriate for the physician to suggest that in addition to medical support, the mother seek counseling from a lactation consultant experienced in induced lactation. Day-by-day contact for verbal support may be helpful, and these needs may be beyond the scope of a busy office practice. The nurse practitioner may be invaluable in this situation, particularly if home visits are made.

Ensuring that the child grows appropriately is the responsibility of the pediatrician; however, this task is best carried out in a nonthreatening way so the mother can concentrate on nurturing and nourishing the infant.[15] Monitoring the usual growth parameters of weight and height as well as the patterns of voiding and stooling is essential.

RELACTATION

The need to relactate exists in a number of circumstances, including the following:

1. A sick or premature infant cannot be fed initially or at all until several weeks or months old (Fig. 19-3).
2. An infant is weaned prematurely because of illness in the infant or in the mother.
3. An infant who was not previously breastfed develops an allergy or food intolerance.
4. A mother who has lactated weeks, months, or years earlier wants to nurse an adopted infant.
5. A mother who is nursing a biologic child wants to nurse an adopted child (without benefit of pregnancy).

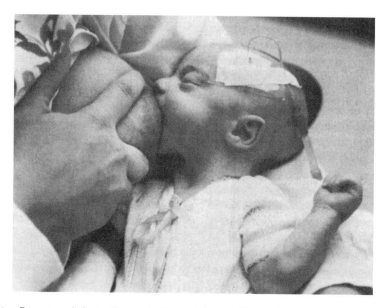

Figure 19-3.   Premature infant at breast: infant weighed 1300 g at time of photograph.

Historical reviews provide many examples of infants suckled in times of crisis by women who have not lactated for years. The process of reestablishing lactation under these circumstances is generally easier than that of nonpuerperal lactation. Investigations have shown that a breast that has been previously primed by pregnancy to respond to prolactin will produce milk more readily.

An early unpublished report of relactation describes a woman who had breastfed her first child for 9 months and was midterm with a second pregnancy. Then the woman experienced the births and finally the deaths of two premature infants, never nursing them. Then she breastfed two adopted infants. The first adoptee was 6 weeks old when the mother began breastfeeding. She had full milk supply within 3 months and nursed for 9 months. Nursing required supplementary formula for the infant at first, but the volume of supplementation was gradually reduced. Three years later, she adopted a 2-week-old infant. She had to entice the infant with honey on the nipple, expressed milk, and spoon feedings. The mother used oxytocin nasal spray to obtain let-down the first few weeks.

This infant was also fully breastfed for months. These protocols have not been tested with placebo-controlled blinded studies and reflect the experience of a number of practitioners.

Psychological factors

Although the general process of nipple stimulation, having the infant suckle the breast, and setting the stage for lactation is similar, the woman who has experienced successful lactation previously may have not only the physiologic but also the psychological edge. As Jelliffe had said, "Breastfeeding is a confidence game."[18]

A prospective study of mothers whose infants were in the neonatal intensive care unit in Durham, North Carolina, was reported by Bose and associates.[5] The profile of the mothers is listed in Table 19-3. Mother and baby were admitted to the clinical research unit, where they were assisted with relactating, including help using the Lact-Aid. The infant's nutritional intake was recorded. Mother and infant were discharged when the mother was comfortable with the Lact-Aid and

TABLE 19-3   Historical and clinical data of mothers in relactation study

Case no.	Gestational age	Time from delivery to entry into study (days)	Time from last lactation to entry into study (days)	Postpartum breast involution*	Time to first breast milk (days)	Time to half breast milk supply† (days)	Time to complete relactation (days)
1	Term	10	10	None	1	4	8
2	Term	120	120	Incomplete	4	20	28
3‡	Twins, 31 wk	49	49	Complete	7	28	Never
4	32 wk	70	42	Complete	7	39	Never
5	28 wk	150	135	Complete	9	Never	Never
6	32 wk	30	16	None	4	17	58
7	Term (adopted)	5 yr	5 yr	Complete	21	Never	Never

*Mothers were asked if their brassiere size was different from that before this pregnancy.
†Estimated on the basis of a decrease in formula intake.
‡Ceased to suckle her infants after 28 days in the study to return to full-time employment.
From Bose CL, D'Ercole J, Lester AG, et al: Relactation by mothers of sick and premature infants. Pediatrics 67:565, 1981.

725

feeding was established (about 3 days). Follow-up occurred every week or two. All but one infant were initially reluctant to suckle, but all received their entire nutritional intake at the breast, with or without Lact-Aid, within the first week of the study. Most of the mothers had trouble initiating suckling, with the most significant factor being the length of separation from their infant and not degree of prematurity, postnatal age, weight, or feeding regimen. Nipple tenderness occurred in all mothers, but it was transient. All the mothers (except number seven, who was an adoptive mother) produced milk in 1 week, with maximum milk production occurring from 8 to 58 days, proportional to the time since delivery.

Although it was done with a small population, this study established some important information. Given appropriate techniques and support, many women appear to be able to relactate, and premature infants can learn to breastfeed after initial bottle feeding.

A retrospective study of relactation was reported by Auerbach and Avery[2] in which 366 women responded with a completed questionnaire out of over 500 contacted from a list of names obtained from manufacturers' lists, magazine ads, and requests to breastfeeding support groups. The bias was in favor of well-educated, affluent women who had probably obtained their lactation goals. The population included those who had untimely weaning ($n = 174$), following delivery of low-birth-weight infants ($n = 117$), and following hospitalization of mother or baby or both ($n = 75$).

The infant's willingness to nurse was related to previous suckling experience, but responses in the first week of effort were not directly correlated with ultimate successful suckling. Fifty percent of mothers were able to discontinue supplementing in 1 month, and 24% were never able to eliminate supplements completely. Once established, the nursing patterns were similar to those of ordinary breastfeeding. The authors[2] point out that keeping the baby hungry in the mistaken notion that the infant will nurse more often and for longer periods does not help and may negatively influence outcome. For the pro-

fessional, it is of interest that fewer than 10% of respondents felt that they had received helpful advice from health care professionals.

Relactation in mothers of children over 12 months of age was reported.[34,40] Six Australian children 12 to 18 months of age had been weaned by the mother with no further stimulus to the breast, then were reinitiated to breastfeeding. The length of time without breastfeeding ranged from 1 week to 6 months (Table 19-4). All the children had been actively weaned and initiated the suckling, although the mothers did not forcibly resist. All the mothers reestablished milk supplies and nursed for 48 months to 5 years.[34,40]

Tandem nursing

Tandem nursing an adoptive child is a phenomenon in which the adoptive mother is still nursing a biologic child and puts an adopted infant to the breast and intends to nourish the newcomer totally. Usually the older child is a toddler and feeding only a few times a day or for comfort and receiving the major nourishment from other food and drink. In biologic tandem nursing, the milk returns to colostrum-like constituency with the birth of the new baby; in the absence of a pregnancy, however, the milk volume may increase with increased nipple stimulus while the constituents do not change. Data on milk constituents beyond a year post partum or in the case of relactation have been noted earlier. In most cases reported anecdotally, the adopted infant is several weeks or months old, so the absence of colostrum is less of a problem. On the other hand, the active state of lactation in terms of immediate availability of milk is actually an advantage.

An additional concern, as in any situation of tandem nursing, is the development of the younger child. The physician will need to be alert to these issues in counseling the family and ensuring adequate total nutrition for the adopted child.

Eighteen respondents to the survey on adoptive nursing by Auerbach and Avery[3] reported tandem-nursing experiences. Eleven of these mothers were able to discontinue supplements totally (two within

		Length of		Evidence of	How long from	
Case no.	Age of child	time off breast	Methods	presence of milk	relactation to weaning	Age at final weaning
1	48 mo	4 mo	Child suckled from breast	Child verbally reported presence of milk	After milk appeared	48 mo
			Mother relaxed, not anxious over outcome	Mother saw whitish milk		
2	12 mo	1 wk	Child took four feeds daily	Milk had not quite dried up	1 yr	2 yr
3	20½ mo	2½ mo	Mother gave in to demands of child and suckled her	Mother noticed child's swallowing while breastfeeding	>10 mo	Some time after 2½ yr
4	2 yr	1 mo	Child suckled from both breasts avidly	Mother saw the milk Flow was enough to soak the bed next morning Mother heard swallowing	Approx. 1 yr	>3 yr
5	>3 yr	6 wk	Child suckled from both breasts	Mother saw the milk Mother noticed swallowing	Approx. 2 yr	5 yr
6	Approx. 2 yr	Approx. 6 mo	Mother attached child to breast to demonstrate	Mother began to feel let-down of milk	12 mo	Almost 3 yr

From Phillips N: Relactation in mothers of children over 12 months. J Trop Pediatr 39:45, 1993.

the first month). Most of the infants were started on solids by 4½ months, which may be the most effective method of supplementing if nutritional value is maintained. For the physician, it is important to be knowledgeable about *tandem adoptive nursing* and to support the family accordingly.

Drugs to induce relactation

Some medications that have been tried in relactation seem to work only when the breast has been primed by mammogenesis, that is, by pregnancy.

TRH (Thyroliberin) has been used by Tyson[42] and others to induce lactation (see Table 19-1). Each woman in the study was primed with estrogens beforehand. TRH stimulates the pituitary to release both thyrotropin-stimulating hormone (TSH) and prolactin. Drugs that produce a decrease in hypothalamic catecholamines, such as phenothiazines, reserpine, meprobamate, amphetamines, and α-methyldopa, cause an increase in prolactin secretion by blocking hypothalamic prolactin inhibitory factor (PIF).

The feasibility of pharmacologically manipulating puerperal lactation was demonstrated by Canales and associates[9] using bromocriptine and TRH sequentially. They suppressed lactation using bromocriptine orally for 8 days in four mothers whose infants were premature or ill and could not be nursed. These mothers did not lactate during this time. On the eighth day, they were given TRH intravenously and then orally daily for 4 days (8th to 12th postpartum days). On the 14th day, they initiated breastfeeding by putting the infant to the breast. Prolactin levels were measured from the day of birth. Levels were depressed by bromocriptine and rose when the TRH was given. The mothers subsequently nursed successfully.

Bose and associates[5] also studied TRH and the basal and stimulated serum prolactin concentrations. Prolactin concentrations were measured followed by levels at 15 and 30 minutes after intravenous infusion of 200 μg of TRH. Prolactin levels were also measured before and after suckling at weekly intervals. Serum prolactin levels rose 15 minutes after infusion of TRH (Table 19-5). The absolute rise in prolactin concentrations did not appear to be related to establishment of milk production. The change over time in the basal prolactin levels was not predictably related to lactation progress.

Lactation can be reestablished with metoclopramide, according to Sousa and associates.[38] Metoclopramide is a derivative of procainamide, as is sulpiride (see Chapter 16). Studies done by McNeilly and associates[25] showed that metoclopramide and sulpiride are potent stimulators of prolactin release. These authors demonstrated marked increase in prolactin when metoclopramide is given, as noted earlier in this chapter. Sousa and associates[38] used metoclopramide to reestablish lactation in women who had experienced diminished milk supply. All five mothers experienced increased production of milk when 10 mg was given orally every 8 hours for 7 to 10 days. No side effects were noted, although this drug is known to cause cardiac arrhythmias and extrapyramidal signs in some adults. No side effects were noted in the infants either, but the level of drug was not measured in the milk. The results were encouraging, but further study is needed to determine the minimum dosage necessary to produce the effect and the amount passed into the milk. The summation of the data on patients treated by Sousa and associates[38] is recorded in Table 19-6.

In a controlled double-blind study with a placebo, Lewis and associates[24] found no difference in the success rate of induced lactation in 10 patients medicated with 10-mg metoclopramide orally three times daily for 7 days compared with 10 matched patients medicated with lactose capsules. Successful lactation was attributed to the special advice and support provided equally for these women by the nursery staff. Before conducting the study, these authors measured the amount of drug that appeared in the milk of 10 women after a single 10-mg dose of metoclopramide given orally at 7 to 10 days post partum. The mean 2-hour postdose plasma level was 68.5 ± 29.6 ng/mL. The simultaneous mean concentration in the breast milk was 125.7 ± 41.7 ng/mL. If the infant consumed a liter of milk a day, the dose to the infant would be calculated at 130 mg or 45 mg/kg, a subtherapeutic dose. These data do not address possible accumulation in the infant, however, when multiple doses are given to the mother.

Domperidone has a better track record anecdotally for stimulating lactation but has not been studied in induced lactation or relactation. Herbals such as fenugreek have not been studied for this purpose either but could be used as an adjunct to protocol.

SPECIAL DEVICES

Although many mechanical devices have been developed since Roman times to augment lactation and give other feeding opportunities, lactation-supplementing devices provide a unique ability to adequately nourish an infant while it is suckling at the inadequately lactating breast (Fig. 19-4). The suckling stimulates the mother's own supply. On the other hand, the infant continues to suckle the breast because milk is available. The devices have been carefully engineered to provide a source of milk that is obtained by suckling, not by gravity. The capillary tube through which the milk flows can be placed along the human nipple without interfering with suckling. The plastic containers that serve as reservoirs for the supplemental milk are sterilizable or disposable. The milk is naturally warmed by hanging the bag beside the mother's breast, as shown in Figure 19-4. See Appendix F for a full description.

TABLE 19-5   **Basal and stimulated serum prolactin concentrations (ng/ml)**

Case no.	TRH stimulation		Suckling stimulation: presuckling/postsuckling					
	Basal	15 min/30 min	1st wk*	2nd wk	3rd wk	4th–5th wk	6th–7th wk	8th–9th wk
1	179.2	611.1/423.5	136.9/155.4	72.3/123.8	—	—	—	—
2	38.7	80.9/70.3	17.2/119.3	38.6/214.3	16.6/180.6	186.2/244.5	—	—
3	19.9	89.6/77.3	17.9/23.5	—	—	—	—	—
4	9.5	89.9/63.4	12.5/12.7	—	7.0/437.6	5.5/47.3	—	—
5	13.9	40.6/36.3	21.1/58.2	37.8/82.0	38.3/57.7	77.2/98.5	24.6/54.2	—
6	31.7	335.6/274.7	9.5/11.4	—	16.5/18.4	11.8/16.3	7.8/13.3	—
7	43.6†	78.8/69.9	8.8/59.6	17.0/77.7	—	—	34.4/147.1	19.2/60.5

*Suckling test performed on day 1 or 2 of study.

†In this mother, suckling test was done first, followed 1 hour later by thyrotropin-releasing hormone (TRH) infusion; thus, 8.8 is the true basal concentration.

From Bose CL, D'Ercole J, Lester AG, et al: Relactation by mothers of sick and premature infants. Pediatrics 67:565, 1981.

				Length of			Education
Case no.	Age of mother (yr)	Age of infant (mo)	Daily dose (mg)	treatment (days)	Side effects	Results	level of mother
1	27	2	30	6	None	Increase in milk volume; infant not weaned	University
2	25	10	30	10	None	Same as above	University
3	29	1	20	7	None	Same as above	High school
4	35	3	30	7	None	Same as above	University
5	20	2	20	7	None	Same as above	High school

TABLE 19-6   Data regarding mothers taking metoclopramide

From Sousa PLR, Barros FC, Pinheiro GNM, et al: Reestablishment of lactation with metoclopramide. J Trop Pediatr Environ Child Health 21:214, 1975.

Gradual weaning from the supplementer can be provided by putting less and less in the container each day. Thus, the infant can obtain milk from the breast in increasing amounts because the nipple stimulation affects milk production.

An increasing number of mothers want to nurse their sick premature infants; however, it is often not possible for the infant to breastfeed for weeks. Meanwhile, the mother may pump but only obtain minimal volume. When the infant is finally ready for discharge from the hospital, it is mandatory that the baby continue to receive reliable nourishment every day. Starving the infant into submission is inappropriate and dangerous. A lactation supplementer is an excellent alternative.

For years, mothers of premature and sick infants have been assisted in breastfeeding their infants in preparation for discharge from the hospital and during the early weeks at home by using dropper feeding, complementary feeds by bottle after each breastfeeding, or solids. The success rate was low and the aggravation for the mother often insurmountable.

Weaning from the device is usually not a problem for most of the infants. It was a problem, however, for an occasional mother who could not nurse without the supplementer even though it contained less than an ounce of formula per feeding and the breast was supplying the rest. Because the mother may use this as a "crutch," careful anticipatory counseling should address this issue.

Special equipment should be started with a full understanding of its role in nourishment of the infant as well as with a plan for weaning from it that begins the first day. Weaning should be appropriate to the infant's age and nutritional needs. The nourishment provided should be donor human milk or regular-strength formula, 20 kcal/oz, and not just water, sugar water, or diluted formula. Starvation, even for a day or so, in a premature infant compromises growth, especially of the brain. An infant who has been in the intensive care nursery is in special jeopardy (see Fig. 14-3).

Several alternative devices have been suggested by professionals interested in the transient supplementation of lactation while a mother increased her milk supply for her full-term baby. Usually in these situations, lactation failure has been the result of inadequate initial advice. The devices are rigged from readily available feeding tubes and syringes but lack the special engineering and safety features of the supplementer. Special precautions are advised when employing such handmade equipment to avoid milk aspiration by the infant, which is the chief hazard. Because they will allow milk to flow without sucking, they do not stimulate the infant to suck. Other devices, such as hand pumps and a variety of electric pumps, which are useful in initiating relactation or induced lactation as well as in puerperal nursing, are illustrated in Chapter 21.

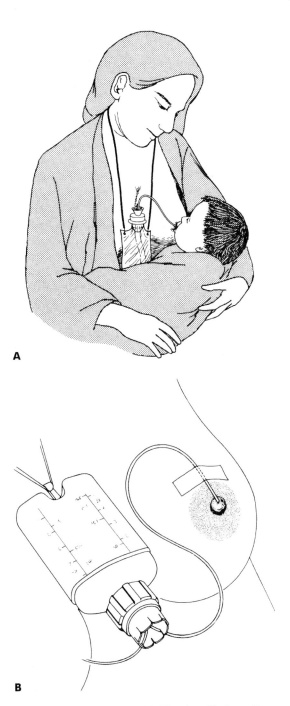

Figure 19-4. **A,** Lact-Aid Nursing Trainer System (Lact-Aid International, Inc.). **B,** Supplemental Nursing System (SNS) by Medela, which provides additional nourishment to infant while suckling at underproducing breast.

SUMMARY

Careful medical management of the adopted infant who is breastfed is important. Many times the prenatal care of this infant as a fetus in utero and the biologic mother has not been optimal. Any failure in growth should be identified quickly so that appropriate supplementation can be provided. In cases of relactation to provide for sick or premature infants, close follow-up is mandatory. A child who does not have a powerful suck may well appear to be very content yet be underfed. This situation was clearly described by Gilmore and Rowland,[17] who reported three cases of malnutrition while breastfeeding, attributed to the failure of the mother to recognize signs of growth failure and dehydration.

Relactation and induced lactation are special events requiring the positive support of medical personnel.[46] The physician can serve as a well-informed stable resource in a process that will require considerable effort and commitment by the participants and will go better if there is an experienced board certified lactation consultant available as a supporter. The pediatrician is responsible for monitoring adequate growth, nutrition and adjustment of the child.

Mother-initiated preparation

1. Nipple stimulation: hand massage and nipple exercise, hand pump, electric "milkers"
2. Diet supplementation: fluids and calories, especially protein
3. Reading, learning, and communication with others with similar experience

Physician-initiated preparation

1. Knowledgeable, sympathetic support
2. Preparatory hormones and lactogogues to promote mammogenesis for prescription
3. Induction of let-down: oxytocin nasal drops to initiate or enhance let-down
4. Counseling about breast preparation and diet supplementation in the context of total care of the mother and the infant
5. Use of lactation-supplementing devices

WET NURSING OR CROSS-NURSING

Although feeding an infant by one who is not the mother is an established means of sustaining life, it has been uncommon in Western cultures since the 1930s. There were no medical contraindications provided the nursing woman was in good health, was infection free, and was taking no medications. The threat of human immunodeficiency virus (HIV) infection has altered the risk. In special cases, surrogate nursing would be acceptable by individual arrangement, with HIV testing in both mother and infant. The chief obstacle had been psychological or social. Actually, women who are trying to develop a supply of milk when their own infant cannot nurse because of prematurity or illness would be greatly benefited by having a vigorous, normal suckling infant nurse at their breasts.

In contemporary society, the term *cross-nursing* has replaced *wet nursing* to disassociate the phenomenon from the negative historical connotations.[21] In cross-nursing the mother continues to breastfeed her own child in addition to the child she takes for a feeding or two per day. The circumstances described in the report by Krantz and Kupper[21] usually involve babysitting arrangements, which may be daily and formal or random and informal. They interviewed three women involved in a mutual agreement for babysitting purposes. The mothers were married and well educated. The babies were female and 4 months old. The mothers reported no physical effects on the babies. The behavioral reactions of the babies were "looking puzzled" and being disturbed if the surrogate mother spoke. Some difficulty was noticed in let-down, and all three mothers noted a difference in the way each baby suckled.

Another purpose of cross-nursing is for maternal benefit, wherein an experienced, vigorous infant is nursed by a woman whose own baby is unable to give proper stimulus to milk production. This has been done by private arrangement and has not caused any known problems. Usually the normal newborn is younger than 2 months. Cross-nursing has also been used to stimulate lactation in adoptive nursing. In this situation, the infants are exchanged to stimulate the adoptive mother's breasts and also to show the adopted infant that milk comes from breasts and how to suckle at the breast.

Cross-nursing had been used in neonatal intensive care units by mothers to encourage their own milk production. It is usually a private arrangement between mothers who have babies to nourish. A mother of an immature infant who cannot be put to the breast sought out a friend who was actively feeding a full-term infant and borrowed the infant to stimulate her production. An infant who needs to learn how to suckle correctly after weeks of bottle feeding or no feeding may benefit from being nursed by a fully lactating woman. The best pump is always a suckling infant.

The hazards to cross-nursing are undocumented but worthy of consideration. The physical problems are the potential for infection, either of mother or of baby; interruption of milk supply for the mother's own baby; and the difference in composition of milk if babies are of different chronologic or conceptual ages. The psychological hazards could include failure of mother to let-down, refusal of infant to nurse (which does occur when infants are introduced to the phenomenon after 4 months of age), and negative impact on siblings and the household environment. The long-range effects are not documented.

Reasonable caution is certainly appropriate, taking care to ensure that the cross-nursing mother is healthy and well nourished without any general or local infection, not taking any medications, and not smoking. The infants should probably be close in age to the mother's own baby and also free of infection, especially thrush. If this were a commercial venture in a public daycare setting, regulations of certification, screening for tuberculosis, syphilis, hepatitis, cytomegalovirus, herpesvirus, HIV, and other infectious agents would be in order. Documents of liability might be required with signed consent forms.

Perhaps as breastfeeding knowledge and understanding reach a greater number of professionals and women, such opportunities may be more common. At present, it is significant to recognize cross-nursing as a viable option, as long as appropriate infection precautions are taken. The hospital or physician cannot be the agent of arrangement.

REFERENCES

1. Arya DK, Taylor WS: Lactation associated with fluoxetine treatment. Aust NZ J Psychiatry 29:697, 1995.
2. Auerbach KG, Avery JL: Relactation: A study of 366 cases. Pediatrics 65:236, 1980.
3. Auerbach KG, Avery JL: Induced lactation: A study of adoptive nursing by 240 women. Am J Dis Child 135:340, 1981.
4. Avery JL: Induced lactation: A Guide for Counseling and Management. Denver, Resources in Human Nurturing, Int., 1979.
5. Bose CL, D'Ercole J, Lester AG et al: Relactation by mothers of sick and premature infants. Pediatrics 67:565, 1981.
6. Brown RE: Some nutritional considerations in times of major catastrophe. Clin Pediatr 11:334, 1972.
7. Brown RE: Breastfeeding in modern times. Am J Clin Nutr 26:556, 1973.
8. Brown RE: Relactation: An overview. Pediatrics 60:116, 1977.
9. Canales ES, Lasso P, Murrieta S, et al: Feasibility of suppressing and reinitiating lactation in women with premature infants. Am J Obstet Gynecol 128:695, 1977.
10. Caron RW, Janh GA, Deis RP: Lactogenic actions of different growth hormone preparations in pregnant and lactating rats. J Endocrinol 142:535, 1994.
11. Cohen R: Breastfeeding without pregnancy. Pediatrics 48:996, 1971 (letter).
12. Cowie AT, Forsyth IA, Hart IC: Hormonal control of lactation. Monographs in Endocrinology, vol. 15. New York, Springer-Verlag, 1980.
13. Creel SR, Monfort SL, Wildt DE, et al: Spontaneous lactation is an adaptive result of pseudopregnancy. Nature 351:660, 1991.
14. Ehernkranz RA, Ackerman BA: Metoclopramide effect on faltering milk production by mothers of premature infants. Pediatrics 78:614, 1986.
15. Evans TJ, Davies DP: Failure to thrive at the breast: An old problem revisited. Arch Dis Child 52:974, 1977.
16. Funk and Wagnalls' Standard Dictionary, International Edition, Vol. II. New York, Funk and Wagnalls, 1960.
17. Gilmore HE, Rowland TW: Critical malnutrition in breast fed infants. Am J Dis Child 132:885, 1978.
18. Jelliffe DB: Hormonal control of lactation. In Schams D (ed): Breast Feeding and the Mother. Ciba Foundation Symposium No. 45. Amsterdam, Elsevier, 1976.
19. Kleinman R, Jacobson L, Hormann E, et al: Protein values of milk samples from mothers without biologic pregnancies. J Pediatr 97:612, 1980.
20. Kramer P: Breastfeeding of adopted infants. Br Med J 310:188, 1995 (letter).
21. Krantz JZ, Kupper NS: Cross-nursing: wet-nursing in a contemporary context. Pediatrics 67:715, 1981.
22. Kulski JK, Hartmann PE, Saint WJ, et al: Changes in the milk composition of non-puerperal women. Am J Obstet Gynecol 139:597, 1981.
23. Larson BL: Lactation: A Comprehensive Treatise. IV. The Mammary Gland/Human Lactation/Milk Synthesis. New York, Academic Press, 1978.
24. Lewis PJ, Devenish C, Kahn C: Controlled trial of metoclopramide in the initiation of breastfeeding. Br J Clin Pharmacol 9:217, 1980.
25. McNeilly AS, Thorner MO, Volans G, et al: Metoclopramide and prolactin. Br Med J 2:729, 1974.
26. Mead M: Sex and Temperament in Three Primitive Societies. New York, Dell, 1963.
27. Mobbs GA, Babbage NF: Breastfeeding adopted children. Med J Aust 2:436, 1971.
28. Nemba K: Induced lactation: A study of 37 non-puerperal mothers. J Trop Pediatr 40:240, 1994.
29. Newman J, Pitman T: The Ultimate Breastfeeding Book of Answers. Roseville, CA, Prima Publishing/Random House, 2000, p 338.
30. Newton M, Egli GE: The effect of intranasal administration of oxytocin on the let-down of milk in lactating women. Am J Obstet Gynecol 76:103, 1958.
31. Packer C, Lewis S, Pusey A: A comparative analysis of non-offspring nursing. Animal Behav 43:265, 1992.
32. Patil SP, Niphadkar PV, Bapat MM: Allergy to fenugreek (Trigonella foenum graecum). Ann Allergy Asthma Immunoe 78:297, 1997.
33. PDR for Herbal Preparation, 2nd ed. Montvale, NJ, Medical Economics Co., 2000.
34. Phillips V: Relactation in mothers of children over 12 months. J Trop Pediatr 39:45, 1993.
35. Raphael D: Breast feeding the adopted baby. In Raphael D: The Tender Gift: Breast Feeding. New York, Schocken, 1976.
36. Selye H, McKeown T: The effect of mechanical stimulation of the nipples on the ovary and the sexual cycle. Surg Gynecol Obstet 59:886, 1934.

37. Slome C: Non-puerperal lactation in grandmothers. J Pediatr 49:550, 1956.

38. Sousa PLR, Barros FC, Pinheiro GNM, et al: Reestablishment of lactation with metoclopramide. J Trop Pediatr Environ Child Health 21:214, 1975.

39. Thearle MJ, Weissenberger R: Induced lactation in adoptive mothers. Aust NZ J Obstet Gynecol 24:283, 1984.

40. Thorley V: Relactation and induced lactation: What the exceptions can tell us. Birth Issues 6:24, 1997.

41. Turkington RW: Human prolactin. Am J Med 53:389, 1972.

42. Tyson JE: Mechanisms of puerperal lactation. Symposium on pregnancy. Med Clin North Am 61:153, 1977.

43. Vorherr H: The Breast: Morphology, Physiology and Lactation. New York, Academic Press, 1974.

44. Vorherr H: Human lactation and breast feeding. In Larson BL (ed): Lactation. New York, Academic Press, 1978.

45. Waletzky LR, Herman EC: Relactation. Am Fam Pract 14:69, 1976.

46. Waterson T: Any questions? Br Med J 310:780, 1995.

20

$\mathcal{R}$eproductive function during lactation

FERTILITY

Although gonadotropic and ovarian function during lactation have been investigated, the major body of knowledge has been collected about the postpartum return of the menstrual cycle and ovulation in the woman who is lactating compared with the nonlactating woman.

Lactational amenorrhea

The amenorrhea of lactation has been attributed to an imperfect balance of hypothalamoanteropituitary function and gonadotropin secretion. However, the complex process by which lactation inhibits ovulation and the menstrual cycle is incompletely understood. Frequent suckling, which results in high prolactin levels, is closely associated with altered luteinizing hormone (LH) secretion and amenorrhea.[72]

Figure 20-1 illustrates the usual menstrual cycle and gonadotropic control. The key points include the following:

1. Follicular development is initiated by pituitary gonadotropin follicle-stimulating hormone (FSH).

2. Continued growth requires FSH and estradiol from the growing follicle in response to LH, which is released in a pulsatile fashion from the pituitary.
3. At midcycle, an increase in estradiol triggers the release of preovulatory surges of LH and FSH.
4. The follicle secretes predominantly progesterone (luteinization).
5. The oocyte is released 36 hours later.

Gonadotropin-releasing hormone (Gn-RH), through pulsatile release from the hypothalamus, stimulates the release of LH. Estrogen increases Gn-RH secretion, and the combination of progesterone and estrogen decreases it.[72]

In lactation the pulsatile secretion of Gn-RH is altered, suggesting that suckling affects ovarian activity at the hypothalamic Gn-RH generator.[72] The follicular development is suppressed because of suppression of estradiol. Ultrasound studies show the absence of medium-size or large follicles during lactation.[72] The period of lactational amenorrhea depends on suckling (Figs. 20-2 to 20-4).

The levels of gonadotropin in all postpartum women for the first weeks of the postpartum period are decreased, which substantiates the theory of

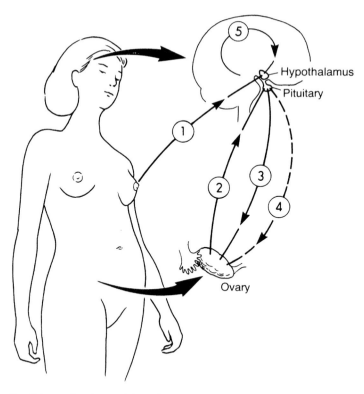

Figure 20-1. Possible mechanisms of lactational amenorrhea: Nervous impulse from nipple produces not only a rise in prolactin (1) but also changes in hypothalamic sensitivity to ovarian steroid feedback (2) and changes in gonadotropin-releasing hormone (Gn-RH) (3), leading to changes in pituitary release of luteinizing hormone (LH) and follicle-stimulating hormone (FSH) (4). Suckling may also stimulate release of β-endorphin (5), thus suppressing Gn-RH from hypothalamus. (Redrawn from Winikoff B, Semeraro P, Zimmerman M: Contraception during Breastfeeding: A Clinician's Source Book. New York, Population Council, 1988.)

postpartum ovarian refractoriness. In the first 2 weeks post partum, low levels of FSH are found in urine and plasma. Beling and associates[6] report estrogen excretion to be low with a linear increase during the first 5 to 8 weeks. When lactating postpartum women are given intramuscular gonadotropins, urinary steroids do not increase, according to studies by Zarate and associates.[109] The prolactin-cell predominance may be responsible for the decreased activity of the pituitary-ovarian axis post partum.

Myometrial and endometrial involution are also considered to reduce fertility. Animal studies have shown that the release of FSH and LH is inhibited by intense suckling. In addition, animals in whom the nipple is stimulated while the milk ducts have been tied off still show a suppression of estrous and menstrual cycles. Selye and McKeown[93] concluded that interruption of sexual cyclicity during lactation is a result of the suckling and not of the secretory activity of the mammary gland. The more the suckling stimulus in frequency and duration, the more consistent is the suppression of ovulation.[72]

In a longitudinal study of 48 women, endocrine profiles were assessed with morning blood samples from the first postpartum month until the recovery of ovulation.[26,27] Additional samples were drawn throughout 24 hours at the end of the third postpartum

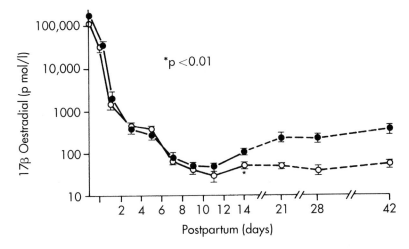

Figure 20-2.   17β- Estradiol levels in postpartum period in lactating (*open circles*) and nonlactating (*dots*) women. Levels in lactating women vary with intensity of suckling. (From Neville MC: Regulation of mammary development and lactation. In Neville MC, Neifert MR (eds): Lactation: Physiology, Nutrition, and Breastfeeding. New York, Plenum, 1983.)

month in 10 of the exclusively nursing amenorrheic women. Prolactin, LH, FSH, estradiol (E_2), progesterone, cortisol, and dehydroepiandrosterone sulfate were measured. In response to suckling, there was a smaller increase in prolactin and higher levels of E_2 in women who ovulated within 6 months post partum compared with those who had not. Diaz and associates[26-28] suggest that this may explain some of the variability in duration of lactational amenorrhea. The greater prolactin response

to suckling associated with longer amenorrhea may result from higher sensitivity to the breast-hypothalamus-pituitary system.[28]

Prolactin and dopamine

The relationship between lactational infertility and physiologic hyperprolactinemia is not clear. In an extensive study of prolactin levels in lactating women, Tay and associates[97] measured the pattern

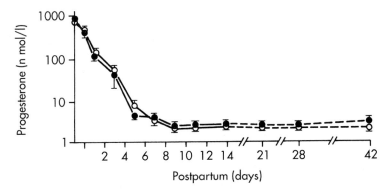

Figure 20-3.   Progesterone levels in postpartum period in lactating (*open circles*) and nonlactating (*dots*) women. (From Neville MC: Regulation of mammary development and lactation. In Neville MC, Neifert MR (eds): Lactation: Physiology, Nutrition, and Breastfeeding. New York, Plenum, 1983.)

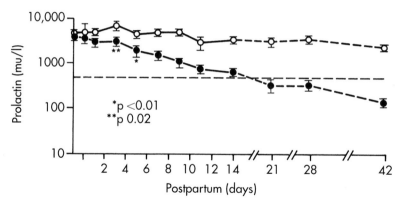

Figure 20-4. Prolactin levels in postpartum period in lactating (*open circles*) and nonlactating (*dots*) women. Levels in lactating women vary with intensity of suckling. (From Neville MC: Regulation of mammary development and lactation. In Neville MC, Neifert MR (eds): Lactation: Physiology, Nutrition, and Breastfeeding. New York, Plenum, 1983.)

of prolactin secretion in relation to suckling and the return of ovarian activity. Blood samples were drawn at 10-minute intervals for 24 hours at 4 and 8 weeks and when weaning was initiated and suckling reduced, at first menses and in the follicular phase of the first menstrual cycle after weaning. Mothers fed their infants on their usual pattern, with no restrictions or alterations, in an effort to replicate natural lactation.

These data confirmed that during frequent suckling, prolactin levels remain high with little decline between feeds. When suckling became less frequent, prolactin dropped to baseline levels between feeds but surged when suckling was initiated (see Chapter 3). The natural increase in prolactin at night was evident only after weaning. Prolactin response also declined greatly in association with suckling after the return of menses. This occurred about 33.6 weeks (± 3.5 weeks) post partum. No relationship was seen between the duration of amenorrhea and plasma prolactin levels over a day, at night, or throughout lactation. The timing of the introduction of solids was strongly correlated with the duration of amenorrhea. The authors concluded that no exact link exists between release of prolactin during lactation and the duration of lactational infertility in breastfeeding women.[97]

The inhibition of dopamine secretion from the hypothalamus has been associated with the neural impulses from stimulation of the nipple during lactation. Normally, dopamine inhibits the secretion of prolactin, and conversely, when dopamine is inhibited, prolactin rises. Two pathways of ovulation inhibition are possible as a result of the rise in prolactin. One is a lack of responsiveness to ovarian steroids of the hypothalamic-pituitary axis of the lactating woman, leading to nonpulsatile release of pituitary gonadotropins, FSH, and LH, which in turn results in absent or reduced ovarian activity. FSH may actually be higher at some points; LH is nonpulsatile. The second possible pathway is through the impaired ovarian response to gonadotropins. It is possible that both pathways function as a result of prolactin surges (see Fig. 20-1).[13]

Return of menses

Clinically, the perceptible measurement of the return of fertility is the onset of menstruation. Return of reproductive function varies, depending on the length and degree of lactation. Most studies do not, in fact, report the completeness of lactation, that is, whether the infant is totally breastfed or is also receiving solid foods or supplemental bottles.[43] By the end of the third month, only 33% of lactating women have had a menstrual period, whereas 91% of nonlactating women have had at least one period.[44]

In 72 fully breastfeeding women studied prospectively from 42 days post partum, vaginal bleeding was recorded daily if it occurred. Almost half the women had some bleeding or spotting between 6 and 8 weeks post partum. Those who experienced this bleeding eventually menstruated and ovulated earlier than those who did not, but differences were not significant. Seven women had ovarian follicular development before day 56, but neither bleeding nor follicular development was associated with ovulation in the first 8 weeks. The authors stated it was unlikely that vaginal bleeding in a fully breastfeeding woman indicates a return to fertility before 8 weeks.[101,102]

The period of lactational amenorrhea does offer a measure of conception protection for 3 months. The nonlactating woman has a return of her period at 25 days at the earliest, a return of ovulation at 25 to 35 days, and a 5% chance of regaining fertility before 6 weeks post partum. In a detailed study of 130 women in Chile, Diaz and associates[29] found the cumulative probability of pregnancy at the end of 6 months post partum in women who were exclusively nursing and amenorrheic to be 1.8%. For exclusively nursing women who had a return of menses, it was 27.2%, and for those partially nursing it was 40.5%.

Perez and associates[83] diagnosed the first post-partum ovulation by endometrial biopsy, basal body temperature, vaginal cytologic evaluation, and cervical mucus in a group of 200 women in a prospective study. The dates of first ovulation, first menses, and nursing status were analyzed. No woman ovulated before day 36, whether lactating or not. The intensity and length of nursing affected the date when ovulation occurred. About 78% of the women ovulated before the first menses, but only 12 pregnancies occurred with first ovulation. Of the 170 women who breastfed, 24 ovulated while completely nursing, 49 while partially nursing, and 97 after weaning.

Although many investigators continue to evaluate the impact of lactation on ovulation and menstruation, the fundamental observations remain the same[3,35,51] (Table 20-1). Available data on return of ovulation and menstruation can be summarized as follows[104]:

TABLE 20-1 Relative risk of ovulation in relation to breastfeeding frequency*

Average number of feeds per day	Relative risk
0	1.0
1	0.62
2	0.43
3	0.28
4	0.19
5	0.12
6	0.08
7	0.05
8	0.04
9	0.02
10	0.01

*Breastfeeding episodes per day before ovulation: $p < 0.0001$
From Gray RH, Campbell O, Eslamic S, et al: The return of ovarian function during lactation: Results of studies from the United States and the Philippines. In Biomedical and Demographic Determinants of Reproduction. Oxford, Clarendon, 1993.

I. Nursing mothers
   A. Earliest possible menstruation is 4 to 6 weeks post partum (pp).
   B. Ovulation before end of amenorrhea varies 14% to 75%.
   C. The longer the first menses is delayed, the more likely the first cycle will be ovulatory.
   D. Continued suckling and elevated prolactin levels produce inadequate luteal function in first cycles.
   E. Exclusive breastfeeding (day and night): return of menses
      1. 9% to 30% in 3 months
      2. 19% to 53% in 180 days
II. Nonnursing mothers
   A. Earliest possible menstruation is 4 weeks pp.
   B. Most women are menstruating by third month pp.
   C. Return of menstruation
      1. 6 weeks pp—40%
      2. 12 weeks pp—65%
      3. 24 weeks pp—90%
   D. Earliest possible ovulation is 3½ to 5 weeks pp.

E. Ovular cycles occur in about 50% with first menstrual period pp.

F. Early pp ovulation may occur late in menstrual cycle: shortening of secretory phase and greater tendency toward irregular menses.

G. Return of ovulation
 1. 6 weeks pp—15%
 2. 12 weeks pp—40%
 3. 24 weeks pp—75%

III. Amenorrheic nonnursing mothers: return of ovulation
 A. 12 weeks pp—20%
 B. 16 weeks pp—40%

Milk composition during the ovulatory menstrual cycle

Acute changes in the composition of milk during the ovulatory menstrual cycle in lactating women were studied by Hartmann and Prosser[40] involving women during lactational amenorrhea, taking oral contraceptives, and during an ovulatory menstrual cycle. Samples of milk were collected from each breast at each feed for each day for 28 days.

During the ovulatory menstrual cycle, two acute changes occurred. For the 5 to 6 days before ovulation and the 6 to 7 days after ovulation, the sodium and chloride values changed from 4.6 mM Na and 11.1 mM Cl to 10.1 and 22.0, respectively, while lactose and potassium decreased. The concentrations of lactose, Cl, K, and Na remained relatively constant during lactational amenorrhea, anovulatory menstrual cycles, and for those women taking oral contraceptives. The authors conclude that an increase in the permeability of the mammary epithelium was effected by changes related to ovulation. Perhaps the first acute change in composition is associated with the final stages of follicle maturation and the second with the regression of the corpus luteum during the ovulatory menstrual cycle (Figs. 20-5 and 20-6).

Breastfeeding and birth interval

Data collected where women practice more intensive breastfeeding show more prolonged lactational amenorrhea as a result of more prolonged total breastfeeding.[55] Nutritional status has virtually no effect on amenorrhea, except in the extremes. In a study of Guatemalan women, maternal energy supplements did not shorten length of lactational amenorrhea; however, supplementing their breastfed infant did shorten amenorrhea by reducing suckling. A difference exists between postpartum and nutritional amenorrhea: *true nutritional amenorrhea* is predictable on the basis of the height/weight ratio; lactational amenorrhea is hormonal, and when it occurs, nutrition has only a trivial role.[34,55]

Among !Kung hunter-gatherers, long intervals pass between births, which has puzzled investigators because the tribes are well nourished, have low fetal wastage, and do not employ contraceptives or prolonged abstinence. The !Kung eat only what

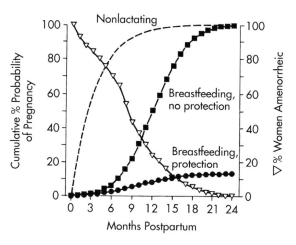

Figure 20-5. Cumulative probability of pregnancy during breastfeeding. ———, Nonlactating women of normal fertility having unprotected intercourse; ■, breastfeeding women having unprotected intercourse throughout 24 months of lactation; ●, breastfeeding women having unprotected intercourse only during lactational amenorrhea and adopting effective contraceptive measures at resumption of menstruation. Percentage of women in lactational amenorrhea by month post partum (▽) is also shown. (From Short RY, Lewis PR, Renfree MB, et al: Contraceptive effects of extended lactational amenorrhoea: Beyond the Bellagio consensus. Lancet 337:715, 1991.)

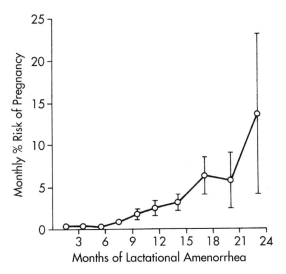

Figure 20-6. Monthly percentage probability of pregnancy during lactational amenorrhea with estimated standard errors. With cumulative percentage probability of pregnancy by months post partum for these three groups of women, 50% of nonlactating women would be pregnant in less than 3 months, and 85% would be pregnant by 6 months. (From Short RY, Lewis PR, Renfree MB, et al: Contraceptive effects of extended lactational amenorrhoea: Beyond the Bellagio consensus. Lancet 337:715, 1991.)

they hunt and gather. They have no agriculture. They are lean, spare people. They have late menarche (about 16 years of age), first pregnancy at age 18, and early menopause at about 40, leaving 24 reproductive years during which they produce 4.4 children, which, with some perinatal deaths, exactly replaces their society. This compares with industrial society, where productive years begin at 11 and end at 51. Konner and Worthman[54] report that the !Kung have unusual temporal patterns of nursing characterized by highly frequent nursing bouts with short space between nursings. The !Kung nurse several times an hour with only 15 minutes at most between bouts, which last only 15 to 120 seconds each. Serum estradiol and progesterone levels are correspondingly low. Infants are always in the immediate proximity of their mothers

until they are weaned, at about 3½ years, during a new sibling's gestation.

In Nigeria the effect of duration and frequency of breastfeeding on postpartum amenorrhea is comparable in that Nigerians breastfeed for 16.5 months with a frequency of 4.5 times a day. The mean length of amenorrhea is 12.5 months. Amenorrheic mothers who were lactating had lower levels of serum estradiol and lactic dehydrogenase (LDH). A significant association was seen between hyperprolactinemia with amenorrhea. The incidence of amenorrhea declined parallel to that of the hyperprolactinemia.[23]

When fertility post partum during lactation was studied in Edinburgh, suckling was the most important factor inhibiting the return to ovulation.[80] Suckling duration was the first factor to discriminate the mothers who experienced early ovulation. Those mothers who ovulated while breastfeeding had all introduced two or more supplementary feeds per day and had reduced suckling to under six times a day, with 60 minutes or less suckling time per day. The basal prolactin levels were below 600 µU/L. The mothers who did not ovulate until after 40 weeks post partum breastfed longest, suckled most intensely, maintained night feeds longest, and introduced supplementary feeds most slowly.[43] The prolactin levels remained substantially above 600 µU/L.

Suckling disrupts the normal pulsatile pattern of hypothalamic Gn-RH secretion which causes a reduction in LH secretion from the pituitary. Because FSH returns to its normal cyclic pattern early in lactation, ovarian follicles may develop. But until suckling declines, the follicles fail to secrete enough estradiol to cause a LH surge and ovulation. In addition, there is little evidence to support a role for nutrition in this paradigm.[71]

Another review of the effects of hormonal contraceptives on lactation by Hull[45] concludes that a significant number of reports indicate decrease in milk yield. The description of severe growth failure[34] in the nursling, even leading to "contraceptive marasmus," in Egypt and Tunisia is cause for concern.

Most large studies of birth interval and its relationship to method of feeding have been conducted in developing countries. However, Rosner and Schulman[89] reported on 112 Orthodox Jewish women from metropolitan New York with 266 birth experiences. The women strictly adhered to biblical and Rabbinic law that prohibits birth control. They were well-nourished, middle-class, educated women who breastfed on demand (210 infants) for a mean duration of 10.7 months, with 177 of the infants receiving formula less than once a week. Significant positive correlations were found with duration of lactational amenorrhea, which increased as duration of breastfeeding increased. Delay in starting solids, continuation of night feedings, and postponement of other liquid feeds all were associated with prolongation of birth interval. The investigators found a longer mean duration of lactational amenorrhea (8.6 months) and mean birth interval (22 months) than other studies because of the more intensive feeding patterns (Table 20-2).[89]

Lactational amenorrhea method

The Bellagio Consensus Conference[21] on breastfeeding as a family-planning method established that a mother who is fully or nearly fully breastfeeding her infant and remains amenorrheic will have more than 98% protection from pregnancy in the first 6 months post partum.[19,48] In a large prospective study of duration of lactational anovulation and amenorrhea in well-nourished Australian women—members of the Nursing Mothers' Association of Australia who breastfed for a long time—Short and associates[95] found that breastfeeding alone is not an effective form of contraception because all the women resumed ovulation while still breastfeeding. They compared breastfeeding women who had unprotected sex with breastfeeding women who had unprotected sex only during lactational amenorrhea and adopted other contraceptive measures after resumption of menstruation. Only 1.7% became pregnant during the first 6 months of amenorrhea, only 7% after 12 months, and 13% after 24 months.[83] Only one woman in a study of 422 middle-class urban women in Chile became pregnant using the lactational amenorrhea method (LAM) as the only method of pregnancy avoidance in the first 6 months,[26,50] a protective rate of 99.5% (see Figs. 20-5 and 20-6).

TABLE 20-2 **Comparison of studies of breastfeeding and its relationship to birth interval when practiced in absence of birth control**

Study	Mean duration of breastfeeding (mo)	Mean lactational amenorrhea (mo)	Mean birth interval (mo)
Bonte and van Balen[10]	N/A	15.2	25.2
Berman et al[8]	7.0	7.1	21.6
Prema et al[85]	19.8	11.1	23.8
Perez[82]*	4.0	3.03†	N/A
Gioiosa[36]	10.27	N/A	21.92
Rosner and Schulman[89]	10.74	8.56	21.95
Adnan and Bakr[3]	36.0	12.0	N/A
Howie et al[43]	10.0	8.1	N/A
Ojofeitimi[80]	16.5	12.5	N/A

N/A. Not available
*Women did introduce family planning after menses return or after supplementation after 6 months.
†First postpartum ovulation.
Modified from Rosner AE, Schulman SK: Birth interval among breastfeeding women not using contraceptives. Pediatrics 86:747, 1990.

Although it has long been recognized that breastfeeding has an effect on fertility, the mechanism is only beginning to be explored. The use of LAM for child spacing is based on the natural infertility associated with lactation, especially during the early months post partum, which are associated with frequent around-the-clock suckling.[53] Infertility is the result of hormonal suppression during lactation.[105]

Menses as an indicator of ovulation has been studied with data collected not only on onset of menses but on urinary hormone assays. Among women who menstruated before 6 months post partum, 67% of cycles were anovulatory, and the lag between anovular first menses and subsequent ovulation was 15.7 weeks.[31] On the other hand, after 6 months post partum, the proportion of anovular first menses declined to 22%, and the lag to ovulation declined to 7.3 weeks. Comparing all menstrual episodes, the mean interval between first observed menses and ovulation was 8.4 weeks the first 6 months and only 0.1 week after 6 months post partum.

A significant distinction should be made between token breastfeeding with early solids and more rigid feeding schedules and the ad lib breastfeeding around the clock with no solids until the infant is 6 months old. The amount and frequency of sucking are closely related to the continued amenorrhea in most women. When a totally breastfed infant sleeps through the night at an early age, requiring no suckling for 6 hours or so at night, the suppressive effect on menses diminishes. It has also been shown that if the infant uses a pacifier rather than receiving nonnutritive sucking at the breast, the suppression of ovulation is diminished.[64]

The degree of fertility inhibition associated with breastfeeding has decreased remarkably since the time of hunter-gatherers, cautions Diaz.[27] She points out that fertility rates vary; population and socioeconomic factors, urbanization, and nutrition all influence not only breastfeeding patterns but associated ovarian quiescence. Lactational amenorrhea can provide protection against pregnancy for the first 6 months even in well-nourished women who are giving the infant some supplemental foods (Fig. 20-7).[56-61]

For women who practice LAM, the efficacy is remarkably good (Table 20-3). Table 20-4 details the reestablishment of menses in breastfeeding women using LAM. *Bellagio and Beyond: Breastfeeding and LAM in Reproductive Health* was published as a final report in 1997 of the many years of work worldwide involving the use of LAM.[21] It was concluded that the efficacy of LAM is well established in prospective studies. Policy support is still needed to institute an additional method that increases the family-planning choices of postpartum women.[20]

Gray and associates[38] studied a population of women in Baltimore in comparison to a group from Manila. Those in the Baltimore group were older, more educated, and more frequently employed and had fewer children. Women in Manila breastfed more frequently (at 10 weeks post partum: 11.4 feeds in Manila versus 7.1 feeds in Baltimore). The mean duration of amenorrhea was 31.7 weeks versus 26.3 weeks, and mean delays before first ovulation were 38 versus 27 weeks (Manila versus Baltimore). The frequency of suckling episodes was most strongly associated with ovulation in the Baltimore population, where small declines in breastfeeding were sufficient to permit the return of ovarian activity. Women in Manila, in contrast, maintained high suckling rates even when solids were introduced. More Baltimore women (49%) than Manila women (31%) ovulated before 6 months. There was no simple algorithm, however, to predict ovulation.[35]

The effects of age at introduction of complementary foods to breastfed infants on duration of lactational amenorrhea in Honduran women were reported by Dewey and associates.[25] Introducing foods at 4 months significantly affected the likelihood of amenorrhea at 6 months but not thereafter. This effect was not seen, however, if breastfeeding frequency was maintained. The most significant determination of lactational amenorrhea was time spent breastfeeding (minutes per day), which was negatively associated with the infant's energy intake from complementary foods.

Ask the mother:

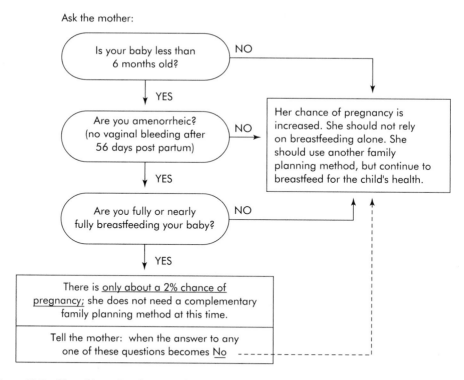

Figure 20-7. Use of lactational amenorrhea method (LAM) for child spacing during first 6 postpartum months.

TABLE 20-3 Life table analysis of lactational amenorrhea method (LAM) efficacy*

Month	No. of pregnancies	WM	WMAC	R × 100	P × 100
1	0	384	384	0.00	0.00
2	0	327	711	0.00	0.00
3	0	272	983	0.00	0.00
4	0	243	1226	0.00	0.00
5	0	224	1450	0.00	0.00
6	1	221	1671	0.45	0.45

WM, Number of women using LAM; WMAC, cumulative women-months of use; R × 100, monthly risk of conception; P × 100, cumulative risk of conception.
*Characteristics of women: Mean age (SEM, range) was 27.1 years (5.0, 18 to 39). Mean parity (SEM, range) was 2.0 (1.0, 1 to 5). 23.6% of the women had primary education, and only 5.4% had completed university studies.
From Perez A, Labbok MH, Queenan JT: Clinical study of the lactational amenorrhoea method for family planning. Lancet 339:968, 1992.

TABLE 20-4   Life table of reestablishment of menses among exclusively breastfeeding women using lactational amenorrhea method (LAM)*

Month	Bleeding	WM	WMAC	R × 100	P × 100
1	0	384	384	0.00	0.00
2	8	327	711	2.45	2.42
3	18	272	983	6.62	8.67
4	11	243	1226	4.55	12.72
5	10	224	1450	4.46	16.53
6	6	221	1671	2.73	18.78

WM, Number of women using LAM; WMAC, cumulative women-months of use; R × 100, monthly bleeding risk; P × 100, cumulative risk of bleeding.
*Characteristics of women: mean age (SEM, range) was 27.1 years (5.0, 18 to 39); mean parity (SEM, range) was 2.0 (1.0, 1 to 5); 23.6% of women had primary education, and only 5.4% had completed university studies.
From Perez A, Labbok MH, Queenan JT: Clinical study of the lactational amenorrhoea method for family planning. Lancet 339:968, 1992.

CONTRACEPTION DURING LACTATION

Natural family planning

Although lactation provides protection early in the postpartum period, a woman who is not exclusively breastfeeding around the clock and who is seriously concerned about avoiding conception should be informed of her options. If she does not want to use contraceptives—medications or devices—she should be instructed in the external signs of ovulation. Most studies of lactation indicate that the initial menses occurs before the onset of adequate ovulation and the luteal phase. The risk of pregnancy during lactational amenorrhea, however, in the first 6 months is less than 1% when LAM is combined with the basal thermal method or secretion surveillance. Unplanned pregnancy rates rise among breastfeeders after menses return compared with the rates for those who use thermal or secretion surveillance methods when not lactating. The increased pregnancy rate was related to poor compliance and understanding of the "rules" of the method.[39]

The *symptothermal method* of fertility awareness during lactation was studied in Canada.[81]

A special postpartum chart was designed to record morning temperature, cervical mucus, and other signs of fertility/infertility in relation to dates and postpartum days. The intensity of the breastfeeding was also recorded. There were 54 breastfeeding experiences in 47 women whose ages ranged from 20 to 39. Parity ranged from 1 to 7 with an average of 3.3. The duration of full breastfeeding averaged 3.6 months (range 3 weeks to 8 months). The duration of partial breastfeeding ranged from 2 to 28 months with an average of 8.8 months. These mothers found that in general they could predict their fertile times with accuracy while breastfeeding. During times of weaning or change in suckling pattern, special caution was suggested during which the mothers watched for signs of first ovulation.

The effectiveness of periodic abstinence for lactating women shows that long periods of lactational infertility can be identified by either lack of mucus or continuous unchanging mucus flow.

Cervical mucus accepts, filters, prepares, and releases sperm for successful transport to the egg for fertilization. The advancing sperm must penetrate the mucous structure or the small interstices between the mucous macromolecules. The interstices are largest in the periovulatory phase of the menstrual cycle.[88] As ovulation resumes, irregular mucous patterns that are difficult to interpret occur and therefore require prolonged abstinence. A pregnancy rate with this method was 9.1 per 100 women-years. Because two thirds of the 82 women studied were totally breastfeeding, many of the ensuing postpartum cycles may have been anovulatory or had an inadequate luteal phase, thus helping to keep the pregnancy rate low.

Studies of cervical secretions alone (mucous patterns) during lactation have indicated that the same signs in mucus are reliable during lactation. Charting is carried out in the usual manner, and feedings are also recorded. A woman who is following her pattern post partum should be seen every 2 weeks for guidance until her pattern is well documented. The couple should make careful observations of when (1) the infant sleeps through the night, (2) the mother reduces the number of breastfeedings, (3) the infant begins solid foods, (4) the infant begins other liquids or a bottle, and (5) illness occurs in either mother or baby. Abstinence is advised until the situation is clear. If there has been no prior ovulation or menstruation when weaning begins, ovulation may occur quite quickly.[14]

Figure 20-8 illustrates temperature, mucus, and cervical assessments during lactation.

Although contraceptive methods such as barrier methods and "the pill" have a statistically better record in avoiding pregnancy, that is a moot point for the woman for whom these methods are not an option for religious, ethical, moral, or medical grounds.[4] It is therefore important that the clinician be as well informed about natural child spacing as possible so the best advice can be provided. Ideally, the woman has used natural family planning before the pregnancy, so she is familiar with her own patterns, but it is more urgent that she knows how to check her mucus, her cervix, and her temperature and is not trying to learn about her fertility signs during lactation. Natural-family-planning programs across the United States are gaining experience with lactating women using the ovulation method and are available to assist lactating women. Further information can be obtained from the National Office of Natural Family Planning, 8514 Bradmoor Drive, Bethesda, MD 20817-3810, (301) 897-9323, if no local office is available; www.boma-usa.org and www.teenstar.org are the Web sites for the Billings Ovulation Method Association, USA.

In a carefully designed study conducted in Chile by Perez[82] at the Pontificia Universidad Católica de

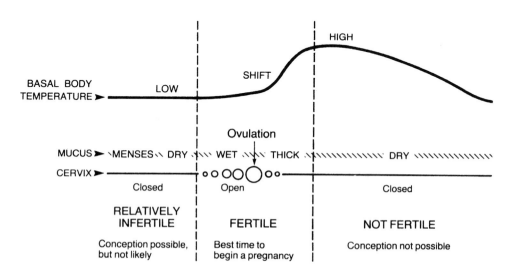

Figure 20-8. Temperature, mucus, and cervical assessments during lactation to identify ovulation. (Courtesy of National Family Planning of Rochester, New York.)

Chile Department of Obstetrics and Gynecology and by members of the faculty at Johns Hopkins University School of Hygiene and Public Health, 419 postpartum women were enrolled in the Natural Family Planning Program and taught the method and how to record their observations. The purpose was to define cervical mucus patterns in relation to time since delivery, time of first bleed, frequency of feeding, introduction of supplements and solid foods, and time of weaning. The diaries of 110 women with detailed records were selected for critical evaluation. Forty-nine have been reported and the preliminary observations evaluated by Barker.[4] Two characteristics of mucus (sensation and observation) were charted each day along with the women's breastfeeding pattern. Only seven women had used natural family planning previously. No woman menstruated before 4 months post partum, when 10% did have first menses. Fifty percent of the women detected mucus by the fourth month, and not until the seventh month had 50% had first menses. Mucus was observed about 2 months before first menses. As women moved from total breastfeeding to partial and to complete weaning, the duration of episodes of mucus increased. Duration of mucus approached normal on weaning.

Rural women exposed to a breastfeeding education program prenatally and postpartum breastfed more and used fewer bottles than the comparison group, who had no training about lactational infertility.[92] However, no difference was seen in postpartum amenorrhea. No measures of ovulation or pregnancy were made. Rural women tend to breastfeed optimally naturally.

The natural suppression of ovulation during early lactation and the concomitant amenorrhea induced by exclusive or nearly exclusive breastfeeding provide 98% or higher protection against pregnancy. Three conditions are necessary: amenorrhea, intensive breastfeeding day and night, and up to 6 months of exclusive breastfeeding post partum. LAM can be used to time the introduction of any complementary method (barrier, etc.) (Fig. 20-9); it is not just for users of natural family planning.

Touch sensitivity and ovulation

In search of a simple method of identifying ovulation during lactation, Drife[30] measured urinary pregnanediol and estrogen and breast sensitivity in six breastfeeding and six bottle feeding normal women. Two-point discrimination and touch sensitivity were measured. The mean duration of amenorrhea among breastfeeders was 24.3 weeks (range 14 to 35 weeks) and among bottle feeders 7.5 weeks (range 6 to 14 weeks). Findings, however, were not diagnostic of ovulation. Touch sensitivity tended to decrease as lactation progressed over months. The change is so gradual and difficult to detect that it has no practical value in determining ovulation.[30]

Oral contraceptives and lactation

The significant issues related to lactation and the use of oral contraceptives are the potentially adverse effects of oral contraceptives on milk production, uterine involution, and growth and development of the breastfed infant.[79] Curtis[22] reported a single case of breast enlargement in a breastfed male infant whose mother began taking norethynodrel with ethinyl estradiol 3-methyl ether (Enovid) on the third day post partum. Breast enlargement began on the third week of life. The mother had noted her milk was not as "rich" and started supplements the second week. Nursing was discontinued at about 4 weeks of age, and the breasts of the infant returned to normal in 2 to 3 weeks. The additional risks to the mother of thromboembolism, hypertension, and cancer have also been discussed extensively in the literature. These occurred with the early high-dose products.

The data on oral contraceptives available have been well reviewed by Vorherr.[103,104] He summarizes the information by noting that preparations containing 2.5 mg or less of a 19-norprogestogen and 50 µg or less of ethinyl estradiol or 100 µg or less of mestranol present no hazard to mother or infant. He further points out that milk yield can be decreased with larger doses of combination oral contraceptives containing estrogen and 5 to 10 mg of progestogen per dose. Only two studies of many suggest any variation

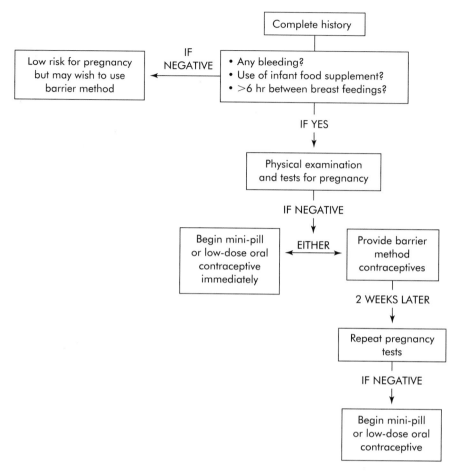

Figure 20-9. Algorithm for initiating contraceptive treatment in a breastfeeding woman. (See references 56, 57, and 69.) (Modified from Winikoff B, Semeraro P, Zimmerman M: Contraception during Breastfeeding: A Clinician's Source Book. New York, Population Council, 1988; Labbok M: Breastfeeding and contraception. N Engl J Med 308:51, 1983.)

in the content of the milk (protein, fat, and calcium) resulting from oral contraceptives.[91,96]

Toddywalla and associates[100] reported the effect of injectable contraceptives as well as oral combinations on milk production. They found an increase in the protein content of the milk and a slight increase in quantity from the group given injection of 150 mg of medroxyprogesterone (Depo-Provera) every 3 months. The group receiving 300 mg of medroxyprogesterone every 6 months showed significant increase in quantity but a decrease in

protein, fat, and calcium as compared with control subjects (who used mechanical means of contraception).[96] The secretion of hormones in human milk is poorly documented, with only a few infants studied in each hormone combination.[18] In all cases, a small but measurable amount was found in the milk. Unfortunately, measurements in the infant's serum are not reported.

The impact of the distribution of oral contraceptives on breastfeeding and pregnancy status in rural Haiti indicated that it did not alter breastfeeding patterns in women who began the pills at 8 to 9 months post partum.[11] Pregnancy prevalence also decreased as a result.[109]

Studies of pregestin-only pills (POP) beginning at 6 weeks post partum showed that POP does not suppress gonadotropins nor does it affect ovarian follicular development. The contraceptive effect is believed mediated through local actions of the endometrium and cervix as in normally menstruating women.[84]

Implants and injections

The recommendation for contraceptive use during lactation is the progestin-only products (Norplant System, Depo-Provera injections and minipills, progestin once-only pills). Use of these methods has not been associated with adverse effects on infant growth or development and may even increase the volume of milk (Table 20-5).[2,68,106,107]

In a study of the effects of levonorgestre (LNG) (Norplant) in breast milk on thyroid activity, Bassol and associates compared infants of mothers with the implant and those of women assigned to IUD use, the hormones (LNG) in the breast milk significantly decreased the infants TSH levels at 3 months and lower at 6 months of age.[5] The higher the LNG levels, the lower the TSH in the infant. It is recommended that the progestin-only method not be initiated until 6 weeks post partum on the premise that the theoretic danger to the infant from exogenous steroids has passed by this time. The practice of injecting Depo-Provera immediately after delivery can interfere with the establishment of lactation, which is dependent upon the dramatic natural decline in progesterone post partum.

Steroids are not bound well in plasma and not well conjugated by the liver or excreted by the immature kidneys of the neonate. Exogenous hormones may compete for receptor sites with natural ones in the liver, brain, or other tissues. As the infant's liver and kidneys mature, these issues disappear.[49] Medications that also contain estrogen suppress milk production.[108] With the many alternatives available, it should never be necessary to discontinue breastfeeding to initiate contraception.[47]

The growth and development of breastfed infants whose mothers received implants of Norplant

TABLE 20-5   Effects of contraceptive agents on milk yield and infant development

Agent	Milk yield	Effect on infant
Combined estrogen/progestin	Moderate inhibitory effect Shorter breastfeeding Milk concentration unchanged Small amount of steroid in milk	Slower weight gain No long-term effects
Progestin only Minipill (Micronor, Nory-D) Other products	No effect on volume No effect on duration	No effect on weight gain No reported long-term effects
Injectable depot medroxy-progesterone acetate (DMPA), Depo-Provera and norethindrone enanthate (NET-EN, NORIS-TERAT)	Breastfeeding lasts longer ? Change in milk: protein increased, fat decreased Steroid present in milk	No long-term effects
Norplant System	No effect Small amount of steroid in milk	Normal growth No long-term effects
Vaginal rings containing natural hormone progesterone	No significant differences	No effect on growth Long-term effects under study

Modified from Winikoff B. Semeraro P. Zimmerman M: Contraception during Breastfeeding: A Clinician's Source Book. New York. Population Council, 1987.

containing levonorgestrel or injections of norethindrone enanthate were studied and compared with those whose mothers used intrauterine devices (IUDs).[42] The breastfeeding performance was similar. The infants were also similar in growth rate, development, and general health. Similarly, a group of mothers were given a vaginal ring that released 10 mg of "natural" progesterone every 24 hours, producing a maternal serum level of 4 ng/mL, which results in only a minimal amount in the milk and which is not absorbed by the infant gut. These infants also had normal growth and development and remained in good health.[94]

Ovulation method, luteinizing hormone releasing hormone, and home tests

Pregnancy rates and fertility-related behavior of users of the *ovulation method* (OM) were studied prospectively in Kenya and Chile in two groups of breastfeeding women.[61] The rate of unplanned pregnancy was less than 1% in the first 6 months. The rate of unplanned pregnancies increased once menses had begun and supplementary food was added to the infant's diet. The rates were compared with the rates among nonlactating women who were also using ovulation method (OM) to avoid pregnancy. The breastfeeding women had followed the method closely, although clients who had not used OM before the pregnancy had an increased incidence of unplanned pregnancy.

Risk of ovulation during lactation was studied by Gray and associates[37] in Baltimore and in Manila. During the first 6 months post partum, amenorrheic women had a low risk of ovulation (below 10%) with a partial breastfeeding and a 1% to 5% risk with exclusive breastfeeding with either frequent short feeds or infrequent longer feeds. This would have resulted in a pregnancy rate of 2% and 1%, respectively.

One of the difficulties of studying the use/effectiveness and continuation of natural-family-planning methods is that terms have always been imprecise and markers have been different between studies.[90] The method is very effective when properly used

(failure rate 3.4%) but unforgiving when use is imperfect (failure rate 84.2% in the first year).[46]

Luteinizing hormone releasing hormone (LH-RH) agonist for contraception has also been tested in nine fully breastfeeding women beginning 6 weeks post partum. They received 300 μg LH-RH agonist (buserelin) intranasally once a day for the duration of their breastfeeding. Urinary excretion of LH, estrone, and pregnanediol was compared with that of nine control breastfeeding women. No ovulation occurred in the treated group, and seven of the nine untreated control subjects had one to six ovulations. LH-RH has potential as a safe, acceptable method of contraception while breastfeeding, according to Fraser and associates.[33]

Home tests to monitor fertility are available; however, women must be tested during lactation and especially during the transition period when breastfeeding frequency and feeding duration are changing. Ovarian follicular dynamics can be accurately monitored through the noninstrumented analysis of daily estrone conjugates in urine samples at home.[63] Readings can be affected by urine osmolarity, either high or low, giving false positive or false negative results, respectively. Controlling intake of fluids would guard against this.

Two algorithms for initiating contraceptive treatment are illustrated in Figures 20-7 and 20-9.

Intrauterine devices and other contraceptive methods

Various alternatives to oral contraceptives do exist and have different degrees of reliability. The IUDs (95% to 98% effective), cervical caps and diaphragms (85% to 88% effective), condoms (80% to 85% effective), and vaginal suppositories, jellies, or creams (80% effective) have no known contraindication during breastfeeding, because no chemicals are absorbed. The only contraceptive that is 100% effective is abstinence.

A study of 2271 postpartum women who had IUDs inserted between 1976 and 1981 and were followed for 6 to 12 months was reported with careful attention to details of lactation.[17] Data were analyzed separately for IUDs inserted immediately after birth (within 10 minutes of placental expulsion). The results of this analysis indicate that IUD insertion for breastfeeding women would be appropriate either immediately after delivery or later (42 days or more post partum). When inserted immediately post partum, the delta loop and delta T were modified by adding projections of chromic sutures, which help the device remain in the uterus. The sutures biodegrade in 6 weeks, leaving a standard device in place. These authors report that breastfeeding is not a contraindication to IUD insertion, with no increased expulsion rate.[42] Conversely, the presence of an IUD has no adverse effect on lactation. The appropriate time for insertion should be selected to predate anticipated ovulation but guarantee patient compliance. A study showed that the use of the TCu-380A IUD in breastfeeding women resulted in fewer insertion-related complaints and lower removal rates for bleeding and pain over 12 months post partum than in nonbreastfeeders. No intrauterine perforations were reported in either group.[32] Copper IUDs are usually smaller, so there is little problem with the effects of let-down on the uterus.

A group of 32 women hospitalized for uterine perforation necessitating transperitoneal IUD removal and a matched control group of 497 women who had worn IUDs uneventfully were compared.[41] Of the women in the study, 97% were post partum compared with 68% of the control subjects. Of the parous study group, 42% were lactating, and of the parous control subjects, 7% were lactating when the IUD was inserted. The risk of perforation was 10 times greater in the lactating than in the nonlactating women, unrelated to time of the insertion post partum. In another group hospitalized for difficult transcervical IUD removal, the risk was 2.3 times greater for lactating women. The authors recommend caution, not abandonment of the procedure, during lactation, because they believe the IUD is the best form of artificial contraception during lactation. Because of problems with the Dalkon shield, IUDs were generally unavailable in the United States in 1986 and 1987, although in other parts of the world they were still in use. In 1989 a copper-T device became available again. The ideal candidate is a woman who wants

reversible contraception to space births or limit size of the family, especially breastfeeding parous women in a monogamous relationship.

The Technical Guidance/Competence Group of the United States Agency for International Development (USAID) and World Health Organization (WHO)[99] recommends IUD insertion immediately post partum as soon as the placenta is removed, whether by vaginal or cesarean delivery. They point out it must be done by a specially trained physician. From 10 minutes to 48 hours after delivery, however, the expulsion rate is high. If this window of opportunity is missed or no urgency exists, it is best to wait. Although immediate insertion is possible, a copper-T device may be safely inserted 4 or more weeks post partum in breastfeeding women. Using the withdrawal technique minimizes the risk of perforation. Other IUDs should not be inserted until 6 weeks post partum.

Use of *barrier* and *spermicidal products* are alternative contraceptive methods during early lactation before hormonal methods or IUDs are introduced. These coital-dependent methods have no effect on lactation. The lubrication provided by the spermicidally treated condoms have the advantage of contributing lubrication when the hypoestrogenic vagina is exceptionally dry in association with lactation. A spermicide is more effective with a condom but is adequate early post partum, when relative infertility is present. A *diaphragm* cannot be adequately fitted for 6 to 8 weeks post partum, so it is not recommended during this period with or without lactation.

Abstinence

Many cultures and societies place taboos on sexual intercourse for the nursing mother as an effective means of spacing children. Usually there are no medical contraindications to sexual relationships during lactation. In a study on contraceptive use in the United States, Ford and Labbok[35] reported that among white women, 34% were not sexually active in the first month post partum, 12.5% in the second month, and 4.3% during the third month. Among black women in the survey, 25% were not sexually active in the first month, 8.1% the second, and 4.2% the third. Contraceptive use among those sexually active was absent in 16% in the first postpartum month and 12.2% and 13.8%, respectively, in the second and the third postpartum months among whites. Among blacks, 27.3% used no method the first month, and 22.7% and 22.3%, respectively, used no method the second and third months.

SEX AND THE NURSING MOTHER

Sexual arousal associated with suckling

If one examines the normal adult female in regard to the menstrual cycle, sexual intercourse, pregnancy, childbirth, and lactation, one observes that these events are all influenced by the interaction of the same hormones—not only estrogen, progesterone, testosterone, FSH, and LH, but oxytocin and prolactin as well. The breast is known to respond during all these phases, enlarging before menstruation, during pregnancy, before orgasm, and during lactation. The nipples also respond during these phases. Furthermore, the uterus contracts during childbirth, orgasm, and lactation. Body temperature rises during ovulation, childbirth, orgasm, and lactation. As pointed out in Chapter 3, *oxytocin* is a critical element in the let-down reflex during lactation. Oxytocin levels also rise during orgasms and labor, and oxytocin causes the uterus to contract and the nipples to become erect. Newton and Newton[76] report other similarities, including sensory perception and emotional reactions, in women during these events. The psychophysiologic similarities between lactation and coitus are as follows:

1. The uterus contracts.
2. The nipples become erect.
3. Breast stroking and nipple stimulation occur.
4. The emotions experienced involve skin changes (vascular dilatation and raised temperature).
5. Milk let-down (or ejection) reflex can be triggered.

6. The emotions experienced may be closely allied.
7. An accepting attitude toward sexuality may be related to an accepting attitude to breastfeeding (and vice versa).

Women also report hot flashes in association with some feeds, especially at night. This phenomenon has been studied by Marshall and associates,[66] who looked at oxytocin effect. Initiation of breastfeeding was accompanied by an increase in skin conductance resulting in increased skin temperature, especially of the breast. The pattern is similar to menopausal hot flashes.

Given the biologic and hormonal similarities of lactation to the other events in the sexual cycle of the adult female, it is not surprising that some women experience some form of sexual gratification during suckling on certain occasions. In a study of 111 parturient women, only 24 of whom breastfed, Masters and Johnson[67] reported that sexual arousal was experienced during suckling on some occasions. The exact incidence of this response is unknown, but it is believed to be uncommon. Nursing mothers may have an element of guilt surrounding these experiences and underreport. That guilt may lead to early weaning in some cases. For some women, the breasts are highly erogenous. The handling and manipulation of the breast necessary during lactation by both mother and infant can, in the right but unpremeditated circumstances, be stimulating. Clearly, the majority of women who enjoy breastfeeding have no feelings or responses to the stimulation of the breast that could be construed as sexual arousal, although they enjoy breastfeeding and the intimacy with their infant that it provides.

The erotic response to nursing the infant has no significance in terms of being normal or abnormal. The decline of breastfeeding because of feelings of shame, modesty, embarrassment, and distaste has been reported by Bentovin[7] and interpreted as indicating that breastfeeding is viewed as a forbidden sexual activity. For such women, any sexual allusions and excitement accompanying breastfeeding are not permissible and cause shame. Such attitudes are more common in lower social groups and need to be considered in counseling mothers about breastfeeding prepartum or when premature weaning takes place. Major changes in the number of women who breastfeed may not be possible until society can accept the breast in its relationship to nurturing the infant and also as an object of less sexual ambivalence.

The sensuousness of breastfeeding has been the topic of discussion in popular women's magazines as more has been written about women and their bodies. For the well-educated, well-read woman who breastfeeds her infant because she intellectually arrives at the decision, such discussions are an avenue of increased knowledge. Others may still be uncomfortable about breastfeeding if it is apt to be "pleasurable." The physician may sense this discomfort in a patient prenatally by her responses to bodily change during pregnancy. Cultural attitudes are an important part of this response and are deeply ingrained in an individual by the time she reaches the age of parenting. Professionals need to be sensitive to the patient and cautious about imposing cultural change on a patient while still being alert to needs for information and openness. A woman who experiences any erogenous reaction to breastfeeding, especially with an older child who may inadvertently roll the nipple while feeding, should not be criticized, but the phenomenon should be explained and discussed openly by the physician.

Sexual activity of the nursing mother

A review of the limited data available on lactating women in the Masters and Johnson study[67] does indicate that in their group of 111 postpartum women, the nursing mothers were more eager than nonnursing mothers to resume sexual relations post partum. The data were independent of the fear of pregnancy. They report that this interest was apparent 2 to 3 weeks post partum. Individual reports through a questionnaire indicate that 30% of nursing mothers believed their sexual relationships were improved and 2.5% believed they were worse post partum. The individual testimonies of nursing mothers indicate they had a better feeling about

themselves as well as their relationships with their husbands and family in general. In a study of sexual behavior during pregnancy and lactation, Kenney[51] reported that the desire returned by 4 weeks for most women, long before they thought it was safe. The longer they had been married and the more children, the sooner the interest returned and the sooner they felt it was safe. No change in interest or enjoyment occurred with weaning.

In studies of recovery after childbirth, the longer duration of breastfeeding (more than 5 months) has been associated with a longer duration of awareness of perineal damage (dyspareunia) during intercourse and a longer amenorrheic period in some women.[2] High prolactin levels and decreased libido have also been observed in women with evidence of continued vaginal discomfort. In the clinical study of lactational amenorrhea in 422 women in Chile, however, Perez and associates[83] recorded the incidence of intercourse to be one to two times a week, beginning 4 weeks post partum.

The frequency of coitus during breastfeeding was studied in four sites: Birmingham, United Kingdom; Montreal, Canada; Sydney, Australia; and Manila, the Philippines. The frequency was lower than reported in other studies of married women, ranging from 4 to 30 episodes a month while averaging three to five times a month. Rates were not correlated with number of children but were related to maternal age, being slightly more frequent in younger women. The resumption of coital activity in these populations was more variable, with a median of 8 weeks post partum, with 75% resuming activities by the end of the third postpartum month. Thus "normal" encompasses a broad range, according to the authors.[101]

More general observations indicate that although some women may have increased interest in sexual relations while nursing, others may experience no interest at all for 6 months or so. Whether this results from the satiation of the mother's needs for intimate relationship and stimulus through nursing, general fatigue, or fear of pregnancy is debatable.[76] Sexual stimulus may trigger the ejection reflex, and milk ejection may have a negative effect on some men. A practical solution to spraying milk during lovemaking is feeding the infant or expressing some milk beforehand. The total knowledge of nursing and suckling as a biologic phenomenon will help couples understand such reactions and thus avoid inappropriate psychological responses.

The conflict in some adult men over their role in regard to the nursing mother's breasts is usually a result of guilt or upbringing. There is no need to advise against fondling the lactating breast during lovemaking, although physicians have often imposed rigid restrictions on sexual activity in the lactating woman. No scientific basis for such restriction exists, and no difference in the incidence of infection and mastitis is associated with such activity. Unusually restrictive protocols are often imposed on patients without medical indication. Bradley[12] recommends, in fact, oral and manual manipulation of the breasts by the husband during both pregnancy and lactation to prevent sore nipples.

It is helpful to discuss with the lactating woman that the hormonal effect on the vagina may be excessive dryness with an increase in dyspareunia. With the abrupt withdrawal of gonadotropins and ovarian hormones and elevation of prolactin at the time of delivery of the infant and placenta, the vaginal epithelium becomes thin and atrophic.[98] Normally the vagina and ectocervix are lined with stratified squamous epithelium, which is multilayered and protective. It is also very responsive to ovarian hormones. The greatest maturation and thickness occur around ovulation in response to peak estrogen secretion. During pregnancy, progesterone inhibits the maturation of the epithelial cells. The vaginal lining retains its thickness, but cells do not fully mature because the effect of progesterone overtakes the effect of estrogen on the epithelium and cervical mucus; both hormones are abundant during pregnancy.

The lowered ovarian hormones that cause vaginal dryness and lack of cervical mucus during lactation lead to discomfort during intercourse. The dryness responds to locally applied lubricants and tends to improve over time. A sudden change may actually reflect ovulation. The breast that is being stimulated by feeding frequently may not be as sensitive during lovemak-

ing. Usually this, too, is transient. The physician should perhaps remind the mother that some adjustment to attend to the father's needs may be necessary.

NURSING DURING PREGNANCY AND TANDEM NURSING

Pregnancy can and does occur while a woman is lactating. When it does occur, it produces a number of questions. There is no need to wean the first infant from the breast, which is often ordered by the physician. It is possible to lactate throughout pregnancy and then to have two infants at the breast post partum. This is now sufficiently common to be called *tandem nursing*.

The amount of nourishment provided the first infant at the breast depends on age and other supplements. When the infant at the breast is only a few months old when pregnancy occurs, there is some rationale to continue breastfeeding for the benefit of the infant until it is time to wean to solids and other liquids at 6 months of age or so. This child will be about a year old when the new infant arrives and, if still at the breast, may have demands in excess of the mother's ability to provide. Concern has been expressed that the older infant will take much of the nourishment needed by the new infant. In some societies, it is believed that a suckling infant will "take the spirit" from the newly conceived fetus; thus, weaning is mandated once pregnancy is confirmed in these communities.

The milk produced immediately post partum by the mother who never stopped nursing appears to be colostrum. The kangaroo has been observed to have a teat with mature milk for the older offspring and a teat for the new offspring who requires significantly different nourishment. Such a provision does not exist for the human. Mothers who want to maintain both infants at the breast have shown that it can be done without any apparent effect on the nourishment of the new infant. Counseling of such a mother should take into account the mother's resources to receive adequate rest, nourishment, and psychological support to withstand the added demand on her, physically and mentally.

If the first child is older and will be well beyond a year of age when the new infant arrives, the need for physical nourishment is minimal, and continuation at the breast is more for the security and psychological benefits. This is referred to as *comfort nursing* and may continue for several years (see Chapter 10). Abrupt weaning should be avoided, and consideration should be given to the impact of separation when the mother is confined during the birth of the new infant. This is an argument for 12-hour hospitalization for delivery for women who request it. The first few days of colostrum are most vital for the new infant, and the supply is not infinite; therefore, priorities need to be set concerning the older child. The new baby should be nursed first. Some older infants reject the colostrum.

The growth rate of children weaned during a subsequent pregnancy was compared with that of children weaned at the same age from nonpregnant mothers in a longitudinal study in Bhutan by Bohler and Bergstrom,[9] who followed 113 children closely for the first 3 years of life. The period of overlap for lactation and pregnancy was 5 months (median), increasing by 1 week for each month reduction in birth interval. When a child stopped breastfeeding during the mother's subsequent pregnancy, the growth rate was reduced during the last months before termination of breastfeeding compared with children weaned at the same age from nonpregnant mothers and with children who continued to breastfeed.

In a study of 503 La Leche League members, Newton and Theotokatos[77] reviewed breastfeeding during pregnancy practices and found that 69% of the breastfeeding children weaned spontaneously when the mother became pregnant. Many of the children may have been at an age to wean even without an intercurrent pregnancy.

Moscone and Moore[75] conducted a questionnaire survey of 57 women who were concurrently pregnant and breastfeeding. The main reasons given for continuing breastfeeding after conception involved the emotional needs of the breastfeeding child; 43% of the children continued to breastfeed throughout pregnancy and after birth of the sibling. The main reason for mother-initiated weaning was breast and nipple pain. When the child weaned during the pregnancy, it occurred during the second trimester and seemed to be associated with diminished milk production. Three pregnancies terminated in spontaneous abortions (a rate higher than in the general population, 5%). The ages of the children at onset of pregnancy varied from 4 to 42 months. The feeding pattern was one to eight times a day for less than 5 minutes to more than 30 minutes.

IMPACT OF NURSING DURING PREGNANCY

Among rural Guatemalan women who were part of a nutrition supplementation trial, 253 women of the 504 pregnancies had another pregnancy overlap while breastfeeding (50.2%); 41.4% of these concurrent pregnancy and lactation mothers continued to breastfeed into the second trimester and 3.2% into the third trimester. These "overlap" mothers received more supplements. The authors stated that overlap resulted in short recuperative periods (<6 months) requiring increased supplement intake and reduced maternal fat stores. The energetic stresses and short recovery time did not significantly affect fetal growth. It appeared the mother buffers the energy stress protecting fetal growth.[74]

Significant decreases in bone mineral density do occur during breastfeeding when calcium demands are the greatest. These changes are reversible and do not persist after a subsequent pregnancy according to Prentice, who has studied calcium utilization and reproduction related osteoporosis extensively. She indicates that extended periods of breastfeeding and closely spaced pregnancies are unlikely to have a lasting effect on bone mineral status and osteoporosis when the mother is healthy and well nourished. Although short birth intervals and breastfeeding during pregnancy further deplete fat stores in the malnourished mother, healthy well nourished women fare well and replenish their stores during a subsequent pregnancy.[74]

Infant health

Although pregnancy during lactation can cause flavor and volume changes that lead to early weaning, the milk still provides immunologic benefits. This is clearly demonstrated by Bohler among women in Bhutan where abrupt weaning caused diarrhea, stunted growth, illness, and even death. Work in India showed that overlapping breastfeeding and pregnancy in a malnourished mother produced growth retardation in the older child. Healthy infants in the United States derive significant nutritional and immunologic benefit in the second year and beyond, however. The risk to the nursling depends on child's age, other diet, and the amount of human milk available.

Fetal health

The nutritional status of the mother is key to adequate fetal growth. Varying results of fetal growth patterns are reported related to mother's nutritional status prior to pregnancy. A significant issue is viability of the pregnancy. Breastfeeding stimulus triggers oxytocin release and concern focuses on the potential for initiating uterine contractions and fetal loss. Studies of oxytocin sensitivities in pregnancy and the state of oxytocin receptors during early pregnancy is graphically illustrated in Figure 3-10. The uterus is very insensitive until close to 40 weeks in most women. It is well documented that nipple stimulation is as effective as intravenous pitocin for inducing labor at term.

Risk of fetal loss or preterm labor

Retrospective studies of fetal loss and preterm loss suggest that breast stimulus could be the source in some women. Regan, head of the Miscarriage Clinic in London, states that once a pregnancy is clinically detectable, breastfeeding should pose no added risk of pregnancy loss. She knows of no reason to link breastfeeding and miscarriage. Most obstetricians caution against sex during pregnancy in a woman with a history of fetal loss or premature birth. Breast stimulus is equally proscribed in such circumstances. Twin pregnancies and other multiples are considered high risk and weaning is usually recommended if the mother is nursing.

The stimulus is not exactly equal. In addition, the nursling will be nursing several times a day every day.

The decision to continue nursing when the new pregnancy is normal with no factors for a high-risk pregnancy should rest with the comfort level of the mother and child. The breast pain can be improved by wearing a supportive bra and repositioning during breastfeeding. The decrease in volume of milk is usually not remediable, but milk usually returns toward the end of pregnancy and is completely regenerated at delivery.[78]

In a study of 68 Peruvian women who breastfed during pregnancy and 65 who had not breastfed during the pregnancy, Marquis and associates reported that on day 2 post partum the breastfeeders had higher concentrations of lactose and lysozyme but lower lactoferrin than the nonbreastfeeders. At 1 month, IgA was lower among breastfeeders. The infants of the breastfeeders were five times as likely to have respiratory symptoms ($p < 0.05$) in these early weeks.[65]

Women who were 2 months pregnant and weaning their infant showed a progressive loss of secretory activity by the mammary gland seemingly due to an inhibition of milk secretion that overrides the stimulus provided by the infant. These results were compared to milk of women weaning without pregnancy.[86]

Many of the changes in child-rearing practices in recent years have increased the freedom and response to human needs. Carried to extremes, instant gratification becomes a right rather than a privilege. Sometimes a mother may need help in seeing that she need not feel guilty if she decides to wean the older child. If it is only an occasional feeding or suckling experience for added security, especially when security is threatened by the arrival of a new infant, it may be tolerable in terms of endurance for the mother, and she may agree willingly. When, however, continuing nursing becomes a strain or is painful or stressful, she should feel free to stop. When the mother feels real resentment toward the older child who is nursing, it is time to wean gently but firmly. If such a situation can be anticipated, it is probably easier for the older child to be weaned before delivery of the new infant.

Sore nipples are the most stressful symptom during pregnancy and may be the first sign of the new pregnancy as the hormonal milieu changes. There is no specific treatment, although having the toddler repositioned at the breast may ease the discomfort. If the toddler is old enough to understand, asking him or her to nurse more gently or "more softly" may help. The soreness may last for the first trimester or for the entire pregnancy until the new baby is born.

Decision: sorting out personal feelings

Little is in the medical literature about nursing during pregnancy and tandem nursing. The mother must make up her own mind if there are no medical contraindications. Much depends on the age of the child, the nursing pattern, and the nutritional and emotional needs of the child. Medical indications to wean during pregnancy are uterine bleeding, signs of preterm labor, or failure to gain enough weight during pregnancy.

Tandem nursing for some women is too much "touching" especially when the infant and toddler are a year or more apart in age. Nursing twins or triplets presents a similar situation for some mothers.

As with any such decisions to wean, it is best for the physician to work this out in frank discussion with the mother (and father, if available) so that any misgivings, resentment, or feeling of failure can be dealt with openly. Many patients automatically suspect the physician of being antagonistic to breastfeeding if the physician suggests weaning. Even when the reason is purely but urgently medical, discussion should be open and include options and alternatives and their risks. Weaning is part of the baby's growing up, but it is sometimes part of the mother's moving on as well.

While tandem nursing requires ordinary hygiene, it is usually not necessary to limit each child to one breast as infections or colds have spread before the first symptom. There are a few precautions. If one child has thrush, assigning one breast may keep it under control. If the older child develops a herpetic lesion or cold sore, he or she must not nurse. The newborn could acquire a potentially fatal herpes infection.

The dilemma of tandem nursing and weaning the older child has been dealt with in other societies with various manipulations, such as painting the breast with pepper or bitter herbs to make it taste terrible. The mother may leave the child with other caregivers. The provision of love and affection during this difficult adaptation for the child is what makes the difference between a traumatic occasion and a step toward growing up. Equally important is the provision of some opportunity for the mother to express her concerns and doubts during the process to her physician, who should be neither judgmental nor unduly rigid in the medical care plan.

Reading for parents

One book recommended for parents is *Adventures in Tandem Nursing (Breastfeeding During Pregnancy and Beyond)* by Hillary Flower, La Leche League International, Schaumburg, Illinois, 2003.

REFERENCES

1. Abdulla KA, Elwan S, Salem H, et al: Effect of early post-partum use of the contraceptive implants, Norplant(Rx), on the serum levels of immunoglobulins of the mothers and their breastfed infants. Contraception 32:261, 1985.
2. Abraham S, Child A, Ferry J, et al: Childbirth recovery. Med J Aust 152:9, 1990.
3. Adnan AM, Bakr SA: Postpartum lactational amenorrhoea as a means of family planning in the Sudan: A study of 500 cases. J Biosoc Sci 15:9, 1983.
4. Barker DC: Use of natural family planning by breastfeeding women. In Shivanandan M (ed): Breastfeeding and Natural Family Planning. Fourth International Symposium

on Natural Family Planning. Chevy Chase, MD, KM Associate Publishers, 1985.

5. Bassol S, Nava-Hernandez MP, Hernandez-Morales C, et al: Effects of levonorgestrel implant upon TSH and LH levels in male infants during lactation. Int J Gynaecol Obstet 76:273, 2002.

6. Beling CG, Frandsen VA, Josimovich JB: Pituitary and ovarian hormone levels during lactation. Acta Endocrinol 155(suppl):40, 1971.

7. Bentovin A: Shame and other anxieties associated with breastfeeding. In Ciba Foundation Symposium No. 45: Breastfeeding and the Mother. Amsterdam, Elsevier, 1976.

8. Berman ML, Hanson K, Hellman IL: Effect of breastfeeding on postpartum menstruation, ovulation and pregnancy on Alaskan Eskimos. Am J Obstet Gynecol 114:524, 1972.

9. Bohler E, Bergstrom S: Child growth during weaning depends on whether mother is pregnant again. J Trop Pediatr 42:104, 1996.

10. Bonte M, van Balen H: Prolonged lactation and family spacing in Rwanda. J Biosoc Sci 1:97, 1969.

11. Bordes A, Allman J, Verly A: The impact on breastfeeding and pregnancy status of household contraceptive distribution in rural Haiti. Am J Publ Health 72:835, 1982.

12. Bradley RA: Husband-Coached Childbirth. New York, 1965, Harper & Row, 1965.

13. Brambilla F, Sirtori CM: Gonadotropin-inhibiting factor in pregnancy, lactation and menopause. Am J Obstet Gynecol 109:599, 1971.

14. Brown RE: Breast-feeding and family planning: a review of relationships between breast-feeding and family planning. Am J Clin Nutr 35:162, 1982.

15. Buckley KM: Long-term breastfeeding: nourishment or nurturance? J Hum Lact 17:304, 2001.

16. Chayen B, Tejani N, Verma U: Induction of labor with an electric breast pump. J Reprod Med 31:116, 1986.

17. Cole LP, McCann MF, Higgins JE, et al: Effects of breast-feeding on IUD performance. Am J Publ Health 73:384, 1983.

18. Committee on Drugs, American Academy of Pediatrics: Breastfeeding and contraception. Pediatrics 68:138, 1981.

19. Consensus statement: Breastfeeding as a family planning method. Lancet 2:1204, 1988.

20. Cooney KA, Koniz-Booher P, Coly S: Taking the first steps: The lactational amenorrhea method, a decade of experience. Georgetown University, Washington, DC, Institute for Reproductive Health, 1977.

21. Cooney KA, Nahmias SR: Bellagio and beyond: Breastfeeding and LAM in reproductive health. Georgetown University, Washington, DC, Institute for Reproductive Health, 1997.

22. Curtis EM: Oral-contraceptive feminization of a normal male infant. Obstet Gynecol 23:295, 1964.

23. Delvoye P, Demaegd M, Nyampeta U, et al: Serum prolactin, gonadotropins, and estradiol in menstruating and amenorrheic mothers during two years' lactation. Am J Obstet Gynecol 130:635, 1978.

24. Dewey KG: Does maternal supplementation shorten the duration of lactational amenorrhea? Am J Clin Nutr 64:377, 1996.

25. Dewey KG, Cohen RJ, Rivera LL, et al: Effects of age at introduction of complementary foods to breast-fed infants on duration of lactational amenorrhea in Honduran women. Am J Clin Nutr 65:1403, 1997.

26. Diaz S, Aravena R, Cardenas ME, et al: Contraceptive efficacy of lactational amenorrhea in urban Chilean women.Contraception 43:335, 1991.

27. Diaz S, Cardenas H, Brandeis A, et al: Early difference in the endocrine profile of long and short lactational amenorrhea. J Clin Endocrinol Metab 72:196, 1991.

28. Diaz S, Jackanicz TM, Herreros C, et al: Fertility regulation in nursing women. VIII. Progesterone plasma levels and contraception efficacy of a progesterone-releasing vaginal ring. Contraception 32:603, 1985.

29. Diaz S, Peralta O, Juez G, et al: Fertility regulation in nursing women. I. The probability of conception in full nursing women living in an urban setting. J Biosoc Sci 14:329, 1982.

30. Drife JO: Breast sensitivity and lactational amenorrhoea. Br J Obstet Gynecol 95:824, 1988.

31. Eslami SS, Gray RH, Apelo R, et al: The reliability of menses to indicate the return of ovulation in breastfeeding women in Manila, the Philippines. Stud Fam Plan 21:243, 1990.

32. Farr G, Rivera R: Interactions between intrauterine contraceptive device use and breastfeeding status at time of intrauterine contraceptive device insertion: Analysis of TCu-380A acceptors in developing countries. Am J Obstet Gynecol 167:144, 1992.

33. Fraser HM, Dewart PJ, Smith SK, et al: Luteinizing hormone releasing hormone agonist for contraception in breast-feeding women. J Clin Endocrinol Metab 69:996, 1989.

34. Frisch RE, McArthur JW: Difference between postpartum and nutritional amenorrhea. Science 203:921, 1979.

35. Ford K, Labbok M: Contraceptive usage during lactation in the United States: an update. Am J Publ Health 77:79, 1987.

36. Gioiosa R: Incidence of pregnancy during lactation in 500 cases. Am J Obstet Gynecol 70:162, 1955.

37. Gray RH, Campbell OM, Apelo R, et al: Risk of ovulation during lactation. Lancet 335:25, 1990.

38. Gray RH, Campbell O, Eslamic S, et al: The return of ovarian function during lactation: Results of studies from the United States and the Philippines. In Biomedical Demographic Determinants. Oxford, 1993, Clarendon.

39. Gross BA: Is the lactational amenorrhea method a part of natural family planning? Biology and policy. Am J Obstet Gynecol 165:2014, 1991.

40. Hartmann PE, Prosser CG: Acute changes in the composition of milk during the ovulatory menstrual cycle in lactating women. J Physiol 324:21, 1982.

41. Hartwell S, Schlesselman S: Risk of uterine perforation among users of IUD. Obstet Gynecol 61:31, 1983.

42. Heikkila M, Luukkainen T: Duration of breastfeeding and development of children after insertion of a levonorgestrel-releasing intrauterine contraceptive device. Contraception 25:279, 1982.

43. Howie P, McNeilly A, Houston M, et al: Fertility after childbirth: Infant feeding patterns, basal PRL levels, and postpartum ovulation. Clin Endocrinol 17:315, 1982.

44. Howie P, McNeilly A, Houston M, et al: Fertility after childbirth: Postpartum ovulation and menstruation in bottle and breastfeeding mothers. Clin Endocrinol 17:323, 1982.

45. Hull VJ: The effects of hormonal contraceptives on lactation: Current findings, methodological considerations and future priorities. Stud Fam Plann 12:134, 1981.

46. Kambic RT: Natural family planning use—Effectiveness and continuation. Am J Obstet Gynecol 165:2046, 1991.

47. Kennedy KI, Labbok MH, Van Look PFA: Consensus statement: Lactational amenorrhea method for family planning. Int J Gynecol Obstet 54:55, 1996.

48. Kennedy KI, Rivera R, McNeilly AS: Consensus statement on the use of breastfeeding as a family planning method. Contraception 39:477, 1989.

49. Kennedy KI, Short RV, Tully MR: Premature introduction of progestin-only contraceptive methods during lactation. Contraception 55:347, 1997.

50. Kennedy KI, Visness CM: Contraceptive efficacy of lactational amenorrhoea. Lancet 339:227, 1992.

51. Kenney JA: Sexuality of pregnant and breastfeeding women. Arch Sex Behav 2:215, 1973.

52. Kent JC, Cox ML, Owens RA, et al: Breast volume and milk production during extended lactation in women. Exper Physiol 84:435, 1999.

53. Kippley S: Breastfeeding and Natural Child Spacing. New York, Harper & Row, 1976.

54. Konner M, Worthman C: Nursing frequency, gonadal function, and birth spacing among !Kung hunter-gatherers. Science 207:788, 1980.

55. Kurz KM, Habicht J-P, Rasmussen KM: Influences of maternal nutrition and lactation on length of postpartum amenorrhoea. J Trop Pediatr 37(suppl):15, 1991.

56. Labbok M: Breastfeeding and contraception. N Engl J Med 308:51, 1983.

57. Labbok M: Contraception during lactation: Considerations in advising the individual and in formulating program guidelines. In Potts M, Thapa S, Herbertson MA: Breastfeeding and Fertility. J Biosoc Sci suppl 9, 1985 (Galton Foundation).

58. Labbok M, Koniz-Booker P, Goney K, et al: Guidelines for Breastfeeding, LAM, and Family Planning. Washington, DC, Institute for Reproductive Health, 1992.

59. Labbok MH, Laukaran VH: Breastfeeding and family planning. In Sciarra JJ: Gynecology and Obstetrics. Philadelphia, Lippincott, 1994.

60. Labbok MH, Peréz A, Valdés F, et al: The lactational amenorrhea method (LAM): A postpartum introductory family

planning method with policy and program implications. Adv Contracept 10:93, 1994.

61. Labbok MH, Stallings RY, Shah F, et al: Ovulation method use during breastfeeding: is there an increased risk of unplanned pregnancy? Am J Obstet Gynecol 165:2031, 1991.

62. Laskey MA, Prentice A: Bone mineral changes during and after lactation. Obstet Gynecol 94:608, 1999.

63. Lasley BL, Shideler SE, Munrol CJ: A prototype for ovulation detection: Pros and cons. Am J Obstet Gynecol 165:2003, 1991.

64. Lewis PR, Brown JB, Renfree MB, et al: The resumption of ovulation and menstruation in a well-nourished population of women breastfeeding for an extended period of time. Fertil Steril 55:529, 1991.

65. Marquis GS, Penny ME, Zimmer JP, et al: An overlap of breastfeeding during late pregnancy is associated with subsequent changes in colostrum's composition and morbidity rates among Peruvian infants and their mothers. Community and International Nutrition. J Nutr 133:2585, 2003.

66. Marshall WM, Cumming DC, Fitzsimmons GW: Hot flushes during breastfeeding? Fertil Steril 57:1349, 1992.

67. Masters WH, Johnson VE: Human Sexual Response. Boston, Little, Brown, 1966.

68. McCann MF, Potter LS: Progestin-only oral contraception: A comprehensive review. Contraception 50:S1, 1994.

69. McCann M, Liskin LK, Piotrow PT, et al: Breastfeeding, fertility, and family planning. Popul Rep J 24:J-552, 1984.

70. McNeilly AS: Lactation and fertility. J Mammary Gland Biol Neoplasia 2:291, 1997.

71. McNeilly AS: Lactational control of reproduction. Reprod Fertil Dev 13:583, 2001.

72. McNeilly AS, Glasier AF, Howie PW, et al: Fertility after childbirth: Pregnancy associated with breastfeeding. Clin Endocrinol 18:167, 1983.

73. McNeilly AS, Glasier AF, Howie PW: Endocrine control of lactational infertility. In Dobbin J (ed): Maternal Nutrition and Lactational Infertility. New York, Vevey/Raven, 1985.

74. Merchant K, Martorell R, Haas J: Maternal and fetal responses to the stresses of lactation concurrent with pregnancy and of short recuperative intervals. Am J Clin Nutr 52:280, 1990.

75. Moscone SR, Moore MJ: Breastfeeding during pregnancy. J Hum Lact 9:83, 1993.

76. Newton N, Newton M: Psychologic aspects of lactation. N Engl J Med 277:1179, 1967.

77. Newton N, Theotokatos M: Breast-feeding during pregnancy in 503 women: Does psychobiological weaning mechanism exist in humans? Emotion Reprod 20B:845, 1979.

78. Nichols-Johnson V: Tandem nursing: Before and after. ABM News Views 2:6, 1996.

79. Nilsson S, Mellbin T, Hofvander Y, et al: Long-term follow-up of children breastfed by mothers using oral contraceptives. Contraception 34:443, 1986.

80. Ojofeitimi EO: Effect of duration and frequency of breast-feeding on postpartum amenorrhea. Pediatrics 69:164, 1982.

81. Perez A: Lactational amenorrhea and natural family planning. In Hafez ESE (ed): Human Ovulation: Mechanisms, Prediction, Detection, and Induction. Amsterdam, North-Holland, 1979.

82. Perez A: Natural family planning: Postpartum period. Int J Fertil 26:219, 1981.

83. Perez A, Labbok MH, Queenan JT: Clinical study of the lactational amenorrhoea method for family planning. Lancet 339:968, 1992.

84. Perheentupa A, Critchley HO, Illingworth PJ, et al: Effect of progestin-only pill on pituitary-ovarian axis activity during lactation. Contraception 67:467, 2003.

85. Prema K, Naidu AN, Kumari SN: Lactation and fertility. Am J Clin Nutr 32:1298, 1979.

86. Prosser CG, Saint L, Hartmann PE: Mammary gland function during gradual weaning and early gestation in women. Aust J Exp Biol Med Sci 62:215, 1984.

87. Pyper CM: Fertility awareness and natural family planning. Eur J Contracept Reprod Health Care 2:131, 1997.

88. Queenan JT, Jennings VH, Spieler JM, et al: Natural family planning: Current knowledge and new strategies for the 1990s. Georgetown University, Washington, DC, Institute for Reproductive Health, 1993.

89. Rosner AE, Schulman SK: Birth interval among breastfeeding women not using contraceptives. Pediatrics 86:747, 1990.

90. Saadeh R, Benboozid D: Breastfeeding and child-spacing: Importance of information collection for public health policy. Bull WHO 68:625, 1990.

91. Sas M, Gellen JJ, Dusitsin N, et al: An investigation on the influence of steroidal contraceptives on milk lipid and fatty acids in Hungary and Thailand. Contraception 33:159, 1986.

92. Savina G, Kennedy K: The effect of a breastfeeding educational program on lactational amenorrhea in the Philippines. Stud Fam Plan 20:203, 1989.

93. Selye H, McKeown T: The effect of mechanical stimulation of the nipples on the ovary and the sexual cycle. Surg Gynecol Obstet 59:856, 1934.

94. Shaaban MM: Contraception with progestogens and progesterone during lactation. J Steroid Biochem Molec Biol 40:705, 1991.

95. Short RV, Lewis PR, Renfree MB, et al: Contraceptive effects of extended lactational amenorrhoea: Beyond the Bellagio consensus. Lancet 337:715, 1991.

96. Tankeyoon M, Dusitsin N, Chalapati S, et al: Effects of hormonal contraceptives on milk volume and infant growth. Contraception 30:505, 1984.

97. Tay CCK, Glasier AF, McNeilly AS: Twenty-four-hour patterns of prolactin secretion during lactation and the relationship to suckling and the resumption of fertility in breast-feeding women. Hum Reprod 11:950, 1996.

98. Taylor RS: Physiology of the vagina and cervix in breast-feeding women. In Shivanandan M (ed): Breastfeeding and Natural Family Planning. Fourth International Symposium on Natural Family Planning. Chevy Chase, MD, KM Associate Publishers, 1985.

99. Technical Guidance/Competence Group, USAID/WHO: Family planning methods: New guidance. Population Report XXIV, No. 2. Baltimore, Johns Hopkins School of Public Health, 1996.

100. Toddywalla VS, Joshi L, Virkar K: Effect of contraceptive steroids on human lactation. Am J Obstet Gynecol 127:245, 1977.

101. Visness CM, Kennedy KI: The frequency of coitus during breastfeeding. Birth 24:253, 1997.

102. Visness CM, Kennedy KI, Gross BA, et al: Fertility of fully breast-feeding women in the early postpartum period. Obstet Gynecol 89:164, 1997.

103. Vorherr H: The Breast: Morphology, Physiology and Lactation. New York, Academic Press, 1974.

104. Vorherr H: Human lactation and breast feeding. In Larson BL (ed): Lactation: A Comprehensive Treatise. New York, Academic Press, 1978.

105. Wade K, Sevilla F, Labbok M: Integrating the lactational amenorrhea method into a family planning program in Ecuador. Stud Fam Plan 25:162, 1994.

106. World Health Organization Task Force for Epidemiological Research on Reproductive Health: Progestogen-only contraceptives during lactation. I and II. Infant development. Contraception 50:55, 1994.

107. Winikoff B, Semeraro P, Zimmerman M: Contraception during breastfeeding: A clinician's source book. New York, Population Council, 1988.

108. Zacharias S, Aguilera E, Assenzo JR, et al: Effects of hormonal and nonhormonal contraceptives on lactation and incidence of pregnancy. Contraception 33:203, 1986.

109. Zarate A, Canales ES, Soria J, et al: Ovarian refractoriness during lactation in women: Effect of gonadotropin stimulation. Am J Obstet Gynecol 112:1130, 1972.

21

$\mathcal{T}$he collection and storage
of human milk and human
milk banking

The human milk bank has entered another era. The interest in providing human milk for infants with special needs, especially premature infants, has increased, but the concerns regarding donor milk have also escalated. Regulatory bodies have decreed that donor milk must be pasteurized. Milk banks have recognized the need for donors being carefully screened and women at high risk for certain infection eliminated.

When there are risks associated with using even the mother's own milk for a given baby, the risk/benefit ratio is determined. Because of the effects of heating, cooling, freezing, and storing milk, some of the most valued and precious qualities are diminished or destroyed; feeding the milk fresh or at least fresh frozen and not heated preserves most of the constituents. The value of the milk produced by women who deliver prematurely has been discussed in Chapter 14. There are no reported cases of infection acquired from milk provided by a milk bank in compliance with the standards prescribed by the Human Milk Banking Association of North America (HMBANA).

HISTORICAL PERSPECTIVE

When wet nursing was the immediate alternative feeding to replace the mother's own milk and no safe ways were available to store milk of any species, no human milk banks existed. As pasteurization became available and formulas based on milk from other species increased in popularity, the pool of human milk diminished. "Wet nurses" were increasingly difficult to locate and often were not safe sources because of wet-nurse lifestyle, risk of infections, and poor nutrition. It had already been clearly demonstrated in the early 20th century that infants who did not receive their mother's milk had six times the risk of dying in the first year of life (see Chapter 1).

The impetus behind milk banks at the turn of the 20th century was actually the medical profession's desire to remove the control of infant feeding from wet nurses and separate the product (human milk) from the producer. Pediatricians anxious to improve the prognosis for infants deprived of their own mother's milk for medical and social reasons developed a means of storing human milk for general use for sick infants. The first milk bank was opened in Vienna in 1900. The first one in the United States was established 10 years later at the Massachusetts Infant Asylum, where wet nurses had been the only sources of human milk.[30] In 1919 the first human milk bank was founded in Germany in Magdeburg by Dr. Marie-Elise Kayser. In 1934 she wrote guidelines that were used throughout Europe for the creation and operation of milk banks.[63]

Early attempts at providing donor milk depended on casual screening of donors for tuberculosis, syphilis, and various acute contagious diseases.[46] There was little investigation of human milk, but the dairy industry was rigorous in its attempt to store and market bovine and other mammalian milks. This technology was applied on a small scale, but other human milk banks appeared after Denny and Talbot created the one in Boston. The American Academy of Pediatrics (AAP) established its first formal guidelines for human milk banks in 1943.[11,12] Similar guidelines were provided in other countries. After World War II, milk banks were mandated on both sides of the Berlin Wall. In 1959 the Federal Republic of Germany (West Germany) had 24 milk banks and the German Democratic Republic had 62.[63] The numbers gradually decreased.

As technology advanced in newborn care and in infant nutrition, science replaced nature. The interest in human milk faded and with it the call for banked human milk in the 1960s and into the 1970s. Experience in Rochester with short-gut syndrome and malabsorption syndromes, however, resulted in the development of a registry of lactating women who donated fresh milk when needed. A milk bank was developed with donors providing frozen milk on a regular basis. By 1975, five large commercial milk banks were operating in Britain. Milk banks also sprang up across the United States. The system thrived with the establishment in 1985 of the HMBANA, which not only facilitated communications among banks, but also began to investigate processes, develop uniform policies, and most important, provide professional and public education.[69]

The threat of human immunodeficiency virus (HIV) and hepatitis, the return of tuberculosis, and drug abuse have cast a long shadow on milk banks in the United States, resulting in the closure of all but seven in North America and five in the United States (see Appendix H). In Europe, milk banking has been key in the nourishment of premature and other high-risk infants. The Sorrento Maternity Hospital has supplied 50,000 L of milk from 10,000 donors over 40 years and now provides 700 L a year both locally and across Britain.[5] In 1994 the remaining 18 milk banks in unified Germany supplied about 15,000 L.

Many developing countries, especially in Central and South America, are establishing milk banks as part of national efforts to promote breastfeeding. Studies done in nurseries in Guatemala have shown a marked decrease in mortality and morbidity rates by providing every infant with human milk, especially colostrum.[13] The United Nations Children's Fund (UNICEF) has encouraged and supported such efforts.[74]

The First International Congress on Human Milk Banking: A Vision of the Future was held in Brazil in 2000, sponsored by the Brazilian Association of Milk Banks. There are 154 milk banks in Brazil. Representatives from South America, France, United Kingdom, North America, and the Caribbean attended. All the milk banks do heat and process the milk. Some serum screen donors but not all. None pay donors but some do provide pumps.[68]

STORING HUMAN MILK

It is often necessary to store milk for infants, especially in the hospital. The storage of human milk involves two types of milk: mother's milk and donor milk. The distinction becomes important in how the milk is stored and prepared for the infant. It is also important because many states have developed codes for donor milk but fortunately have not regulated mother's milk as yet. Certain guidelines are appropriate for each milk. Indications for use of such milk were alluded to in other chapters but are briefly summarized here.

Mother's milk for a healthy infant

The conditions under which a mother collects and stores milk while at work are not always ideal. At home, at work, or at school, milk should be collected with clean equipment, stored in sterile containers (dishwasher cleaned and dried suffices), and handled with just-washed hands. The limits of temperature and time are an important consideration.

To assess microbial growth and stability of milk protein and lipid at varying temperatures and for varying lengths of time, Hamosh and associates[32] collected samples from 16 healthy women with healthy babies who were exclusively breastfed. Sampling was done early in lactation (1 month post partum) and late in lactation (5 to 6 months post partum). The milk pH decreased from 7.02 ± 0.20 to 5.16 ± 0.26 after 24 hours of storage at 38° C (100° F), and significant differences in pH occurred at all temperatures at 24 hours or longer. Proteolysis was minimal at 15° C (59° F) and 25° C (77° F) but became apparent at 38° C at 24 hours. Lipolysis was marked in the first 24 hours at all temperatures compared with freshly expressed milk. Bacterial growth or normal flora was minimal at 15° C at 24 hours, low at 25° C at 8 hours, and higher at 38° C by 4 hours.

The authors concluded that storage of human milk is safe at 15° C for 24 hours and 25° C room temperature for 4 hours and should not be stored at 38° C. Proteins appear to maintain their structure and function in short-term storage. The marked lipolysis appears to slow bacterial growth at the same time.[32]

Pasteurizing breast milk at home

Many women face the dilemma of discarding milk pumped when they had a *Candida* infection of the breast before it was diagnosed. Freezing does not destroy *Candida*. It has been suggested that milk could be "pasteurized" at home for use at home by the mother's own infant. The following steps are those utilized by Nancy Powers, MD* for her patients, recognizing that there is no control over

---

*Nancy G. Powers, MD, Medical Director of Lactation Services, Wesley Medical Center, Wichita, KS.

the temperature. Mothers, however, who wish to salvage this milk must follow these steps:

> Pour all milk into a large saucepan, and place over medium heat on your stove.
>
> Using a candy thermometer, gradually bring the milk up to a temperature of 145° F (62.5° C).
>
> Watch closely, and stir often, keeping milk at this temperature for 30 minutes.
>
> Milk can then be poured into appropriate storage containers.
>
> Label each container with the baby's name amd the date and time of pasteurization.
>
> Freeze the pasteurized milk in dishwasher-clean containers until ready for use.
>
> *Do not boil the milk* (boiling occurs at 212° F or 100° C).

If performed correctly, this process will decrease nutritional and immunologic components by about 30%, but will destroy *all* microorganisms.

See Protocol 7 in Appendix P for more information.

Mother's milk for a sick infant

The following situations are common scenarios for the use of mother's own milk.

1. The mother plans to breastfeed the infant ultimately but needs to provide pumped milk until the infant can be put to the breast.
2. The infant requires the special nutritional benefits of human milk (as with those infants who are recovering from intestinal surgery) but cannot nurse at the breast.
3. The infant weighs 1500 g or less and has difficulty digesting and absorbing other milks and is usually fed by nasogastric tube.

Appendix H lists guidelines for handling mother's milk for hospital use.

Donor milk

The following scenarios are common reasons for obtaining donor milk.

1. The infant is at risk of infection or necrotizing enterocolitis. Although effects are not

clearly demonstrated with mature milk, fresh colostrum is held to be especially protective and may be collected from low-risk, carefully screened mothers.

2. The infant has a gastrointestinal anomaly or other reasons for intestinal tract surgery, especially short-gut syndrome.
3. The physician believes the infant would benefit from the nourishment in human milk because of prematurity, especially if the infant weighs less than 1500 g.
4. The mother is temporarily unable to nourish a breastfed infant completely. It may be that the mother's supply is inadequate when she first puts the infant to the breast after weeks of pumping or when the mother has been ill or hospitalized. Usually these infants are already at home.
5. Donor milk is an excellent transition from parenteral nutrition when mother's milk is not available. It allows earlier weaning from parenteral solution—earlier than formula is known to be tolerated.
6. Metabolic disorders, especially amino acid disorders, respond well because of the physiologic profile of human milk (decreased casein, tyrosine, and phenylalanine). In addition, human milk is protective against infection, which may be a serious complication of these disorders.
7. Pooled samples of donor milk are prepared as a dried preparation for addition to fresh mother's milk to increase the calorie and nutrient value for high-risk premature infants whose requirements exceed those available with unsupplemented human milk.
8. The older infant or child has unique feeding difficulties usually characterized by an inability to tolerate any oral nourishment except human milk (e.g., the child dying of HIV infection).

Structure of a milk bank

Most informal and casual milk banks operating in conjunction with a neonatal intensive care unit

(NICU) have disappeared.[58] NICUs may provide a deep freeze for storage of mother's own milk for use by her infant. They store it for feeding of the infant and do not process it at all except to culture random samples for contamination. Most do not permit "donating" milk to other infants except by private arrangements between the two mothers with physician's approval. No feeding is given an infant in the hospital without a physician's order. Smaller public milk banks have phased out since state legislation or local medical practice standards have mandated strict surveillance of samples and pasteurization.

A few large, well-established banks continue to operate in the United States and around the world. A network of these milk banks meets and shares information through the HMBANA.[4,69,*] Copies of the association's guidelines for milk storage are available for a fee. HMBANA works closely with the Food and Drug Administration (FDA) concerning FDA regulations for human tissues and fluids. Appendix H provides the 2003 guidelines.

The Mother's Milk Bank (MMB) of the Institute for Medical Research in San Jose, California, was established in 1974. It has a full-time coordinator and a medical director, provides milk for hundreds of infants, and contributes to the fund of knowledge on human milk. Because the milk is provided to patients only by physician's prescription, it is reimbursable by health insurance carriers of California. MMB has developed procedures and policies regarding milk collection, storage, and processing. This is described in detail by Asquith and associates[4] and documented with an extensive bibliography. The MMB has prepared and keeps current a comprehensive manual for the organization and operation of a modern human milk bank, which is available to health care facilities. It is also a member of HMBANA, which can provide the names and addresses of other centers (Fig. 21-1).

The state of New York passed an amendment to the public health law in 1980 in which it was declared policy that any and all infants requiring human breast milk be assured access to sufficient quantities of

---

*HMBNA, c/o Mother's Milk Bank, Wakemed, 3000 New Bern Ave, Raleigh, NC 27610

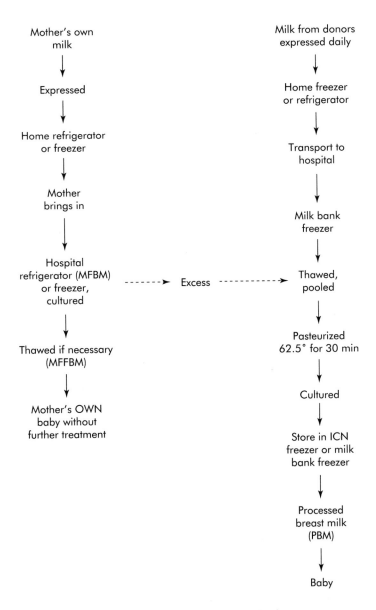

Figure 21-1. Flowchart of human milk bank process.

wholesome human breast milk donated by concerned lactating mothers on a continued and systematic basis (see Appendix L for entire law). New York State has regulations, which have the force of law, governing human milk banks. They address construction, medical direction, donor qualifications, milk collection and storage, maintenance of records, and milk distribution. They are available over the Internet in Part 52, Subpart 52-9, of Title 10 (Health) of the New York Code of Rules and Regulations, which can be accessed from the NY State Department of Health's Public Web site at http://www.health.state.ny.us/

nysdoh/phforum/nycrr10.htm (see Appendix H for reference).

The recommendations for the expansion of the human-milk-banking system have not gone without challenge from neonatologists. They offer sincere concerns about the risk/benefit ratio because alteration during storage and contamination may detract from the value of the original product for the mother's own infant. They caution that the cavalier feeding of unsterile unsupplemented breast milk to premature infants may produce iatrogenic problems. Mothers who pump and save milk for their own infants should follow the instructions/guidelines for storing mother's own milk (see Appendix P).

Qualifications of donors

A mother who is willing to donate milk should be healthy and fulfill the following qualifications (Box 21-1):

1. Normal pregnancy and delivery
2. Serologically negative for syphilis, hepatitis B surface antigen (HBsAg), cytomegalovirus (CMV), and HIV
3. No infection, acute or chronic (i.e., not at high risk)
4. Not taking medications, smoking, or using excessive alcohol
5. Capable of carrying out sterile technique
6. If donating for other infants, own child is healthy and without jaundice

A directive from the Department of Health and Social Security (DHSS) in Great Britain mandated HIV testing for donors to milk banks, and it was observed that the list of 19 established milk banks dwindled to six.[5] The Sorrento Maternity Hospital, however, in accordance with the DHSS directive, screened all donors for HIV antibodies. Only four mothers of 470 potential donors have refused to be tested, contrary to fears that the ruling would discourage donating.[5]

The donor should not be taking medications, including certain oral contraceptives and any nonprescription medications, regularly, such as aspirin or acetaminophen. Her infant should be well and should not have had neonatal jaundice. If the mother is donating only for her own infant, the

---

BOX 21-1 Screening and exclusion of human milk donors

Donor screening procedures

1. Donors answer questions on a verbal health history screening form. Primary health care providers for the prospective donor and her infant are asked for verification of health.
2. Donors are tested serologically for:
   a. HIV-1 and HIV-2
   b. HTLV-1 and HTLV-II
   c. Hepatitis B
   d. Hepatitis C
   e. Syphilis
3. Repeat donors are treated as new donors with each pregnancy.
4. Milk banks will cover the cost of the serologic screening if the tests are done by the milk bank.

Reasons for excluding a donor

- Receipt of a blood transfusion or blood products within last 12 months.
- Receipt of an organ or tissue transplant within last 12 months.
- Regular use of more than 2 ounces of hard liquor or its equivalent in a 24-hour period
- Regular use of over-the-counter medications or systemic prescriptions (replacement hormones and some birth control hormones are acceptable)
- Use of megadose vitamins or pharmacologically active herbal preparations
- Total vegetarians (vegans) who do not supplement their diet with vitamins
- Use of illegal drugs
- Use of tobacco products
- Silicone breast implants
- History of hepatitis, systemic disorders of any kind, or chronic infections (e.g., HIV, HTLV, TB)

HIV, Human immunodeficiency virus; HTLV, human T-cell leukemia virus; TB, tuberculosis.
Modified from Arnold LDW: How North American donor banks operate: Results of a survey. I. J Hum Lact 13:159, 1997.

---

state of the infant's health does not prevent her from donating. Any time the donor becomes ill, however, she should discard milk from the previous 24-hour period and not save milk until the illness is over if the milk is to be donated.

Discarding milk during maternal illness is the most difficult regulation to which a mother must adhere. The desire to contribute may overshadow the mother's understanding of the risk it poses for an infant not her own receiving such milk.

The one limiting factor in donating milk is that the woman must be lactating. Becoming a professional donor of milk today is highly unlikely. The amount of protein has been noted to be lower after 6 months of lactation; thus, it is advisable to limit a given mother's contributions to 6 months or, at most, 8 months post partum. There is always the theoretical risk of a donor mixing her collections with cow milk. This can be tested for bovine protein.

Technique for collection

Whether collecting for a mother's own infant or for other uses, it is of prime importance to maintain cleanliness and minimize bacteria in the process of collection. The mother should be instructed in washing her hands and her breasts before handling the equipment or pumping.

The two major ways of collecting are letting the milk drip while the infant nurses on the other side and pumping or manually expressing the milk.[27,29,65] Drip milk is acceptable for one's own infant when it is used as an occasional tide-over feeding in the mother's temporary absence; however, it is not appropriate for donor milk. Dripped milk has been found to have lower caloric value and a much higher incidence of contamination. Pumped milk has a higher fat content than dripped or manually expressed milk, and in most individuals the volume is also greater. Any equipment used, such as hand pumps, tubing, and collecting bottles, should be sterile. If an electric pump is used, the parts that come in contact with the milk should be sterile or disposable (Fig. 21-2). Many hospitals own electric pumps, or one may be rented from a local rental company. Some women can pump large volumes of fat-rich milk manually, and for them, manual expression would be acceptable on a case-by-case basis.

The hospital or the bank should provide a program of education for the donors. Milk samples should be cultured initially to ensure proper tech-

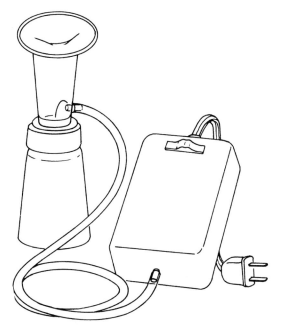

Figure 21-2. Purse-sized electric pump. This type of breast pump is serviceable for women who are fully lactating.

nique and the absence of significant contamination. Then samples should be sent for culture on a random basis. Studies have shown that milk collected at home has a higher contamination rate than that collected while the same donor is hospitalized or with equipment maintained by the hospital. Collection at the hospital also avoids the transportation problem.

Many hospitals use the 4-oz sterile water-nursing bottles packaged by formula companies for collections by discarding the water at the time of collection and then filling them with milk. This can be very costly if the hospital is paying for feeding supplies. Other programs suggest the use of 50-mL plastic centrifuge tubes,* which are presterilized and have tight-fitting tops. These tubes have the advantage of more appropriate volume and easy measurability and sterility. Ideally the hospital or milk bank provides a

---

*No. 25330, manufactured by Corning Glass Works.

uniform container. Soft plastic bags are not recommended. If a woman wants to donate a large amount of previously collected and frozen milk that suddenly becomes available (infant weans or dies), this milk is a valuable resource and can be handled separately with culturing and pasteurization if the milk bank has a protocol for accepting such milk.[1-3]

Zinaman and associates[80] evaluated the efficacy of various methods of removing milk from the breast. Electric pumping (White River model) was clearly more effective in raising the maternal prolactin levels and increasing the volume of milk when compared with hand pumping and manual expression. The study did not compare various brands of pumps. A hospital may own a breast pump that is 10 or 20 years old, however, which may not have safety features that are built into current models. Problems of contamination are a significant issue because old models may not protect against milk backing up into the motor or tubing normally thought to be free of milk and of potential contamination. Care must be taken to check each machine and follow directions for its proper use. Old vacuum extraction pumps should be discarded.

The use of most of the modern electric pumps with their disposable tubing and collecting vessels makes mechanical pumping the most efficient and cleanest of the methods. In addition, the milking action of an electric pump produces more physiologic stimulus to the breast. Most electric pumps provide attachments for pumping both breasts simultaneously. With double pumping, overall production is increased, and time for pumping may be cut in half.

Bank milk collected by manual expression is less likely to be contaminated than that collected by hand pumps, even when pumps are boiled or placed in an electric dishwasher.[41,70] The rubber bulb of the hand pump, resembling a bicycle horn, retains milk and bacteria and should not be used. "Nesty cups," which are placed inside the brassiere to collect milk drippings between feedings, have been associated with the greatest contamination and are not recommended. Some women develop mastitis using small hand pumps.[22]

Donowitz and associates[15] reported contaminated breast milk as the source of *Klebsiella* bacteremia in an NICU. Unpasteurized human milk from a single donor fed through nasogastric and nasoduodenal tubes to sick newborns was found to be contaminated from the safety overflow bottle and tubing of the electric breast pump maintained in the NICU. This part of the tubing and equipment should be sterilized or disposed of between collections according to the manufacturer's instructions. Strict attention to sterilization of equipment is imperative. Older electric pumps that do not have a built-in mechanism to prevent milk from getting into the permanent "works" should be discarded, and only pumps with disposable or cleanable parts and a safety valve should be used.

The bacteriologic benefit to discarding the first 5 to 10 mL of milk pumped from the breast remains disputed.[9] Some banks require that their donors follow instruction for discarding the first 5 to 10 mL of milk expressed at each pumping and each breast. When a donor is collecting for long-term storage, this may be appropriate. When a mother is collecting for her own baby and her volume is meager, discarding 10 mL may be counterproductive. This is particularly important initially, when early colostrum and milk are less in total volume but high in value to the infant. At home, later, when production is abundant and technique may be less stringent, discarding 2 to 3 mL might be appropriate. This will allow a clean collection without washing the breast before pumping, which is associated with sore nipples in some women.

Collection and storage containers

Colostrum was reported by Goldblum and associates[29] to impart greater stability to its components than did mature milk. None of the cellular or humoral immunologic factors investigated was diminished when colostrum was stored at 4° C (39° F) for 24 hours in any of the containers (Table 21-1).

The effect of the container on the stability of the constituents of milk was investigated by Garza and associates.[26] Pyrex and polypropylene containers were found not to interact with water-soluble and

TABLE 21-1   **Effect of container type on milk constituents**

Constituent	Pyrex	Polypropylene	Polyethylene bags	Polyethylene (rigid)
Colostrum	Constituents stable	When refrigerated	24 hours in all	Containers
Mature milk				
Cells	Stick to glass	Maintain phagocytosis	Stable	Stable
Fat-soluble vitamins	No effect	No effect	—	—
Micronutrients	No effect	No effect	—	—
Secretory IgA	—	—	Lower	Stable
Difficult to handle	—	—	Very	—
			Spill easily	
Recommend for	Highly	No	No	Yes
donor milk				

fat-soluble nutrients such as vitamin A, zinc, iron, copper, sodium, and protein nitrogen. Polyethylene bags were found to spill easily, to be harder for mothers to fill without contamination, and to be difficult to handle in the nursery. The containers also leaked and punctured easily, resulting in 60% lower secretory immunoglobulin A (sIgA) levels because of adherence to the material. It appears that rigid polypropylene plastic containers may have a significant advantage in maintaining the stability of all constituents in human milk collections and may be easier and safer to handle.

Paxson and Cress[55] have reported a significant difference in the survival of the leukocytes when the milk is collected and stored in plastic containers rather than glass, because the cells apparently stick to the glass. The phagocytosis of these cells, however, is not affected by the container. The researchers further demonstrated that varying the osmolarity or protein concentration does not alter the number or the phagocytosis of the cells. Because they believe the main reason for feeding preterm infants human milk is for the protection against infection, they suggest nasogastric feedings instead of nasojejunal feeding (to maintain pH in the acid range; in the small bowel, the pH is 6.5 to 8). The milk is collected in sterile plastic containers and maintained in the refrigerator until it is fed to the infant, avoiding heating, freezing, and alkaline solutions (see Table 21-1).

Storage and testing of milk samples

Fresh refrigerated unsterilized mother's milk can be used for 48 hours following collection. If the milk is to be used fresh chilled, it should be refrigerated at home and brought in promptly for use within 48 hours. If it is to be frozen, this should be done immediately at $-18°$ C ($0°$ F) (standard home freezer) or in top of a refrigerator freezer. The milk stored in the latter should be deep frozen within 24 hours if it is to be stored any length of time. The milk kept at $-18°$ C can be kept for 6 months. Freezing and thawing, which can occur in a freezer that is part of a refrigerator, significantly alter the energy content and predispose to separation of the fat layer. Therefore, milk stored in the freezer compartment of a refrigerator-freezer with separate doors should be placed well back in the freezer (not in door) and stored only 1 month. In the hospital or at a bank, all samples should be labeled with name of donor, date, and time. Milk is stored in the freezer in such a way that the oldest milk is used first, and all milk of a single donor is kept together and used only for the infant of that mother.

When a hospitalized mother is contributing fresh milk to her own infant, it is usually not cultured. Pumping is usually done with the help of the nursing staff, and colostrum seems to be more resistant to contamination.[14] Once a mother has been discharged home and she is producing mature milk, however, random sample culturing of her milk samples every week or two is a mechanism for checking milk-expression technique.[19] NICUs have found that random testing improves technique in general.

Because using the fresh milk from the mother to feed a premature infant is becoming commonplace, it is important to be aware of the bacteria cultured from fresh samples during refrigeration.[6] Samples pumped by hand pump and manually expressed were cultured at zero time and after 48 and 120 hours of refrigeration by Sosa and Barness.[62] Although 8 of 41 samples had no growth, the others had the same bacteria on skin and nipple as appeared in the milk (Table 21-2). Concentration was low and decreased over time (Table 21-3), which is attributed to the bacterial inhibitory factors present in milk and suggests that refrigeration of carefully collected breast milk is a safe method for over 48 hours. Guidelines for collection and use of mother's own milk appear in Appendix H.

Standards for raw donor milk

The FDA and the Centers for Disease Control and Prevention (CDC) do not recommend use of donor milk without heat treatment.[69] Rare children, however, require fresh donor milk and cannot tolerate the heat-treated product. For these infants, the guidelines should be carefully followed. These spe-

TABLE 21-2 Positive bacterial cultures from 41 breastfeeding mothers

| Bacterial groups* | No. (%) of cultures | |
	Skin and nipple	Milk
Staphylococcus epidermidis	77 (94)	29 (71)
Streptococcus	17 (21)	6 (15)
Propionibacterium	10 (12)	5 (12)
Staphylococcus aureus	4 (5)	—
Pseudomonas aeruginosa	2 (2)	—
Klebsiella pneumoniae	1 (1)	2 (5)

*Two or more organisms were identified in several skin, nipple, and milk cultures.

TABLE 21-3 Positive rate of breast milk cultures over time

| Cultures | Time of refrigeration (hr) | | |
	0	48	120
Positive	33	27	11
Negative	8	14	30
	—	—	—
Total	41	41	41

From Sosa R. Barness L: Bacterial growth in refrigerated human milk. Am J Dis Child 141:111, 1987.

cial donors must be meticulously screened and monitored for high-risk behaviors. Parents of the infant recipient should sign an informed consent.

All raw donor milk should be screened microbiologically before use. No generally accepted microbiologic criteria exist for such milk except that no potential pathogens should be present.[10] Such pathogens include *Staphylococcus aureus*, β-hemolytic streptococci, *Pseudomonas* species, *Proteus* species, and *Streptococcus faecalis*. Some milk that cannot be fed raw can be pasteurized.[76]

Other guidelines include the following[69]:
1. Each pool of milk shall have a sterile sample taken for bacteriologic screening.
2. Only milk from pools with less than 10^4 CFU/mL of normal skin flora (e.g., coagulase negative staphylococcus, diphtheroids, *Staphyloccus epidermis*, or *Streptococcus viridans*) will be acceptable to dispense raw. The presence of any pathogens is unacceptable.

Standards for pasteurization of donor milk

Milk suitable for pasteurization should meet the following minimum standards[76]:
1. A total aerobic count that does not exceed 1×10^6 CFUs/mL
2. *S. aureus* that does not exceed 1×10^3 CFUs/mL; risk of feeding heat-treated enterotoxins when *S. aureus* exceeds 1×10^6 CFUs/mL

3. Presence of organisms defined as being of fecal origin not exceeding 1×10^4 CFUs/mL
4. Presence of organisms not part of normal flora not exceeding 1×10^7 CFUs/mL
5. Presence of no unusual organisms such as *Pseudomonas aeruginosa*, spore-bearing aerobes, or spore-bearing anaerobes

Heat treatment

When human milk was pasteurized at 73° C (163° F) for 30 minutes, minimal immunoglobulins A and G (IgA, IgG), lactoferrin, lysozyme, and C3 complement remained. When the temperature was kept at 62.5° C (144.5° F) for 30 minutes, there was a loss of 23.7% of the lysozyme, 56.8% of the lactoferrin, and 34% of the IgG, but no loss of IgA, according to work done by Evans and associates.[20] Similar studies of heat treatments of graded severity were carried out by Ford and associates.[21] The findings were similar. Pasteurization at 62° C for 30 minutes (*Holder method*) reduced IgA by 20% and destroyed IgM and lactoferrin. Lysozyme was stable at 62.5° C but destroyed at 100° C, as was lactoperoxidase and the ability to bind folic acid against bacterial uptake. Growth of *Escherichia coli* increased when introduced into heated milk. Vitamin B_{12}-binding capacity declined progressively with increasing temperature of the heat treatment.[24]

The effects of the Holder method on antiinfective agents were reviewed by Orloff and associates,[53] who concluded that high temperatures destroyed much of the bacteriostatic effect of human milk, thus decreasing the benefit to the infant. These data raise the question of whether any heat treatment might not increase the risk of enteric infection in the infant. Ford and associates[21] suggest that for batch processing, however, 62.5° C for 30 minutes may be the method of choice.

The alterations of the lymphocyte and antibody content after processing were studied by Liebhaber and associates.[40,41] They, too, found significant changes with heat, including a decrease in total lymphocyte count and in specific antibody titer to *E. coli*.

Welsh and May[73] discuss antiinfective properties of breast milk and provide two tables (Tables 21-4 and 21-5) to demonstrate the stability of the antibacterial and antiviral properties of human milk.

Low-temperature short-time pasteurization of human milk was reported by Wills and associates[77] using the Oxford human milk pasteurizer. Heating at 56.0° C for 15 minutes destroyed over 99% of the inoculated organisms, which included *E. coli*, *S. aureus*, and group B β-hemolytic streptococci. The remaining activity of antimicrobial proteins after different time/temperature treatments is shown in Table 21-6.

High-temperature short-time (HTST) (72° or 87° C up to 15 seconds) treatment of human milk inoculated with endogenous bacteria and CMV rendered the milk bacteria-free in 5 seconds and CMV-free in 15 seconds.[28] Folic acid and vitamins B_1, B_2, B_6, and C were not affected. Bile salt-stimulated lipase (BSSL) was inactivated by these conditions. Lactoferrin and IgA and sIgA antibody activity were stable at 72° C (162° F) for 15 seconds. Lysozyme concentration and enzymatic activity were increased, suggesting that lysozyme may be sequestered in the milk (Tables 21-7 and 21-8).

The effect of temperature on transforming growth factors TGF-α and TGF-$β_2$ human milk concentrations during pasteurization, at temperatures commonly used by donor milk banks, slightly decreased TGF-α concentrations but not milk TGF-$β_2$ with little difference when temperature was increased to 71° C.[47]

Pasteurization

Recommended pasteurization of human milk for banks follows these steps[69]:

1. All containers shall be tightly closed with new caps to prevent contamination of milk during heat treatment.
2. Heat processing
   a. Aliquots of milk shall be processed by completely submerging the containers in a well-agitated or shaking water bath preheated to a minimum of 63° C.
   b. A control bottle containing the same amount of milk or water as the most filled container of milk in the batch shall be

TABLE 21-4   Antibacterial factors in breast milk

Factor	Shown in vitro to be active against	Effect of heat
Bifid* growth factor	Enterobacteriaceae, enteric pathogens	Stable to boiling
Secretory IgA	*Escherichia coli, E. coli* enterotoxin; *Clostridium tetani, Corynebacterium diphtheriae, Streptococcus pneumoniae, Salmonella, Shigella*	Stable at 56°C for 30 min; some loss (0%–30%) at 62.5°C for 30 min; destroyed by boiling
C1 to C9	Effect not known	Destroyed by heating at 56°C for 30 min
Lactoferrin	*E. coli, Candida albicans*	Two thirds destroyed at 62.5°C for 30 min
Lactoperoxidase	*Streptococcus, Pseudomonas, E. coli, Salmonella typhimurium*	Not known; presumably destroyed by boiling
Lysozyme	*E. coli, Salmonella, M. lysodeikticus*	Stable at 62.5°C for 30 min; activity reduced 97% by boiling for 15 min
Lipid (unsaturated fatty acid)	*Staphylococcus aureus*	Stable to boiling
Milk cells	By phagocytosis: *E. coli, C. albicans* By sensitized lymphocytes: *E. coli*	Destroyed at 62.5°C for 30 min

Lactobacillus bifidus/Bifidobacterium bifidum.
From Welsh JK, May JT: Anti-infective properties of breast milk. J Pediatr 93:1, 1979.

TABLE 21-5   Antiviral factors in breast milk

Factor	Shown in vitro to be active against	Effect of heat
Secretory IgA	Polio virus types 1, 2, 3; coxsackie-virus types A9, B3, B5; Echo virus types 6, 9; Semliki Forest virus, Ross River virus, rotavirus	Stable at 56°C for 30 min; some loss (0%–30%) at 62.5° for 30 min; destroyed by boiling
Lipid (unsaturated fatty acids and monoglycerides)	Herpes simplex, Semliki Forest virus, influenza, dengue, Ross River virus, murine leukemia virus, Japanese B encephalitis virus	Stable to boiling for 30 min
Nonimmunoglobulin macromolecules	Herpes simplex, vesicular stomatitis virus	Destroyed at 60°C; stable at 56°C for 30 min; destroyed by boiling for 30 min
	Rotavirus	Unknown
Milk cells	Induced interferon activity against Sendai virus; ? sensitized lymphocytes; ? phagocytosis	Destroyed at 62.5°C for 30 min

From Welsh JK, May JT: Anti-infective properties of breast milk. J Pediatr 93:1, 1979.

TABLE 21-6   Remaining activity of antimicrobial proteins after pasteurization of human milk

Temperature/time	IgA (%)	Lactoferrin (%)	Lysozyme (%)
72.0° C/15 sec	67	27	67
62.5° C/5 min	77	59	96
56.0° C/15 min	90	91	100

fitted with a calibrated thermometer to register milk temperature during heat processing. The control bottle should follow the same process as the rest of the batch at all times.

c. The thermometer shall be positioned such that approximately 25% of the milk volume is below the measuring point of the thermometer.

d. The monitored aliquot shall be placed into the water bath after all other aliquots, and shall be positioned centrally among the treated aliquots.

e. After the temperature of the monitored control bottle has reached a minimum of 62.5° C, the heat treatment shall continue for 30 minutes. Milk shall not reach a core temperature higher than 63° C.

Viruses in human milk

The dilemma of CMV is a significant one, because the virus does pass into the milk. In a study of postpartum women, CMV was recovered from the genital tract in 10%, from the urine in 7%, from the saliva in 2%, and from the breast milk in 30%. CMV does persist after storage at 4° C and − 20° C (39° and −4° F) in some specimens.[64] It is destroyed at 62.5° C after 30 minutes.[16] Donor milk should be accepted only from CMV-negative mothers. Mothers who are seropositive may be permitted to provide for their own infants because they continue to provide the antibody protection as well.

Hepatitis virus also passes into milk, and donors should therefore be screened and be seronegative.

The question of having seropositive women feed their own infants is discussed in Chapter 17.

The acquired immunodeficiency syndrome (AIDS) virus has been identified in human milk.[67,78] Most banks require that donors be HIV negative, but because seropositivity may take months to develop, some mechanism for excluding high-risk donors should be in place. On the other hand, some think that donors should not be screened. Holding all milk samples for several months may not be practical, and pasteurizing all milk may decrease the value of the nutrient. Some AIDS experts are concerned that the threat may seriously alter the future of milk banks.[42] It has been demonstrated that heat treatment kills the virus when milk is inoculated experimentally.[17]

The virus associated with HIV and human T-cell leukemia virus (HTLV) were incubated at temperatures from 37° to 60° C, and the virus titer was determined over time by a microculture infectivity assay. It required 32 minutes at 60° C to reduce the virus titer.[45] Using the HMBANA standard of 62.5° C for 30 minutes totally destroyed the viruses. No virus could be recovered after the process even with repeated subculturing. Human milk contains one or more components that inactivate HIV-1 but that are not toxic for the cells in which the virus replicates.[53] These components are under study and are probably lipids.

Lyophilization and freezing

The impact of lyophilization was similar to that of heating, showing a decrease in total lymphocyte count and in immunoglobulin concentration and specific antibody titer to E. coli. (Lyophilization is the creation of a stable preparation of a biologic substance by rapid freezing and dehydration of the frozen product under high-vacuum freeze drying.)

Freezing specimens up to 4 weeks showed no change in IgA or E. coli antibody titer, although the lymphocyte count was decreased. The technique involved freezing to − 23° C (−9° F) and thawing at 1, 2, 3, and 4 weeks. Although cells were present after freezing, they showed no viability when tested with the trypan blue stain exclusion method.

TABLE 21-7 Effect of high-temperature short-time (HTST) pasteurization on selected vitamins in human milk

	Time (sec)							
	0		**1**		**3**		**15**	
	$\bar{X} \pm SD$	n	$\bar{X} \pm SD$	n	$\bar{X} \pm SD$	n	$\bar{X} \pm SD$	n
Vitamin B$_1$ (μg/mL)	0.104 ± 0.013	9						
72° C			0.098 ± 0.005	3	0.091 ± 0.008	3	0.088 ± 0.009	3
87° C			0.084 ± 0.011*	3	0.095 ± 0.027	3	ND	
Vitamin B$_2$ (μg/mL)	0.724 ± 0.132	9						
72° C			0.75 ± 0.08	3	0.70 ± 0.09	3	0.56 ± 0.07	3
87° C			0.66 ± 0.13†	3	0.72 ± 0.22	3	ND	3
Vitamin B$_6$ (μg/mL)	0.237 ± 0.081	9						
72° C			0.27 ± 0.05	3	0.26 ± 0.025	3	0.22 ± 0.012	3
87° C			0.25 ± 0.07	3	0.26 ± 0.02	3	ND	
Folic acid (μg/mL)	0.106 ± 0.020	9						
72° C			0.089 ± 0.005‡	3*	0.065 ± 0.018	3	0.101 ± 0.012	3
87° C			0.088 ± 0.008	3	0.080 ± 0.023	3	ND	
Vitamin C (μg/mL)	9.2 ± 2.4	9						
72° C			11.2 ± 1.2	3	21.5 ± 3.0*	3	8.7 ± 1.7	3
87° C			16.0 ± 4.9*	3	22.5 ± 13.3	3	ND	3

*$p < 0.07$.
†$p < 0.001$.
‡$p < 0.04$.
From Goldblum RM, Dill CW, Albrecht TB et al: Rapid high-temperature treatment of human milk. J. Pediatr 104:380, 1984.

TABLE 21-8 **Effect of high-temperature short-time (HTST) pasteurization on immunologic proteins in human milk**

	Time (sec)							
	0		**1**		**3**		**15**	
	X̄ ± SD	**n**	**X̄ ± SD**	**n**	**X̄ ± SD**	**n**	**X̄ ± SD**	**n**
Lactoferrin (mg/mL)	0.67 ± 0.10	8						
72° C			0.95 ± 0.21	2	0.58 ± 0.2	3	0.83 ± 0.05	3
87° C			0.50 ± 0.02	3	0.50 ± 0.2	3	0.47 ± 0.17	2
Lysozyme (µg/mL)	15.0 ± 8.7	8						
72° C			86.0 ± 3.5*	2	78.0 ± 16.0	3†	59.0 ± 7.0*	3
87° C			86.0 ± 9.1*	3	59.0 ± 9.0	3†	36.0 ± 7.7	2
Total IgA (mg/mL)	0.37 ± 0.08	8						
72° C			0.37 ± 0.07	2	0.25 ± 0.06	3	0.3 ± 0.04	3
87° C			0.06 ± 0.04*	3	0.04 ± 0.02	3†	0.05 ± 0.03	2
sIgA Ab (reciprocal titer)	10.0 ± 4.8	7						
72° C			10.2 ± 12.4	2	10.6 ± 4.8	2	15.0 ± 3.5	3
87° C			<1	3	<1	2	<1	2

n. Number of experiments.
* $p < 0.01$.
† $p < 0.05$.
From Goldblum RM, Dill CW, Albrecht TB, et al: Rapid high-temperature treatment of human milk. J Pediatr 104:380, 1984.

The storage of human milk at 4° C (39° F) for 48 hours caused a decrease in the concentration of milk macrophages and neutrophils but not of the lymphocytes, which also maintained their activity, according to Pittard and Bill.[56] The loss of cells may be desirable if the graft versus host reaction in a premature infant who is possibly immunodeficient is of concern.

Evans and associates[20] reported their results with 3-month storage at −20° C and of freeze drying and reconstitution (lyophilization). They found no significant change in lactoferrin, lysozyme, IgA, IgG, and C3 after 3-month freezing but a small loss of IgG after lyophilization (Table 21-9).

Nutritional consequences

Initially the focus in processing human milk was the effect on its unique antiinfective properties,[29,34] but attention has been given to the nutritional consequences as well.[59] Storage for 24 hours did not affect vitamin A, zinc, iron, copper, sodium, or protein nitrogen concentrations at 37° C.[66,75] Ascorbic acid levels decreased greatly when stored at 37° C and 4° C at 24 and 48 hours. (They remained stable for 4 hours.) Other investigators have found that ascorbic acid levels drop 40% with heating.[26,66]

Levels of unsaturated fatty acids apparently are also affected by heating and cold storage, but the data need clarification.[49] It is anticipated that heating or freezing and thawing are capable of damaging membranes surrounding milk fat globules.[59] The fat globule could then undergo fragmentation and allow greater access of milk lipases to triglycerides. The percentages of polyunsaturated fatty acids, linoleic ($C_{18:2}$) and linolenate ($C_{18:3}$), decreased after both heating and freezing, while monounsaturates and saturated fatty acids were unaffected.[72] When milk is stored at −11° C over 48 hours, release of fatty acids progresses over time with an increase in the proportion of free $C_{18:2}$, $C_{20:4}$, and other long-chain polyenic acids. No measurable lipolysis occurred when milk was stored at −70° C. The higher the temperature and the longer the time, the greater is the accumulation of free fatty acids.[37] Other investigators have confirmed this, concluding the lipoprotein lipase and

BSSL remain fully active at −20° C but not −70° C with or without presence of serum. Berkow and associates[7] therefore recommend that milk be stored at −70° C. Other enzymes were not affected by freezing and storing except lactoperoxidase, which lost activity (Tables 21-10 and 21-11).

Because the nourishment of low-birth-weight (LBW) infants has been the purpose of many milk banks, the ability of preterm infants to utilize treated bank milk is relative. Pasteurization at 62.5° C for 30 minutes was reported not to influence nitrogen absorption or retention in LBW infants.[59] When raw, pasteurized, and boiled human milks were fed to very LBW (VLBW) (less than 1.3 kg) preterm infants in three separate consecutive weeks, fat absorption was reduced by one third in the heat-treated group. There was a reduction in the amount of nitrogen retained in the heat-treated group as well, although the absorption was unaffected. The absorption and retention of calcium, phosphorus, and sodium were unaffected by heating or freezing. The mean weight gain was greater by one third when the infants were fed raw human milk.[75,76]

Pasteurization decreased vitamin B_{12} by about 50% and folate-binding capacity by 10%[51] (see Table 21-11). Sterilization (100° C for 20 minutes), on the other hand, had similar effects on vitamin B_{12} binding and completely inactivated folate binding.[66] Vitamins A, D, E, B_2, and B_6, choline, niacin, and pantothenic acid were barely affected by pasteurization, whereas thiamine was reduced up to 25%, biotin up to 10%, and vitamin C up to 35%.[71]

Refrigeration at 4° to 6° C for 72 hours allows little bacterial growth and causes no change in nutrients or infection-protective properties. Freezing does have some effect on both, and the milk can be kept for months, whereas heating has significant effect, and the milk still requires freezing for storage. Experience feeding donated raw milk to newborns has shown no ill effects if carefully monitored, according to Björksten and associates.[8] Quick freezing and frozen storage do not significantly affect levels of biotin, niacin, folic acid, vitamin E, and the fat-soluble vitamins. Photooxidation and absorption by the container or tubing are always a consideration. Vitamin C is reduced by both these processes.[25]

TABLE 21-9   Effect of deep freezing (3 mo) at −20° C and lyophilization of human milk proteins (mg/dL milk)

	Raw milk (mean ± SE)	Deep-frozen milk			Lyophilized milk		
		Mean ± SE	Mean as % raw	p	Mean ± SE	Mean as % raw	p
α_1-Antitrypsin (16 samples)	2.38 ± 0.3	1.98 ± 0.2	83.2	<0.05	2.22 ± 0.3	93.3	>0.1
IgA (8 samples)	9.55 ± 0.84	9.25 ± 0.83	96.9	>0.1	9.33 ± 0.74	97.7	>0.1
IgG (16 samples)	0.42 ± 0.05	0.42 ± 0.04	100	>0.1	0.33 ± 0.04	78.6	<0.05
Lactoferrin (11 samples)	332 ± 71.7	338 ± 57.4	102	>0.1	363 ± 79	109.3	>0.1
Lysozymes (11 samples)	5.1 ± 1.26	4.6 ± 0.67	90.2	>0.1	4.8 ± 1.19	94.1	>0.1
C3 (16 samples)	1.35 ± 0.13	1.26 ± 0.11	93.3	>0.1	1.27 ± 0.13	94.1	>0.1

From Evans TJ, Ryley HC, Neale LM, et al: Effect of storage and heat on antimicrobial proteins in human milk. Arch Dis Child 53:239, 1978.

TABLE 21-10   Storage of human milk and protein N concentrations (mg N/dL)

	Storage temperature		
Storage time (hr)	37° C	4° C	−72° C
4	187 ± 8*	181 ± 7*	
24	183 ± 7*†	178 ± 5*†	186 ± 8†
48	189 ± 8*	178 ± 5*	

Mean ± 1 SM ($n = 11$)
*Effects from temperature significant when samples stored at 37° and 4° C are compared ($p < 0.05$. $F = 9.3$)
†Comparison of storage temperature effects on samples stored only for 24 hr not significant ($p > 0.05$. $F = 1.4$)
From Garza C, Johnson CA, Harrist R, et al: Effects of methods of collection and storage on nutrients in human milk. Early Hum Dev 6:295, 1982.

The effect of heating and freezing on the various constituents of human milk has been studied by a number of investigators. Their data should be considered before deciding how to store milk for special purposes.

Routine analysis of the nutrient value of milk samples is often not practical, so gross screening by creamatocrit has been done by some banks and nurseries. A method of infrared (IR) analysis using a Milko-Scan 104 IR Analyzer (A/S Foss Electric) has been described by Michaelsen and associates.[48] It is simpler and more rapid than previous methods. These investigators found a linear correlation between IR results and the standard reference

TABLE 21-11   Thermal destruction of milk components (follows first-order reaction kinetics)

	D value* at 60° C (sec)	Z value†
IgA	4.9×10^4	5.5°C
Lactoferrin	2.4×10^3	4.7°C
Thiamine	7.7×10^5	28.4°C
Folic acid	1.9×10^4	6.4°C

*90% degradation at 60° C in seconds.
†Temperature change to alter degradation rate by a factor of 10.
Modified from Morgan JN, Toledo RT, Eitenmiller RR, et al: Thermal destruction of immunoglobulin A, lactoferrin, thiamin, and folic acid in human milk. J Food Sci 51:348, 1986.

methods of Kjeldahl for nitrogen (protein), Roese Gottlieb for fat, and bomb calorimetry for energy. These techniques were used on all incoming milk and on the outgoing pooled milk.

All the milk from the same mother was thawed, pooled, and stirred vigorously on arrival at the bank. A 10-mL sample was taken and stored at −5° C until analysis. Samples were collected every 2 weeks and were analyzed up to 2 to 3 weeks after expression. For the 2554 collections of milk contributed by 224 women, the mean protein content was 9 g/L and the fat was 39 g/L. The greater the body mass index of the mother, the greater was the protein and fat content.

The authors suggest that by selecting the milk with the highest protein content (12 g/L), a high-protein milk can be created with a higher energy content (725 kcal/L) for use in the VLBW infant. Furthermore, they recommend pooling milk from up to five mothers to decrease the variability in nutrient levels.[48]

At the Hvidovre Milk Bank in Copenhagen, monitoring of the macronutrients in donor milk is part of the bank's quality assurance standards, and donors are discontinued if their milk protein content falls below 8 g/L. Their milk was viewed adequate for their own baby but not for high-risk infants, especially premature infants.

Creamatocrit

Testing milk for protein, fat, and carbohydrate is not necessary and is costly and time consuming. However, Lucas and associates[43] have suggested a quick method of analysis. It involves standard hematocrit microtubes and a centrifuge. The percentage of cream, or "creamatocrit," is read from the capillary tube. Fat and energy content have a linear relationship, as follows:

$$\text{Fat (g/L)} = (\text{Creamatocrit [\%]} - 0.59) / 0.146$$

$$\text{kcal/L} = 290 + (66.8 \times \text{Creamatocrit [\%]})$$

Accuracy is within 10%.

The Research Institute for Health Sciences provides the following formula for calculating the fat and energy content of milk using the measurement of the creamatocrit (%)[60]:

$$Fat\ (g/L) = (6.24 \times Creamatocrit\ [\%]) - 3.08$$

$$[r = 0.98, 95\%\ confidence\ limit = \pm\ 4.39\ g/L]$$

$$kcal/dL = (5.57 \times Creamatocrit\ [\%]) + 45.13$$

$$[r = 0.92, 95\%\ confidence\ limit = \pm 12.61\ kcal/dL]$$

Studies done comparing energy value calculated by creamatocrit with energy value from percentage of carbon, as measured by Manchester bomb calorimeter using pooled pasteurized milk samples, were somewhat inaccurate compared with data obtained by creamatocrit on fresh or fresh-frozen samples.[61]

The methodology was validated with further analysis by Lemons and associates,[39] who repeated the studies and confirmed actual measurements of total fat and caloric content. Because the protein and lactose content remains relatively constant over time, the variation in fat content is the primary constituent affecting caloric value of the milk. Neither freezing for up to 2 months nor pasteurization affected the creamatocrit. There was no evidence of fat globule degradation during storage that affected the test.

Special cautions while performing this simple test should include the following:

- Use a representative, well-mixed sample.
- Complete a sample of pumping from at least one breast; do not take just a spot sample.
- Use a well-mixed 24-hour sample.
- Use tube at least three-fourths filled; seal one end.
- Centrifuge for 15 minutes in standard table-top centrifuge.

A new technology, the Creamatocrit Plus, has been reported by Meier and colleagues.* the devide is a special centrifuge to spin and calculate the creamatocrit. It automatically calculates the fat and calorie content.

---

*Meier PP, Engstrom JL, Zuleger JL, et al: The Creamatocrit Plus™: A new centrifuge for measuring creamatocrits with mother's milk. Funded by and available from Separation Technology, Inc., Altamonte Springs, FL, www.separationtechnology.com.

Ultrasonic homogenization

Pooling specimens of human milk may not result in a milk of uniform fat content after storage. The separation of fat during processing, storage, and administration by continuous nasogastric infusion, whether by gravity flow or continuous mechanical pump, results in significant loss of fat and variation in the milk received (47.4% of fat with slow infusion and 16.8% with fast infusion).

Homogenization by ultrasonic treatment was studied by Martinez and associates,[44] who found that changes in fat concentration during infusion and loss of fat during administration, caused by the fat sticking to the container and tubes, were eliminated. Furthermore, the fat-soluble vitamins are preserved. Because 31% of iron, 15% of copper, 12% of zinc, 10% of calcium, and 2% of magnesium sulfate are in the fat fraction of both human and cow milk, preserving the fat is essential to maximizing nutrient intake from human milk, especially in compromised infants. Tube feedings have been noted to reduce vitamins B_2, B_6, A, and C in human milk.

Ultrasonic homogenization was accomplished in this study by subjecting the milk to treatment in a Tekmar Sonic Disruptor TSD-P 250 (Tekmar Co., Cincinnati, OH). The homogenization time (2, 4, or 8 minutes) is a function of the volume of milk and intensity of vibration. The procedure should be done with milk in an ice bath.

Microwave effects

The milk should be thawed in the refrigerator, and each bottle should be used completely within 24 hours. Defrosting in the microwave oven may lead to separation of layers, and microwaves decrease vitamin C content. The greatest danger of microwaving is that the milk heats and the container does not, so that an infant could be burned or the milk significantly overheated.

The effects of microwave radiation on human milk have been much debated. The only nutritional effect identified has been the lowering of the vitamin C level. Lysozyme activity, total IgA, and specific IgA to *E. coli* serotypes 01, 04, and 06 were

TABLE 21-12	**Impact of microwaving on antiinfective factors in human milk**[*]			
	No.	Control	Low microwave	High microwave
Lysozyme activity (μg/mL)	22	23.7 ± 4.0	19.2 ± 3.4 $p < .005$	0.9 ± 0.72 $p < .0005$
Total IgA (mg/dL)	22	73.3 ± 16.1	48.9 ± 15.8 NS[†]	1.55 ± 1.54 $p < 0.0005$
Antigen-specific antigen to *E. coli* serotype				
01	22	100%	91 ± 9.2[‡]	24.9 ± 10.0[‡]
04	22	100%	90.3 ± 6.5 [‡]	12.3 ± 3.7[‡]
06	22	100%	79.8 ± 5.7[‡] $p < 0.005$	17.1 ± 3.6[‡] $p < 0.0005$

[*]Results are mean ± SE. All significant differences were also confirmed by the Fisher's protected least significant difference test.
[†]Not significant.
[‡]Percent of control.
From Quan R, Yang C, Rubinstein S, et al: Effects of microwave radiation on anti-infective factors in human milk. Pediatrics 89:667, 1992.

tested in 22 freshly frozen milk samples before and after heating for 30 seconds at low-power and high-power settings of the microwave oven.[57] Additional samples were tested at microwave low (20° to 25° C), medium (60° to 70° C), and high (98° C or higher) powers before the addition of *E. coli* suspension. Microwaving at high temperatures (72° to 98° C) greatly decreased all the tested antiinfective factors (Table 21-12). *E. coli* growth at 98° C or higher was 18 times that of untreated thawed human milk. Low temperatures did not affect total IgA or specifics IgA to *E. coli* serotypes 01 and 04 or specifics IgA to *E. coli* serotype 06. At only 20° to 25° C, the growth of *E. coli* was five times that of the untreated thawed milk.[57]

In the experimental laboratories, the microwaves are carefully controlled. In the home, they vary tremendously. Ovensen and associates admitted that the temperature had to stay under 60° C (140° F). Above that, antibodies were decreased and at 77° C (170° F), they were totally destroyed. Vitamins B_1 and E were apparently stable, but they did not test for vitamin C. Kerner and associates state very clearly that IgA, sIgA, and lysozyme were affected by microwaving at 14° to 25° C (i.e., lower temperatures). Time is important because even at 30% power the temperature will increase over time.

Microwaving clearly interferes with the antiinfective properties of human milk: the higher the temperature, the greater the effect (Table 21-13).

Specialty milks

New technologies offer the potential for providing specialty milks. Simple homogenization would preserve the fat, as noted; however, because of the presence of active enzymes, once the fat membrane is ruptured by homogenization, the milk should be used promptly to prevent excessive fat breakdown. Lyophilization or freeze drying is an opportunity to concentrate the nutrients without increasing the volume. Adding a freeze-dried aliquot to liquid human milk would be preferable to using the commercial bovine-based products. In Denmark, infrared analysis of milk donations is used to provide high-protein or high-fat pools of milk. In Canada and the United States, some banks identify donors with dairy-free diets for specific infants.[1-3]

Contamination with cow milk

Donor milk is at risk for being contaminated with cow milk by the donor. The California Mother's Milk Bank checks its contributions with a simple test directed at precipitating the casein. They mix 1 mL of donor milk with 1 mL of 8 *N* sulfuric acid and 8 mL

TABLE 21-13   Impact of microwaving on *Escherichia coli* growth in human milk at 3 ½ hours*

	No.	Colony count
Control	10	$8.4 \pm 2.7 \times 10^7$
Low microwave	10	$43.9 \pm 11.4 \times 10^{7\dagger}$
Medium microwave	10	$90.1 \pm 24.1 \times 10^{7\ddagger}$
High microwave	10	$152 \pm 43 \times 10^{7\ddagger}$

*Results are mean ± SE. All significant differences were also confirmed by the Fisher's protected least significant difference test.
†$p = 0.005$ compared with control.
‡$p = 0.001$ compared with control.
From Quan R, Yang C, Rubinstein S, et al: Effects of microwave radiation on anti-infective factors in human milk. Pediatrics 89:667, 1992.

of water, and let it sit at room temperature for 5 hours. If cow milk is present, it will precipitate.[52]

Changing flavors of stored milk

Women have reported to the lactation study center that their fresh-frozen breast milk smells sour and even rancid and is rejected by their infant. Although a slightly soapy odor had sometimes been noted, it had never been reported to be harmful or to be rejected by the infant. This soapy smell has been attributed to a change in the lipid structure associated with the freeze-thaw effects of the self-defrost cycle in the freezer-refrigerator.

The cases reported to the center, however, have suggested true lipid breakdown is associated with the rancid smell. The speculation was that some women have more lipase activity than others, as noted in the study of lipase and hyperbilirubinemia. Some mothers reported that their milk began to smell as soon as it cooled, whether refrigerated or frozen. Others have noted that their stockpile of milk, meticulously stored in anticipation of returning to work, was rancid and rejected by their infant. When these mothers heated their milk to a scald (not boiling) immediately after collection and then quickly cooled and froze it, the effect was not apparent, and their infants accepted the heat-treated milk. That process inactivated the lipase and halted the process of fat digestion. On the other hand, scalding rancid milk will not improve the flavor or smell.

Financial aspects

Established milk banks have various financial structures.[5] Charges can include fees for equipment rental and for processing milk. Certainly the hospital should recover costs of collecting and processing. Precedent for this has been set in the United States. Because some states have passed legislation mandating the availability of human milk for all babies who need it, reimbursement and funds must be available for its proper handling.

All banks have a minimal charge that partially covers the cost of processing, such as labor, equipment, and supplies. As with blood banks, the recipient is not charged for the milk itself. Third-party payers do reimburse for this, and Women, Infants, and Children (WIC) programs also provide this reimbursement in more and more states.

The recommendations from the State of New York (see Appendix L) suggest that the monitoring of standards of a hospital-based bank be absorbed into existing hospital surveillance. Free-standing banks would be monitored by the state and local health departments. Economic analysis indicates that the primary costs would be administrative overhead costs. The human milk supply is considered a donated product. Also acknowledged are staff costs, minimal equipment costs, and laboratory costs, as well as costs to the state health department to administer the system. Much consideration is being given to limiting banks to hospital settings, where health professionals and equipment are readily available.

The average processing fee charged by milk banks in the United States begins at $2.50 per ounce, although it does not totally cover costs.[3] No infant is refused access for lack of funds, and banks cover their costs by various methods, including donations, subsidies, and grants. With proper physician orders and paperwork, most third-party payers cover the cost of bank breast milk.

BREAST-PUMPING EQUIPMENT

As noted earlier, several types of breast-pumping devices have provoked questions of the sterility of milk collected. Additional issues need to be considered, including efficiency, ease of use, potential for breast trauma, availability, and cost. A good pump should be capable of completely emptying the breast and of stimulating production. It should be clean and easy to keep clean, contamination free, easy to use, and atraumatic.

Hand pumps

The "bicycle horn" pump has been marketed in drugstores for years without instructions for use or cleaning. At the museum at the Corning Glass Works in Corning, NY, a glass and rubber hand pump made by Davol circa 1830 is on display next to glass baby bottles and pewter nipples. The current model is the same, except the glass has been replaced by plastic. The dangers of this pump are legion but can be summarized by saying the milk is contaminated, a spray of milk can go directly into the bulb, the pump requires constant emptying, and it can be quite traumatic to the nipple, areola, and breast and predispose to mastitis.[22]

Modifications of the bicycle horn pump insert a removable collecting bottle in place of the well. The modification permits feeding the infant directly from the collecting vessel by placing a nipple on it. Milk does not wash back over the breast, and pumping is not interrupted for emptying. The bulb still may harbor bacteria because it is difficult to clean. The limitations of the effect of creating a simple vacuum and applying a simple, rigid, sharp-edged flange against the breast are still present. This pump is satisfactory for temporary use, but it takes time to become proficient in its use, and it may never create enough pressure to be effective. Another model (Nurture) with a special flexible silicone funnel overcomes these problems and is available from White River Natural Technologies, Inc. Figure 21-3 illustrates application of the flange. This model uses a cylinder for suction and collection.

The cylindric pumps are two all-plastic cylindric tubes that fit inside one another to create a vacuum. A rigid flange to accommodate the nipple and areola is at the top of the inner tube, which also has a gasket for tight fit at the other end. The outer tube collects the milk and is adapted for use as a feeding

unit when a nipple is screwed on top. The mother creates the vacuum by pulling the outer tube and creates rhythm by alternating pushing the outer tube in and out (Fig. 21-4). It is simple, easy to clean, and the milk is usable directly from the collecting cylinder with a nipple attached. This pump is excellent in the hands of an experienced, dextrous mother. The product has several manufacturers, and models differ slightly. Some have a choice of flanges. The only precaution is that 220 mm Hg of negative pressure can be produced if the cylinder is drawn at least three quarters of the way out when empty or when there is fluid (pumped milk) in the cylinder. The pressure desired can be achieved by pulling out the cylinder only a fraction. Most cylinder pumps are marked by the manufacturer to indicate degree of a cycle.

The Lloyd-B pump has a trigger handle adapted to a flange mechanism that empties into a collection jar the size of a baby-food jar (not a baby bottle). It does have a vacuum relief switch; however, the entire mechanism requires a certain dexterity and a rather large hand to operate. It is portable and also easily cleaned. No parts harbor bacteria.

Electric mechanical pumps

Battery-operated pumps are available, but they have all the disadvantages of most battery-operated devices and in most cases are not sufficiently powerful to stimulate the breast adequately. They are ineffective for women whose infants are not feeding at the breast, such as premature infants or those hospitalized in an NICU. These small hand pumps work for some fully lactating women and have no trouble with volume but need a pump that fits in their purse for use while at work or school.

Small, purse-size electric pumps may be effective for the fully lactating woman (see Fig. 21-2). They have an advantage over a manually powered hand pump in that the electric power frees one hand for the mother to stroke the breast and encourage let-down. If flow is going well, the hand is free to perform other tasks, such as read, telephone, or write, not an insignificant advantage for a busy, working, breastfeeding woman. Most small electric models have a small hole in the flange

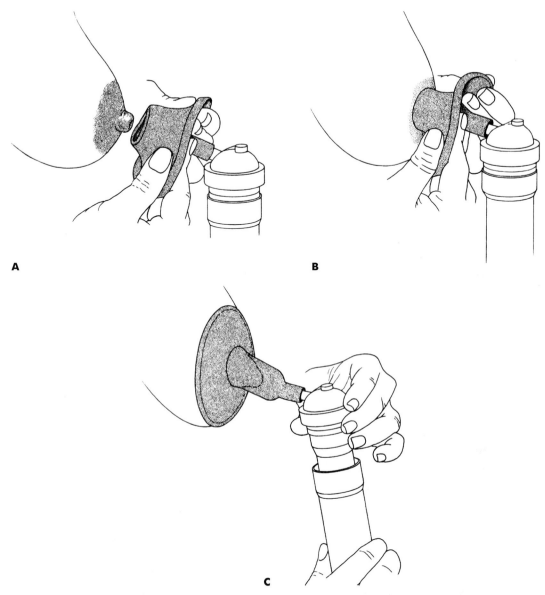

Figure 21-3. A, Step 1. Apply soft flange to ensure proper positioning and comfort. Evert flange back over base. Soft flange has advantage of close application and gentle massaging (milking) of areola and nipple to create a teat. **B,** Step 2. Apply everted flange squarely over nipple for careful placement, and fold flange back over areola. **C,** Step 3. Attach flange to hand pump or electric pump.

base that must be closed with a finger to develop the suction, as in many hospital suctioning devices. This also gives the mother control over the pressure. By rhythmically opening and closing the hole with the finger, the operator can simulate

milking action that is very effective in extracting milk. The manufacturers, unfortunately, do not always point this out.

Hand-held mechanical devices may not be enough for the woman trying to build up a supply

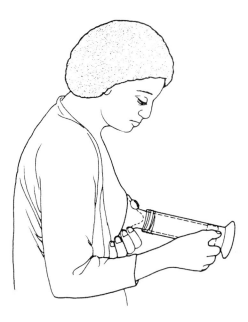

Figure 21-4.   Cylindric pump in use.

when the infant cannot stimulate the breast directly. A new mother may become quite discouraged at the low volume of her production and discontinue the process. Part of the management of a sick infant is to be sure that the mother's milk production is also progressing. Most hospitals provide a lactation consultant for lactating women with babies in the NICU or have trained the unit's nursing staff to provide assistance. Large NICUs in the United States provide a room with electric pumps for the mothers of NICU infants to learn how to pump their milk and breastfeed their infants. This is a key resource for any NICU as appropriate nourishment is key in NICU survival.

Full-size electric pumps are the most efficient because the motor applies the mechanical effort. The mother can concentrate on applying the cup to her breast, massaging the breast, and relaxing so that adequate let-down can take place. All electric pumps are not equal, and some guidance is needed to be sure that the mother understands the principles involved. Nursery staff should be familiar with the equipment. The pumps are no challenge to skilled NICU nurses, who are adept

at handling much more complicated electronic equipment.

A pump that cycles pressure instead of maintaining constant negative pressure will be less likely to cause petechiae or internal trauma to the breast. The ultimate effect of pressure also depends on the length of time the pressure is applied. Tissue cannot withstand sustained high pressure. Pressure sustained for 2 seconds or at a rate of 30 pumps per minute is considered maximum time or minimum rate.[18] Negative pressures should have a governing mechanism to avoid excessive pressures. Mean sucking pressures of most normal full-term infants range from -50 to -155 mm Hg/in^2, with a maximum up to -220 mm Hg/in^2. Manufacturers recommend about 200 mm Hg/in^2 to initiate flow in most women.

A careful study by Johnson[35] of over 1000 patients at the University of Texas using a variety of pumps has confirmed some facts about pumps. The amount of negative pressure possible and the control mechanisms were recorded (Tables 21-14 and 21-15).

An increasing number of pumps on the market have similar designs, but each has its special nuances. A standard electric pump capable of cycling pressures to 220 mm Hg (2.5 to 8.5 psi/Hg) is usually required to stimulate production de novo, that is, when an infant is unavailable to suckle directly as a small premature infant on a ventilator in the NICU. Smaller electric pumps are effective in pumping milk at work when this is done daily. The various hand models can be used for the occasional pumping.[23]

Breast pumps have been identified repeatedly as the source of infection.[50] Improvement in design with a safety trap between the collecting vessel and the machine to prevent milk getting into the mechanism is important. In addition, all equipment that comes in contact with milk or the breast should be sterilizable or disposable. The well-designed electric pump properly used is the best system for stimulating lactation and increasing volume.

In the hospital, as with all special equipment, it is advisable to select the best equipment to fill the needs of that hospital and then purchase the same

(Text continued on p.32)

TABLE 21-14   Electric pumping devices

Mechanical pump	Advantages	Disadvantages
All mechanical pumps	More efficient than hand or battery powered Can rent Should be covered by insurance Well serviced by company	Expensive
Hollister-Egnell	Rhythmic vacuum Stimulates nursing Helpful in initiating let-down Simulates rhythm of suckling Disposable tubing and collecting cups Has double-pumping capability Accessory equipment readily available	

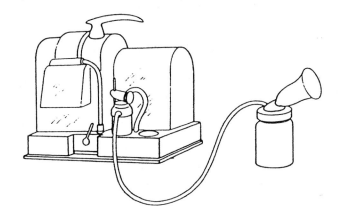

Gomco/Sorenson	Good visibility
	Good collection vessel
		Adapted from suction
		  apparatus
		Poor cup design—painful
		Operates on negative
		  pressure
		Continuous negative pressure
		  can run too high
		Finger control of T-tube
		  needed to cycle vacuum
		Hard to control
		Not good for long use
		Noisy

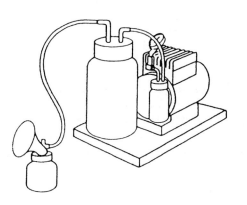

(Continued)

TABLE 21-14   Electric pumping devices—cont'd

Mechanical pump	Advantages	Disadvantages
Medela	Comfortable Automatic cycling Adjustable vacuum Double or single pump	
Classic electric breast pump Heavy duty for hospital use (available to rent)		

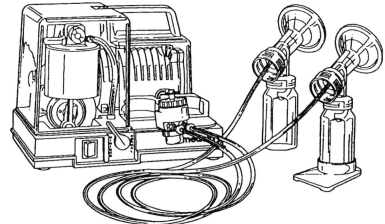

Lactina Select electric breast
pump
Light, portable, economical

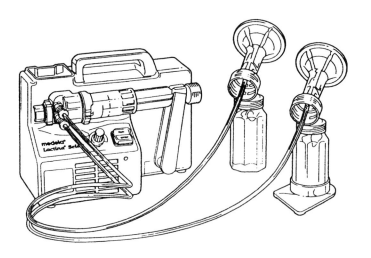

TABLE 21-14	Electric pumping devices—cont'd	
Mechanical pump	**Advantages**	**Disadvantages**
White River Concepts electric breast pump	Flexible silastin flange (Soft-Cup Funnel) Automatic cycling Variable vacuum control Minimal assembly Sturdy carrying case Hospital grade/rental grade Single or double pump kits Easy to clean between rentals Model 9050	Simple appearance

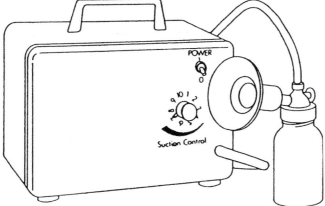

Attachment for double pumping also available

TABLE 21-14   Electric pumping devices—cont'd

Mechanical pump	Advantages	Disadvantages
Automatic breast pump (for use with hospital wall suction)	Flexible silastin flange (Soft-Cup Funnel) Automatic cycling, variable vacuum Single patient use at bedside Minimizes possibility of user cross contamination Single or double pumping capability Adjustable from low to high levels Low maintenance Impact-resistant internal components Convenient and sanitary bedside pumping Can be rented in most countries	Limited to hospital use

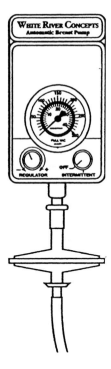

TABLE 21-15	**Hand pumping devices**	
Hand pump	**Advantages**	**Disadvantages**
Bicycle horn	Inexpensive Portable	Difficult to clean Bulb retains bacteria Works as vacuum No instructions Can cause trauma Not appropriate for donor milk Milk washes back over nipple Requires constant emptying Not recommended
Evenflo	Inexpensive	Difficult to clean; bulb harbors bacteria even when boiled
White River	Pliable flange Can feed baby from collecting container Works well for less experienced mother with good let-down No milk contacts mechanism	

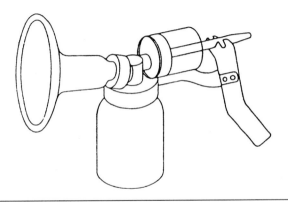

(Continued)

TABLE 21-15	**Hand pumping devices—cont'd**	
Hand pump	**Advantages**	**Disadvantages**
Cylindric: two all-plastic cylindric tubes fit inside one another to create vacuum; inner tube has flange at top and rubber or nylon gasket	Less expensive than electric Portable Can feed baby from collecting container Easily cleaned and sterilized	Requires some dexterity Works as vacuum with some rhythm Rigid flange Can achieve >220 mm Hg of pressure Must follow instructions

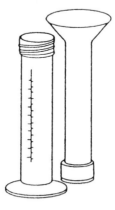

Lloyd: glass flange attached to collecting jar; trigger handle mechanism creates vacuum; has vacuum relief switch	Less expensive than electric Portable Can be cleaned No milk contacts mechanism	Handle difficult to squeeze Hand becomes cramped Awkward Large breast and nipple may hit flange Transfer of milk to feeding unit necessary

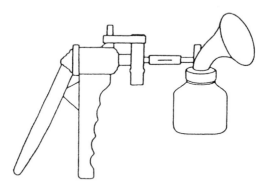

TABLE 21-15   Hand pumping devices—cont'd

Hand pump	Advantages	Disadvantages
Ameda-Egnell, one handed	Spring-loaded handle Each pumping action requires only one motion of energy per pump Squeeze provides suction "Ergonomically" correct Avoids muscle cramping Cleans easily	Awkward 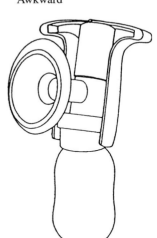
Battery operated (several brands available)	One-handed operation Portable Milk collected in feeding container Intermittent suction release bar Adequate in good lactator who wants to pump a little once a day or less	Not adequate to stimulate production Limited pressure curve Need infant to be feeding at most feeds to stimulate breast

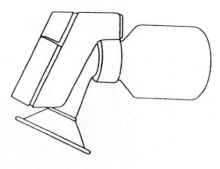

model so that staff can learn how to use it properly and can instruct the patient.

Similarly, the equipment should be checked on a routine basis, cleaned, and bacteriologically tested. Accessory equipment (disposable) can be resterilized for the same patient but not for a second patient.

Although attention is usually given to the pressure mechanisms, equally important is the cup or flange that is applied to the breast. The diameter and depth of the flare are fixed for the hand pumps and the Gomco electric pump, but a choice is offered for the Egnell, Medela, and White River pumps (Fig. 21-5). The nipple should have room to be drawn out, and the flange should be adequate to transmit pressure or milking action to the collecting

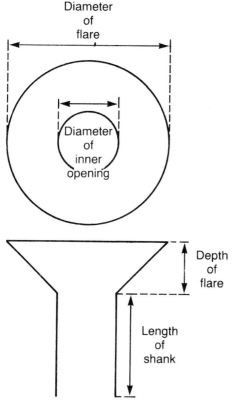

Figure 21-5. Measurement of nipple cups. (From Johnson CA: An evaluation of breast pumps currently available on the American market. Clin Pediatr 22:40, 1983.)

ampullae under the areola. The hand pumps are too small; however, bigger is not always better, and a mother may find that the smaller model of the two offered may be more suited physiologically to her anatomy. This feature does not correlate directly with overall size of the breast. The ideal range is 68- to 82-mm outer diameter and 35- to 40-mm depth of flare (see Fig. 21-5).[35] The White River and the Nurture silicone funnels adapt well to all sizes and shapes because of their flexibility. Instructions for the White River soft flange suggest moistening the flange with milk or water to allow the nipple and areola to adapt well to the flange and the shaft.

The relative efficacy of four methods of human milk expression was measured by Green and associates.[31] The electric pump (Egnell) enabled mothers to pump significantly more milk with higher fat content in the 10-minute time allotted for the study than did the Lloyd-B, the Evenflo hand pump, or manual expression, all three of which were about equal in efficacy.

To test the effect on milk ejection, an electric pump was programmed to cycle 45 to 125 times per minute with vacuums between 45 to 273 mm Hg. The time it took for milk to be ejected was determined by ultrasound of the opposite breast measuring the dilation of lactiferous ducts. Ejection occurred between 136 ± 12 to 104 ± 10 seconds. This compares with ejection time when the infant suckles at 56 ± 4 seconds. The vacuum affected the volume of milk but not the time of ejection.[36]

To understand the ability of various pumps to stimulate lactation and enhance milk volume in the maintenance of lactation, Zinaman[79] and associates[80] studied milk yield, prolactin levels, and oxytocin. Twenty-three women exclusively breastfeeding were randomly assigned to use three different pumping methods serially and compare them with the suckling effectiveness of their infants. Blood samples were collected every 10 minutes from a previously inserted intravenous line controlled with a heparin lock. An electric pump (White River), pulsatile on medium settings of 180 mm Hg and autocycled at 40 pumps per minute, was used with double setup. The Medela manual pump was cycled by the user at 40 times per minute; pressures of 220 mm Hg were used

15 minutes on both breasts simultaneously. The Gentle Expressions battery-operated pump achieved suction levels of 110 mm Hg and was cycled 6 to 10 times per minute by the subject, individually pumping each side for 15 minutes. Hand expression was performed by the Marmet method. Testing was done over 7 days, at 10 AM, at least 2½ hours after the infant's last feeding. Blood was collected at −15, 0, 10, 20, 30, 40, 50, and 60 minutes. Serum prolactin and plasma oxytocin tests were performed simultaneously on all samples, which had been previously separated and frozen.

Prolactin levels were highest with the pulsatile electric pump compared with those of the infant's suckling, actually exceeding levels created by the infant. The hand pumps were similar to hand expression, with the battery-operated pump achieving the lowest levels (Figs. 21-6 and 21-7). No difference was seen in the oxytocin response, although the levels increased before feeding when the baby fed but not when the breast was pumped (Table 21-16). The mean volumes obtained were similar, with the pulsatile electric pump reaching 175 mL over 60 minutes, the manual pump 125 mL over 60 minutes, the battery-operated pump 110 mL over 60 minutes, and hand expression 75 mL

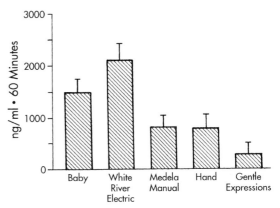

Figure 21-7. Serum prolactin results, with breast stimulation calculated as mean net area under curves for each of five methods. Data given as mean ± SEM. (Modified from Zinaman MJ, Hughes V, Queenan JT et al: Acute prolactin, oxytocin responses and milk yield to infant suckling and artificial methods of expression in lactating women. Pediatrics 89:437, 1992.)

over 60 minutes. Marked differences were seen in the pumps' ability to produce an acute and sustained response, and differences in time were required to achieve the ultimate volume (Fig. 21-8). The differences were related to the method of pumping (i.e., electric, battery operated, manual) and not to comparison of brands.

The universal availability of a double collecting system so both breasts are "pumped" simultaneously greatly enhances production and saves time.

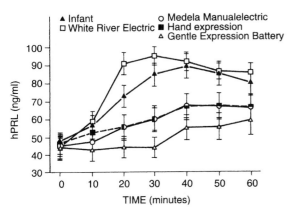

Figure 21-6. Mean human serum prolactin (hPRL) levels for each of five expression methods. Data given as mean ± SEM. (Modified from Zinaman MJ, Hughes V, Queenan JT, et al: Acute prolactin, oxytocin responses and milk yield to infant suckling and artificial methods of expression in lactating women. Pediatrics 89:437, 1992.)

TABLE 21-16	Oxytocin results[*]	
Method	**Mean net AUC**	**SEM**
Infant	224.7	75.4
White River Electric	174.1	41.3
Medela Manual	218.5	157.5
Hand expression	140.5	66.5
Gentle Expressions Battery	186.7	67.6

[*]Levels of plasma oxytocin with breast stimulation calculated as mean net area under the curves (AUC) for each of the five methods over the 60-minute sampling session. No significant differences were noted.
From Zinaman M, Hughes V, Queenan JT, et al: Acute prolactin, oxytocin responses and milk yield to infant suckling and artificial methods of expression in lactating women. Pediatrics 89:437, 1992.

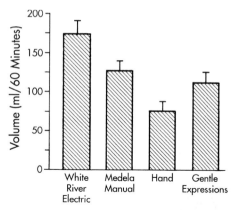

Figure 21-8. Mean milk volumes obtained with breast stimulation for four of the five expression methods (infant not included). Data given as mean ± SEM. (Modified from Zinaman MJ, Hughes V, Queenan JT et al: Acute prolactin, oxytocin responses and milk yield to infant suckling and artificial methods of expression in lactating women. Pediatrics 89:437, 1992.)

Breast pump efficiency was studied by Hartmann and colleagues,[33] utilizing a procedure for objective determination of breast pump efficiency by measuring milk removal from one breast over a 5-minute period in 30 women using an electric breast pump (vacuum pattern of Medela Classic). They compared these data with breastfeeding characteristics. They determined each woman's breastfeeding characteristics by collecting milk samples before and after each feed from each breast by either manual breast pump (Medela AG) or hand expression, by test weighing the infant, measuring degree of fullness and direct measurement of breast volume, all techniques standardized in their laboratory. The authors concluded that pump efficiency can be measured if maternal characteristics and the amount of milk in the breast available to be expressed are known. The proportion of available milk expressed varied greatly between mothers.

A complete assessment of all the pumps readily available on the market and details about other equipment for breastfeeding are provided in the *Breastfeeding Product Guide* by Kittie Frantz.[23]

REFERENCES

1. Arnold LDW: The statistical state of human milk banking and what's in the future. J Hum Lact 7:25, 1991.
2. Arnold LDW: How North American donor milk banks operate: Results of a survey. I. J Hum Lact 13:159, 1997.
3. Arnold LDW: How North American donor milk banks operate: Results of a survey. II. J Hum Lact 13:234, 1997.
4. Asquith MT, Pedrotti PW, Stevenson DK, et al: Clinical uses, collection, and banking of human milk. Clin Perinatol 14:173, 1987.
5. Balmer SE, Wharton BA: Human milk banking at Sorrento Maternity Hospital, Birmingham. Arch Dis Child 67:556, 1992.
6. Beerens H, Romond C, Neut C: Influence of breastfeeding on the bifid flora of the newborn intestine. Am J Clin Nutr 33:2434, 1980.
7. Berkow SE, Freed LM, Hamosh M, et al: Lipases and lipids in human milk: Effects of freeze-thawing and storage. Pediatr Res 18:1257, 1984.
8. Björksten B, Burman LG, DeChateau P, et al: Collecting and banking human milk: To heat or not to heat? Br Med J 281:765, 1980.
9. Carroll L, Osman M, Davies DP: Does discarding the first few milliliters of breast milk improve the bacteriological quality of bank breast milk? Arch Dis Child 55:898, 1980.
10. Carroll L, Osman M, Davies DP, et al: Bacteriological criteria for feeding raw breast-milk to babies on neonatal units. Lancet 2:732, 1979.
11. Committee on Mother's Milk, American Academy of Pediatrics: Operation of mother's milk bureaus. J Pediatr 23:112, 1943.
12. Committee on Nutrition, American Academy of Pediatrics: Human milk banking. Pediatrics 68:854, 1980.
13. Cruz JR, Gil L, Cano F, et al: Protection by breastfeeding against gastrointestinal infection and disease in infancy. In Atkinson SA, Hanson LA, Chandra RK (eds): Nutrition, Infection and Infant Growth in Developed and Emerging Countries. Saint John's, Newfoundland, Canada, Arts Biomedical Publishers, 1990.
14. Davidson DC, Poll RA, Roberts G: Bacteriological monitoring of unheated human milk. Arch Dis Child 54:760, 1979.
15. Donowitz LG, Marsik FJ, Fisher KA, et al: Contaminated breast milk: A source of Klebsiella bacteremia in a newborn intensive care unit. Rev Infect Dis 3:716, 1981.
16. Dworsky M, Stagno S, Pass RF, et al: Persistence of cytomegalovirus in human milk after storage. J Pediatr 101:440, 1982.
17. Eglin RP, Wilkinson AR: HIV infection and pasteurization of breast milk. Lancet 1:1093, 1987.

18. Egnell E: The mechanics of different methods of emptying the female breast. J Swed Med Assoc 40:1, 1956.

19. Eidelman AI, Szilagyi G: Patterns of bacterial colonization of human milk. Obstet Gynecol 53:550, 1979.

20. Evans TJ, Ryley HC, Neale LM, et al: Effect of storage and heat on antimicrobial proteins in human milk. Arch Dis Child 53:239, 1978.

21. Ford JE, Law BA, Marshall VM, et al: Influence of heat treatment of human milk on some of its protective constituents. J Pediatr 90:29, 1977.

22. Foxman B, D'Arcy H, Gillespie B: Lactation mastitis: Occurrence and medical management among 946 breastfeeding women in the United States. Am J Epidemiol 155:115, 2002.

23. Frantz K: Breastfeeding Product Guide. Sunland, CA, Geddes Productions, 1994.

24. Freier S, Faber J: Loss of immune components during the processing of human milk. In Williams AF, Baum J (eds): Human Milk Banking. Nestle Nutrition. New York, Vevey/Raven, 1984.

25. Friend BA, Shahani KM, Long CA, et al: The effect of processing and storage on key enzymes, B vitamins, and lipids of mature human milk. I. Evaluation of fresh samples and effects of freezing and frozen storage. Pediatr Res 17:61, 1983.

26. Garza C, Johnson CA, Harrist R, et al: Effects of methods of collection and storage on nutrients in human milk. Early Hum Dev 6:295, 1982.

27. Gibbs JH, Fisher C, Bhattacharya S, et al: Drip breast milk: Its composition, collection and pasteurization. Early Hum Dev 1:227, 1977.

28. Goldblum RM, Dill CW, Albrecht TB, et al: Rapid high-temperature treatment of human milk. J Pediatr 104:380, 1984.

29. Goldblum RM, Goldblum AS, Garza C, et al: Human milk banking. II. Relative stability of immunologic factors in stored colostrum. Acta Paediatr Scand 71:143, 1982.

30. Golden J: From wet nurse directory to milk bank: The delivery of human milk in Boston, 1909-1927. Bull His Med 62:589, 1988.

31. Green D, Moye L, Schreiner RL, et al: The relative efficacy of four methods of human milk expression. Early Hum Dev 6:153, 1982.

32. Hamosh M, Ellis LA, Pollock DR, et al: Breastfeeding and the working mother: Effect of time and temperature of short-term storage on proteolysis, lipolysis, and bacterial growth in milk. Pediatrics 97:492, 1996.

33. Hartmann PE, Mitoulas LR, Gurrin LC: Physiology of breastmilk expression using an electric breast pump. J Nutr 131:3016S, 2001.

34. Hernandez J, Lemons P, Lemons J, et al: Effect of storage processes on the bacterial growth-inhibiting activity of human breast milk. Pediatrics 63:597, 1979.

35. Johnson CA: An evaluation of breast pumps currently available on the American market. Clin Pediatr 22:40, 1983.

36. Kent JC, Ramsay DT, Doherty D, et al: Response of breasts to different stimulation patterns of an electric breast pump. J Hum Lact 19:179, 2003.

37. Lavine M, Clark RM: Changing patterns of free fatty acids in breast milk during storage. J Pediatr Gastroenterol Nutr 6:769, 1987.

38. Lawrence RA: Commentary. In Foxman B, D'Arcy H, Gillespie B: Lactation mastitis: Occurrence and medical management among 946 breastfeeding women in the United States. Am J Epidemiol 155:115, 2002.

39. Lemons JA, Schreiner RL, Gresham EL: Simple method for determining the caloric and fat content of human milk. Pediatrics 66:626, 1980.

40. Liebhaber M, Lewiston NJ, Asquith MT, et al: Alterations of lymphocytes and antibody content of human milk after processing. J Pediatr 91:897, 1977.

41. Liebhaber M, Lewiston NJ, Asquith MT, et al: Comparison of bacterial contamination with two methods of human milk collection. J Pediatr 92:236, 1978.

42. Lucas A: Human milk banks. Lancet 1:103, 1982.

43. Lucas A, Gibbs JAH, Lyster RLJ, et al: Creamatocrit: Simple clinical technique for estimating fat concentration and energy value of human milk. Br Med J 1:1018, 1978.

44. Martinez FE, Desai ID, Davidson AGF, et al: Ultrasonic homogenization of expressed human milk to prevent fat loss during tube feeding. J Pediatr Gastroenterol Nutr 6:593, 1987.

45. McDougal JS, Martin LS, Cort SP, et al: Thermal inactivation of the acquired immunodeficiency syndrome virus, human T lymphotropic virus-III/lymphadenopathy-associated virus, with special reference to antihemophilic factor. J Clin Invest 76:875, 1985.

46. McEnery G, Chattopadhyay B: Human milk bank in a district general hospital. Br Med J 2:794, 1978.

47. McPherson RJ, Wagner CL: The effect of pasteurization on TGFα and TGFβ2 concentrations in human milk. Adv Exp Med Biol 501:359, 2001.

48. Michaelsen KF, Skafte L, Badsberg JH, et al: Variation in macronutrients in human bank milk: Influencing factors and implications for human milk banking. J Pediatr Gastroenterol Nutr 11:229, 1990.

49. Moffatt PA, Lammi-Keefe CJ, Ferris AM, et al: Alpha and gamma tocopherols in pooled mature human milk after storage. J Pediatr Gastroenterol Nutr 6:225, 1987.

50. Moloney AC, Quoraishi AH, Parry P, et al: A bacteriological examination of breast pumps. J Hosp Infect 9:169, 1987.

51. Morgan JN, Toledo RT, Eitenmiller RR, et al: Thermal destruction of immunoglobulin A, lactoferrin, thiamin, and folic acid in human milk. J Food Sci 51:348, 1986.

52. Mother's Milk Unit, California Transplant Bank: Procedures and Protocols. San Jose, CA, The Mother's Milk Bank, The Institute for Medical Research, 1988.

53. Orloff SL, Wallingford JC, McDougal JS: Inactivation of human immunodeficiency virus type I in human milk: Effects of intrinsic factors in human milk and of pasteurization. J Hum Lact 9:300, 1993.

54. Ovesen L, Jakobsen J, Leth T, et al: The effect of microwave heating on vitamins B1 and E, and linoleic and linolenic acids, and immunoglobulins in human milk. Int J Food Sci Nutr 47:427, 1996.

55. Paxson CI, Cress CC: Survival of human milk leukocytes. J Pediatr 94:61, 1979.

56. Pittard WB, Bill K: Human milk banking: effect of refrigeration on cellular components. Clin Pediatr 20:31, 1981.

57. Quan R, Yang C, Rubinstein S, et al: Effects of microwave radiation on anti-infective factors in human milk. Pediatrics 89:667, 1992.

58. Reynolds GJ, Lewis-Jones DI, Isherwood DM, et al: A simplified system of human milk banking. Early Hum Dev 7:281, 1982.

59. Schmidt E: Effects of varying degrees of heat treatment on milk protein and its nutritional consequences. Acta Paediatr Scand Suppl 296:41, 1982.

60. Silprasert A, Dejsarai W, Keawvichit R, et al: Effect of storage on the creamatocrit and total energy content of human milk. Hum Nutr Clin Nutr 40C:31, 1986.

61. Smith L, Bickerton J, Pilcher G, et al: Creamatocrit, carbon content, and energy value of pooled banked human milk: implications for feeding preterm infants. Early Hum Dev 11:75, 1985.

62. Sosa R, Barness L: Bacterial growth in refrigerated human milk. Am J Dis Child 141:111, 1987.

63. Springer S: Human milk banking in Germany. J Hum Lact 13:65, 1997.

64. Stagno S, Reynolds DW, Pass RF: Breast milk and the risk of cytomegalovirus infection. N Engl J Med 302:1073, 1980.

65. Stocks RJ, Davies DP, Carroll LP, et al: A simple method to improve the energy value of bank human milk. Early Hum Dev 8:175, 1983.

66. Sunshine P, Asquith MT, Liebhaber M: The effects of collection and processing on various components of human milk. In Frier S, Eidelman AI (eds): Human Milk: Its Biological and Social Value. Amsterdam, Excerpta Medica, 1980.

67. Thiry L, Sprecher-Goldberger S, Jonckheer T, et al: Isolation of AIDS virus from cell-free breast milk of three healthy virus carriers. Lancet 2:891, 1985.

68. Tully MR: Excelencia em bancos de leite humano: Uma visao do futuro—the First International Congress on Human Milk Banking. J Hum Lact 17:51, 2001.

69. Tully MR, Jones F: Guidelines for the Establishment and Operation of a Donor Human Milk Bank. Raleigh, NC, Human Milk Banking Association of North America, 2003.

70. Tyson JE, Edwards WH, Rosenfeld AM, et al: Collection methods and contamination of bank milk. Arch Dis Child 57:396, 1982.

71. Van Zoeren-Grobben D, Schrijver J, Van Den Berg H, et al: Human milk vitamin content after pasteurisation, storage or tube feeding. Arch Dis Child 62:161, 1987.

72. Wardell JM, Hill CM, D'Souza SW: Effect of pasteurization and of freezing and thawing human milk on its triglyceride content. Acta Paediatr Scand 70:467, 1981.

73. Welsh JK, May JT: Anti-infective properties of breast milk. J Pediatr 93:1, 1979.

74. WHO/UNICEF joint statement: Meeting on infant and young child feedings. J Nurs Midwife 25:31, 1980.

75. Williamson S, Finucane E, Ellis H, et al: Effect of heat treatment of human milk on absorption of nitrogen, fat, sodium, calcium, and phosphorus by preterm infants. Arch Dis Child 53:555, 1978.

76. Williamson S, Hewitt JH, Finucane E, et al: Organisation of bank of raw and pasteurised human milk for neonatal intensive care. Br Med J 1:393, 1978.

77. Wills ME, Han VEM, Harris DA, et al: Short-time low-temperature pasteurisation of human milk. Early Hum Dev 7:71, 1980.

78. Ziegler JB, Cooper DA, Johnson RO, et al: Post-natal transmission of AIDS-associated retrovirus from mother to infant. Lancet 1:896, 1985.

79. Zinaman MJ: Breast pumps: Ensuring mother's success. Contemp Obstet Gynecol 32:55, 1988.

80. Zinaman MJ, Hughes V, Queenan JT, et al: Acute prolactin, oxytocin responses and milk yield to infant suckling and artificial methods of expression in lactating women. Pediatrics 89:437, 1992.

22

Breastfeeding support groups and community resources

Certain changes in cultural aspects of Western civilization have contributed to the widespread use of artificial feedings for human infants as well as to the changing structure of the family. Urbanization has been associated not only with industrialization but also with the separation of generations. This has produced the nuclear family. *Nuclear families* are smaller, mobile, isolated families often stranded in a large urban population. In a nuclear family, the young couple and their new infant are totally without personal human resources. That is, no one cares enough to give individual support to the family. There is no one to turn to and from whom to receive advice, encouragement, and support.

HISTORICAL PERSPECTIVE

Rites de passage were described by the French author Van Gennep[34] as the ceremonies and rituals that mark special changes in people's lives. The list includes marriage, motherhood, birth, death, circumcision, graduation, ordination, and retirement. In our present culture, support exists for most of these events except birth and motherhood. The most critical rite of passage in a woman's life, Raphael[25] points out, is when she becomes a mother. Raphael further distinguishes this period of transition with the term *matrescence,* "to emphasize the mother and to focus on her new life-style." Traditional cultures herald a mother giving birth, whereas our culture announces the birth of an infant. The former highlights the mother, the latter the infant. Matrescence is a time of coddling. In preindustrial societies, the mother is coddled for some time after birth, having only the responsibility of the infant's care while the mother's needs are met by doulas. Mothering the mother should be part of the postpartum support for a new mother.

A number of other forces added momentum to the bottle feeding trend that began in the 1920s, when manufacturers finally were able to mass-produce an inexpensive container and rubber nipple with which to feed infants inexpensively. *Pediatrics* was a new specialty to guard the health of children. The stress was on measuring and calculating. Physicians seemed more secure when they could prescribe nutrition. The rise in the female labor force has also been credited with having an impact on the method of feeding infants, who were no longer brought everywhere with the mother to be nursed but instead were left behind to be bottle fed. The technology of the infant food industry was a continuing influence on nutritional thinking of both medical and lay groups.

Breastfeeding was never totally abandoned. There was always a group of women who prepared themselves for childbirth and read and researched feeding and nutrition and chose to breastfeed.[22] In the mid-1940s, Dr. Edith Jackson began the Rooming-In Project in New Haven, Connecticut. Families in New Haven who sought "childbirth without fear" and an opportunity to room-in with their infants usually chose to breastfeed. In the rooming-in unit, breastfeeding was often "contagious" because one mother successfully nursing would encourage others to try. Hospital stays averaged 5 to 7 days, during which time the mother-infant couple was cared for as a pair. About 70% of the patients left this hospital breastfeeding. The national average at that time (1945–1955) was less than 25%.

Students and staff who were exposed to the philosophy of this unit went to many parts of the country, taking with them tremendous commitment to prepared childbirth and nurturing through breastfeeding. The classic article on the management of breastfeeding by Barnes and associates[2] was published as a result of counseling hundreds of nursing mothers. The students of Jackson inoculated many hundreds of hospitals and communities with a zeal for breastfeeding.

DEVELOPMENT OF MOTHER SUPPORT GROUPS

The need remained for nuclear families to have access to support and conversation about healthy infants, mothering, and breastfeeding.[6] The La Leche League, developed by a group of seven mothers to meet these needs, was established in Franklin Park, Illinois, in 1957. The original intent was to provide other nursing mothers with information, encouragement, and moral support. There are now thousands of local chapters and a network of 32,000 state and regional coordinators who all synchronize their activities with the headquarters now in Schaumburg, Illinois. La Leche League International's 4000 groups are in 66 countries, including the United States, Canada, parts of

Europe, New Zealand, and Africa, and other parts of the world.[13]

An excellent publication, *The Womanly Art of Breastfeeding*,[13] was prepared by the original group of mothers involved in the La Leche League. The publication was revised for the 25th anniversary of the organization in 1982, and in celebration of the 40th anniversary in 1997, the 6th edition was published. The 7th edition was released in 2004. La Leche League continues to provide information and updated publications about common questions that arise during lactation. Local groups offer classes to prepare mothers to breastfeed. They help with suggestions about the nitty-gritty details of preparation, nutrition, clothing, and mothering in general. They also provide every mother with a telephone counselor. To be qualified to serve as a counselor to another mother, a member must demonstrate knowledge and expertise in breastfeeding as well as an understanding of how to counsel and render support. "Telephone mothers" do not give medical advice and are instructed to tell a troubled mother to call her own physician for such advice. Interested local physicians provide medical expertise for the group when a medical opinion is appropriate. The league provides support for mothers to reduce the time the physician needs to spend counseling on the nonmedical aspects of lactation. Most information needed by the new mother is not medical.

In the decades that this support system has been in place, no good substitute for this mother-to-mother program has evolved, because a woman needs a true *doula*.

Similar programs have been developed in more than 70 other countries. A well-established and respected program in Norway is Ammehjelpen International Group; in Australia, the Nursing Mothers' Association of Australia; and in the United Kingdom, the National Childbirth Trust.

Sociologist Alice Ladas[14] studied women who attended La Leche League preparation classes and compared them with a similar group who attempted to breastfeed but did not have this preparation. She was able to demonstrate clearly that the women who attended such programs had more confidence and seemed to benefit from receiving accurate, up-to-date, and relevant information as well as receiving individual and group support.[15]

Silverman and Murrow[30] studied league activities and concluded that group dynamics are important and feelings of normalcy are reinforced. The information and experience were shown to be important, but the support from the group had far greater influence on success in breastfeeding.[33] Meara[18] reports similar observations on league activities in a nonsupportive culture.

A follow-up study of breastfeeding in Oxford was carried out by Sloper and associates.[31] They observed that significantly more mothers went home breastfeeding, mothers nursed longer, and solid foods were started later when support was provided. The authors attribute this shift to the change in advice and support given in the hospital and at home visits.

The Breastfeeding Association of South Africa is a nongovernmental, nonprofit voluntary organization founded in 1978 by South Africans for the express needs of South African women. Their special problems and solutions are well described by Bergh.[3] Support groups for all of life's events, especially those covering health, have become a common feature (there are more than 150 parent support groups). In the field of perinatal care, there are groups for infertile couples; couples who are expecting; those who have experienced pregnancy loss, loss of a premature infant, or loss of a term baby; those who had a cesarean birth; and so on. Physicians should be aware of the groups that function in their community and the policies and philosophies they embrace.

The International Childbirth Education Association also provides resources for the new family in many countries. Its program makes preparation and training available for couples during pregnancy and afterward as parents. Its scope embraces the entire childbirth concept, of which breastfeeding is part.

Adolescents need special support to improve the outcome of their pregnancies, to encourage them to breastfeed, and to establish the special relationship with and commitment to their infants. A study done in the Breastfeeding Educated and

Supported Teen (BEST) Club in Melbourne, Florida, looked at the impact of specific breastfeeding education provided by a lactation consultant in group classes. Teens were randomly assigned to the program or as a control; ethnicity and age were not significant factors. Of the 43 adolescents in the education group, 28 (65%) initiated breastfeeding, but of the 48 control subjects without education, only 7 (14.6%) initiated breastfeeding ($p < 0.001$). The authors concluded that targeted education makes a difference in adolescents.[35]

When a similar study was performed involving low-income women, a community based program studied a hospital, home visit, and telephone support system provided by a community health nurse and a peer counselor for 6 months. After random assignment, those receiving intervention, breastfed longer. The infants had fewer sick visits and use of medicines than the group with "standard care." The cost of the program per mother was $301, which was offset by the savings on the cost of formula and health care.[24]

In another study, adult women without a personal breastfeeding support system at home were randomized to receive support or not. The support group received support in the hospital and at home from a practicing midwife in the community. She visited in the hospital daily and was available by pager continually. After discharge, she telephoned within 72 hours and then weekly for 4 weeks. At home, the participants had access to the midwife by phone and pager. One home visit was made the first week and then as necessary. In the supported group, 26 of 26 were still breastfeeding at 1 month, but only 17 of 25 (68%) in the unsupported group were breastfeeding, proving that intensive professional support works. No costs of the program were provided.[21]

Active support outreach clearly impacts the duration of breastfeeding and ultimately saves health care dollars. Such programs can be included in private practice.

Some carefully researched and accurate videotapes cover the subject of perinatal experiences, including breastfeeding (e.g., VIDA's tape, entitled "Baby"). Some done by popular TV personalities, however, reflect only an individual's experience, with little substance. A list of videos is given in Appendix N.

COMMUNITY RESOURCES

Most hospitals provide training in preparation for childbirth. Part of the program is about the new infant and how to plan for neonatal care. These programs often serve as the initial stimulus to consider breastfeeding. Many such programs are given by the hospital lactation staff.

When a large HMO looked at 5213 new mothers enrolled in a commercial managed care plan, by telephone survey at 4 to 6 month post partum, 75% had breastfed for some time. Of these, 75% breastfed for more than 6 weeks. Breastfeeding for more than 6 weeks was associated with level of education, employment status (part-time 84%), and adequacy of postpartum information. Health plans and employees should consider promoting breastfeeding, concluded the authors.[8]

Because hospitals have become competitive and are marketing their services, many are developing birthing centers and are trying to capture the attention of the childbearing public with special services. These services often include classes on child rearing, including breastfeeding. Physicians should investigate the programs and printed materials distributed by the hospitals where their patients deliver. Many pediatricians are coping with the flood of patient information from conflicting sources by printing up an office manual (desktop printers make this quite feasible). This is especially helpful if the patients give birth at more than one hospital or more than one lay advocacy group is active in the community. Hospital procedures and policies can influence the success or failure of breastfeeding mothers.[29] Pediatricians should be aware of the policies at the hospital(s) with which they are associated.

In a few short decades, we have gone from a paucity of support groups and resource literature to an overwhelming flood. Health care books and childbearing and family-rearing advice books are cascading off the press, written by everyone from qualified experts to poorly informed freelance writers. Some are written by health care professionals who have personal experience in childbearing. The pediatrician should be familiar with a few good references for parents and provide a list for patients in the practice.

The Young Women's Christian Association (YWCA) in most communities may also provide preparation for childbirth. Its classes usually provide programming that appeals to young and unwed women, a group in need of services rarely provided by other sources.

The Visiting Nurses Association and the public health nurses on the staff of the local county health department are special resources particularly skilled at counseling new mothers with their infants. They can provide valuable information to the physician who is working with an infant who fails to thrive at the breast by witnessing the breastfeeding scene at home. As discharge from the hospital occurs earlier and earlier, the pediatrician should consider employing nurse practitioners who are prepared to make housecalls immediately after births.

Many other organizations, local and national in scope, have the perinatal period and the family as their focus. Many of these are also interested in promoting breastfeeding as part of their overall goals.

The World Health Organization (WHO) and United Nations International Children's Education Fund (UNICEF) have joined in an international effort to create a supportive atmosphere in hospitals around the world by developing the Baby Friendly Hospital Initiative (see Chapter 1 and Appendix K). Both WHO and UNICEF provide international support for breastfeeding, especially in developing countries.

A list of breastfeeding support groups can be found in Appendix K.

Government organizations

The U.S. government has taken an active interest in the promotion of breastfeeding as well. In the goals for national health prepared by a multidisciplinary task force in 1978, it is stated that by 1990, 75% of infants leaving the hospital shall be breast-fed and at 6 months of age at least 35% will still be breastfeeding.[23] The rates in 1990 fell short of the goals, and they were thus restated to be achieved by the year 2000, extending to 50% the number to still be breastfeeding at 5 to 6 months. The goals for 2010 include 75% breastfeeding at hospital discharge, 50% at 6 months, and at least 25% breastfeeding at 1 year.

The plan of action to reach these goals has included the development of a Healthy Mothers–Healthy Babies Program. Also, a national committee for the promotion of breast-feeding includes representation from major pro-fessional organizations of physicians, dietitians, social service workers, nurses, nurse midwives, and hospital administrators. A major thrust of the national effort has been through the Women, Infants, and Children program (WIC), in which mothers are being encouraged to breastfeed and are given nutrition and practical lactation man-agement instruction and support. An instruction manual is available for WIC workers.[9]

The surgeon general conducted a national workshop on breastfeeding and human lactation in Rochester, New York, in June 1984 to develop recommendations for national policy. A publi-cation from the workshop was available from the U.S. Government Printing Office in Washing-ton, DC. A follow-up workshop was held in Washington, DC, in 1985, gathering the represen-tatives of the major official national organizations for obstetrics, pediatrics, and family physicians, including the credential organizations for physi-cians, nurses, nurse midwives, and dietitians. The organizations responded to a request to have each approve a model statement in support of breast-feeding. This was accomplished by January 1987. The organizations have also undertaken a review of curriculum within their discipline to ensure adequate education, training, and accreditation regarding human lactation and breastfeeding for their members. Although there have been improvements and certifying examinations have incorporated questions about breastfeeding and

human lactation, curriculum development in most institutions has lagged behind.

Issues of rural health have begun to include those surrounding birth and the infant's welfare. Programs are being developed to increase breast-feeding among rural women. Although the inci-dence of breastfeeding has increased among well-educated, self-motivated middle Americans, the number of impoverished, less well-educated women who breastfeed remains small. Progress is being made, community by community, by dedi-cated health care workers, dietitians, and WIC staff. Health professionals often serve as a catalyst in developing such programs but should always be ready to serve as knowledgeable, supportive con-sultants to the effort of others.[11]

Grants and other incentives provided by public and private sources have enlarged the communica-tions network in states where breastfeeding remains minimal. Groups such as the Healthy Mothers–Healthy Babies Program maximize com-munications between resource programs and offer opportunities to share ideas, logos, publications, and strategies that work. Information about these resources is available from the Healthy Mothers–Healthy Babies Coalition.

The U.S. Department of Agriculture's breastfeed-ing program, through the WIC's Nutrition Program, has launched a major effort announced first during International Breastfeeding Week in August 1997 in Washington, DC, to increase breastfeeding initiation and duration throughout the 50 states. The program, Best Start, includes social marketing research, a media campaign, a staff support kit, a breastfeeding resource guide, a training conference, and continu-ing education and technical assistance. WIC has been made a permanent national health and nutrition program; and breastfeeding was written into the leg-islation (see Chapter 1). The program even mandates that every WIC agency must have accommodations for employees breastfeeding their infants to pump and store their milk.[28]

In order to fulfill a mandate of the Innocenti Declaration signed in 1990 in Italy by representa-tives of 90 countries including Audrey Nora, MD, assistant surgeon general of the United States, a group of interested breastfeeding supporters and advocates met in Florida in January 1996. The declaration states that each member country should have a national breastfeeding committee, and many countries had complied.

The United States Breastfeeding Committee

A small group of breastfeeding advocates met to discuss the need for coordination of breastfeeding activities in the United States. After conducting an intensive needs assessment, the National Alliance for Breastfeeding Advocacy (NABA) was formed to address needs not being met by organizations, government agencies, or individuals. NABA convened the first National Breastfeeding Leadership Roundtable (NBLR) in January 1996 to determine if another organization was needed to move breastfeeding forward in this country. Working on the international model, the formation of this committee, if successful, would satisfy one of the four operational targets set forth by the 1990 Innocenti Declaration. This was to establish a multisectoral national breastfeeding committee composed of representatives from relevant government departments, nongovernmental organizations, and health professional associations in every country.

It was agreed at that meeting of 19 breastfeeding leaders to do four things: (1) to support ongoing breastfeeding projects in the United States; (2) to develop a strategic plan for breastfeeding in the United States; (3) to formalize NBLR into the U.S. Breastfeeding Committee (USBC); and finally, (4) to establish the organization of the USBC and its leadership, the NBLR. The organization continued to meet twice a year and in January 1998 voted to declare itself, with the encouragement of Assistant Surgeon General Audrey Nora, MD, the United States Breastfeeding Committee.

The USBC is a collaborative partnership of organizations. The mission of the committee is to protect, promote, and support breastfeeding in the United States. The USBC exists to assure the rightful place of breastfeeding in society. Major organizations include but are not limited to the American College of Obstetricians and Gynecologists (ACOG), the American Academy of Pediatrics (AAP), the American Academy of Family Practice (AAFP), the La Leche League International (LLLI), the International Lactation Consultant Association (ILCA), and Wellstart and the National Alliance for Breastfeeding Advocacy (NABA). The National Institutes of Health (NIH), Maternal and Child Health Bureau of the Health Resources Division of the U.S. Department of Health and Human Serives (MCHB), Women's Health, and the Centers for Disease Control (CDC) also participate. The USBC's Web site is: http:// www.usbreastfeeding.org.

Wellstart International

A program to extend the scope of global breastfeeding promotion was launched by Wellstart International in a cooperative agreement with U.S. Agency for International Development (AID). Wellstart International, a private, nonprofit organization headquartered in San Diego, grew out of clinical and teaching experiences at the University of California, San Diego Medical Center in the late 1970s.[20] In 1983, in response to a clear need to improve the breastfeeding knowledge of health professionals, a Lactation Management Education (LME) program was initiated with funding from AID. Almost 400 participants of the LME program now form a network of Wellstart Associates in 28 countries.

In late 1991, Wellstart joined in a cooperative agreement with AID to expand and diversify its global breastfeeding promotion activities.[20] The Expanded Promotion of Breastfeeding (EPB) can work in any country at the request of the local AID mission. Wellstart continues to provide educational information for the training of physicians, nurses, and dietitians.

Other lactation centers have been created in health care facilities, such as the program developed by Neifert in Denver. The purpose of these programs is to provide consultation services for mothers as well as education, training, and information for health care workers. Efforts have been made to change hospital policy regarding breastfeeding to increase the success rate.[17] A very impressive program was initiated in the Philippines by Relucio-Clavano.[26] She has not only increased the incidence of breastfeeding but also lowered the morbidity rate from sepsis, diarrhea, and malnutrition.

Best Start—the concept of social marketing

Using the concept of social marketing, Bryant and associates[4] have designed an approach to promoting breastfeeding that utilizes the counseling strategies, educational materials, policies, and community-based activities that form the Best Start Program. *Social marketing* "combines the principles of commercial marketing with health education to promote a socially beneficial idea, practice or product."[4] Typically, a well-articulated program involves a combination of mass media, print materials, personal counseling, and community-based activities.

Best Start is an innovative program that grew out of a project involving focus-group interviews, which were used to identify the determinants of infant feeding decisions and the most effective strategies. Focus-group interviews, according to Bryant and associates,[4] "are small group discussions, guided by a trained moderator, which provide insights into the participants' perceptions, attitudes, and opinions on a designated topic." The composition of the group and the discussions are carefully planned to encourage relationships and disclosure by creating a permissive, nonthreatening environment. Motivations and perceived barriers related to breastfeeding as well as social network influences on feeding choice were identified.

From these findings, a multifaceted breastfeeding promotion campaign was designed for new mothers, family members, health professionals, and the community at large. The Best Start Program has proved to be extremely successful (see Appendices K and N) and has been replicated by others very successfully using the materials developed by Best Start, which are available for an at-cost fee.

Utilizing strategies developed in social marketing and segmentation modeling for health communication, Best Start developed a multimedia program, Loving Support Makes Breastfeeding Work, and has provided a training manual to educate staff in the use of the Best Start visual resources. These materials are also available for a small fee. This program was the substance of the WIC National Breastfeeding Promotion Project launched in April 1997.[1,5]

When the Loving Support Program was evaluated at the Mississippi WIC Program with a cross-sectional study utilizing a questionnaire, 202 health care providers responded (104 nurses and 98 physicians). A greater proportion of nurses than physicians actually mentioned the health benefits of breastfeeding to their patients or helped with breastfeeding management or referred mothers to lactation consultants. The authors concluded that the Loving Support Program was effective but more effort should be made to address physicians' needs.

Breastfeeding and Human Lactation Study Center

The Lactation Study Center of the University of Rochester School of Medicine and Dentistry (NY) encourages and promotes human lactation and breastfeeding through physician education and support. The goal is to provide information that will help the practitioner encourage and support breastfeeding for all patients. Information is available to the health care professional by telephone (see Appendix K). Originally federally funded and established at the request of the surgeon general in 1984, the center now depends on private grants and donations from users. The drug information line operates Monday through Friday from 9 AM to 4 PM EST. Physician consultation is available by call back.

LACTATION CONSULTANTS

For years, many medical and nursing professionals have served as lactation consultants ready to respond to any colleague's request for knowledge and expertise. With the great national movement to embrace breastfeeding, however, a new type of lactation consultant is evolving from the vast pool of women who have served in local mother-to-mother programs to help others breastfeed. The health care professional needs to ensure that the lactation resources available in the community are truly of professional quality and background and that the individuals have obtained the proper certification and licensure. Counseling on any topic is a special skill requiring more than personal experience with the situation.

The International Board of Lactation Consultant Examiners (IBLCE) was developed as a separate organization by the La Leche League International to credential individuals who want to counsel about breastfeeding.[12,*] Those who successfully complete the IBLCE certification process, which includes a written examination, are entitled to use the designation IBCLC (International Board Certified Lactation Consultant) after their names. The IBLCE has defined lactation consultants as "allied health care providers who possess the necessary skills, knowledge, and attitudes to facilitate breastfeeding." These lactation consultants perform as employees in some situations and as independent contractors in states where the medical practice act allows such activity. A lactation consultant should have professional liability insurance coverage and a license to practice in the health field in the state. Nurses, midwives, nurse practitioners, and dietitians are usual candidates. Some physicians have taken the examination.

The International Lactation Consultants Association (ILCA) stated, "A lactation consultant is a health care professional whose scope of practice is focused upon providing education and management to prevent and solve breastfeeding problems and to encourage a social environment that effectively supports the breastfeeding mother/infant dyad." ILCA has published Standards of Practice for Lactation Consultants, which is available in print (see Appendix K).

---

*7309 Arlington Blvd. Suite 300, Falls Church, VA 22042-0348 USA; 703-560-7330 (tel), 703-560-7332 (fax).

Lactation specialist as member of health care team

Modern medicine has developed a team approach to the management of many patient populations, such as elderly or handicapped persons.[16] A team approach also is used in the management of many categories of diseases, such as cancer and diabetes. A health care team provides medical service for the family during the perinatal period. This team includes an obstetrician and a pediatrician or a family physician; nurse midwives; nurses working in prenatal care, obstetrics, neonatal care, and public health; social workers; dietitians; and when a problem develops, perinatologists, neonatologists, and the skilled team from the perinatal center. These team members are well educated and extensively trained professionals. Together they have lowered the morbidity and mortality rates of childbirth. The long-range prognosis for the intact survival of infants has been significantly improved.

Thus, medical progress has occurred concomitantly with the isolation of the nuclear family. The result is a medically successful birth to a family poorly prepared emotionally and socially to cope. The family is inadequately prepared to take over when the mother and infant are discharged from the hospital and instantly placed on their own without a transitional period of adjustment with close support and supervision.

Lactation specialists become a very important addition to the health care team, replacing the traditional family support system. Specialists not only must know their role as counselors interacting with the family, but also must understand how they interface with other members of the health care team. The professional team members are beginning to understand the importance of lactation specialists and how to work most effectively with them. Some physicians, however, provide a nurse practitioner, whose role is to fill that gap between medical care and family support. The nurse practitioner is usually skilled in well-baby care, especially breastfeeding, and in the era of early postpartum discharge home, may make housecalls within 48 hours of arrival home.

Lactation consultants will quickly earn the respect of the health care team if they communicate openly with them, support the mother in a positive manner, and encourage a relationship of mutual trust and respect between the mother and the team.[16]

PEER COUNSELING

Peer counseling is part of a system developed by health care providers and health educators to change personal health behavior.[32] It is an adaptation of a cultural technique that has been used for generations, wherein the family provided a personal advocate or omsbudsman to help the individual carry out good health practices. In lay midwifery, for example, members of the group attended a woman throughout pregnancy, delivery, and postpartum period. The important point is that the peer counselor is a member of the *same* sociocultural group as the recipient, is selected for leadership qualities and experience, and is trained in the special issues.

Public health programs have used peer counselors to encourage women to seek prenatal care or well-child care for their children. Other programs have provided peer counselors for individuals with hypertension, diabetes, or other chronic diseases to help the patient access health care and carry out instructions for treatment. This concept has been applied to the WIC program.[32] A model program was developed in south Georgia in the mid-1980s by Wanda Grogan, PhD, and was very effective in encouraging women to carry out health care advice, to keep appointments for health care, and appropriately to breastfeed their infants.[27] This system has been expanded to many parts of the country.

The most successful programs involve the peer in all health issues so that the relationship between counselor and client continues. These peer programs are integrated with efforts to improve health habits in general and especially those associated with childbearing. The best programs train community counselors to support women through pregnancy, delivery, and early child rearing, of which breastfeeding is a part. This type of program encourages the development of a relationship that lasts several years.

Because the lowest incidence and duration of breastfeeding are among low-income women and among black mothers, a peer-support program among these clients would have the highest probability of success.[27] Using the same model for training candidates that has been developed for other health projects will facilitate initiating the program. The local WIC program or health department is ideal to undertake a peer-support program because the permanent, full-time staff are knowledgeable about nutrition and lactation and can provide continuity when peer counselors leave the program and new ones need training. This stability is essential to developing some consistency and permanency for the system. The WIC program supports women from early pregnancy through postpartum and early infancy periods.

Because a peer counselor is an individual from the social or cultural community who is selected because of good health behaviors and an innate ability to help others and gain respect, a peer counselor for breastfeeding is a respected member of the community or neighborhood, is of the same or similar ethnic background and of similar educational and economic level, and has breastfed one or more children. The tremendous success of the La Leche League was based on peer counseling among well-educated, white, middle-class American women.

To effect a change among WIC women and the target populations of the U.S. health goals for the year 2010 (low-income, black, and minority women), peer counselors will have to come from these groups. The WIC programs have developed a means to identify and train women from the neighborhood to serve as models of successful breastfeeding. A program limited to breastfeeding has the disadvantage of being very limited in scope; the client has to have several other individuals with whom to relate about nonbreastfeeding issues.

Some physician practices have employed (yes, peer counselors *should* be trained and paid) peer counselors very successfully to take over some of the role of the health care professional who lacks the time to relate on an even plane with a client of different educational or socioeconomic status. Well-established peer-counseling programs may even inspire the counselors to obtain further training as nurses' aides or licensed practical nurses.

Peer support programs have been developed in Britain and Canada. In a randomized control trial of a telephone-based peer support intervention there was increased duration of breastfeeding and increased satisfaction with experience.[17] Women valued the support of a counselor in another study in London and South Essex, but the impact on duration was not as dramatic, probably because mothers had to ask for help after discharge and they were not routinely contacted.[10]

The peer counselor will complement the work of the health professionals but should never replace the role of the health care provider.

Who shall counsel?

Among those working closely with people in critical life situations, some people make good counselors and some equally good people are not appropriate as counselors and should have other jobs in the organization.[16]

Counseling is a profession, and professional counselors are carefully screened, educated, and trained. Therefore, individuals who help mothers breastfeed should be screened, educated, and trained as well. They should have the following special abilities:

   To listen
   To avoid judgment
   To understand other lifestyles
   To admit it when they do not know
   To seek appropriate help from professionals
   To recognize incompatibility in a given
      relationship

In the past few decades, peer counseling has become widespread and has been successful, not only with breastfeeding and childbirth, but also with chronic disease such as cystic fibrosis and with devastating illnesses such as cancer. The first fact that all these groups have had to acknowledge is that just because one has experienced a life event, one is not automatically qualified to counsel others experiencing similar situations.

The candidate must first put personal experiences into perspective and understand the motivation for seeking this counseling role. Counseling is an opportunity to help by listening, and being a *sympathetic listener* is the most important quality. This is not a time to talk about the counselor's pregnancies. The counselor cannot have a personal agenda and press personal views or lifestyle on the mother being counseled, nor should counseling be used as a personal platform to promote organizational biases.

The counselor must understand that assuming a place on the health care team demands time and effort. One must be available at the convenience and need of the client, even when this is inconvenient to the counselor.

Learning to help mothers

The suggestions to guide a counselor in training must be general guidelines about *attitude*. The emphasis is on listening, encouraging a mother to talk, and ultimately helping her to solve her own problem by understanding it. Professional counselors are trained using didactic sessions, role play, and supervisory sessions until skills are developed. Continued reinforcement of philosophy and techniques forms the basis of growth and improvement. The lay counselor should attend counselor-training sessions provided by the parent organization and work closely with the supervisor. Sharing counseling situations with others with more experience will give further insight. Returning to the reference materials again and again will bring to light new thoughts that have been read before but not truly assimilated initially because of lack of experience.

The peer counselor does not provide medical advice. The counselor can encourage the mother to contact her physician. When the infant is doing poorly or is sick, the pediatrician should be consulted promptly. The rare condition of failure to thrive while breastfeeding is increasing in frequency, paralleling the increased incidence of breastfeeding.

It has serious implications for the infant and for the continuation of breastfeeding unless treatment is initiated promptly by the physician. The physician is powerless to help if not consulted. When the infant's problem is identified and it is prudent to continue breastfeeding, the counselor can be an invaluable asset in supporting and reassuring the mother.

Maternal problems such as mastitis should respond well if treated early, but recurrent mastitis may develop when home remedies are substituted for proper treatment. The role of the counselor in such situations is significant. Encouraging the mother to seek medical care promptly is most important. Reinforcing medical advice will further enhance its effectiveness. For example, if rest is prescribed, the counselor can help the mother to understand how critical rest is to recovery and then help her determine how she is going to cope at home with family responsibilities and a newborn and still rest.

The role of the counselor is support of the mother. The counselor should work in concert with the medical health care team as a team player, not as a competitor or as an adversary, but as a *facilitator*. The mission of the team is successful lactation, a satisfying mothering experience, and a healthy infant. The health care team will continue to be responsible for the family long after lactation has been discontinued. The confidence and trust developed between the health team and family will be critical to lasting success. The counselor should be remembered as a gentle facilitator and a caring support person who was there through the rite of passage of matrescence.

A physician working with a lactation counselor or consultant needs to recognize this specialist's skills and limitations. As in other, similar situations, the physician is the leader of the health care team and carries the ultimate responsibility.

REFERENCES

1. Albreht TL, Bryant C: Advances in segmentation modeling for health communication and social marketing campaigns. J Health Communications 1:65, 1996.
2. Barnes GR, Lethin AN, Jackson EB, et al: Management of breastfeeding. JAMA 151:192, 1953.
3. Bergh A-M: The role of a nongovernmental organization in breast feeding education. J Nutr Educ 19:117, 1987.
4. Bryant CA, Coreil J, D'Angelo SL, et al: A strategy for promoting breastfeeding among economically disadvantaged women and adolescents. NAACOGS Clin Issues Perinatal Women's Health Nurs 3:723, 1992.
5. Bryant CA, Verbal M: The Best Start Approach to Breastfeeding Promotion: Training Manual. Tampa, Best Start, 1997.
6. Ciba Foundation: Breast Feeding and the Mother: Symposium No. 45. Amsterdam, Elsevier, 1976.
7. Dennis CL, Hodnett E, Gallop R, Chalmers B: The effect of peer support on breast-feeding duration among primiparous women: A randomized controlled trial. Can Med Assoc J 166:21, 2002.
8. Deshpande AD, Gazmararian JA: Breast-feeding education and support: Association with the decision to breast-feed. Eff Clin Pract 3:116, 2000.
9. Food and Nutrition Service, U.S. Department of Agriculture: Promoting Breastfeeding: A Guide for Health Professionals Working in the WIC and CSF Programs. Washington, DC, USDA, 1983.
10. Graffy J, Taylor J, Williams A, Eldridge S: Randomised controlled trial of support from volunteer counselors for mothers considering breast feeding. BMJ 328:26, 2004; accessed at www.bmj.com.
11. Gussler J, Bryant C: Helping Mothers Breastfeed: Program Strategies for Minority Communities. Health Action Papers, Vol. I. Lexington, Lexington Fayette County Health Department, University of Kentucky Medical Behavioral Sciences Department, 1984.
12. International Board of Lactation Consultant Examiners, 2315 Wickersham Cove, Germantown, TN 38138.
13. La Leche League International: The Womanly Art of Breastfeeding, 7th ed. Franklin Park, IL, La Leche League, 1997.
14. Ladas AK: How to help mothers breast feed. Clin Pediatr 9:702, 1970.
15. Ladas AK: Breastfeeding: The less viable option. J Trop Pediatr 18:318, 1972.
16. Lawrence RA: Introduction. In Lauwers J, Woessner C (eds): Counseling the Nursing Mother: A Reference Handbook for Health Care Providers and Lay Counselors. Wayne, NJ, Avery, 1983.
17. Lewis L: Successful breastfeeding programs for low-income, minority mothers. Publ Health Currents 22:1, 1982.
18. Meara H: A key to successful breastfeeding in a nonsupportive culture. J Nurse Midwifery 21:20, 1976.

19. Mitra AK, Khoury AJ, Carothers C, et al: The loving support breastfeeding campaign: Awareness and practices of health care providers in Mississippi. J Obstet Gynecol Neonate Nurs 32:753, 2003.

20. Naylor A, Wester R: Providing professional lactation management consultation. Clin Perinatol 14:33, 1987.

21. Porteous R, Kaufman K, Rush J: The effect of individualized professional support on duration of breastfeeding: A randomized controlled trial. J Hum Lact 16:303, 2000.

22. Pryor K: Nursing Your Baby. New York, Harper & Row, 1973.

23. Public Health Service: Implementation plans for attaining the objectives for the nation. In Healthy People 2000: National Health Promotion and Disease Prevention Objectives. DHHS Pub. No. (PHS) 91-50213. Washington, DC, U.S. Government Printing Office, 1991.

24. Pugh LC, Milligan RA, Frick KD, et al: Breastfeeding duration, costs, and benefits of a support program for low-income breastfeeding women. Birth 29:95, 2002.

25. Raphael D: The Tender Gift: Breast Feeding. New York, Schocken, 1976.

26. Relucio-Clavano N: The results of a change in hospital practices. Assignment Child 55/56:139, 1981.

27. Report of the Surgeon General's Workshop on Breastfeeding and Human Lactation. DHHS Pub. No. HRS-D-MC 84-2. Washington, DC, U.S. Government Printing Office, 1984.

28. Schwartz JB, Popkins BA, Tognetti J, et al: Does WIC participation improve breastfeeding practices? Am J Publ Health 85:729, 1995.

29. Scrimshaw SCM: The cultural context of breastfeeding in the United States. In Report of the Surgeon General's Workshop on Breastfeeding and Human Lactation. DHHS Pub. No. HRS-D-MC 84-2. Washington, DC, U.S. Government Printing Office, 1984.

30. Silverman PR, Murrow HG: Caregiver during critical role in the normal life cycle. Unpublished report. Boston, Harvard Medical School, 1978.

31. Sloper KS, Elsden E, Baum JD: Increasing breast feeding in a community. Arch Dis Child 52:700, 1977.

32. Spisak S, Gross SS: Second follow-up report: The Surgeon General's Workshop on Breastfeeding and Human Lactation. Washington, DC, National Center for Education in Maternal and Child Health, 1991.

33. Thompson M: The effectiveness of mother-to-mother help: Research on the La Leche League International program. Birth Fam J 3:1, Winter 1976–1977.

34. Van Gennep A: Rites of Passage. London, Routledge & Kegan Paul, 1960 (translated by MB Vizedom and GL Caffee).

35. Volpe, EM, Bear M: Enhancing breastfeeding initiation in adolescent mothers through the breastfeeding educated and supported teen (BEST) club. J Hum Lact 16:196, 2000.

$\mathscr{E}$ducating and training the medical professional

The 1984 Surgeon General's Workshop on Breastfeeding and Human Lactation[17] was the first national meeting to focus exclusively on breastfeeding. The breastfeeding strategies developed at that workshop are still being used as the United States and the world move toward the breastfeeding objectives set in *Healthy People 2010: National Health Promotion and Disease Prevention Objectives*.[9]

Although many of the objectives have been addressed, the education of the health care professional remains a challenge.[12] A second meeting of the National Planning Committee of the Surgeon General's Workshop convened in Washington, DC, in 1985 to address the issue of that education.[19] The leaders of major professional organizations attended, including the American College of Obstetricians and Gynecologists, American Academy of Pediatrics, American Academy of Family Physicians, National Association of Pediatric Nurse Practitioners, American Dietetic Association, Nurses of American College of Obstetricians and Gynecologists, National Association of Nurse-Midwives, and National Board of Medical Examiners. These organizations developed and ratified a policy in support of educating and certifying its membership in human lactation and breastfeeding. Discussion was initiated about developing a curriculum appropriate to each professional level of training and specialization.

CONTINUING EFFORTS

Work continues in scattered ad hoc special presentations that may or may not have some affiliation with a medical school or hospital. However, no central unified program has been developed to change the curriculum at the seat of learning: U.S. medical schools and nursing schools.

The second follow-up report of the surgeon general's workshop in 1991 noted several accomplishments.[19] Although many respondents thought that lack of support or encouragement from physicians and nurses was a continuing barrier, no substantive progress had been made in developing curricula or credentialing. Excellent programs have been provided by Wellstart International[21,23] for teams consisting of a physician, a nurse, and a nutritionist from the same institution with co-sponsorship by the University of California at San Diego or the University of Hawaii. Wellstart's programs have been international, and they provide resources around the world. Many other universities have served as co-sponsors for a program, seminar, or workshop in their own geographic area. However, the programs have not been integrated into the total medical school curriculum or the training in a residency program, and they are not taught by any medical school faculty at all levels of training.

The failure of medical schools to address the issue of education about the breast and training in the clinical issues of breastfeeding has been addressed at the University of Texas at San Antonio by Newton.[14] He initiated a program on the obstetric service for medical students and residents. He also reported the results of his national survey of medical schools' curricula: 55% of the 127 U.S. obstetric and pediatric departments had no didactic lectures for medical students. Of obstetric and pediatric residencies, 30% provided no didactic lectures to their students. Most programs relied on clinical opportunities for learning.

When Freed and associates[8] investigated the attitudes and education of pediatric house staff concerning breastfeeding, they found that third-year residents did not know any more than interns about the subject. Furthermore, only personal experience seemed to provide any in-depth knowledge about simple problems, such as sore nipples. Freed[4] suggests that we "preach what we teach": that breastfeeding education for physicians should focus on (1) *knowledge* regarding techniques and problem solving to become a good counselor; (2) *outcome expectations,* that is, breastfeeding results in healthier children; and (3) *efficacy expectations,* the confidence that physicians themselves can be effective counselors and influence the incidence and duration of breastfeeding.

THE PROBLEM

Breastfeeding is important to infants and their mothers for nutritional, immunologic, psychological, and other health reasons. U.S. health goals strive to increase the incidence and duration of breastfeeding. Little formal education is provided on the topic in medical schools and residency training programs. No planned curricula or testing mechanisms are available.

Breastfeeding has another unique problem of interest to the lay public, who have become very involved. Many nonphysicians have become involved in training. Some attempts at educating physicians have been made by nonphysicians and sometimes by non–health care professionals.[2,3] The message to the medical student is that understanding and encouraging breastfeeding are not in the physician's job description. When other care providers give presentations to medical students or residents, it is assumed the provider is describing the work for information only and not for its role in the physician's work. Childbirth is of great interest to the lay public and to consumer advocacy groups as well, but they do not provide the physicians' training in childbirth. This training is provided by skilled specialists who have doctoral degrees, residency training, board certification, and in many cases, additional fellowship training and subspecialty certification, which are minimal qualifications for medical school faculty.

How much do residents and physicians know about managing breastfeeding? The data suggest the answer is "very little." In a study of obstetric residents, Freed and associates[5] mailed a survey to more than 600 residents, and 64% responded. Only 38% had any education from the faculty about breastfeeding and indicated what little they knew came from other residents and nurses. All participants agreed, however, that they should have a role in the management of breastfeeding for their patients. A survey of 87 of a possible 108 (81%) pediatric residents evenly distributed among levels I, II, and III in a large hospital reported that level III residents were no more competent than their PL-1 counterparts.[7] If they or their spouse breastfed, they were more confident in their knowledge base. No differences were found between men and women or between those breastfed or not breastfed as an infant.[7,8]

The knowledge, training, and attitudes of obstetricians concerning the management of breastfeeding was evaluated by the American College of Obstetricians and Gynecologists (ACOG).[15] A survey was sent to 1200 fellows of the college, and 397 practitioners responded. Obstetricians considered counseling their patients and managing breastfeeding care an important part of their clinical responsibilities. They felt very qualified to treat mastitis, prescribe maternal medications, and advise their lactating patients about contraception. They were less confident about educating their patients about breastfeeding and solving any problems. Personal breastfeeding experience for the women was a predictor of confidence. Four of 10 physicians felt their training was inadequate in lactation.[15]

A subsequent study confirmed that residents' knowledge was low and their misinformation disturbingly high.[7] The authors concluded that residency training programs must provide comprehensive education on breastfeeding to prepare residents to meet the needs of patients and other parents. Another study of pediatricians in training given a 15-minute self-administered and anonymous questionnaire resulted in 53% participation (29 respondents).[22] On a 6-point scale of support of breastfeeding, the group achieved 2.6 (1 being most supportive), revealing an attitude barely above neutral. They achieved only 53% on the management questions, and their confidence in their skills was low, confirming the need for didactic and clinical training in breastfeeding.

The effect of an educational intervention about breastfeeding on the knowledge, confidence, and behaviors of pediatric resident physicians was evaluated using before and after questionnaires. Their behaviors in the clinical setting were also measured before and after an interactive multimedia curricular intervention to increase their knowledge about common lactation issues. The investigators also telephoned the mothers after the clinic visit. Acceptable management went from 22% to 65% after the training. The resident physicians especially improved in assessing breastfeeding adequacy and the correct management of problems (Figs. 23-1 and 23-2).[10]

A national survey of 1099 family medicine residents, 71% of whom responded, indicated that they thought they should be involved in breastfeeding promotion and support.[6] They demonstrated significant deficits, however, in knowledge about benefits and clinical management. These same investigators also polled practitioners regarding their beliefs and knowledge base.[7] The results indicated a similar level of support and lack of knowledge.

Others have investigated the level of knowledge of physicians in training in other countries. A self-administered questionnaire was returned by 76 (84%) obstetric residents in metropolitan areas of South Korea.[11] Korean breastfeeding rates have decreased, especially among well-educated women; the rate was only 17% in 1994. The questionnaire responses indicated that the residents were neutral about breastfeeding. They considered themselves very competent to handle breastfeeding situations, but they scored only 38% on the management quiz.

Improved breastfeeding education clearly is needed in obstetrics, pediatrics, and family medicine, the physicians who should be most involved in supporting and promoting breastfeeding.

THE SOLUTION

To begin to solve this educational problem, a curriculum should be developed. It should span all four years of medical school and be carefully woven into the fabric of medical school for all students and of the residency years for those specializing in obstetrics, pediatrics, and family medicine.

The program should be taught by physicians who are qualified faculty members recognized by their peer group and certified by specialty examining boards. The classes should be part of the total curriculum and not something a student can elect to do only in the fourth year, when most of the assignments are by electives. Graduate physicians in practice rarely will go to a teaching day exclusively on breastfeeding, and they rarely attend programs directed at a broad-based audience of nonphysicians. It does not serve their educational needs when they are also responsible for keeping up to date on the constant flow of advancements in every branch of medicine.

Breastfeeding topics should become part of a well-rounded continuing education program that includes a number of other important issues, such as infectious diseases, endocrine problems, growth, development, and perinatology. When breastfeeding is included in programs on infant nutrition and presented by a physician, it will gain the status it needs.

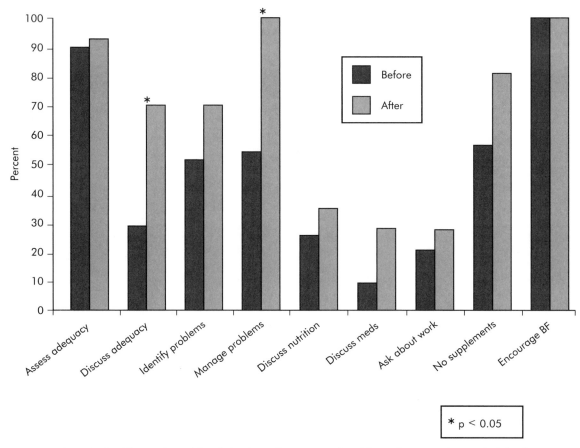

Figure 23-1. Change in resident behaviors: Percentage of residents demonstrating each behavior before and after the educational intervention. BF, breastfeeding. (From Hillenbrand KM, Larsen PG: Effect of educational intervention about breastfeeding on the knowledge, confidence, and behaviors of pediatric resident physicians. Pediatrics 110:e59, 2002.)

SUGGESTED CURRICULUM FOR MEDICAL STUDENTS

Utilizing as a model the present program at the University of Rochester School of Medicine, Rochester, New York, the following schedule is suggested as a starting point for instilling knowledge about human lactation and breastfeeding into the traditional curriculum of all medical students.

First-year students have a 16-week program in *human nutrition,* which meets weekly for a 2-hour session. Breastfeeding is presented in the section on child nutrition, and the discussion provides information about the reasons breastfeeding and human milk are superior to formula feeding. The lecture is didactic but is followed by discussion. At least two questions about the composition and benefits of human milk are on the final examination.

Second-year students have a 12-week program in the last half of the year on *women's health issues.* The class meets for 4 hours once a week to explore a variety of topics, including hormonal maturation, menarche, sex, contraception, child-

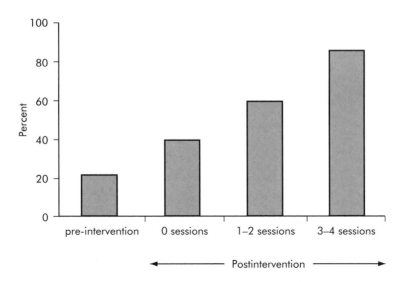

Figure 23-2. Percentage of residents with "acceptable performance" of desired behaviors (at least 6 of 9) compared with number of session attended. (From Hillenbrand KM, Larsen PG: Effect of educational intervention about breastfeeding on the knowledge, confidence, and behaviors of pediatric resident physicians. Pediatrics 110:e59, 2002.)

bearing, menopause, and the breast. A 4-hour session is about the breast. The first 2 hours of the session are dedicated to the use of the breast, that is, the anatomy and physiology of lactation. At least two questions on the final examination for this course are about lactation. The second 2 hours cover pathology, including augmentation mammoplasty, reduction mammoplasty, and benign and malignant tumors.

The third year begins with the general clerkship, wherein skills in history taking and physical examination are sharpened. A separate session taught by faculty from obstetrics and gynecology concentrates on *breast and pelvic examinations.* It is expected that all students, residents, and practitioners will always make these examinations part of the physical examination of women.

Third-year medical students spend 6 weeks on *obstetrics and gynecology,* usually half of which is spent on obstetrics, treating patients prenatally, intrapartum, at delivery, and post partum. Breastfeeding is part of that continuum, from the discussion of infant feeding prenatally through the postpartum checks for physiologic engorgement and the mother's questions about her afterpains, for example.

The third-year student also spends 6 weeks on the *pediatric service,* half on the ward and half in the outpatient and emergency service. While in clinic, each student spends a week of mornings in the newborn nursery going crib to crib, checking the newborn's adaptation to extrauterine life. The student also examines infants and talks to mothers. Observing a feeding is part of all discharge examinations and mandatory if the infant is breastfed. The student learns about the breastfed infants' feeding and weight patterns and early lactation. The student learns to identify problems and treat them.

The weeks in the clinic provide additional experience when seeing well babies. The students are exposed to the early weeks and months of breastfeeding and learn about infant weight gain and any problems that arise. The preceptors are experienced, board-certified pediatricians. The daily lecture series, which starts the day for all the residents and students assigned to the outpatient service, is directed at reviewing routine clinical issues. At least 1 in 10 lectures is about breastfeeding. Students are encouraged to visit their patients while they breastfeed and to accompany the mother-baby nurse when assisting the nursing dyad. They also attend the breastfeeding classes for mothers given by the lactation consultants, who are the health educators. The student also makes rounds with the lactation consultants who are college-prepared nurses and board-certified lactation consultants (IBCLC).

Fourth-year medical students have a few required courses—a surgical subspecialty, emergency medicine, and a clinical clerkship—but the rest of the year is given to electives. A student may elect extra time in the newborn nursery or the outpatient service or even at the Lactation Study Center. Summer fellowships are available to medical students throughout the 4 years to do a research project with a faculty member. One or two students a year are selected to work with the Lactation Study Center. A small stipend, which covers living expenses, is provided by the medical school. Reports of the questions on the national board examination confirm that human lactation and breastfeeding are included. (The recent FLEX examination had nine questions about breastfeeding and human lactation.)

Residents in obstetrics and pediatrics are assigned to the nursery and receive experience in managing the breastfeeding newborn. The obstetric house officer receives additional experiences by following patients prenatally and post partum. Formal lectures are also provided in the Grand Round Series of both departments. Special lectures directed specifically at the house officer on topics in breastfeeding and lactation are scheduled (e.g., drugs in breast milk, mastitis, failure to thrive).

The breastfeeding and lactation curriculum for the medical student is not unlike the approach to studying other organ systems, such as the cardiovascular system or the renal system. It includes the anatomy, physiology, biochemistry, pharmacology, normal function, pathology, and finally the clinical application in a wide range of clinical settings.

Expertise and leadership issues

As in other medical issues, the physician also learns about interacting with the patient and the family and studies all the psychosocial implications. When a medical school offers a visible clinical and research program that focuses attention on a subject, it improves the image of the subject matter. Cancer centers, poison centers, and sports medicine clinics are examples of how certain medical problems have been elevated to positions of importance in education and training by pooling resources and expertise. The Breastfeeding and Human Lactation Study Center at the University of Rochester School of Medicine has served as an information center, a resource of expertise for the educational matrix, and an ongoing research program that allows students, residents, and fellows to develop their own investigational work. Wellstart provides a similar focus of resources at the University of California at San Diego. Newton's work in East Carolina University Medical School, Neifert's at the University of Colorado at Denver, and that of many others are examples of medical school-based programs that are developing models for physician training.

The greatest obstacle to initiating a self-sustaining program on human lactation in medical schools is the need for *leadership* among the faculty. At least one interested, knowledgeable, credible faculty member must emerge to develop the curriculum so that it becomes part of the permanent learning plan. Faculty more recently trained are more interested in breastfeeding than senior faculty trained in the heyday of formula feeding. If there is a parallel training program in the nursing school, an appropriate division of labor can occur at the clinical interface.

The physician does not put the infant to the breast; that is the responsibility of the mother-baby nurse. The physician does, however, have to understand the process so that problems in clinical outcome can be solved. The nurse does not choose the medications prescribed to a lactating woman, but should understand the importance of lactation in those selections. The mother should be reminded to notify her internist that she is lactating. The health management of breastfeeding and lactation is a team effort, and it is the job of the physicians, nurses, and nutritionists working in perinatal medicine to assist in the process.

Wellstart program

Wellstart International[23] has developed a multidisciplinary approach to breastfeeding education that includes various health professionals, such as nurses, midwives, nutritionists, and physicians. The training materials are predicated on training the team together. This model works well when an institution can send a team simultaneously to the training with the intent that the team members will return and each train members of their own discipline, thus ensuring credible expertise across medicine, nursing, and nutrition. Naylor and associates[13] point out that "for the continuum of health care and the safety of the mother and infant, the physician has the final responsibility for diagnosis and medical management, including the treatment of illnesses, lactation problems and growth abnormalities." The authors agree that the material must be integrated into courses that already exist, whether in traditional didactic curricula or problem-based models. Table 23-1 presents the curriculum recommended in the Wellstart model, and Box 23-1 provides the model's breastfeeding policy for hospitals.

CURRICULUM FOR NURSES' TRAINING IN BREASTFEEDING AND LACTATION

A number of programs have been developed for the training of the health professional.[18,20] According to their titles, they have been developed by nurses for nurses or by nutritionists for nutritionists. Several of these programs were sponsored by the Maternal and Child Health Bureau, and their materials are available through the National Center for Education in Maternal and Child Health. *Lactation Education for Health Professionals,* edited by Rodriguez-Garcia, Schaefer, and Yunes of the Pan American Health Organization of the World Health Organization, provides an excellent description of such a program.[18] This text is directed at nursing school faculty. The target audience is undergraduate nursing students, although the text could serve

as a guide for postgraduate and continuing education programs. The well-trained student will be able to teach the mother optimal breastfeeding and weaning techniques. The student will also be able, within the scope of the total health team, to promote, maintain, and protect breastfeeding.[16]

The learning objectives for the nurse include being able to do the following:
- Apply acquired knowledge and skills.
- Assist mothers in initiating and continuing breastfeeding.
- Promote breastfeeding.
- Organize and conduct breastfeeding education seminars for other members of the nursing staff.
- Plan and implement breastfeeding services in clinical sites.

A training guide for experienced health care professionals has been prepared by Best Start and Bryant and Roy.[1] The work is culturally sensitive and is based on a thorough study of social marketing. Using this guide, health care professionals will be able to do the following:
- Identify the common factors that deter disadvantaged women from breastfeeding.
- Develop strategies for helping these women overcome these barriers.
- Develop strategies for identifying and building on the factors that make breastfeeding appealing to these women.

Other resources for education and training are listed in Appendix N. Nursing schools should seek the same quality in their lactation resources as they have in all other phases of nursing. When the professional nursing certifying organizations develop appropriate certification for lactation throughout perinatal nursing to accompany the certification already established for labor and delivery, normal newborn, postpartum care, and other areas, the curriculum will come into place quickly.

The Ontario Public Health Association, Toronto, Canada, has developed a series of modules covering the basic essential information regarding breastfeeding, which it recommends be incorporated into the undergraduate curricula of all health care professionals who work with

TABLE 23-1	**Wellstart International curriculum for breastfeeding management**	
Level I (awareness)	**Level II (generalist)**	**Level III (specialist)**
Module A: scientific basis		
Discuss, in general terms, findings from basic and social sciences of lactation	*Apply findings from basic and social sciences to breastfeeding and lactation issues:*	*Critique findings from basic and social sciences and evaluate their applicability to clinical management issues:*
1. Describe general benefits of breastfeeding for infant.	1.1 Describe unique properties of human milk for human infants.	1.1 Discuss in detail components of human milk and their functions.
	1.2 Describe advantages of preterm milk for preterm infant.	1.2 Describe in detail suitability of preterm human milk for preterm infant.
2.1 Describe general benefits of breastfeeding for mother.	2.1 Summarize impact of lactation on maternal nutritional status.	2.1 Critically review current literature on impact of lactation on maternal health status.
2.2 Describe benefits of breast-feeding for community.	2.2 Discuss effect of lactation on fertility.	2.2 Discuss current research and controversies related to lactational infertility.
3. Identify mammary structures involved in milk production and transfer.	3.1 Diagram anatomic structures of breast.	3. Describe normal and abnormal development of breast from fetal life through lactation and involution.
	3.2 Describe structural changes in breast during pregnancy and lactation.	
4. Describe process of milk production and removal.	4. Describe physiology of milk production, removal, and involution.	4. Describe synthesis of human milk at cellular level.
5. Describe ways that suckling process differs between breastfeeding and bottle feeding.	5. Describe anatomic development and physiology of suckling process.	5. Describe structural and functional factors related to oral-motor dysfunction.
6. Describe, in general terms, impact of maternal nutrition on lactation.	6. Describe specific impact of maternal diet and nutritional status on quantity and quality of milk produced.	6. Critically review current literature on impact of maternal nutrition on lactation.
7. Describe growth pattern of breastfed infant.	7. Summarize current knowledge on normal growth parameters of breastfed infants.	7. Critique scientific literature on infant growth and its applicability to breastfed infants.
8. Describe relative impact of age, ethnicity, socioeconomic status, and geographic region on breast-feeding rates in your country.	8. Identify local sources of data on breastfeeding trends.	8. Identify and interpret national and international trends in breastfeeding incidence and duration.
9. Identify cultural and psychosocial factors that impact breastfeeding rates.	9. Describe ways in which cultural beliefs, societal influences, and community practices impact breastfeeding in local community.	9. Critique and interpret research on cultural and psychosocial aspects of breastfeeding.

TABLE 23-1	Wellstart International curriculum for breastfeeding management—cont'd	
Level I (awareness)	**Level II (generalist)**	**Level III (specialist)**
Module B: clinical management		
Provide clinical care consistent with initiation and maintenance of lactation:	*Provide routine clinical support for successful initiation and maintenance of lactation and prevention and management of common clinical problems:*	*Provide clinical support/develop protocols for successful initiation and maintenance of lactation in high-risk/complicated situations:*
1. Identify factors that contribute to breastfeeding decision.	1.1 Provide breastfeeding care that is sensitive to cultural influences.	1.1 Same as level II.
	1.2 Assist expectant mother with breastfeeding decision.	1.2 Same as level II.
2. Conduct breastfeeding history and examination of breasts.	2. Use breast examination as opportunity to reassure woman she can breastfeed her infant.	2. Same as level II.
3.1 Identify components of anticipatory guidance for all women.	3. Provide anticipatory guidance targeted to specific needs of expectant mother and breast-feeding dyad.	3. Provide anticipatory guidance to pregnant women with unusual or high-risk conditions.
3.2 Identify components of anticipatory guidance and support for women with special needs.		
4. Recognize impact of intrapartum and immediate postpartum procedures/medications on lactation.	4. Provide intrapartum and immediate postpartum care that supports successful lactation.	4. Develop and implement intrapartum care protocols that facilitate breastfeeding for high-risk mother-infant dyads.
5. Recognize correct attachment and effective suckling at breast.	5. Provide postpartum care that supports successful lactation.	5. Same as level II.
6. Recognize when and how lactation needs to be maintained during separation, and refer mother for assistance.	6. Assist mother to maintain lactation during separation from her infant.	6. Provide consultation regarding banking and use of human milk in special circumstances.
7. Discuss basic nutrition recommendations for lactating woman.	7. Assess lactating woman for nutritional risk and refer appropriately.	7. Assess and manage breastfeeding mother with complicated nutritional needs.
8. Describe current recommendations for introducing complementary foods and supplements.	8. Provide guidance regarding introduction of complementary foods.	8. Manage complex lactation-related issues associated with introduction of complementary foods.
9. Discuss causes and prevention of common breastfeeding problems.	9. Manage uncomplicated problems seen in breastfed infant.	9.1 Assess and manage complex dysfunctional suckling patterns.
		9.2 Assess and manage lactation in infants with persistent slow growth.
10. Recognize that infants with special health care needs can breastfeed.	10. Facilitate breastfeeding for infant with special health care needs.	10. Facilitate successful lactation in infant with complex health care needs.

(Continued)

TABLE 23-1	**Wellstart International curriculum for breastfeeding management—cont'd**	
Level I (awareness)	**Level II (generalist)**	**Level III (specialist)**

Module B: clinical management—cont'd

11. Same as 9.	11. Manage uncomplicated breastfeeding problems of mother.	11. Facilitate successful lactation in mother with complex breastfeeding problems.
12. Prescribe/recommend medications and treatment options compatible with lactation.	12. Facilitate successful lactation in mother with medical conditions or receiving treatments.	12. Provide consultation to colleagues and breastfeeding mothers regarding support of breastfeeding for mothers with complex health problems.
13. Discuss family-planning options for lactating woman.	13.1 Counsel lactating woman about contraceptive options.	13.1 Same as level II.
	13.2 Provide anticipatory guidance and problem solving regarding lactation and sexuality.	13.2 Same as level II.
14. Same as 6.	14. Counsel woman about maintaining lactation while returning to work/school.	14. Same as level II.

Module C: professional practice issues

1.0 Coordinate services with, and provide appropriate referral to, other professionals, lay persons, and community groups:	*1.0 Coordinate care consistent with multidisciplinary approach:*	*1.0 Provide leadership in development and implementation of a team approach to lactation management:*
1.1 Identify various professionals who contribute to support and management of breastfeeding mother/infant pair.	1.1 Describe and explain philosophy of multidisciplinary approach to care.	1.1 Evaluate own team situation in terms of philosophy and decision-making structure.
1.2 Discuss, in general terms, roles of various professionals as members of lactation management team.	1.2 Define one's own role on lactation management team.	1.2 Identify specific strategies for change in own team activities.
1.3 Identify community and professional groups and activities that promote breastfeeding.	1.3 Work within team to coordinate lactation services and ensure continuity of care.	1.3 Provide leadership for multidisciplinary lactation management team.
1.4 Make appropriate referrals for women needing assistance with breastfeeding.	1.4 Develop linkages among appropriate community and professional groups to support breastfeeding.	1.4 Develop team protocols to promote accurate, consistent, and continuous care to breastfeeding families at critical periods.
2.0 Support policies that promote breastfeeding:	*2.0 Advocate for policies that support breastfeeding:*	*2.0 Develop policies/positions on breastfeeding-related issues:*
2.1 Discuss your professional organization's policy statements regarding breastfeeding.	2.1 Debate ethical issues affecting breastfeeding promotion and support.	2.1 Formulate a position on ethical issues that affect breastfeeding.
2.2 Discuss your country's policies and goals for breastfeeding.	2.2 Analyze effect of hospital and health service policies on actual breastfeeding practice.	2.2 Formulate positions on current national or international policies/initiatives that affect breastfeeding.

TABLE 23-1	Wellstart International curriculum for breastfeeding management—cont'd		
Level I (awareness)	**Level II (generalist)**		**Level III (specialist)**

Module C: professional practice issues—cont'd

Level I (awareness)	Level II (generalist)	Level III (specialist)
	2.3 Analyze local, state, or national policy issues affecting breastfeeding promotion and support.	2.3 Participate in effecting policy changes.
	3.0 *Apply change theory and adult learning principles to breast-feeding promotion:*	3.0 *Provide leadership in development, implementation, and evaluation of programs that support and promote breastfeeding:*
	3.1 Discuss strategies for over-coming resistance to change.	3.1 Compare and contrast change theories.
	3.2 Apply principles of adult learning to development of educational session on breast-feeding.	3.2 Describe program planning process and program evaluation techniques as they pertain to lactation programs.
	3.3 Plan a teaching session on breastfeeding.	3.3 Apply adult learning principles, change theory, and program plan-ning principles to development of lactation programs in any of fol-lowing areas: • Health professional education and training • Health care practice • Population/community level interventions
	3.4 Critique breastfeeding-related teaching materials.	

From Wellstart International and the University of California, San Diego: Lactation Management Curriculum: A Faculty Guide for Schools of Medicine, Nursing and Nutrition, 4th ed. San Diego, Wellstart International, 1998.

childbearing families. Breastfeeding resource material can be accessed on their Web site at www.hc-sc.gc.ca. Their contact information is in Appendix K.

Postgraduate learning opportunities for nurses and lactation consultants

Numerous programs across the United States are geared toward nurses and often are provided by nurses. Many of these focus on curricula designed to assist the participant in passing the certifying examination provided by the International Board of Lactation Consultant Examiners (IBLCE). Post-graduate teaching for lactation consultants is provided by the International Lactation Consultants Association (ILCA) and by independent profes-sional groups. La Leche League International also provides programs for all levels of interest, from the lay public to professionals, including a physician's seminar.

BOX 23-1   Wellstart International model hospital breastfeeding policies for full-term normal newborn infants

Definition and purpose: To promote a philosophy of maternal and infant care that advocates breastfeeding and supports the normal physiologic functions involved in this maternal-infant process. The goal is to ensure that all families who elect to breastfeed their infants will have a successful and satisfying experience.

1. Hospital administrative, medical, nursing and nutrition staff should establish a strategy that promotes and supports breastfeeding through the formation of an interdisciplinary team responsible for the implementation of hospital policies and provision of ongoing educational activities.
2. All pregnant women should receive information before delivery regarding the benefits and management of breastfeeding.
3. Every mother should be allowed to have a close companion stay with her continuously throughout labor.
4. Infants are to be put to breast as soon after birth as feasible for both mother and infant. This is to be initiated in either the delivery room or the recovery room, and every mother is to be instructed in proper breast-feeding technique and reevaluated before discharge.
5. Breastfeeding mother-infant couples are to room-in together on a 24-hour basis.
6. The infant is to be encouraged to nurse *at least* 8 to 12 times or more in 24 hours, for a minimum of 8 feedings per 24 hours.
7. Specific timing at the breast is not necessary. Infants usually fall asleep or release the nipple spontaneously when satiated.
8. Infants should spontaneously finish at the first breast, then should be encouraged to try the second breast at each feed.
9. If a feeding at the breast is incomplete or ineffective, the mother should be instructed to begin regular expression of her breasts in conjunction with continued assistance by an experienced staff member. The colostrum or milk obtained by expression should be given to the baby.
10. No supplementary water or milk is to be given unless specifically ordered by a physician or nurse practitioner.
11. Pacifiers are not to be given to any breastfeeding infant unless specifically ordered by a physician or nurse practitioner. The use of bottle nipples and nipple shields should be discouraged.
12. Breastfeeding mothers are to have breasts examined for evidence of lactation or breastfeeding problems at least once every nursing staff shift.
13. Discharge gift packs offered to breastfeeding mothers should contain only noncommercial materials that provide educational information and promote breastfeeding.
14. All breastfeeding mothers are to be advised to arrange for an appointment for their baby's first checkup within 1 week after discharge.
15. At discharge, each mother is to be given a phone number to call for breastfeeding assistance.
16. Policies 1, 2, 4, and 10 through 15 apply when mothers and babies are separated. Mothers who are separated from their babies are to be instructed on how to maintain lactation.

From Naylor AJ, Creer AE, Woodward-Lopez G, et al: Lactation management education for physicians. Semin Perinatol 18:525, 1994.

Postgraduate learning opportunities by medical groups for physicians

Postgraduate educational opportunities are one of the major goals of the Academy of Breastfeeding Medicine (ABM), an international organization founded in 1994 and limited to physicians from all disciplines and physician trainees. The ABM holds an annual meeting with plenary sessions, workshops, and submitted papers and posters on the wide range of topics involving breastfeeding and human lactation. ABM's mission is to encourage and support breastfeeding, especially through physician education.

The Milk Club is a group that meets in conjunction with the American Pediatric Society, Society for Pediatric Research, and Ambulatory Pediatric Association. Their mission is to bring new science in the field to the attention of all investigators. The format is usually a symposium with discussion and a poster session.

The International Society for Research in Human Milk and Lactation is an organization of investigators who meet annually in conjunction with the Federation of American Societies for Experimental Biology and meet biannually and independently at international sites to discuss current knowledge of laboratory and clinical research. Membership is limited to qualified investigators in the field. Appendix K provides the addresses for these organizations.

The American Academy of Pediatrics (AAP), American College of Obstetricians and Gynecologists, and American Academy of Family Practice all have increased their programming about human lactation at their annual and regional meetings. The AAP established a Work Group on Breastfeeding and approved its statement in support of breastfeeding, published in *Pediatrics* in December 1997. The statement makes the following 12 major recommendations for pediatricians[24]:

1. Promote and support breastfeeding enthusiastically. In consideration of the extensive published evidence for improved outcomes in breastfed infants and their mothers, a strong position on behalf of breastfeeding is justified.
2. Become knowledgeable and skilled in both the physiology and the clinical management of breastfeeding.
3. Work collaboratively with the obstetric community to ensure that women receive adequate information throughout the perinatal period to make a fully informed decision about infant feeding. Pediatricians should also use opportunities to provide age-appropriate breastfeeding education to children and adults.
4. Promote hospital policies and procedures that facilitate breastfeeding. Electric breast pumps and private lactation areas should be available to all breastfeeding mothers in the hospital, on both ambulatory and inpatient services. Pediatricians are encouraged to work actively toward eliminating hospital practices that discourage breastfeeding (e.g., infant formula discharge packs, separation of mother and infant).
5. Become familiar with local breastfeeding resources (e.g., Special Supplemental Nutrition Program for Women, Infants, and Children (WIC) clinics; lactation educators and consultants; lay support groups; breast pump rental stations) so that patients can be referred appropriately. When specialized breastfeeding services are used, pediatricians need to clarify for mothers the pediatrician's essential role as the infant's primary medical caregiver. Effective communication among the various counselors who advise breastfeeding women is essential.
6. Encourage routine insurance coverage for necessary breastfeeding services and supplies, including breast pump rental and the time required by pediatricians and other licensed health care professionals to assess and manage breastfeeding.
7. Promote breastfeeding as a normal part of daily life, and encourage family and societal support for breastfeeding.
8. Develop and maintain effective communications and collaboration with other health care providers to ensure optimal breastfeeding education, support, and counseling for mother and infant.
9. Advise mothers to return to their physicians for a thorough breast examination when breastfeeding is terminated.
10. Promote breastfeeding education as a routine component of medical school and residency education.
11. Encourage the media to portray breastfeeding as positive and the norm.
12. Encourage employers to provide appropriate facilities and adequate time in the workplace for breast pumping.

The statement has been updated and published in 2004. It includes the additional AAP recommendation for vitamin D to be given to breastfed infants by two months of age because of a deficiency of sunlight exposure in present lifestyles. The dose is 200 IU of vitamin D daily by mouth after 2 months. The original work group on breastfeeding of the AAP became a committee and is now a full-fledged Section on Breastfeeding of the AAP. Members of the AAP are welcome to join. The section is the sponsor of the Program on Breastfeeding in Pediatric Offices, which is now offered to the American College of Obstetricians and Gynecologists and all obstetricians as well as to the American Academy of Family Practice and its members. The section has also prepared a speaker's kit on breastfeeding with a Power Point presentation for the physician to present his or her own lecture in the practice area.

The section has authored a book for parents edited by Joan Meek, MD, and a handbook for physicians edited by Richard Schanler, MD.

SUMMARY

To establish breastfeeding and human lactation as an integral part of medical student education, the topic should be inserted into the present curriculum at the appropriate natural points, whether it is a class on anatomy, physiology, nutrition, endocrinology, women's health, or infant care. The class should be taught by recognized faculty who also teach the other parts of the subject material. Finally, the material should be included in the examination for the subject. Much remains to be learned in modern medicine, and lactation should be part of it.

REFERENCES

1. Bryant CA, Roy M: Best Start Training Manual: Breastfeeding for Healthy Mothers, Healthy Babies. Tampa, Best Start, 1990.
2. Department of Human Services, WIC State Agency: District of Columbia Breastfeeding Peer Counselor Program: Training Manual. Washington, DC, Department of Health and Human Services, 1990.
3. Food and Nutrition Service, U.S. Department of Agriculture: Promoting Breastfeeding in WIC: A Compendium of Practical Approaches. Alexandria, VA, Nutrition and Technical Services Division, USDA, 1988.
4. Freed GL: Breastfeeding: Time to teach what we preach. JAMA 269:243, 1993.
5. Freed GL, Clark SJ, Cefalo RC, et al: Breast-feeding education of obstetrics-gynecology residents and practitioners. Am J Obstet Gynecol 173:1607, 1995.
6. Freed GL, Clark SJ, Curtis P, et al: Breast-feeding education and practice in family medicine. J Fam Pract 40:263, 1995.
7. Freed GL, Clark SJ, Lohr JA, et al: Pediatrician involvement in breast-feeding promotion: A national study of residents and practitioners. Pediatrics 96:490, 1995.
8. Freed GL, Jones MTM, Fraley JK: Attitudes and education of pediatric house staff concerning breastfeeding. South Med J 85:484, 1992.
9. Healthy People 2010: National Health Promotion and Disease Prevention Objectives, DHHS Pub. No. (PHS) 91-50213. Washington, DC, U.S. Government Printing Office, 2000.
10. Hillenbrand KM, Larsen PG: Effect of an educational intervention about breastfeeding on the knowledge, confidence, and behaviors of pediatric resident physicians. Pediatrics 110:e59, 2002.
11. Kim HS: Attitudes and knowledge regarding breast-feeding: A survey of obstetric residents in metropolitan areas of South Korea. South Med J 89:684, 1996.
12. Lawrence RA: Review of the Surgeon General's Workshop on Breastfeeding and Human Lactation. Presented at American Public Health Association meetings, San Diego, November 1984.
13. Naylor AJ, Creer AE, Woodward-Lopez G, et al: Lactation management education for physicians. Semin Perinatol 18:525, 1994.
14. Newton E: Breastfeeding/lactation and the medical school curriculum. J Hum Lact 8:122, 1992.
15. Power ML, Locke E, Chapin J, et al: The effort to increase breast-feeding: Do obstetricians, in the forefront, need help? J Reprod Med 48:72, 2003.
16. Powers NG, Naylor AJ, Wester RA: Hospital policies: Crucial to breastfeeding success. Semin Perinatol 18:517, 1994.
17. Report of the Surgeon General's Workshop on Breastfeeding and Human Lactation, DHHS Pub. No. HRS-D-MC 84-2. Washington, DC, U.S. Government Printing Office, 1984.
18. Rodriguez-Garcia R, Schaefer LA, Yunes J: Lactation education for health professionals. Washington, DC, Pan American Health Organization, 1990.

19. Spisak S, Gross SS: Second Follow-Up Report: The Surgeon General's Workshop on Breastfeeding and Human Lactation. Washington, DC, National Center for Education in Maternal and Child Health, 1991.

20. Tully MR, Overfield ML: Educating health professionals for breastfeeding support. SPRANS Grant. Athens, University of Georgia, 1986.

21. Wellstart International: Model Hospital Breastfeeding Policies for Full-Term Normal Newborn Infants. San Diego, Wellstart, 1990.

22. Williams EL, Hammer LD: Breastfeeding attitudes and knowledge of pediatricians-in-training. Am J Prev Med 11:26, 1995.

23. Woodward-Lopez G, Creer AE (eds): Lactation Management Curriculum: A Faculty Guide for Schools of Medicine, Nursing and Nutrition, 4th ed. San Diego, Wellstart International and University of California at San Diego, 1994.

24. Working Group on Breastfeeding, American Academy of Pediatrics: Breastfeeding and the use of human milk. Pediatrics 100:1035, 1997.

Composition of human milk

TABLE A-1   Composition of human colostrum and mature breast milk

Constituent (per 100 mL)	Colostrum 1–5 days	Mature milk >30 days
Energy (kcal)	58	70
Total solids (g)	12.8	12.0
Lactose (g)	5.3	7.3
Total nitrogen (mg)	360	171
Protein nitrogen (mg)	313	129
Nonprotein nitrogen (mg)	47	42
Total protein (g)	2.3	0.9
Casein (mg)	140	187
α-Lactalbumin (mg)	218	161
Lactoferrin (mg)	330	167
IgA (mg)	364	142
Amino acids (total)		
Alanine (mg)	—	52
Arginine (mg)	126	49
Aspartate (mg)	—	110
Cystine (mg)	—	25
Glutamate (mg)	—	196
Glycine (mg)	—	27
Histidine (mg)	57	31
Isoleucine (mg)	121	67
Leucine (mg)	221	110
Lysine (mg)	163	79
Methionine (mg)	33	19
Phenylalanine (mg)	105	44
Proline (mg)	—	89
Serine (mg)	—	54
Threonine (mg)	148	58
Tryptophan (mg)	52	25
Tyrosine (mg)	—	38

Continued

TABLE A-1	Composition of human colostrum and mature breast milk—cont'd	
Constituent (per 100 mL)	**Colostrum 1–5 days**	**Mature milk >30 days**
Amino acids (total)—cont'd		
Valine (mg)	169	90
Taurine (free) (mg)	—	8
Urea (mg)	10	30
Creatine (mg)	—	3.3
Total fat (g)	2.9	4.2
Fatty acids (% total fat)		
12:0 tauric	1.8	5.8
14:0 myristic	3.8	8.6
16:0 palmitic	26.2	21.0
18:0 stearic	8.8	8.0
18:1 oleic	36.6	35.5
18:2, n-6 linoleic	6.8	7.2
18:3, n-3 linolenic	—	1.0
C_{20} and C_{22} polyunsaturated	10.2	2.9
Cholesterol (mg)	27	16
Vitamins		
Fat soluble		
Vitamin A (retinol equivalents) (µg)	89	67
β-Carotene (µg)	112	23
Vitamin D (µg)	—	0.05
Vitamin E (total tocopherols) (µg)	1280	315
Vitamin K (µg)	0.23	0.21
Water soluble		
Thiamin (µg)	15	21
Riboflavin (µg)	25	35
Niacin (µg)	75	150
Folic acid (µg)	—	8.5
Vitamin B_6 (µg)	12	93
Biotin (µg)	0.1	0.6
Pantothenic acid (µg)	183	180
Vitamin B_{12} (ng)	200	26
Ascorbic acid (mg)	4.4	4.0
Minerals		
Calcium (mg)	23	28
Magnesium (mg)	3.4	3.0
Sodium (mg)	48	18
Potassium (mg)	74	58
Chlorine (mg)	91	42
Phosphorus (mg)	14	15
Sulphur (mg)	22	14

TABLE A-1 Composition of human colostrum and mature breast milk—cont'd		
Constituent (per 100 mL)	Colostrum 1–5 days	Mature milk >30 days
Trace elements		
Chromium (ng)	—	50
Cobalt (μg)	—	1
Copper (μg)	46	25
Fluorine (μg)	—	16
Iodine (μg)	12	11
Iron (μg)	45	40
Manganese (μg)	—	0.6±
Nickel (μg)	—	2
Selenium (μg)	—	2.0
Zinc (μg)	540	120

Data from multiple references (see Chapter 4). Figures have been averaged.

$\mathcal{D}$ietary guidance during lactation

GENERAL GUIDELINES

1. Follow nutrition guide for regular food plan during pregnancy.
2. Eat a wide variety of foods, including milk and milk products and eggs.
3. If no milk is allowed, use a supplement of 4 μg of vitamin B_{12} daily. If goat or soy milk is used, partial supplementation may be needed.
4. If no milk is taken, also use supplements of 1200 mg of calcium and 400 IU of vitamin D daily. Partial supplementation will be necessary if fewer than four servings of milk and milk products are consumed.
5. Select a variety of plant foods (especially nuts, grains, legumes, and seeds) to obtain "complete" proteins by complementary combinations.
6. Use iodized salt.
7. At least 1800 kcalories per day are needed in the diet to meet the minimum requirements of vitamins and minerals for lactation.

Normal serum values for breastfed infants

TABLE C-1   Serum chemical values of normal breastfed infants*

Concentration/100 mL of serum	Age 28 days			Age 56 days			Age 84 days			Age 112 days		
	N	Mean	SD	N	Mean	SD	N	Mean	SD	N	Mean	SD
Males												
Total protein (g)	22	5.87	0.50	36	5.96	0.42	29	6.16	0.57	51	6.29	0.51
Albumin (g)	22	4.02	0.35	36	4.14	0.34	29	4.27	0.39	51	4.38	0.40
Globulins (g)												
alpha$_1$	22	0.14	0.03	36	0.17	0.03	29	0.18	0.03	51	0.17	0.04
alpha$_2$	22	0.53	0.10	36	0.60	0.11	29	0.74	0.14	51	0.81	0.19
beta	22	0.61	0.11	36	0.67	0.13	29	0.69	0.20	51	0.67	0.11
gamma	22	0.57	0.14	36	0.38	0.09	29	0.28	0.08	51	0.26	0.10
Cholesterol (mg)	21	139	31	32	153	34	25	133	32	47	145	26
Triglycerides (mg)	18	122	36	32	106	57	25	170	76	46	148	57
Urea nitrogen (mg)	43	8.5	3.2	49	6.6	2.1	47	7.0	2.7	51	7.3	4.2
Calcium (mg)	41	10.2	0.8	47	10.3	1.0	42	10.4	0.8	48	10.3	0.8
Phosphorus (mg)	43	6.6	0.7	49	6.4	0.7	47	6.2	0.5	49	6.2	0.7
Alkaline phosphatase[†]	31	22	6	40	21	7	35	21	8	44	18	7
Magnesium (mg)	40	2.0	0.2	47	2.1	0.2	45	2.2	0.2	50	2.2	0.2

Females

	n	Mean	SD	n	Mean	SD	n	Mean	SD	n	Mean	SD
Total protein (g)	18	6.04	0.40	27	5.86	0.44	21	6.21	0.57	42	6.31	0.62
Albumin (g)	18	4.07	0.27	27	4.03	0.35	21	4.29	0.37	42	4.36	0.42
Globulins (g)												
alpha$_1$	18	0.15	0.02	27	0.17	0.04	21	0.17	0.03	42	**0.19**	0.04
alpha$_2$	18	0.55	0.07	27	0.65	0.12	21	0.74	0.18	42	0.78	0.17
beta	18	0.70	0.18	27	0.63	0.11	21	0.71	0.13	42	0.67	0.16
gamma	18	0.57	0.10	27	0.38	0.10	21	0.30	0.06	42	**0.31**	0.10
Cholesterol (mg)	13	**180**	35	25	157	37	20	**155**	29	40	**165**	36
Triglycerides (mg)	9	**157**	43	24	112	53	18	195	56	38	**170**	52
Urea nitrogen (mg)	37	8.3	2.3	33	6.4	2.2	40	6.4	2.2	42	6.6	3.5
Calcium (mg)	37	10.3	0.8	33	10.3	0.8	40	10.3	0.8	42	10.7	0.7
Phosphorus (mg)	39	6.9	0.8	33	6.4	0.8	40	6.1	0.7	42	6.1	0.7
Alkaline phosphatase	31	19	5	28	17	5	32	17	5	36	17	5
Magnesium (mg)	39	2.0	0.4	32	2.0	0.2	40	2.1	0.2	41	2.1	0.3

*Bold figures indicate that value is greater than the corresponding value for infants of the opposite sex and that the difference is statistically significant at the 95% level of confidence.

†King-Armstrong units.

From Fomon SJ, Filer LJ, Thomas LN, et al: Growth and serum chemical values of normal breastfed infants. Acta Paediatr Scand Suppl 202:1, 1970.

Drugs in breast milk and the effect on the infant

The extensive list of drugs in Table D-1 is provided to assist the clinician in making judgments about management for specific drugs in an individual mother and her infant. The clinician is referred to Chapter 11 for the discussion of risks and benefits. It is also important to point out that the significance of a given blood level would vary with the pH and the binding capacity of the maternal plasma protein, which may differ for various ethnic and racial groups. Furthermore, it is a matter of not merely understanding the pharmacokinetics of a specific drug, but also understanding the physiology of milk production and, most critically, understanding the absorption and excretion of the drug by the newborn, which changes with conceptual and chronologic age.

The drugs have been grouped by their major use to provide an opportunity to compare therapeutic choices and select the medication that is best for both mother and infant. Under each drug name, three ratings have been provided. First is the AAP number, if they were rated by the Committee on Drugs of the American Academy of Pediatrics (AAP), which has published lists of drugs that may transfer into human milk since 1983. When no Arabic number is listed, a dash indicates that the compound was not included in

the AAP list. The following numbers and definitions are used by the AAP committee:

1. Drugs that are contraindicated during breastfeeding
2. Drugs of abuse that are contraindicated during breastfeeding
3. Radioactive compounds that require temporary cessation of breastfeeding
4. Drugs whose effect on nursing infants is unknown but may be of concern
5. Drugs that have been associated with significant effects on some nursing infants and should be given to nursing mothers with caution
6. Maternal medication usually compatible with breastfeeding
7. Food and environmental agents that have an effect on breastfeeding

Because several additional references and scoring systems have been created, two other major systems have been included.

Hale's (H) scoring is approximately the reverse of the AAP:

L1 Safest
L2 Safer
L3 Moderately safe

L4   Possibly hazardous
L5   Contraindicated

Weiner's code of breastfeeding safety is as follows:

S   Safe
NS   Not safe
U   Unknown

This appendix has been grouped into drugs used in different medical situations, thus providing the physician an opportunity to select the safest drug for a specific purpose. The classifications are grouped by use, and drugs under each class are presented alphabetically. The drug can also be found in the main index of the book for easy location. Only the most significant references have been included to conserve space.

The classifications of the drugs listed are as follows:

   Analgesics and antiinflammatory (nonnarcotic)
   Anesthetics (inhalation, intravenous, and oral)
   Anticoagulants and coagulants
   Anticonvulsants and sedatives
   Antihistamines
   Antiinfective agents
   Antineoplastics and antimetabolites
   Autonomic and cardiovascular drugs
   Dermatologic preparations
   Diagnostic materials and procedures; radioactive isotopes
   Diuretics
   Environmental agents
   Gastrointestinal agents
   Heavy metals and other elements
   Hormones, antithyroid, contraceptives
   Narcotics and antiaddiction drugs
   Psychotropic and mood-altering drugs
   Vitamins
   Miscellaneous

The continued update and expansion of the drug information resource has been carried out by the Lactation Study Center staff. In the interest of space, references older than 1985 have been deleted. Please refer to the fourth edition of the text to access them.

Table D-2 lists herbs and their possible effects on the mother and infant during pregnancy and lactation. This table is also accompanied by a list of relevant references.

TABLE D-1   Relationship of drugs to breast milk and effect on infant

Drugs and ratings*	Oral availability (%)	Peak plasma time (hr)	Plasma protein bound (%)	Volume of distribution (L/kg)
Analgesics and antiinflammatory (nonnarcotic)				
Acetaminophen AAP 6 H L1 W S	88 ± 15	0.16–1	0–25	0.8–1.36
Antipyrine H L5 W —	99		Negligible	
Aspirin AAP 5 H L3 W S?	58.5 ± 12.5		49–70	0.15 ± 0.03
Auranofin AAP — H — W U	15–25	Within 2	60	0.045
Aurothioglucose AAP — H — W —			90–99	
Azapropazone AAP 6 H — W —		2–6	99.5	0.125 ± 0.025
Butorphanol AAP 6 H L3 W S	~5 44–113 nasal	0.15–1.5 nasal	80	5
Celecoxib AAP — H L3 W —		2.8	97	5.71
Colchicine AAP 6 H L4 W S		1.25	31	0.7

Milk/plasma (M/P) ratio	Adult dose in milk (%)	Maximum amount in milk (mg/L)	Comments and references
0.2–1.9	0.04–1.85	15	In milk: 0.05%–0.7% of newborn therapeutic dose; mean 0.888 mg/L, peak 2 hr. Active metabolite: paracetamol. Only drug found in milk; both drug and metabolite found in the infant's urine. Brand names: Tylenol, Excedrin, Darvocet, Comtrex, etc. (67, 181, 360)
1	0.56–2.38	30	Use in ear drops. In milk: half-life 11.6 ± 5.4 hr. (118)
0.03–1.0	0.5–21	42.6	High first-pass hepatic metabolism. Exposure in utero may increase rate of maturation of metabolic process. In milk: 0.06%–25% of newborn therapeutic dose, peak 6 ± 3 hr. Brand names: Bayer, Anacin, Bufferin, Excedrin, Fiorinal, Empirin, etc. (181, 477, 514)
Found in rodent milk, and gold is excreted into human milk			Brand name: Ridaura (181, 393)
0.01–0.2	20	10.2	Antirheumatic. In milk: peak 5 ± 1 hr. Gold has been found in the infant's red blood cells and serum. Some believe it is incompatible with breastfeeding. Brand name: Solganal. (181, 376, 393, 420, 477)
	0.04–1.5		Almost completely absorbed. (30, 477)
0.7–1.9		0.004	1% of newborn dose in milk. Given during labor, it crosses the placenta. Brand name: Stadol. (393, 448, 477)
~1			Cox-2 inhibitor, NSAID. Brief dosing ok/long range? Probably a little in the milk. Brand name: Celebrex.
>1		0.003	One report of a woman who took drug as long-term therapy through pregnancy and 0.6 mg twice a day while lactating. No apparent effects on a 6-month-old. Brand name: ColBenemid. (181, 326, 348, 477)

Continued

TABLE D-1 **Relationship of drugs to breast milk and effect on infant—cont'd**

Drugs and ratings*	Oral availability (%)	Peak plasma time (hr)	Plasma protein bound (%)	Volume of distribution (L/kg)
Analgesics and antiinflammatory (nonnarcotic)—cont'd				
Diclofenac AAP — H L2 W S?	58 ± 14	0.5–4	99–99.9	0.335 ± 0.215
Diflunisal AAP — H L3 W S?	>99	2.5 ± 0.5	99.9 ± 0.01	0.1 ± 0.01
Dipyrone AAP 6 H — W —				
Etodolac AAP — H L3 — W U	At least 80	1.2–2	95–>99	0.84–3.1 active S enantiomer
Fenbufen AAP — H — W —	86	1.5 ± 0.5	98–99	3
Fenoprofen AAP — H L2 W U	82.5 ± 2.5	1–2	99	0.08–0.1
Flufenamic acid AAP 6 H — W —		1.5–6	>90	
Flunisolide AAP — H L3 W U	8–78 Mean 20			1.96 ± 0.46
Fluocortolone AAP — H — W —	78–89	1.4 ± 0.2	80	0.84 ± 0.16

Milk/plasma (M/P) ratio	Adult dose in milk (%)	Maximum amount in milk (mg/L)	Comments and references
	1.2	0.01	Completely and rapidly absorbed with extensive first-pass metabolism. Food delays absorption but does not decrease amount taken in. Rectal and oral parameters are the same. 48% protein bound in human skim milk. Has four active metabolites whose presence in milk is unknown. Brand name: Voltaren. (18, 393, 455, 496, 505, 550)
0.02–0.07			A difluorophenyl derivative of aspirin whose half-life is dose dependent. The percentage protein bound decreases at concentrations greater than 100 mg/L. Brand name: Dolobid. (181, 393, 477)
			Analgesic. Brand name: Metamizole.
			Food delays absorption. Brand name: Lodine. (33, 228)
0.006–0.02	<0.75		Absorption delayed but not decreased when taken with food. Has two active metabolites that have longer half-lives than drug. (20, 477)
0.017			Food delays and reduces absorption. Brand name: Nalfon. (67, 393, 455, 477)
<0.01			Maternal plasma level is 50 times greater than infant's. Mean plasma concentration in nursing infant is 0.43 µg/L. Brand name: Arlef. (477)
			Extensive first-pass metabolism. Not known whether excreted into milk; other corticosteroids are. Brand names: Nasalide, AeroBid. (7, 393)
			The metabolite is less active. (455)

Continued

TABLE D-1   Relationship of drugs to breast milk and effect on infant—cont'd

Drugs and ratings*	Oral availability (%)	Peak plasma time (hr)	Plasma protein bound (%)	Volume of distribution (L/kg)
Analgesics and antiinflammatory (nonnarcotic)—cont'd				
Flurbiprofen AAP — H L2 W S	Almost completely absorbed orally	0.5–4	99	0.1
Gold salts AAP 6 H L5 W NS?	20–25 (auranofin)	3–6	95	0.1
Ibuprofen AAP 6 H L1 W S	>80	1.5 ± 0.5	>99	0.15 ± 0.02
Indomethacin AAP 6 H L3 W S	85–122 37–112 rectal	2 ± 1	90–99.6	0.12–1.57
Ketoprofen AAP — H L3 W S?	92 ± 7	1.25 ± 0.75	99.2 ± 0.1	0.15 ± 0.03
Ketorolac tromethamine AAP 6 H L2 W U?	80–100	0.33–1	99.1–99.3	0.11–0.33
Mefenamic acid AAP 6 H — W S		1–3	High	
Nalbuphine AAP — H L3 W S	16 ± 8	0.3		3.8 ± 1.1
Naproxen AAP 6 H L3, L4 for chronic use W —	74–99	1–4	98.2 ± 4.5	0.16 ± 0.02

Milk/plasma (M/P) ratio	Adult dose in milk (%)	Maximum amount in milk (mg/L)	Comments and references
0.008–0.03	0.25	0.08	Metabolites are inert. Drug not detected in most milk samples. Peak plasma concentration, but not amount absorbed, reduced when taken with food. Bioavailability from suppositories similar to tablets. Brand name: Ansaid. (86, 464)
0.02–0.3			Antiarthritic. At least 10% appears in milk and accumulates in infant. AAP says it is safe, but others feel it is risky. Brand names: Ridaura, Myochrysine, Solganol, Myocrisin.
	<0.8	<0.05	Metabolites are inert. Food slows absorption. Half-life and % protein bound show nonlinear kinetics probably caused by saturable plasma-binding protein. Brand names: Advil, Motrin, Rufen, Dristan, Nuprin, etc. (20, 181, 464, 550)
0.01–1.48	0.07–0.98	4	Food delays absorption. In milk: 66%–133% of newborn dose. Bioavailability in premature infant: 13%. Brand name: Indocin. (39, 50, 51, 181, 281, 393, 410, 455, 477, 517, 521)
		Trace	Brand name: Orudis. (181, 393, 455, 477)
0.015–0.037	0.16–0.4	0.008	Food decreases rate but not extent of absorption. Brand name: Toradol. (7, 69, 550)
0.23	0.036–0.8		Infant able to excrete drug via urine. No evidence for drug accumulation. Brand name: Ponstel. (393, 477)
	<1		Has active metabolites. Brand name: Nubain. (181, 393, 477)
0.01	0.26–1.1	2.37	In milk: less than 0.5%–2% of newborn therapeutic, peaks at 4 hr. 0.26% of a chronic user's dose recovered in infant's urine. Food delays absorption. Brand names: Anaprox, Naprosyn. (7, 17, 20, 181, 393, 455, 501, 525)

Continued

TABLE D-1 **Relationship of drugs to breast milk and effect on infant—cont'd**

Drugs and ratings*	Oral availability (%)	Peak plasma time (hr)	Plasma protein bound (%)	Volume of distribution (L/kg)
Analgesics and antiinflammatory (nonnarcotic)—cont'd				
Nefopam AAP 6 H — W —				
Noscapine AAP 6 H — W —	30	1.5 ± 0.5		
Olsalazine AAP — H L3 W U	1–3	0.5–2	99.5	
Oxaprozin AAP — H L3 W U	95	3–5	99.9	Large
Oxyphenbutazone AAP — H — W —			95.7 ± 3.3	Small
Pentazocine AAP — H L3 W U	18 ± 8	0.5–4	60–65	5.6
Phenacetin AAP — H — W —	0–49		30–52.7	1.5
Phenylbutazone AAP 6 H — W —	80–100 rectal availability 77% of oral availability	2.5 ± 1.4	97 ± 2	0.14 ± 0.05
Piroxicam AAP 6 H L2 W S	99	2–3 after oral dose 5–6 after rectal dose	99.3 ± 0.2	0.12–0.15

Milk/plasma (M/P) ratio	Adult dose in milk (%)	Maximum amount in milk (mg/L)	Comments and references
			CNS analgesic.
0.15–0.88	0.5		Extensive first-pass metabolism. In milk: peak 1.5 ± 0.5 hr. (20, 246, 373)
			Two molecules of 5-aminosalicylic acid (ASA) joined by an azo bond. Most of it is split into two ASA in the colon. Brand name: Dipentum. (278, 527)
			Brand name: Daypro. (393)
0.1–0.8			Drug was found in the milk of 2 of 55 women. No known effect of drug in milk. (181, 477)
			Well absorbed from GI tract with extensive first-pass metabolism. Brand names: Talacen, Talwin. (7, 393, 455, 477)
0.16–1.02	0.05		Active metabolite: acetaminophen. Average amount in milk: 0.071 mg/L. (67, 455, 477)
0.1–0.91	0.4	6.3	Two active metabolites; dose-dependent kinetics. In newborn, plasma protein bound: 85%–90%, volume of distribution 0.2–0.25 L/kg, plasma half-life 21–34 hr. Brand name: Butazolidin. (67, 181, 393)
0.01–0.03	6.75 ± 3.25	0.22	One nursing infant was studied: drug not detected in infant's plasma. In milk: peak 4 hr. Brand name: Feldene. (20, 375, 393, 455)

Continued

TABLE D-1	**Relationship of drugs to breast milk and effect on infant—cont'd**			
Drugs and ratings[*]	**Oral availability (%)**	**Peak plasma time (hr)**	**Plasma protein bound (%)**	**Volume of distribution (L/kg)**
Analgesics and antiinflammatory (nonnarcotic)—cont'd				
Propoxyphene AAP 6 H L2 W S	23–35	2.25 ± 0.25		
Rofecoxib AAP — H L3 W —	97	2–3	87	1.3
Salicylic acid AAP — H — W —	95 ± 6	2.3 ± 0.1	70 ± 20	0.13–0.2
Sulindac AAP — H — W U	89 ± 1	1–4	92–96	2
Suprofen AAP 6 H — W —	92	1.25 ± 0.75	99.2 ± 0.2	
Tolmetin AAP 6 H L3 W U	>90	0.34–1	99.6 ± 0.1	0.54 ± 0.07
Tramadol AAP — H L3 W S?	68 after single dose 90–100 after multiple doses	1.6–2	4–20	3.3
Valdecoxib AAP — H — W U	83	3	98	

Milk/plasma (M/P) ratio	Adult dose in milk (%)	Maximum amount in milk (mg/L)	Comments and references
0.5		1	Extensive hepatic first-pass metabolism. In milk: less than 0.3% of newborn therapeutic dose, maximum amount of active metabolite, norpropoxyphene: 169.1 µg/mL. M/P ratio based on one mother-infant pair. Brand name: Darvon, Wygesic. (67, 393, 455)
			Cox-2 inhibitor, NSAID analgesic. Brief dosing ok/long-term dosing unknown. Estimates are less than 5% passes to milk. Brand name: Vioxx.
0.03–0.4	11.6 ± 9.4	38	Aspirin metabolite with dose-dependent kinetics. Amount bound to plasma protein decreases as amount in plasma increases. In neonate: half-life greater than 7 hr. In milk: average amount 0.924 mg/L, peaks at 3 hr; 0.1% of maternal dose excreted in 12 hr. Metabolic acidosis reported in 16-day-old when mother took drug every 4 hr. Brand names: Viranol, Salactic, Sal-Plant, Paplex, SalAc, Occlusal, etc. (20, 50, 181, 455)
Excreted into rat's milk			Food decreases rate and extent of absorption. Brand name: Clinoril. (181, 393, 455, 477)
0.005–0.014	0.7	0.23	On empty stomach, rapidly and completely absorbed. With food, oral availability is less. Does not accumulate to any extent. In milk: peak 1.5 ± 0.5 hr. 10% is bound to milk proteins. (20, 393, 455)
0.005–0.007	0.3	0.18	Completely absorbed. In milk: peak 0.67–1 hr. Active metabolite formed. Brand name: Tolectin. (20, 67, 181, 393)
	0.1		% availability: IM 100; rectal 78. Brand name: Ultram. (284)
			Cox-2 antagonist, NSAID analgesic. Not found in rodent milk. Brand names: Valdecoxib, Bextra.

Continued

TABLE D-1	**Relationship of drugs to breast milk and effect on infant—cont'd**			

Drugs and ratings*	Oral availability (%)	Peak plasma time (hr)	Plasma protein bound (%)	Volume of distribution (L/kg)
Anesthetics				
Alfentanil AAP — H L2 W S			80.9–96.3	0.8 ± 0.3
Bupivacaine AAP — H L2 W S		0.15–1.5	90 ± 5	1.2 ± 0.4
Chloroform AAP 6 H — W —				
Fentanyl AAP 6 H L2 W S	0–49	0.33–3	84 ± 2	4 ± 0.4
Halothane AAP 6 H L2 W S				
Ketamine AAP — H — W U	20 ± 7		12	1.8 ± 0.7
Lidocaine AAP 6 H L3 W S	34 ± 12	0.5	55–80	0.2–1.8
Meperidine AAP 6 H L2, L3 if used early post partum W S?	54 ± 19	1.25 ± 0.75	54.5 ± 15.5	4.4 ± 0.9

Milk/plasma (M/P) ratio	Adult dose in milk (%)	Maximum amount in milk (mg/L)	Comments and references
		0.00156	Used in premature infants. Brand name: Alfenta. (181, 286, 287)
	0.1	0.45	Infant exposed during C-section. No drug isolated from the blood of infant whose mother had 0.1% of the dose in her milk. Brand names: Marcaine, Sensorcaine. (28, 65, 222, 393)
			Anesthetic. Considered safe by AAP.
2.1			In colostrum: at peak 0.08–0.97 ng/mL. In milk: peak 0.75 hr. Brand names: Duragesic, Innovar, Sublimaze. (7, 181, 477, 484, 488)
3.5		0.002	In milk: 2 ppm. No symptoms in infants. Mother's exposure may be in working environment (i.e., operating room). Brand name: Fluothane. (395)
			Has metabolites with possible metabolic activity. Brand name: Ketalar. (181, 477)
0.4	0.34	16	Rapidly metabolized in liver. Given to neonates. Depresses prolactin secretion. Brand names: Anestacon, Decadron, Xylocaine. (20, 50, 181, 327, 455, 477, 536, 566)
1–2.5		0.571	In milk: peak 2 hr, less than 3.3% newborn therapeutic dose. Renal excretion of drug and metabolite, which is half as active as drug, is pH dependent. Brand names: Demerol, Mepergan. (67, 181, 350, 358, 480)

Continued

TABLE D-1   Relationship of drugs to breast milk and effect on infant—cont'd

Drugs and ratings*	Oral availability (%)	Peak plasma time (hr)	Plasma protein bound (%)	Volume of distribution (L/kg)
Anesthetics—cont'd				
Methohexital AAP 6 H L3 W —				2.2 ± 0.7
Midazolam AAP 4 H L3 W S	28–72	1.22 ± 0.88	93–97	0.6–6.6
Procaine AAP — H L3 W S?	When given as a local for dental work, it is usually confined to the local area by the addition of adrenalin			
Propofol AAP — H L2 W S?			97–99	2.46–8.09
Sufentanil AAP — H — W S		0.05–1.5	93 ± 1	2.5 ± 1.6
Thiopental AAP 6 H L3 W S			87 ± 6	2.3 ± 0.5
Vecuronium bromide AAP — H — W S	given IV	min	60–90	0.19–0.51
Anticoagulants and coagulants				
Acenocoumarol AAP — H — W —		1–4	98.5	
Aminocaproic acid AAP — H — W U		2	0	0.4

Milk/plasma (M/P) ratio	Adult dose in milk (%)	Maximum amount in milk (mg/L)	Comments and references
0.4–2.5		0.407	Brand name: Brevital. (181, 477)
0.09–0.21		0.7	Undergoes first-pass metabolism. Active metabolite: hydroxymidazolam is less active than the drug and is found in milk in the same amount as parent drug. Drug used in C-sections and in critically ill neonates. Brand name: Versed. (7, 23, 181, 233, 307, 477)
			Brand name: Novocain.
0.6–1.3		0.97	May not have good oral availability in infant. Exposure through breast milk is negligible compared to placental transfer during C-section. Brand name: Diprivan. (104, 182)
Not detected in breast milk after a single dose			80% excreted in 24 hr with only 2% eliminated as unchanged drug. Volume of distribution and half-life increase in neonate. Very lipid soluble. (181, 202, 393)
0.4–0.5		20	Used for C-sections. (23, 181)
			Half-life in maternal plasma: 0.52–1.92 hr. Metabolite has 50%–70% of the activity of the drug. Brand name: Norcuron. (2, 7, 181, 393, 441)
Not detected in milk of 20 mothers (sensitivity 15 ng/mL)			Food delays absorption. Brand name: Sintrom. (154)
			Completely absorbed from GI tract. Brand name: Amicar. (7, 477)

Continued

TABLE D-1   Relationship of drugs to breast milk and effect on infant—cont'd

Drugs and ratings*	Oral availability (%)	Peak plasma time (hr)	Plasma protein bound (%)	Volume of distribution (L/kg)
Anticoagulants and coagulants—cont'd				
Dicumarol AAP — H — W —	Slow and incomplete		95–99	0.15
Enoxaparin AAP — H L3 W S?	Inactivated in the GI tract			
Ethyl biscoumacetate AAP — H — W —			90	0.079 ± 0.021
Heparin AAP — H L1 W S	0		95	0.058 ± 0.010
Phenindione AAP 5 H — W —				
Tranexamic acid AAP — H — W —	34–38.5 Low absorption through rectum			
Warfarin AAP 6 H L2 W S	93 ± 8	1–9	97–99	0.14 ± 0.06
Anticonvulsants and sedatives				
Barbiturate AAP 6 H — W —				
Carbamazepine AAP 6 H L2 W S?	70–85	4–8	73–90	1.4 ± 0.4

Milk/plasma (M/P) ratio	Adult dose in milk (%)	Maximum amount in milk (mg/L)	Comments and references
0.01–0.02	0.5	2	Not measurable in all milk samples. Has been associated with bleeding in breastfed infants. (181, 393)
			A heparin of 4500 average molecular weight. Brand name: Lovenox. (67, 393)
0.013–0.8	0.1	1.7	Hemorrhage around umbilical stump and cephalhematoma reported. No adverse effects found in the nursing infants of 22 mothers taking the drug. Brand name: Tromexan. (67, 477)
Not excreted into human milk			(181, 393, 477)
		5	Not used in U.S. Amount in milk dose related. Breast milk a major route of excretion. Reports of serious hemorrhaging in the infant. (67)
	0.018 ± 0.006		Brand name: Cyklokapron. (455, 477)
<0.2	<4.4		Excretion into milk varies. In 13 mothers taking 2–12 mg/day, less than 25 ng/mL found in milk. Brand name: Coumadin. (17, 181, 329, 393, 477)
			Short-acting forms clear quickly. Phenobarbital more prolonged. Requires liver metabolism.
0.2–0.69	2.5–4.9	4.8	Amount in nursing infant's serum about 0.004 mg/L. One report of transient cholestatic hepatitis in a nursing baby. Plasma level of metabolite, carbamazepine-10, 11-epoxide is 10%–50% that of the drug. Metabolite's kinetics are oral availability: 90% ± 11%; M/P ratio: 0.53–1.8; maximum amount in breast milk: 2 mg/L. Brand name: Tegretol. (20, 48, 67, 119, 161, 181, 315, 393, 410, 547)

Continued

TABLE D-1   Relationship of drugs to breast milk and effect on infant—cont'd

Drugs and ratings*	Oral availability (%)	Peak plasma time (hr)	Plasma protein bound (%)	Volume of distribution (L/kg)
Anticonvulsants and sedatives—cont'd				
Clonazepam AAP — H L3 W NS?	98 ± 31	1.5 ± 0.5	86 ± 0.5	1.5–4.4
Divalproex AAP — W S	Drug dissociates into valproic acid in the GI tract			
Ethosuximide AAP 6 H L4 W S	100 ± 10	3 ± 1	0	0.72 ± 0.16
Gabapentin AAP S H L3 W S?	53–60	2–3.2	<3	0.7–1
Glutethimide AAP — H — W —	Erratic	1–6	47.3–59.3	
Lamotrigine AAP — H L3 W S?	98 ± 5	2.75 ± 1.2	55	1.15 ± 0.25
Magnesium sulfate AAP 6 H L1 W S	25–40		30	
Oxcarbazepine AAP — H L3 W S?		1–4	67	
Pentobarbital AAP — H L3 W S	94 ± 11		55	1

Milk/plasma (M/P) ratio	Adult dose in milk (%)	Maximum amount in milk (mg/L)	Comments and references
0.33	2.5	0.013	In milk: peak 4 hr. Brand name: Klonopin. (181, 393, 467, 477)
			Brand name: Depakote. (393)
0.5–1.1	13–30	80	Half-life lower in children; varies in neonates. In nursing infant's serum: 15–40 mg/L. Drug not bound to protein in milk. Infants may be sedated. Brand name: Zarontin. (17, 20, 38, 67, 181, 315, 410, 455, 477)
			Brand name: Neurontin. (53, 404)
1	0.5	0.27	In milk: peak 8–12 hr. Active metabolite: 4-hydroxygluthimide. Brand name: Doriden. (20, 393, 477)
			Brand name: Lamictal. (53, 184, 404)
0.6–2.1	0.5		M/P ration in women not taking the drug: 2.1; in women taking the drug: 1.9. Brand names: Eldertonic, Vicon Forte. (20, 67)
0.5			Amount in milk comes from the study of one patient. Active metabolite, 10-hydroxycarbazepine, is 30%–47% protein bound, systemic availability of metabolite increases 17% when the drug is taken with food. (80, 129)
	Excreted into human milk		0.17 mg/L was detected in milk 19 hr after a 100-mg dose taken daily for 32 days. Depends on the liver for detoxification, so may accumulate in newborn. Plasma half-life is dose dependent. Brand name: Nembutal. (67, 393, 455, 477)

Continued

TABLE D-1   Relationship of drugs to breast milk and effect on infant—cont'd

Drugs and ratings*	Oral availability (%)	Peak plasma time (hr)	Plasma protein bound (%)	Volume of distribution (L/kg)
Anticonvulsants and sedatives—cont'd				
Phenobarbital AAP 5 H L3 W S?	97 ± 14	3 ± 1	20–60	0.63 ± 0.12
Phenylethylmalonamide AAP — H — W —	91 ± 4		8 ± 1	0.69 ± 0.1
Phenytoin AAP 6 H L2 W S	89 ± 16		89 ± 23	0.675 ± 0.075
Primidone AAP 5 H L3 W NS?	92 ± 18		19	0.67 ± 0.6
Sodium bromide AAP 6,7 H — W —				
Topiramate AAP — H L3 W S	75–80	1.8–4.3	9–17	0.6–0.8
Valproic acid AAP 6 H L2 W S	100 ± 10	1–4	80–95	0.22 ± 0.07
Valpromide AAP — H — W —				1

Milk/plasma (M/P) ratio	Adult dose in milk (%)	Maximum amount in milk (mg/L)	Comments and references
0.2–1	1.5	33	In milk: 4%–100% of newborn therapeutic dose. If mother's plasma level >30 mg/L, infant may be excessively sleepy. One case of methemoglobinemia reported. Drug is active metabolite of primidone. Brand names: Donnatal, Kinesed, Tedral, Quadrinal. (119, 315, 455, 477)
0.5–1			Active metabolite of primidone with increased half-life in neonate. (119, 181)
0.13–2	1.4–7.2	18	No problem breastfeeding if mother's plasma concentration is in therapeutic range. Decreased oral availability in newborn. In milk: peak 3.5 ± 0.5 hr; 2%–40% of newborn therapeutic dose. Brand name: Dilantin. (17, 20, 50, 67, 119, 181, 315, 327, 359, 393, 395, 410, 422, 455, 467)
0.18–1	2.1 ± 0.7	10	15%–25% of dose converted to phenobarbital. Phenylethylmalonamide also a metabolite. Infant may be drowsy. Bleeding may result from hypoprothrombinemia. Brand name: Mysoline. (20, 129, 181, 315, 329, 410, 477)
		66	No longer available in the US. Rash and drowsiness reported after breastfeeding. Absorption through skin and transfer to milk is a concern if mother works in a photographic laboratory. (39, 67)
	Excreted in rat milk		Elimination is faster in children. Brand name: Topamax. (53)
0.05–0.42	1.8	12	In milk: 0.05%–11.3% of newborn therapeutic dose. Neonate has good clearance and poorly absorbs drug orally. Brand name: Depakene. (20, 67, 119, 181, 256, 315, 367, 547)
			81% ± 11% metabolized to valproic acid. If taken orally, not found in the plasma, only metabolite is. (52)

Continued

TABLE D-1   Relationship of drugs to breast milk and effect on infant—cont'd

Drugs and ratings[*]	Oral availability (%)	Peak plasma time (hr)	Plasma protein bound (%)	Volume of distribution (L/kg)
Antihistamines				
Azatadine AAP — H — W —	Anticholinergic action may suppress lactation; administer after nursing 4			
Brompheniramine AAP — H L3 W —		3.1 ± 1.1		11.7 ± 3.1
Brompheniramine maleate AAP — H — W —		1–5		11.7
Cetirizine AAP — H L2 W —	70	0.5–1.2	93	0.7
Chlorpheniramine AAP — H L3 W —	41 ± 16	4.25 ± 1.75	70 ± 3	3.2 ± 0.3
Chlorpheniramine maleate AAP — H — W —	25–60	4 ± 2	69–72	2.5–3.2
Clemastine AAP 5 H L4 W —		3.5 ± 1.5		
Dexbrompheniramine AAP 6 H — W —	Dexbrompheniramine maleate is well absorbed from GI tract			
Diphenhydramine AAP — H L2 W —	72 ± 25	1–4	75–98.5	6.2 ± 2.9

Milk/plasma (M/P) ratio	Adult dose in milk (%)	Maximum amount in milk (mg/L)	Comments and references
			Readily absorbed from GI tract. Brand name: Trinalin. (7, 393)
	Half-life in milk: 24.9 ± 9.3 hr		Has two active metabolites.
			Well absorbed from GI tract. Active metabolite: brompheniramine. Brand names: Bromfed, Dimetane, Dristan. (7)
			Does not have anticholinergic activity. Half-life is shorter in children. Brand name: Zyrtec. (84, 117, 478)
	Excreted into human milk		Clearance negatively correlated with age. Other reports of volume of distribution: children 4.3–7 L/kg, adults 5.9–11.7 L/kg. (181, 477, 500)
			Oral availability: tablets, 25%–45%; solution, 35%–60%. Volume of distribution in children: 3.8 L/kg. Brand name: Chlor-Pro. (7)
0.25–0.5	29.5 ± 20.5	0.01	Drug not detected in infant's plasma. Infant may be irritable and drowsy. Brand name: Tavist. (67, 393, 477)
			Related to brompheniramine. (7, 393)
	Excreted into human milk		Metabolism shows ethnic variation. Volume of distribution greater and amount protein bound less in Orientals than Caucasians. In rats, amount received through milk is quite low, but the M/P ratio varies from 3.85 to 9.54. Brand name: Benadryl. (7, 67, 123, 181, 455, 477)

Continued

TABLE D-1   Relationship of drugs to breast milk and effect on infant—cont'd

Drugs and ratings*	Oral availability (%)	Peak plasma time (hr)	Plasma protein bound (%)	Volume of distribution (L/kg)
Antihistamines—cont'd				
Fexofenadine AAP 6 H L2 W —				
Flunarizine AAP — H L4 W —	85–86	2–4	90–99	43–78
Levocabastine AAP — H L2 W —	100–120	2	55	1.14
Loratadine AAP 6 H L2 W —				
Promethazine AAP — H L2 W —	25 ± 10 Well absorbed from GI tract; rapidly metabolized	2.8 ± 1.4	76–80	13.4 ± 3.6
Roxatidine AAP — H — W —		1.3 ± 0.7		1.7–3.2
Trimeprazine AAP — H L3 W —				
Tripelennamine AAP — H L4 W —		2–3		
Triprolidine AAP 6 H L1 W —	Erratic	2 ± 1.2		

Milk/plasma (M/P) ratio	Adult dose in milk (%)	Maximum amount in milk (mg/L)	Comments and references
0.04–0.77			In milk: peak 4.25 ± 2.36 hr; half-life 14.15 ± 5.44 hr. Brand name: Allegra.
	Excreted into dog's milk		Elimination half-life after one dose is 17–18 days. (477)
			Availability: intranasal 60%–80%; ocular, 30%–60%; topically absorption incomplete. As nasal spray, amount in milk <3.5 µg/day. (111)
1.2	0.01	0.0292	In milk: worst case, drug + metabolite, 1.1% of adult dose on mg/kg basis. Brand name: Claritin. (212)
	Passage into human milk expected		Increases serum prolactin level. Brand names: Phenergan, Mepergan. (67, 455)
			Taken as roxatidine acetate. Greater than 95% orally absorbed; almost completely deacetylated to roxatidine. In vitro, 6%–7% plasma protein bound. (294, 344)
	Low level found in human milk		May cause galactorrhea. Brand name: Temaril. (67)
	Has been isolated from bovine milk		Well absorbed orally. Brand name: PBZ. (7, 67)
0.5–1.2	0.06–0.2	0.004	In milk: peak 1.5 ± 0.5 hr. Transdermal patch: plasma peak 14.4 ± 9.9 hr. Brand name: Actified. (20, 324)

Continued

TABLE D-1	Relationship of drugs to breast milk and effect on infant—cont'd			

Drugs and ratings*	Oral availability (%)	Peak plasma time (hr)	Plasma protein bound (%)	Volume of distribution (L/kg)
Antiinfective agents				
	May change intestinal flora of baby and sensitize for later allergic reaction			
Acyclovir AAP 6 H L2 W S	15–50	1.5–2.5	9–33	0.69 ± 0.19
Amantadine AAP — H L3 W —	50–100	4	67	6.6 ± 1.5
Amikacin AAP — H L2 W —	Poor absorption	1 after IM	<10	0.08–0.48
Aminosalicylic acid (para) AAP — H L3 W —		1.5–2	15	0.2
Amoxicillin AAP 6 H L1 W —	70.9–105.5	1.5 ± 0.5	17–20	0.29 ± 0.11
Amphotericin B AAP — H L3 W —	<10 Poor absorption		90–95	3–4.4
Ampicillin AAP — H L1 W —	62 ± 17	1.5	22 ± 7	0.21–0.7
Azithromycin AAP — H L2 W —	37–40	1–4	7–50 Negatively correlated with serum concentration	23–31
Azlocillin AAP — H — W —	Poor absorption		28 ± 6	0.22 ± 0.06

Milk/plasma (M/P) ratio	Adult dose in milk (%)	Maximum amount in milk (mg/L)	Comments and references
0.6–4.1	5.6 ± 4.4	5.81	Oral availability decreases with dose. Baby gets <1–2 mg/day. In milk: peak 3–10 hr, half-life 2.8 hr. Minimal absorption through skin. Brand name: Zovirax. (20, 67, 119, 181, 276, 335, 455, 492, 529)
Excreted into human milk in low amounts			May lower maternal prolactin levels. Brand name: Symmetrel. (67, 181, 393, 455, 477)
Trace			In milk: peak 5 ± 1 hr. Given to premature infants. Renal function most significant factor in drug elimination. Brand name: Amikin. (20, 67, 181, 255, 377, 477, 564)
0.016	0.25–0.5	1.1	In milk: peak 3 hr. (20, 181, 477)
0.013–0.043	0.7	1.3	In milk: 0.18% of calculated newborn therapeutic dose. Dose-dependent oral availability. Brand names: Amoxil, Augmentin. (7, 20, 181, 410, 477, 538)
			Used in infants. Brand names: Abelect, Amphotec, Fungizone. (7, 32, 181, 410, 433, 455, 477)
0.01–0.58	0.05–0.4	1	In milk: 0.14%–0.4% newborn therapeutic dose, reaches a plateau at 2–6 hr. In neonates: half-life increases, 7%–12% plasma protein bound, oral availability increases. An active metabolite of pivampicillin and bacampicillin. Brand name: Unasyn. (50, 63, 67, 181, 309, 410)
		2.8	Average tissue half-life is 1–4 days. Given directly to 20 children between the ages of 7 months and 2 years. No side effects were noted. Brand name: Zithromax. (97, 218, 254, 268, 297, 392, 548)
Low			Half-life dose dependent, increases from beginning to end of treatment. Given to neonates and premature infants. Brand name: Azlin. (181, 377, 393, 477)

Continued

TABLE D-1	Relationship of drugs to breast milk and effect on infant—cont'd			

Drugs and ratings*	Oral availability (%)	Peak plasma time (hr)	Plasma protein bound (%)	Volume of distribution (L/kg)
Antiinfective agents—cont'd				
Aztreonam AAP 6 H L2 W —	Poor absorption	1.5 after IM	56	0.21
Bacampicillin AAP — H — W —	87 ± 22	0.8 ± 0.1		
Carbenicillin AAP — H L1 W —	<10		50–60	0.18–0.2
Cefaclor AAP — H L2 W —	90	0.5–2	25	0.36
Cefadroxil AAP 6 H L1 W —	78–90	1–3	18–20	0.17–0.3
Cefamandole nafate AAP — H — W —	Not absorbed orally	1.25 ± 0.75	73.5 ± 6.5	0.16 ± 0.05
Cefatrizine AAP — H — W —	55–77	2	58	
Cefazolin AAP 6 H L1 W —	Not absorbed orally	1.5 ± 0.5 after IM	77.5 ± 7.5	0.12 ± 0.03
Cefixime AAP — H L2 W —	30–50	2–6	65–70	0.103 ± 0.008
Cefmenoxime AAP — H — W —	Not absorbed orally			0.12

Milk/plasma (M/P) ratio	Adult dose in milk (%)	Maximum amount in milk (mg/L)	Comments and references
0.002–0.009	2.35 ± 0.35	0.4	In milk: peak 3–6 hr. Used in premature infants. Brand name: Azactam. (20, 102)
			In GI tract, converted to ampicillin. Brand name: Spectrobid. (393, 455)
0.02	0.001		Not well absorbed from GI tract. Given to neonates. In milk: 0.03% of newborn dose, peak 4 hr, 1 hr after 1-g dose, 0.265 µg/mL found. Brand name: Geocillin. (19, 20, 181, 377, 410, 455, 477)
		0.21	Food delays absorption. Brand name: Ceclor. (67, 181, 364, 393, 455)
0.009–0.02	0.4	2.4	Saturable GI and renal tubular reabsorption; both affect amount of drug in the system. In milk: peak 5–7 hr; larger doses peak later. Brand name: Duricef. (7, 67, 177, 181, 334, 393, 477)
0.02		0.46	85%–89% rapidly hydrolyzed to cefamandole. Half-life longer in neonates. Brand name: Mandol. (7, 67, 181, 377, 393, 477)
Excreted into human milk			(455, 500)
0.02–0.023	0.075	1.5	Detected in milk, when given IV not IM. Given to premature infants. In milk: maximum amount 0.9% of newborn therapeutic dose; peak 3 hr. Brand names: Ancef, Kefzol. (20, 67, 181, 377, 393)
Excreted into human milk			Third generation cephalosporin. Absorption limited, food delays it. Given to 2-month-olds. Brand name: Suprax. (7, 334, 393, 500)
1.1–1.6			Competes with bilirubin. (374)

Continued

TABLE D-1   Relationship of drugs to breast milk and effect on infant—cont'd

Drugs and ratings[*]	Oral availability (%)	Peak plasma time (hr)	Plasma protein bound (%)	Volume of distribution (L/kg)
Antiinfective agents—cont'd				
Cefonicid AAP — H — W —	Not absorbed orally		96–98	0.11 ± 0.01
Cefoperazone AAP — H L2 W —	<10		77.5 ± 12.5	0.25 ± 0.15
Ceforanide AAP — H — W —	Not absorbed orally	1 after IM	80–82	0.14 ± 0.04
Cefotaxime AAP 6 H L2 W —		0.5	40 ± 10	0.33 ± 0.12
Cefotetan AAP — H L2 W —	Not absorbed orally	1.5–3 after IM	76–91	0.194
Cefotiam hexitil AAP — H — W —			40	0.3
Cefoxitin AAP 6 H L1 W —	Not absorbed orally		61.5 ± 11.5	0.31 ± 0.12
Cefpodoxime AAP — H L2 W —		2.9 ± 0.8	18–50	
Cefpodoxime proxetil AAP — H L2 W —	Food increases bioavailability; esterases in the intestinal wall convert this prodrug to the active compound cefpodoxime (see above)			

Milk/plasma (M/P) ratio	Adult dose in milk (%)	Maximum amount in milk (mg/L)	Comments and references
0.002		0.3	In milk: average amount 0.16 mg/L. Brand name: Monocid. (181)
	0.9		Brand name: Cefobid. (67, 181, 377, 477)
Excreted into human milk			Brand name: Precef. (67, 181, 393, 500)
0.02–0.21	0.3	1.6	In milk: maximum found, 0.1%–0.2% of the newborn dose; peak 2.5 ± 0.5 hr. Brand name: Claforan. (20, 21, 251, 393)
		0.59	Plasma protein binding inversely related to plasma drug concentration. In milk: peak 4 hr. Brand name: Cefotan. (7, 67, 181, 393)
			Hydrolyzed in the GI tract to cefotiam (plasma protein bound: 44.5% ± 2.1%) with the main metabolite being cyclohexanol (plasma protein bound: 53.1% ± 0.8%). (35, 477)
	0.16	2	Not all women excrete drug into milk. In milk: peak 4 ± 3 hr. Given to neonates. Brand name: Mefoxin. (19, 20, 67, 181, 377, 393)
		0.12	A cephalosporin used in infants 6 months old. (24, 428)
			Brand name: Vantin. (428)

Continued

TABLE D-1 Relationship of drugs to breast milk and effect on infant—cont'd

Drugs and ratings[*]	Oral availability (%)	Peak plasma time (hr)	Plasma protein bound (%)	Volume of distribution (L/kg)
Antiinfective agents—cont'd				
Cefprozil AAP 6 H L1 W —	90	1–3.5	36–45	
Ceftazidime AAP 6 H L1 W —	<10		21 ± 6	0.23 ± 0.02
Ceftibuten AAP — H L2 W —	90–94	1.96 ± 1.12	63	0.21 ± 0.03
Ceftizoxime AAP — H — W —	1		23–65	0.36 ± 0.19
Ceftriaxone AAP 6 H L2 W —		0.5–1	<60–95 Saturable	0.1–0.2
Cefuroxime AAP — H L2 W —	Poor		27–50	0.19 ± 0.04
Cefuroxime axetil AAP — H L2 W —	38 ± 17	2.5 ± 1.5		
Cephacetrile AAP — H — W —	Not absorbed orally		23 ± 3	0.6
Cephalexin AAP — H L1 W —	90 ± 9	1–2	13.5 ± 3.5	0.26 ± 0.03

Milk/plasma (M/P) ratio	Adult dose in milk (%)	Maximum amount in milk (mg/L)	Comments and references
0.05–5.67	0.3	3.4	About 95% absorbed. Food does not affect absorption. In milk: peak 6 hr. Brand name: Cefzil. (393, 446, 449, 450, 451, 452, 551)
		7.6	In milk: peak 1 hr. In prematures and neonates: half-life 2.9–14.2 hr, volume of distribution 0.53 ± 0.12 L/kg. Brand names: Ceptaz, Fortaz, Tazicef, Tazidime. (181, 339, 377, 393, 455, 477, 497)
			Absorption slightly decreased by food. Six women given 200 mg, no drug detected in milk; assay limit of 1 mg/L. (35, 143, 252)
0.01		0.35 ± 0.08	Brand name: Cefizox. (67, 181, 410, 455)
0.03–0.04	0.7	7.89	Saturable plasma protein binding. In milk: half-life IM 17.3 hr, IV 12.8 hr, peak 5.5 ± 1.5 hr. Brand names: Rocephin, Bourqet. (19, 20, 61, 67, 181, 377, 393, 477)
	Excreted into human milk		Brand names: Kefurox, Zinacef. (7, 67, 181, 262, 377, 393)
	A prodrug for cefuroxime		Food and milk increase absorption by 50%. More orally bioavailable than cefuroxime. Brand name: Ceftin. (7, 35, 234, 393, 500)
	Excreted into human milk		Given to premature infants. (7, 500)
0.008–0.14	0.85 ± 0.35	5.23	In milk: peak 4.5 ± 0.5 hr, completely gone by 8 hr, maximum 0.04%–0.4% newborn therapeutic dose. Absorption less in the first few months of life. Food lowers plasma peak at 2 hr. Brand name: Keflex. (20, 35, 67, 181, 334, 393, 477)

Continued

TABLE D-1	**Relationship of drugs to breast milk and effect on infant—cont'd**		

Drugs and ratings*	Oral availability (%)	Peak plasma time (hr)	Plasma protein bound (%)	Volume of distribution (L/kg)
Antiinfective agents—cont'd				
Cephaloridine AAP — H — W —	Poor oral absorption	1 after IM	10–30	0.2
Cephalothin AAP — H L2 W —	Negligible	0.75 ± 0.25 after IM	66 ± 6	0.26 ± 0.11
Cephapirin AAP — H L1 W —	0	0.75 ± 0.25	55 ± 11	0.21 ± 0.06
Cephradine AAP — H L1 W —	85 ± 29	0.75	11.5 ± 5.5	0.25 ± 0.01
Chloramphenicol AAP 4 H L4 W —	75–90	1	53 ± 5	0.94 ± 0.06
Chloroquine AAP 6 H L3 W —	67–114 Absorption not complete	1.6–5.3	61 ± 9	100–1000
Chlortetracycline AAP — H — W —	25–30		55	1.2
Cilastatin AAP — H — W —			35–40	0.2 ± 0.03
Cinoxacin AAP — H — W —			63	0.25–0.33

Milk/plasma (M/P) ratio	Adult dose in milk (%)	Maximum amount in milk (mg/L)	Comments and references
	Excreted into human milk		Serum bioavailability: 76%. Not metabolized. (477, 500)
0.051–0.57	0.4	0.62	Higher volume of distribution in baby. In milk: maximum 0.05%–0.09% of newborn dose. Peak: 1–2 hr. (20, 51, 67, 181, 393, 410)
0.068–0.5		0.64	Amount in cow milk: 5 ppb. (89, 181, 393, 477)
0.12–1.3	0.005	0.7	Food in GI tract delays uptake; amount absorbed is the same. Over 90% of drug excreted by kidneys within 6 hr. In milk: peak 1 hr. Brand names: Anspor, Velosef. (20, 181, 334, 393, 455, 477)
0.05–0.73	1.3–7.4	26	In milk: 0.2%–25% of newborn dose, peak 3.5 ± 2.5 hr. Possible idiosyncratic bone marrow depression. Brand name: Chloromycetin. (19, 20, 50, 67, 89, 181, 393)
0.268–9	0.55–4.2	0.319	In milk: peak 2.2–7 hr, half-life 5.5 ± 0.7 days, upper limit is 4.2% of maternal dose. Metabolite also found in milk. Level in maternal saliva about the same as in milk. Brand name: Aralen. (4, 7, 20, 67, 181, 365, 498)
0.125–1	0.7 ± 0.2	4.1	Oral availability reflects GI absorption. In cow milk: 2000 ppb. Brand name: Aureomycin. (20, 67, 89, 455, 463, 477)
			Combined with antibiotics because it is an inhibitor of renal dipepidase. (75, 181, 393)
			(181, 393, 477)

Continued

TABLE D-1   Relationship of drugs to breast milk and effect on infant—cont'd

Drugs and ratings*	Oral availability (%)	Peak plasma time (hr)	Plasma protein bound (%)	Volume of distribution (L/kg)
Antiinfective agents—cont'd				
Ciprofloxacin AAP 6 H L3 W —	52–86	1–2.4	20–40	1.74–5
Clarithromycin AAP — H L2 W —	50–55	0.5–6	42–70	
Clavulanic acid AAP — H — W —	31–99	0.75–2	19.5 ± 9.5	0.2
Clindamycin AAP 6 H L3 W —	86 ± 1	0.5–1.5	93.6 ± 0.2	1.1 ± 0.3
Clofazimine AAP 4 H L3 W U	45–70			
Cloxacillin AAP — H L2 W —	41.5 ± 17.5	1.25 ± 0.25	94.1 ± 1.1	0.094 ± 0.015
Colistimethate AAP — H — W —	Not absorbed orally			
Colistin AAP — H — W —	GI absorption negligible			
Cycloserine AAP 6 H L3 W —	70–90			

Milk/plasma (M/P) ratio	Adult dose in milk (%)	Maximum amount in milk (mg/L)	Comments and references
0.85–2.14		3.79	Four less active metabolites from 15% of dose. Milk decreases uptake. Causes arthropathy in immature animals and teens with cystic fibrosis. Has been given directly to two preterm infants. In milk: plateaus at 4–12 hr. Pump 4 hr after last pill, feed 6 hr after last pill. Previously not approved by AAP. Brand name: Cipro. (100, 169, 179, 270, 298, 305, 354, 393, 515, 533)
Excreted into animal milk			Food slightly delays absorption and metabolism but does not affect overall availability. Higher doses have longer half-lives. Kinetics in infants published. Brand name: Biaxin. (91, 159, 174, 393)
Excreted into human milk			Brand name: Augmentin. (106, 455, 477, 535)
0.1–3	4.1 ± 1.3	4	Absorption not decreased by food. 400 ppb in cow milk. In milk: 1%–7.6% of newborn therapeutic dose; peak 2–4 hr. Brand name: Cleocin. (7, 20, 67, 89, 181, 393, 455, 477)
1,7			Antimicrobial for leprosy. Does pass into milk. Stains tissues, causes hyperpigmentation. Use alternative during lactation. Brand name: Lamprene.
	9		Oral absorption delayed if taken with food. 100 ppb in cow milk. Brand names: Cloxapen, Tegopen. (89, 181, 349, 359, 393, 455, 477)
0.17–0.18			Hydrolized to colistin in vitro and in vivo. Brand name: Coly-Mycin. (67)
0.17–0.18	0.07	0.9	Brand name: Coly-Mycin. (393)
0.31–1.18	0.6	19	From milk, a nursing infant would ingest up to 11.3% of the usual pediatric dose. The average M/P ratio is 0.72. Antituberculosis drug. Brand name: Seromycin.

Continued

TABLE D-1   Relationship of drugs to breast milk and effect on infant—cont'd

Drugs and ratings*	Oral availability (%)	Peak plasma time (hr)	Plasma protein bound (%)	Volume of distribution (L/kg)
Antiinfective agents—cont'd				
Dapsone AAP 6 H L4 W —	93 ± 8	6 ± 2	70–80	1.09 ± 0.18
Demeclocycline AAP — H — W —	66		70–95	1.8
Dicloxacillin AAP — H L1 W —	38–85	1 ± 0.8	89–96	0.095 ± 0.026
Didanosine AAP — H — W —	19–43	0.25–2	<5	0.87 ± 0.33
Dirithromycin AAP — H L3 W —	6–14	4.8 ± 2.6	15–30	109 ± 69
Doxycycline AAP — H L3, L4 if used chronically W —	94 ± 1	2.9 ± 0.9	88 ± 5	0.75 ± 0.32
Enoxacin AAP — H L4 W —	70–90	1.9 ± 1	18–54	1.6–2.9
Erythromycin AAP 6 H L1 W —	37.5 ± 27.5	3	66 ± 24	0.89 ± 0.55
Ethambutol AAP 6 H L2 W —	77 ± 8	2–4	<5–22	1.6 ± 0.2

Milk/plasma (M/P) ratio	Adult dose in milk (%)	Maximum amount in milk (mg/L)	Comments and references
0.22–0.67	11.95 ± 2.35		Two acetylation phenotypes in the population. Drug and primary metabolite found in milk. One case report in which both mother and baby had compensating hemolytic anemia. (20, 133, 135, 181, 393, 453, 477)
0.7		1.4	Oral availability reflects absorption through GI tract. Drug is given to infants. Drug remains in milk for 3 days after dose. Brand name: Declomycin. (455, 463, 477)
Small amount found in human milk			Has been used to treat mastitis without stopping nursing. Brand names: Dynapen, Dycill, Pathocil. (181, 349, 455, 477)
			Bioavailability reduced by half when taken with food. Brand name: Videx. (7, 146, 228, 260, 447)
	65		Brand name: Dynabac. (454)
0.3–0.4		0.77	Bioavailability not altered by food. Brand names: Doryx, Vibramycin, Monodox. (67, 181, 477)
			Absorption not decreased by food. Brand name: Penetrex. (219, 270, 298, 516, 532)
0.02–1.6	0.1–2.1	6.2	Maximum absorption on an empty stomach. Possible jaundice if infant less than 1 month old. In milk: peak 4 hr, 0.1%–0.25% of newborn therapeutic dose. Brand names: Benzamycin, E-Mycin, Pediazole. (20, 66, 67, 181, 431, 455, 477)
1		4.6	In milk: 1%-5.7% of newborn therapeutic dose. Brand name: Myambutol. (181, 393, 477)

Continued

TABLE D-1 Relationship of drugs to breast milk and effect on infant—cont'd

Drugs and ratings*	Oral availability (%)	Peak plasma time (hr)	Plasma protein bound (%)	Volume of distribution (L/kg)
Antiinfective agents—cont'd				
Famciclovir AAP — H L2 W —	77 ± 8	Not detected in plasma or urine		
Fleroxacin AAP — H — W —	99 ± 14	0.2–6	27.5 ± 4.5	1.4 ± 0.34
Fluconazole AAP 6 H L2 W —	90	1–3	10–15	0.85 ± 0.15
Flucytosine AAP — H — W —	88.5 ± 10.5	1–2	2–4	0.68 ± 0.04
Fosfomycin AAP — H L3 W —	10–58	2.2 ± 0.9	0	1.5
Gentamicin AAP — H L2 W —	Negligible		0–30	0.34 ± 0.15
Griseofulvin AAP — H L2 W —	95	4 when fasting		1.5
Halofantrine AAP — H — W —	Oral absorption poor and variable	3–27	>98	1.1–9.7
Hydroxychloroquine AAP 6 H L2 W —	Absorption 25%–100% from tablet; mean: 70	2.3–6	62.5 ± 2.5	

Milk/plasma (M/P) ratio	Adult dose in milk (%)	Maximum amount in milk (mg/L)	Comments and references
See active metabolite, penciclovir			Brand name: Famvir. (393, 402)
0.62		4.5	Food does not affect absorption. In milk: peak 2–6 hr. half-life 7.18–8.97 hr. (105, 298, 460, 489, 555)
0.46–1		2.93	80% of dose recovered in urine unchanged. Oral availability independent of pH of stomach and food in GI tract. In milk: peaks by 2 hr. In premature infants: half-life 43.3–187.3 hr; volume of distribution 1.05–1.48 L/kg. Brand name: Diflucan. (7, 56, 107, 156, 173, 188, 210, 393, 409, 537, 543)
			Half-life slightly longer in premature infants. Given to neonates. Brand name: Ancobon. (7, 32, 181, 455)
0.1			Drug has poor solubility and is degraded by stomach acid. Food significantly reduces oral absorption. Brand name: Monural. (45, 477)
0.08–0.57		0.78	In neonate may see appreciable GI absorption. In milk: 0.012%–0.9% of the neworn therapeutic dose. Brand names: Garamycin, G-myticin. (7, 50, 87, 172, 181, 377, 393, 397, 410)
Not excreted into human milk			Absorption from GI tract varies considerably. There are good and poor absorbers. Brand names: Fulvicin, Grisactin. (7, 393, 455, 477)
			Oral availability increased by food. (74, 245, 264)
5.5	0.0003–2	1.46	If chronically used by mother, may cause retinal damage in infant. Percentage of adult dose in chart based on data from two women. Brand name: Plaquenil. (498)

Continued

TABLE D-1   Relationship of drugs to breast milk and effect on infant—cont'd

Drugs and ratings*	Oral availability (%)	Peak plasma time (hr)	Plasma protein bound (%)	Volume of distribution (L/kg)
Antiinfective agents—cont'd				
Imipenem AAP — H L2 W —	Not absorbed orally		<10–20	0.23 ± 0.05
Isoniazid AAP 6 H L3 W —	90	1–2	0	0.67 ± 0.15
Ivermectin AAP — H L3 W —		3–6	93.2 ± 4.4	11.1 ± 4.2
Kanamycin AAP 6 H L2 W S?	Oral absorption poor		0	0.26 ± 0.05
Ketoconazole AAP 6 H L2 W S		1.5 ± 0.5	99 ± 0.1	2.4 ± 1.6
Levofloxacin AAP H L3 W U	99	1–2	24–38	1.25
Lincomycin AAP — H L3 W S		3 ± 1	72	0.5
Lindane AAP — H L3 W S?		6–8		
Lomefloxacin AAP — H L3 W U	92–100 absorbed	0.7–2	17.5 ± 7	1.5–2.5

Milk/plasma (M/P) ratio	Adult dose in milk (%)	Maximum amount in milk (mg/L)	Comments and references
			Brand name: Primaxin. (181, 456, 477)
0.5–3	2.3	16.6	In milk: 6.3%–25% newborn therapeutic dose, peak 3 hr. Not detected in infant's blood, but found in urine. Oral absorption decreased by food. Active metabolite: M/P ratio 1; peaks in milk at 5 hr. Brand names: INH, Rifamate. (50, 67, 181)
0.18–0.97 at peak: 0.18–0.37		0.0206	Bioavailability of tablet vs. solution is 60%. Mean amount in milk: 9.85 ± 0.38 ng/mL. Brand name: Stromectol. (181, 183, 363, 370)
0.05->1	0.95	18.4	IM serum peak: 1 hr with 100% bioavailability. In milk: 30% of newborn therapeutic dose, peak 1 hr. Serum half-life in infant is inversely related to age. Brand name: Kantrex. (67, 181, 377)
0.38	0.3–1.4	0.22	Oral absorption varies considerably. Extensively metabolized in the liver to inactive products. Oral availability decreases as pH of stomach increases. Brand name: Nizoral. (7, 56, 173, 181, 286, 333, 389, 393)
Secretion into breast milk is expected as with other fluoroquinolones			Brand name: Levaquin. (393)
0.13–2.25	0.026–0.6	2.4	Brand name: Lincocin. (20, 67, 89, 393, 477)
		0.08	Used as a cream, lotion, or shampoo. Through milk, maximum daily intake 62.07 µg/kg. Brand name: Kwell. (67, 235, 236, 393)
			Food decreases rate but not amount absorbed. Amount in serum proportional to dose. Probably safer than cipro. Brand name: Maxaquin. (219, 285, 474, 527, 555)

Continued

TABLE D-1   Relationship of drugs to breast milk and effect on infant—cont'd

Drugs and ratings[*]	Oral availability (%)	Peak plasma time (hr)	Plasma protein bound (%)	Volume of distribution (L/kg)
Antiinfective agents—cont'd				
Mebendazole AAP — H L4 W U	2–22	0.5–7.25	90	2
Mefloquine AAP — H L2 W S	85–89	33.6 ± 12	98.2-98.4	25.27 ± 9.75
Methacycline AAP — H — W —	58	2–3	80-95	
Methenamine AAP — H— W S		1.5 ± 0.5		0.63 ± 0.12
Methicillin AAP — H L3 W S	Negligible		39 ± 2	0.43 ± 0.1
Metronidazole AAP4 H L2 W —	80–100 Availability: intravaginally 19–81, usually 20; ointment 3–10	0.25–4 oral 4–24 vaginal 17 ± 9.6 ointment	<1–20	0.52–1.1
Mezlocillin AAP — H — W —	Negligible		16–42	0.25
Miconazole AAP — H L2 W —	25–30		90–99	20
Minocycline AAP — H L2 acute use, L4 chronic W —	95–100	2	70–76	1.3 ± 0.2

Milk/plasma (M/P) ratio	Adult dose in milk (%)	Maximum amount in milk (mg/L)	Comments and references
		0.005	May inhibit lactation (one case, with circumstantial evidence). Brand name: Vermox. (7, 181, 455, 477)
0.13-0.27	3.2 ± 0.6	0.31	In milk: maximum 0.14 mg/kg. During lactation, plasma clearance and volume of distribution about 50% less than after weaning. Elimination half-life of drug: 6–28 days. Brand name: Lariam. (60, 134, 244, 379, 455, 477)
0.5		2.6	Oral absorption about 60% in a fasting adult. Food and/or milk reduces normal GI absorption by 50% or more. (7, 181, 455, 463)
0.88-1.08	8.3	1.1	In milk: 0.07%–0.6% of the newborn therapeutic dose, peak 1 hr. Brand names: Hiprex, Urex. (20)
A small amount found in milk			Brand name: Staphcillin. (50, 181, 410, 477)
0.45–1.8	0.13–36	60	In milk: 1.3%–75% newborn therapeutic dose, amount secreted is dose dependent, peak 2.25 ± 1.75 hr. AAP recommends mother take 2 g orally, discard milk for 12–24 hr. Brand names: Flagyl, MetroGel, Protostat. (7, 20, 67, 181, 275, 383, 455, 566)
Low amount detected in human milk			Given to neonates. Brand name: Mezlin. (181, 241, 377, 393, 477)
			About 50% of oral dose is absorbed from GI tract. Used in infants. Brand name: Monistat. (7, 393, 455, 477)
		0.8	May turn milk black. Brand name: Minocin. (181, 463, 477)

Continued

TABLE D-1   Relationship of drugs to breast milk and effect on infant—cont'd

Drugs and ratings*	Oral availability (%)	Peak plasma time (hr)	Plasma protein bound (%)	Volume of distribution (L/kg)
Antiinfective agents—cont'd				
Moxalactam AAP 6 H — W —	Negligible	0.5–2	45–67	0.25 ± 0.08
Nafcillin AAP — H L1 W —	33 ± 3		87–90	0.63 ± 0.3
Nalidixic acid AAP 6 H L4 W —	60 50%–100% absorbed	1–2	82–97	1
Netilmicin AAP — H L3 W —			<10	0.2 ± 0.02
Nitrofurantoin AAP 6 H L2 W —	99 Food increases absorption		20–60	0.8
Norfloxacin AAP — H L3 W —	30–80 Milk reduces absorption	1–2	10–15	3.2 ± 1.4
Novobiocin AAP — H — W —		2.5 ± 0.5		
Nystatin AAP — H L1 W —	Sparingly absorbed in GI tract			
Ofloxacin AAP 6 H L3 W —	70–100	1.5–3	8–30	1.25 ± 0.25
Oxacillin AAP — H — W —	55 ± 25		91.6–96	0.33 ± 0.09

Milk/plasma (M/P) ratio	Adult dose in milk (%)	Maximum amount in milk (mg/L)	Comments and references
	0.6	6	IM availability 70%–100%. In milk: up to 1.7% of newborn therapeutic dose. Brand name: Moxam. (7, 20, 181, 377, 410, 477)
A small amount found in milk			Variable oral absorption. Increased oral availability in neonates. Brand name: Unipen. (181, 377, 455, 477)
0.08–0.13	0.3	4	Decreased oral availability in neonate. Caution needed in G6PD-deficient infants. Brand name: NegGram. (20, 67, 393, 532)
Small amount found in human milk			Given to neonates. Brand name: Netromycin. (181, 377, 393)
0.3–2	0.6	0.5	Caution needed in G6PD-deficient infants. Brand names: Macrodantin, Furadantin. (20, 181, 393)
In milk, not detected after a single 200-mg dose			Food may delay, not reduce absorption. Brand names: Chibroxin, Noroxin. (7, 181, 270, 295, 532)
0.1–0.25	0.15	7	Drug may be given to infants directly. In cow milk: 50 ppb. Brand name: Albamycin. (7, 67)
Not excreted into human milk			Can be given to infants directly. Brand names: Mycolog, Mycostatin, Mytrex. (393)
0.98–1.66		2.41	Food delays peak plasma time. Brand names: Floxin, Ocuflox. (125, 179, 192, 270, 295, 502, 532, 533, 556)
Excreted into human milk in low concentrations			Displaces bilirubin from albumin in neonates. Brand names: Bactocill, Prostaphlin. (67, 377, 477)

Continued

TABLE D-1	**Relationship of drugs to breast milk and effect on infant—cont'd**			

Drugs and ratings*	Oral availability (%)	Peak plasma time (hr)	Plasma protein bound (%)	Volume of distribution (L/kg)
Antiinfective agents—cont'd				
Oxytetracycline AAP — H — W —	58		20–40	1.5
Pefloxacin AAP — H — W —	80–110	1–3	20–30	1.4 ± 0.3
Penciclovir AAP — H L3 W —		0.9 ± 0.5	<20	1.08 ± 0.17
Penicillin G AAP — H L1 W —	15–30	0.75 ± 0.25	60 ± 10	0.1–0.3
Penicillin V AAP — H — W —	60	0.75	75–89	0.25–0.51
Pentamidine AAP — H — W —	Negligible Poor GI absorption			16 ± 9
Permethrin AAP — H L2 W —	Used as a topically applied 5% cream; 2% or less is absorbed through the skin			
Piperacillin AAP — H L2 W —	Not absorbed orally		16–48	0.17–0.37
Praziquantel AAP — H L3 W —	80	2 ± 1		
Pyrazinamide AAP — H L3 W —	Well absorbed orally	2	50	

Milk/plasma (M/P) ratio	Adult dose in milk (%)	Maximum amount in milk (mg/L)	Comments and references
		3	In cow milk: 2000 ppb. Oral availability reflects absorption from GI tract. Brand names: Terra-Cortril, Terramycin, Urobiotic. (89, 455, 463, 477)
0.75–1.04		3.54	Norfloxacin is the active metabolite. (179, 219, 226, 270, 295, 455)
Drug is concentrated in rat milk			Drug given IV. A metabolite of famciclovir. (158, 393)
0.016–0.37	0.8	0.036	Oral availability: best on empty stomach, increased in neonate. In milk: 0.005%–0.4% of newborn therapeutic dose, peak 2–4 hr. Brand name: Bicillin. (20, 89, 181, 359, 377, 393, 410, 455, 477)
0.016–0.13	0.2		Kinetics may differ in woman with mastitis. In neonate: 65% plasma protein bound. Brand name: Pen-Vee. (50, 308, 349, 393, 455, 477)
			Has been detected in some tissues for up to a year. Brand names: Pentam, Nebupent. (181, 331)
			Rapidly metabolized in the body to inactive products. (393)
Passage into human milk after IM is minute			Amount in milk is below any therapeutic or toxic level. Brand names: Pipracil, Zosyn. (257, 377, 393)
0.25–0.28	0.13		Infant receives, through milk, 69 μg/kg/day. In milk: peak 6 ± 4 hr. Brand name: Biltricide. (20, 477)
0.036	0.5–1.4	1.5	In milk: peak 3 hr. (20, 477)

Continued

TABLE D-1   Relationship of drugs to breast milk and effect on infant—cont'd

Drugs and ratings*	Oral availability (%)	Peak plasma time (hr)	Plasma protein bound (%)	Volume of distribution (L/kg)
Antiinfective agents—cont'd				
Pyrethrin AAP — H — W —	Poorly absorbed through the skin and metabolized rapidly			
Pyrimethamine AAP 6 H L1 W —	Well absorbed orally	4.7 ± 3.25	87 ± 1	2.9 ± 0.5
Quinine AAP 6 H L2 W —	99 ± 10	1–6	93 ± 3	1.8 ± 0.4
Rifampin AAP 6 H L2 W —	99	3 ± 1	80–90	0.97 ± 0.36
Rosaramicin AAP — H — W —				3.78
Roxithromycin AAP — H — W —		2–2.5	96	
Streptomycin AAP 6 H L3 W —	GI absorption poor	1 after IM	48 ± 14	0.18 ± 0.11
Sulbactam AAP 6 H — W —	Minimal	Rapid IV/IM		
Sulfacetamide AAP — H — W —	Readily absorbed from GI tract			

Milk/plasma (M/P) ratio	Adult dose in milk (%)	Maximum amount in milk (mg/L)	Comments and references
			Brand name: RID. (181)
0.2–0.66	31.2 ± 14.4	3.3	In milk: peak 6 hr, found up to 48 hr after last dose, enough drug to cure an infant less than 6 months old, 62%–66% of the newborn therapeutic dose. Brand names: Daraprim, Fansidar. (67, 135, 181, 393, 477)
0.14	0.05	2.2	In milk: peak 0.5–6 hr. At therapeutic doses, no effect on infant except rare thrombocytopenia. If at risk for G6PD, do not breastfeed until it is ruled out. Brand name: Quinamm. (67, 181, 455, 541)
0.19–0.6	0.05	4.9	Given to infants. In milk: 0.57%–60% of therapeutic dose. If taken with food, plasma peak is delayed 1–2 hr. May turn milk orange. Brand names: Rifadin, Rifamate, Rimactane. (67, 181, 477)
0.12	0.0025–0.2		In milk: peak 3±1 hr. Positive correlation between breast milk volume and milk clearance. Infant gets 6.7 μg/kg/day. (20)
	<0.05		In milk: drug appears by 2 hr. Within 12 hr, 0.14 mg of a 300-mg dose is found in milk. (57, 83, 356)
0.12–1	0.5	30	In milk: 0.3%–1.3% newborn dose. (67, 181)
			Antibiotic. Beta-lactamase inhibitor given IV or IM, not orally bioavailable. Given to infants. Brand name: Unasyn.
0.08–1.3		66	(393)

Continued

TABLE D-1 **Relationship of drugs to breast milk and effect on infant—cont'd**

Drugs and ratings*	Oral availability (%)	Peak plasma time (hr)	Plasma protein bound (%)	Volume of distribution (L/kg)
Antiinfective agents—cont'd				
Sulfadiazine AAP — H — W —	99		54 ± 4	0.29 ± 0.04
Sulfamethazine AAP — H — W —		2–4	80	0.2
Sulfamethoxazole AAP 6 (listed with trimethoprim) H L3 W —	96 ± 14	2.5 ± 1.5	63.5 ± 6.5	0.21 ± 0.02
Sulfanilamide AAP — H — W —				
Sulfapyridine AAP 6 H — W —				
Sulfasalazine AAP 5 H L3 W —	10–30 absorbed in small intestine	1.5–6		1
Sulfathiazole AAP — H — W —				
Sulfisoxazole AAP 6 H L2 W —	96 ± 14	2.5 ± 1.5	88–92.6	0.13–0.35
Teicoplanin AAP — H — W —	Not absorbed orally		87.6–90.8	0.6–2.78

Milk/plasma (M/P) ratio	Adult dose in milk (%)	Maximum amount in milk (mg/L)	Comments and references
0.21			An infant over 1 month can better clear the drug. Brand name: Microsulfon. (67, 181, 477)
	Excreted into human milk		Food delays absorption. (7, 477)
0.06	0.45		In milk: about 1.2% of newborn dose. In first month, displaces bilirubin. Contraindicated in G6PD-deficient infants. Cow milk: 50 ppb. Brand names: Gantanol, Bactrim, Septra. (67, 89, 94, 181, 477)
0.5–1.2	1.6	94	In milk: may persist several days after mother stops taking it. Avoid in first month as it displaces bilirubin. Significant therapeutic doses not found in milk. Brand name: AVC. (67)
0.4–1	0.12	130	A metabolite of sulfasalazine. Caution in infant with jaundice or G6PD. (28, 40, 477)
0.3–0.6	4.1 ± 2.9	2.5	Active metabolites: sulfapyridine and 5-aminosalicylic acid. If jaundice develops, postpone nursing till it clears. Bloody diarrhea can develop. Brand name: Azulfidine. (20, 64, 67, 278, 393, 477, 498)
0.33–0.7		77	A vaginal cream or tablet. In milk: 5 mg/L after maternal dose of 3 g/day. Some reports of diarrhea and rash in infants when mother took drug. Caution if jaundice occurs. Brand names: Sultrin, Trysul. (67, 393, 477)
0.06–1	0.45	1.1	In milk: 33%–50% of newborn therapeutic dose. Jaundice may develop. Avoid in infants with G6PD. Brand names: Gantrisin, Pediazole. (50, 67, 89, 181, 393, 477)
			Given to newborns. (11, 37, 113, 466)

Continued

TABLE D-1   Relationship of drugs to breast milk and effect on infant—cont'd

Drugs and ratings*	Oral availability (%)	Peak plasma time (hr)	Plasma protein bound (%)	Volume of distribution (L/kg)
Antiinfective agents—cont'd				
Temafloxacin HCl AAP — H — W —	62–93	2.7 ± 1.9	26	1.53–1.83
Terconazole AAP — H L3 W —				
Tetracycline AAP 6 H L2 W —	72.5 ± 22.5	2	20–75	1.5 ± 0.08
Thiabendazole AAP — H L3 W —	100	1–2		
Ticarcillin AAP 6 H L2 W —	0	0.5–1.25 after IM	45–65	0.21 ± 0.03
Tinidazole AAP 4 H — W —	108 ± 47			
Tobramycin AAP — H L3 W —	GI absorption poor	1 ± 0.5	<10	0.25–0.33
Trimethoprim AAP 6 H L3 W —	99	2.5 ± 1.5	44–45	1.8 ± 0.2
Valacyclovir AAP — H L1 W —	Converted to acyclovir, the active compound			
	54	1.5		
Vancomycin AAP — H L1 W —	Not absorbed orally		10–55	0.39 ± 0.06

Milk/plasma (M/P) ratio	Adult dose in milk (%)	Maximum amount in milk (mg/L)	Comments and references
			Absorption not affected by food. (187, 382, 393, 477)
	Excreted into rat milk		As vaginal suppository amount absorbed, 5%–16%, is proportional to dose. Does not accumulate in body. Brand name: Terazol. (7, 393)
0.2–1.5	0.03–4.8	8	In infant: drug negligibly absorbed, undetected in serum. In milk: probably chelated by calcium, peak 4 hr. In cow milk: 2000 ppb. Brand name: Achromycin. (7, 20, 67, 89, 181, 393, 455, 463, 477)
	Excreted into cow milk		Brand name: Mintezol. (7, 13, 181)
	<0.09		Brand names: Timentin, Ticar. (7, 20, 181, 194, 377, 393, 477, 535)
0.62–1.39	1		(20, 455)
		0.6	In milk: 0%–2.4% of newborn therapeutic dose, peak 4 hr. Brand name: TobraDex. (67, 181, 377, 393, 477)
1.25		5.5	In children: decreased half-life. In milk: peak 2.5 ± 0.5 hr, amount related to dose. Newborn absorbs 0.75–1 mg daily. Brand names: Bactrim, Septra, Trimpex. (67, 181, 477)
0.6–4.1			Compared with taking acyclovir, the relative bioavailability of acyclovir from taking this drug is 3.3–5.5 times greater. Brand name: Valtrex (393)
Approximately 1		12.7	Given to newborns. Brand name: Vancocin. (67, 181, 289, 377, 393, 477)

Continued

TABLE D-1   Relationship of drugs to breast milk and effect on infant—cont'd

Drugs and ratings*	Oral availability (%)	Peak plasma time (hr)	Plasma protein bound (%)	Volume of distribution (L/kg)
Antiinfective agents—cont'd				
Zidovudine AAP — H — W —	63 ± 13	0.1–2 Food delays peak	<25–38	1.6 ± 0.6
Antineoplastics and antimetabolites				
Allopurinol AAP 6 H L2 W —	90 ± 9			0.6
Azathioprine AAP — H L3 W —	60 ± 31		30	0.81 ± 0.65
Bleomycin AAP — H — W —				0.27 ± 0.09
Busulfan AAP — H L5 W —	Oral absorption is slow and almost complete			0.99 ± 0.23
Carmustine AAP — H — W —	Rapidly absorbed			3.3 ± 1.7
Chlorambucil AAP — H L5 W —	87 ± 20	1	99	0.86 ± 0.81
Cisplatin AAP 6 H L4 W —	Negligible		Extensive	0.28 ± 0.07
Cyclophosphamide AAP 1— H L5 W —	74 ± 22	1	13–20	0.78 ± 0.57

Milk/plasma (M/P) ratio	Adult dose in milk (%)	Maximum amount in milk (mg/L)	Comments and references
			Brand name: Retrovir. (181, 186, 393, 546)
0.9–1.4		1.4	Drug not found in infant's plasma. Active metabolite, alloxanthine (oxipurinol): maternal plasma peak 4.5 hr; M/P ratio 2.4–3.89; maximum in milk 53.7 mg/L; 6.6 mg/L found in infant's plasma. Brand name: Zyloprim. (242, 442, 455, 477)
Small amount excreted into human milk			Metabolite: mercaptopurine. Half-life 0.6 hr. Should clear in 3 hr. Brand name: Imuran. (41, 181, 393)
			Brand name: Blenoxane. (181, 393, 477)
			Half-life 2.6 hr. Should clear in 13 hr. Brand name: Myleran. (181, 393, 477)
			Brand names: BiCNU, Gliadel. (181, 393, 477)
			When taken with food, peak value reduced by 50%, the extent of absorption by 25%. Half-life 1.3 hr. Should clear in 7 hr. Brand name: Leukeran. (181, 353, 393, 477)
AAP states not found in milk		0.9	Half-life 25–72 hr. Complete clearance in 3–15 days. Brand name: Platinol. (20, 67, 181, 410, 477)
Excreted into human milk			Is activated in liver. Metabolites in maternal plasma for up to 72 hr. Half-life 7.5 hr. Clearance in 37 hr. Brand name: Cytoxan. (181, 332, 393, 477)

Continued

TABLE D-1   Relationship of drugs to breast milk and effect on infant—cont'd

Drugs and ratings[*]	Oral availability (%)	Peak plasma time (hr)	Plasma protein bound (%)	Volume of distribution (L/kg)
Antineoplastics and antimetabolites—cont'd				
Cytarabine AAP — H L5 W —	20 ± 1		13	3 ± 1.9
Dacarbazine AAP — H — W —	Oral absorption poor			0.88–1.74
Doxorubicin AAP 1 H L5 W —	5	0.5	50–85	9–66
Estramustine phosphate AAP — H — W —	44 ± 5	2.2 ± 0.2		
Etoposide AAP — H — W —	17–72	0.5–4	96 ± 0.4	0.36 ± 0.15
Fluorouracil AAP — H L5 W —	0–74		8–12	0.25 ± 0.12
Gallium citrate AAP 3 H L4 W —	5			1.27
Hydroxyurea AAP — H L2 W —	>80			
Idarubicin AAP — H — W —	30.5 ± 18.5	1–6	97	63.9
Ifosfamide AAP — H — W —	85–100	1–2		0.34–0.64

Milk/plasma (M/P) ratio	Adult dose in milk (%)	Maximum amount in milk (mg/L)	Comments and references
			Brand name: Cytosar-U. (181, 393, 477)
			Brand name: DTIC-Dome. (7, 78, 393, 477)
4.4	1.3	0.24	In milk: detectable up to 72 hr, peak 24 hr, no platinum found. Brand name: Adriamycin. (7, 20, 67, 181, 410, 479)
			Metabolically activated by extensive first-pass metabolism. Brand name: Emcyt. (393)
			Oral availability decreases at doses greater than 200 mg. Brand name: VePesid. (181, 477)
			When used topically, <5%–10% absorbed. Brand names: Efudex, Fluoroplex. (7, 181, 399, 455, 477)
			Half-life 3 days. Clearance 15 days. Brand name: Ganite. (228, 504)
		8.4	Half-life > 40 days. Brand name: Hydrea. (67, 393, 490)
			Pharmacokinetics not affected by food. Not detected in plasma after 72 hr. Active metabolite, idarubicinol, detected for up to 7 days. Brand name: Idamycin. (82, 138, 216, 429, 486)
	Excreted into human milk		Metabolically activated in liver. Some evidence that drug has dose-dependent kinetics. Brand name: Ifex. (108, 291, 393, 455)

Continued

TABLE D-1 **Relationship of drugs to breast milk and effect on infant—cont'd**

Drugs and ratings[*]	Oral availability (%)	Peak plasma time (hr)	Plasma protein bound (%)	Volume of distribution (L/kg)
Antineoplastics and antimetabolites—cont'd				
Melphalan AAP — H — W —	71 ± 23			0.45 ± 0.15
Mercaptopurine H L5 W U	5–37	2–2.5	19	0.56 ± 0.38
Methotrexate AAP 1 H L3 (acute), L5 (chronic) W NS	36–88 Can be saturated	1.5 ± 0.5		0.55 ± 0.19
Tamoxifen H L5 W U	30	3–7	>99	~20
Autonomic and cardiovascular drugs				
Autonomic drugs				
Acebutolol AAP 5 H L3 W S	37 ± 12	1–4	11–29	1–3.8
Albuterol H L1 W S	50	1–4	7–8	2.5
Alprenolol	1–15	1 ± 0.5	85 ± 3	3.3 ± 1.2
Amphetamine AAP 2 H L5 W NS	>95		15	0.6
Atorvastatin calcium AAP — H L3 W U	12–30	1–2	98	8

Milk/plasma (M/P) ratio	Adult dose in milk (%)	Maximum amount in milk (mg/L)	Comments and references
			Food reduces absorption. Brand name: Alkeran. (181, 353, 477)
Excreted into breast milk			Active metabolite of azathioprine. Food reduces absorption. When first-pass metabolism inhibited by allopurinol, oral availability is 60%. Brand name: Purinethol. (7, 9, 181, 288, 353, 455)
0.04–0.1	0.93	0.003	Food delays absorption. In milk: peak 10 hr. Brand names: Folex, Rheumatrex. (20, 181, 353, 393, 455, 477)
			Brand name: Nolvadex. (7, 209, 299, 393)
1.9–10 mean: 7.1	3.5	4.123	Beta blocker. Risk of hypotension, bradycardia, tachypnea, and/or drowsiness. Active metabolite, diacetolol: poorly absorbed from GI tract; M/P ratio 1.5–24.7 (mean 12.2). If mother's dose exceeds 400 mg/day or her renal function is impaired, baby may receive a therapeutic dose through the milk. Brand name: Sectral. (7, 20, 62, 99, 181, 258, 407, 436)
			Beta agonist. As an inhaler, bioavailability is 2%–15%. Brand names: Airet, Proventil, Ventolin. (7, 214, 336, 393, 477)
			Extensive hepatic first-pass metabolism, which exhibits debrisoquine polymorphism. Dose-dependent bioavailability. (130, 181, 196, 359, 494)
2.8–7.5	6.1 ± 0.1	0.138	Baby's urinary excretion 0.001%–0.003% of mother's. Stimulation (jitteriness, irritability, sleepiness) may be seen in nursing infants. Half-life depends on pH of urine. Brand name: Adderall. (20, 410, 477)
			Cholesterol-lowering agent. Brand name: Lipitor.

Continued

TABLE D-1   Relationship of drugs to breast milk and effect on infant—cont'd

Drugs and ratings*	Oral availability (%)	Peak plasma time (hr)	Plasma protein bound (%)	Volume of distribution (L/kg)
Autonomic and cardiovascular drugs—cont'd				
Atropine AAP 6 H L3 W U	50		14–50	3–3.3
Dobutamine W U				0.2 ± 0.8
Domperidone AAP 6 H L2 W —	12–18	0.5–1	92	5–6
Dopamine H L2 W NS	Low	5 min Oral drug rapidly metabolized in GI tract		
Edrophonium W S				1.1 ± 0.2
Ephedrine W S H L4	85%	2.12 ± 0.75		
Ergonovine H L3 W —	60%	0.5–3		
Ergotamine AAP 5 H L4 W NS?	2–5 Low	0.5–3		1.8
Hyoscyamine AAP — H L3 W S?	Well absorbed		50	

Milk/plasma (M/P) ratio	Adult dose in milk (%)	Maximum amount in milk (mg/L)	Comments and references
		1	Antidysrhythmic/cardiac arrest. Drug is racemic mixture of S (active) and R (inactive) isomers. May inhibit lactation. Brand names: Arco-Lase, Donnatal, Lomotil, Urised. (5, 50, 181, 477)
			Pressor/inotrope. Not effective orally; rapidly metabolized in liver to inactive products. Brand name: Dobutrex. (20, 277)
0.03–0.6	0.05	2.6	Not available in USA per FDA. (20, 277)
			Pressor/inotrope. Not absorbed by infant. Given to pediatric patients. Suggested to inhibit prolactin release. (7, 393, 438)
			Given by injection. Ionized at physiologic pH; not expected to be excreted into milk. Brand names: Enlon-Plus, Tensilon. (67, 181, 393)
	Excreted into human milk		Pressor/inotrope. Case report of mother with a 3-month-old who took a long-acting preparation. Child became irritable and changed sleeping pattern; returned to normal after mother stopped taking the drug. Half-life 3–5 hr. Brand name: Marax. (67)
	Excreted into human milk		Abrupt drop in prolactin levels at 30 min with normal levels returning by 2.5 hr. Brand name: Ergotrate. (498)
	Excreted into human milk		Vomiting, diarrhea, convulsions in infant when mother took drug for migraines. May inhibit lactation. Half-life 21 hr. Caffeine increases absorption and peak plasma concentration by a factor of 2. Brand names: Cafergot, Ergomar, Wigraine. (7, 181, 393, 455, 477)
	Traces found in breast milk		Food does not affect absorption. Brand names: Cystospaz, Urised. (7)

Continued

TABLE D-1   Relationship of drugs to breast milk and effect on infant—cont'd

Drugs and ratings*	Oral availability (%)	Peak plasma time (hr)	Plasma protein bound (%)	Volume of distribution (L/kg)
Autonomic and cardiovascular drugs—cont'd				
Labetalol AAP 6 H L2 W S	10–80	0.33–2	45–55	2–16
Mepenzolate bromide H — W U	Completely ionized in GI tract and not absorbed			
Mepindolol H — W —	82 ± 11		40–60	
Methylergonovine (methylergometrine) L2 (acute) L4 (chronic) W S	60	0.5–3	36	
Neostigmine H — W S	1–20	0.5	15–25	0.7 ± 0.3
Oxprenolol AAP 6 H — W —	24–60 About 90% absorbed	0.75 ± 0.25	80–92	1.1–1.3
Pindolol H — W U	86 ± 21	1.75 ± 0.25	47 ± 7	2.3 ± 0.9
Propantheline bromide H — W U		1		
Propranolol AAP 6 H L2 W S	2–54	2.5 ± 0.5	87 ± 6	2.8–4.9

Milk/plasma (M/P) ratio	Adult dose in milk (%)	Maximum amount in milk (mg/L)	Comments and references
0.4–2.6	0.004–0.07	0.662	Beta blocker. Food increases oral availability. Extensive first-pass metabolism. If mother takes 330–800 mg/day, a mean of 33 ng/mL in milk. Recovered in some infants, not all. Half-life 6–8 hr. In milk: peak 2.7 ± 0.6 hr. Brand names: Normodyne, Trandate. (20, 46, 67, 122, 166, 181, 353, 393, 410, 455)
			Brand name: Cantil. (7, 393)
0.35–0.61	0.1–1.1	0.095	Recovered in 20% of nursing infants whose mothers took the drug. (20, 393, 455)
0.3	4.6		Quickly disappears into the tissues. Half-life 20–30 min. Brand name: Methergine. (20, 455)
Not detected in breast milk			Poorly absorbed from GI tract. Ionized at physiologic pH. Brand name: Prostigmin. (7, 181, 455, 477)
0.14–0.49	0.45–1.5	0.47	(20, 166, 455, 477)
1.6			Beta blocker. Food does not alter oral availability. Brand name: Visken. (166, 181, 258, 393, 407, 436, 455)
			Rapidly metabolized to inactive products. Uncontrolled data: no measurable amounts found in human milk. Activity of long-acting dose not studied. Brand name: Pro-Banthine. (393, 477)
0.05–2	0.05–1	0.16	Beta blocker. 99% absorbed from GI tract. More available if taken with food. In milk: peak 3.5 ± 1.5 hr; 0.4%–6% newborn therapeutic dose; risk of an effect dose almost nonexistent. 5%–10% of Caucasians poor metabolizers. Brand names: Inderal, Inderide. (17, 20, 50, 153, 155, 181, 455)

Continued

TABLE D-1	**Relationship of drugs to breast milk and effect on infant—cont'd**			
Drugs and ratings[*]	Oral availability (%)	Peak plasma time (hr)	Plasma protein bound (%)	Volume of distribution (L/kg)
Autonomic and cardiovascular drugs—cont'd				
Pseudoephedrine AAP 6 H L3 (acute), L4 (chronic) W S	Almost 100% absorbed	1		
Pyridostigmine AAP 6 H L2 W U	19 ± 15			1.1 ± 0.3
Salbutamol W —	See albuterol; it is the same drug with two different names			
Scopolamine AAP 6 H L3 W S?	27 ± 12	0.88 ± 0.13		1.4 ± 0.7
Sumatriptan succinate AAP 6 H L3 W S?	14	12 min (IM)	14–21	1.34–2.34
Terbutaline AAP 6 H L2 W S	12–40 52% absorbed from GI tract	1–4	14–25	1.4 ± 0.4
Terfenadine AAP 6 H — W —				
Timolol AAP 6 H L2 W S?	30–95	1–3	60 ± 3	2.4 ± 1.2
Cardiovascular drugs				
Amiodarone AAP 4 H L5 W NS	3–100 Incomplete absorption	1.5–10	95–99	66 ± 44

Milk/plasma (M/P) ratio	Adult dose in milk (%)	Maximum amount in milk (mg/L)	Comments and references
2–3.9	3.2 ± 2.8	0.33	Report of a 3-month-old with excessive irritability that cleared up when mother stopped taking a decongestant with this and dexbrompheniramine in it. Half-life 4 hr. In milk: peak 1.25 ± 0.25 hr. May decrease milk production (Hale) Brand names: Actifed, Advil, Dristan, etc. (20, 67, 393)
0.22–4	0.05–0.12	0.025	Poor absorption from gut. Half-life 3.3 hr. In milk: peak 3.75 ± 0.25 hr. Drug not detected in nursing infants. Brand names: Mestinon, Regonol. (20, 181, 455)
			Beta agonist.
Excreted into human milk in minute amounts			Half-life 2.9 hr. Brand names: Atrohist, Ballatal, Donnatal. (181)
4.1–5.7	0.21	0.113	An ergotamine derivative. Half-life 1.3 hr. In milk: peak 1.7–3.5 hr. By 8 hours, almost no drug in milk. (110, 393, 538, 553)
1.04–2.9	0.45 ± 0.25	0.005	Beta agonist. Food decreases oral availability. Substantial first-pass metabolism. Half-life 14 hr. In milk: peak 4 hr. Not detected in nursing infant. Brand names: Brethine, Bricanyl, (20, 92, 181, 393, 455)
			The maximum level of infant exposure would not exceed 0.45% of maternal dose. Would not result in infant plasma levels.
0.25–1.73	3.3	0.088	Beta blocker used for hypertension and glaucoma. When used as eyedrop solution, 1.5 hr after dose, M/P ratio is 6.02. Half-life 4 hr. Brand names: Blocadren, Timoptic. (20, 166, 181, 393, 455, 477)
0.4–13	37	16.4	Antidysrhythmic/cardiac arrest. Terminal half-life: 8–120 days. In milk: 8%–50% of newborn dose. Concern: might affect infant's thyroid. Brand name: Cordarone. (20, 67, 160, 180, 181, 393, 394, 455, 468, 513)

Continued

TABLE D-1 **Relationship of drugs to breast milk and effect on infant—cont'd**

Drugs and ratings*	Oral availability (%)	Peak plasma time (hr)	Plasma protein bound (%)	Volume of distribution (L/kg)
Autonomic and cardiovascular drugs—cont'd				
Amlodipine besylate H L3 W U	52–88 Completely absorbed from GI tract	8.9 ± 3.7	95.5–98	21.4 ± 4.4
Amrinone W —	93 ± 12	0.5–2	35–49	1.3 ± 0.3
Aprindine W —	85–95		96	4–16
Atenolol AAP 5 H L3 W NS	56 ± 30	1–4	5–16	0.95 ± 0.15
Benazepril W — H L3 (L4 in neonate)	17	0.5–0.7 in fasting state 2–4 with food	95–97	
Betaxolol H L3 W U	80–90	2–4	45–60	4.9–9.8
Bretylium W U	12–37		0–8	5.9 ± 0.8
Cadralazine W —	80	0.5–1.3	25.9	0.7–1
Captopril AAP 6 H L4 (neonatal), L3 > 1 mo of age W S	63.5 ± 1.5 60–75 orally absorbed	1 ± 0.5	30 ± 6	0.81 ± 0.18
Carteolol HCl H L3 W U	85–90	2 ± 1	20–30	
Cibenzoline (cifenline) W U	83–90	1–3	50–60	4.1–7.3

Milk/plasma (M/P) ratio	Adult dose in milk (%)	Maximum amount in milk (mg/L)	Comments and references
			Calcium-channel blocker. Food does not alter oral availability. Extensively metabolized in the liver. Half-life 30–50 hr. Brand names: Norvasc, Lotrel. (231, 253, 322, 343)
			There are fast and slow acetylators. Brand name: Inocor. (181)
			Dose-dependent half-life. Exhibits debrisoquine polymorphic metabolism. (47, 274, 455, 477)
1.3–6.8	12.45 ± 6.75	1.8	Beta blocker. Half-life 6 hr. In milk: peak 5 ± 3 hr. In serum and urine of some breastfed infants. Serum level 0.1% of mothers. Limited absorption decreased by food. One report of beta blocker effect in infant. Brand names: Tenoretic, Tenormin. (7, 17, 20, 181, 247, 320, 327, 436, 455, 477)
0.01 drug and metabolite	0.04 of drug 0.1 of active metabolite		Antihypertensive/ACE inhibitor. At least 37% of this prodrug is absorbed from GI tract. Brand names: Lotensin, Captropril. (34, 301, 302, 445)
2.5–3.0			Beta blocker. Food does not alter rate or extent of absorption. When used ophthalmically risk of effective intake by breastfed infant extremely low. Half-life 14–22 hr. Brand names: Betoptic, Kerlone. (7, 76, 99, 406, 482)
	Excreted into human milk		Antidysrhythmic. Brand name: Bretylol. (9, 181, 274, 455)
			Slow and fast acetylators. Has active metabolite. (72, 282, 318)
0.006–0.6	0.002–0.014	0.008	ACE inhibitor. Food decreases absorption by 30%–40%. Half-life 2.2 hr. In milk: peak 3.8 ± 0.6 hr; 0.1% of newborn dose. Brand names: Capoten, Capozide. (20, 165, 181, 362, 393, 455, 477, 526)
	Excreted into rat milk		Beta blocker. Food in GI tract slows absorption but does not affect extent. Brand name: Cartrol. (166, 393)
			(204, 274, 306, 323, 352)

Continued

TABLE D-1   Relationship of drugs to breast milk and effect on infant—cont'd

Drugs and ratings*	Oral availability (%)	Peak plasma time (hr)	Plasma protein bound (%)	Volume of distribution (L/kg)
Autonomic and cardiovascular drugs—cont'd				
Clofibrate W U	95 ± 10	4–6	95–98 Lower when plasma concentration is >200 mg/L	0.11 ± 0.02
Clonidine H L3 W NS?	87 ± 12 Available in transdermal patches	3–5	20	3.32 ± 1.5
Deserpidine W —				
Diazoxide W U	86–96		94 ± 14 Can be saturated	0.21 ± 0.02
Digitoxin AAP 6 W U	84–93		90–97	0.54 ± 0.14
Digoxin AAP 6 H L2 W S	40–100	1.5–3	20–40	5.17–7.35
Dilevalol W —	10–33	0.85 ± 0.15	68–77	17–25
Diltiazem AAP 6 W S?	24–90 80%-90% absorbed orally	2–4	70–86	3–8
Diprafenone W —	50-mg dose 11 ± 1 150-mg dose 33 ± 26	1.35 ± 0.15	98.45 ± 0.55	1.23 ± 0.28
Dipyridamole H L3 W S?	52 ± 23		95–99	

Milk/plasma (M/P) ratio	Adult dose in milk (%)	Maximum amount in milk (mg/L)	Comments and references
	Excreted into animal milk		Data are for active metabolite. Drug used in neonates to treat jaundice. Brand name: Atromid-S. (7, 171, 181, 393, 477)
1.5–4.0	7.9 ± 0.1	0.002	Antiadrenergic agent. In milk: up to 10% of newborn therapeutic dose. Hypotension not observed in nursing infants; drug found in their serum at mean levels less than in mother's serum. Half-life 20–24 hr. ?↓ milk production. Brand names: Catapres, Combipres, Duraclon. (20, 67, 148, 181, 205, 393, 455, 477)
	Excreted into human milk		Antihypertensive. Predicted that may cause prolactin increases. Brand names: Enduronyl, Harmonyl, Oreticyl. (393)
			Antihypertensive. Brand names: Hyperstat, Proglycem. (181, 393, 477)
			Active metabolite: digoxin. Brand name: Crystodigin. (181, 327, 455)
0.45–1.0	0.07–14	0.0019	Antidysrhythmic. In milk: 0.06%–0.3% newborn therapeutic dose, peak 4–6 hr. Half-life 39 hr. Not detected in nursing infant's plasma. Brand name: Lanoxin. (19, 20, 46, 50, 239, 327, 410, 453)
0.31–0.46		0.149	Optical isomer of labetalol. Absorption through GI tract 100% with dose-dependent hepatic metabolism. In milk: peak 1 hr. (122, 166, 167, 168)
0.98–1.0	0.9	0.22	Calcium-channel blockers. Drug undergoes hepatic metabolism. In milk: peak 2.5 ± 0.5 hr. Brand names: Cardizem, Dilacor, Tiazac. (7, 20, 77, 181, 327, 393, 410, 413, 455, 499)
			First-pass metabolism can be saturated, so oral availability is dose dependent. (510)
	Amount in human milk too low to measure		Vasodilator, antiplatelet. Brand name: Persantine. (67, 307, 455)

Continued

TABLE D-1   **Relationship of drugs to breast milk and effect on infant—cont'd**

Drugs and ratings*	Oral availability (%)	Peak plasma time (hr)	Plasma protein bound (%)	Volume of distribution (L/kg)
Autonomic and cardiovascular drugs—cont'd				
Disopyramide AAP 6 H L2 W S?	83 ± 11	0.5–3	35–95	0.59 ± 0.15
Doxazosin W U H L4	65 ± 14	3 ± 2.1	98–99	0.97
Enalapril AAP 6 H L2 W S?	41 ± 15 53%–74% of dose absorbed	0.5–1.5	<50	1.7 ± 0.7
Enalaprilat W —	5%–12% orally absorbed	2–5	5	
Encainide W U H L3	30 ± 19	1.1 ± 0.6	70 ± 6	3.6 ± 1
Enoximone W —	53–60	0.75–6	1–15	9.23 ± 6.81
Esmolol H L3 W —		15 min	55	1.9 ± 1.3
Felodipine H L3 W U	4.4–36	0.34–3	99.64 ± 0.08	9.7 ± 4
Flecainide AAP 6 H L4 W S	50–95	0.5–6	32–60	5–13.4

Milk/plasma (M/P) ratio	Adult dose in milk (%)	Maximum amount in milk (mg/L)	Comments and references
0.4–1.07	6.8 ± 0.2	4.4	Antiarrhythmic. Active metabolite, *N*-monodesalkyl disopyramide: M/P ratio 2.7–8.5, maternal plasma level 10% that of drug. Half-life 8–12 hr. Drug found in blood of some nursing infants. Both drug and metabolite found in the infant's urine. Amount protein bound in milk and plasma is concentration dependent. Brand name: Norpace. (17, 20, 67, 181, 220, 248, 327, 393, 406, 408, 455)
			Antiadrenergic. Completely absorbed with first-pass metabolism. Half-life 9–22 hr. Significant accumulation during chronic administration. Brand name: Cardura. (121, 250, 372, 406)
0.14–0.78		0.002 Not found in all milk samples	ACE inhibitor. Food does not influence absorption. A prodrug for enalaprilat (see below). Half-life 35 hr. Brand names: Vasotec, Vaseretic. (67, 165, 181, 230, 303, 393, 455)
0.02–0.11		0.00172	Active metabolite of enalapril. (67, 302, 393)
1		0.4	Antiarrhythmic. Tabular data for the 93% of U.S. population who are fast metabolizers. Slow metabolizers: oral availability 83% ± 19%, plasma level 20 times that of fast metabolizers. Metabolites formed are more active than the drug. Half-life 2–36 hr. Maximum amount of one of the metabolites (ODE) in milk is 0.2 mg/L. Brand name: Enkaid. (67, 323, 416, 417, 477, 539)
			Rapidly absorbed orally with significant first-pass metabolism. Food increases absorption, with peak being achieved earlier. (462, 465, 524)
			Beta blocker. Half-life approximately 9 min. Available IV. Brand name: Brevibloc. (247, 393)
			Calcium-channel blocker. Complete absorption; first-pass metabolism. Half-life 11–16 hr. Flavonoids in grapefruit juice inhibit its oxidation; oral availability when taken with grapefruit juice instead of water or orange juice: 164%–469%. Brand name: Plendil. (25, 126, 130)
0.8–4.6		1.68	Antiarrhythmic. Half-life 7–22 hr. In milk: peak 3–6 hr. Exhibits debrisoquine polymorphic metabolism. Brand name: Tambocor. (7, 248, 317, 393, 477, 558)

Continued

TABLE D-1 Relationship of drugs to breast milk and effect on infant—cont'd

Drugs and ratings*	Oral availability (%)	Peak plasma time (hr)	Plasma protein bound (%)	Volume of distribution (L/kg)
Autonomic and cardiovascular drugs—cont'd				
Fosinopril L4 (neonatal), L3 > 1 mo W U	29–36	3	95	
Guanabenz W U	70–80 absorbed with extensive hepatic metabolism	2–5	90	93–191
Guanethidine W U	Individual variation in absorption and metabolism			
Hydralazine AAP 6 H L2 W S	26–55	0.5–2	85–89	5.45 ± 5.15
Ketanserin W —	50	0.5–2	95.1 ± 0.36	3.3–6.2
Lorcainide W —	1–65	1–2	85 ± 5	11.79 ± 7.15
Losartan H L4 (neonatal), L3 W —	25–35	About 1	98.7	
Methyldopa AAP 6 H L2 W S	8–62 Due to absorption parameters	1–4	1–16	0.28–1.4
Metoprolol AAP 6 H L3 W S	42.5 ± 18.5	0.5–2	8–12	4.55 ± 1.05
Mexiletine AAP 6 H L2 W S	87 ± 13	2–4	50–75	4.9–9.5

Milk/plasma (M/P) ratio	Adult dose in milk (%)	Maximum amount in milk (mg/L)	Comments and references
Excreted into human milk			ACE inhibitor. Almost completely hydrolyzed to active metabolite whose oral availability is 25%-29%. Brand name: Monopril. (101, 225, 228, 229, 345)
			Antiadrenergic. Prolactin level in serum not affected. Brand name: Wytensin. (7, 477)
Not in significant therapeutic doses in human milk			Antiadrenergic. Brand names: Esimil, Ismelin. (393, 477)
0.49–1.4	0.8	0.76	Antihypertensive. In milk: 0.3%–3% of newborn therapeutic dose, peak 2 hr. Half-life 1.5–8 hr. Oral availability higher in slow acetylators. First-pass metabolism may be saturated in rapid acetylators. Brand names: Apresazide, Apresoline, Ser-Ap-Es. (20, 67, 181, 455, 477)
			Absorption not affected by food in GI tract. (390, 477)
			Saturable first-pass metabolism gives dose-dependent oral availability: 100 mg 1%–4%; 200 mg 35%–65%. (181, 469, 477)
Both drug and potent metabolite appear in rat milk at a significant level			ACE-like antihypertensive. Half-life 4–9 hr. Brand name: Cozaar. (341)
0.19–0.34	0.02–0.09	1.36	Antihypertensive, Half-life 1½ hr. In milk: peak 3–6 hr, 0.04%–2.7% of newborn dose. With maternal dose of 750–2000 mg/day, 0.1–0.9 mg/mL excreted into milk. Found in plasma in 1 of 3 infants. Recovered from infant's urine. Brand names: Aldoclor, Aldomet, Aldoril. (20, 181, 393, 410, 477)
2–4.8	1.7–5	0.225	Beta blocker. Near complete absorption with first-pass metabolism: metabolites active. Food increases oral availability. Shows debrisoquine-type polymorphism. Increased half-life in neonate. Half-life 3–7 hr. In milk: peak 4 ± 2 hr. Brand name: Toprol. (149, 240, 259)
0.78–2	0.6–2.8	0.959	Antiarrhythmic. 10% of Caucasians lack enzyme to metabolize drug. Food delays absorption, lowers peak level. In milk: 0.6%–2.4% newborn dose. Half-life 9.2 hr. Brand name: Mexitil. (20, 180, 327, 393, 411, 512)

Continued

TABLE D-1   Relationship of drugs to breast milk and effect on infant—cont'd

Drugs and ratings[*]	Oral availability (%)	Peak plasma time (hr)	Plasma protein bound (%)	Volume of distribution (L/kg)
Autonomic and cardiovascular drugs—cont'd				
Minoxidil AAP 6 H L3 W U	90	Within 1	0	2.7 ± 0.7
Moricizine W —	30–40	0.5–3	88 ± 7	11.6 ± 6.71
Nadolol AAP 6 H L4 W S?	34 ± 5	2–4	16–30	2.1 ± 1
Nicardipine W U	8.7–45	0.5–2.25	89–99.5	1.13 ± 0.51
Nifedipine AAP 6 H L2 W S?	31–92	45 min	90–98	1.45 ± 0.75
Nimodipine AAP — H L2 W S?	10–20	0.5–1.5	98	0.94–2.3
Nitrendipine AAP — H L2 W —	5–30 Increased when taken with grapefruit juice	0.33–3	98	2.3–9.5
Nitroglycerin AAP — H L4 W U	<1			3.3 ± 1.2
Penbutolol AAP — H — W U	92.5 ± 2.5	2–3	89 ± 9	

Milk/plasma (M/P) ratio	Adult dose in milk (%)	Maximum amount in milk (mg/L)	Comments and references
0.67–1.13	2.5	0.042	Vasodilator/antihypertensive. Half-life 3.5 hr. In milk: peak 1 hr. Brand name: Loniten. (19, 20, 181, 393, 410, 477)
			Antidysrhythmic. Some active metabolites. Well absorbed with extensive first-pass metabolism. Brand name: Ethmozine. (1, 150, 223, 453)
2–8	4.5 ± 2.5	0.44	Beta blocker. In milk: 2%–7% of newborn dose, peak 6 hr. Half-life 20 hr. Brand names: Corgard, Corzide. (19, 20, 67, 181, 247, 327, 393, 410, 436)
Excreted into rat milk			Calcium-channel blocker. 90%–100% absorbed; extensive first-pass metabolism. Food in GI tract lowers availability, delays plasma peak. Brand name: Cardene. (165, 193, 328, 393, 455)
1	0.00163 ± 0.00125	0.053	Calcium-channel blocker. In milk: less than 5% of effective dose, peak 0.75 ± 0.25 hr. In rapid absorber, drug peak 0.5 hr; in slow absorber, peak 4 hr. Half-life 2–7 hr. Total amount absorbed is the same. Oral availability when taken with grapefruit juice. 108%–169% of oral availability when taken with water. Brand names: Adalat, Procardia. (43, 67, 118, 136, 181, 200, 377, 387, 393, 440, 455)
~1	0.008–0.3	0.0047	Calcium-channel blocker. Half-life 9 hr. Complete absorption with first-pass metabolism. Brand name: Nimotop. (7, 200, 253, 393, 496, 507)
0.5–1.4	0.095	0.007	Calcium-channel blocker. Half-life 8–11 hr. In milk: peak 2.5 ± 1.5 hr. (26, 200, 471, 472, 541)
			Vasodilator. Little found in milk. Half-life in maternal plasma: 1–4 min. (67, 506)
			Brand name: Levatol. (99, 166, 393, 455, 477)

Continued

TABLE D-1   Relationship of drugs to breast milk and effect on infant—cont'd

Drugs and ratings*	Oral availability (%)	Peak plasma time (hr)	Plasma protein bound (%)	Volume of distribution (L/kg)
Autonomic and cardiovascular drugs—cont'd				
Pentoxifylline AAP — H L2 W NS?	19 ± 13 Nearly completely absorbed from the GI tract	1 ± 0.6	0	2.4 ± 1.2
Perindopril AAP — H — 　W U	66–95 Food decreases it by 35%	0.6–1.2	60	0.22
Pinacidil AAP — H — W —	57.1 ± 13.7	1 and 4–6	39–65	1.25 ± 0.25
Pindolol AAP — H — W U	86 ± 21	1.75 ± 0.25	47 ± 7	2.3 ± 0.9
Pirmenol AAP — H — W —	83 ± 24	1–2	83–90	1.93 ± 1.17
Prazosin AAP — H L4 W S	43–82	1–3	94 ± 3.1	0.6 ± 0.13
Procainamide AAP 6 H L3 W S	83 ± 16	0.66–2	16 ± 5	1.9 ± 0.3
Propafenone AAP — H L2 W U	5–15	1–5.68	77–97	3 ± 1.4

Milk/plasma (M/P) ratio	Adult dose in milk (%)	Maximum amount in milk (mg/L)	Comments and references
0.25–1.49	0.17	0.074	In milk: peak 2 hr. Metabolites I, IV, V appear in milk. M/P ratio: I, 0.53–0.99; IV, 0.27–0.81; V, 0.64–1.62. Half-life 0.4–1.6 hr. Drug and metabolites stable in breast milk frozen for 3 weeks. Viscosity. Brand name: Trental. (20, 67, 181)
	<0.02		ACE inhibitor. Drug has weak activity; metabolite, perindoprilat, potent. Metabolite: poorly absorbed from GI tract; plasma peak 3–4 hr; plasma protein bound 10%–20%; volume of distribution 0.16 L/kg. In plasma, 19% ± 7% of drug is metabolite. Brand name: Aceon. (405, 503)
			Available in a control-release tablet. (163)
1.6			Beta blocker. Bioavailability not altered if taken with food. Brand name: Visken. (166, 181, 258, 393, 407, 436, 455)
			(176, 323, 352)
		0.018	Antihypertensive. Bioavailability unchanged if taken with food. Extensive first-pass metabolism. Half-life 2–3 hr. In milk: 1%–4% of newborn therapeutic dose. Brand name: Minizide. (7, 181, 258, 393, 520)
1–7.3	1.5 ± 0.5	10.2	Antiarrhythmic. Rapid acetylators make *N*-acetylprocainamide. M/P ratio 1:6.2. Half-life (3 hr) of drug and metabolite 3–4 times longer in infant than adult. In milk: 2.2% of newborn therapeutic dose. Brand name: Procanbid. (181, 327, 406, 408, 410, 477)
	0.03	0.032	Antiarrhythmic. Bioavailability increased greatly by food. Over 95% absorbed. Half-life 2–10 hr. Good and poor metabolizers. In milk: 47 ng/mL of active metabolite. Brand name: Rythmol. (170, 198, 211, 293, 323, 352, 353, 393, 437, 455)

Continued

TABLE D-1   Relationship of drugs to breast milk and effect on infant—cont'd

Drugs and ratings*	Oral availability (%)	Peak plasma time (hr)	Plasma protein bound (%)	Volume of distribution (L/kg)
Autonomic and cardiovascular drugs—cont'd				
Quinidine AAP 6 H L2 W U			72.5 ± 22.5	2.7 ± 1.2
Recainam AAP — H — W —	39–106	1.2–5.4		1.4 ± 0.4
Sotalol AAP 6 H L3 W U	77.5 ± 17.5	2–4	0	1.3–2.4
Terazosin H L4 W U	82–90	1.3 ± 0.9	90–94	0.8 ± 0.18
Tocainide AAP — H — W U	89 ± 5	0.5–2	2–22	1.6–3.8
Urapidil AAP — H — W —	78 ± 6	0.75 ± 0.25	76–80	0.87 ± 0.29
Verapamil AAP 6 H L2 W S	10–27 Oral absorption >90%	0.5–2	84–91.3	4.7 ± 2.5
Dermatologic preparations				
Acitretin AAP 6 H —	36–95 Food increases availability	0.9–4.6	Extensive	
Calcipotriene AAP — H — W —		Same as calcipotriol (see below)		

Milk/plasma (M/P) ratio	Adult dose in milk (%)	Maximum amount in milk (mg/L)	Comments and references
0.71–0.91	4.1	8.2	Antiarrhythmic. In milk: 3.5%–10% of newborn therapeutic dose. Half-life 6–8 hr. Sulfate peaks in plasma at 1–1.5 hr, with oral availability of 80% ± 15%. Gluconate peaks at 3–4 hr, with oral availability of 71% ± 17%. May suppress prolactin secretion. Brand names: Quinaglute, Quinidex. (20, 115, 145, 181, 327, 383, 536, 558)
			(274, 511)
2.2–8.8	20–30	20.2	Beta blocker. Half-life 12 hr. Food alters availability. Brand name: Betapace. (99, 152, 197, 274, 366, 430, 477)
			Antihypertenive. Plasma peak when taken with food: 2.2 ± 1.1 hr. Total amount absorbed is unaffected. Half-life 9–12 hr. Brand name: Hytrin. (181, 316, 393, 470)
2.143–3.043			Food delays absorption and decreases peak values. Brand name: Tonocard. (7, 181, 352, 411, 455, 477, 549)
			100% absorbed orally. (59, 258, 401, 487)
0.23–0.94	0.01–0.835	0.026	Calcium-channel blocker. In milk: peak 1.25 ± 0.25 hr, not detected 38 hr after treatment stopped. Half-life 3–7 hr. Active metabolite: norverapamil. Brand names: Calan, Isoptin, Verelan. (7, 8, 20, 181, 203, 238, 274, 323, 329, 393, 434, 477)
0.093–0.18			Steady state milk level: 30–40 ng/mL. (272, 419)
			(342)

Continued

TABLE D-1 Relationship of drugs to breast milk and effect on infant—cont'd

Drugs and ratings[*]	Oral availability (%)	Peak plasma time (hr)	Plasma protein bound (%)	Volume of distribution (L/kg)
Dermatologic preparations—cont'd				
Calcipotriol AAP — H — W —	Less than 1% systemically absorbed; rapidly metabolized to inactive products			
Etretinate AAP — H L5 W —	50	2–6	98–>99	2
Isotretinoin AAP — H L5 W NS		3.2	99.9	7
Tretinoin AAP — H L3 W U	Minimal absorption occurs after topical application			
Diagnostic materials and procedures; radioactive isotopes[†]				
Copper 64 AAP 3 H L4 W —	12.7			2
Diatrizoate meglumine AAP 6 H — W u	Poorly absorbed from GI tract		<5	
Fluorescein AAP 6 H L3 W —	99			
Gadopentetic acid, Gadopentetate dimeglumine AAP 6 H L2	0.80	Immediate		
Gallium 67 AAP 3 H L4 W —				

[†]**Radioactive isotopes**: Nursing should be discontinued until radioactivity is no longer excreted into the milk. Have milk tested if possible. Times to stop breastfeeding are advisory.

Milk/plasma (M/P) ratio	Adult dose in milk (%)	Maximum amount in milk (mg/L)	Comments and references
		(342)	
Excreted into human milk			Stored in adipose tissue; absorption enhanced by milk or fatty foods. Brand name: Tegison. (67, 181, 272, 393, 477)
Concentrated in milk			Brand name: Accutane. Vitamin A derivative for acne contraindicated in pregnancy. (181, 273, 393)
			Vitamin A derivative applied to skin. May be taken orally. 70% absorbed. Brand name: Retin. (67)
			Half-life 12.7 hr. Clearance 64 hr. Radioactive isotope.
Not found in human breast milk			Used on newborn eyes. Brand names: Gastrogralin. Renovist, Hypaque, Angiovist. (7)
0.5		8.826	In milk: peak 6 hr; half-life 62 hr. Decrease in neonatal renal clearance along with accumulation in milk may present toxic problems for infant. (312, 455)
			Gadolinium. Radiocontrast agent (MRI). Does not enter milk. Brand name: Magnevist Galodiamide (Omniscan).
Excreted into human milk			Discontinuing nursing for 72 hr usually sufficient. Half-life 78.3 hr. (425)

Continued

TABLE D-1 Relationship of drugs to breast milk and effect on infant—cont'd

Drugs and ratings[*]	Oral availability (%)	Peak plasma time (hr)	Plasma protein bound (%)	Volume of distribution (L/kg)
Diagnostic materials and procedures; radioactive isotopes—cont'd				
Indium 111 AAP 3 H L4 W —	2.8 days	Immediate (IV)		
Iodine is concentrated in human milk. Always potential for interference with normal thyroid function.				
Iodine 123 AAP 3 H — W —				
Iodine 123 hippuran AAP 3 H — W —			5 ± 1.9	
Iodine 125 AAP 3 H — W —				
Iodine 131 AAP 3 H — W —				
Iodine 131 hippuran AAP — H — W —				
Iodine 131 macroaggregate AAP — H — W —				
Iohexol AAP 6 H L2 W —	4 ± 2		<5	0.35–0.83
Ipanoic acid AAP 6 H L2 W —				

Milk/plasma (M/P) ratio	Adult dose in milk (%)	Maximum amount in milk (mg/L)	Comments and references
			Radioactive isotope. Small amount left at 20 hr.
	<10		May contain up to 4.6% of ^{124}I, whose physical half-life is 4.2 days with a half-life in milk of 3.5 days. See References for debate on how long to stop nursing, or have milk tested. (128, 208)
	1.2–3.5		In milk: half-life 3.5 hr. Effective secretion half-life is 2.2–5.8 hr. Breast should be pumped for 24 hr. (338, 421)
	Excreted into human milk		Radioactivity may be found in milk for 2 weeks. Some say stop breastfeeding for 3–4 weeks. Have milk tested for isotope. (312)
40–65	2–46		In milk: half-life 4 ± 1.8 hr; peak 6 hr; excreted for 2–14 days. Suggestions: (1) give infant 60–100 mg KI, nurse, give mother isotope, discard next three pumpings of milk; (2) discard milk for 8 days; (3) if test dose used, discard milk for 36 hr; if diagnostic dose used, discard milk for 2 weeks. (128, 329, 424)
	1.8–4.9		In milk: peak first day at an average of 0.37 nCi/mL. Discontinue breastfeeding for 24 hr. (421)
	Excreted into human milk		4.2–2.8 nCi/mL peaking in milk probably at 24 hr after dose. Half-life in milk: 20 hr. Discontinue breastfeeding for 10–12 days.
	0.5		Radiopaque. In milk: 0.2% of pediatric dose, half-life 33.5 ± 18.5 hr. Brand name: Omnipaque. (355, 393)
	0.08	29.9	Radiopaque. In milk: peak 5–19 hr; compound is inert. Brand name: Telepaque. (67)

Continued

TABLE D-1   Relationship of drugs to breast milk and effect on infant—cont'd

Drugs and ratings*	Oral availability (%)	Peak plasma time (hr)	Plasma protein bound (%)	Volume of distribution (L/kg)
Diagnostic materials and procedures; radioactive isotopes—cont'd				
Iothalamate AAP — H — W —				
Metrizamide AAP 6 H L2 W —		0–7	0	
Metrizoate AAP 6 H L2 W —	Nil	< 2	<5	
Radioactive sodium AAP 3 H L5				
Technetium 99m Tc AAP 3 H L4				
Technetium 99m MMA AAP — H — W S?			22	
Technetium pertechnetate AAP — H — W —				
Technetium 99m plasmin AAP — H L4 W —	100			
Technetium 99m RBC AAP — H — W —				

Milk/plasma (M/P) ratio	Adult dose in milk (%)	Maximum amount in milk (mg/L)	Comments and references
Contains iodine, which appears in human milk			Used in organ-specific tests. May cause transient metabolic taste in milk.
	0.02	214	In milk: 0.02% of dose recovered in 44.3 hr. If given to mother IV, 94% excreted in her urine in 24 hr. (7, 67, 393, 554)
	<0.2		Radiocontrast agent. Not absorbed from milk. Minimal in milk. Brand name: Isopaque.
Can be detected in milk after 96 hr			In milk: 0.5%–1.3% of dose/L, peak 2 hr. (329)
3–5.2			In milk: half-life 35 ± 0.5 hr; amount and its kinetics depend on what molecule carries the label. (208)
	0.2–5.4		In milk: half-life 4.6 hr; peak 4 hr; maximum amount found 150 nCi/mL. If infant nursed just before dose, 4 hr later the milk will contain 60% of total activity. Suggestions: (1) feed just before dose, discard the next three fractions, (2) stop breastfeeding for 24 hr. (338, 421)
	0.07%–33% of the radioactivity found in milk		In milk: from mother who got 10 mCi: 6.5% after 24 hr, 0.177% after 46 hr, none after 70 hr. (337, 426)
	1.75 ± 0.25		Half-life <6 hr. Clearance in mother <30 hr.
	0.006–1		Binding to maternal RBC very stable. 0.000005 of ingested activity excreted into breast milk. (421)

Continued

TABLE D-1   Relationship of drugs to breast milk and effect on infant—cont'd

Drugs and ratings*	Oral availability (%)	Peak plasma time (hr)	Plasma protein bound (%)	Volume of distribution (L/kg)
Diagnostic materials and procedures; radioactive isotopes—cont'd				
Thallium 201 H L4 W —				
Tuberculin test AAP — H L2 W —	OK to do when mother is lactating			
X-rays	No effect on breastfeeding and lactation			
Diuretics				
Amiloride AAP — H — W U	54 ± 7	3–4	40	17 ± 4
Bendroflumethiazide AAP 6 H L4 W S		2.3	94	1.18 ± 0.31
Bumetanide H L3 W U	66 ± 11	0.5–2	94–97	0.19 ± 0.09
Canrenone AAP — H — W —		2–4	94 ± 4	
Chlorothiazide AAP 6 H L3 W S	9–56		94.6 ± 1.3	0.2 ± 0.08
Chlorthalidone AAP 6 H L3 W S?	64 ± 10		75 ± 1	3.9 ± 0.8
Dyphylline AAP 6 H L3 W —		0.75		

Milk/plasma (M/P) ratio	Adult dose in milk (%)	Maximum amount in milk (mg/L)	Comments and references
Concentrated in human milk			In milk: effective half-life has two components: 1.13 and 15.1 days. Infant gets radiation by being held by mother. (347)
			Tuberculin-sensitive mothers can immunize their infants through breast milk. Immunity may last several years.
Excreted into animal milk			May suppress lactation.
			Food interferes with oral absorption. Brand names: Midamor, Moduretic. (7, 181, 393, 477)
Excreted into human milk			Used to suppress lactation. Brand name: Corzide. (39, 477)
			Brand name: Bumex. (50, 164, 181, 393, 453, 477)
0.51–0.72	0.2	0.2	Active metabolite of spironolactone and potassium canrenoate. (67, 393)
0.05–0.25		1	Absorption from GI tract incomplete, dose dependent, and saturable. In milk: peak 7.5 ± 2.5 hr, 0.4%–1% of new-born therapeutic dose. Brand names: Aldoclor, Diupres, Diuril. (7, 67, 181, 477)
0.03–0.05	6.7	36	Drug sequestered in RBC. In milk: excreted slowly, 0.75%–7.5% of newborn therapeutic dose. Term baby might get 180 µg/day. Brand names: Combipres, Tenoretic, Thalitone. (6, 20, 181, 477)
2			Brand names: Dylline, Lufyllin. (393)

Continued

TABLE D-1   Relationship of drugs to breast milk and effect on infant—cont'd

Drugs and ratings*	Oral availability (%)	Peak plasma time (hr)	Plasma protein bound (%)	Volume of distribution (L/kg)
Diuretics—cont'd				
Ethacrynic acid AAP — H L3 W U	Well absorbed from GI tract		Largely bound to plasma proteins	
Furosemide AAP — H L3 W S?	11–90	1–5	91–99	0.07–0.35
Hydrochlorothiazide AAP 6 H L2 W S	72 ± 17	1.5–5	58 ± 17	1.53–4.19
Hydroflumethiazide AAP — H — W —	50		95	
Spironolactone AAP 6 H L2 W S	25 ± 9		94 ± 4	
Torsemide (Torasemide) AAP — H L3 W U	76–92	1	97–99	0.09–0.31
Triamterene AAP — H L3 W U	52 ± 18	3	61 ± 2	13.4 ± 4.9
Environmental agents				
Cadmium AAP 7 H — W —				

Milk/plasma (M/P) ratio	Adult dose in milk (%)	Maximum amount in milk (mg/L)	Comments and references
			Brand name: Edecrin. (393, 477)
	Excreted into some human milk		Food delays absorption. In milk: not found in all samples. Given to neonates. Brand name: Lasix. (41, 50, 67, 164, 181, 393, 477)
0.25–0.43		0.43	In milk: average amount 80 ng/mL, <0.02%–4% of newborn therapeutic dose, peak 7.5 ± 2.5 hr. Food in GI tract increases absorption. No drug found in infant (<1 ng/mL) when mother took 50 mg. Brand names: Aldactazide, Aldoril, Apresazide, Capozide, Esimil, HydroDIURIL, Inderide, Lopressor, Maxzide, etc. (67, 90, 181, 455, 477)
	Excreted into human milk		Brand name: Diucardin. (393, 455, 477)
		0.104	80% of drug converted to canrenone. In milk: 0.3%–6% of newborn therapeutic dose. Oral availability of film-coated tablets 25%–30% higher than uncoated ones. Brand names: Aldactazide, Aldactone. (20, 41, 67, 393, 455, 565)
			(164, 455, 476)
	Excreted into animal milk		(181, 393, 455, 477)
0.1		0.786	About 10 times more absorbed through GI tract by neonate than by adult. Smokers have 2–3 times more in their milk than nonsmokers. Exposure of infants of smoking or nonsmoking mothers is far below that of formula fed infants. (395, 403, 457)

Continued

TABLE D-1   Relationship of drugs to breast milk and effect on infant—cont'd

Drugs and ratings*	Oral availability (%)	Peak plasma time (hr)	Plasma protein bound (%)	Volume of distribution (L/kg)
Environmental agents—cont'd				
Carbon disulfide				
AAP —				
H —				
W —				
Chlordane				
AAP 7				
H —				
W —				
DDE (Dichlorodiphenyl chloroethane)				
AAP —				
H —				
W —				
DDT (Dichlorodiphenyl trichloroethane)				
AAP 7				
H —				
W —				
Dieldrin				
AAP 7				
H —				
W —				
Heptachlor				
AAP —				
H —				
W —				
Heptachlorepoxide				
AAP 7				
W —				
Hexachlorobenzene				
AAP 7				
H —				
W —				
Methylmercury				
AAP —				
H —				
W —				

Milk/plasma (M/P) ratio	Adult dose in milk (%)	Maximum amount in milk (mg/L)	Comments and references
1		0.306	Neurovascular and cardiovascular volatile solvent toxin that can be found on the hands and clothes of mother. (395)
	Range in human milk is 0–66 ng/g, mean 6 ng/g		Metabolized to oxychlordane. In milk: peak 1–7 weeks after exposure.
6–7			A stable metabolite of DDT. In colostrum: 0.168–3.175 mg/kg. In mature milk: 0.011–2.86 mg/kg. (243, 385, 395, 418)
6–7		0.83	In milk: in general population, 20–830 µg/L, mean 100 µg/L or 4 mg/kg. Maximum daily intake of infant: 33.78 µg/kg of body weight. No need to test milk unless inordinate exposure. (235, 236, 313, 418, 509)
6		0.007	Found in permanently mothproofed garments. In milk: in general population, 2–7 µg/L or 0.05 mg/kg. Still found in milk in usual quantities months after spraying. (313, 509)
	Range in human milk is 0–13 ng/g, mean 1 ng/g		In milk: peak 1 day after spraying. The 1970 FOA/WHO level for amount allowed in cow milk is 5 times higher than the mean level in human milk reported by Matuo of 0.001 mg/kg. (313, 509)
		0.07	Amount generally found in human milk is 2–9 µg/L. In milk: peak 4–5 weeks after spraying. (509)
	Excreted into human milk		Allowed in cow milk at 0.02 ppm. Significant amount found in milk of Turkish women 25 years after massive contamination of grain seeds. Symptoms in nursing infants: skin rash, diarrhea, vomiting, dark urine, neurotoxicity, and death. (6, 385, 509)
0.086–0.9			In milk: half-life 70 days. (329)

Continued

TABLE D-1 Relationship of drugs to breast milk and effect on infant—cont'd

Drugs and ratings*	Oral availability (%)	Peak plasma time (hr)	Plasma protein bound (%)	Volume of distribution (L/kg)
Environmental agents—cont'd				
Polybrominated biphenyl AAP 7 H — W —				
Polychlorinated biphenyl AAP 7 H — W —				
Tetrachloroethylene AAP 7 H — W —				
Gastrointestinal agents				
Bisacodyl AAP — H L2 W —	Not absorbed from the GI tract			
Casanthranol AAP — H — W S				
Cascara sagrada AAP 6 H L3 W —				
Cimetidine AAP 6 H L2 W S	58–89	0.75–1.5	19 ± 6	2.85 ± 1.45
Cisapride AAP 6 H L2 W S?	40–50	1–2	98	2.4
Danthron AAP 6 H — W —				

Milk/plasma (M/P) ratio	Adult dose in milk (%)	Maximum amount in milk (mg/L)	Comments and references
3–131.7		0.036	Concentrated in fat. The more in mother's milk, the greater the amount in the child's adipose tissue. If mother at risk, milk should be tested. (395)
4–10		4.091	Concentrated in fat. The more in mother's milk, the greater the amount in the child's adipose tissue. If mother at risk, milk should be tested. (124, 395, 509)
3.3		0.01	1 hour after exposure at a cleaning plant, mother had 10 ppm in milk, child developed severe jaundice. Detectable in milk for 2 weeks. (395, 554)
			Brand name: Dulcolax. (9)
Low amount found in human milk; can cause colic and diarrhea in infant			Brand name: Peri-Colace. (67)
High			May increase bowel activity in infant. Brand name: Milk of Magnesia. (393)
1.6–12	5.2 ± 0.2	6	In milk: 2%–2.5% of newborn therapeutic dose. Has produced galactorrhea. Theoretically may suppress infant's gastric activity, inhibit drug metabolism, and produce CNS stimulation. These effects not reported. Time taking drug and nursing. Brand name: Tagamet. (20, 85, 137, 277, 294)
0.05–0.063	0.1		Food slightly enhances absorption. Nursing infant gets 600–800 times lower dose through milk than the normal therapeutic dose for infants. Brand name: Propulsid. (215, 277)
Excreted into human milk			Absorbed to a limited extent. May increase bowel activity in infant.

Continued

TABLE D-1	Relationship of drugs to breast milk and effect on infant—cont'd			

Drugs and ratings*	Oral availability (%)	Peak plasma time (hr)	Plasma protein bound (%)	Volume of distribution (L/kg)
Gastrointestinal agents—cont'd				
Diphenoxylate HCl AAP — H L3 W —		2–3		4.6
Esomeprazole magnesium AAP — H — W —	90 with repeated daily dose	1.5	> 97	~16
Famotidine AAP — H L2 W U	45 ± 14	1–4	17 ± 7	0.94–1.42
Lansoprazole AAP — H L3 W S?	>85 Absolute bioavailability	1.48 ± 0.99		
Loperamide AAP 6 H L2 W S	40	2.5–5	97	
Metformin AAP — H L3 W S	50	2.75	Minimal	3.7
Metoclopramide AAP 4 H L2 W S	32–97	1.6–3	13–44	3.4 ± 1.3
Nizatidine AAP — H L2 W S?	70–90	1–3	35 ± 3	1.2 ± 0.5

Milk/plasma (M/P) ratio	Adult dose in milk (%)	Maximum amount in milk (mg/L)	Comments and references
	Rapidly produced active metabolite excreted into human milk		Bioavailability of tablet is 90% of liquid. Brand names: Lomotil, Lonox. (7, 67, 278, 393, 477)
			Inhibits gastric acid secretion. Is L isomer of omeprazole; acts like omeprazole. Should be safe. Brand name: Nexium.
0.41–1.78		0.072	Minimal first-pass metabolism. Decreased oral availability because of incomplete absorption. Calculated amount in milk (assuming intake of 600–800 mL) is 0.14 mg/day. Brand names: Pepcid, Mylanta. (67, 85, 131, 181, 277, 294, 296, 393)
			Proton pump inhibitor. Delayed release capsules. Found in rat milk. Human milk? Not approved for children younger than 1 year. Acid liable, extensively degraded in stomach, so enteric capsules are used. Brand name: Prevacid. (114)
			Brand name: Imodium. (7, 278, 393, 477)
1			Oral hypoglycemic agent for diabetes. Brand names: Glucophage, Glucovance, Diabex, Diaformin, Diguanil, Gen-Metformin, Glycon.
0.543–4.062	8 ± 3.3	0.157	In milk: peak 1–2 hr 10%–31% newborn therapeutic dose. Found in plasma of 1 of 5 infants studied. May see sedation, poor feeding. Brand name: Reglan. (7, 20, 181, 277, 319, 393)
	<0.1		Metabolite 60% as active as drug. In milk: peak 1–2 hr; mean amount at 12 hr 96.1 ± 31 mg. Experiments in rats show growth depression in pups. Brand names: Nizatidine, Axid. (181, 277, 294, 296, 361, 393)

Continued

TABLE D-1   Relationship of drugs to breast milk and effect on infant—cont'd

Drugs and ratings*	Oral availability (%)	Peak plasma time (hr)	Plasma protein bound (%)	Volume of distribution (L/kg)
Gastrointestinal agents—cont'd				
Omeprazole AAP — H L2 W S?	25–100	0.5–3.5	95.5 ± 0.5	0.19–0.45
Ondansetron AAP — H L2 W U	52–62	0.75–3	4–10	
Pantoprazole AAP — H — W —	77	2.5 hr with 40-mg dose	98	0.32
Prochlorperazine AAP — H L3 W U	4.8–25.3	3.4–9.9		5.8–17.1
Ranitidine AAP — H L2 W S?	39–87	0.5–3	10–19	1.3 ± 0.4
Senna AAP 6 H L3 W S	Drug not absorbed from GI tract; active metabolite is rhein			
Simethicone AAP — H — W S				
Trimethobenzamide AAP — H L4 W U	60% of IM			
Heavy metals and other elements				
Aluminum AAP — H — W —	Greater than 95% ingested aluminum is excreted in feces			

Milk/plasma (M/P) ratio	Adult dose in milk (%)	Maximum amount in milk (mg/L)	Comments and references
			Proton pump inhibitor. Reduces gastric acid secretion. Omeprazole is very acid sensitive with half-life of 10 minutes at a pH of 4. Little (< 10%) in milk. Should be safe in lactation. Undergoes first-pass metabolism to active compound. Brand name: Prilosec. (93, 221, 227, 311, 423, 455, 477)
			Brand name: Zofran. (95, 325)
			Active ingredient pantoprazole sodium sesquihydrate inhibits gastric secretion. Proton pump inhibitor similar to omeprazole. Brand name: Protonix.
Excretion into milk not significant after therapeutic dose			Galactorrhea reported in some women. Increases serum prolactin levels. Brand name: Compazine. (231, 477)
0.25–7		3	Decreases gastric acidity. Amount in milk varies widely. IM availability: 90%–100%. Cimetidine is rated "6." Brand name: Zantac. (7, 67, 85, 181, 277, 294, 393, 477)
			Active metabolite, rhein, found in milk at 27 ng/mL or 0–4086 ng/day. Some suggestion that older preps might affect the infant's bowel function. Brand names: Perdiem, Senokot. (67, 141)
			Acts locally, little absorbed. Based on inert silicone which is present in many medications as inert ingredient. Brand name: Phazyme (Mylicon).
			Brand name: Tigan. (7)
			Amount in breast milk less than in drinking water and soy or cow milk formula. (54, 395, 531)

Continued

TABLE D-1	**Relationship of drugs to breast milk and effect on infant—cont'd**			
Drugs and ratings*	Oral availability (%)	Peak plasma time (hr)	Plasma protein bound (%)	Volume of distribution (L/kg)
Heavy metals and other elements—cont'd				
Antimony AAP 6 H — W —				
Chromium AAP — H L3 W —				
Copper AAP — H — W —				
Fluoride AAP 7 H L2 W —		2		
Iron AAP — H L1 W —				
Lead AAP 7 H L5 W —	5–10			
Mercury AAP 7 H L5 W —				
Zinc AAP — H L3 W —				
Hormones, antithyroid, contraceptives, steroids				
Acetohexamide AAP — H L3 W U			75	0.2

Milk/plasma (M/P) ratio	Adult dose in milk (%)	Maximum amount in milk (mg/L)	Comments and references
			Considered safe by AAP.
Excreted into human milk			In multiple vitamins. In milk: about 0.4 µg/L, half-life 6 ± 1 hr. Allowable daily intake is 5–15 µg/day.
Excreted into human milk			Maternal elimination fairly rapid. Maternal homeostatic mechanisms should prevent excess transfer during lactation. Prolactin levels increase.
0.21–0.32	0.19	0.008	In milk: peak 2 hr, 0–0.35 ppm reflects level in local water supply. Frequency of dental caries equal in breastfed infants and infants receiving formula diluted with fluorinated water. (20, 532)
Excreted into human milk			
0.02–1		0.35	Higher uptake in infant than mother. Strongly bound to hemoglobin so not much gets into milk. Formula may have higher concentration. Not found in milk when maternal level <40 mg%. (6, 201, 329, 385, 455, 554)
0.03–1		0.54	Toxicity caused by lactation transfer reported. In milk: 0.93 ± 0.23 ppb. (329, 385)
Excreted into human milk			Essential dietary element. Homeostatic mechanisms of mother prevent excess transfer to milk.
			Brand name: Dymelor (7, 393, 477)

Continued

TABLE D-1   Relationship of drugs to breast milk and effect on infant—cont'd

Drugs and ratings*	Oral availability (%)	Peak plasma time (hr)	Plasma protein bound (%)	Volume of distribution (L/kg)
Hormones, antithyroid, contraceptives, steroids—cont'd				
Beclomethasone dipropionate AAP — H L2 W —			87	
Betamethasone AAP — H L3 W U	72	1–3	64 ± 6	1.4 ± 0.3
Carbetocin AAP 6 H — W —				
Carbimazole AAP 6 H L3 W —				
Chlormethiazole AAP — H — W —	12 ± 3		64	
Chlorotrianisene AAP — H — W NS				
Chlorpropamide AAP — H L3 W NS	99 ± 9	3 ± 1	90–96.6	0.09–0.27
Clogestone AAP 6 H — W —				
Clomiphene AAP — H L4 W U				Large

Milk/plasma (M/P) ratio	Adult dose in milk (%)	Maximum amount in milk (mg/L)	Comments and references
			Given to neonates. Brand name: Vancenase. (7, 9, 386, 393)
			Half-life in human milk is 5.6 ± 0.8 hr. Can use in a limited area as a cream. (181, 266)
			A long-acting oxytocin analog.
0.58–0.9	27		Active metabolite: methimazole. Average concentration in milk: 182 ± 25 µg/L. Dose of 5–15 mg/day appears safe for nursing. In milk: peak 1 hr. (20, 96, 427)
0.73		3.23	Extensive first-pass metabolism. Detected in blood of 3 of 27 infants. (455, 477)
	Excreted into human milk		Has estrogenic effect but does not change consistency of milk. May suppress lactation. Brand name: Tace.
	Excreted into human milk		In milk: after 5 hr, 5 mg/L. How quickly mother eliminates it depends on pH of urine. Brand name: Diabinese. (181, 393, 455, 477)
			Contraceptive. Should be safe in lactation. Mothers have taken it up to 3 years with no effect in the baby.
			Taking fertility drug and nursing gives the body two opposite stimuli. Brand name: Serophene, Clomid. (491)

Continued

TABLE D-1   Relationship of drugs to breast milk and effect on infant—cont'd

Drugs and ratings*	Oral availability (%)	Peak plasma time (hr)	Plasma protein bound (%)	Volume of distribution (L/kg)
Hormones, antithyroid, contraceptives, steroids—cont'd				
Cortisone AAP — H — W U				
Cyclosporine AAP 1 H L3 W S?	2–89 Mean: 30 More absorbed if taken with food	1–8	91–98	2.9–8
Dexamethasone AAP — H L3 W U	53 ± 40		68 ± 3	1.163 ± 0.88
Dienestrol AAP — H — W NS?	Possible decrease in milk volume and its nitrogen and protein content			
Diethylstilbestrol AAP — H L5 W NS	Possible decrease in milk volume and its nitrogen and protein content			
Epinephrine AAP — H L4 W U				
Estradiol AAP 6 H L3 W S				
Estrogen AAP 6 H L3 W S				
Ethinyl estradiol AAP 6 W S	20–65	2.1 ± 0.99		3.79 ± 0.83

Milk/plasma (M/P) ratio	Adult dose in milk (%)	Maximum amount in milk (mg/L)	Comments and references
	Excreted into human milk		Probably okay to use as replacement therapy in Addison's disease or if used as a one-time shot in a joint (it is depot, not systemic). Brand name: Cortone. (477)
0.17–0.4		0.263	Drug extensively metabolized. It consists of 11 amino acids. Not absorbed if given by enema. 16 µg/L found in breast milk 22 hr after last dose. Brand name: Sandimmune. (3, 142, 147, 181, 261, 292, 295, 393, 432, 562)
	Excreted into human milk		Some, not all, studies show drug induces prolactin suppression. Concern about interface with endogenous steroid production. Brand name: Decadron. (36, 181, 393)
			(67, 393)
			(15, 67)
	Destroyed in GI tract of infant		Brand names: EpiPen, Sensorcaine. (393)
	0.004–<10		In milk: peak 7 ± 4 hr. Brand names: Emcyt, Estrace. (20, 67)
	0.1		May alter the quality and quantity of milk.
0.25	0.16 ± 0.14		In milk: peak 2 hr. May alter the quality and quantity of milk. In many birth control medications. (20, 393, 443)

Continued

TABLE D-1	Relationship of drugs to breast milk and effect on infant—cont'd			

Drugs and ratings*	Oral availability (%)	Peak plasma time (hr)	Plasma protein bound (%)	Volume of distribution (L/kg)
Hormones, antithyroid, contraceptives, steroids—cont'd				
Ethynodiol AAP — H L1 W —	Data for active metabolite: norethisterone			
Fluoxymesterone AAP — H — W—				
Fluticasone propionate AAP — H L3 W —		<1		
Glipizide AAP — H L3 W U	95–99	1.95 ± 1.45	98.5 ± 0.5	0.17 ± 0.02
Halobetasol propionate AAP — H — W S?	In 96 hr, approximately 3% enters the circulation after topical application			
Hydrocortisone AAP — H L2 W S?	96 ± 20	1.2 ± 0.4	75–95	0.4 ± 0.1
Insulin AAP — H L1 W S			5	
Leuprolide AAP — H L5 W U	Not active when given orally; it is a modified 10 amino acid compound			
Levonorgestrel AAP 6 H L1 W —	87 ± 9	1–4	50	1.75 ± 0.45

Milk/plasma (M/P) ratio	Adult dose in milk (%)	Maximum amount in milk (mg/L)	Comments and references
	0.02–0.07	0.00084	Rapidly metabolized to norethisterone, which peaks in milk at 4–8 hr. Brand name: Demulen.
	Suppresses lactation		Brand name: Halotestin. (393)
			87%–100% excreted in the feces. 3%–40% as inactive metabolite. Brand name: Flonase. (10, 73)
			Brand name: Glucotrol. (181, 393, 477)
			Brand name: Ultravate. (393)
	Excreted into human milk		Drug exhibits dose-dependent kinetics. Rectal availability: $2 \pm 1\%$. Brand name: Westcort. (115, 330, 477)
	Not excreted into human milk		(477)
			Brand name: Lupron. (181, 393)
0.072–0.365	1.1	0.0005	Does not undergo first-pass metabolism or affect milk production. Brand names: Norplant, Levlen, Triphasil. (20, 157, 314, 443, 444, 455, 477)

Continued

TABLE D-1	Relationship of drugs to breast milk and effect on infant—cont'd			
Drugs and ratings[*]	**Oral availability (%)**	**Peak plasma time (hr)**	**Plasma protein bound (%)**	**Volume of distribution (L/kg)**
Hormones, antithyroid, contraceptives, steroids—cont'd				
Levothyroxine AAP 6 H L1 W S	50–80			
Liothyronine AAP — H L2 W U	95		>99	0.5
Medroxyprogesterone AAP 6 H L1, L4 if used first 3 days postpartum W S	<10		94	0.6
Mestranol AAP — H — W NS				
Methimazole AAP 6 H L3 W S?	93	1.5 ± 0.5	0	0.6
Methylprednisolone AAP — H L2 W S?	49–81		78 ± 3	1.2 ± 0.2
Mometasone furoate AAP — H L3 W S?	When used as a topical ointment, after 8 hr of contact, about 0.7% is systemically absorbed of the 0.1% ointment			
Norethindrone AAP — H L1 W S	64 ± 8		80	4
Norethynodrel AAP 6 H L2 W —				

Milk/plasma (M/P) ratio	Adult dose in milk (%)	Maximum amount in milk (mg/L)	Comments and references
		0.043	May increase milk production. Not a problem as a replacement hormone. Brand names: Levothroid, Synthroid. (7, 67)
0.36		0.005	Brand names: Cytomel, Triostat. (67, 393, 477)
0.2–1	0.86–5		Increased prolactin level before and after sucking. When 3-month injection given, no decrease in amount of milk produced; 6-month injection had a strong negative effect. Brand names: Amen, Cycrin, Depo-Provera. (20, 140, 237, 477)
	1.4		May interfere with quality and quantity of milk. Brand names: Norethin, Norinyl, Ortho-Novum. (20, 393)
0.3–1.28	0.47–16.6	0.207	In milk: peak 2.5 ± 1.5 hr. Brand name: Tapazole. (20, 67, 96, 181, 455)
			Oral availability may be saturated. Brand name: Solu-Medrol. (181, 213, 455, 477)
			Brand name: Elocon. (393)
0.1–0.26	0.02–2.12	0.016	Higher levels in milk when taken with norgestrel. In milk: peak 6 ± 2 hr, some decrease of fat and calcium. Brand name: Micronor. (20, 67, 393, 410, 429, 455, 477)
	1.1		May decrease quality and quantity of milk. (393)

Continued

TABLE D-1   Relationship of drugs to breast milk and effect on infant—cont'd

Drugs and ratings*	Oral availability (%)	Peak plasma time (hr)	Plasma protein bound (%)	Volume of distribution (L/kg)
Hormones, antithyroid, contraceptives, steroids—cont'd				
Norgestrel AAP — H — W S		2		
Norsteroids AAP 6 H — W —				
Oxycodone AAP — H L3 W U, analgesic	60 ± 20	0.75–4.17		1.83–3.65
Oxytocin AAP — H L2 W S		Destroyed in the stomach		
Phenformin AAP — H — W —			12–20	5–10
Prednisolone AAP 6 H L2, L4 for chronic high doses W S?	82 ± 13	1–4 Drug concentration dependent	65–95	0.2–1.3
Prednisone AAP 6 H L2, L4 for chronic high doses W S	80 ± 11		75 ± 2	0.97 ± 0.11
Progesterone AAP 6 H L3 W S	Low	6	99	
Propylthiouracil AAP 6 H — W S	78 ± 15		80	0.4

Milk/plasma (M/P) ratio	Adult dose in milk (%)	Maximum amount in milk (mg/L)	Comments and references
0.1–0.2	2.8	0.5	In milk: peak 2 hr; if taken alone, below detection level by 4 hr; if taken with norethisterone, high level in milk for 24 hr. Brand names: Lo/Ovral, Ovrette. (20, 67, 393)
			Appears in breast milk. Considered safe by the AAP.
3.4		0.226	In milk: peak 1.75 ± 0.25 hr. Structurally related to codeine and morphine. (67, 181, 400)
	Excreted into human milk		Enhances let-down reflex; does not necessarily increase amount of milk. Brand names: Pitocin, Syntocinon. (393)
	Minimal amount excreted into human milk		No effects seen in infants. Fast and slow metabolizers exist. (477)
0.05–0.25	0.06–3.6	0.3	Active form of prednisone. In milk: peak 1 hr, half-life 23 hr. At a high dose of 80 mg/day, infant gets less than 0.1% of dose, less than 10% of the child's own endogenous cortisol production. Brand names: Blephamide, Pediapred. (20, 67, 181, 393, 410, 477)
0.05–0.25	0.15 ± 0.11	0.042	Active metabolite: prednisolone. Brand name: Deltasone. (20, 67, 162, 181)
			Progestational agent. In low dose, progesterone-only oral contraceptives are ok. Brand names: Crinone, Prometrium, Cyclogest, Gesterol, Gestone.
0.1–0.77	0.03–2.6	0.9	In milk: peak 1.5 hr. In infant, get baseline levels of T_3, T_4, TSH before and 6 weeks after mother starts taking medication. (20, 67, 96, 181, 455, 477)

Continued

TABLE D-1	Relationship of drugs to breast milk and effect on infant—cont'd			
Drugs and ratings*	Oral availability (%)	Peak plasma time (hr)	Plasma protein bound (%)	Volume of distribution (L/kg)
Hormones, antithyroid, contraceptives, steroids—cont'd				
Tolbutamide AAP 6 H L3 W S	93 ± 10	3.5 ± 0.5	93 ± 4	0.1–0.25
Triamcinolone AAP — H L3 W U				1.39–2.11 The higher the dose, the lower the volume of distribution
Vasopressin AAP — H L3 W S	Negligible			
Narcotics and antiaddiction drugs				
Cocaine AAP 2 H L5 W NS	30–40	0.5–2	91	1.2–3
Codeine AAP 6 H L3 W S	12–84	0.5–2	7	1.1–3.3
Dextromethorphan AAP — H L1 W S		1.6		
Disulfiram AAP — H L5 W U	80%–95% absorbed from the GI tract			8.2
Heroin AAP 2 H L4 W —	Excreted into human milk in sufficient quantities to cause addiction in the infant			
Hydrocodone bitartrate AAP — H L3 W S	Well absorbed from GI tract	1.3		

Milk/plasma (M/P) ratio	Adult dose in milk (%)	Maximum amount in milk (mg/L)	Comments and references
0.09–0.4	18	20	Fast and slow metabolizers exist. Percent plasma protein bound is concentration dependent. Watch for jaundice. Brand name: Orinase. (20, 181, 378, 393, 477)
	Excreted into human milk		Brand names: Aristocort, Azmacort, Kenalog, Mycolog, Mytrex, Nasacort. (477)
		0.001	Brand name: Pitressin. (67, 410)
	Significant level excreted into human milk		57% ± 19% intranasally available. No drug or metabolite found in milk after 36 hr or in infant's urine after 60 hr. In rats, M/P ratio >1. (44, 181, 544)
1.3–2.5	5 ± 2	179	About 10% metabolized to morphine. Chinese metabolize less drug than Caucasians. In milk: half-life 2–2.5 hr, peak 1.25 ± 0.25 hr, 1.5% of newborn therapeutic dose, average amount 0.14 mg/L. Brand name: Calcidrine. (20, 181, 391, 455, 554, 562, 563)
			The *d* isomer of codeine analog levorphanol. 5%–10% of Caucasians are poor metabolizers. (181, 458)
			Brand name: Antabase. (7, 393, 477)
			(67)
			Chemically related to codeine and morphine. (7, 393, 477)

Continued

TABLE D-1   Relationship of drugs to breast milk and effect on infant—cont'd

Drugs and ratings*	Oral availability (%)	Peak plasma time (hr)	Plasma protein bound (%)	Volume of distribution (L/kg)
Narcotics and antiaddiction drugs—cont'd				
Hydromorphone AAP — H L3 W S	51–52 Rectal availability 36			
Lysergic acid diethylamide (LSD) AAP — H L5 W —	Expected to be excreted into human milk; ergot, a structurally related compound is found in milk			
Marijuana AAP 2 H L5 W —				
Methadone AAP 6 H L3 W S	79 ± 21	1.8–3.8	89 ± 1.4	4.13–13.4
Morphine AAP 6 H L3 W S	15–64		38 ± 5	2.2–5.5
Naloxone AAP — H — W S	2 91% of drug absorbed			2.1–3
Naltrexone AAP — H L3 W U	5–40	0.8 ± 0.2	20–21	16.1 ± 5.2
Nicotine (smoking) AAP — H 3 (therapeutic patch) W S	30–>90		4.9 ± 2.8	2.6 ± 0.9

Milk/plasma (M/P) ratio	Adult dose in milk (%)	Maximum amount in milk (mg/L)	Comments and references
			Very closely related to morphine. Brand name: Dilaudid. (393, 455)
			Rapidly absorbed and distributed throughout body. Half-life is not dose dependent. (67, 181)
>1			Metabolite: THC. In infants: found in urine and stool, at risk of inhaling smoke when held while mother is smoking. In animals, makes structural changes in nurslings' brain cells. (14, 329)
0.3–1.5	2.2	5.6	In milk: peak 2–6 hr. No signs in infants if mother getting less than 20 mg/24 hr. Above that, withdrawal may be a problem. Suggested that mother get her daily dose after the evening feeding, supplement with a bottle at the next feeding. (6, 19, 66, 67, 181, 393, 455, 477, 554)
0.23–5.07	0.8–12	0.1	High first-pass metabolism. In infant: found in plasma when not detected in milk 108 hr after mother's last dose; elimination half-life is increased. Amount in milk too variable to treat withdrawal symptoms. May cause galactorrhea and prolactin increase. Brand names: Astramorph, MSIR, Roxanol. (7, 50, 181, 207, 350, 414, 455, 492)
			91% of drug is absorbed, but hepatic metabolism destroys most of it. Brand names: Narcan, Talwin. (181, 393, 477)
			Brand name: Trexan. (181, 393)
0.3–9.6		0.6	In milk: peak 0.165 hr; half-life 1.53 ± 0.25 hr. May suppress lactation. Decreased response of prolactin and oxytocin to suckling. Active metabolite, continine, excreted into milk. Nicotine replacement therapy is considered compatible with breastfeeding. (6, 20, 103, 181, 300, 439, 485)

Continued

TABLE D-1   Relationship of drugs to breast milk and effect on infant—cont'd

Drugs and ratings*	Oral availability (%)	Peak plasma time (hr)	Plasma protein bound (%)	Volume of distribution (L/kg)
Narcotics and antiaddiction drugs—cont'd				
Phencyclidine (PCP) AAP 2 H L5 W —	72			
THC (tetrahydrocannabinol) AAP 2 H L5 W —	4–12 2%–50% availability if smoked		95	8.9 ± 4.2
Psychotropic and mood-altering drugs				
Alprazolam AAP 4 H L3 W NS	92 ± 17	0.3–6	71 ± 3	0.72 ± 0.12
Amitriptyline AAP 4 H L2 W S?	48 ± 11 High hepatic metabolism	4	98.8 ± 0.8	15 ± 3
Amoxapine AAP 4 H L2 W U	99	1.5	90	
Bupropion AAP 4 H L3 W S?	60–80 Extensive hepatic metabolism	1–2	>80	Very large
Buspirone AAP — H L3 W U	7.25 ± 5.75	1.1 ± 0.4	95	5.31
Caffeine AAP 6 H L2 W S	99 ± 14	0.5 ± 0.25	29 ± 14	0.5 ± 0.1
Chloral hydrate AAP 6 H L3 W NS?		0.5		1.5 ± 0.5

Milk/plasma (M/P) ratio	Adult dose in milk (%)	Maximum amount in milk (mg/L)	Comments and references
	Excreted into human milk		Animal studies show M/P ratio as 10. In one case, mother's last dose was 40 days previous and milk had 3.9 ng/mL. (455)
8–8.4		0.34	Δ-9-Tetrahydrocannabinol, an active metabolite of marijuana. Infants may have decreased motor development. (14, 16, 67)
	Excreted into human milk		Withdrawal symptoms seen in an infant when mom stopped taking the drug. Metabolite is half as active as drug. Brand name: Xanax. (7, 181, 191, 393, 477, 498)
0.5–1.69	0.8 ± 0.2	0.15	Galactorrhea or prolactin increase reported. Not detected in infant's urine or serum detection limit, 5 ng/mL. In milk: peak 1.5 hr. Brand names: Elavil, Etrafon, Limbitrol, Triavil. (20, 67, 71, 79, 181, 393)
0.21	<0.07	<0.02	Active metabolite, in milk: maximum amount 168 ng/ml, M/P ratio 0.45–0.86. Brand name: Asendin. (20, 67, 393)
2.49–8.72		0.189	One report of a woman taking the drug and no drug or metabolite found in the infant's plasma. Brand name: Wellbutrin. (68, 227, 393, 455)
	Excreted in rat milk		Extensively metabolized. Brand name: BuSpar. (393)
0.48–0.9	0.66–2.3	28.6	In milk: peak 0.5–2 hr, average amount 0.846 mg/L, half-life 6.1 ± 4.4 hr. Ability to metabolize it developed by 3–4.5 months of age. After 100 mg, not found in baby's urine. (20, 50, 67, 178, 181, 290, 351, 530)
0.09–3	0.6–2	15	Trichloroethanol is metabolite to which effects are attributed. In milk: 0%–15% newborn therapeutic dose, peak 0.75 hr, trace amounts after 10 hr. (12, 20, 67, 181, 269)

Continued

TABLE D-1 Relationship of drugs to breast milk and effect on infant—cont'd

Drugs and ratings*	Oral availability (%)	Peak plasma time (hr)	Plasma protein bound (%)	Volume of distribution (L/kg)
Psychotropic and mood-altering drugs—cont'd				
Chlordiazepoxide AAP — H L3 W S?	100		96 ± 5.8	0.3 ± 0.03
Chlorpromazine AAP 4 H L3 W S?	32 ± 19	2	95–98	9.9–254.3
Chlorprothixene AAP 4 H L3 W —	41 ± 21			
Citalopram hydrobromide AAP — H L3 W S?	80	2–4	80	12
Clomipramine AAP 4 H L2 W U	36–68	3–5	96.5–98.6	16.6 ± 4.9
Clorazepate AAP — H — W U				0.33 ± 0.17
Clozapine AAP 4 H L3 W U	12–90 Mean 50–60	1–6	95	5
Desipramine AAP 4 H L2 W S	33–68 Well absorbed, high first-pass metabolism	4–6	86.55 ± 4.45	20 ± 3

Milk/plasma (M/P) ratio	Adult dose in milk (%)	Maximum amount in milk (mg/L)	Comments and references
Excreted into human milk			In first weeks of life, may contribute to jaundice. Conflicting reports of drowsiness. Brand names: Libritabs, Limbitrol, Librium, Menrium. (39, 181, 393, 410, 477)
0.3≥1	0.07–0.2	0.3	Rapidly and completely absorbed; high hepatic metabolism. Galactorrhea, increase in serum prolactin level reported. Drowsiness and lethargy in infant. In 11 mothers taking an average of 200 mg/day, no ill effects were seen in the infants. In milk: 0.05%–0.26% of newborn therapeutic dose, peak 2 hr. Brand name: Thorazine. (6, 20, 71, 181, 189, 267, 410, 477)
1.2–2.6	0.12 ± 0.04	18.75	In milk: peak 4.25 ± 0.25 hr. Active metabolite M/P ratio 0.5–0.8. Causes galactorrhea, prolactin increase. Brand name: Taractan. (20, 67, 455)
1.16–3			Antidepressant. Does get into milk. Two cases of somnolent infants. Measurable in infant. Brand name: Celexa (Cipramil).
0.76–1.62	0.4	0.624	Well absorbed from GI tract. Up to 50% first-pass metabolism yielding active metabolite. Hydroxylation of drug and metabolite under debrisoquin/sparteine control; 10%–20% of Caucasians cannot break down either. Not detected in infant's serum. Brand name: Anafranil. (7, 29)
Excreted into human milk			A prodrug for desmethyldiazepam. Brand name: Tranxene. (181, 393, 500)
2.79–4.32		0.116	High first-pass hepatic metabolism. Produces little or no prolactin increase. Brand name: Clozaril. (31, 393)
0.4–1.2	1	0.328	Neither drug nor metabolite recovered from nursing infant's serum or urine. 5%–10% of Caucasians are poor metabolizers. Metabolite of imipramine. Its metabolite is excreted into milk: M/P ratio 1.63: maximum amount found 327 ng/mL. Brand name: Norpramin. (7, 20, 67, 79, 155, 181, 393, 455, 477, 483, 552)

Continued

TABLE D-1   Relationship of drugs to breast milk and effect on infant—cont'd

Drugs and ratings[*]	Oral availability (%)	Peak plasma time (hr)	Plasma protein bound (%)	Volume of distribution (L/kg)
Psychotropic and mood-altering drugs—cont'd				
Desmethyldiazepam AAP — H — W —	99 ± 6		97.25 ± 0.25	0.78 ± 0.12
Dextroamphetamine AAP — H L4 W NS		2		
Diazepam AAP 4 H L3, L4, if used chronically W S?	100 ± 14		90–98	0.7–4.7
Dichloralphenazone AAP — H — W —	Body reduces drug to trichloroethanol, which produces CNS effect			
Dothiepin AAP 4 H L2 W —				70
Doxepin AAP 4 H L5 W NS?	13–45			20 ± 8
Escitalopram AAP — H — W —	80	5	56	
Ethanol AAP 6 H L3 W S	90 ± 10			0.54 ± 0.05
Fenfluramine AAP — H — W —	89 ± 10		34	

Milk/plasma (M/P) ratio	Adult dose in milk (%)	Maximum amount in milk (mg/L)	Comments and references
0.08–0.53		0.085	A metabolite of clorazepate, pinazepam, prazepam, and diazepam. Metabolizes to oxazepam. Higher in evening milk and morning plasma. (181, 410, 480)
2.8–7.5			In infant: amphetamine in the urine, insomnia, or stimulation not seen. Brand names: Biphetamine, Dexedrine. (67, 393)
0.1–2.7	2–12	0.6	In infant: sedation if fed 4 hr but not 8 hr after dose. More in evening milk when plasma levels are lower. In milk: 1.7%–3.8% therapeutic pediatric dose. Brand name: Valium. (17, 20, 50, 58, 67, 315, 410, 477, 480)
			(67)
0.33–1.59	0.15–0.58	0.475	Drug not detected in infant's serum. (20, 67, 477, 552)
0.3–2.39	0.01–2.2	0.029	Estimated that infant gets 71 μg/day. One report of a very sedated infant when mother took 25 mg 3 times a day. In milk: peak 4–5 hr. Active metabolite: M/P ratio 0.12:2.35; 11 ng/mL found in milk. Brand names: Adapin, Sinequan. (7, 20, 67, 181, 410, 455)
			Antidepressant. Selective serotonin reuptake inhibitor (SSRI). Does pass into milk. Two cases of somnolence in breastfed infants. Brand name: Lexapro.
0.777–1.41	1–19.5	5600	Milk may smell of it. High amounts may suppress lactation. Infant can't metabolize it. Metabolite, acetaldehyde, not excreted into milk. In milk: peak 0.5–1 hr. (19, 20, 67, 181, 271, 321, 395)
			Mediates release of prolactin. Excreted rapidly if urine pH less than 5. Brand name: Pondimin. (393, 455, 477)

Continued

TABLE D-1 **Relationship of drugs to breast milk and effect on infant—cont'd**

Drugs and ratings*	Oral availability (%)	Peak plasma time (hr)	Plasma protein bound (%)	Volume of distribution (L/kg)
Psychotropic and mood-altering drugs—cont'd				
Flunitrazepam AAP — H L3, L4 if used chronically W —	85		77–79	3.3 ± 0.6

Fluoxetine
AAP 4
H L2 in older infants,
  L3 if used in
  neonatal period
W S, conditionally
	>60–80
	Drug almost
	completely
	absorbed
		6–8	80–95	35 ± 21

Fluphenazine AAP — H L3 W —		1.5–2	>99	20–>30
Flurazepam AAP — H L3 W U		0.75 ± 0.25	97	
Fluvoxamine maleate AAP4 H L2 W S	94	2–12	77	5.1
Haloperidol AAP4 H L2 W S?	60 ± 18		92 ± 2	18 ± 7
Hydroxyzine AAP — HL1 W U		2 ± 0.9		19.5 ± 9.7
Imipramine AAP 4 H L2 W —	19–68	1–2	85–95	20–40

Milk/plasma (M/P) ratio	Adult dose in milk (%)	Maximum amount in milk (mg/L)	Comments and references
0.6–0.9			No significant binding to milk proteins. (18, 181, 477, 558)
0.29–0.88	3.3–13.9	0.181	In milk: maximum of active metabolite 0.199 mg/L. Recovered from infant's blood: drug 0–61 ng/mL, metabolite 57–58 ng/mL. Twelve reports of mothers taking the drug and breastfeeding. Possible connection with one case of colic. Otherwise, no adverse effects reported. Brand name: Prozac. (81, 181, 195, 217, 232, 384, 393, 481)
Excreted into human milk			Galactorrhea seen.
			Brand name: Dalmane. (7, 181, 393)
0.29	0.5	0.09	Not metabolized to active products. One case report of nursing mother taking the drug; no unwanted effects seen in infant. Brand name: Luvox. (195, 546, 559)
0.6–0.7	0.15–2	0.032	In milk: 1.3%–10% of newborn calculated dose, 2–5 ng/mL if mother has 12–30 mg/day. Causes prolactin increase. In animals if dose 1 mg/kg, nurslings have behavioral abnormalities. These effects not seen in humans. Brand name: Haldol. (20, 67, 181, 368, 522)
			Half-life is shorter in children. Active metabolite is cetirizine. Brand name: Atarax, Vistaril. (393)
0.08–1.0	0.1	1	Active metabolite: desipramine. Reported to cause galactorrhea and prolactin increase. Completely absorbed from GI tract. Brand name: Tofranil. (7, 20, 79, 181, 410, 455)

Continued

TABLE D-1	**Relationship of drugs to breast milk and effect on infant—cont'd**			
Drugs and ratings[*]	**Oral availability (%)**	**Peak plasma time (hr)**	**Plasma protein bound (%)**	**Volume of distribution (L/kg)**
Psychotropic and mood-altering drugs—cont'd				
Lithium AAP 5 H L4 W S?	95 ± 5	2–4	0	0.79 ± 0.31
Lorazepam AAP 4 H L3 W S?	64–109	2	91 ± 2	1.3 ± 0.2
Lormetazepam AAP — H — W —	70–80			
Maprotiline AAP — H L3 W U	36–67	9–16	88	22.6–52
Meprobamate AAP — H L3 W S		2		
Mesoridazine AAP 4 H L4 W U				>30
Methyprylon AAP 6 H — W —		1.5 ± 0.5	60	
Mirtazapine AAP — H L3 W U	50 Completely absorbed	2	85	
Moclobemide AAP — H L3 W —	27–70	0.58–3.17	50	0.81–1.5
Nefazodone AAP — H L4 W NS?	20 Completely absorbed; decreased 20% by food	1	>99	0.22–0.87

Milk/plasma (M/P) ratio	Adult dose in milk (%)	Maximum amount in milk (mg/L)	Comments and references
0.24–0.66	1.8	4	Infant's serum level: 10%–50% of mother. Inhibits cAMP, which is significant for brain growth. Cyanosis, poor muscle tone, and ECG changes seen in nursing infants. Brand names: Eskalith, Lithobid. (20, 79, 181, 455)
0.148–0.257	2.2	0.082	Infant toxicity observed at times. Increased half-life in neonate. Brand name: Ativan. (20, 181, 393, 410, 455)
Est. 0.06	<0.1–0.35		Drug and metabolite found in infant's plasma. Metabolite: M/P ratio 0.04. (20, 455)
1–1.5		0.2	Slowly but completely absorbed from GI tract. In milk: peak 8 hr. Brand name: Ludiomil. (7, 67, 393, 455, 477)
2–4			In milk: 96% of newborn dose; peak 4 hr. Galactorrhea seen in some women. Brand names: Equagesic, Miltown, PMB, Equanil. (393, 477)
Minimal amount excreted into human milk			May cause galactorrhea or prolactin increase. Brand name: Serentil.
Excreted into human milk			May see sedation and poor feeding in infant. Brand name: Noludar. (181, 329)
			Brand name: Remeron. (393)
0.69–0.72	0.057 ± 0.02		In milk: peak 3 hr. More than 95% absorbed with hepatic metabolism. Stimulates the release of prolactin in men. (42, 398, 435)
			Brand name: Serzone. (393, 534)

Continued

TABLE D-1   Relationship of drugs to breast milk and effect on infant—cont'd

Drugs and ratings*	Oral availability (%)	Peak plasma time (hr)	Plasma protein bound (%)	Volume of distribution (L/kg)
Psychotropic and mood-altering drugs—cont'd				
Nitrazepam AAP — H L3 W —	78 ± 16		87 ± 1	1.9 ± 0.3
Nortriptyline AAP 4 H L2 W S	46–59	10	92 ± 2	18 ± 4
Oxazepam AAP — H L3 W S?	97 ± 11		97.8 ± 2.3	0.6 ± 0.2
Paroxetine AAP 4 H L2 W S?		0.5–11	95	
Perphenazine AAP 4 H L3 W U				
Pinazepam AAP — H — W —	Active metabolite desmethyldiazepam, not drug, found in human milk			
Prazepam AAP 4 H L3 W —				14.4 ± 5.1
Protriptyline AAP — H — W S	77–93		92 ± 0.6	22 ± 1
Quazepam AAP 4 H L2 W —		2.5 ± 0.5		

Milk/plasma (M/P) ratio	Adult dose in milk (%)	Maximum amount in milk (mg/L)	Comments and references
0.18–0.6	<1	0.015	Not detected in infant's plasma. (80, 181, 307, 559)
0.6–3.71	0.53	0.404	Extensive first-pass metabolism; 5%–10% of Caucasians are poor metabolizers. Not detected in infant's serum. Brand names: Pamelor, Aventyl. (20, 67, 69, 155, 181, 255)
0.1–0.33	0.001	0.03	Also metabolite of prazepam and diazepam. Detected in urine of infant exposed to high doses through milk. In milk: half-life 12 hr. Brand name: Serax. (67, 79, 127, 181, 410, 477, 558)
1			Extensive first-pass metabolism; can be partially saturated. Absorption not affected by food. Usual plasma peak: 4.8–5.6 hr. Brand name: Paxil. (109, 518)
0.7–1.1	0.1	0.003	Increases serum prolactin levels. One report: mother taking drug, infant grew normally. Brand names: Etrafon, Triavil, Trilafon. (371, 477)
>1			A prodrug for desmethyldiazepam. Metabolized ultimately to 3-hydroxyprazepam and oxazepam. Brand name: Centrax. (6, 181)
	Excreted into human milk		Predicted to cause galactorrhea and prolactin increase. Brand name: Vivactil. (181, 393, 500)
4.13	0.02–5.8	0.216	Levels of drug and active metabolite decline at same rate in plasma and milk. In milk: peak 3 ± 1 hr. Brand name: Doral. (20)

Continued

TABLE D-1	**Relationship of drugs to breast milk and effect on infant—cont'd**			
Drugs and ratings*	Oral availability (%)	Peak plasma time (hr)	Plasma protein bound (%)	Volume of distribution (L/kg)
Psychotropic and mood-altering drugs—cont'd				
Raclopride AAP — H — W —	65 ± 15	0.45 ± 0.2	94–96	1.1 ± 0.4
Remoxipride AAP — H — W —	96	1.25 ± 0.75	81 ± 3	0.41 ± 0.31
Risperidone AAP — H L3 W U	66–70	0.8 ± 0.3	90	1.1
Secobarbital AAP 6 H L3 W S		2–4	30–50	1.5
Sertraline AAP 4 H L2 W S?		4–8.5	98–99	>20
Temazepam AAP 4 H L3 W NS?	98.4 ± 15.6	1–3	96–97.6	1.06 ± 0.31
Theobromine AAP — H — W —		2.3 ± 0.8	20 ± 5	0.63 ± 0.19
Thioridazine AAP — H L4 W U			99	>30
Tranylcypromine AAP — H — W U	Inhibits lactation			

Milk/plasma (M/P) ratio	Adult dose in milk (%)	Maximum amount in milk (mg/L)	Comments and references
			Increases serum prolactin levels. (340)
			Acid urine enhances excretion; basic urine delays it. Low doses decrease prolactin concentration; high doses increase it. (22, 340, 543)
			Increase in prolactin levels. Data given for good metabolizers. 6%–8% of Caucasians and a low percentage of Asians are poor metabolizers. Brand name: Risperdal. (224, 393)
Small amounts excreted into human milk			Oral dose: about 90% absorbed. Brand names: Tuinal, Seconal. (7, 393, 477)
			Extensive first-pass metabolism. Metabolite has 10% the activity of the drug. Drug usually not recovered from infant's serum; metabolite found at level of <2 ng/ml. Four nursing infants had normal platelet levels of 5-hydroxytryptamine. Brand name: Zoloft. (139, 346, 393, 552)
0.09–0.63	4.7	0.028	Level of drug in infant's plasma: 7 µg/L. Metabolite of diazepam. Brand name: Restoril. (127, 181, 282, 336, 393, 477, 500)
0.6–1.06	20	7.5	Usual source is chocolate. In milk: peak 4.5 ± 2.5 hr. half-life 4–8 hr. If mother consumes more than a pound per day, may see irritability or increased bowel activity in infant. (6, 19, 20, 554)
Excreted into human milk			Galactorrhea reported in some women. Percent plasma protein bound is concentration dependent. Brand name: Mellaril. (477)
Excreted into human milk in insignificant amounts			Brand name: Parnate. (393)

Continued

TABLE D-1   Relationship of drugs to breast milk and effect on infant—cont'd

Drugs and ratings*	Oral availability (%)	Peak plasma time (hr)	Plasma protein bound (%)	Volume of distribution (L/kg)
Psychotropic and mood-altering drugs—cont'd				
Trazodone AAP 4 H L2 W S	81 ± 29	1.34 ± 0.84 on empty stomach 2.03 ± 1.51 if taken with food	89–98	1.0 ± 0.3
Triazolam AAP — H L3 W U	44	1.25 ± 0.32	80–91.6	1.1 ± 0.4
Trichloroethanol AAP — H — W —			38 ± 3	
Trifluoperazine AAP 4 H — W S?				>30
Venlafaxine AAP — H L3 W U	12.6 At least 92% absorbed 45 for extended release	1–2	27 ± 2	7.5 ± 3.7
Zopiclone AAP — H L2 W —	75–80	0.5–4	45	1.5
Vitamins				
Dihydrotachysterol (vitamin D) AAP — H — W S?				
Folic acid AAP 6 H L1 W S				
Pyridoxine AAP — H L2, L4 in high doses W S				

Milk/plasma (M/P) ratio	Adult dose in milk (%)	Maximum amount in milk (mg/L)	Comments and references
0.09–0.2	0.0065–1.1		In milk: peak 2 hr. Brand name: Desyrel. (7, 20, 79, 181, 357, 393, 523)
	Excreted into human milk		Sublingual availability: 53%. Brand name: Halcion. (55, 181, 393, 415, 477, 500)
0.125–2.4		2.7	Active metabolite of dichloralphenazone and chloral hydrate. In milk (when taken as chloral hydrate): peak 3.37 ± 2.63 hr, 2.4% of the adult dose. (20, 67)
	Excreted into human milk		Excretion into milk not significant after therapeutic doses. Galactorrhea reported in some women. There is an increase in serum prolactin levels. Brand name: Stelazine. (393)
			Extensive first-pass metabolism. Active metabolite: percent plasma protein bound 30 ± 12; volume of distribution 5.7 ± 1.8 L/kg; peaks in plasma at 1–2 hr. Brand name: Effexor (393)
0.39–0.63	1.2		In milk: peak 1–6 hr; in most women 2–3 hr. (310)
	Excreted into human milk		Concern about hypercalcemia. Monitor calcium in infant's serum and urine. Brand name: DHT. (67)
0.02–0.23	0.1	0.141	Preferentially excreted into milk. (67, 393)
0.25	Amount in milk directly proportional to mother's intake		Large amounts may inhibit lactation. In milk: peak 5.5 ± 2.5 hr. Brand names: Beelith, Mega-B, Lurline. (67, 388)

Continued

TABLE D-1   Relationship of drugs to breast milk and effect on infant—cont'd

Drugs and ratings*	Oral availability (%)	Peak plasma time (hr)	Plasma protein bound (%)	Volume of distribution (L/kg)
Psychotropic and mood-altering drugs—cont'd				
Riboflavin (vitamin B$_2$) AAP 6 H L1 W S	Complete	Rapid		
Thiamin (vitamin B$_1$) AAP 6 H — W S				
Vitamin B$_{12}$ (cyanocobalamin) AAP 6 H L1 W —	Variable	2		
Vitamin D AAP 6 H L3 W S	Variable			
Vitamin K$_1$ AAP 6 H — W —				
Miscellaneous				
Acetazolamide AAP 6 H L2 W S	>90	Within 2	91.5 ± 4.5	0.2
Aflatoxin AAP 7 H — W —				
Aminophylline AAP 6 HL 3 W S	99	1.75 ± 1.25	61 ± 12	
Aspartame AAP 7 H L1, L5 if used in infants with phenylketonuria W —	Complete	2–3		

Milk/plasma (M/P) ratio	Adult dose in milk (%)	Maximum amount in milk (mg/L)	Comments and references
			Maternal supplement is safe. Brand names: Abdec, Accomin.
			Vitamin. Necessary during lactation. Wide margin of safety.
			Vitamin supplement. Necessary for vegans. Brand names: Anacobin, Cytacon, Rubramin
			Vitamin D supplement is safe upto 4000 IU daily to mother. Brand names: Calciferol, Delta-D, Calcijex, Drisdol, Hytakerol, Radiostol.
			Vitamin. Given to neonates. May need to be repeated. Infant formula contains 100 times that in human milk.
0.25–0.3	0.06–1.9	2.1	Amount in maternal plasma about 30 times the amount in neonate's plasma. Brand name: Diamox. (20, 432, 477)
			Any of several carcinogenic mycotoxins that are produced, especially in stored agricultural crops (as peanuts) by molds (as *Aspergillus flavus*). No effect on lactation per AAP.
			Active metabolite: theophylline. (393, 455)
			Artificial sweetener. Mothers should limit their daily intake while nursing because it increases phenylalanine levels in milk. Brand name: NutraSweet.

Continued

TABLE D-1   Relationship of drugs to breast milk and effect on infant—cont'd

Drugs and ratings[*]	Oral availability (%)	Peak plasma time (hr)	Plasma protein bound (%)	Volume of distribution (L/kg)
Miscellaneous—cont'd				
Azelaic acid AAP — H L3 W —		2		
Baclofen AAP 6 H L3 W S		2–3	30	
Bromocriptine AAP 5 H L5 W NS	65 ± 25	1–3	92.5 ± 2.5	3.4
Carisoprodol AAP — H L3 W NS?				
Chlorhexidine gluconate AAP — H L2 W S?	Poorly absorbed	0.5		
Cromolyn AAP — H L1 W S?	1 Little gastric absorption		70	0.32 ± 0.06
Cyclobenzaprine AAP — H L3 W U	52	3–8	93	
Doxapram AAP — H — W —	35–86	2.4		3.5
Enprofylline AAP — H — W —	Oral absorption complete Rectal availability 89%	0.5	47	

Milk/plasma (M/P) ratio	Adult dose in milk (%)	Maximum amount in milk (mg/L)	Comments and references
			Percutaneous absorption: at 8 hr, 8.1% absorbed from gel; 3%–3.6% from aqueous solution. Mostly dissociated at physiologic pH. (49, 151, 393)
0.66	0.1–5.4		In milk: peak 4 hr; half-life 5.6 hr. Absorption decreases as dose decreases. Elimination from milk delayed 3 hr in relation to serum. (20, 393, 477)
Excreted into human milk			Suppresses prolactin secretion. Extensive first-pass metabolism. Hyperprolactinemic mothers taking drug can breastfeed successfully. Brand name: Parlodel. (185, 249, 263, 477)
2–4			Brand name: Soma. (393)
			Can cause allergic reactions. Brand names: Hibiclens, Peridex, Hibistat. (369, 393)
			After eye treatment, 0.03% absorbed. 10% or less absorbed from an inhaled dose. Brand names: Intal, Gastrocrom. (181, 190, 393, 477)
			Well absorbed orally. Structurally related to tricyclic antidepressants. Concern about SIDS if it gets into milk. Brand name: Flexeril. (7, 393, 455)
			Used in premature infants where it is poorly absorbed orally. Brand name: Dopram. (27, 393, 477)
0.67–0.98	10		Some binding may occur to milk proteins, 90% excreted renally by mother. Dose to infant: 1.32 mg/kg/day. (179)

Continued

TABLE D-1	**Relationship of drugs to breast milk and effect on infant—cont'd**			

Drugs and ratings*	Oral availability (%)	Peak plasma time (hr)	Plasma protein bound (%)	Volume of distribution (L/kg)
Miscellaneous—cont'd				
Fava beans AAP 7 H — W —				
Guaifenesin AAP — H — W U	Readily absorbed from the GI tract			
Hexachlorophene AAP 7 H L4 W S	Complete			
Interferon-alpha N$_3$ AAP 6 H L3 W —	Low	Immediate		0.44
Lanolin AAP — H — W —	If used on nipples, there is a concern about the presence of pesticides			
Levodopa AAP — H L4 W U	35			
Methocarbamol AAP — H L3 W U	Oral absorption complete Extensive first-pass metabolism	1–2		
Methylmethacrylate AAP 7 H — W —				
Metocurine iodide AAP — H — W —			35 ± 6	0.35 ± 0.04

Milk/plasma (M/P) ratio	Adult dose in milk (%)	Maximum amount in milk (mg/L)	Comments and references
			Problem if mother or infant has G6PD deficiency.
A small, insignificant amount is excreted into milk			(393)
			Antiseptic scrub. Should not be used on nipples. Brand names: Septisol, Phisohex, Septi-soft, Dermalex, Sapoderm, pHisoHex.
			Immune modulator, antiviral. Not absorbed orally, of little or no risk to infant. Brand names: Alferon N, Interferon Alpha, Peg-Intron.
			(98)
			May suppress prolactin levels. Brand names: Dopar, Sinemet, Larodopa, Atamet. (455, 477)
Minimal amount excreted into animal milk			Too little in milk to produce any effects. Brand name: Robaxin, Robaxisal. (7)
			Does pass into milk.
			Brand name: Metubine. (2, 181, 393)

Continued

TABLE D-1   Relationship of drugs to breast milk and effect on infant—cont'd

Drugs and ratings*	Oral availability (%)	Peak plasma time (hr)	Plasma protein bound (%)	Volume of distribution (L/kg)
Miscellaneous—cont'd				
Monosodium glutamate (MSG) AAP 7 H — W —				
Olopatadine AAP — H — W S?	Low exposure when used as eye drops; plasma concentration			<0.5–1.3 ng/mL
Papaverine AAP — H — W —	23 ± 6	2	91 ± 4	1.5
Povidone-iodine AAP 6 H L4 W —				
Pravastatin AAP — H L3 W NS?	17–18	0.7–1.6	43–55	0.67 ± 0.21
Probenecid AAP — H— W S	100		89 ± 6	0.17 ± 0.03
Rubella vaccine AAP — H L2 W U				
Silicone AAP 7 H L3 (breast implants) W —				
Sulfinpyrazone AAP — H — W —	99		98.3 ± 0.5	0.74 ± 0.23

Milk/plasma (M/P) ratio	Adult dose in milk (%)	Maximum amount in milk (mg/L)	Comments and references
			No reports of effects on the milk.
			(393)
			Extensive first-pass metabolism. Bioavailability of slow-release tablets: 68% and 89%. (455, 477)
8–25	15		Increase of iodine in the milk and a shift in concentration of neonatal TSH when used on or by mother. Brand names: Betadine, Massengill. (88, 106, 112)
	<0.4	0.047	In milk: peak 3.3 ± 0.8 hr. Oral absorption: 34%. Food in GI tract reduces bioavailability. Brand name: Pravachol. (381, 393, 459)
			Dose-dependent half-life. Brand name: Benemid. (181, 477)
	Live, attenuated virus gets into milk		Infant may have serologic evidence of disease but does not exhibit severe symptoms. Does not enhance or suppress subsequent response to vaccine in early childhood. (265, 393)
			Determined by FDA to be safe and not enter breast milk. Esophageal dysmotility from implants unproven. Found in foods and medicines.
			Brand name: Anturane. (181)

Continued

TABLE D-1 **Relationship of drugs to breast milk and effect on infant—cont'd**

Drugs and ratings[*]	Oral availability (%)	Peak plasma time (hr)	Plasma protein bound (%)	Volume of distribution (L/kg)
Miscellaneous—cont'd				
Theophylline AAP 6 H L3 W S?	65–100	1.5 ± 0.5	55 ± 15	0.5 ± 0.16
Thiouracil AAP 6 H — W —				
Tiapamil AAP — H — W —	15–40		75	
Tubocurarine AAP — H — W S?			50 ± 8	0.39 ± 0.14
Zafirlukast AAP — H L3 W S?		2–4	>99	
Zolpidem AAP 6 H L2 W S	67 ± 4	0.5–2	92	

[*]Ratings for each drug represent three classification systems: American Academy of Pediatrics (AAP), Hale (H), and Weiner (W). See text for a complete listing of categories in each system. A dash indicates that the drug is not listed in that system.

cAMP, cyclic adenosine monophosphate; CNS, central nervous system; C-section, cesarean section; ECG, electrocardiogram; GI, gastrointestinal; G6PD, glucose-6-phosphate dehydrogenase; IM, intramuscular; IV, intravenous; MRI, magnetic resonance imaging; NSAID, nonsteroidal antiinflammatory drug; RBC, red blood cell; SIDS, sudden infant death syndrome; T_3, triiodothyronine; T_4, thyroxine; TSH, thyroid-stimulating harmone.

© The Lactation Study Center, Rochester, New York.

Milk/plasma (M/P) ratio	Adult dose in milk (%)	Maximum amount in milk (mg/L)	Comments and references
0.45–1.08	<1–15	8	In milk: peak 1–3 hr; half-life 6 ± 2 hr; 6.7%–20% newborn therapeutic dose. Extremely low clearance in infants less than 6 months old. Brand names: Marax, Quibron, Theolair. (6, 17, 20, 50, 67, 172, 175, 181, 455, 461, 477, 493)
			Propylthiouracil is the safer choice.
0.36–0.6			Is extensively bound to tissues. (206)
			(2, 181, 477)
0.2			Extensive first-pass metabolism. Food decreases mean bioavailability by 40%. Brand name: Accolate. (393)
0.11–0.18	0.005–0.019		Most of the drug excretion into milk occurs in the first 3 hr. Brand name: Ambien. (144, 396, 455)

REFERENCES

1. Abramowicz M: Moricizine for cardiac arrhythmias. Med Lett Drugs Ther 32:99, 1990.
2. Agoston S, Vandenbrom RHG, Wierda JMKH: Clinical pharmacokinetics of neuromuscular blocking drugs. Clin Pharmacokinet 22:94, 1992.
3. Akagi H, Reynolds A, Hjelm M: Cyclosporin A and its metabolites: Distribution in blood and tissues. J Int Med Res 19:1, 1991.
4. Akintonwa A, Gbajumo SA, Mabadeje AFB: Placental and milk transfer of chloroquine in humans. Ther Drug Monit 10:147, 1988.
5. Ali-Melkkila T, Kanto J, Iisalo E: Pharmacokinetics and related pharmacodynamics of anticholinergic drugs. Acta Anaesthesiol Scand 37:633, 1993.
6. American Academy of Pediatrics, Committee on Drugs: The transfer of drugs and other chemicals into human milk. Pediatrics 108:776, 2001.
7. American Hospital Formulary Service: AHFS Drug Information. Bethesda, MD, American Society of Hospital Pharmacists, 1993.
8. Anderson P, Bondesson U, Mattiasson I, et al: Verapamil and norverapamil in plasma and breast milk during breast-feeding. Eur J Clin Pharmacol 31:625, 1987.
9. Anderson PO: Drug use during breast-feeding. Clin Pharm 10:594, 1991.
10. Andersson P, Brattsand R, Dahlstrom K, et al: Oral availability of fluticasone propionate. Br J Clin Pharmacol 36:135, 1993.
11. Antony KK, Lewis EW, Kenny MT, et al: Pharmacokinetics and bioavailability of a new formulation of teicoplanin following intravenous and intramuscular administration to humans. J Pharm Sci 80:605, 1991.
12. Anyebuno MA, Rosenfeld CR: Chloral hydrate toxicity in term infant. Dev Pharmacol Ther 17:116, 1991.
13. Arenas RV, Johnson NA: Liquid chromatographic fluorescence method for multiresidue determination of thiabendazole and 5-hydroxythiabendazole in milk. J AOAC Int 78:642, 1995.
14. Asch RH, Smith CG: Effects of 9-THC, the principal psychoactive component of marijuana, during pregnancy in the rhesus monkey. J Reprod Med 31:1071, 1986.
15. Assies J: Hyperprolactinaemia in diethylstilboestrol-exposed women. Lancet 337:983, 1991.
16. Astley SJ, Little RE: Maternal marijuana use during lactation and infant development at one year. Neurotoxicol Teratol 12:161, 1990.
17. Atkinson HC, Begg EJ: Prediction of drug concentrations in human skim milk from plasma protein binding and acid-base characteristics. Br J Clin Pharmacol 25:495, 1988.
18. Atkinson HC, Begg EJ: The binding of drugs to major human milk whey proteins. Br J Clin Pharmacol 26:107, 1988.
19. Atkinson HC, Begg EJ: Prediction of drug distribution into human milk from physiochemical characteristics. Clin Pharmacokinet 18:151, 1990.
20. Atkinson HC, Begg EJ, Darlow BA: Drugs in human milk: Clinical pharmacokinetic considerations. Clin Pharmacokinet 14:217, 1988.
21. Aujard Y, Brion F, Jacqz-Aigrain E, et al: Pharmacokinetics of cefotaxime and desacetylcefotaxime in the newborn. Diagn Microbiol Infect Dis 12:87, 1989.
22. Awad AG, Lapierre YD, Jostell K-G, et al: Selective dopamine D2 antagonist and prolactin response in acute schizophrenia: Results from remoxipride studies. Progr Neuropsychopharmacol Biol Psychiatry 14:769, 1990.
23. Bach V, Carl P, Ravlo O, et al: A randomized comparison between midazolam and thiopental for elective cesarean section anesthesia. III. Placental transfer and elimination in neonates. Anesth Analg 68:238, 1989.
24. Backhouse C, Wade A, Williamson P: Multiple dose pharmacokinetics of cefpodoxime in young adult and elderly patients. J Antimicrob Chemother 26(suppl E):29, 1990.
25. Bailey DG, Spence JD, Munoz C, et al: Interaction of citrus juices with felodipine and nifedipine. Lancet 337:268, 1991.
26. Bailey DG, Arnold JMO, Strong HA, et al: Effect of grapefruit juice and naringin on nisoldipine pharmacokinetics. Clin Pharmacol Ther 54:589, 1993.
27. Bairam A, Akramoff-Gershan L, Beharry K, et al: Gastrointestinal absorption of doxapram in neonates. Am J Perinatol 8:110, 1991.
28. Baker PA, Schroeder D: Interpleural bupivacaine for postoperative pain during lactation. Anesth Analg 69:400, 1989.
29. Balant-Gorgia AE, Gex-Fabry M, Balant LP: Clinical pharmacokinetics of clomipramine. Clin Pharmacokinet 20:447, 1991.
30. Bald R, Bernbeck-Betthauser E-M, Spahn H, et al: Excretion of azapropazone in human breast milk. Eur J Clin Pharmacol 39:271, 1990.
31. Baldessarini RJ, Frankenburg FR: Clozapine: A novel antipsychotic agent. N Engl J Med 324:746, 1991.
32. Baley JE, Meyers C, Kliegman RM, et al: Pharmacokinetics, outcome of treatment, and toxic effects of amphotericin B and 5-fluorocytosine in neonates. J Pediatr 116:791, 1990.
33. Balfour JA, Buckley MMT: Etodolac: A reappraisal of its pharmacology and therapeutic use in rheumatic diseases and pain states. Drugs 42:274, 1991.
34. Balfour JA, Goa KL: Benazepril: A review of its pharmacodynamic and pharmacokinetic properties, and therapeutic efficacy in hypertension and congestive heart failure. Drugs 42:511, 1991.
35. Barr WH, Lin C-C, Radwanski E, et al: The pharmacokinetics of ceftibuten in humans. Diagn Microbiol Infect Dis 14:93, 1991.

36. Bartha L, Nagy GM, Kiem DT, et al: Inhibition of suckling-induced prolactin release by dexamethasone. Endocrinology 129:635, 1991.

37. Bassetti D, Cruciani M: Teicoplanin therapy in children: A review. Scand J Infect Dis 72(suppl):35, 1990.

38. Bauer J, Uhlig B, Schrell U, et al: Exhaustion of postictal serum prolactin release during status epilepticus. J Neurol 239:175, 1992.

39. Beall MH: Advising the nursing mother about her medications. Contemp Pediatr 5:67, 1988.

40. Beaulac-Baillargeon L, Allard G: Distribution of indomethacin in human milk and estimation of its milk to plasma ratio in vitro. Br J Clin Pharmacol 36:413, 1993.

41. Beeley L: Drugs and breastfeeding. Clin Obstet Gynecol 13:247, 1986.

42. Begg EJ, Atkinson HC, Duffull SB: Prospective evaluation of a model for the prediction of milk: Plasma drug concentrations from physiochemical characteristics. Br J Clin Pharmacol 33:501, 1992.

43. Bennett PN, Humphries SJ, Osborne JP, et al: Use of sodium aurothiomalate during lactation. Br J Clin Pharmacol 29:777, 1990.

44. Benowith NL: Clinical pharmacology and toxicology of cocaine. Pharmacol Toxicol 72:3, 1993.

45. Bergan T, Thorsteinsson SB, Albini E: Pharmacokinetic profile of fosfomycin trometamol. Chemotherapy 39:297, 1993.

46. Berlin CM: Advances in pediatric pharmacology and toxicology. Adv Pediatr 34:411, 1987.

47. Berlin CM Jr: Drugs in breastfeeding. Pediatrics 95:957, 1995.

48. Bertilsson L, Tomson T: Clinical pharmacokinetics and pharmacological effects of carbamazepine and carbamazepine-10,11-epoxide: An update. Clin Pharmacol Ther 11:177, 1986.

49. Bertuzzi A, Gandolfi A, Salinari S, et al: Pharmacokinetic analysis of azelaic acid disodium salt: a proposed substrate for total parenteral nutrition. Clin Pharmacokinet 20:411, 1991.

50. Besunder JB, Reed MD, Blumer JL: Principles of drug biodisposition in the neonate: A critical evaluation of the pharmacokinetic-pharmacodynamic interface. I. Clin Pharmacokinet 14:189, 1988.

51. Besunder JB, Reed MD, Blumer JL: Principles of drug biodisposition in the neonate: A critical evaluation of the pharmacokinetic-pharmacodynamic interface. II. Clin Pharmacokinet 14:261, 1988.

52. Bialer M: Clinical pharmacology of valpromide. Clin Pharmacokinet 20:114, 1991.

53. Bialer M: Comparative pharmacokinetics of the newer antiepileptic drugs. Clin Pharmacokinet 24:441, 1993.

54. Bishop NJ: Aluminum in infant feeding: Is it a problem? Eur J Clin Nutr 46(suppl 4):S37, 1992.

55. Bixler EO, Kales A, Manfredi RL, et al: Next-day memory impairment with triazolam use. Lancet 337:827, 1991.

56. Blum RA, D'Andrea DT, Florentino BM, et al: Increased gastric pH and the bioavailability of fluconazole and ketoconazole. Ann Intern Med 114:755, 1991.

57. Boeckh M, Lode H, Hoffken G, et al: Pharmacokinetics of roxithromycin and influence of H_2-blockers and antacids on gastrointestinal absorption. Eur J Clin Microbiol Infect Dis 11:465, 1992.

58. Borgatta L, Jenny RW, Gruss L: Clinical significance of methohexital meperidine and diazepam in breast milk. J Clin Pharmacol 37:186, 1997.

59. Bottorff MB, Hoon TJ, Rodman JH, et al: Pharmacokinetics and pharmacodynamics of urapidil in severe hypertension. J Clin Pharmacol 28:420, 1988.

60. Boudreau EF, Fleckenstein L, Pang LW, et al: Mefloquine kinetics in cured and recrudescent patients with acute falciparum malaria and in healthy volunteers. Clin Pharmacol Ther 48:399, 1990.

61. Bourget P, Quinquis-Desmaris V, Fernandez H: Ceftriaxone distribution and protein binding between maternal blood and milk postpartum. Ann Pharmacother 27:294, 1993.

62. Boutroy MJ, Bianchetti G, Dubruc C, et al: To nurse when receiving acebutolol: Is it dangerous for the neonate? Eur J Clin Pharmacol 30:737, 1986.

63. Branebjerg PE, Heisterberg L: Blood and milk concentration of ampicillin in mothers treated with pivampicillin and in their infants. J Perinat Med 15:555, 1987.

64. Branski D, Kerem E, Gross-Kieselstein E, et al: Bloody diarrhea: A possible complication of sulfasalazine transferred through human breast milk. J Pediatr Gastroenterol Nutr 5:316, 1986.

65. Brashear WT, Zuspan KJ, Lazebnik N, et al: Effect of ranitidine on bupivacaine disposition. Anesth Analg 72:369, 1991.

66. Bree F, Houin G, Barre J, et al: Binding to alpha-1-acid glycoprotein and relevant apparent volume of distribution. Prog Clin Biol Res 300:321, 1989.

67. Briggs GC, Freeman RK, Yaffe SJ: Drugs in Pregnancy and Lactation, 6th ed. A Reference Guide to Fetal and Neonatal Risk. Philadelphia, Lippincott, Williams & Wilkins, 2002.

68. Briggs GG, Samson JH, Ambrose PJ, et al: Excretion of bupropion in breast milk. Ann Pharmacother 27:431, 1993.

69. Brixen-Rasmussen L, Halgrener J, Jorgensen A: Amitriptyline and nortriptyline excretion in human breast milk. Psychopharmacology (Berl) 76:94, 1982.

70. Brocks DR, Jamali F: Clinical pharmacokinetics of ketorolac tromethamine. Clin Pharmacokinet 23:415, 1992.

71. Brodie MJ, Feely J: Adverse drug interactions. Br Med J 296:845, 1988.

72. Brunel P, Lecaillon JB, Guyene TT, et al: Influence of acetylator status on the haemodynamic effects and pharmacokinetics of cadralazine in healthy subjects. Br J Clin Pharmacol 29:503, 1990.

73. Bryson HM, Faulds D: Intranasal flucticasone propionate: A review of its pharmacodynamic and pharmacokinetic properties, and therapeutic potential in allergic rhinitis. Drugs 43:760, 1992.

74. Bryson HM, Goa KL: Halofantrine: A review of its anti-malarial activity, pharmacokinetic properties and therapeutic potential. Drugs 43:236, 1992.

75. Buckley MM, Brogden RN, Barradell LB, Goa KL: Imipenem/cilastatin: A reappraisal of its antibacterial activity, pharmacokinetic properties and therapeutic efficacy. Drugs 44:408, 1992.

76. Buckley MMT, Goa KL, Clissold SP: Ocular betaxolol: A review of its pharmacological properties, and therapeutic efficacy in glaucoma and ocular hypertension. Drugs 40:75, 1990.

77. Buckley MMT, Grant SM, Goa KL, et al: Diltiazem: A reappraisal of its pharmacological properties and therapeutic use. Drugs 39:757, 1990.

78. Buesa JM, Urrechaga E: Clinical pharmacokinetics of high dose DTIC. Cancer Chemother Pharmacol 28:475, 1991.

79. Buist A, Norman TR, Dennerstein L: Breastfeeding and the use of psychotropic medication: A review. J Affective Disord 19:197, 1990.

80. Bulau P, Paar WD, von Unruh GE: Pharmacokinetics of oxcarbazepine and 10-hydroxy-carbazepine in the newborn child of an oxcarbazepine-treated mother. Eur J Clin Pharmacol 34:311, 1988.

81. Burch KJ, Wells BG: Fluoxetine/norfluoxetine concentrations in human milk. Pediatrics 89:676, 1992.

82. Camaggi CM, Strocchi E, Carisi P, et al: Idarubicin metabolism and pharmacokinetics after intravenous and oral administration in cancer patients: A crossover study. Cancer Chemother Pharmacol 30:307, 1992.

83. Campa M, Zolfino I, Senesi S, et al: The penetration of roxithromycin into human skin. J Antimicrobial Chemother 26:87, 1990.

84. Campoli-Richards DM, Buckley MMT, Fitton A: Cetirizine: A review of its pharmacological properties and clinical potential in allergic rhinitis, pollen-induced asthma, and chronic urticaria. Drugs 40:762, 1990.

85. Campoli-Richards DM, Clissold SP: Famotidine: Pharmacodynamic and pharmacokinetic properties and a preliminary review of its therapeutic use in peptic ulcer disease and Zollinger-Ellison syndrome. Drugs 32:197, 1986.

86. Cefali EA, Poynor WJ, Sica D, et al: Pharmacokinetic comparison of flurbiprofen in end-stage renal disease subjects and subjects with normal renal function. J Clin Pharmacol 31:808, 1991.

87. Celiloglu M, Celiker S, Guven H, et al: Gentamicin excretion and uptake from breast milk by nursing infants. Obstet Gynecol 84:263, 1994.

88. Chanoine JP, Boulvain M, Bourdoux P, et al: Increased recall rate at screening for congenital hypothyroidism in breastfed infants born to iodine overloaded mothers. Arch Dis Child 63:1207, 1988.

89. Charm SE, Chi R: Microbial receptor assay for rapid detection and identification of seven families of antimicrobial drugs in milk: Collaborative study. J Assoc Off Anal Chem 71:304, 1988.

90. Chen T-M, Chiou WL: Large differences in the biological half-life and volume of distribution of hydrochlorothiazide in normal subjects from eleven studies. Int J Clin Pharmacol Ther Toxicol 30:34, 1992.

91. Chu S-Y, Park Y, Locke C, et al: Drug-food interaction potential of clarithromycin, a new macrolide antimicrobial. J Clin Pharmacol 32:32, 1992.

92. Chung KF, Barnes PJ: Treatment of asthma. Br Med J 294:103, 1987.

93. Clissold SP, Campoli-Richards DM: Omeprazole: A preliminary review of its pharmacodynamic and pharmacokinetic properties, and therapeutic potential in peptic ulcer disease and Zollinger-Ellison syndrome. Drugs 32:15, 1986.

94. Cockerill FR, Edson RS: Trimethoprim-sulfamethoxazole. Mayo Clin Proc 66:1260, 1991.

95. Colthup PV, Felgate CC, Palmer JL, et al: Determination of ondansetron in plasma and its pharmacokinetics in the young and elderly. J Pharm Sci 80:868, 1991.

96. Cooper DS: Antithyroid drugs: To breast-feed or not to breast-feed. Am J Obstet Gynecol 157:234, 1987.

97. Cooper MA, Nye K, Andrews JM, et al: The pharmacokinetics and inflammatory fluid penetration of orally administered azithromycin. J Antimicrob Chemother 26:533, 1990.

98. Copeland CA, Raebel MA, Wagner SL: Pesticide residue in lanolin. JAMA 261:242, 1989.

99. Coumel P, Leclercq JF, Escoubet B: Beta-blockers: Use for arrhythmias. Eur Heart J 8(suppl A):41, 1987.

100. Cover DL, Mueller BA: Ciprofloxacin penetration into human breast milk: A case report, DICP. Ann Pharmacother 24:703, 1990.

101. Criscuoli M, Lippi A, Mengozzi G: Pharmacokinetics and pharmacodynamics of idrapril in rats, dogs, and humans. Drug Metab Dispos 21:835, 1993.

102. Cuzzolin L, Fanos V, Zambreri D, et al: Pharmacokinetics and renal tolerance of aztreonam in premature infants. Antimicrob Agents Chemother 35:1726, 1991.

103. Dahlstrom A, Lundell B, Curvall M, et al: Nicotine and cotinine concentrations in the nursing mother and her infant. Acta Paediatr Scand 79:142, 1990.

104. Dailland P, Cockshott ID, Lirzin JD, et al: Intravenous propofol during cesarean section: placental transfer, concentrations in breast milk, and neonatal effects—A preliminary study. Anesthesiology 71:827, 1989.

105. Dan M, Weidekamm E, Sagiv R, et al: Penetration of fleroxacin into breast milk and pharmacokinetics in lactating women. Antimicrob Agents Chemother 37:293, 1993.

106. Davies BE, Coates PE, Clarke JGN, et al: Bioavailability and pharmacokinetics of clavulanic acid in healthy subjects. Int J Clin Pharmacol Ther Toxicol 23:70, 1985.

107. Debruyne D, Ryckelynck J-P: Clinical pharmacokinetics of fluconazole. Clin Pharmacokinet 24:10, 1993.

108. Dechant KL, Brogden RN, Pilkington T, et al: Ifosfamide/mesna: A review of its antineoplastic activity, pharmacokinetic properties and therapeutic efficacy in cancer. Drugs 42:428, 1991.

109. Dechant KL, Clissold SP: Paroxetine: A review of its pharmacodynamic and pharmacological properties, and therapeutic potential in depressive illness. Drugs 41:225, 1991.

110. Dechant KL, Clissold SP: Sumatriptan: A review of its pharmacodynamic and pharmacokinetic properties and therapeutic efficacy in the acute treatment of migraine and cluster headache. Drugs 43:776, 1992.

111. Dechant KL, Goa KL: Levocabastine: A review of its pharmacological properties and therapeutic potential as a topical antihistamine in allergic rhinitis and conjunctivitis. Drugs 41:202, 1991.

112. Delange F, Chanoine JP, Abrassart C, et al: Topical iodine, breastfeeding, and neonatal hypothyroidism. Arch Dis Child 63:106, 1988.

113. Del Favero A, Patoia L, Rosina R, et al: Pharmacokinetics and tolerability of teicoplanin in healthy volunteers after single increasing doses. Antimicrob Agents Chemother 35:2551, 1991.

114. Delhotal-Landes B, Flouvat B, Duchier J, et al: Pharmacokinetics of lansoprazole in patients with renal or liver disease of varying severity. Eur J Clin Pharmacol 45:367, 1993.

115. De Mey C, Enterling D, Brendel E, et al: Pharmacokinetics and pharmacodynamics of single oral doses of ibopamine, quinidine, and their combination in normal man. Eur J Clin Pharmacol 34:415, 1988.

116. Derendorf H, Mollmann H, Barth J, et al: Pharmacokinetics and oral bioavailability of hydrocortisone. J Clin Pharmacol 31:473, 1991.

117. Desager JP, Horsmans Y, Harvengt C: A pharmacokinetic evaluation of the second-generation H_1-receptor antagonist cetirizine in very young children. Clin Pharmacol Ther 53:431, 1993.

118. Dickinson TH, Egan JM, Abernethy DR: Effects of nifedipine on hepatic drug oxidation. Pharmacology 36:405, 1988.

119. Dodson WE: Special pharmacokinetic considerations in children. Epilepsia 28(suppl):S56, 1987.

120. Don PC, Kizner R: Excretion of acyclovir in human breast milk. J Am Acad Dermatol 25:342, 1991.

121. Donnelly R, Elliott HL, Meredith PA, et al: Concentration-effect relationships and individual responses to doxazosin in essential hypertension. Br J Clin Pharmacol 28:517, 1989.

122. Donnelly R, Macphee GJA: Clinical pharmacokinetics and kinetic-dynamic relationships of dilevalol and labetalol. Clin Pharmacokinet 21:95, 1991.

123. Dostal LA, Schwetz BA: Determination of diphenhydramine in rat milk and plasma and its effects on milk composition and mammary gland nucleic acids. J Pharm Sci 78:423, 1989.

124. Drijver M, Duijkers TJ, Kromhout D, et al: Determinants of polychlorinated biphenyls (PCBs) in human milk. Acta Paediatr Scand 77:30, 1988.

125. Dudley MN, Marchbanks CR, Flor SC, et al: The effect of food or milk on the absorption kinetics of ofloxacin. Eur J Clin Pharmacol 41:569, 1991.

126. Dunselman PHJM, Edgar B: Felodipine clinical pharmacokinetics. Clin Pharmacokinet 21:418, 1991.

127. Dusci LJ, Good SM, Hall RW, et al: Excretion of diazepam and its metabolites in human milk during withdrawal from combination high dose diazepam and oxazepam. Br J Clin Pharmacol 29:123, 1990.

128. Dydek GJ, Blue PW: Human breast milk excretion of iodine-131 following diagnostic and therapeutic administration to a lactating patient with Graves' disease. J Nucl Med 29:407, 1988.

129. Eadie MJ: Formation of active metabolites of anticonvulsant drugs: A review of their pharmacokinetic and therapeutic significance. Clin Pharmacokinet 21:27, 1991.

130. Ebihara A, Fujimura A: Metabolites of antihypertensive drugs: An updated review of their clinical pharmacokinetic and therapeutic implications. Clin Pharmacokinet 21:331, 1991.

131. Echizen H, Ishizaki T: Clinical pharmacokinetics of famotidine. Clin Pharmacokinet 21:178, 1991.

132. Edgar B, Bailey D, Bergstrand R, et al: Acute effects of drinking grapefruit juice on the pharmacokinetics and dynamics of felodipine and its potential clinical relevance. Eur J Clin Pharmacol 42:313, 1992.

133. Edstein MD, Rieckmann KH: Lack of effect of proguanil on the pharmacokinetics of dapsone in healthy volunteers. Chemotherapy 39:235, 1993.

134. Edstein MD, Veenendaal JR, Hyslop R: Excretion of mefloquine in human breast milk. Chemotherapy 34:165, 1988.

135. Edstein MD, Veenendaal JR, Newman K, et al: Excretion of chloroquine, dapsone, and pyrimethamine in human milk. Br J Clin Pharmacol 22:733, 1986.

136. Ehrenkranz RA, Ackerman BA, Hulse JD: Nifedipine transfer into human milk. J Pediatr 114:478, 1989.

137. Ehrinpreis MN, Dhar R, Narula A: Cimetidine-induced galactorrhea. Am J Gastroenterol 84:563, 1989.

138. Eksborg S, Soderberg M, Nilsson B, et al: Plasma pharmacokinetics of idarubicin and its 13-hydroxy-metabolite after intravenous and oral administration under fasting and non-fasting conditions. Acta Oncol 29:921, 1990.

139. Epperson CN, Anderson GM, McDougle CJ: Sertraline and breast-feeding. N Engl J Med 336:1189, 1997.

140. Etienne M-C, Milano G, Rene N, et al: Improved bioavailability of a new oral preparation of medroxyprogesterone acetate. J Pharm Sci 80:1130, 1991.

141. Faber P, Strenge-Hesse A: Relevance of rhein excretion into breast milk. Pharmacology 36:212, 1988.

142. Fahr A: Cyclosporin clinical pharmacokinetics. Clin Pharmacokinet 24:472, 1993.

143. Fassbender M, Lode H, Schaberg T, et al: Pharmacokinetics of new oral cephalosporins, including a new carbacephem. Clin Infect Dis 16:646, 1993.

144. Fattapposta F, Sanarelli L, Valle E, et al: A double-blind study of the effects of zolpidem, a new imidazopyridine hypnotic, on contingent negative variation in patients with situational insomnia. Curr Ther Res 48:766, 1990.

145. Fattinger K, Vozeh S, Ha HR, et al: Population pharmacokinetics of quinidine. Br J Clin Pharmacol 31:279, 1991.

146. Faulds D, Brogden RN: Didanosine: A review of its antiviral activity, pharmacokinetic properties and therapeutic potential in human immunodeficiency virus infection. Drugs 44:94, 1992.

147. Faulds D, Goa KL, Benfield P: Cyclosporin: A review of its pharmacodynamic and pharmacokinetic properties, and therapeutic use in immunoregulatory disorders. Drugs 45:953, 1993.

148. Fauler J, Verner LJ: The pharmacokinetics of clonidine in high dosage. Eur J Clin Pharmacol 45:165, 1993.

149. Feliciano NR, Bouvet AA, Redalieu E, et al: Pharmacokinetic and pharmacodynamic comparison of an osmotic release oral metoprolol tablet and the metoprolol conventional tablet. Am Heart J 120:483, 1990.

150. Fitton A, Buckley MMT: Moricizine: A review of its pharmacological properties, and therapeutic efficacy in cardiac arrhythmias. Drugs 40:138, 1990.

151. Fitton A, Goa KL: Azelaic acid: A review of its pharmacological properties and therapeutic efficacy in acne and hyperpigmentary skin disorders. Drugs 41:780, 1991.

152. Fitton A, Sorkin EM: Sotalol: An updated review of its pharmacological properties and therapeutic use in cardiac arrhythmias. Drugs 46:678, 1993.

153. Fleishaker JC, Desai N, McNamara J: Factors affecting the milk-to-plasma drug concentration ratio in lactating women: Physical interactions with protein and fat. J Pharm Sci 76:189, 1987.

154. Fondevila CG, Meschengieser S, Blanco A, et al: Effect of acenocoumarine on the breast-fed infant. Thromb Res 56:29, 1989.

155. Fonne-Pfister R, Meyer UA: Xenobiotic and endobiotic inhibitors of cytochrome P-450dbl function, the target of the debrisoquine/sparteine type polymorphism. Biochem Pharmacol 37:3829, 1988.

156. Force RW: Fluconazole concentrations in breast milk. Pediatr Infect Dis J 14:235, 1995.

157. Fotherby K: Pharmacokinetics of gestagens: Some problems. Am J Obstet Gynecol 163:323, 1990.

158. Fowles SE, Pierce DM, Prince WT, et al: The tolerance to and pharmacokinetics of penciclovir (BRL 39 123A), a novel antiherpes agent, administered by intravenous infusion to healthy subjects. Eur J Clin Pharmacol 43:513, 1992.

159. Fraschini F, Scaglione F, Demartini G: Clarithromycin clinical pharmacokinetics. Clin Pharmacokinet 25:189, 1993.

160. Freedman MD, Somberg JC: Pharmacology and pharmacokinetics amiodarone. J Clin Pharmacol 31:1061, 1991.

161. Frey B, Schubinger G, Musy JP: Transient cholestatic hepatitis in a neonate associated with carbamazepine exposure during pregnancy and breastfeeding. Eur J Pediatr 150:136, 1990.

162. Frey BM, Frey FJ: Clinical pharmacokinetics of prednisone and prednisolone. Clin Pharmacokinet 19:126, 1990.

163. Friedel HA, Brogden RN: Pinacidil: A review of its pharmacodynamic and pharmacokinetic properties, and therapeutic potential in the treatment of hypertension. Drugs 39:929, 1990.

164. Friedel HA, Buckley MMT: Torasemide: A review of its pharmacological properties and therapeutic potential. Drugs 41:81, 1991.

165. Frishman WH: Comparative pharmacokinetic and clinical profiles of angiotensin-converting enzyme inhibitors and calcium antagonists in systemic hypertension. Am J Cardiol 69:17C, 1992.

166. Frishman WH, Lazar EJ, Gorodokin G: Pharmacokinetic optimisation of therapy with beta-adrenergic blocking agents. Clin Pharmacokinet 20:311, 1991.

167. Fujimura A, Ohashi K, Tsuru M, et al: Clinical pharmacology of dilevalol. I. Comparison of the pharmacokinetic and pharmacodynamic properties of dilevalol and labetalol after a single oral administration in subjects. J Clin Pharmacol 29:635, 1989.

168. Fujimura A, Ohashi K, Tsuru M, et al: Clinical pharmacology of dilevalol. II. The pharmacokinetic, pharmacodynamic and tolerance studies of dilevalol during repeated administration in healthy subjects. J Clin Pharmacol 29:643, 1989.

169. Fulton B, Moore LL: Comment: Ciprofloxacin excretion into breast milk, DICP. Ann Pharmacother 24:1122, 1990.

170. Funck-Brentano C, Kroemer HK, Lee JT, et al: Drug therapy. N Engl J Med 322:518, 1990.

171. Gabilan JC, Benattar C, Lindenbaum A: Clofibrate treatment of neonatal jaundice. Pediatrics 86:647, 1990.

172. Gal P: Therapeutic drug monitoring in neonates: Problems and issues. Drug Intell Clin Pharm 22:317, 1988.

173. Galgiani JN: Fluconazole, a new antifungal agent. Ann Intern Med 113:177, 1990.

174. Gan VN, Chu S-Y, Kusmiesz HT, et al: Pharmacokinetics of a clarithromycin suspension in infants and children. Antimicrob Agents Chemother 36:2478, 1992.

175. Gardner MJ, Schatz M, Zeiger R, et al: Longitudinal effects of pregnancy on the pharmacokinetics of theophylline. Eur J Clin Pharmacol 31:289, 1987.

176. Garg DC, Jallad NS, Singh S, et al: Efficacy and pharmacokinetics of oral pirmenol, a new anti-arrhythmic drug. J Clin Pharmacol 28:812, 1988.

177. Garrigues TM, Martin U, Peris-Ribera JE, et al: Dose-dependent absorption and elimination of cefadroxil in man. Eur J Clin Pharmacol 41:179, 1991.

178. Giacoia GP, Jungbluth GL, Jusko WJ: Effect of formula feeding on oral absorption of caffeine in premature infants. Dev Pharmacol Ther 12:205, 1989.

179. Giamarellou H, Kolokythas E, Petrikkos G, et al: Pharmacokinetics of three newer quinolones in pregnant and lactating women. Am J Med 87(suppl 5A):49S, 1989.

180. Gill J, Heel RC, Fitton A: Amiodarone: An overview of its pharmacological properties, and review of its therapeutic use in cardiac arrhythmias. Drugs 43:69, 1992.

181. Gilman AG, Rall TW, Nies AS, et al (eds): The Pharmacological Basis of Therapeutics, 8th ed. New York, Pergamon Press, 1990.

182. Gin T, Yau G, Jong W, et al: Disposition of propofol at caesarean section and in the postpartum period. Br J Anaesth 67:49, 1991.

183. Goa KL, McTavish D, Clissold SP: Ivermectin: A review of its antifilarial activity, pharmacokinetic properties and clinical efficacy in onchocerciasis. Drugs 42:640, 1991.

184. Goa KL, Ross SR, Chrisp P: Lamotrigine: A review of its pharmacological properties and clinical efficiency in epilepsy. Drugs 46:152, 1993.

185. Godo G, Koloszar S, Szilagyi I, et al: Experience relating to pregnancy, lactation, and the after-weaning condition of hyperprolactinemic patients treated with bromocriptine. Fertil Steril 51:529, 1989.

186. Good SS, Koble CS, Crouch R, et al: Isolation and characterization of an ether glucoronide of zidovudine, a major metabolite in monkeys and humans. Drug Metab Dispos 18:321, 1990.

187. Granneman GR, Guay DRP: The influence of age on the pharmacokinetics of temafloxacin. Am J Med 91(suppl 6A):71S, 1991.

188. Grant SM, Clissold SP: Fluconazole: A review of its pharmacodynamic and pharmacokinetic properties, and therapeutic potential in superficial and systemic mycoses. Drugs 39:877, 1990.

189. Green AI, Brown WA: Prolactin and neuroleptic drugs. Neurol Clin 6:213, 1988.

190. Greenberger PA, Patterson R: The management of asthma during pregnancy and lactation. Clin Rev Allergy 5:317, 1987.

191. Greenblatt DJ, Wright CE: Clinical pharmacokinetics of alprazolam: Therapeutic implications. Clin Pharmacokinet 24:453, 1993.

192. Guay DRP, Opsahl JA, McMahon FG, et al: Safety and pharmacokinetics of multiple doses of intravenous ofloxacin in healthy volunteers. Antimicrob Agents Chemother 36:308, 1992.

193. Guerret M, Cheymol G, Hubert M, et al: Simultaneous study of the pharmacokinetics of intravenous and oral nicardipine using a stable isotope. Eur J Clin Pharmacol 37:381, 1989.

194. Guglielmo BJ, Flaherty JF, Batman R, et al: Comparative pharmacokinetics of low and high-dose ticarcillin. Antimicrob Agents Chemother 30:359, 1986.

195. Guimaraes FS: Fluoxetine and fluvoxamine. Br J Hosp Med 45:146, 1991.

196. Guttendorf RJ, Wedlund PJ: Genetic aspects of drug disposition and therapeutics. J Clin Pharmacol 32:107, 1992.

197. Hackett LP, Wojnar-Horton RE, Dusci LJ, et al: Excretion of sotalol in breast milk. Br J Clin Pharmacol 29:277, 1990.

198. Haefeli EW, Vozeh S, Ha HR, et al: Comparison of the pharmacodynamic effects of intravenous and oral propafenone. Clin Pharmacol Ther 48:245, 1990.

199. Hale TW: Medications and Mother's milk, 10th ed. Amarillo, TX, Pharmasoft Publishing, 2002.

200. Hall ST, Harding SM, Evans GL, et al: Clinical pharmacology of lacidipine. J Cardiovasc Pharmacol 17:S9, 1991.

201. Hallen IP, Oskarsson A: Dose dependent transfer of 203lead to milk and tissue uptake in suckling offspring studied in rats and mice. Pharmacol Toxicol 73:174, 1993.

202. Hansdottir V, Hedner T, Woestenborghs R, et al: The CSF and plasma pharmacokinetics of sufentanil after intrathecal administration. Anesthesiology 74:264, 1991.

203. Harder S, Thurmann P, Siewert M, et al: Pharmacodynamic profile of verapamil in relation to absolute bioavailability: investigations with a conventional and a controlled-release formulation. J Cardiovasc Pharmacol 17:207, 1991.

204. Harron DWG, Brogden RN, Faulds D, et al: Cibenzoline: A review of its pharmacological properties and therapeutic potential in arrhythmias. Drugs 43:734, 1992.

205. Hartikainen-Sorri AL, Heikkinen JE, Koivisto M: Pharmacokinetics of clonidine during pregnancy and nursing. Obstet Gynecol 69:598, 1987.

206. Hartmann D, Lunell NO, Friedrich G, et al: Excretion of tiapamil in breast milk. Br J Clin Pharmacol 26:183, 1988.

207. Hasselstrom J, Sawe J: Morphine pharmacokinetics and metabolism in humans: Enterohepatic cycling and relative contribution of metabolites to active opioid concentrations. Clin Pharmacokinet 24:344, 1993.

208. Hedrick WR, DiSimone RN, Keen RL: Radiation dosimetry from breast milk excretion of radioiodine and pertechnetate. J Nucl Med 27:1569, 1986.

209. Herrlinger C, Braunfels M, Fink E, et al: Pharmacokinetics and bioavailability of tamoxifen in healthy volunteers. Int J Clin Pharmacol Ther Toxicol 30:487, 1992.

210. Heykants J, Van Peer A, Lavrijsen K, et al: Pharmacokinetics of oral antifungals and their clinical implications. Br J Clin Pharmacol 44(suppl 71):50, 1990.

211. Hii JTY, Duff HJ, Burgess ED: Clinical pharmacokinetics of propafenone. Clin Pharmacokinet 21:1, 1991.

212. Hilbert J, Radwanski E, Affrime MB, et al: Excretion of loratadine in human breast milk. J Clin Pharmacol 28:234, 1988.

213. Hill MR, Szefler SJ, Ball BD, et al: Monitoring glucocorticoid therapy: A pharmacokinetic approach. Clin Pharmacol Ther 48:390, 1990.

214. Hochhaus G, Mollmann H: Pharmacokinetic/pharmacodynamic characteristics of the beta-2-agonists terbutaline,

salbutamol and fenoterol. Int J Clin Pharmacol Ther Toxicol 30:342, 1992.

215. Hofmeyr GJ, Sonnendecker EWW: Secretion of the gastrokinetic agent cisapride in human milk. Eur J Clin Pharmacol 30:735, 1986.

216. Hollingshead LM, Faulds D: Idarubicin: A review of its pharmacodynamic and pharmacokinetic properties, and therapeutic potential in the chemotherapy of cancer. Drugs 42:690, 1991.

217. Hollister LE, Claghorn JL: New antidepressants. Annu Rev Pharmacol Toxicol 32:165, 1993.

218. Hopkins S: Clinical safety and tolerance of azithromycin in children. J Antimicrob Chemother 31(suppl E):111, 1993.

219. Hooper DC, Wolfson JS: Fluoroquinolone antimicrobial agents. N Engl J Med 324:384, 1991.

220. Hoppu K, Neuvonen PJ, Korte T: Disopyramide and breast feeding. Br J Clin Pharmacol 21:533, 1986.

221. Howden CW: Clinical pharmacology of omeprazole. Clin Pharmacokinet 20:38, 1991.

222. Howell P, Davies W, Wrigley M, et al: Comparison of four local extradural anaesthetic solutions for elective caesarean section. Br J Anaesth 65:648, 1990.

223. Howrie DL, Pieniaszek HJ, Fogoros RN, et al: Disposition of moracizine (Ethomozine) in healthy subjects after oral administration of radiolabelled drug. Eur J Clin Pharmacol 32:607, 1987.

224. Huang M-L, Van Peer A, Woestenborghs R, et al: Pharmacokinetics of the novel antipsychotic agent risperidone and the prolactin response in healthy subjects. Clin Pharmacol Ther 54:257, 1993.

225. Hui KK, Duchin KL, Kripalani KJ, et al: Pharmacokinetics of fosinopril in patients with various degrees of renal function. Clin Pharmacol Ther 49:457, 1991.

226. Humbert G, Brumpt I, Montay G, et al: Influence of rifampin on the pharmacokinetics of pefloxacin. Clin Pharmacol Ther 50:682, 1991.

227. Hussar DA: New drugs of 1989. Am Pharm NS30:27, 1990.

228. Hussar DA: New drugs of 1991. Am Pharm NS32:37, 1992.

229. Hussar DA: New drugs of 1992. Am Pharm NS33:20, 1993.

230. Huttunen JK, Gronhagen-Riska C, Fybrquist F: Enalapril treatment of a nursing mother with slightly impaired renal function. Clin Nephrol 31:278, 1989.

231. Isah AO, Rawlins MD, Bateman DN: Clinical pharmacology of prochlorperazine in healthy young males. Br J Clin Pharmacol 32:677, 1991.

232. Isenberg KE: Excretion of fluoxetine in human breast milk. J Clin Psychiatry 51:169, 1990.

233. Jacqz-Aigrain E, Daoud P, Burtin P, et al: Pharmacokinetics of midazolam during continuous infusion in critically ill neonates. Eur J Clin Pharmacol 42:329, 1992.

234. James NC, Donn KH, Collins JJ, et al: Pharmacokinetics of cefuroxime axetil and cefaclor: relationship of concentrations in serum to MICs for common respiratory pathogens. Antimicrob Agents Chemother 35:1860, 1991.

235. Jani JP, Patel JS, Shah MP, et al: Levels of organochlorine pesticides in human milk in Ahmedabad, India. Int Arch Occup Environ Health 60:111, 1988.

236. Jemaa Z, Sabbah S, Bouguerra ML: Preliminary study of organochlorine residues in human milk and cord blood. Acta Biol Hung 38:93, 1987.

237. Johansson E, Odlind V: The passage of exogenous hormones into breast milk: Possible effects. Int J Gynecol Obstet 25(suppl):111, 1987.

238. John DN, Fort S, Lewis MJ, et al: Pharmacokinetics and pharmacodynamics of verapamil following sublingual and oral administration to healthy volunteers. Br J Clin Pharmacol 33:623, 1992.

239. Johnson BF, Wilson J, Johnson J, et al: Digoxin pharmacokinetics and spirapril, a new ace inhibitor. J Clin Pharmacol 31:527, 1991.

240. Jonkers RE, Koopmans RP, Portier EJG, et al: Debrisoquine phenotype and the pharmacokinetic and beta-2 receptor pharmacodynamics of metoprolol and its enantiomers. J Pharmacol Exp Ther 256:959, 1991.

241. Jungbluth GL, Wirth FH Jr, Rubio TT, et al: Developmental pharmacokinetics of mezlocillin in 4 newborn infants. Dev Pharmacol Ther 11:317, 1988.

242. Kamilli I, Gresser U, Schaefer C, et al: Allopurinol in breast milk. Adv Exp Med Biol 309A:143, 1991.

243. Kanja LW, Skaare JU, Ojwang SBO, et al: A comparison of organochlorine pesticide residues in maternal adipose tissue, maternal blood, cord blood, and human milk from mother/infant pairs. Arch Environ Contam Toxicol 22:21, 1992.

244. Karbwang J, Bangchang KN, Bunnag D, et al: Pharmacokinetics and pharmacodynamics of mefloquine in Thai patients with acute falciparum. Bull World Health Organ 69:207, 1991.

245. Karbwang J, Milton KA, Bangchang KN, et al: Pharmacokinetics of halofantrine in Thai patients with acute uncomplicated falciparum malaria. Br J Clin Pharmacol 31:484, 1991.

246. Karlsson MO, Dahlstrom B, Eckernas SA, et al: Pharmacokinetics of oral noscapine. Eur J Clin Pharmacol 39:275, 1990.

247. Kassner JT: Beta blockers. Clin Tox Rev 12:1, 1989.

248. Kates RE: Metabolites of antiarrhythmic drugs: Are they clinically important? Rational Drug Ther 20:1, 1986.

249. Katz E, Schran HF, Weiss BE, et al: Increased circulating levels of bromocriptine after vaginal compared with oral administration. Fertil Steril 55:882, 1991.

250. Kaye B, Cussans NJ, Faulkner JK, et al: The metabolism and kinetics of doxazosin in man, mouse, rat and dog. Br J Clin Pharmacol 21:19S, 1986.

251. Kearns GL, Jacobs RF, Thomas BR, et al: Cefotaxime and desacetylcefotaxime pharmacokinetics in very low birth weight neonates. J Pediatr 114:461, 1989.

252. Kelloway JS, Awni WM, Lin CC, et al: Pharmacokinetics of ceftibuten-cis and its trans metabolite in healthy volunteers and in patients with chronic renal insufficiency. Antimicrob Agents Chemother 35:2267, 1991.

253. Kelly JG, O'Malley K: Clinical pharmacokinetics of calcium antagonists. Clin Pharmacokinet 22:416, 1992.

254. Kelsey JJ, Moser LR, Jennings JC, et al: Presence of azithromycin breast milk concentrations: A case report. Am J Obstet Gynecol 170:1375, 1994.

255. Kenyon CF, Knoppert DC, Lee SK, et al: Amikacin pharmacokinetics and suggested dosage modifications for the preterm infant. Antimicrob Agents Chemother 34:265, 1990.

256. Kilpatrick CJ, Moulds RFW: Anticonvulsants in pregnancy. Med J Aust 154:199, 1991.

257. Kinzig M, Sorgel F, Brismar B, et al: Pharmacokinetics and tissue penetration of tazobactam and piperacillin in patients undergoing colorectal surgery. Antimicrob Agents Chemother 36:1997, 1992.

258. Kirsten R, Nelson K, Molz KH, et al: Influence of food intake on the bioavailability of urapidil in healthy volunteers. Int J Clin Pharmacol 27:298, 1989.

259. Klotz U, Ogbuokiri JE, Okonkwo PO: Ivermectin binds avidly to plasma proteins. Eur J Clin Pharmacol 39:607, 1990.

260. Knupp CA, Milbrath R, Barbhaiya RH: Effect of time of food administration on the bioavailability of didanosine from a chewable tablet formulation. J Clin Pharmacol 33:568, 1993.

261. Kolars JC, Awni WM, Merion RM, et al: First-pass metabolism of cyclosporin by the gut. Lancet 338:1488, 1991.

262. Konishi K, Suzuki H, Hayashi M, et al: Pharmacokinetics of cefuroxime axetil in patients with normal and impaired renal function. J Antimicrob Chemother 31:413, 1993.

263. Kremer JAM, Rolland R, Van der Heijden PFM, et al: Lactation inhibition by a single injection of a new depot-bromocriptine. Br J Obstet Gynaecol 97:527, 1990.

264. Krishna S, ter Kuile F, Supanaranond W, et al: Pharmacokinetics, efficacy and toxicity of parenteral halofantrine in uncomplicated malaria. Br J Clin Pharmacol 36:585, 1993.

265. Krogh V, Duffy LC, Wong D, et al: Postpartum immunization with rubella virus vaccine and antibody response in breastfeeding infants. J Lab Clin Med 113:695, 1989.

266. Kubota K, Lo ES, Huttinot G, et al: Plasma concentrations of betamethasone after topical application of betamethasone 17-valerate: Comparison with oral administration. Br J Clin Pharmacol 37:86, 1994.

267. Lader M: Clinical pharmacology of antipsychotic drugs. J Int Med Res 17:1, 1989.

268. Lalak NJ, Morris DL: Azithromycin clinical pharmacokinetics. Clin Pharmacokinet 25:370, 1993.

269. Lambert GH, Muraskas J, Anderson CL, et al: Direct hyperbilirubinemia associated with chloral hydrate administration in the newborn. Pediatrics 86:277, 1990.

270. Lamp KC, Bailey EM, Rybak MJ: Ofloxacin clinical pharmacokinetics. Clin Pharmacokinet 22:32, 1992.

271. Lancaster FE, Selvanayagam PF, Hsu LL: Lactational ethanol exposure: Brain enzymes and 3(H)spiroperidol binding. Int J Dev Neurosci 4:151, 1986.

272. Larsen FG, Jakobsen P, Eriksen H, et al: The pharmacokinetics of acitretin and its 13-cis-metabolite in psoriatic patients. J Clin Pharmacol 31:477, 1991.

273. Larsen FG, Nielsen-Kudsk F, Jakobsen P, et al: Pharmacokinetics and therapeutic efficacy of retinoids in skin diseases. Clin Pharmacokinet 23:42, 1992.

274. Latini R, Maggioni AP, Cavalli A: Therapeutic drug monitoring of antiarrhythmic drugs: Rationale and current status. Clin Pharmacokinet 18:91, 1990.

275. Lau AH, Lam NP, Piscitelli SC, et al: Clinical pharmacokinetics of metronidazole and other nitroimidazole anti-infectives. Clin Pharmacokinet 23:328, 1992.

276. Lau RJ, Emery MG, Glainsky RE: Unexpected accumulation of acyclovir in breast milk with estimation of infant exposure. Obstet Gynecol 69:468, 1987.

277. Lauritsen K, Laursen LS, Rask-Madsen J: Clinical pharmacokinetics of drugs used in the treatment of gastrointestinal diseases. I. Clin Pharmacokinet 19:11, 1990.

278. Lauritsen K, Laursen LS, Rask-Madsen J: Clinical pharmacokinetics of drugs used in the treatment of gastrointestinal diseases. II. Clin Pharmacokinet 19:94, 1990.

279. Laursen LC, Borga O, Ljungholm K, et al: Transfer of enprofylline into breast milk. Ther Drug Monit 10:150, 1988.

280. Leal-Cerro A, Garcia-Luna PP, Pereira JL, et al: Ketoconazole: A new type of agent in the treatment of hypercholesterolemia? Horm Metab Res 22:398, 1990.

281. Lebedevs TH, Wojnar-Horton RE, Yapp P, et al: Excretion of indomethacin in breast milk. Br J Clin Pharmacol 32:751, 1991.

282. Lebedevs TH, Wojnar-Horton RE, Yapp P, et al: Excretion of temazepam in breast milk. Br J Clin Pharmacol 33:204, 1992.

283. Lecaillon JB, Dubois JP, Darragon T, et al: Pharmacokinetics of cadralazine in a large group of hypertensive patients chronically treated with cadralazine: Advantage over a conventional study in a small group of patients. Ther Drug Monit 13:103, 1991.

284. Lee CR, McTavish D, Sorkin EM: Tramadol: A preliminary review of its pharmacodynamic and pharmacokinetic properties, and therapeutic potential in acute and chronic pain states. Drugs 46:313, 1993.

285. Leigh DA, Harris C, Tait S, et al: Pharmacokinetic study of lomefloxacin and its effect on the faecal flora of volunteers. J Antimicrob Chemother 27:655, 1991.

286. Lemmens HJM, Burm AGL, Bovill JG, et al: Pharmacodynamics of alfentanil. Anesthesiology 76:65, 1992.

287. Lemmens HJM, Burm AGL, Hennis PJ, et al: Influence of age on the pharmacokinetics of alfentanil: Gender dependence. Clin Pharmacokinet 19:416, 1990.

288. Lennard L: The clinical pharmacology of 6-mercaptopurine. Eur J Clin Pharmacol 43:329, 1992.

289. Leonard MB, Koren G, Stevenson DK, et al: Vancomycin pharmacokinetics in very low birth weight neonates. Pediatr Infect Dis J 8:282, 1989.

290. Leonard TK, Watson RR, Mohs ME: The effects of caffeine on various body systems: A review. J Am Diet Assoc 87:1048, 1987.

291. Lewis LD: Ifosfamide pharmacokinetics. Invest New Drugs 9:305, 1991.

292. Li G, Treiber G, Meinshausen J, et al: Is cyclosporin A an inhibitor of drug metabolism? Br J Clin Pharmacol 30:71, 1990.

293. Libardoni M, Piovan D, Busato E, et al: Transfer of propafenone and 5-OH-propafenone to foetal plasma and maternal milk. Br J Clin Pharmacol 32:527, 1991.

294. Lin JH: Pharmacokinetic and pharmacodynamic properties of histamine H_2-receptor antagonists: Relationship between intrinsic potency and effective plasma concentrations. Clin Pharmacokinet 20:218, 1991.

295. Lindholm A: Factors influencing the pharmacokinetics of cyclosporine in man. Ther Drug Monit 13:465, 1991.

296. Lipsy RJ, Fennerty B, Fagan TC: Clinical review of histamine-2 receptor antagonists. Arch Intern Med 150:745, 1990.

297. Lode H: The pharmacokinetics of azithromycin and their chemical significance. Eur J Clin Microbiol Infect Dis 10:807, 1991.

298. Lode H, Hoffken G, Boeckh M, et al: Quinolone pharmacokinetics and metabolism. J Antimicrob Chemother 26(suppl B):41, 1990.

299. Lucas BD Jr, Purdy CY, Scarim SK, et al: Terfenadine pharmacokinetics in breastmilk in lactating women. Clin Pharmacol Ther 57:398, 1995.

300. Luck W, Nau H: Nicotine and cotinine concentrations in the milk of smoking mothers: influence of cigarette consumption and diurnal variation. Eur J Pediatr 146:21, 1987.

301. MacDonald N-J, Elliot HL, Hughes DM, et al: A comparison in young and elderly subjects of the pharmacokinetics and pharmacodynamics of single and multiple doses of benazepril. Br J Clin Pharmacol 36:201, 1993.

302. MacDonald N-J, Sioufi A, Howie CA, et al: The effects of age on the pharmacokinetics and pharmacodynamics of single oral doses of benazerpril and enalapril. Br J Clin Pharmacol 36:205, 1993.

303. MacFadyen RJ, Meredith PA, Elliot HL: Enalapril clinical pharmacokinetics and pharmacokinetic-pharmacodynamic relationships. Clin Pharmacokinet 25:274, 1993.

304. MacGregor TR, Sardi ED: In vitro protein binding behavior of dipyridamole. J Pharm Sci 80:119, 1991.

305. Martell M, de Ben S, Weinberger M, et al: Growth and development in preterm infants receiving fluoroquinolones. J Perinat Med 24:287, 1996.

306. Massarella JW, Khoo KC, Aogaichi K, et al: Effect of renal impairment on the pharmacokinetics of cibenzoline. Clin Pharmacol Ther 43:317, 1988.

307. Matheson I, Lunde PKM, Bredesen JE: Midazolam and nitrazepam in the maternity ward: Milk concentrations and clinical effects. Br J Clin Pharmacol 30:787, 1990.

308. Matheson I, Samseth M, Loberg R, et al: Milk transfer of phenoxymethylpenicillin during puerperal mastitis. Br J Clin Pharmacol 25:33, 1988.

309. Matheson I, Samseth M, Sande HA: Ampicillin in breast milk during puerperal infections. Eur J Clin Pharmacol 34:657, 1988.

310. Matheson I, Sande HA, Gaillot J: The excretion of zopiclone into breast milk. Br J Clin Pharmacol 30:267, 1990.

311. Maton PN: Omeprazole. N Engl J Med 324:965, 1991.

312. Mattern J, Mayer PR: Excretion of fluorescein into breast milk. Am J Ophthalmol 109:598, 1990.

313. Matuo YK, Lopes JNC, Casanova IC, et al: Organochlorine pesticide residues in human milk in the Ribeirao Preto Region, State of Sao Paulo, Brazil. Arch Environ Contam Toxicol 22:167, 1992.

314. McCann MF, Moggia AV, Higgins JE, et al: The effects of a progestin-only oral contraceptive (Levonorgestrel 0.03 mg) on breastfeeding. Contraception 40:635, 1989.

315. McCormick KB: Pregnancy and epilepsy: Nursing implications. J Neurosci Nurs 19:66, 1987.

316. McNeil JJ, Drummer OH, Raymond K, et al: The influence of food on the oral bioavailability of terazosin. Br J Clin Pharmacol 32:775, 1991.

317. McQuinn RL, Pisani A, Wafa S, et al: Flecainide excretion in human breast milk. Clin Pharmacol Ther 48:262, 1990.

318. McTavish D, Young RA, Clissold SP: Cadralazine: A review of its pharmacodynamic and pharmacokinetic properties, and therapeutic potential in the treatment of hypertension. Drugs 40:543, 1990.

319. Meadow WL, Bui KC, Strates E, et al: Metoclopramide promotes enteral feeding in preterm infants with feeding intolerance. Dev Pharmacol Ther 13:38, 1989.

320. Mehvar R, Gross ME, Kreamer RN: Pharmacokinetics of atenolol enantiomers in humans and rats. J Pharm Sci 79:881, 1990.

321. Mennella JA, Beauchamp GK: The transfer of alcohol to human milk. N Engl J Med 325:981, 1991.

322. Meredith PA, Elliott HL: Clinical pharmacokinetics of amlodipine. Clin Pharmacokinet 22:22, 1992.

323. Michelson EI, Dreifus LS: Newer antiarrhythmic drugs. Med Clin North Am 72:275, 1988.

324. Miles MV, Balasubramanian R, Pittman AW, et al: Pharmacokinetics of oral and transdermal triprolidine. J Clin Pharmacol 30:572, 1990.

325. Milne RJ, Heel RC: Ondansetron: therapeutic use as an antiemetic. Drugs 41:574, 1991.

326. Milunsky JM, Milunsky A: Breast-feeding during colchicine therapy for familial Mediterranean fever. J Pediatr 119:164, 1991.

327. Mitani GM, Steinberg I, Lien EJ, et al: The pharmacokinetics of antiarrhythmic agents in pregnancy and lactation. Clin Pharmacokinet 12:253, 1987.

328. Modi NB, Veng-Pedersen P, Graham DJ, et al: Application of a system analysis approach to population pharmacokinetics and pharmacodynamics of nicardipine hydrochloride in healthy males. J Pharm Sci 82:705, 1993.

329. Mofenson HC, Caraccio TR: Lactation pharmacology 1987. Pediatr Pharmacol Toxic News 6:47, 1987.

330. Mollmann H, Barth J, Mollmann C, et al: Pharmacokinetics and rectal bioavailability of hydrocortisone acetate. J Pharm Sci 80:835, 1991.

331. Monk JP, Benfield P: Inhaled pentamidine: An overview of its pharmacological properties and a review of its therapeutic use in *Pneumocystis carinii* pneumonia. Drugs 39:741, 1990.

332. Moore MJ: Clinical pharmacokinetics of cyclophosphamide. Clin Pharmacokinet 20:194, 1991.

333. Moretti ME, Ito S, Koren G: Disposition of maternal ketoconazole in breast milk. Am J Obstet Gynecol 173:1625, 1995.

334. Morrow JD: The oral cephalosporin: A review. Am J Med Sci 303:35, 1992.

335. Morse GD, Shelton MJ, O'Donnell AM: Comparative pharmacokinetics of antiviral nucleoside analogues. Clin Pharmacokinet 24:101, 1993.

336. Motwani JG, Lipworth BJ: Clinical pharmacokinetics of drugs administered buccally and sublingually. Clin Pharmacokinet 21:83, 1991.

337. Mountford PJ, Coakley AJ: Breast milk radioactivity following injection of ^{99m}Tc-pertechnetate and ^{99m}Tc-glucoheptonate. Nucl Med Commun 8:839, 1987.

338. Mountford PJ, Coakley AJ: Secretion of radioactivity in breast milk following administration in hippuran. Br J Radiol 62:388, 1989.

339. Mouton JW, Horrevorts AM, Mulder PGH, et al: Pharmacokinetics of ceftazidime in serum and suction blister fluid during continuous and intermittent infusions in healthy volunteers. Antimicrob Agents Chemother 34:2307, 1990.

340. Movin-Osswald G, Nordstrom A-L, Hammarlund-Udenaes M, et al: Pharmacokinetics of raclopride formulations: Influence of prolactin and tolerability in healthy male volunteers. Clin Pharmacokinet 22:152, 1992.

341. Munafo A, Christen Y, Nussberger J, et al: Drug concentration response relationships in normal volunteers after oral administration of losartan, an angiotensin II receptor antagonist. Clin Pharmacol Ther 51:513, 1992.

342. Murdoch D, Clissold SP: Calcipotriol: A review of its pharmacological properties and therapeutic use in psoriasis vulgaris. Drugs 43:415, 1992.

343. Murdoch D, Heel RC: Amlodipine: A review of its pharmacodynamic and pharmacokinetic properties, and therapeutic use in cardiovascular disease. Drugs 41:478, 1991.

344. Murdoch D, McTavish D: Roxatidine acetate: A review of its pharmacodynamic and pharmacokinetic properties, and its therapeutic potential in peptic ulcer disease and related disorders. Drugs 42:240, 1991.

345. Murdoch D, McTavish D: Fosinopril: A review of its pharmacodynamics and pharmacokinetic properties and therapeutic potential in essential hypertension. Drugs 43:123, 1992.

346. Murdoch D, McTavish D: Sertraline: A review of its pharmacodynamic and pharmacokinetic properties, and therapeutic potential in depression and obsessive-compulsive disorder. Drugs 44:604, 1992.

347. Murphy PH, Beasley CW, Moore WH, et al: Thallium-201 in human milk: Observations and radiological consequences. Health Phys 56:539, 1989.

348. Muzaffar A, Brossi A: Chemistry of colchicine. Pharmacol Ther 49:105, 1991.

349. Nathwani D, Wood MJ: Penicillins: A current review of their clinical pharmacology and therapeutic use. Drugs 45:866, 1993.

350. Naumberg EG, Meny RG: Breast milk opioids and neonatal apnea. Am J Dis Child 142:11, 1988.

351. Nehlig A, Debry G: Consequences on the newborn of chronic maternal consumption of coffee during gestation and lactation: a review. J Am Coll Nutr 13:6, 1994.

352. Nestico PF, Morganroth J, Horowitz LN: New antiarrhythmic drugs. Drugs 35:286, 1988.

353. Neuvonen PJ, Kivisto KT: The clinical significance of food-drug interactions: A review. Med J Aust 150:36, 1989.

354. Neuvonen PJ, Kivisto KT, Lehto P: Interference of dairy products with the absorption of ciprofloxacin. Clin Pharmacol Ther 50:498, 1991.

355. Nielsen ST, Matheson I, Rasmussen JN, et al: Excretion of iohexol and metrizoate in human breast milk. Acta Radiol 28:523, 1987.

356. Nilsen OG, Aamo T, Zahlsen K, et al: Macrolide pharmacokinetics and dose scheduling of roxithromycin. Diagn Microbiol Infect Dis 15:71S, 1992.

357. Nilsen OG, Dale O: Single dose pharmacokinetics of trazodone in healthy subjects. Pharmacol Toxicol 71:150, 1992.

358. Nissen E, Widstrom A-M, Lilja G, et al: Effects of routinely given pethidine during labour on infants' developing breastfeeding behaviour: effects of dose-delivery time interval and various concentrations of pethidine/norpethidine in cord plasm. Acta Paediatr 86:201, 1997.

359. Notarianni LJ: Plasma protein binding of drugs in pregnancy and in neonates. Clin Pharmacokinet 18:20, 1990.

360. Notarianni LJ, Oldham HG, Bennett PN: Passage of paracetamol into breast milk and its subsequent metabolism by the neonate. Br J Clin Pharmacol 24:63, 1987.

361. Obermeyer BD, Bergstrom RF, Callaghan JT, et al: Secretion of nizatidine into human breast milk after single and multiple doses. Clin Pharmacol Ther 47:724, 1990.

362. O'Dea RF, Mirkin BL, Alward CT, et al: Treatment of neonatal hypertension with captopril. J Pediatr 113:403, 1988.

363. Ogbuokiri JE, Ozumba BC, Okonkwo PO: Ivermectin level in human breastmilk. Eur J Clin Pharmacol 45:389, 1993.

364. Oguma T, Yamada H, Sawaki M, et al: Pharmacokinetic analysis of the effects of different foods on absorption of cefaclor. Antimicrob Agents Chemother 35:1729, 1991.

365. Ogunbona FA, Onyeji CO, Bolaji OO, et al: Excretion of chloroquine and desethylchloroquine in human milk. Br J Clin Pharmacol 23:473, 1987.

366. O'Hare MF, Murnaghan GA, Russell CJ, et al: Sotalol as a hypotensive agent in pregnancy. Br J Obstet Gynaecol 87:814, 1980.

367. Ohdo S, Nakano S, Ogawa N: Circadian changes of valproate kinetics depending on meal condition in humans. J Clin Pharmacol 32:822, 1992.

368. Ohkubo T, Shimoyama R, Sugawara K: Measurement of haloperidol in human breast milk by high-performance liquid chromatography. J Pharm Sci 81:947, 1992.

369. Okano M, Nomura M, Hata S, et al: Anaphylactic symptoms due to chlorhexidine gluconate. Arch Dermatol 125:50, 1989.

370. Okonkwo PO, Ogbuokiri JE, Ofoegbu E, et al: Protein binding and ivermectin estimations in patients with onchocerciasis. Clin Pharmacol Ther 53:426, 1993.

371. Olesen OV, Bartels U, Poulsen JH: Perphenazine in breast milk and serum. Am J Psychiatry 147:1378, 1990.

372. Oliver RM, Upward JW, Dewhurst AG, et al: The pharmacokinetics of doxazosin in patients with hypertension and renal impairment. Br J Clin Pharmacol 29:417, 1990.

373. Olsson B, Bolme P, Dahlstrom B, et al: Excretion of noscapine in human breast milk. Eur J Clin Pharmacol 30:213, 1986.

374. Onks DL, Harris JG, Robertson AF: Cefmenoxine and bilirubin: Competition for albumin binding. Pharmacol Toxicol 68:329, 1991.

375. Ostensen M, Matheson I, Laufen H: Piroxicam in breast milk after long-term treatment. Eur J Clin Pharmacol 35:567, 1988.

376. Ostensen M, Skavdal K, Myklebust G, et al: Excretion of gold into human breast milk. Eur J Clin Pharmacol 31:251, 1986.

377. Paap CM, Nahata MC: Clinical pharmacokinetics of antibacterial drugs in neonates. Clin Pharmacokinet 19:280, 1990.

378. Page MA, Boutagy JS, Shenfield GM: A screening test for slow metabolisers of tolbutamide. Br J Clin Pharmacol 31:649, 1991.

379. Palmer KJ, Holliday SM, Brogden RN: Mefloquine: A review of its antimalarial activity, pharmacokinetic properties and therapeutic efficacy. Drugs 45:430, 1993.

380. Pan H, Fleiss P, Moore L, et al: Excretion of pravastatin, an HMG CoA reductase inhibitor, in breast milk of lactating women. J Clin Pharmacol 28:942, 1988.

381. Pan HY, DeVault AR, Wang-Iverson D, et al: Comparative pharmacokinetics and pharmacodynamics of pravastatin and lovastatin. J Clin Pharmacol 30:1128, 1990.

382. Pankey GA: Temafloxacin: An overview. Am J Med 91(suppl 6A):166S, 1991.

383. Passmore CM, McElnay JC, Rainey EA, et al: Metronidazole excretion in human milk and its effect on the suckling neonate. Br J Clin Pharmacol 26:45, 1988.

384. Pato MT, Murphy DL, DeVane CL: Sustained plasma concentrations of fluoxetine and/or norfluoxetine four and eight weeks after fluoxetine discontinuation. J Clin Psychopharmacol 11:224, 1991.

385. Paul M, Himmelstein J: Reproductive hazards in the workplace: What the practitioner needs to know about chemical exposures. Obstet Gynecol 71:921, 1988.

386. Pavord I, Knox A: Pharmacokinetic optimisation of inhaled steroid therapy in asthma. Clin Pharmacokinet 25:126, 1993.

387. Penny WJ, Lewis MJ: Nifedipine is excreted in human milk. Eur J Clin Pharmacol 36:427, 1989.

388. Pepperell RJ: Suppression of lactation. Med J Aust 144:37, 1986.

389. Pershing LK, Corlett J, Jorgensen C: In vivo pharmacokinetics and pharmacodynamics of topical ketoconazole and miconazole in human stratum corneum. Antimicrob Agents Chemother 38:90, 1994.

390. Persson B, Heykants J, Hedner T: Clinical pharmacokinetics of ketanserin. Clin Pharmacokinet 20:263, 1991.

391. Persson K, Hammarlund-Udenaes M, Mortimer O, et al: The postoperative pharmacokinetics of codeine. Eur J Clin Pharmacol 42:663, 1992.

392. Peters DH, Friedel HA, McTavish D: Azithromycin: A review of its antimicrobial activity, pharmacokinetic properties and clinical efficacy. Drugs 44:750, 1992.

393. Physicians' Desk Reference. Montvale, NJ, Medical Economics, 1998.

394. Plomp TA, Vulsma T, de Vijlder JJM: Use of amiodarone during pregnancy. Eur J Obstet Gynecol Reprod Biol 43:201, 1992.

395. Poitrast BJ, Keller WC, Elves RG: Estimation of chemical hazards in breast milk. Aviat Space Environ Med 59:A87, 1988.

396. Pons G, Francoual C, Guillet P, et al: Zolpidem excretion in breast milk. Eur J Clin Pharmacol 37:245, 1989.

397. Pons G, Rey E, d'Athis P, et al: Gentamicin monitoring in neonates. Ther Drug Monit 10:421, 1988.

398. Pons G, Schoerlin MP, Tam YK, et al: Moclobemide excretion in human breast milk. Br J Clin Pharmacol 29:27, 1990.

399. Port RE, Edler L, Herrmann R, et al: Pharmacokinetics of 5-fluorouracil after short systemic infusion: Plasma level at the end of the distribution phase as an indicator of the total area under the plasma concentration-time curve. Ther Drug Monit 13:96, 1991.

400. Poyhia R, Seppala T, Olkkola KT, et al: The pharmacokinetics and metabolism of oxycodone after intramuscular and oral administration to healthy subjects. Br J Clin Pharmacol 33:617, 1992.

401. Prichard BNC, Tomlinson B, Renondin JC: Urapidil, a multiple-action alpha-blocking drug. Am J Cardiol 64:11D, 1989.

402. Pue MA, Pratt SK, Fairless AJ, et al: Linear pharmacokinetics of penciclovir following administration of single oral doses of famciclovir 125, 250, 500, and 750 mg to healthy volunteers. J Antimicrob Chemother 33:119, 1994.

403. Radisch B, Luck W, Nau H: Cadmium concentrations in milk and blood of smoking mothers. Toxicol Let 36:147, 1987.

404. Ramsay RE: Advances in the pharmacotherapy of epilepsy. Epilepsia 34(suppl 5):S9, 1993.

405. Resplandy G, Genissel P: Pharmacokinetics of perindipril in high-risk populations. J Cardiovasc Pharmacol 18(suppl 7):S9, 1991.

406. Rey AM, Grauer K, Gums JG: Newer antihypertensive agents. Postgrad Med 89:75, 1991.

407. Riant P, Urien S, Albengres E, et al: High plasma protein binding as a parameter in the selection of beta blockers for lactating women. Biochem Pharmacol 35:4579, 1986.

408. Ribeiro C, Longo A: Procainamide and disopyramide. Eur Heart J 8(suppl A):11, 1987.

409. Ripa S, Ferrante L, Prenna M: Pharmacokinetics of fluconazole in normal volunteers. Chemotherapy 39:6, 1993.

410. Rivera-Calimlim L: The significance of drugs in breast milk. Clin Perinatol 14:51, 1987.

411. Rizzon P, Di Biase M, Favale S, et al: Class 1B agents lidocaine, mexiletine, tocainide, phenytoin. Eur Heart J 8(suppl A):21, 1987.

412. Robert J: Clinical pharmacokinetics of idarubicin. Clin Pharmacokinet 24:275, 1993.

413. Roberts D, Honcharik N, Sitar DS, et al: Diltiazem overdose: Pharmacokinetics of diltiazem and its metabolites and effect of multiple dose charcoal therapy. Clin Toxicol 29:45, 1991.

414. Robieux I, Koren G, Vandenbergh H, et al: Morphine excretion in breast milk and resultant exposure of a nursing infant. Clin Toxicol 28:365, 1990.

415. Robin DW, Lee MH, Hasan SS, Wood AJJ: Triazolam in cirrhosis: Pharmacokinetics and pharmacodynamics. Clin Pharmacol Ther 54:630, 1993.

416. Roden DM, Wood AJJ, Wilkinson GR, et al: Disposition kinetics of encainide and metabolites. Am J Cardiol 58:4C, 1986.

417. Roden DM, Woosley RL: Clinical pharmacokinetics of encainide. Clin Pharmacokinet 14:141, 1988.

418. Rogan WJ, Gladen BC, McKinney JD, et al: Polychlorinated biphenyls (PCBs) and dichlorodiphenyl dichloroethene (DDE) in human milk: Effects on growth, morbidity, and duration of lactation. Am J Publ Health 77:1294, 1987.

419. Rollman O, Pihl-Lundin I: Acitretin excretion into human breast milk. Acta Derm Venereol (Stockh) 70:487, 1990.

420. Roony TW, Lorber A, Veng-Pedersen P, et al: Gold pharmacokinetics in breast milk and serum of a lactating woman. J Rheumatol 14: 1120, 1987.

421. Rose MR, Prescott MC, Herman KJ: Excretion of iodine-123-hippuran, technetium-99m-red blood cells, and technetium-99m-macroaggregated albumin into breast milk. J Nucl Med 31:978, 1990.

422. Rosenbaum DH, Rowan AJ, Tuchman L, et al: Comparative bioavailability of a generic phenytoin and dilantin. Epilepsia 35:656, 1994.

423. Rowbotham DJ: Omeprazole: A useful new agent? Br J Anaesth 65:607, 1990.

424. Rubow S, Klopper J: Excretion of radioiodine in human milk following a therapeutic dose of I-131. Eur J Nucl Med 14:632, 1988.

425. Rubow S, Klopper J, Scholtz P: Excretion of gallium 67 in human breast milk and its inadvertent ingestion by a 9-month-old child. Eur J Nucl Med 18:829, 1991.

426. Rubow S, Klopper J, Wasserman H, et al: The excretion of radiopharmaceuticals in human breast milk: Additional data and dosimetry. Eur J Nucl Med 21:144, 1994.

427. Rylance GW, Woods CG, Donnelly MC, et al: Carbimazole and breastfeeding. Lancet 1:928, 1987.

428. Saathoff N, Lode H, Neider K, et al: Pharmacokinetics of cefpodoxime proxetil and interactions with an antacid and an H2 receptor antagonist. Antimicrob Agents Chemother 36:796, 1992.

429. Sahlberg BL: The characterization of sulphated metabolites of norethindrone in human milk after oral administration of contraceptive steroids. J Steroid Biochem 26:481, 1987.

430. Samoil D, Grubb BP, Temesy-Armos PN: Sotalol: A new agent for the treatment of ventricular arrhythmias. Am J Med Sci 307:49, 1994.

431. Samples JR, Meyer SM: Use of ophthalmic medications in pregnant and nursing women. Am J Ophthalmol 106:616, 1988.

432. Sandborn WJ, Strong RM, Forland SC, et al: The pharmacokinetics and colonic tissue concentrations of cyclosporine after IV, oral, and enema administration. J Clin Pharmacol 31:76, 1991.

433. Sanders SW, Buchi KN, Goddard MS, et al: Single-dose pharmacokinetics and tolerance of a cholesteryl sulfate complex of amphotericin B administered to healthy volunteers. Antimicrob Agents Chemother 35:1029, 1991.

434. Sasaki M, Tateishi T, Ebihara A: The effects of age and gender on the stereoselective pharmacokinetics of verapamil. Clin Pharmacol Ther 54:278, 1993.

435. Scheinin M, Koulu M, Karhuvaara S, et al: Evidence that the reversible MAO-A inhibitor moclobemide increases prolactin secretion by a serotonergic mechanism in healthy male volunteers. Life Sci 47:1491, 1990.

436. Schimmel MS, Eidelman AI, Wilschanski MA, et al: Toxic effects of atenolol consumed during breastfeeding. J Pediatr 114:476, 1989.

437. Schlepper M: Propafenaone: A review of its profile. Eur Heart J 8(suppl A):27, 1987.

438. Schwartz PH, Eldadah MK, Newth CJL: The pharmacokinetics of dobutamine in pediatric intensive care unit patients. Drug Metab Dispos 19:614, 1991.

439. Schwartz-Bickenbach D, Schulte-Hobein B, Abt S, et al: Smoking and passive smoking during pregnancy and early infancy: Effects on birth weight, lactation period, and cotinine concentration in mother's milk and infant's urine. Toxicol Lett 35:73, 1987.

440. Shaheen O, Zmeili S, Al-Qussuois Y, et al: Pharmacokinetics and pharmacodynamics of two commercial oral nifedipine products. Int J Clin Pharmacol Ther Toxicol 29:337, 1991.

441. Shanks CA, Avram MJ, Fragen RJ, et al: Pharmacokinetics and pharmacodynamics of vecuronium administered by bolus and infusion during halothane or balanced anesthesia. Clin Pharmacol Ther 42:459, 1987.

442. Shapiro TA, Were JBO, Danso K, et al: Pharmacokinetics and metabolism of allopurinol riboside. Clin Pharmacol Ther 49:506, 1991.

443. Shenfield GM, Griffin JM: Clinical pharmacokinetics of contraceptive steroids: An update. Clin Pharmacokinet 20:15, 1991.

444. Shikary ZK, Betrabet SS, Patel ZM, et al: Transfer of levonorgestrel administered through different drug delivery systems from the maternal circulation into the newborn infant's circulation via breastmilk. Contraception 35:477, 1987.

445. Shionoiri H, Ueda S-I, Minamisawa K, et al: Pharmacokinetics and pharmacodynamics of benazepril in hypertensive patients with normal and impaired renal function. J Cardiovascular Pharmacol 20:348, 1992.

446. Shukla UA, Pittman KA, Barbhaiya RH: Pharmacokinetic interactions of cefprozil with food, propantheline, metoclopramide, and probenecid in healthy volunteers. J Clin Pharmacol 32:725, 1992.

447. Shyu WC, Knupp CA, Pittman KA, et al: Food-induced reduction in bioavailability of didanosine. Clin Pharmacol Ther 50:503, 1991.

448. Shyu WC, Pittman KA, Robinson DS, et al: The absolute bioavailability of transnasal butorphanol in patients experiencing rhinitis. Eur J Clin Pharmacol 45:559, 1993.

449. Shyu WC, Pittman KA, Wilber RB, et al: Pharmacokinetics of cefprozil in healthy subjects and patients with renal impairment. J Clin Pharmacol 31:362, 1991.

450. Shyu WC, Shah VR, Campbell DA, et al: Excretion of cefprozil into human breast milk. Antimicrob Agents Chemother 36:938, 1992.

451. Shyu WC, Shah VR, Campbell DA, et al: Oral absolute bioavailability and intravenous dose-proportionality of cefprozil in humans. J Clin Pharmacol 32:798, 1992.

452. Shyu WC, Wilber RB, Pittman KA, et al: Pharmacokinetics of cefprozil in healthy subjects and patients with hepatic impairment. J Clin Pharmacol 31:372, 1991.

453. Siddoway LA, Schwartz SL, Barbey JT, et al: Clinical pharmacokinetics of moricizine. Am J Cardiol 65:21D, 1990.

454. Sides GD, Cerimele BJ, Black HR, et al: Pharmacokinetics of dirithromycin. J Antimicrob Chemother 31(suppl C):65, 1993.

455. Sietsema WK: The absolute oral bioavailability of selected drugs. Int J Clin Pharmacol Ther Toxicol 27:179, 1989.

456. Signs SA, Tan JS, Salstrom S-J, et al: Pharmacokinetics of imipenem in serum and skin window fluid in healthy adults after intramuscular or intravenous administration. Antimicrob Agents Chemother 36:1400, 1992.

457. Sikorski R, Paszkowski T, Radomanski T, et al: Cadmium contamination of early human milk. Gynecol Obstet Invest 27:91, 1989.

458. Silvasti M, Karttunen P, Happonen P, et al: Pharmacokinetic comparison of a dextromethorphan-salbutamol combination tablet and a plain dextromethorphan tablet. Int J Clin Pharmacol Ther Toxicol 28:268, 1990.

459. Singhvi SM, Pan HY, Morrison RA, et al: Disposition of pravastatin sodium, a tissue-selective HMG-CoA reductase inhibitor, in healthy subjects. Br J Clin Pharmacol 29:239, 1990.

460. Singlas E, Leroy A, Sultan E, et al: Disposition of fleroxacin, a new trifluoroquinolone, and its metabolites: Pharmacokinetics in renal failure and influence of haemodialysis. Clin Pharmacokinet 19:67, 1990.

461. Skopnik H, Bergt U, Heimann G: Neonatal theophylline intoxication: Pharmacokinetics and clinical evaluation. Eur J Pediatr 151:221, 1992.

462. Skoyles JR, Sherry KM: Pharmacology, mechanisms of action and uses of selective phosphodiesterase inhibitors. Br J Anaesth 68:293, 1992.

463. Smilack JD, Wilson WR, Cockerill FR: Tetracyclines, chloramphenicol, erythromycin, clindamycin, and metronidazole. Mayo Clin Proc 66:1270, 1991.

464. Smith IJ, Hinson JL, Johnson VA, et al: Flurbiprofen in post-partum women: Plasma and breast milk disposition. J Clin Pharmacol 29:174, 1989.

465. Smith NA, Kates RE, Lebsack C, et al: Clinical pharmacology of intravenous enoximone: Pharmacodynamics and pharmacokinetics in patients with heart failure. Am Heart J 122:755, 1991.

466. Smithers JA, Kulmala HK, Thompson GA, et al: Pharmacokinetics of teicoplanin upon multiple-dose intravenous administration of 3, 12, and 30 milligrams per kilogram of body weight to healthy male volunteers. Antimicrob Agents Chemother 36:115, 1992.

467. Soderman P, Matheson I: Clonazepam in breast milk. Eur J Pediatr 147:212, 1988.

468. Somani P: Basic and clinical pharmacology of amiodarone: Relationship of antiarrhythmic effects, dose and drug concentrations to intracellular inclusion bodies. J Clin Pharmacol 29:405, 1989.

469. Somani P, Fraker TD, Temesy-Armos PN: Pharmacokinetic implications of lorcainide therapy in patients with normal and depressed cardiac function. J Clin Pharmacol 27:122, 1987.

470. Somberg JC, Achari R, Laddu AR: Terazosin: Pharmacokinetics and the effect of age and dose on the incidence of adverse events. Am Heart J 122:901, 1991.

471. Soons PA, Grib C, Breimer DD, Kirch W: Effects of acute febrile infectious diseases on the oral pharmacokinetics and effects of nitrendipine enantiomers and of bisoprolol. Clin Pharmacokinet 23:238, 1992.

472. Soons PA, Mulders TMT, Uchida E, et al: Stereoselective pharmacokinetics of oral felodipine and nitrendipine in healthy subjects: Correlation with nifedipine pharmacokinetics. Eur J Clin Pharmacol 44:163, 1993.

473. Soons PA, Van den Berg G, Danhof M, et al: Influence of single- and multiple-dose omeprazole treatment on nifedipine pharmacokinetics and effects in healthy subjects. Eur J Clin Pharmacol 42:319, 1992.

474. Sorgel F, Kinzig M: Pharmacokinetics of gyrase inhibitors. I. Basic chemistry and gastrointestinal disposition. Am J Med 94(suppl 3A):44S, 1993.

475. Sorgel F, Naber KG, Kinzig M, et al: Comparative pharmacokinetics of ciprofloxacin and temafloxacin in humans: A review. Am J Med 91(suppl 6A):51S, 1991.

476. Spahn H, Knauf H, Mutschler E: Pharmacokinetics of torasemide and its metabolites in healthy controls and in chronic renal failure. Eur J Clin Pharmacol 39:345, 1990.

477. Speight TM, Holford NHG (eds): Avery's Drug Treatment, 4th ed. Auckland, Adis International, 1997.

478. Spencer CM, Faulds D, Peters DH: Cetirizine: A reappraisal of its pharmacological properties and therapeutic use in selected allergic disorders. Drugs 46:1055, 1993.

479. Speth PAJ, Van Hoesel QGCM, Haanen C: Clinical pharmacokinetics of doxorubicin. Clin Pharmacokinet 15:15, 1988.

480. Spigset O: Anaesthetic agents and excretion in breast milk. Acta Anaesthesiol Scand 38:94, 1991.

481. Spiller HA, Morse S, Muir C: Fluoxetine ingestion: A one year retrospective study. Vet Hum Toxicol 32:153, 1990.

482. Stagni G, Davis PJ, Ludden TM: Human pharmacokinetics of betaxolol enantiomers. J Pharm Sci 80:321, 1991.

483. Stancer HC, Reed KL: Desipramine and 2-hydroxydesipramine in human breast milk and the nursing infant's serum. Am J Psychiatry 143:1597, 1986.

484. Steer PL, Biddle CJ, Marley WS, et al: Concentration of fentanyl in colostrum after an analgesic dose. Can J Anaesth 39:231, 1992.

485. Steldinger R, Luck W: Half lives of nicotine in breast milk of smoking mothers: Implications for nursing. J Perinat Med 16:261, 1988.

486. Stewart DJ, Grewaal D, Green RM, et al: Bioavailability and pharmacology of oral idarubicin. Cancer Chemother Pharmacol 27:308, 1991.

487. Storck J, Kirsten R: Binding of urapidil to human serum albumin: Dependency on free fatty acid concentration. Int J Clin Pharmacol Ther Toxicol 29:204, 1991.

488. Streisand JB, Varvel JR, Stanski DR, et al: Absorption and bioavailability of oral transmucosal fentanyl citrate. Anesthesiology 75:223, 1991.

489. Stuck AE, Kim DK, Frey FJ: Fleroxacin clinical pharmacokinetics. Clin Pharmacokinet 22:116, 1992.

490. Sylvester RK, Lobell M, Teresi ME, et al: Excretion of hydroxyurea into milk. Cancer 60:2177, 1987.

491. Szutu M, Morgan DJ, McLeish M, et al: Pharmacokinetics of intravenous clomiphene isomers. Br J Clin Pharmacol 27:639, 1989.

492. Taddio A, Klein J, Koren G: Acyclovir excretion in human breast milk. Ann Pharmacother 28:585, 1994.

493. Takagi K, Yamaki K, Nadai M, et al: Effect of a new quinolone, sparfloxacin, on the pharmacokinetics of theophylline in asthmatic patients. Antimicrobial Agents Chemother 35:1137, 1991.

494. Tam YK: Individual variation in first-pass metabolism. Clin Pharmacokinet 25:300, 1993.

495. Tartara A, Galimberti CA, Manni R, et al: Differential effects of valproic acid and enzyme-inducing anticonvulsants on nimodipine pharmacokinetics in epileptic patients. Br J Clin Pharmacol 32:335, 1991.

496. Terhaag B, Gramatte T, Hrdlcka P, et al: The influence of food on the absorption of diclofenac as a pure substance. Int J Clin Pharmacol Ther Toxicol 29:418, 1991.

497. Tessin I, Thiringer K, Trollfors B, et al: Comparison of serum concentrations of ceftazidime and tobramycin in newborn infants. Eur J Pediatr 147:405, 1988.

498. Tett SE: Clinical pharmacokinetics of slow-acting antirheumatic drugs. Clin Pharmacokinet 25:392, 1993.

499. Thiercelin JF, Necciari J, Caplain H, et al: Development and pharmacokinetics of a new sustained-release formulation of diltiazem. J Cardiovasc Pharmacol 16(suppl):S31, 1990.

500. Thoman ME: Drug toxicology and breast-feeding. Pediatr Basics 57:2, 1991.

501. Todd PA, Clissold SP: Naproxen: A reappraisal of its pharmacology, and therapeutic use in rheumatic diseases and pain states. Drugs 40:91, 1990.

502. Todd PA, Faulds D: Ofloxacin: A reappraisal of its antimicrobial activity, pharmacology and therapeutic use. Drugs 42:825, 1991.

503. Todd PA, Fitton A: Perindopril: A review of its pharmacological properties and therapeutic use in cardiovascular disorders. Drugs 42:90, 1991.

504. Todd PA, Fitton A: Gallium nitrate: A review of its pharmacological properties and therapeutic potential in cancer-related hypercalcaemia. Drugs 42:261, 1991.

505. Todd PA, Sorkin EM: Diclofenac sodium: A reappraisal of its pharmacodynamic and pharmacokinetic properties, and therapeutic efficacy. Drugs 35:244, 1988.

506. Todd PA, Goa KL, Langtry HD: Transdermal nitroglycerin (glyceryl trinitrate): A review of its pharmacology and therapeutic use. Drugs 40:880, 1990.

507. Tonks AM: Nimodipine levels in breast milk. Aust N Z J Surg 65:693, 1995.

508. Trautner K, Einwag J: Influence of milk and food on fluoride bioavailability from NaF and Na$_2$FPO$_3$ in man. J Dent Res 68:72, 1989.

509. Travis CC, Hattemer-Frey HA, Arms AD: Relationship between dietary intake of organic chemicals and their concentrations in human adipose tissue and breast milk. Arch Environ Contam Toxicol 17:473, 1988.

510. Trenk D, Wagner F, Sachs W, et al: Pharmacokinetic characterization of the antiarrhythmic drug diprafenone in man. Eur J Clin Pharmacol 37:313, 1989.

511. Troy SM, Cevallos WH, Conrad KA, et al: The absolute bioavailability and dose proportionality of intravenous and oral dosage regimens of recainam. J Clin Pharmacol 31:433, 1991.

512. Turgeon J, Fiset C, Giguere R, et al: Influence of debrisoquine phenotype and of quinidine on mexiletine disposition in man. J Pharmacol Exp Ther 259:789, 1991.

513. Unger J, Lambert M, Jonckheer MH, et al: Amiodarone and the thyroid: pharmacological, toxic and therapeutic effects. J Intern Med 233:435, 1993.

514. Unsworth J, d'Assis-Fonseca A, Beswick DT, et al: Serum salicylate levels in a breastfed infant. Ann Rheum Dis 46:638, 1987.

515. Vance-Bryan K, Guay DRP, Rotschafer JC: Clinical pharmacokinetics of ciprofloxacin. Clin Pharmacokinet 19:434, 1990.

516. Van der Auwera P, Stolear JC, George B, et al: Pharmacokinetics of enoxacin and its oxometabolite following intravenous administration to patients with different degrees of renal impairment. Antimicrob Agents Chemother 34:1491, 1990.

517. Vanhaesebrouck P, Thiery M, Leroy JG, et al: Oligohydramnios, renal insufficiency, and ileal perforation in preterm infants after intrauterine exposure to indomethacin. J Pediatr 113:738, 1988.

518. van Harten J: Clinical pharmacokinetics of selective serotonin reuptake inhibitors. Clin Pharmacokinet 24:203, 1993.

519. Van Hecken AM, Depre M, De Schepper PJ, et al: Lack of effect of flunarizine on the pharmacokinetics and pharmacodynamics of sumatriptan in healthy volunteers. Br J Clin Pharmacol 34:82, 1992.

520. Vanholder R, Van Landschoot N, De Smet R, et al: Drug protein binding in chronic renal failure: Evaluation of nine drugs. Kidney Int 33:996, 1988.

521. van Hoogdalem EJ, de Boer AG, Breimer DD: Pharmacokinetics of rectal drug administration. II.

Clinical applications of peripherally acting drugs and conclusions. Clin Pharmacokinet 21:110, 1991.

522. Van Putten T, Marder SR, Mintz J: Serum prolactin as a correlate response to haloperidol. J Clin Psychopharmacol 11:357, 1991.

523. Verbeeck RV, Ross SG, McKenna EA: Excretion of trazodone in breast milk. Br J Clin Pharmacol 22:367, 1986.

524. Vernon MW, Heel RC, Brogden RN: Enoximone: A review of its pharmacological properties and therapeutic potential. Drugs 42:997, 1991.

525. Vree TB, Van den Biggelaar-Martea M, Verwey-Van Wissen CPWGM, et al: The pharmacokinetics of naproxen, its metabolite O-desmethylnaproxen, and their acylglucuronides in humans: Effect of cimetidine. Br J Clin Pharmacol 35:467, 1993.

526. Wadworth AN, Brogden RN: Quinapril: A review of its pharmacological properties, and therapeutic efficacy in cardiovascular disorders. Drugs 41:378, 1991.

527. Wadworth AN, Fitton A: Olsalazine: A review of its pharmacodynamic and pharmacokinetic properties, and therapeutic potential in inflammatory bowel disease. Drugs 41:647, 1991.

528. Wadworth AN, Goa KL: Lomefloxacin: A review of its antibacterial activity, pharmacokinetic properties and therapeutic use. Drugs 42:1018, 1991.

529. Wagstaff AJ, Faulds D, Goa KL: Aciclovir: A reappraisal of its antiviral activity, pharmacokinetic properties and therapeutic efficacy. Drugs 47:153, 1994.

530. Wakamatsu A, Umetsu M, Motoya H, et al: Change of plasma half-life of caffeine during caffeine therapy for apnea in premature infants. Acta Paediatr Jpn 29:595, 1987.

531. Walker JA, Sherman RA, Cody RP: The effect of oral bases on enteral aluminum absorption. Arch Intern Med 150:2037, 1990.

532. Walker RC, Wright AJ: The quinolones. Mayo Clin Proc 62:1007, 1987.

533. Walker RC, Wright AJ: The fluoroquinolones. Mayo Clin Proc 66:1249, 1991.

534. Walsh AES, Hockney RA, Campling G, et al: Neuroendocrine and temperature effects of nefazodone in healthy volunteers. Biol Psychiatry 33:115, 1993.

535. Walstad RA, Hellum KB, Thurmann-Nielsen E, et al: Pharmacokinetics and tissue penetration of timentin: A simultaneous study of serum, urine, lymph, suction blister, and subcutaneous thread fluid. J Antimicrob Chemother 17(suppl C):71, 1986.

536. Wang X, Sato N, Greer MA, et al: Quinidine inhibits prolactin secretion induced by thyrotropin-releasing hormone, high medium potassium or hyposmolarity in GH4C1 cells. J Pharmacol Exp Ther 256:135, 1991.

537. Weiner CP, Buhimschi C: Drugs for Pregnant and Lactating Women. Philadelphia, Churchill Livingstone, 2004.

538. Weintrub PS, Chapman A, Piecuch R: Renal fungus ball in a premature infant successfully treated with fluconazole. Pediatr Infect Dis J 13:1152, 1994.

539. Westphal JF, Deslandes A, Brogard JM, et al: Reappraisal of amoxicillin absorption kinetics. J Antimicrob Chemother 27:647, 1991.

540. Wettrel G, Anderson KE: Cardiovascular drugs. I. Antidysrhythmic drugs. Ther Drug Monit 8:59, 1986.

541. White NJ: Antimalarial pharmacokinetics and treatment regimens. Br J Clin Pharmacol 34:1, 1992.

542. White WB, Yeh SC, Krol GJ: Nitrendipine in human plasma and breast milk. Eur J Clin Pharmacol 36:531, 1989.

543. Widerlov E, Termander N, Nilsson MI: Effect of urinary pH on the plasma and urinary kinetics of remoxipride. Eur J Clin Pharmacol 37:359, 1989.

544. Wiest DB, Fowler SL, Garner SS, et al: Fluconazole in neonatal disseminated candidiasis. Arch Dis Child 66:1002, 1991.

545. Wiggins RC, Rolsten C, Ruiz B, et al: Pharmacokinetics of cocaine: Basic studies of route, dosage, pregnancy and lactation. Neurotoxicology 10:367, 1989.

546. Wilde MI, Langtry HD: Zidovudine: An update of its pharmacodynamic and pharmacokinetic properties, and therapeutic efficacy. Drugs 46:515, 1993.

547. Wilde MI, Plosker GL, Benfield P: Fluvoxamine: An updated review of its pharmacology, and therapeutic use in depressive illness. Drugs 46:895, 1993.

548. Wilder BJ: Pharmacokinetics of valproate and carbamazepine. J Clin Psychopharmacol 12:64S, 1992.

549. Wildfeuer A, Laufen H, Leitold M, et al: Comparison of the pharmacokinetics of three-day and five-day regimens of azithromycin in plasma and urine. J Antimicrob Chemother 31(suppl E):51, 1993.

550. Wilson JH: Breast milk tocainide levels. J Cardiovasc Pharmacol 12:497, 1988.

551. Wischnik A, Manth SM, Lloyd J, et al: The excretion of ketorolac tromethamine into breast milk after multiple oral dosing. Eur J Clin Pharmacol 36:521, 1989.

552. Wiseman LR, Benfield P: Cefprozil: A review of its antibacterial activity, pharmacokinetic properties, and therapeutic potential. Drugs 45:295, 1993.

553. Wisner KL, Perel JM, Findling RL: Antidepressant treatment during breast-feeding. Am J Psychiatry 153:1132, 1996.

554. Wojnar-Horton RE, Hackett LP, Yapp P, et al: Distribution and excretion of sumatriptan in human milk. Br J Clin Pharmacol 41:217, 1996.

555. Wolff MS: Lactation. In Paul M (ed): Occupational and Environmental Reproductive Hazards: A Guide for Clinicians. Baltimore, Williams & Wilkins, 1993.

556. Wolfson JS, Hooper DC: Pharmacokinetics of quinolones: Newer aspects. Eur J Clin Microbiol Infect Dis 10:267, 1991.

557. Wong FA, Flor SC: The metabolism of ofloxacin in humans. Drug Metab Dispos 18:1103, 1990.

558. Woosley RL, Funck-Brentano C: Overview of the clinical pharmacology of antiarrhythmic drugs. Am J Cardiol 61:61A, 1988.

559. Wretlind M: Excretion of oxazepam in breast milk. Eur J Clin Pharmacol 33:209, 1987.

560. Wright S, Dawling S, Ashford JJ: Excretion of fluvoxamine in breast milk. Br J Clin Pharmacol 31:209, 1991.

561. Yee GC, McGuire TR: Pharmacokinetic drug interactions with cyclosporin. Part I. Clin Pharmacokinet 19:319, 1990.

562. Yue QY, Hasselstrom J, Svensson JO, et al: Pharmacokinetics of codeine and its metabolites in Caucasian healthy volunteers: Comparisons between extensive and poor hydroxylators of desbrisoquine. Br J Clin Pharmacol 31:635, 1991.

563. Yue QY, Svensson JO, Sjoqvist F, et al: A comparison of the pharmacokinetics of codeine and its metabolites in healthy Chinese and Caucasian extensive hydroxylators of debrisoquine. Br J Clin Pharmacol 31:643, 1991.

564. Yusuff NT, York P, Chrystyn H, et al: Improved bioavailability from a spironolactone beta-cyclodextrin complex. Eur J Clin Pharmacol 40:507, 1991.

565. Zaske DE, Strate RG, Kohls PR: Amikacin pharmacokinetics: Wide interpatient variation in 98 patients. J Clin Pharmacol 31:158, 1991.

566. Zeisler JA, Gaarder TD, DeMesquita SA: Lidocaine excretion in breast milk. Drug Intell Clin Pharm 20:691, 1986.

567. Zschiesche M, Focke N, Hoffmann C, et al: Bioavailability of metronidazole vaginal tablets (Vagimid). Int J Clin Pharmacol Ther Toxicol 30:485, 1992.

TABLE D-2 Herbs: use during pregnancy and lactation

Herb common name/rating*	Synonyms	Active ingredient	Uses	Present in milk	Safety/efficacy
Aloe vera AAP— H L3 W—	*Aloe barbadensis, A. capensis, vera*	Polysaccharide, glucomannan	Wound healing and small burns	Unknown, probably none when applied to skin	Orally is a strong purgative; oral dosing not recommended during lactation. Dermal use ok. (11, 12)
Blessed thistle AAP— H L3 W—		Many chemicals and volatile oils	Gastrointestinal symptoms	Unknown	This is not a galactogogue. It is a different plant from milk thistle. No known toxicity. (11)
Cannabis AAP 2 H L5 W—	Marijuana	Δ9-Tetrahydrocannabinol (THC)	Sedative, hallucinogen	Yes	Remains in infant's system for weeks, especially in fat. (11)
Chamomile AAP— H L3 W—	*Matricaria recutita,* Aster Aceae family	Terpenoids (coumarins), flower heads	Antiinflammatory, carminative, antiseptic, sedative (all unproved)	Unknown	Potential for allergic reaction. Animal studies question safety in pregnancy and lactation.
Cohosh (black) AAP— H L4 W—	*Cimicifuga racemosa,* black cohosh, black snakeroot, found in Lydia Pinkham's compound	Estrogenic compounds, tannins, terpesoids, use roots and rhizome	Dysmenorrhea, dyspepsia, rheumatism, menopause	Unknown	May cause hypotension; could decrease milk production.? Efficacy and safety in lactation.
Cohosh (blue) AAP— H L5 W—	*Caulophyllum,* blue cohosh, squaw root	Roots and rhizome, methylcytosine, caulosaponin	Uterine stimulant, emmenagogue, increased blood pressure, like nicotine, induces labor	Unknown	Safety of concern, can constrict coronary vessels, leaves and seeds are known to be toxic.
Comfrey AAP— H L5 W—	*Symphytum officinale*	Roots and rhizome and leaves, allantoin, hepatotoxic, pyrrolizidine alkaloids	"Wonder drug," heals wounds, used as poultice, used as tea	Yes	Veno-occlusive disease causing hepatic failure. Banned in many countries; unsafe. (11, 27)

Herb	Parts/Active ingredients	Uses	Safe in lactation	Comments
Echinacea AAP— H L3 W—	*Echinacea angustifolia*, coneflower	Whole plant, flowers, dried roots	Immunostimulant, antiinfective, tested for upper respiratory infections	Unknown	Has been studied—effective in short courses, not continual use. No known toxicity; probably safe during lactation. (11, 12)
Evening primrose AAP— H L3 W—	*Oenothera biennis*	Biennis, oil from seeds, cis-gamma-linoleic acid (GLA), a precursor of prostaglandin E₁, essential fatty acids (EFA)	Lower cholesterol, lower blood pressure, lower dysmenorrhea, mastalgia, eczema	Yes	Efficacy—conflicting reports. Safety, +/− probably in small amounts. Supplements increase EFA in milk. (9)
Fennel AAP— H L4 W—	*Foeniculum vulgare*	Dried ripe fruit, volatile oil, transanethole estrogenic effect	Carminative, loosen phlegm, galactogogue, increase libido	Probable	Volatile oil can be toxic; use only fruits (seeds). Because of estrogenic effect, its reputation as a galactogogue is questioned. (11)
Fenugreek AAP— H L3 W—	*Trigonella foenumgraecum*, Greek hayseed	Dried ripe seeds, disgenin and alkaloids smell like maple syrup	Hypoglycemia, galactogogue, anticoagulant, see text	Probable	Risk cross allergy to chrysanthemum family. Probably in milk—infants smell of maple syrup. No studies of efficacy. (11)
Garlic AAP— H L3 W—	Lily family: *Allium sativum*, poor man's treacle, clove garlic, common garlic, allium, stinking rose	Allin, ajoens	Has 125 different uses, some contradictory, both high and low blood pressure, antibacterial, antithrombotic, lower cholesterol	Yes	Can cause colic in breastfed infant. Can enhance warfarin. Not tolerated by some infants.
Ginkgo AAP— H L3 W—	*Ginkgo biloba*	Flavones and glycosides, seeds ginkgotoxin, ginkgo biloba extract (GBE), leaves for tea	Herbal antioxidant	Unknown	Placebo-controlled studies suggest no efficacy in young adults. Use in elderly more effective.

Continued

TABLE D-2 Herbs: use during pregnancy and lactation—cont'd

Herb common name/rating	Synonyms	Active ingredient	Uses	Present in milk	Safety/efficacy
Ginseng AAP— H L3 W—	Panax ginseng (*P. quinquefolius*), Asian ginseng	Root and extracts	Panacea, cure-all, adaptogen, strengthening, increasing mental capacity	Unknown	Too much has been written, with considerable conflict of opinion. Ginseng abuse syndrome (GAS); research done mostly by manufacturers. Safety—not long-term use; efficacy questionable. (11, 12)
Grapefruit seed extract AAP— H— W—		Flavonols	Antimicrobial inhibits intestinal cytochrome 450		Noted to have antiinfection, antiviral, antibacterial, and antifungal effects. Grapefruit is known to contain quinine, especially in the bitter skin and section fibers. Recommended as an extract for use by direct application on sore nipples. If it has antiinfectious properties, it should be effective when traumatized nipples have become infected. (27)
Kava AAP— H L5 W—	Pipermethysticum, Kew, tonga	Roots/rhizomes, dihydropyrones with central nervous system activity, kavapyrones	Inebriation, muscle relaxants, alternative to penzodiapams	Unknown	Unsafe in pregnancy and lactation. Numbs the mouth; nauseating. Causes yellow discoloration of the skin, hair, nails. (11, 12)
Milk thistle (holy thistle) (not blessed thistle) AAP— H L3 W—	*Silybum marianum*, St. Mary's thistle	Fruits, flavolignans, inhibits oxidative damage to cells	Protective effect, concentrates in the liver	Unknown	Galactogogue. Problem—can cause allergy; low oral bioavailability. Probably safe. (11)

Panax (see Ginseng)

Sage AAP— H L4 W—	*Salvia officinalis*	Fresh leaves and fresh flowering aerial parts, dried leaves, and oils prepared as extracts and teas	Loss of appetite, inflammation of mouth and pharynx, excessive perspiration	Unknown	Contraindicated in pregnancy.
St. John's wort AAP— H L3 W—	*Hypericum perforatum*	Naphthodianthrones, phloroglucinols	Depression	Unknown	Can cause photosensitivity. Risk of self-medication for a serious psychiatric problem.
Valerian root AAP— H— W—	*Valeriana officinalis*, all-heal, amantilla, setwell, setewale, capon's tail, heliotrope, vandal root	Liquid, tablets, tea, volatile oil	Nervousness and insomnia	Unknown	Not recommended.

REFERENCES

1. Abbot PJ: Comfrey: Assessing the low-dose health risk. Med J Aust 149:678, 1988.

2. American Academy of Pediatrics, Committee on Drugs: The transfer of drugs and other chemicals into human milk. Pediatrics 108:776, 2001.

3. Awang DVC: Maternal use of ginseng and neonatal androgenization. JAMA 265:1828, 1991.

4. Bach N, Thung SN, Schaffner F: Comfrey herb tea-induced hepatic veno-occlusive disease. Am J Med 87:97, 1998.

5. Bach N, Thung SN, Schaffner F: Comfrey herb tea-induced hepatic veno-occlusive disease. Am J Med 87:97, 1989.

6. Barr RG: Herbal teas for infantile colic. J Pediatr 123:669, 1993.

7. Briggs GC, Freeman RK, Yaffe SJ: Drugs in Pregnancy and Lactation, 6th ed. A Reference Guide to Fetal and Neonatal Risk. Philadelphia, Lippincott, Williams & Wilkins, 2002.

8. Burger RA, Torres AR, Warren RP, et al: Echinacea-induced cytokine production by human macrophages. Int J Immunopharmacol 19: 371, 1997.

9. Cant A, Shay J, Horrobin DF: The effect of maternal supplementation with linoleic and gamma-linoleic acids on the fat composition and content of human milk: A placebo-controlled trial. J Nutr Sci Vitaminol (Tokyo) 37:573, 1991.

10. Doughty C, Walker A, Brenchley J: Herbal mind altering substances: An unknown quanity? Emerg Med J 21:253, 2004.

11. Foster S, Tyler VE: Tyler's Honest Herbal: A Sensible Guide to the Use of Herbs and Related Remedies. New York, The Haworth Herbal Press, 1999.

12. Hale TW: Medications and Mother's Milk, 10th ed. Amarillo, TX, Pharmasoft Publishing, 2002.

13. Huggins KE: Fenugreek: One remedy for low milk production. The Medela Messenger Winter 15:16, 1998.

14. Huxtable RJ, Luthy J, Zweifel U: Toxicity of comfrey-pepsin preparations. N Engl J Med 315:1095, 1986.

15. Kopec K: Herbal medications and breastfeeding. J Hum Lact 15:157, 1999.

16. Koren G, Randor S, Martin S, Danneman D: Maternal ginseng use associated with neonatal androgenization. JAMA 264:2866, 1990.

17. Koupparis LS: Harmless herbs: A cause for concern. Anaesthesia 55:101, 2000 (correspondence).

18. Linde K, Ramirez G, Mulrow CD, et al: St. John's Wort for depression—An overview and meta-analysis of randomised clinical trials. BMJ 313:253, 1996.

19. McRae S: Elevated serum digoxin levels in a patient taking digoxin and Siberian ginseng. Can Med Assoc J 155:293, 1996.

20. Mullins RJ: Echinacea-associated anaphylaxis. Med J Aust 168:170, 1998.

21. Nice F, Coghlan RJ, Birmingham: Which herbals are safe to take while breastfeeding? Here's a guide to popular herbs and their potential risk to nurslings. Personal communication (e-mail).

22. Patil SP, Niphadkap PV, Bapat MM: Allergy to fenugreek (Trigonella foenum graecum). Ann Allergy Asthma Immunol 78:297, 1997.

23. Physicians Desk Reference for Herbal Medicines, 2nd ed. Montvale, New Jersey, Medical Economics Co., 2000.

24. Ramsay HM, Goddard W, Gill S, Moss C: Herbal creams used for atopic eczema in Birmingham, UK illegally contain potent corticosteroids. BMJ 88:2056, 2003.

25. Rengers B, Foote J: Fenugreek: An aid to lactation? Breastfeeding Update 5:3,1997.

26. Ridker PM, McDermott WV: Hepatotoxicity due to comfrey herb tea. Am J Med 87:701, 1989.

27. Rotblatt M, Ziment I: Evidence-Based Herbal Medicine. Philadelphia, Hanley and Belfus, 2002.

28. Roulet M, Laurini R, Rivier L, Calame A: Hepatic veno-occlusive disease in newborn infant of a woman drinking herbal tea. Pediatr 112:433, 1988.

29. Sewell AC, Mosandl A, Bohles H: False diagnosis of maple syrup urine disease owing to ingestion of herbal tea. N Engl J Med 341:769, 1999.

30. Stickel F, Poschl G, Seitz HK, et al: Acute hepatitis induced by greater celandine (Chelidonium majus). Scand J Gastroenterol 38:565, 2003.

31. U.S. Food and Drug Administration: FDA advises dietary supplement manufacturers to remove comfrey products from the market. Rockville, MD, U.S. Food and Drug Administration 2001.

32. Weiner CP, Buhimschi C: Drugs for Pregnant and Lactating Women. New York, Churchill Livingstone, 2004.

33. Wilasrusmee C, Kittur S, Shah G, et al: Immunostimulatory effect of Silybum marianum (milk thistle) extract. Med Sci Monit 8:BR439, 2002.

Precautions and breastfeeding recommendations for selected maternal infections

TABLE E-1 Precautions and breastfeeding recommendations for selected maternal infections*

Organism, syndrome, or condition[†‡]	Empiric precautions[§]	Breastfeeding acceptable[‖]	Compatibility of medications with breastfeeding[¶]
Adenoviruses			
Conjunctivitis	Contact		
Upper/lower respiratory infections	Droplet	Yes[#]	
Gastroenteritis	Standard		
Amebiasis			
Entamoeba histolytica			
Intestinal	Standard	Yes	Iodoquinol, paromomycin, metronidazole, tinidazole
Extraintestinal	Standard	Yes	
Anthrax			
Bacillus anthracis (cutaneous, inhalation, gastrointestinal)	Standard	Yes	Ciprofloxacin
Arboviruses			
Arthropod-borne infections, meningoencephalitis, hemorrhagic fevers, hepatitis	Standard	Yes	
California encephalitis	Standard	Yes	
Colorado tick fever	Standard	Yes	
Dengue fever	Standard	Yes	
Eastern equine encephalitis	Standard	Yes	
Japanese encephalitis	Standard	Yes	
St. Louis encephalitis	Standard	Yes	
Yellow fever	Standard	Yes	
Arcanobacterium haemolyticus			
Pharyngitis, skin infections	Standard	Yes	Erythromycin, clindamycin, chloramphenicol, tetracycline
Ascaris lumbricoides			
Gastrointestinal infections, pneumonitis	Standard	Yes	Pyrantel pamoate, mebendazole, albendazole, piperazine
Aspergillosis			
Bronchopulmonary, sinus, or invasive infections	Standard	Yes	Amphotericin B, flucytosine, rifampin
Astroviruses			
Gastroenteritis	Standard, but contact for incontinent individuals	Yes	

Disease / Organism	Breastfeeding	Precautions	Drugs
Babesiosis			
Babesia microti			
Subacute/chronic febrile illness	Yes	Standard	Clindamycin, quinine
Blastocystis hominis			
Gastrointestinal infection	Yes	Standard	Metronidazole
Blastomyces dermatitidis			
Pulmonary, cutaneous, or invasive infection	Yes	Standard	Amphotericin B, ketoconazole, itraconazole
Borrelia			
Relapsing fever			
Borrelia hermsii	Yes	Standard (tick-borne)	Penicillin, erythromycin
Borrelia recurrentis	Yes	Contact (louse-borne)	Tetracycline, chloramphenicol
Borrelia turicatae	Yes	Standard (tick-borne)	Doxycycline
Botulism			
Clostridium botulinum			
Hypotonia, progressive weakness, toxin-mediated paralysis	Yes	Standard	
Breast abscess (see Mastitis)			
Staphylococcus aureus Enterobacteriaceae *Streptococcus pyogenes*	Yes (after 24 hr if no drainage into breast milk; discard breast milk for first 24 h after surgery)	Contact (24 hr)	First-generation cephalosporin, amoxicillin/clavulanate, ampicillin/sulbactam
Brucellosis			
Febrile illness with variable manifestations	Yes (after 48 hr of therapy in the mother; discard breast milk for 48 hr)	Standard	Doxycycline. TMP-SMX, rifampin, gentamicin, streptomycin, tetracycline
Brucella abortus *Brucella melitensis* *Brucella suis*	Yes	Contact (for draining wounds)	
Caliciviruses			
Gastroenteritis	Yes	Standard, but contact for incontinent individuals	
Campylobacter			
Gastrointestinal infection	Yes	Standard, but contact for incontinent individuals	Erythromycin, ciprofloxacin
Campylobacter fetus *Campylobacter jejuni*			
Candidiasis			
Mucocutaneous infection, vulvovaginitis, invasive infections	Yes (therapy for the infant simultaneous with mother's therapy)**	Standard	Topical agents, fluconazole, ketoconazole, itraconazole, amphotericin B, flucytosine
Candida albicans			

Continued

TABLE E-1 Precautions and breastfeeding recommendations for selected maternal infections*—cont'd

Organism, syndrome, or condition[†‡]	Empiric precautions[§]	Breastfeeding acceptable[‖]	Compatibility of medications with breastfeeding[¶]
Candida krusei			
Candida tropicalis			
Cat-scratch disease			
Skin infection, regional lymphadenitis, and rarely, invasive infection *Bartonella henselae*	Standard	Yes	TMP-SMX, rifampin, ciprofloxacin, gentamicin, doxycycline, erythromycin
Chlamydia			
Chlamydia pneumoniae Pharyngitis, pneumonia	Standard	Yes	Tetracycline, erythromycin azithromycin, clarithromycin
Chlamydia psittaci Psittacosis, pneumonia, rarely invasive infection	Standard	Yes	
Chlamydia trachomatis Urethritis, vaginitis, endometritis, salpingitis, lymphogranuloma venereum (LGV), conjunctivitis, pneumonia	Standard	Yes (consider treating the infant)	Erythromycin, azithromycin, clarithromycin, doxycycline, tetracycline, sulfisoxazole
Clostridia			
Clostridium botulinum Toxin-mediated paralysis	Standard	Yes	
Clostridium difficile Antimicrobial-associated diarrhea, pseudomembranous colitis	Contact	Yes	Metronidazole, vancomycin
Clostridium perfringens Food poisoning, wound infection, gas gangrene, myonecrosis	Standard	Yes	Penicillin, chloramphenicol, clindamycin, metronidazole
Coccidioides immitis Pulmonary, invasive infections rarely, extrapulmonary	Standard, but contact for draining lesions	Yes	Amphotericin B, fluconazole, itraconazole
Conjunctivitis			
Adenovirus	Contact	Yes	
Chlamydia trachomatis	Standard	Yes	Tetracycline, doxycycline, erythromycin
Neisseria gonorrhoeae	Standard	Yes[††]	Penicillin, ceftriaxone

Disease/Organism	Precautions	Breast-feeding	Treatment
Cryptococcus neoformans			
Meningitis, pneumonia	Standard	Yes	Amphotericin B, flucytosine
Cryptosporidiosis			
Cryptosporidium parvum			
Diarrhea	Contact	Yes	Paromomycin, azithromycin
Cytomegalovirus (CMV)			
Asymptomatic infection	Standard	Yes (for full-term infants)	
Infectious mononucleosis	Standard	No (for premature or immunodeficient infants, do not give expressed breast milk)	
Dengue fever			
Acute febrile illness, hemorrhagic fever	Standard	Yes	
Diphtheria			
Corynebacterium diphtheriae			
Membranous nasopharyngitis	Droplet (DI)	Yes (with infant receiving chemoprophylaxis-P)	Erythromycin, penicillin
Obstructive laryngotracheitis	Droplet (DI)		
Cutaneous infection, toxin-mediated myocarditis, or neurologic disease	Contact (cover lesions)	No (only if skin lesion involves breast)	
Diarrhea			
Campylobacter fetus	Standard	Yes	TMP-SMX
Campylobacter jejuni	Standard	Yes	Erythromycin, ciprofloxacin
Escherichia coli (0157:H7)	Contact	Yes	None indicated
Giardia lamblia	Standard	Yes	Furazolidone, metronidazole
Rotavirus	Contact	Yes	
Salmonella enteritidis	Standard	Yes	
Shigella boydii	Contact	Yes	Ciprofloxacin, norfloxacin, TMP-SMX
Shigella dysenteriae	Contact	Yes	Ciprofloxacin, norfloxacin, TMP-SMX
Shigella flexneri	Contact	Yes	Ciprofloxacin, norfloxacin, TMP-SMX
Shigella sonnei	Contact	Yes	Ciprofloxacin, norfloxacin, TMP-SMX
Vibrio cholerae	Standard	Yes	Ciprofloxacin, doxycycline
Vibrio parahaemolyticus	Standard	Yes	None

Continued

TABLE E-1 Precautions and breastfeeding recommendations for selected maternal infections*—cont'd

Organism, syndrome, or condition[†‡]	Empiric precautions[§]	Breastfeeding acceptable[‖]	Compatibility of medications with breastfeeding[¶]
Yersinia enterocolitica	Standard	Yes	Ciprofloxacin, norfloxacin, ceftriaxone, TMP-SMX, doxycycline
Yersinia pseudotuberculosis	Standard	Yes	
Ebola virus	Contact, droplet, and airborne	No (do not give expressed breast milk)	
Encephalitis			
Enteroviruses	Standard	Yes	
Lyme disease (*Borrelia burgdorferi*)	Standard	Yes	Ceftriaxone, doxycycline, amoxicillin
Rabies	Standard	No (BM+)	Rabies immune globulin, rabies vaccine
Endometritis, pelvic inflammatory disease			
Anaerobic organisms	Standard	Yes	Clindamycin, metronidazole, cefoxitin, cefmetazole
Chlamydia trachomatis	Standard	Yes	Erythromycin, azithromycin, tetracycline
Enterobacteriaceae	Standard	Yes	Ampicillin, aminoglycosides, cephalosporins
Group B streptococci	Standard	Yes (after 24 hr of therapy, breast milk is ok; observation)	Penicillin, cephalosporin, macrolides
Mycoplasma hominis	Standard	Yes	Clindamycin, tetracycline
Neisseria gonorrhoeae	Standard	Yes[††]	Ceftriaxone, spectinomycin, doxycycline, azithromycin
Ureaplasma urealyticum	Standard	Yes	Erythromycin, azithromycin, clarithromycin, tetracycline
Enteroviruses			
Myocarditis: respiratory, gastrointestinal, skin, central nervous system, and eye infections	Adults: standard Children: contact		
Coxsackievirus		Yes	
Echovirus		Yes	
Polioviruses		Yes	

Epstein-Barr virus			
Infectious mononucleosis, broad range of infections	Standard	Yes	
Erythema infectiosum			
Parvovirus B19	Standard	Yes	
Food poisoning			
Bacillus cereus			
Toxin mediated	Standard	Yes	
Clostridium perfringens			
Toxin mediated	Standard	Yes	
Escherichia coli (0157:117)			
Enterohemorrhagic	Contact	Yes	
Hepatitis A	Standard	Yes (immune serum globulin and hepatitis A vaccine for the infant)	
Norwalk virus	Standard	Yes	
Salmonella enteritidis	Standard	Yes	
Shigella	Contact	Yes	Ciprofloxacin, TMP-SMX
Staphylococcus aureus			
Enterotoxin	Standard	Yes	
Gastroenteritis (see Diarrhea or Food Poisoning)			
Giardiasis			
Giardia lamblia	Standard, no contact with incontinent individuals	Yes	Furazolidone, metronidazole
Gonorrhea			
Genital, pharyngeal, conjunctival, or disseminated infection			
Neisseria gonorrhoeae	Standard	Yes††	Ceftriaxone, ciprofloxacin, spectinomycin, azithromycin, doxycycline
Haemophilus influenzae			
Meningitis, epiglottitis, pneumonia, cellulitis, sinusitis, bacteremia	Droplet	Yes (24 hr after initiating therapy in mother; BM+; P** if infant has not been fully immunized, observation)	Cefotaxime, ceftriaxone, ampicillin

Continued

TABLE E-1 Precautions and breastfeeding recommendations for selected maternal infections*—cont'd

Organism, syndrome, or condition[†‡]	Empiric precautions[§]	Breastfeeding acceptable[‖]	Compatibility of medications with breastfeeding[¶]
Hantavirus			
Pulmonary syndrome, hemorrhagic fever with renal syndrome	Standard	Yes	Intravenous ribavirin is investigational
Hemorrhagic fevers			
African hemorrhagic fever			
Ebola virus	Contact	No	
Marburg virus			
Dengue virus (1–4)	Standard	Yes (expressed breast milk is ok)	
Hantavirus	Standard	Yes (expressed breast milk is ok)	
Lassa fever	Contact	No (no expressed breast milk)	Intravenous ribavirin
Yellow fever	Standard	Yes (expressed breast milk is ok)	Vaccine
Hepatitis[††]			
A Acute only	Standard, but contact for incontinent individuals	Yes (after immune serum globulin [ISG] and vaccine)	
B Chronic hepatitis, cirrhosis, hepatocellular carcinoma	Standard	Yes (after hepatitis B immune globulin [HBIG] and vaccine)	
C Chronic hepatitis, cirrhosis, hepatocellular carcinoma	Standard	Yes	
D Associated with hepatitis B	Standard	Yes (after HBIG and vaccine)	
E Severe disease in pregnant women	Standard	Yes	
G	Standard	Inadequate data	
Herpes viruses			
Cytomegalovirus (CMV) Asymptomatic, infectious mononucleosis–like syndrome: severe disease in the immunodeficient person	Standard	Yes for full-term infants No for premature or immunodeficient infants (infant of CMV-negative mother should not receive milk from CMV-positive mothers)	Ganciclovir, foscarnet
Epstein-Barr virus Asymptomatic, infectious mononucleosis, associated with chronic fatigue syndrome, African Burkitt's lymphoma, and nasopharyngeal carcinoma	Standard	Yes	

Disease	Precautions	Breastfeeding	Treatment
Herpes simplex Types 1, 2 (HSV$_{1,2}$)			
Mucocutaneous	Contact	Yes (in the absence of breast lesions)	Acyclovir, valacyclovir, famciclovir
Neonatal	Contact		
Encephalitis	Standard		
Varicella-zoster virus (VZV)**			
Varicella	Airborne	No (expressed breast milk is ok in the absence of lesions on the breast)	Acyclovir, valacyclovir, famciclovir
Zoster	Standard in normal patient	Yes (covered lesions, with none involving the breast)	
	Airborne/contact in immunocompromised individuals	No, VZIG for the exposed infant, especially less than 1 month of age**	
Human herpes virus 6 (HHV-6)			
Roseola (exanthema subitum, sixth disease), acute febrile illness	Standard	Yes	
Histoplasmosis	Standard	Yes	Amphotericin B, ketoconazole, fluconazole, itraconazole
Human immunodeficiency viruses (HIV)**			
HIV-1	Standard	Yes/no**	Little or no available information on antiretrovirals in breast milk
HIV-2	Standard	Yes/no**	
Human T-cell leukemia viruses (HTLV)			
HTLV-1			
T-cell leukemia/lymphoma, myelopathy, dermatitis, adenitis, Sjögren's syndrome	Standard	No**	
HTLV-II			
Myelopathy, arthritis, glomerulonephritis	Standard	No**	
Impetigo	Contact	Yes	Oxacillin, dicloxacillin, erythromycin, first-generation cephalosporins
Infectious mononucleosis (see CMV, EBV)			
Influenza	Droplet	Yes	Amantadine, rimantadine
Junin virus			
Argentine hemorrhagic fever	Contact	No (do not give expressed breast milk)	

Continued

TABLE E-1 Precautions and breastfeeding recommendations for selected maternal infections*—cont'd

Organism, syndrome, or condition[†‡]	Empiric precautions[§]	Breastfeeding acceptable[‖]	Compatibility of medications with breastfeeding[¶]
Lassa fever	Contact	No (do not give expressed breast milk)	Intravenous ribavarin
Legionnaires' disease			
Legionella pneumophila Pneumonia ± gastrointestinal, central nervous system, or renal involvement	Standard	Yes	Erythromycin, rifampin
Leprosy			
Mycobacterium leprae Chronic disease of skin, peripheral nerves, and respiratory mucosa	Standard	Yes	Dapsone, rifampin, clofazimine
Leptospirosis Abrupt febrile illness, often biphasic, with multiple organ involvement			
Leptospira interrogans	Standard	Yes (no mother-infant contact except for breastfeeding)	Penicillin, tetracycline, doxycycline
Leptospira icterohaemorrhagiae *Leptospira canicola*			
Listeria monocytogenes In adults: nonspecific febrile illness; in neonates: meningitis, pneumonia, sepsis, granulomatosis infantisepticum	Standard	Yes	Ampicillin, penicillin, TMP-SMZ
Lyme disease			
Borrelia burgdorferi Multi-staged illness of skin, joint, and peripheral or central nervous system	Standard	Yes, with informed discussion	Ceftriaxone, ampicillin, doxycycline
Lymphocytic choriomeningitis Aseptic meningitis to severe encephalitis, with variable presentation of other symptoms	Standard	Yes	
Malaria	Standard	Yes	Pyrimethamine-sulfadoxine, chloroquine, quinidine, quinine, tetracycline, mefloquine
Marburg virus Hemorrhagic fever	Contact	No (no expressed breast milk)	

Condition/Organism	Precautions	Breastfeeding	Treatment
Mastitis			
Candida albicans	Standard	Yes, with simultaneous treatment of the infant	Nystatin, ketoconazole
Enterobacteriaceae	Standard	Yes	Fluconazole
Staphylococcus aureus	Contact	Yes (after 24 hr of therapy, during which milk must be discarded)	First-generation cephalosporin, dicloxacillin, oxacillin, erythromycin
Group A streptococcus	Contact		
Mycobacterium tuberculosis	Standard (unless there is also pulmonary involvement, then airborne precautions as well)	No breast milk or breastfeeding for 2 weeks of maternal therapy,** consider prophylactic INH for the infant (see Figs. 17-1 and 17-2)	Isoniazid, rifampin, ethambutol, pyrazinamide ethionamide
Measles			
Febrile illness with coryza, conjunctivitis, cough, and an erythematous maculopapular rash	Airborne	Yes (after 72 hr of rash in the mother and after the infant receives ISG, expressed breast milk is ok)	Ribavirin is experimental
Meningitis			
Aseptic meningitis (nonbacterial, viral meningitis)	Standard	Yes	
Fungal meningitis	Standard	Yes	Amphotericin, itraconazole, flucytosine
Haemophilus influenzae	Droplet (for first 24 hr of appropriate therapy and carrier eradication with ceftriaxone or rifampin)	Yes (after 24 hr of maternal therapy, with the infant receiving prophylaxis, P); begin infant vaccination; expressed breast milk is ok	Ceftriaxone, ampicillin, chloramphenicol, rifampin
Neisseria meningitidis	Droplet (24 hr of appropriate therapy and carrier eradication with ceftriaxone or rifampin)	Yes (after 24 hr of maternal therapy, with the infant receiving prophylaxis, P); expressed breast milk is ok	Ceftriaxone, penicillin, chloramphenicol
Streptococcal pneumoniae	Standard	Yes	Ceftriaxone, penicillin, vancomycin
Mumps	Droplet	Yes	
*Mycobacterium tuberculosis***	Standard and airborne	Yes	Antituberculosis medications are acceptable during breastfeeding (see Chapter 17)
Mycoplasma pneumoniae			

Continued

TABLE E-1 Precautions and breastfeeding recommendations for selected maternal infections*—cont'd

Organism, syndrome, or condition[†‡]	Empiric precautions[§]	Breastfeeding acceptable[‖]	Compatibility of medications with breastfeeding[¶]
Bronchitis, pneumonia, pharyngitis, otitis media, and a broad range of unusual manifestations, including central nervous system, cardiac, skin, muscle, and joint involvement	Droplet	Yes	Erythromycin, clarithromycin, azithromycin, tetracycline
Neisseria meningitidis			
Meningitis, meningococcemia	Droplet (for 24 hr of appropriate therapy and carrier eradication with ceftriaxone or rifampin)	Yes (after 24 hr of appropriate therapy, and with prophylaxis for the infant)	Penicillin, ceftriaxone, chloramphenicol, rifampin
Norwalk agent			
Gastroenteritis	Standard	Yes	
Papillomaviruses			
Skin or mucous membrane warts, laryngeal papillomas	Standard	Yes (in the absence of breast involvement)	
Parainfluenzae viruses			
Laryngotracheobronchitis, upper and lower respiratory infections	Standard (contact for infants and children)	Yes	
Parvovirus B19			
Erythema infectiosum, fifth disease, aplastic crisis, arthritis	Standard with erythema infectiosum, droplet for aplastic crisis or infection in patients with hemoglobinopathy or immunodeficiency	Yes	
Pelvic inflammatory disease (see Endometritis)			
Pertussis			
Whooping cough, pneumonia, bronchitis, encephalitis			
Bordetella parapertussis and *Bordetella pertussis*	Droplet (for 5 days of appropriate therapy)	Yes (after 5 days of appropriate therapy and chemoprophylaxis for the infant, expressed breast milk is ok)	Erythromycin, clarithromycin, TMP-SMX
Pneumocystis carinii pneumonitis (PCP)	Standard	Yes, but suspect HIV infection if	Pentamidine, TMP-SMX,

Disease / Organism	Clinical features	Precautions	Breast-feeding	Treatment
			the mother develops PCP and reassess breastfeeding with HIV infection in mind	atovaquone, prednisone
Pneumonia (see specific causative agents)				
Poliomyelitis		Standard	Yes	
Rabies	Severe, progressive central nervous system infection, generally fatal	Standard	No when mother is clinically sick; yes (BM+); yes during postexposure immunization of the mother without symptoms; yes if both mother and infant are receiving postexposure immunization	Rabies immune globulin, rabies vaccine
Rat-bite fever				
Spirillum minus				
Streptobacillus moniliformis		Standard	Yes	Tetracycline, chloramphenicol, streptomycin; Penicillin
Relapsing fever				
Borrelia recurrentis		Standard (tick-borne)	Yes	Tetracycline, doxycycline, TMP-SMX, streptomycin, rifampin
		Contact if louse infested	Yes with simultaneous treatment of mother and infant for lice	
Respiratory syncytial virus	Upper respiratory infection, pneumonia, bronchiolitis	Contact	Yes	Ribavirin
Retroviruses (see Human immunodeficiency viruses 1, 2 and Human T-cell leukemia viruses I. II)				
Rickettsial diseases	Fever, rash, vasculitis; arthropod, louse-borne			
Ehrlichiosis, leukopenia *Ehrlichia chaffensis*		Standard	Yes	Doxycycline, tetracycline
Q fever *Coxiella burnetii*				

Continued

TABLE E-1 Precautions and breastfeeding recommendations for selected maternal infections*—cont'd

Organism, syndrome, or condition[†,‡]	Empiric precautions[§]	Breastfeeding acceptable[‖]	Compatibility of medications with breastfeeding[¶]
Pneumonia, hepatosplenomegaly, endocarditis	Standard	Yes	Doxycycline, tetracycline
Rickettsialpox			
Rickettsia akari			
Scab or eschar, rash, regional lymphadenopathy, self-limited	Standard	Yes	Doxycycline, tetracycline, chloramphenicol
Rocky Mountain spotted fever			
Rickettsia rickettsii	Standard	Yes	Doxycycline, chloramphenicol
Typhus (flea-borne)			
Rickettsia typhi	Standard	Yes	Doxycycline (single dose)
Typhus (louse-borne)			
Rickettsia prowazekii	Standard	Yes	Tetracycline, chloramphenicol
Rotavirus			
Diarrhea, vomiting, "winter vomiting disease"	Contact	Yes	
Rubella virus			
Self-limited, mild exanthem with fever: congenital rubella syndrome	Contact	Yes	
Salmonella (see Diarrhea/gastroenteritis)			
SARS-associated coronavirus, severe acute respiratory syndrome	Droplet	Yes	
Shigella			
Smallpox			
Variola virus (variola major)	Contact, airborne	No (no expressed breast milk)	
Vaccinia virus (smallpox vaccine) secondary contact infection	Contact	Yes, except if breast involved with lesions	
Staphylococcus aureus			
Cellulitis, abscess	Contact	Yes	Oxacillin, dicloxacillin, first-generation cephalosporins, erythromycin, vancomycin
Enterocolitis, diarrhea	Standard	Yes	
Scalded-skin syndrome	Contact	Yes (after 24 hr of effective therapy; discard breast milk for 24 hr)	

Infection/Organism	Precautions	Breastfeeding	Treatment
Toxic shock syndrome	Standard	Yes**	
Methicillin-resistant *S. aureus* (MRSA)	Contact	Yes**	
Staphylococcus epidermidis Opportunistic infections	Standard	Yes	Oxacillin, dicloxacillin, vancomycin
Streptococcus (group A) Cellulitis, pharyngitis, pneumonia, myositis/fasciitis, scarlet fever	Standard	Yes (24 hr after beginning appropriate therapy; discard breast milk for 24 hr)	Penicillin, erythromycin, cephalosporin
	Contact (for extensive skin infection unable to be covered until after 24 hr of therapy)	Yes (24 hr after beginning appropriate therapy; discard breast milk for 24 hr)	
Streptococcus (group B) Urinary tract infection, endometritis, mastitis; infants: sepsis, pneumonia, meningitis, osteomyelitis, arthritis	Standard	Yes** (after 24 hr of effective therapy); for perinatal exposure, high risk, or suspected illness, infant is given empiric therapy	Penicillin, ampicillin
Streptococcus pneumoniae Pneumonia, occult bacteremia, otitis media, sinusitis	Standard	Yes	Penicillin, ceftriaxone, vancomycin, cefotaxime, rifampin
Syphilis *Treponema pallidum* Multisystem, multistage infection with widely varying presentations, congenital infection	Standard	Yes (after 24 hr of effective therapy; discard breast milk for 24 hr)	Penicillin
Open skin lesions of breast or nipples	Contact	No, until 24 hr of effective therapy in mother if open skin lesions involve the breast	Penicillin
Tetanus Exotoxin-mediated severe muscular spasms *Clostridium tetani*	Standard	Yes (age-appropriate vaccination of the child, no tetanus immune globulin [TIG] necessary for infant)	Penicillin, metronidazole

Continued

TABLE E-1 Precautions and breastfeeding recommendations for selected maternal infections*—cont'd

Organism, syndrome, or condition[†‡]	Empiric precautions[§]	Breastfeeding acceptable[‖]	Compatibility of medications with breastfeeding[¶]
Tinea			
Capitis			
Microsporum audouinii	Standard	Yes	Griseofulvin, selenium sulfide shampoo, prednisone
Microsporum canis			
Trichophyton tonsurans			
Corporis, cruris, pedis			
Epidermophyton floccosum	Standard	Yes	Topical agents
Trichophyton canis			
Trichophyton rubrum			
Versicolor			
Malassezia furfur	Standard	Yes	Topical agents, ketoconazole, itraconazole
Toxoplasmosis			
Toxoplasma gondii	Standard	Yes	Pyrimethamine, sulfadiazine
Asymptomatic or mononucleosis-like illness with lymphadenopathy, ocular symptoms; congenital infection			
Toxic shock (see *S. aureus*, *Streptococcus* [group A])	See specific agents		
Toxin-mediated illness			
Bacillus cereus			
Botulism			
Food poisoning			
Staphylococcal scalded-skin syndrome (SSSS)			
Trichinosis			
Trichinella spiralis	Standard	Yes	Mebendazole, thiabendazole, prednisone
Asymptomatic, or may cause myalgia, periorbital edema, myocardial failure, CNS involvement, or pneumonitis			
Trichomonas vaginalis	Standard	Yes	Metronidazole
Vaginitis, urethritis, or asymptomatic infections			

Disease/Organism	Isolation	Reportable	Treatment
Trypanosomiasis			
Trypanosoma brucei			
"Sleeping sickness"; tsetse fly vector (African)	Standard	No	Suramin, pentamidine, eflornithine, melarsoprol
Trypanosoma cruzi			
Chagas' disease (American)	Standard	Yes	Nifurtimox, benznidazole
TT virus			
Hepatitis	Standard	Yes	
Tuberculosis (see Figs. 17-1 and 17-2)			
Tularemia			
Francisella tularensis			
Acute febrile illness with various syndromes; oculoglandular, ulceroglandular, glandular, oropharyngeal, typhoidal, pneumoniae	Standard	Yes	Streptomycin, tetracycline, chloramphenicol
Ureaplasma urealyticum			
Nongonococcal urethritis (NGU), endometritis, pelvic inflammatory disease	Standard	Yes	Doxycycline, erythromycin, azithromycin
Urinary tract infection			
Group B streptococcus (see *Streptococcus* [group B])	Standard	Yes	Ampicillin, aminoglycosides, cephalosporin
Enterobacteriaceal			
Staphylococcus saprophyticus	Standard	Yes	Quinolones
Vaginitis			
Bacterial	Standard	Yes	Metronidazole, clindamycin
Candida albicans (see Candidiasis)			
Trichomonas vaginalis			
Varicella-zoster virus (see Herpes viruses)			
West Nile virus	Standard	Yes	
Asymptomatic, fever, meningoencephalitis			
Whooping cough			
Bordetella parapertusis and *Bordetella pertussis:* see also Adenovirus, *Chlamydia (Chlamydia pneumoniae, Chlamydia trachomatis), Mycoplasma pneumoniae*	Droplet (for 5 days of appropriate therapy and chemoprophylaxis for the infant)	Yes, after 5 days of appropriate therapy, BM+, P	Erythromycin, clarithromycin, TMP-SMX

Continued

TABLE E-1 **Precautions and breastfeeding recommendations for selected maternal infections*—cont'd**

Organism, syndrome, or condition[†‡]	Empiric precautions[§]	Breastfeeding acceptable[‖]	Compatibility of medications with breastfeeding[¶]
Yersinia enterocolitica			
Diarrhea, pseudoappendicitis, focal infections, and bacteremia	Contact precautions for incontinent individuals	Yes	Aminoglycosides, cefotoxine, tetracycline, chloramphenicol
Yersinia pseudotuberculosis			
Fever, rash, abdominal symptoms	Standard	Yes	TMP-SMX

*To ensure that appropriate empiric precautions are always implemented, hospitals must have systems in place to routinely evaluate patients according to these criteria as part of their preadmission and admission care.

[†]Patients with the syndromes or conditions listed may present with atypical signs and symptoms (e.g., pertussis in neonates and adults may not have paroxysmal or severe cough). The clinician's index of suspicion should be guided by the prevalence of specific conditions in the community, as well as clinical judgment.

[‡]The organisms listed are not intended to represent the complete, or even most likely diagnoses, but rather possible etiologic agents that may require additional precautions beyond *standard precautions* until they can be excluded.

[§]These are the usual precautions (Standard, Airborne, Contact, and Droplet), outlined in the text, as proposed by the Centers for Disease Control and Prevention. Symbols for duration of precautions: 24 hours, 24 hours after start of antibiotic therapy. CN, until off antibiotics and culture negative; DI, duration of the illness; PI, period of infectivity.

[‖]Yes means that if in a hospitalized mother and infant, the proposed precautions are followed, breastfeeding is acceptable and may be beneficial to the infant. Any infant breastfeeding during a maternal infection should be observed closely for signs or symptoms of illness.

[¶]See Appendix D and Chapter 11 on medications in breast milk.

[#]Adenovirus types 4 and 7 have been known to cause severe respiratory disease in premature infants or individuals with immunodeficiency or underlying respiratory disease. In certain situations, feeding of expressed breast milk to the infant may not be advisable.

**See text for more complete explanation; *P,* prophylactic antibiotics for the infant with *H. influenzae:* rifampin 10 mg/kg/dose once daily × 4 days for infants less than 1 month of age; rifampin 20 mg/kg/dose once daily × 4 days for infants over 1 month of age (without complete Hib vaccine series, two to three doses of vaccine before 12 months and one after 12 months, one dose after 15 months or two doses between 12 and 14 months). For *Neisseria meningitidis,* give rifampin 10 mg/kg/dose every 12 hours for four doses and 5 mg/kg/dose in children less than 1 month old. Give sulfisoxazole if *N. meningitidis* isolate is sensitive. Alternatively, ceftriaxone 250 mg IM for one dose (125-mg dose for children less than 15 years old) is acceptable. For *Corynebacterium diphtheriae,* give erythromycin 40–50 mg/kg/day × 7 days or a single IM dose of benzathine penicillin G (600,000 U for the child less than 30 kg of weight. For *Bordetella pertussis* or *B. parapertussis,* give erythromycin 40–50 mg/kg/day divided four times a day × 14 days or clarithromycin 15 mg/kg/day in two divided doses × 10 days or TMP-SMX 8 mg/kg of TMP/day and 40 mg/kg of SMX/day in two divided dose × 14 days. *BM+,* although breastfeeding is not acceptable because of exposure risk, giving the mother's expressed breast milk is acceptable.

[††]Breastfeed immediately if mother receives ceftriaxone intramuscularly or intravenously. Breastfed after 24-hr antibiotic therapy for other treatment regiments, with feeding expressed breast milk for the first 24 hours.

Modified from Garner JS: Hospital Infection Control Practices Advisory Committee guidelines for isolation precautions in hospitals. Infect Control Hosp Epidemiol 17:53–80, 1996.

*T*he Lact-Aid Nursing Trainer System

The Lact-Aid Nursing Trainer System is made up of four parts: (1) the body with permanently attached nursing tube, (2) the clamp ring, (3) the extension tube, and (4) the presterilized Lact-Aid bag with 4-oz capacity.

For convenience in filling and assembling the Lact-Aid system, a bag hanger and funnel have been specially designed. Six T-shaped end tabs provide easy attachment to the nursing bra (Figs. F-1 and F-2).

The filled Lact-Aid is attached to the nursing bra or neck cord between the breasts and is positioned so that the supplement cannot siphon out. The presterilized bag is attached to the body by the clamp ring. The infant suckles the tip of the nursing tube and the nipple of the breast at the same

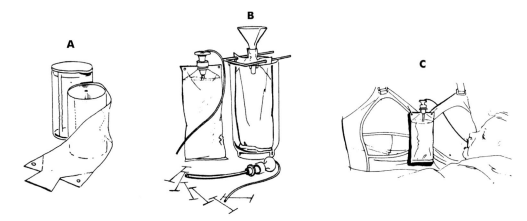

Figure F-1 **A,** Presterilized, disposable bags have 4-oz capacity. **B,** Lact-Aid system includes detailed instruction booklet plus accessories for filling, cleaning, and use. **C,** Filled nursing trainer may be attached directly to the nursing bra as shown or suspended by the neck cord as depicted in Figure 19-4. (From Avery JL: Lact-Aid Nursing Trainer Instruction Book, rev. ed. Athens, TN, Lact-Aid International, Inc, 1983; phone 423-744-9090.)

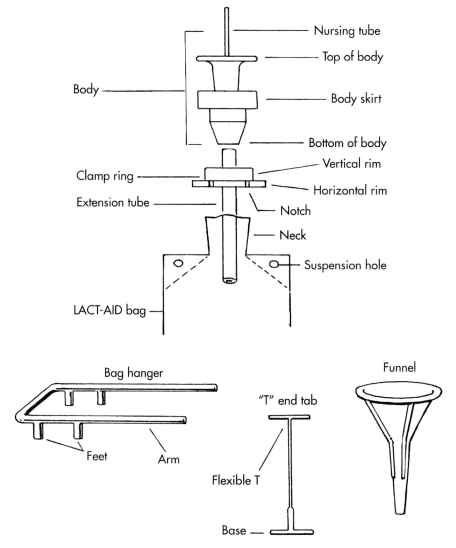

Figure F-2.   Lact-Aid parts. (From Avery JL: Lact-Aid Nursing Trainer Instruction Book, rev. ed. Athens, TN, Lact-Aid International, Inc, 1998; phone 423-744-9090.)

time. As the infant nurses, supplement is drawn from the bottom of the presterilized bag by the extension tube attached to the bottom of the body. This keeps the infant from swallowing any air that might be trapped in the top of the bag. The body has an orifice designed to provide the best rate of flow, slower than milk flows from the breast, but fast enough to keep from overtiring the infant. The nursing tube carries the supplement to the infant's mouth. It is clear, very soft, and flexible and will not cause the infant's mouth or the nipple any discomfort.

When the infant is put to the breast, the flow of supplement rewards the infant's nursing efforts.

This provides a pleasant incentive for the infant to continue nursing, which in turn provides the breasts with suckling stimulation to build up the milk supply. The Lact-Aid is small enough, even when it contains the full 4-oz capacity of supplement, to enable one to nurse discreetly without it showing. It is valuable in adoptive nursing[*] and in infants diagnosed with failure to thrive (see Chapters 12, 14, and 19).

Lactation Supplementer is a similar device made of a rigid plastic container and two tiny plastic tubes, one for each breast. It is is available from Medela.

---

[*]Avery JL: A brief discussion of adoptive nursing: An introduction to the topic, rev. ed. Athens, TN, Lact-Aid International, Inc, 1983; and Avery JL: Induced lactation: A guide for counseling and management, rev. ed. Athens, TN, Lact-Aid International, Inc, P.O. Box 1066, Athens TN 37371-1066 USA.

$\mathscr{M}$anual expression
of breast milk

The health care professional should be familiar with the technique of manual expression and be able to diagnose improper technique.

TECHNIQUE

All breastfeeding women should be familiar with the basic technique of manual expression of milk from the breast, and ideally, this technique is acquired before discharge from the hospital and with the assistance of the nursery or postpartum nursing staff.

Reasons to express breast milk include the following:

1. To initiate flow and assist the infant to grasp the breast properly
2. To encourage production of milk early in lactation when the infant is premature or ill
3. To relieve engorgement
4. To remove milk when it is not possible to nurse the infant at a given feeding
5. To maintain lactation when the infant cannot be fed
6. To pump and save milk for feeding the infant at another time
7. To contribute to a milk bank
8. To pump and discard milk while temporarily on a specific medication

Manual expression is appropriate to initiate the flow before applying a hand pump or an electric pump. Not many women can manually pump large volumes over time without mechanical assistance. The breast should always be massaged and flow initiated before applying any pump.

PROCEDURE

Step 1. *Always* wash hands before handling the breast.

Step 2. Breast massage: whether planning to manually express or mechanically pump, preparing the breast for ejecting the milk facilitates the process. The release of oxytocin and the ejection reflex are stimulated by external stimuli: the baby's cry, a picture of the baby, or gentle handling of the breast. Prolactin release and milk production are stimulated by "sucking" stimulation.

After mother finds a comfortable sitting position and is relaxed, the breast is exposed and gently stroked with the fingertips from periphery to areola (Fig. G-1). As this stroking is intensified, one should avoid slipping the hand across skin and irritating tissues. Gently massage. A warm washcloth soak is also helpful in initiating flow through the ducts. Gentle fingertip massage around all quadrants should follow and be repeated several times during extended mechanical pumping. It should not leave red marks or hurt.

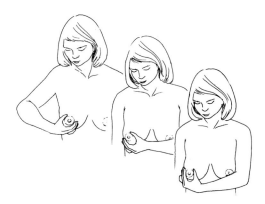

Figure G-1.

Step 3. Position hands on the breast—usually, placing the fingers below and thumb on top is natural for most women. One hand placed above and one hand placed below the areola may be easier when the hand is small compared with breast size. The target area is beyond the ampullae, which are the collecting areas of the main ducts that radiate out from the nipple to the areola. The ampullae are about 3 cm from the nipple base, which may not be at the edge of the areola. Press toward the chest wall and then compress the thumb and fingers together (Fig. G-2). Continue to compress the

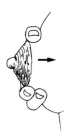

Figure G-2.

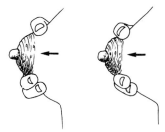

Figure G-3.

breast while moving the hand away from the chest wall in a "milking" action toward the nipple (Fig. G-3). (Avoid pulling, squeezing, or rubbing motions.) Perform this motion in a repeated rhythmic manner at a comfortable but not abrasive rate. Infant suckling does not involve movement (stroking) of the tongue along the elongated areola and nipple, but an undulating motion of the tongue itself. Simulating that motion is the goal of manual expression. This action is similar to a peristaltic motion. The hand should be rotated around the breast to massage and stroke all quadrants, including the periphery and the axillae.

Use one or both hands to find the most productive grasp. Preventing trauma is essential; thus, avoid squeezing, rubbing, or pulling the breast tissue. Every mother develops her own natural pattern, so rigid adherence to methods may be counterproductive. Effectiveness is measured by the comfortable release of milk.

Total emptying of the breast will require 20 to 30 minutes of manual stimulation. Warm compresses, hot showers, or suspending the breast in a bowl of warm water may help, especially if there is engorgement or mastitis. Leaning over and gently shaking the breast may help stimulate flow. Manual expression while leaning over may help empty the lower quadrants.

$\mathcal{T}$he storage of human milk*

ACADEMY OF BREASTFEEDING MEDICINE—HUMAN MILK STORAGE INFORMATION FOR HOME USE FOR HEALTHY FULL-TERM INFANTS

A central goal of the Academy of Breastfeeding Medicine (ABM) is the development of clinical protocols for managing common medical problems that may have an impact on breastfeeding success. These protocols serve only as guidelines for the care of breastfeeding mothers and infants and do not delineate an exclusive course of treatment or serve as standards of medical care. Variations in treatment may be appropriate according to the needs of an individual patient.

*Fully referenced version of the protocol is available from the Academy of Breastfeeding Medicine:

ABM Executive Office
191 Clarksville Road
Princeton Junction, NJ 08550
Toll-free phone: 1 877-836-9947 ext. 25
Permanent tracking telephone: 1 585-275-4354
Local/International phone: 1 609-799-6327
Fax: 1 609-799-7032
E-mail: ABM@bfmed.org
Web site: http://www.bfmed.org

Storage containers

1. Hard-sided containers, such as hard plastic or glass, are the preferred containers for long-term human milk storage. These containers should have an airtight seal.
2. Plastic bags specifically designed for human milk storage can be used for short-term (less than 72 hours) milk storage. Use of plastic bags is not recommended for long-term storage because they may spill, leak, or become contaminated more easily than hard-sided containers, and some important milk components may adhere to the soft plastic and be lost.

General guidelines

1. Hands must be washed prior to expressing or pumping milk.
2. Use containers and pumping equipment that have been washed in hot, soapy water and rinsed thoroughly. If available, cleaning in a dishwasher is acceptable; dishwashers that additionally heat the water may improve cleanliness. If a dishwasher is not available, boiling the containers after washing is recommended. Boiling is particularly important where the water supply may not be clean.
3. Store in small portions to minimize waste. Most breastfed babies take between 2 and

4 oz (60 to 120 mL) of milk when beginning with an alternative feeding method. Storing in 2-oz (60 mL) amounts and offering additional amounts if the baby is still hungry will prevent having to throw away unfinished milk.

4. Consider storing smaller portions (1 to 2 oz [30 to 60 mL] each) for unexpected situations. A small amount of milk can keep a baby happy until mom comes to nurse the baby.

5. Several expressions throughout a day may be combined to get the desired volume in a container. Chill the newly expressed milk for at least 1 hour in the main body of the refrigerator or in a cooler with ice or ice packs, and then add it to previously chilled milk expressed on the same day.

6. Do not add warm breast milk to frozen milk because it will partially thaw the frozen milk.

7. Keep milk from 1 day separate from other days.

8. Do not fill the container; leave some room at the top because breast milk expands as it freezes.

9. Label containers clearly with waterproof labels and ink, if possible.

10. Indicate the date that the milk was expressed, and the child's name (for daycare).

11. Expect that the milk will separate during storage because it is not homogenized. The cream will rise to the top of the milk, and look thicker and whiter. Before feeding, gently swirling the container of milk will mix the cream back through again. Avoid vigorously shaking the milk.

12. The color of milk may vary from day to day, depending on maternal diet. It may look bluish, yellowish, or brownish. Frozen breast milk may also smell different than fresh breast milk. There is no reason not to use the milk if the baby accepts it.

Milk storage guidelines

1. Milk may be kept at room temperature (up to 77° F or 25° C) for 6 to 8 hours.

Temperatures greater than 77° F (25° C) may not be safe for room temperature storage. Containers should be covered and kept as cool as possible; covering the container with a cool towel may keep milk cooler.

2. Milk may be stored in an insulated cooler bag with ice packs for 24 hours.

3. Milk may be safely refrigerated (39° F or 4° C) for up to 5 days. Store milk in the back of the main body of the refrigerator, where the temperature is the coolest.

4. The type of freezer in which the milk is kept determines timetables for frozen milk. Generally, store milk toward the back of the freezer, where the temperature is most constant. Milk stored for the longer durations in the ranges listed below is safe, but there is some evidence that the lipids in the milk undergo degradation resulting in lower quality.

   • Freezer compartment located inside the refrigerator (5° F or −15° C) *2 weeks*
   • Refrigerator/freezer with separate doors (0° F or −18° C) *3 to 6 months*
   • Chest or upright manual defrost deep freezer that is opened infrequently and maintains ideal temperature (−4° F or −20° C) *6 to 12 months*

5. Above guidelines apply only to healthy, full-term infants; guidelines are different for hospitalized, sick, or preterm infants. (See Table H-1 and Box H-1 for guidelines on milk storage.)

Thawing or warming milk

1. The oldest milk should be used first.

2. The baby may drink the milk cool, at room temperature, or warmed.

3. Thaw milk by placing it in the refrigerator the night before use or gently rewarm it by placing the container under warm running water or in a bowl of warm water.

4. Do not let the level of water in the bowl or from the tap touch the mouth of the container.

5. Milk may be kept in the refrigerator for 24 hours after it is thawed.

TABLE H-1	Storage of human milk for home use		
Breast milk	**Room temperature**	**Refrigerator**	**Freezer**
Freshly expressed into closed container	6–8 hr (78°F or lower)	3–5 days (39° F or lower)	2 weeks in freezer compartment inside refrigerator 3 to 6 months in freezer section of refrigerator with separate door 6–12 months in deep freeze (0° F or lower)
Previously frozen—thawed in refrigerator but not warmed or used	4 hr or less (i.e., next feeding)	Store in refrigerator 24 hr	Do not refreeze
Thawed outside refrigerator in warm water	For completion of feeding	Hold for 4 hr or until next feeding	Do not refreeze
Infant has begun feeding	Only for completion of feeding; then discard	Discard	Discard

Developed from Recommendations of The Milk Banking Association of North America, Inc. and current literature. See References, Chapter 21.

6. Never use a microwave oven or stovetop to heat the milk, as these may cause scald spots and will also destroy antibodies.
7. Swirl the container of milk to mix the cream back in, and distribute the heat evenly. Do not stir the milk.
8. Milk left in the feeding container after a feeding should be discarded and not used again.
9. As with all foods, do not refreeze breastmilk once it is thawed or partially thawed.

BOX H-1   Suggestions for milk storage for infant at home

- Wash hands thoroughly.
- Polyethylene bags are acceptable for home use.
- Refrigerate or freeze milk after expressing.
- Use fresh milk whenever possible.
- Freeze milk that will not be used within 2 days.
- Use milk stored in a self-defrosting freezer within 3 months (top of refrigerator).
- Use milk stored in a deep-freeze within 12 months.
- Use the oldest milk first. Date container at time of collection.

HUMAN MILK BANKING AND THE HMBANA

The Human Milk Banking Association of North America (HMBANA) was established in 1985, drawing together representatives of donor milk banks and members of the medical community. The goals of HMBANA are as follows:

1. Provide a forum for networking among experts in the field on issues relating to human milk banking
2. Provide information to the medical community on the benefits and appropriate uses of banked human milk
3. Develop and annually review guidelines for milk banking practices in North America
4. Communicate among member milk banks to ensure adequate supplies for all patients
5. Encourage research into the unique properties of human milk and its uses
6. Act as a liaison between member institutions and governmental regulatory agencies
7. Ensure quality control of donor human milk banking among member banks

through adherence to the mandatory guidelines and periodic inspection of member banks

What is a human milk bank?

A donor human milk bank is a service established for the purpose of collecting, screening, processing, storing, and distributing donated human milk to meet the specific medical needs of individuals for whom human milk is prescribed by physicians. A small processing fee is charged by each milk bank on a per-ounce basis.

How does a human milk bank operate?

Donor human milk banks solicit lactating mothers to donate milk. Donors are carefully screened for health behaviors and tested for communicable diseases before they are accepted as donors.

Donors are taught how to express their milk using sanitary collecting methods.

Donated milk is heat treated to destroy any bacteria or viruses that may be present.

Frozen, heat-treated milk is dispensed to recipients with a medical need for donor milk. A physician's prescription is required.

FREQUENT REASONS FOR PRESCRIBING DONOR MILK

Nutritional uses

Prematurity
Failure to thrive
Malabsorption syndromes
Short-gut syndrome
Renal failure
Feeding intolerance
Inborn errors of metabolism
Postsurgical nutrition
Cardiac problems
Bronchopulmonary dysplasia
Pediatric burn cases

Medicinal/therapeutic uses

Treatment for infectious diseases such as intractable diarrhea, gastroenteritis, infantile botulism, sepsis, pneumonia, and hemorrhagic conjunctivitis
Postsurgical healing (omphalocele, gastroschisis, intestinal obstruction/bowel fistula, colostomy repair)
Immunodeficiency diseases (severe allergies, IgA deficiencies)
Inborn errors of metabolism
Solid-organ transplants (including use for adults)
Noninfectious intestinal disorders (ulcerative colitis, irritable bowel syndrome)

Preventive uses

Necrotizing enterocolitis
Crohn's disease
Colitis
Allergies to bovine and soy milks/feeding intolerance
During immune suppression therapy

DONOR MILK BANKS IN THE UNITED STATES, CANADA, AND MEXICO

Mothers' Milk Bank
751 South Bascom
P. O. Box 5730
San Jose, CA 95150
(408) 998-4550
mothersmilkbank@hhs.co.santaclara.ca.us

Triangle Mothers' Milk Bank
Wake Medical Center
3000 New Bern Avenue
Raleigh, NC 27610
(919) 350-8599
mmould@wakemed.org
abuckley@wakemed.org

Mothers' Milk Bank at
P/SL Medical Center
1719 East 19th Avenue
Denver, CO 80218
(303) 869-1888
mmilkbank@health1.org

Mothers' Milk Bank at Austin
900 E. 30th Street., Ste. 214
Austin, TX 78705
(512) 494-0800
info@mmbaustin.org

Mother's Milk Bank of Iowa
Division of Nutrition
Department of Pediatrics
Children's Hospital of Iowa
University of Iowa Hospitals and Clinics
Iowa City, Iowa 52242
(877) 891-5347 (toll free)
www.uihealthcare.com/milkbank

Mothers' Milk Bank
Special Care Nursery
Christiana Hospital
Christiana Care Health Systems
4755 Ogletown-Stanton Road
Newark, DE 19718
(302) 733-2340 or 1 (800) NICU, ext. 101

Lactation Support Service
BC Childrens' Hospital
4480 Oak Street
Vancouver, BC V6H 3V4, Canada
(604) 875-2282
francesjones@shaw.ca

Banco de Leche Humana
Av. Adalfo Ruiz Cortines #2903
CP 91020
Xalapa, Veracruz, Mexico
52-55-14-4500

Definitions

Donor human milk bank: A donor human milk bank is a service established for the purpose of collecting, screening, processing, storing, and distributing donated human milk to meet the specific needs of individuals for whom human milk is prescribed by health care providers who are licensed to prescribe.

Donor milk: Donor milk is voluntarily given by women other than the biologic mother of the recipient. Donors are not paid.

Fresh-raw milk: Milk stored continuously at approximately 4° C for use not longer than 72 hours after expression.

Fresh-frozen milk: Fresh-raw milk that has been frozen and held at approximately −20° C for not longer than 12 months from date of collection.

Heat-processed milk: Fresh-raw or fresh-frozen milk that has been heated to a minimum of 62.5° C, but no more than 63° C, for 30 minutes, to minimize loss of the unique beneficial properties of the milk.

Pooled milk: Milk received from more than one donor.

Preterm milk: Milk pumped within the first month post partum by a mother who delivered at or before 36 weeks' gestation

DONOR SELECTION

Definition of a donor

1. Acceptable donors shall be healthy lactating women.
2. Use of the following medications is acceptable: insulin, thyroid replacement hormone, nasal sprays, asthma inhalers, topical treatments, eye drops, progestin-only birth control products, and low-dose estrogen birth control products, including Loestrin 1/20, Alesse, Levlite, and Levora. Donors must not be users of nicotine products.
3. The standards of the American Association of Blood Banks for screening donors will be used to determine donor eligibility.
4. Potential donors shall be screened verbally and in writing and given educational materials informing them of the characteristics of the high-risk groups or activities that might

put them at risk for transmitting blood-borne diseases.

Exclusions

1. Potential donors shall be excluded on the basis of the following:
   a. Receipt of a blood transfusion or blood products, except RhoGAM, within the last 12 months
   b. Receipt of an organ or tissue transplant within the last 12 months
   c. Ears or other body parts pierced, tattooing, permanent makeup applied by needle, or an accidental stick with a contaminated needle within the last 12 months
   d. Regular use of more than 2 oz of hard liquor or its equivalent in 24 hours (Institute of Medicine, 1991)
   e. Regular use of over-the-counter medications or systemic prescriptions
   f. Regular use of megadose vitamins or herbal products use as medication, including vitamin/herb combinations
   g. Total vegetarians (vegans) who do not supplement their diet with vitamins
   h. Use of illegal drugs
   i. Use of tobacco products
2. Chronic infections (for example, HIV, HTLV, malaria, and active TB), a history of hepatitis B or C, or a history of cancer other than nonmelanoma skin cancer or cervical cancer in situ will be sufficient to exclude donation of milk.
3. Donors who in the last 12 months had a sexual partner who is at risk for HIV, HTLV, or hepatitis (including anyone with hemophilia or anyone who has used a needle for injection of illegal or non-prescription drugs) will be excluded.
4. Donors will be excluded who in the last 12 months had a sexual partner who in the last 12 months has had tattoos, permanent makeup applied with needles, ear or other body parts pierced, or been accidentally stuck with a contaminated needle.

5. Donors will be excluded if they have ever received human pituitary-derived growth hormone, dura mater (or brain covering) graft, bovine insulin, or had a family history of Creutzfeldt-Jakob disease.
6. Donors are excluded if since 1980 they have spent time that adds up to a total of 5 years in Europe (includes Albania, Austria, Belgium, Bosnia-Herzegovina, Bulgaria, Croatia, Czech Republic, Denmark, Finland, France, Germany, Greece, Hungary, Republic of Ireland, Italy, Liechtenstein, Luxembourg, Macedonia, Netherlands, Norway, Poland, Portugal, Romania, Slovak Republic, Slovenia, Spain, Sweden, Switzerland, UK, and Federal Republic of Yugoslavia).
7. Donors with incarceration for more than 72 consecutive hours are excluded.

Temporary disqualification

Donors shall be instructed to report all infections in the household to the milk bank. After a temporary disqualification, milk donation shall resume at the discretion of the milk bank coordinator.

1. Active donors shall be temporarily disqualified from donating milk under the following conditions:
   a. During any acute infection, including clinical mastitis or monilial and fungal infections of the nipple or the breast
   b. During the 4-week period after a case of rubella or varicella (chickenpox) in the household (starting from when the lesions crust over).
   c. During a reactivation of latent infection with herpes simplex virus (HSV) or varicella zoster of the breast or thorax (starting from when the lesions crust over).
   d. During the 12-hour period after consumption of alcohol (hard liquor, beer, or wine)
   e. During the 30 days after the donor herself or anyone with whom she has household contact has received the smallpox vaccine.

2. Consumption of any over-the-counter or prescription medication, including vitamins, homeopathic remedies, and herbs shall be reported to the milk bank. The milk bank coordinator may temporarily disqualify the donor.
3. Donors who have their ears or other body parts pierced, have tattoos, permanent makeup applied with needles, or are accidentally stuck with a contaminated needle shall be temporarily disqualified from donating for 12 months, and repeat serologic screening shall be required.

Note: Needle acupuncture with sterile, disposable needles shall not disqualify a donor.

For the benefit of the recipient, each donor shall be screened serologically for HIV-1, HIV-2, HTLV, hepatitis C, hepatitis B surface antigen, and syphilis no more than 6 months prior to the first donation. Tests shall be done by a Level 1 CLIA certified laboratory. With any positive result on a diagnostic/confirmatory serologic test a donor is excluded. Any milk from this potential donor which has been held at the milk bank shall be returned to the donor or disposed of as a biohazardous material according to institutional protocols.

Guidelines for the Establishment and Operation of a Donor Human Milk Bank are available in English from HMBANA for a fee. A Spanish translation is also available on request at no additional cost. The guidelines are reviewed and revised annually. For further information or a copy of the guidelines contact:

Mary Rose Tully, MPH, IBCLC
Chair, HMBANA
c/o Mother's Milk Bank
Wake Medical Center
3000 New Bern Ave.
Raleigh, NC 27610
(919) 350 -8599

Recommendations for collection, storage, and handling of a mother's milk for her own infant in the hospital setting can be obtained from the same address.

STANDARDS FOR COLLECTION AND USE OF MOTHER'S OWN MILK WHEN MOTHER AND INFANT ARE SEPARATED*

In a public institution, hospital, daycare center, or health clinic, universal precautions are mandated whenever handling body fluids, including human milk. Gloves shall be worn. Handwashing after exposure should be carried out as soon as gloves are removed. Strict handwashing is required before and after feeding an infant, whether mother's milk or infant formula is used. Bottles of fresh or frozen mother's milk should be returned to the mother by the caregiver even if the infant has begun to feed from the container. The milk should be kept refrigerated except when the infant is being fed. Bottle propping is not permitted.

*Excerpts from Caring for Our Children, National Health and Safety Performance Standards: Guidelines for Out-of-Home Child Care Programs. Aurora, CO, National Resource Center for Health and Safety in Child Care, 1992, pp 74–78, 117–120.

$\mathscr{V}$itamin and mineral supplement needs in normal children in the United States*

GUIDELINES FOR SUPPLEMENTATION

Table I-1 summarizes the following guidelines for the use of supplements in healthy infants and children. The indications for vitamin K and fluoride are discussed in the text only.

Newborn infants

Vitamin K administration to all newborn infants is effective as a prophylaxis against hemorrhagic disease of the newborn. This 1961 recommendation was strongly reaffirmed in 1971 to prevent or minimize the postnatal decline of the vitamin K–dependent coagulation factors (II, VII, IX, and X). Vitamin K_1 is considered the vitamin derivative of choice in a single, intramuscular dose of 0.5 to 1 mg or an oral dose of 1.0 to 2.0 mg. In some instances, the dose may have to be repeated after

1 to 2 weeks and at 4 weeks of age. The more fat in the milk, the higher the vitamin K level. Enhancing fat level in the milk should be encouraged.

Breastfed infants

The renewed emphasis on human milk as an ideal food has raised the question whether breastfed infants require any vitamin or mineral supplements before the introduction of solid foods. This subject bears further discussion, particularly with respect to the most widely used supplements: vitamins A, C, D, and E, iron, and fluoride.

Rickets is uncommon in the breastfed term infant, despite the fact that human breast milk appears to contain small amounts of vitamin D (i.e., about 22 IU/L). One possible explanation is that the vitamin D in breast milk is in the form of an easily absorbed sulfate analogue, but this needs to be confirmed. The antirachitic properties of breast milk seem to be adequate for the normal term infant of a well-nourished mother. However, if the mother's vitamin D nutrition has been inadequate and if the infant does not benefit from adequate ultraviolet light (because of dark skin color, little exposure to

---

*Modified from American Academy of Pediatrics Committee on Nutrition: Vitamin and mineral supplement needs in normal children in the United States. Pediatrics 66:1015, 1980.

| TABLE I-1 | Guidelines for use of supplements in healthy infants and children | | | | |

Child	Multivitamin-multimineral	Vitamin D	Vitamin E	Folate	Iron
Term infants					
Breastfed	0	+	0	0	±[*]
Formula fed with iron fortified	0	0	0	0	0
Preterm infants					
Breastfed[†]	+[†]	+	±[‡]	±[†]	+
Formula fed with iron fortified[†]	+[†]	+	±[‡]	±[†]	+[*]
Older infants (after 6 mo)					
Normal	0	0	0	0	±[‖]
High-risk[§]	+	0	0	0	±
Children					
Normal	0	0	0	0	0
High-risk	+	0	0	0	0
Pregnant teenager					
Normal	±	0	0	±	+
High-risk	+	0	0	+	+

+, a supplement is usually indicated; ± a supplement is possibly or sometimes indicated; 0, a supplement is not usually indicated. Vitamin K for newborn infants and fluoride in areas where there is insufficient fluoride in the water supply are not shown.

[*]Iron-fortified formula or infant cereal is a more convenient and reliable source of iron than a supplement.

[†]Multivitamin supplement (plus added folate) is needed primarily when calorie intake is below approximately 300 kcal/day or when the infant weighs 2.5 kg; vitamin D should be supplied at least until 6 months of age in breastfed infants. Iron should be started by 2 months of age (see text).

[‡]Vitamin E should be in a form that is well absorbed by small, premature infants. If this form of vitamin E is approved for use in formulas, it need not be given separately to formula fed infants. Infants fed breast milk are less susceptible to vitamin E deficiency.

[§]Multivitamin-multimineral preparation (including iron) is preferred to use of iron alone.

[‖]Multivitamin-multimineral preparation (including iron and folate) is preferred to use of iron alone or iron and folate alone.

light, or use of sunscreen on the infant), the infant is at risk for vitamin D deficiency. Supplements of 200 IU of vitamin D daily have been recommended by the American Academy of Pediatrics (AAP) and the Centers for Disease Control and Prevention (CDC) for all breastfed infants, starting at 2 months of age.

Vitamin A deficiency rarely occurs in breastfed infants. Historically, vitamin A supplementation was coupled with vitamin D supplementation because both were provided by cod liver oil. Currently, there is little reason to provide vitamin A supplements; thus, there would be no harm in omitting vitamin A from supplements designed to provide vitamin D for infants who are breastfed. Similarly, there is no evidence that supplementation with vitamin E is needed for the normal breastfed term infant.

Vitamin B_{12} deficiency has been reported in breastfed infants of strict vegetarian mothers but is relatively rare in North America. The report of a 6-month-old infant of a vegan mother with severe megaloblastic anemia and coma is a reminder that the maternal diet strongly influences the concentration of certain water-soluble vitamins in breast milk. Thiamine deficiency can also occur in breastfed infants of thiamine-deficient mothers, but this situation is virtually restricted to infants in developing countries. In the United States, the rare breastfed infants of mothers who are themselves malnourished should receive multivitamin supplements.

Iron deficiency rarely develops before 4 to 6 months of age in breastfed infants because neonatal iron stores can supply the major portion of iron needs during this period. Although breast milk may contain little more than 0.3 mg iron per liter, about half of this iron is absorbed in contrast to the much smaller proportion that is assimilated from other foods. This iron helps to delay the depletion of neonatal iron stores, but other sources of iron are required in midinfancy. In normal breastfed term infants, the addition to the diet of iron-fortified cereal after 6 months of age probably is desirable to supply adequate amounts of iron.

The supplementation of fluoride in the diet of a healthy breastfed infant is no longer recommended by the Academy of Pediatrics. Evidence supports the contention that there is adequate fluoride in human milk, and fluorosis from excessive amounts is a concern.

The Committee on Nutrition* stated in 2003, "It may not be necessary to give fluoride supplements to breastfed infants who are living in an area where water is adequately fluoridated."

Formula fed term infants

Infants consuming adequate amounts of commercial cow milk formulas that are in keeping with the recommendations of the Committee do not need vitamin and mineral supplementation in the first 6 months of life. They do not require supplements during the latter part of the first year if formula continues to be used in appropriate combination with solid foods. After 4 months of age, iron-fortified formula and iron-fortified cereal are convenient sources of iron and are preferable to the use of iron supplements. If powdered or concentrated formula is used, fluoride supplements should be administered only if the community water contains less than 0.3 ppm of fluoride. Ready-to-use formulas are now manufactured with water low in fluoride, and recommendations for fluoride supplementation should be individualized by the pediatrician to provide a total of 0.5 g/day.

Vitamin K deficiency is seen occasionally in infants. It is usually associated with diarrhea and especially with the administration of antibiotics, through a decrease in the synthesis of vitamin K by the intestinal microflora. In the past, the feeding of soy or other nonmilk formulas was associated with vitamin K deficiency and was related in part to the type of oil used in the formula. In 1976 the Committee on Nutrition recommended that all infant formulas, particularly nonmilk formulas, be required to contain an appropriate level of vitamin K.

Preterm infants

The needs of preterm infants for certain nutrients are proportionately greater than those of term infants because of the increased demands of a more rapid rate of growth and less complete intestinal absorption.

During the first weeks of life (before consumption of about 300 kcal/day or reaching a body weight of 2.5 kg), a multivitamin supplement that provides the equivalent of the recommended dietary allowances (RDAs) for term infants should be supplied. The components of this supplement should ideally include vitamin E in a form well absorbed by preterm infants, such as d-α-tocopheryl polyethylene glycol 1000 succinate. Folic acid deficiency has been reported in preterm infants, and folic acid should be included in the regimen. Folic acid is not in liquid multivitamin-multimineral mixes because of its lack of stability. However, because the period of administration will generally be in a hospital, folate can be added to a multivitamin preparation in the hospital pharmacy in a concentration to provide 0.1 mg (the U.S. RDA) per daily dose. The shelf life should be limited to 1 month, and the label should read "shake well" because folate will gradually precipitate. Iron supplementation is best delayed until after the first few weeks of life because extra iron may predispose an infant to anemia when there is insufficient absorption of vitamin E. Neonatal iron stores are still abundant, and iron needs for erythropoiesis are relatively small during the physiologic postnatal decline in hemoglobin concentration.

After several weeks of age, when the infant is consuming more than 300 kcal/day or when the body weight exceeds 2.5 kg, a multivitamin supplement is no longer needed, but it is a convenient

---

*American Academy of Pediatrics Committee on Nutrition: Pediatric Nutrition Handbook, 5th ed. Elk Grove, Ill, American Academy of Pediatrics, 2004.

method for providing the few specific nutrients that still may be required. These nutrients include vitamin D, iron, and possibly folic acid.

There have been sporadic reports of rickets, particularly in breastfed premature infants. This probably results from the low phosphorus content of breast milk, which has only 150 mg/L in contrast to about 450 mg/L in formulas. The condition is also correctable with phosphate supplementation.

However, there is also evidence that vitamin D supplementation is helpful. Iron is required at a level of 2 mg/kg/day beginning at 2 months of age because neonatal iron stores may become depleted earlier than in term infants—before it is appropriate to supply iron in the form of fortified solid foods. Iron-fortified formula also supplies sufficient iron for the prevention of iron deficiency in preterm infants.

$\mathcal{M}$easurements of growth of breastfed infants

Birth to 36 months: Boys
Length-for-age and Weight-for-age percentiles

NAME _____

RECORD # _____

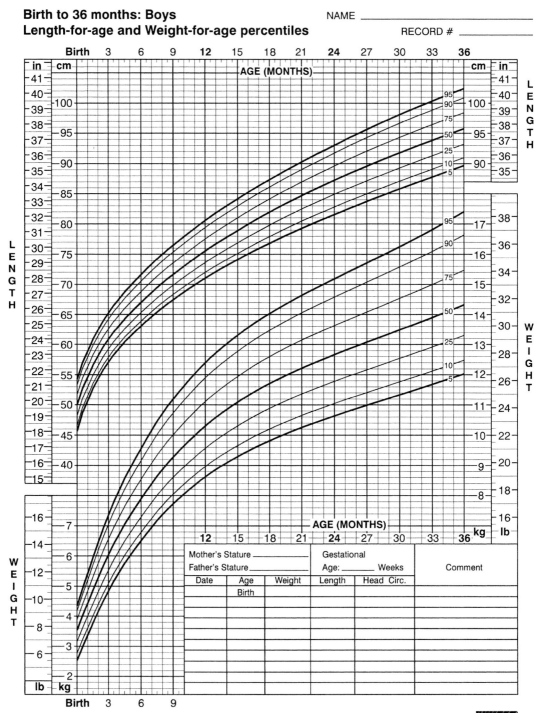

Published May 30, 2000 (modified 4/20/01).
SOURCE: Developed by the National Center for Health Statistics in collaboration with
    the National Center for Chronic Disease Prevention and Health Promotion (2000).
    http://www.cdc.gov/growthcharts

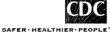

SAFER · HEALTHIER · PEOPLE™

Birth to 36 months: Boys
Head circumference-for-age and
Weight-for-length percentiles

NAME _____

RECORD # _____

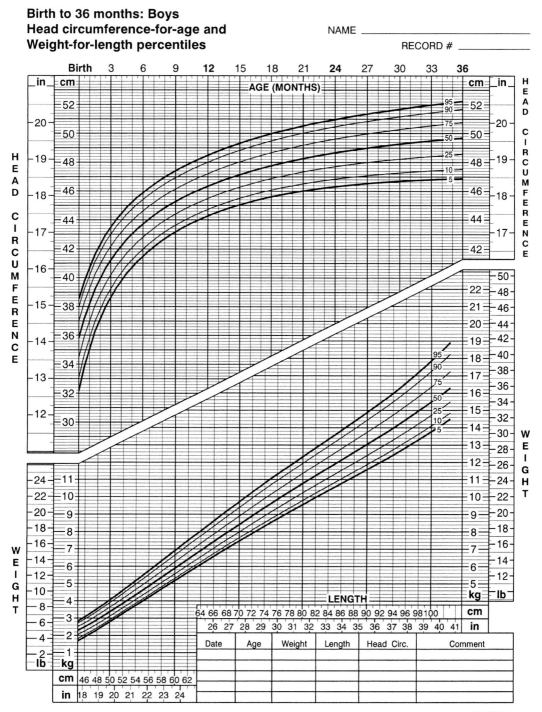

Published May 30, 2000 (modified 10/16/00).
SOURCE: Developed by the National Center for Health Statistics in collaboration with
the National Center for Chronic Disease Prevention and Health Promotion (2000).
http://www.cdc.gov/growthcharts

SAFER · HEALTHIER · PEOPLE™

Birth to 36 months: Girls
Length-for-age and Weight-for-age percentiles

NAME _____

RECORD # _____

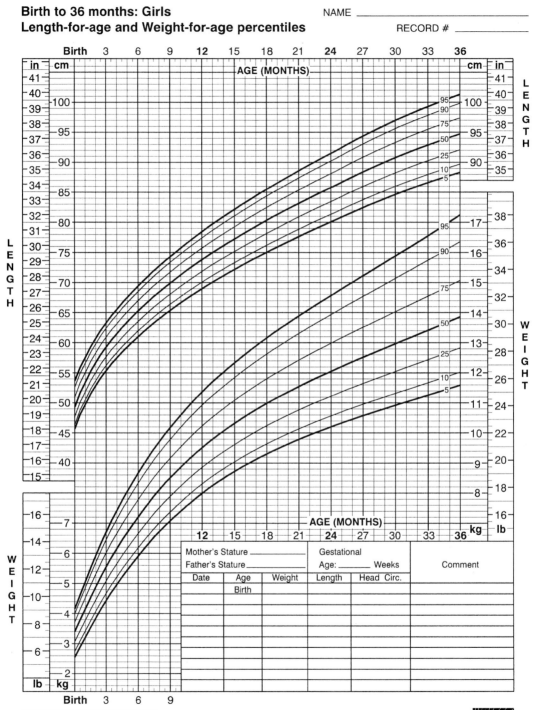

Published May 30, 2000 (modified 4/20/01).
SOURCE: Developed by the National Center for Health Statistics in collaboration with
the National Center for Chronic Disease Prevention and Health Promotion (2000).
http://www.cdc.gov/growthcharts

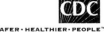

SAFER · HEALTHIER · PEOPLE™

Birth to 36 months: Girls
Head circumference-for-age and
Weight-for-length percentiles

NAME _____

RECORD # _____

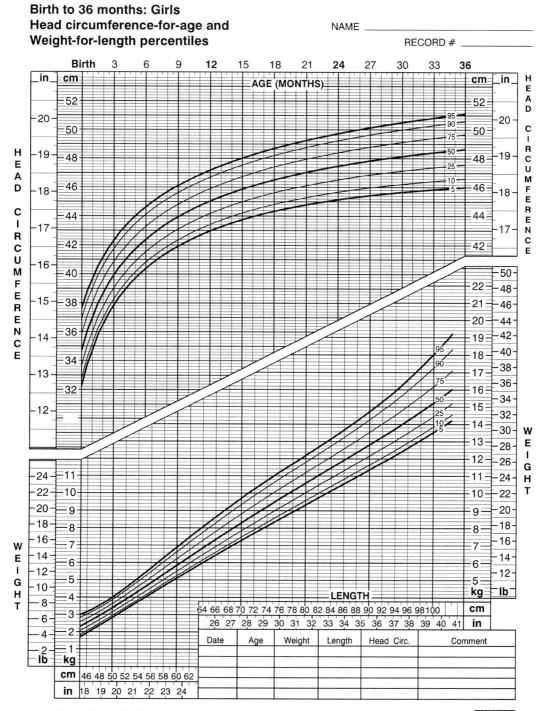

Published May 30, 2000 (modified 10/16/00).
SOURCE: Developed by the National Center for Health Statistics in collaboration with
the National Center for Chronic Disease Prevention and Health Promotion (2000).
http://www.cdc.gov/growthcharts

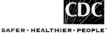

SAFER·HEALTHIER·PEOPLE™

Body mass index-for-age percentiles:

Boys, 2 to 4 years

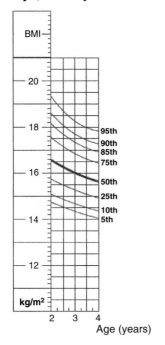

BMI

20

18

95th
90th
85th
75th

16

50th

25th

10th
5th

14

12

kg/m²

2   3   4

Girls, 2 to 4 years

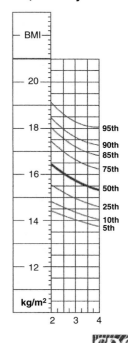

BMI

20

18

95th
90th
85th

75th

16

50th

25th

10th
5th

14

12

kg/m²

2   3   4

Age (years)

Published May 30, 2000.

SOURCE: Developed by the National Center for Heath Statistics in collaboration with the National Center for Chronic Disease Prevention and Health Promotion (2000).

SAFER · HEALTHIER · PEOPLE™

$\mathcal{O}$rganizations that support and provide materials for breastfeeding

GOVERNMENT AGENCIES

Food and Nutrition Information Center
Agricultural Research Service, USDA
National Agricultural Library, Room 105
10301 Baltimore Avenue
Beltsville, MD 20705-2351
(301) 504-5719
Fax: (301) 504-6409
TTY: (301) 504-6856
E-mail: *fnic@nal.usda.gov*
Web site: *http://www.nal.usda.gov/fnic/*

The Center serves the information needs of people interested in human nutrition, nutrition education, food service management, consumer education, and food technology. It acquires and lends books, journal articles, and audiovisual materials dealing with these areas of concern, including breastfeeding research and education.

International Nutrition Communication Service
Education Development Center
55 Chapel Street

Newton, MA 02160
(617) 969-7100

Funded by the U.S. Agency for International Development, the Service provides support and assistance in designing, implementing, and evaluating nutrition training projects in Third World countries. It has also published the *Nutrition Training Manual Catalogue,* which contains reviews of 116 training manuals. The manuals focus on nutrition in developing countries. Breastfeeding training manuals are included.

National Health Information Clearinghouse
PO Box 1133
Washington, DC 20013
(800) 336-4797 (voice, toll-free), (301) 565-4167 (voice)
Fax: (301) 984-4256
E-mail: *info@nhic.org*
Web site: *www.health.gov/NHIC/*

The Clearinghouse helps the public locate health information by identifying health information resources. Health questions are referred to appropriate health agencies that, in turn, respond directly to inquirers.

World Health Organization
Publications Center, USA
49 Sheridan Avenue
Albany, NY 12210
(518) 436-9686
Fax: (518) 436-7433
E-mail: *QCORP@compuserve.com*

Publications available include a statement on infant and young child feeding, a breastfeeding guide for use by community health workers, and a study on patterns of breastfeeding.

PRIVATE EDUCATIONAL AND SUPPORT ORGANIZATIONS

Best Start, Inc.*
4809 E. Busch Blvd., Suite 104
Tampa, FL 33617
(813) 971-2119

Best Start, Inc., is a not-for-profit resource for the social marketing of and training in breastfeeding. The following description is provided by Carol Bryant, Ph.D., executive director.

The Best Start approach calls for local and state coalitions to develop strategies for bringing about institutional and legal changes needed to overcome the barriers created by hospitals, employers, child care facilities, and retailers. For example, the Florida Healthy Mothers, Healthy Babies Coalition has developed a set of model hospital policies and accompanying training module for use in enabling administrators and staff to improve the support that they offer breastfeeding mothers. Efforts are also under way to develop more supportive maternity benefits, provide training for child care providers, and encourage retailers to provide comfortable places for mothers to nurse in department stores and malls.

---

*All materials from Best Start, Inc. available in English and Spanish.

Other components of a comprehensive social marketing approach include community networking, product development, and public information. Outreach to family and friends and the community at large is also important. Classes and activities can be used to provide the community with new information on breastfeeding's advantages and create a more supportive environment for nursing mothers. Many clinic-based programs offer special products such as gift certificates, T-shirts, diapers, shopping bags, and other incentives to breastfeeders. The WIC (Women, Infants, Children) program is also exploring ways to enhance its food package and use other incentives to offset the draw of the free formula. For example, peer counselors can provide valuable support outside the hospital and clinic setting.

Finally, to increase the acceptance of breastfeeding among women, their families, and the public at large, Best Start has developed public service announcements (PSAs) for radio and television. These PSAs attempt to counter the misinformation and lack of confidence many women have, as well as present the many advantages that breastfeeding offers. News releases, newspaper articles, and advocate appearances on talk shows are also used to improve the image of breastfeeding in the wider society.

Clearinghouse on Infant Feeding and Maternal Nutrition
American Public Health Association
1015 Fifteenth Street, NW
Washington, DC 20005
(202) 789-5712

The Clearinghouse serves as a resource primarily for health professionals who work in Third World countries. They also respond to domestic requests as time and staffing permit. They have a large collection of materials of all types on breastfeeding. They make available bibliographies and lists of resources on a variety of topics, and refer inquiries to appropriate sources for information.

Health Education Associates
327 Quaker Meeting House Road
East Sandwich, MA 02537-1300

(888) 888-8077, (508) 888-8044
Mon-Fri 9–5 Eastern Standard Time
Fax: (508) 888-8050

Health Education Associates make available inexpensive pamphlets and other materials as teaching aids on breastfeeding. They sponsor training programs for breastfeeding counseling and promotion techniques.

International Childbirth Education Association
8060 26th Avenue S
Minneapolis, MN 55425-1302
(952) 854-8660
E-mail: *info@icea.org*
Web site: *http://www.icea.org/info.htm*

The association's *Bookmarks* catalog has a large selection of books and inexpensive pamphlets on breastfeeding, childbirth, and parenting. They publish *ICEA News,* with news about childbirth, prenatal, and parenting issues; and *ICEA Review,* which provides in-depth review of current perinatal issues. They also have a resource committee on breastfeeding.

International Lactation Consultant Association
1500 Sunday Drive, Suite 102
Raleigh, NC 27607
(919) 861-5577
Fax: (919) 787-4916
E-mail: *info@ilca.org*
Web site: *www.ilca.org*

The International Lactation Consultant Association (ILCA) provides many member services including newsletters and annual conferences.

Lact-Aid International, Inc.
PO Box 1066
Athens, TN 37371-1066
(423) 744-9090 (orders outside United States, information, and consulting)
(866) 866-1239 (toll-free ordering in the United States)

Fax: (423) 744-9116
E-mail: *feedback@lact-aid.com*
E-mail: *orders@lact-aid.com*
Web site: *www.lact-aid.com*

Lact-Aid International, Inc. formerly published a quarterly journal, *Keeping Abreast, Journal of Human Nurturing.* They make available back issues of the journal and reprints of selected articles. They also produce and market the Lact-Aid Nursing Trainer and specialize in giving information and consultation on specific breastfeeding situations, including prematurity, relactation, adoptive nursing, and failure to thrive.

Also available is a special counseling service: LAMBS (Lact-Aid Mom's Buddies) are peer counselors ready to assist a mother with the same special problem. Resource LAMBS who have personal experience nursing infants with a variety of problems (e.g., cleft palate, Down syndrome) can be reached by calling the Lact-Aid "Warmline."

Lactation Institute and Breastfeeding Clinic
16430 Ventura Blvd. Suite 303
Encino, CA 91436
(818) 995-1913
Fax: (818) 995-0634
Web site: *http://www.lactationinstitute.org/*

La Leche League International, Inc.
1440 North Meacham Road
Schaumburg, IL 60173
(847) 519-7730; (800) LaLeche

La Leche's publications catalog includes a large variety and broad scope of materials for mothers and health professionals to use in promoting and supporting breastfeeding. There is also a directory of League area coordinators by state and foreign country. The coordinators can give information about local support groups.

Nursing Mothers Counsel, Inc.
PO Box 50063
Palo Alto, CA 94303
(408) 272-1448

The Counsel makes available a variety of publications on breastfeeding for mothers and health professionals.

Wellstart International
Corporate Headquarters
PO Box 80877
San Diego, CA 92138-0877
(619) 295-5192
Fax: (619) 574-8159
Helpline: (619) 295-5193
E-mail: *info@wellstart.org*
Web site: *www.wellstart.org*

Wellstart International is a private, nonprofit organization dedicated to the global promotion of healthy families through breastfeeding. Its purpose is to promote breastfeeding for future generations, to expand and share knowledge and understanding of breastfeeding and its benefits to families throughout the world, and to provide leadership for global change.

Wellstart International uses the following methodologies to build on existing resources and ensure quality and sustainability:

Knowledge and skill transfer

Development of health professional faculty as core resources of in-country expertise

Short- and long-term technical assistance, follow-up, and field support

Assessment of infant feeding practices

Program evaluation, impact appraisal, and trends monitoring

Network development and utilization

Policy and economic analyses

Information dissemination, including publications and meetings

Funding support for national program activities

These methodologies are used to spread knowledge, skills, and information in the following subject areas:

Clinical lactation management

Scientific fundamentals of lactation and breastfeeding

Communication and social marketing

Community outreach and mother-to-mother support

Evaluation and research methodologies

Education and training methodologies

Wellstart International has been designated as a WHO Collaborating Center on Breastfeeding Promotion and Protection, with particular emphasis on lactation management education. The organization has also been involved in a variety of global breastfeeding initiatives, including preparation for the Innocenti Declaration, the World Summit for Children, and the Baby-Friendly Hospital Initiative.

OTHER NATIONAL AND INTERNATIONAL BREAST-FEEDING SUPPORT PROGRAMS

For information about Baby-Friendly Hospital Initiative, contact:

Baby Friendly, USA
Karin Cadwell, Ph.D.
Lois Arnold, MPH
327 Quaker Meeting House Road
East Sandwich, MA 02537
(508) 888-8044
Fax: (508) 888-8050
E-mail: *info@babyfriendlyusa.org*
Website: *www.babyfriendlyusa.org*

The World Alliance for Breastfeeding Action (WABA) is a network of organizations and individuals dedicated to protecting, promoting, and supporting breastfeeding as a right of all children and women. For information, contact:

WABA Secretariat
World Alliance for Breastfeeding Action
PO Box 1200
10850 Penang
Malaysia
60-4-884-816
Fax: 60-4-872-655

Other international support organizations:
Ammehejelpen
Postboks 15
Holmen, Oslo 3, Norway

Arbeitsgruppe and Dritte Welt
Postbach 1007
Bern 300, Switzerland

Association for Improvement of Maternity
    Services, Canada/BC
2940 2nd Avenue
Prince George, BC
Canada V2M 1E8
E-mail: *info@aimsbc.org*

Australian Breastfeeding Association (ABA)
PO Box 4000
Glen Iris, Victoria 3146
Australia
(03) 9885 0855, or from outside Australia +61 3
    98850855
Fax: (03) 9885 0866, or from outside Australia +61
    3 98850866
E-mail: *info@breastfeeding.asn.au*
Website: *http://www.breastfeeding.asn.au*

Australian Lactation Consultants' Association Inc.
PO Box 4248
MANUKA ACT 2603
(02) 6295-0384
E-mail: *info@alca.asn.au*
Web site: *www.alca.asn.au*

Baby Milk Action Group
23 St. Andrew's Street
Cambridge, CB2 3AX, UK

Center for Science in the Public Interest
1875 Connecticut Ave. NW
Suite 300
Washington, DC 20009
Main switchboard: (202) 332-9110
Fax: (202) 265-4954
General e-mail address: *cspi@cspinet.org*

National Childbirth Trust
Alexandra House
Oldham Terrace
London, UK
W3 6NH
Breastfeeding line: 0870 444 8708
Enquiries: 0870 444 8707
Administration: 0870 770 3236
Fax: 0870 770 3237
Web site: *www.nctpregnancyandbabycare.com*

War on Want
Fenner Brockway House
37-39 Great Guildford Street
London, UK
SE1 OES
020 7620 1111
Fax: 020 7261 9291
E-mail: *mailroom@waronwant.org*

INTERNATIONAL ORGANIZATION FOR PHYSICIANS

Academy of Breastfeeding Medicine
191 Clarksville Road
Princeton Junction, NJ 08550
(877) 836-9947, ext 25 (toll-free)
(609) 799-6327 (local/international)
(585) 275-4354 (permanent tracking number)
Fax: (609) 799-7032
E-mail: *ABM@bfmed.org*
Web site: *http://www.bfmed.org*

The Academy of Breastfeeding Medicine is a
worldwide organization of physicians dedicated to
the promotion, protection, and support of breastfeeding and human lactation. Its mission is to unite
into one association members of the various medical specialties with this common purpose. The
academy's goals are as follows:
• Physician education
• Expansion of knowledge in both breastfeeding
  science and human lactation
• Facilitation of optimal breastfeeding practices

- Encouragement of the exchange of information among organizations

LACTATION STUDY CENTER

Breastfeeding and Human Lactation Study Center—
Encouraging and Promoting Breastfeeding*
(585) 275-0088, 8 AM to 5 PM EST

The Breastfeeding and Human Lactation Study Center at the University of Rochester Medical Center encourages and promotes human lactation and breastfeeding through physician education and support. The goal is to provide the information that will help the practitioner encourage and support breastfeeding for all patients.

Ruth A. Lawrence, MD, Professor of Pediatrics and of Obstetrics/Gynecology, is responsible for the program's development and operation.

The computer data bank

The core of the Lactation Study Center program is a networked computer system offering physicians information on issues critical to the success of lactation and breastfeeding.

The bibliography data bank, which is constantly updated, provides immediate access to the latest published references on the subject by searching for an article's primary author, for any author, for a word in the title, or by using the keyword code (the keyword categorizes papers by subject areas).

The Center can, for example, look up all papers in the collection discussing "anticonvulsant drugs," using a single keyword that will generate a comprehensive list.

The subject data bank has been divided into major category areas, each of which is summarized from thousands of articles from the medical literature.

The drug data bank includes all the available information about the drug in question, including, if known, its oral availability, whether it appears in the milk, the half-life in maternal plasma and milk, peak time in the maternal plasma and milk, percent protein bound in plasma, percent of adult dose in milk, the maximum amount in a liter of milk, and the ratio of the concentration in milk to the concentration in the maternal plasma.

The biochemistry information can be accessed by the compound name and gives the amount of the compound in various milk fractions; its molecular weight; its solubility properties, including a discussion of the function of the compound in milk; variations related to diet and other factors; the source of the compound; and pertinent references in the literature.

The information on conditions of mother or infant can be identified by name. The information focuses on the effect the condition has on nursing and lactation and what compensatory actions are needed to facilitate the process. The presentation is geared for the professional.

EQUIPMENT COMPANIES

Bailey Medical Engineering
2216 Sunset Drive
Los Osos, CA 93402
(805)528-5781
Fax: (805)528-1461

Hollister
Customer Care Department
2000 Hollister Drive
Libertyville, IL 60048
(847) 918-5882, (800) 323-4060

Kendall
15 Hampshire Street
Mansfield, MA 02048
877-GEL-DISCS

Lact-Aid International, Inc.
PO Box 1066
Athens TN 37371-1066
(423) 744-9090 (orders outside United States, information, and consulting)
(866) 866-1239 (toll-free ordering in the United States)

Maternal Concepts
130 N. Public Street
Elmwood, WI 54740
(800) 310-5817

Medela
PO Box 660
McHenry, IL 60051-0660
(800) 435-8316

Prolac Inc.
10 W. Genesee St.
PO Box 117
Skaneateles, NY 13152
(888) 410-2547

Puronyx, Inc.
990 Park Center Drive, Suite E
Vista, CA 92081
(800) 944-4006

White River Concepts
41715 Enterprise Circle North, Ste 204
Temecula, CA 92590
(909) 296-0081

Whittlestone
PO Box 2237
Antioch, CA 94531
(877) 608-6455

INFORMATION ABOUT EXAMINATION AND CERTIFICATION

Information regarding eligibility to sit the examination for lactation consultants may be obtained by contacting:

International Board of Lactation Consultant Examiners (IBLCE)
7309 Arlington Blvd., Suite 300
Falls Church, VA 22042
(703) 560-7330
Fax: (703) 560-7332
E-mail: *iblce@iblce.org*

Information for physicians as a medical specialist in lactation may be obtained from:

Academy of Breastfeeding Medicine
191 Clarksville Road
Princeton Junction, NJ 08550
(877) 836-9947, ext 25 (toll-free)
(609) 799-6327 (local/international)
Fax: (609) 799-7032
E-mail: *ABM@bfmed.org*
Web site: http://www.bfmed.org

$\mathcal{L}$egislation regarding human milk*

AVAILABILITY OF HUMAN MILK

State of New York

An ACT to amend the public health law, in relation to the availability of human breast milk for infant consumption.

The People of the State of New York, represented in Senate and Assembly, do enact as follows:

Section 1. Legislative findings. The legislature hereby finds and declares that human breast milk, the preferred food for all infants, provides a superior, well tolerated nutritional source because of its unique components. It contains substances, lacking in other forms of infant nutrition, which help control infection and aid in preventing infant disease. For premature infants or those with a low birth weight or infants who are allergic to cow's milk and infant formulas, human breast milk is essential.

It shall be the declared policy of the state of New York that any and all infants requiring human breast milk be assured access to sufficient quantities of wholesome human breast milk, donated by concerned lactating mothers on a continual and systematic basis. The availability of such a supply of human breast milk should be made known to the public so that health providers and families of infants with particular need for human breast milk will be aware of its accessibility.

§2. The public health law is amended by adding a new section twenty-five hundred five to read as follows:

§2505. Human breast milk; collection, storage, and distribution; general powers of the commissioner. The commissioner is hereby empowered to:

(a) adopt regulations and guidelines including, but not limited to donor standards, methods of collection, and standards for storage, and distribution of human breast milk;

(b) conduct educational activities to inform the public and health care providers of the availability of human breast milk for infants determined to require such milk and to inform potential donors of the opportunities for proper donation;

(c) establish rules and regulations to effectuate the provisions of this section.

§3. This act shall take effect immediately.

---

* Excerpts verbatim from relevant legislative acts passed by the States of New York and Florida.

NEW YORK STATE CODE IN SUPPORT OF BREASTFEEDING (ADDED 1984)

Chapter V Subchapter A Article 2 Part 405 Hospitals—minimum standards (statutory authority: public health law § 2803) 405.8 Maternal, child health and newborn services

(10)(i) The hospital, with the advice of the maternity staff, shall formulate a program of instruction and provide assistance for each maternity patient(s) in the fundamentals of (normal) infant care including infant feeding choice and techniques, post-pregnancy care and family planning.

(ii) The hospital shall provide instruction and assistance to each maternity patient who has chosen to breast-feed and shall provide information on the advantages and disadvantages of breast-feeding to women who are undecided as to the feeding method for their infants. As a minimum:

(a) the hospital shall designate at least one person who is thoroughly trained in breast-feeding physiology and management to be responsible for ensuring the implementation of an effective breast-feeding program; and

(b) policies and procedures shall be developed to assist the mother to breast-feed which shall include but not be limited to:

(1) prohibition of the application of standing orders for antilactation drugs;

(2) placement of the infant for breast-feeding immediately following delivery, unless contraindicated;

(3) restriction of the infant's supplemental feedings to those indicated by the medical condition of the infant or of the mother;

(4) provision for the infant to be fed on demand; and

(c) assurance that an educational program has been given as soon after admission as possible which shall include but not be limited to:

(1) the nutritional and physiological aspects of human milk;

(2) the normal process for establishing lactation, including care of breasts, common problems associated with breast-feeding and frequency of feeding;

(3) dietary requirements for breast-feeding;

(4) diseases and medication or other substances which may have an effect on breast-feeding;

(5) sanitary procedures to follow in collecting and storing human milk; and

(6) sources for advice and information available to the mother following discharge.

FLORIDA LEGISLATION— FEBRUARY 1993

House bill no. HB 231, Senate bill no. SB 472

SUBJECT: Encouraging breastfeeding and authorizing breastfeeding in public

1. EFFECT OF PROPOSED CHANGES/ COMMENTS:

This bill would be an endorsement of the importance of Florida infants being breastfed and protect a mother's right to breastfeed whenever and wherever she needs to.

Increasing breastfeeding rates is an international, national and state health priority. Florida has among the lowest breastfeeding rates in the nation. A perceived major barrier for many women to breastfeeding is a fear of embarrassment and harassment when breastfeeding in public. This bill would diminish those fears and make women more secure in their right to breastfeed. More Floridian mothers breastfeeding would lead to decreased infant mortality and morbidity rates. Increased rates of breastfeeding among WIC infants would lead to significant financial savings, due to reduction in illness and associated physician visits, outpatient treatment and hospitalization.

2. ECONOMIC IMPACT AND FISCAL NOTE:
  None

Florida House of Representatives—1993 CS/HB 231

A bill to be entitled

An act relating to breast feeding; encouraging breast feeding and authorizing breast feeding in public; amending ss. 800.02 and 800.03, F.S.; clarifying language and providing that breast feeding a baby does not violate prohibitions against unnatural and lascivious acts or exposure of sexual organs, and reenacting s. 933.18(7)(b) and (c), F.S., relating to search warrants, to incorporate said amendments in references thereto; amending s. 800.04, F.S.; clarifying language and providing that breast feeding a baby does not violate prohibitions against lewd, lascivious, or indecent conduct in the presence of a child; amending s. 847.001, F.S.; providing that breast feeding a baby does not violate prohibitions against obscenity, is not harmful to minors, and does not constitute unlawful nudity or sexual conduct, and reenacting s. 847.0133(1), F.S., relating to protection of minors, to incorporate said amendment in a reference thereto; providing an effective date.

WHEREAS, the Surgeon General of the United States recommends that babies from birth to 1 year of age be breast fed, unless medically contraindicated, in order to attain an optimal healthy start, and

WHEREAS, despite the Surgeon General's recommendation, statistics reveal a declining percentage of mothers who are choosing to breast feed their babies, and

WHEREAS, nearly half of all new mothers are now choosing formula over breast feeding before they even leave the hospital, only 20 percent are still breast feeding when their babies are 6 months old, and only 6 percent are still breast feeding when their babies are 1 year old, and

WHEREAS, breast milk offers better nutrition, immunity, and digestion, and may raise a baby's IQ, in addition to such other benefits as improved mother-baby bonding, and its encouragement has been established as a major goal of this decade by the World Health Organization and UNICEF, and

WHEREAS, the social constraints of modern society militate against the choice of breast feeding and lead new mothers with demanding time schedules to opt for formula feeding for reasons such as embarrassment and the fear of social ostracism or criminal prosecution, and

WHEREAS, the promotion of family values and infant health demand putting an end to the vicious cycle of embarrassment and ignorance that constricts women and men alike on the subject of breast feeding and represents hostility to mothers and babies in our culture based on archaic and outdated moral taboos, and

WHEREAS, any genuine promotion of family values should encourage public acceptance of this most basic act of nurture between mother and baby, and no mother should be made to feel incriminated or socially ostracized for breast feeding her baby, NOW, THEREFORE,

Be It Enacted by the Legislature of the State of Florida:

Section 1. The breast feeding of a baby is an important and basic act of nurture which must be encouraged in the interests of maternal and child health and family values. A mother may breast feed her baby in any location, public or private, where the mother is otherwise authorized to be, irrespective of whether or not the nipple of the mother's breast is covered during or incidental to the breast feeding.

Section 2. Section 800.02, Florida Statutes, is amended to read:

800.02 Unnatural and lascivious act.—A person who commits any unnatural and lascivious act with another person commits a misdemeanor of the second degree, punishable as provided in s. 775.082 or s. 775.083. A mother's breast-feeding of her baby does not under any circumstance violate this section.

Section 3. Section 800.03, Florida Statutes, is amended to read:

800.03 Exposure of sexual organs.—It is unlawful to expose or exhibit one's sexual organs in public or on the private premises of another, or so near thereto as to be seen from such private premises, in a vulgar or indecent manner, or to be naked in public except in any place provided or set apart for that purpose. Violation of this section is a misdemeanor of the first degree, punishable as provided in s. 775.082 or s. 775.083. A mother's breast feeding of her baby does not under any circumstance violate this section.

Section 4. For the purpose of incorporating the amendments to sections 800.02 and 800.03, Florida Statutes, in references thereto, section 933.18(7)(b) and (c), Florida Statutes, are reenacted to read:

933.18 When warrant may be issued for search of private dwelling.—No search warrant shall issue under this chapter or under any other law of this state to search any private dwelling occupied as such unless:

(7) One or more of the following misdemeanor child abuse offenses is being committed there:

(b) Commission of an unnatural and lascivious act with a child, in violation of s. 800.02.

(c) Exposure of sexual organs to a child, in violation of s. 800.03.

If, during a search pursuant to a warrant issued under this section, a child is discovered and appears to be in imminent danger, the law enforcement officer conducting such search may remove the child from the private dwelling and take the child into protective custody pursuant to s. 415.506. The term "private dwelling" shall be construed to include the room or rooms used and occupied, not transiently but solely as a residence, in an apartment house, hotel, boardinghouse, or lodging house. No warrant shall be issued for the search of any private dwelling under any of the conditions herein above mentioned except on sworn proof by affidavit of some creditable witness that he has reason to believe that one of said conditions exists, which affidavit shall set forth the facts on which such reason for belief is based.

Section 5. Section 800.04, Florida Statutes, is amended to read:

800.04 Lewd, lascivious, or indecent assault or act upon or in presence of child.—A person who:

(1) Handles, fondles, or assaults any child under the age of 16 years in a lewd, lascivious, or indecent manner;

(2) Commits actual or simulated sexual intercourse, deviate sexual intercourse, sexual bestiality, masturbation, sadomasochistic abuse, actual lewd exhibition of the genitals, or any act or conduct which stimulates that sexual battery is being or will be committed upon any child under the age of 16 years or forces or entices the child to commit any such act;

(3) Commits an act defined as sexual battery under s. 794.011(1)(b) upon any child under the age of 16 years; or

(4) Knowingly commits any lewd or lascivious act in the presence of any child under the age of 16 years, without committing the crime of sexual battery, commits a felony of the second degree, punishable as provided in s. 775.082, s. 775.083, or s. 775.084. Neither the victim's lack of chastity nor the victim's consent is a defense to the crime proscribed by this section. A mother's breast feeding of her baby does not under any circumstance violate this section.

Section 6. Subsections (3), (5), (7), (11), and (13) of section 847.001, Florida Statutes, are amended to read:

847.001 Definitions.—When used in this chapter:

(3) "Harmful to minors" means that quality of any description, exhibition, presentation, or representation, in whatever form, of nudity, sexual conduct, or sexual excitement when it:

(a) Predominantly appeals to the prurient, shameful, or morbid interest of minors;

(b) Is patently offensive to prevailing standards in the adult community as a whole with respect to what is suitable material for minors; and

(c) Taken as a whole, is without serious literary, artistic, political, or scientific value for minors.

A mother's breast feeding of her baby is not under any circumstance "harmful to minors."

(5) "Nudity" means the showing of the human male or female genitals, pubic area, or buttocks with less than a fully opaque covering; or the showing of the female breast with less than a fully opaque covering of any portion thereof below the top of the nipple; or the depiction of covered male genitals in a discernibly turgid state. A mother's breast feeding of her baby does not under any circumstance constitute

"nudity," irrespective of whether or not the nipple is covered during or incidental to feeding.

(7) "Obscene" means the status of material which:

(a) The average person, applying contemporary community standards, would find, taken as a whole, appeals to the prurient interest;

(b) Depicts or describes, in a patently offensive way, sexual conduct as specifically defined herein; and

(c) Taken as a whole, lacks serious literary, artistic, political, or scientific value.

A mother's breast feeding of her baby is not under any circumstance "obscene."

(11) "Sexual conduct" means actual or simulated sexual intercourse, deviate sexual intercourse, sexual bestiality, masturbation, or sadomasochistic abuse; actual lewd exhibition of the genitals; actual physical contact with a person's clothed or unclothed genitals, pubic area, buttocks, or, if such person is a female, breast; or any act or conduct which constitutes sexual battery or simulates that sexual battery is being or will be committed. A mother's breast feeding of her baby does not under any circumstance constitute "sexual conduct."

$\mathcal{B}$reastfeeding health supervision

TABLE M-1 Overview of breastfeeding health supervision: prenatal to 15 months

Visit	Primary issues	History	Physical assessment	Anticipatory guidance	Interventions
Prenatal	Explore family perceptions Provide accurate information Endorse breastfeeding	Previous experience with breastfeeding Breast-related medical or surgical history Breastfeeding family history	Refer for or offer prenatal breast exam to identify breastfeeding-related concerns	Review issues regarding breastfeeding immediately after birth Refer to breastfeeding support group or classes Provide books or videos to borrow or buy	Avoid nipple preparation techniques that may precipitate premature labor
Newborn	Evaluate delivery events Minimize interference and anxiety Targeted education Identify any need to monitor	Birth history, weight, gestational age Details of first feeding Subsequent feedings Any supplements No wets and stools Mother's condition Family's feelings	Weight loss since birth Newborn exam Oral/motor assessment Note behavioral state State of hydration Maternal breast exam Observe breastfeeding	Breastfeed on cue Baby may show little interest Arouse to feed q 4 h Issues of pacifiers Normal breastfeeding Normal elimination	Supportive nondisruptive care Intervene when indicated Correct latch-on or feeding position problems Treat cause of low milk supply Maintain lactation if maternal-infant separation
At 48–72 hours	Adequacy of milk supply Milk transfer and intake Hydration status Maternal nutrition status	Number and length of feedings Any supplements? Wets and stools per 24 hr Does baby latch on easily and nurse eagerly? Mother's feelings, conditions of breasts, nutrition Family's feelings	Weight gain or loss since birth Newborn exam ? jaundice Oral/motor assessment Access state of hydration Observe breastfeeding Maternal breast exam Consider test weight	Breastfeed on cue Review normal variability of feeds Discourage pacifiers Nighttime feeding Discuss sleeping arrangements Maternal care and nutrition Pros and cons of introducing a bottle Celebrate success or mourn loss	Correct latch-on or feeding position Identify cause and treat low milk supply before supplementing Provide supplemental feeds if necessary Pump breasts if baby not nursing effectively Schedule appropriate follow-up until weight gain adequate and feeding well

Age	Goals	History	Examination	Anticipatory Guidance	Interventions
By 1 month	Sustain mother Adequacy of milk supply and intake	Baby's feeding pattern and no. of feeds? Any supplements? Is newborn feeding on cue? Wets and stools per 24 hr? Mother's feelings, perception of milk supply, condition of breasts, nutrition, plans Family's perceptions	Weight change since birth Should gain 140–196 g/wk Observe breastfeeding Maternal breast exam Newborn examination Consider using test weight	Breastfeed on cue, usually 8–12 feeds per 24 hr Discourage pacifiers Discuss nighttime feedings and sleep Discuss elimination patterns and appetite spurts Exclusive breast milk feedings until ~6 mo Maternal issues, e.g., child care, contraceptives Discuss pumping and storing breast milk Discuss OTC medications	Consider referral to lactation specialist Correct latch-on or feeding position Identify cause and treat low milk supply Supplement may be indicated if weight gain < 140–196 g/wk or has not regained birth weight by 10–14 d Increase feeding frequency to improve milk supply Refer to breastfeeding support group
At 2 months	Maintain commitment Integrate into family lifestyle Determine maternal well-being	Baby's feeding pattern Is baby content with feedings? Any formula or foods? Mother's perception of milk supply, any food restrictions, meds, plans to return to work Family's perceptions	Should be gaining 140–196 g/wk Observe breastfeeding, if indicated Newborn examination	Unrestricted feeding ~8–12 per 24 hr Nighttime feedings Support exclusivity Stool frequency may decrease Teething Maternal issues	Consider referral to lactation specialist Identify cause and treat low milk supply before supplementing Supplement may be indicated if weight gain less than 140–196 g/wk or has not regained birth wt by 10–14 d Vitamin D supplement (200 units/day) if indicated
At 4 months	Sustain exclusivity Sustain duration Interpret changes in behavior	Feeding behavior Feedings other than breast milk Feeding on cue	Weight gain since birth Should be gaining 140–196 g/wk Evidence of teething	Breastfeed 6–12 times per 24 hr Encourage exclusive breast milk feeds until about 6 mo	If baby is growing normally and mother is satisfied with feeding routine,

Continued

TABLE M-1	Overview of breastfeeding health supervision: prenatal to 15 months—cont'd				
Visit	Primary Issues	History	Physical Assessment	Anticipatory Guidance	Interventions
		Family's opinions Mother's health Working and breastfeeding	Assess developmental indicators for solid foods	Discuss signs of readiness for solids Stools may change when solids are introduced Baby's distractibility Teething behavior and management, wearing not indicated when baby cuts teeth Offer supplemental fuids in a cup	no intervention is necessary May use any previously described interventions that are indicated
At 6 months	Celebration Introduction of food Sustain commitment to duration	Feeding behavior Feedings other than breast milk Sleep and night feedings Mother's health Working and breastfeeding Family's opinions	Weight gain since birth Should be gaining 84–140 g/wk May follow lower percentile than expected from standard growth chart Assess developmental indicators of readiness for foods	6–12 feedings per 24 hr Solid foods should not replace breastfeeding Offer fluids in a cup Encourage continued breastfeeding Appropriate dental hygiene Discuss nursing in public and pressure to wean Importance of iron-containing foods Ovulation and menstruation may return when not breastfeeding exclusively	Initiate fluoride supplement if indicated Consider iron supplement for babies who continue to breastfeed exclusively Administer vitamin D supplement if indicated Breastfeeding interventions when and if indicated Refer mother for routine breast exam if weaning
At 9 months	Extended breastfeeding Pressures to wean Behavioral interpretations	Feeding behavior Acceptance of solid foods Mother's interpretation of baby's feeding	Weight gain since birth Should be gaining 34–140 g/wk May follow lower percentile than expected from standard growth	≤6 to ≥12 breastfeeds per 24 hr, some brief Normal breastfeeding behaviors of the older baby Communication behaviors regarding nursing	Breastfeeding interventions when and if indicated Refer mother for routine breast exam if weaning

Age		History	Examination/Laboratory	Counsel	Intervention
		behavior Family's opinions Other concerns	chart Obtain Hgb or Hct	Encourage continued breastfeeding Emphasize the expanding role of the father Discuss nursing in public and pressure to wean Importance of iron-containing foods	Breastfeeding interventions when and if indicated Refer mother for routine breast exam if weaning Baby-led weaning and appropriate weaning techniques for mother
At 1 year	Celebration Continuing to breastfeed Weaning issues	Mother's feelings Baby's feeding pattern Mother's diet Baby's diet other than breast milk Sleeping pattern Family's opinions	Weight gain Consider Hgb or Hct	≤6 to ≥12 breastfeeds per 24 hr, some brief Normal breastfeeding behaviors of the older baby, including nursing for comfort Communication behaviors regarding nursing Encourage continued breastfeeding Discuss weaning options	
At 15 months	Reassurance Support	Breastfeeding behavior Baby's diet Mother's feelings	Weight gain Consider Hgb or Hct	Normal for mother and baby to enjoy nursing Breastfeeding times can be negotiated Any weaning should be gradual and sensitive Encourage a variety of foods	Offer ways for parents to expand their relationship with the child during the weaning period Appropriate weaning techniques

Hgb (hemoglobin) at 9–15 mo, mean = 12.3, lower limit = 11.3; Hct (hematocrit) at 9–15 mo, mean = 35.9, lower limit = 33.0; OTC, over-the-counter.
Modified from Black LS: Incorporating breastfeeding care into daily newborn rounds and pediatric office practice. Pediatr Clin North Am 48: 299, 2001. Excerpted from American Academy of Pediatrics Breastfeeding Health Supervision and Checklists for Breastfeeding Health Supervision. Elk Grove, Ill. American Academy of Pediatrics: copyright American Academy of Pediatrics; with permission.

TABLE M-2 **Breastfeeding developmental milestones: The first year**

Parameter	Birth	2 Wk	1 Mo	2 Mo	4 Mo	6 Mo	9 Mo	12 Mo
Weight	May lose ≈ 8% of birth weight in first 3–4 d	Regains birth weight	Gains 140–196 g/wk, growth follows std chart	—	—	Gains 84–140 g/wk, growth may follow lower percentile on std chart	—	—
Stools	Meconium changing to yellow/greenish black by day 3 or 4	3–4/d, possibly one every feed, color yellow. Can be watery	Frequency ↓ if formula offered	Stools may decrease to one every 3–7 d	—	Stools change when start solid foods	—	—
Feeding	Variable, at least 8–12 per 24 h	—	↑ Predictability 8–12 per 24 h	8 to ≥10 feeds per 24 h	—		≥ 6 to ≤ 12 feeds per 24 h, some brief	—
Night feeding	Wake baby to feed every 3–4 h	Feed on cue, wake for night feeding if sleeps > 5 h	—	Feed on cue if gaining well	—	—	—	—
Feeding devices	Avoid artificial nipples	Discourage pacifiers, may introduce bottle nipple if indicated	—	—	After 4–6 mo offer supplemental fluids in cup	—	—	—
Vitamins and minerals	—	—	—	Vit. D 400 IU/d at any age if indicated	Fluoride if indicated Consider iron sources	Check Hgb/Hct	—	—
Solid foods	—	Effects of mother's diet on infant	—	The effect of what the neighbors fed their infant	The infant looks at what mom is eating	The right time to give the infant solid food	"The baby doesn't like the solid food"	"The baby only wants table

Sleep issues	Unpredictable pattern Importance of night feedings "He wakes up every time I put him down"	Options of where infant will sleep Sleep safety counselling Father can help at night	—	—	Usually content to wake once at night	—	food." "The only thing he will do is nurse." Some may sleep through the night.
Behavior issues	Sleeps too much Infant cues	Doesn't sleep enough Fussiness Colic Appetite spurts	—	Distractibility Teething behavior "The baby likes the bottle better"	—	Focus on developmental tasks may change breastfeeding behavior	Infant "asks" to nurse Nursing for comfort Attachment and independence
Maternal issues	Adequacy of milk supply Sleep Fluids and nutrition Changing relationship with partner Visitors Help with house and sibs Engorgement Sore nipples	Milk supply Breast size returns to prepregnancy appearance Dietary restrictions Nursing in public Contraception	—	Return to work Child care Exercise Dieting OTC meds	Return of ovulation and menstrual cycle	Referral for routine breast exam by mother's physician	Pressure to wean Expanding paternal role —

Modified from Black LS: Incorporating breast feeding care into daily newborn rounds and pediatric office practice. Pediatr Clin North Am 48: 299, 2001.
OTC, over-the-counter; Hgb, hemoglobin at 9–15 mo, mean 12.3, lower limit 11.0; Hct, hematocrit at 9–15 mo, mean 35.9, lower limit 33.0

$\mathcal{R}$esources for education and training

Breastfeeding: A Special Relationship
Eagle Video Productions
2201 Woodnell Drive
Raleigh, NC 27603

Breastfeeding: The Art of Mothering
Alive Productions, Ltd.
PO Box 72
Port Washington, NY 11050

Best Start: For All the Right Reasons
Other materials listed in the Best Start Breast-
feeding Promotion Catalogue
Best Start, Inc.
4809 E. Busch Blvd., Suite 104
Tampa, FL 33617

Breastfeeding Your Preterm Baby
Health Sciences Center for Educational Resources
Distribution Center, SB-56
University of Washington
Seattle, WA 98195
(206) 543-6114

Breastfeeding: Catalogue of products from
projects supported by the Bureau of Maternal and
Child Health and Resources Development, 1989
National Center for Education in Maternal and
Child Health
Georgetown University
Box 571272
Washington, DC 20057-1272

Childbirth Graphics,
a division of WRS Group, Inc.
PO Box 21207
Waco, TX 76702-1207
(800) 299-3366 ext 287

Noodle Soup
4614 Prospect Ave. #421
Cleveland, OH 44103-4314
(800) 795-9295

Vida Health Communications, Inc.
6 Bigelow Street
Cambridge, MA 02139
(800) 550-7047

Wellstart, Inc.
Corporate Headquarters
PO Box 80877
San Diego, CA 92138-0877
(619) 295-5192

$\mathcal{T}$he AAP guideline for hyperbilirubinemia

In July 2004, the Subcommittee on Hyperbili-rubinemia of the American Academy of Pediatrics published the following guideline on the manage-ment of hyperbilirubinemia in newborn infants:

These guidelines emphasize the importance of universal systematic assessment for the risk of severe hyperbilirubinemia, close follow-up, and prompt intervention when indicated. The recom-mendations apply to the care of infants at 35 or more weeks of gestation. These recommendations seek to further the aims defined by the Institute of Medicine as appropriate for health care: safety, effectiveness, efficiency, timeliness, patient-cen-teredness, and equity. They specifically emphasize the principles of patient safety and the key role of timeliness of interventions to prevent adverse out-comes resulting from neonatal hyperbilirubinemia.

The following are the key elements of the recom-mendations provided by this guideline. Clinicians should:

Excerpted from Subcommittee on Hyperbilirubinemia, American Academy of Pediatrics: Management of hyperbilirubinemia in the newborn infant 35 or more weeks' gestation. Pediatrics 114: 297, 2004.

1. Promote and support successful breastfeeding.
2. Establish nursery protocols for the identifica-tion and evaluation of hyperbilirubinemia.
3. Measure the total serum bilirubin (TSB) or transcutaneous bilirubin (TcB) level on infants jaundiced in the first 24 hours (Table O-1).
4. Recognize that visual estimation of the degree of jaundice can lead to errors, particularly in darkly pigmented infants.
5. Interpret all bilirubin levels according to the infant's age in hours.
6. Recognize that infants at less than 38 weeks' gestation, particularly those who are breastfed, are at higher risk of developing hyperbiliru-binemia and require closer surveillance and monitoring.
7. Perform a systematic assessment on all infants before discharge for the risk of severe hyper-bilirubinemia (Table O-2).
8. Provide parents with written and verbal infor-mation about newborn jaundice.
9. Provide appropriate follow-up based on the time of discharge and the risk assessment.
10. Treat newborns, when indicated with pho-totherapy or exchange transfusion (Table O-3).

TABLE O-1	**Laboratory evaluation of the jaundiced infant of 35 or more weeks' gestation**

Indications	Assessments
Jaundice in first 24 h	Measure TcB and/or TSB
Jaundice appears excessive for infant's age	Measure TcB and/or TSB
Infant receiving phototherapy or TSB rising rapidly (i.e., crossing percentiles) and unexplained by history and physical examination	Blood type and Coombs' test, if not obtained with cord blood
	Complete blood count and smear
	Measure direct or conjugated bilirubin
	It is an option to perform reticulocyte count, G6PD, and $ETCO_c$, if available
	Repeat TSB in 4–24 h depending on infant's age and TSB level
TSB concentration approaching exchange levels or not responding to phototherapy	Perform reticulocyte count, G6PD, albumin, $ETCO_c$, if available
Elevated direct (or conjugated) bilirubin level	Do urinalysis and urine culture. Evaluate for sepsis if indicated by history and physical examination
Jaundice present at or beyond age 3 wk, or sick infant	Total and direct (or conjugated) bilirubin level
	If direct bilirubin elevated, evaluate for causes of cholestasis
	Check results of newborn thyroid and galactosemia screen, and evaluate infant for signs or symptoms of hypothyroidism

TABLE O-2   Risk factors for development of severe hyperbilirubinemia in infants of 35 or more weeks' gestation (in approximate order of importance)

Major risk factors
   Predischarge TSB or TcB level in the high-risk zone
   Jaundice observed in the first 24 h
   Blood group incompatibility with positive direct antiglobulin test, other known hemolytic disease
      (e.g, G6PD deficiency), elevated ETCO$_c$
   Gestational age 35–36 wk
   Previous sibling received phototherapy
   Cephalohematoma or significant bruising
   Exclusive breastfeeding, particularly if nursing is not going well and weight loss is excessive
   East Asian race[*]
Minor risk factors
   Predischarge TSB or TcB level in the high intermediate-risk zone
   Gestational age 37–38 wk
   Jaundice observed before discharge
   Previous sibling with jaundice
   Macrosomic infant of a diabetic mother
   Maternal age ≥25 y
   Male gender
Decreased risk (these factors are associated with decreased risk of significant jaundice, listed in order
      of decreasing importance)
   TSB or TcB level in the low-risk zone
   Gestational age ≥41 wk
   Exclusive bottle feeding
   Black race[*]
   Discharge from hospital after 72 h

[*]Race as defined by mother's description.

TABLE O-3	**Example of a clinical pathway for management of the newborn infant readmitted for phototherapy or exchange transfusion**

Treatment
  Use intensive phototherapy and/or exchange transfusion
Laboratory tests
  TSB and direct bilirubin levels
  Blood type (ABO, Rh)
  Direct antibody test (Coombs')
  Serum albumin
  Complete blood cell count with differential and smear for red cell morphology
  Reticulocyte count
  ETCO$_c$ (if available)
  G6PD if suggested by ethnic or geographic origin or if poor response to phototherapy
  Urine for reducing substances
  If history and/or presentation suggest sepsis, perform blood culture, urine culture, and cerebrospinal fluid for
    protein, glucose, cell count, and culture
Interventions
  If TSB ≥25 mg/dL (428 µmol/L) or ≥20 mg/dL (342 µmol/L) in a sick infant or infant <38 wk gestation, obtain
    a type and crossmatch, and request blood in case an exchange transfusion is necessary
  In infants with isoimmune hemolytic disease and TSB level rising in spite of intensive phototherapy or within
    2–3 mg/dL (34–51 µmol/L) of exchange level, administer intravenous immunoglobulin 0.5–1 g/kg over 2 h
    and repeat in 12 h if necessary
  If infant's weight loss from birth is >12% or there is clinical or biochemical evidence of dehydration, recommend
    formula or expressed breast milk. If oral intake is in question, give intravenous fluids.
For infants receiving intensive phototherapy
  Breastfeed or bottle-feed (formula or expressed breast milk) every 2–3 h
  If TSB ≥25 mg/dL (428 µmol/L), repeat TSB within 2–3 h
  If TSB 20–25 mg/dL (342–428 µmol/L), repeat within 3–4 h. If TSB <20 mg/dL (342 µmol/L), repeat in 4–6 h.
    If TSB continues to fall, repeat in 8–12 h
  If TSB is not decreasing or is moving closer to level for exchange transfusion or the TSB/albumin ratio increases,
    consider exchange transfusion
  When TSB is <13–14 mg/dL (239 µmol/L), discontinue phototherapy
  Depending on the cause of the hyperbilirubinemia, it is an option to measure TSB 24 h after discharge to check
    for rebound

Modified from Subcommittee on Hyperbilirubinemia, American Academy of Pediatrics: Management of hyperbilirubinemia in the newborn 35 or more weeks' gestation. Pediatrics 114:297, 2004.

$\mathscr{T}$he Academy of Breastfeeding Medicine protocols

Protocol #1: Guidelines for glucose monitoring and treatment of hypoglycemia in breastfed neonates

PURPOSE

To provide guidelines[1] for the first hours of life for obtaining blood glucose levels in neonates at risk for developing hypoglycemia and to delineate the appropriate interventions for hypoglycemia in the neonate. Clinical management is based on four basic principles: (1) monitoring the infants at highest risk; (2) confirming that plasma glucose concentration is low and is responsible for the clinical manifestations present; (3) demonstrating that the symptoms have responded following glucose therapy with restoration of the blood glucose to normoglycemic levels, and (4) observing and carefully documenting all of these events.[2]

BACKGROUND

Transient hypoglycemia is almost universal in newborn mammals. In healthy, term human infants, even if enteral feedings are withheld, this phenomenon is self-limited and blood glucose concentrations rise.[3–5] This early, self-limited period of hypo-glycemia therefore cannot be considered pathological, and there is little practical value in measuring the blood glucose concentrations of asymptomatic, term normal newborns in the first 2 postnatal hours or beyond.[6,21] After this period, blood glucose concentrations less than 47 mg/dL (2.6 mmol/L) *may* recur in many healthy babies, particularly those who are demand fed with long intervals between feedings and those that are breastfed.[4] However, a marked ketogenic response to low blood glucose concentrations has been demonstrated in these infants, and evidence from animal studies suggests that this response protects neurologic function, as ketone bodies are important glucose-sparing brain fuels.[4,7–9]

The Committee on Fetus and Newborn of the American Academy of Pediatrics states: "No study has shown that the treatment of a transient low blood glucose level offers a better short-term or long-term outcome than the outcome resulting with no treatment. . . . Furthermore, there is no evidence that asymptomatic hypoglycemic infants will benefit from treatment."[10] At least one recent study using recommended breastfeeding management demonstrated clinically insignificant differences in blood glucose levels between breastfed and artificially fed infants.[11,12] Older studies' results, confounded by variations in glucose water supplementation, still found no clinically significant differences in glucose levels[13]; **therefore, monitoring of blood glucose concentrations in healthy, appropriately grown neonates is unnecessary, and potentially harmful to parental well-being and the successful establishment of breastfeeding.**[6,14,15,21]

There is much disagreement as to what constitutes hypoglycemia. Cornblath and Schwartz[2] defined hypoglycemia as a whole blood glucose level of less than 30 mg/dL (1.7 mmol/L) in term infants and less than 20 mg/dL (1.1 mmol/L) in preterm infants.[10] The American Academy of Pediatrics defines hypoglycemia in the first 24 hours as a blood glucose level of less than 22 mg/dL in preterm or low-birth-weight infants weighing less than 2.5 kg or less than 30 mg/dL in a full-term infant.[17] Glucose concentrations in plasma or serum are 10% to 15% higher than in whole blood.[18]

Recent studies have defined hypoglycemia in term infants as a serum glucose level of less than 40–45 mg/dL (2.2–2.5 mmol/L) after the first 24 hours of life.[3,13] A recent consensus meeting concluded that "the rational definition of hypoglycemia was not a specific value, but a continuum of falling glucose levels, creating thresholds for neurologic dysfunction, which may vary from one cause of hypoglycemia or clinical circumstance to another."[19] All agree that bedside glucose oxidase strip tests, whether read by meter or by eye, are too variable and unreliable to establish the diagnosis.[19,20]

In a recent extensive review of the literature by Anthony F. Williams, DPhil, FRCP, commissioned by the World Health Organization,[21] it was recommended that asymptomatic newborns *at risk* for hypoglycemia have their blood glucose concentration maintained at or above 47 mg/dL (2.6 mmol/L), and that symptomatic infants below this level receive intravenous glucose as soon as possible. He further noted that early and exclusive breastfeeding is safe to meet the nutritional needs of healthy

term newborns worldwide and that healthy term newborns who are breastfeeding on demand do not need routine glucose screening or supplementary foods or fluids.

For at-risk newborns who are not able to suckle adequately or whose blood glucose falls below 47 mg/dL, breast milk or an appropriate breast milk substitute should be given by cup or gavage.

Cornblath and Schwartz's current, self-designated conservative definition of hypoglycemia is plasma glucose concentration less than 40 mg/dL (2.2 mmol/L) (whole blood glucose less than 34–36 mg/dL) in the first 24 hours. After 24 hours of age, plasma glucose levels 40–50 mg/dL (2.2–2.8 mmol/dL) can be used. The authors stress that values below these ranges are an indication to raise plasma glucose levels and do not imply neuroglycopenia or neurologic damage. At all ages and gestations, plasma glucose values less than 20–25 mg/dL (1.1–1.3 mmol/L) (whole blood glucose less than 17–22 mg/dL) should be treated by parenteral glucose and monitored at regular intervals.[2]

In summary:

1. Early and exclusive breastfeeding is safe to meet the nutritional needs of healthy term newborns.

2. Monitoring of blood glucose levels in well term newborns is unnecessary.

3. Breastfed infants may have lower blood glucose levels but have higher blood ketone body levels than formula-fed infants, to use as alternative brain fuel.

4. The major determinant of blood glucose concentration is the interval between feeds, but even intervals up to 8 hours are not associated with excessively low glucose concentrations.[4]

5. Bedside glucose oxidase strip tests should not be used as the basis for treatment or screening.

6. Whole blood glucose concentrations are 10% to 15% lower than plasma or serum values.

7. Because institutions may vary in glucose measurement techniques, these guidelines are based on serum (plasma) glucose values with whole blood values in parentheses where appropriate.

8. Symptomatic infants require immediate investigation and treatment and should respond to IV glucose. If the infant does not respond to treatment with glucose, other causes of the symptoms should be sought.

RISK ASSESSMENT/ MANIFESTATIONS

A. Infants most at risk for developing neonatal hypoglycemia include:
 1. Small for gestational age (SGA) (<10th percentile or smaller of discordant twins)
 2. Large for gestational age (LGA) (>90th percentile)
 3. Premature infants (< or = 34 wk) or very low birth weight infants (<1250 g)
 4. Infants of diabetic or massively obese mothers
 5. Significant perinatal asphyxia or respiratory distress
 6. Severe erythroblastosis
 7. Polycythemia
 8. Any infant with microphallus or anterior midline defects
 9. Infants with Beckwith-Wiedemann Syndrome
 10. Twin to twin transfusion
 11. Cold stress
 12. Any infant admitted to the NICU
 13. Any symptomatic infant (see later section)
B. Clinical manifestations of hypoglycemia are never specific and may include
 1. Tremors, irritability, jitteriness, high-pitched cry, exaggerated Moro reflex, seizures, or coma
 2. Lethargy, listlessness, limpness, hypotonia
 3. Cyanosis, apnea, irregular or rapid respirations
 4. Hypothermia, temperature instability
 5. Refusal to suck or difficulty in feeding
Clinical manifestations should subside within minutes or hours in response to adequate treatment with intravenous glucose if hypoglycemia alone is responsible. If they do not, the signs and symptoms may be secondary to other common neonatal problems.

RECOMMENDATIONS

A. Routine glucose monitoring is not indicated in the absence of specific risk factors or clinical signs of possible hypoglycemia.
B. When performed, measurement of serum glucose should be STAT and have a rapid turn-around time.
C. Timing of glucose measurements:
 1. At 4 to 6 hours of age[21] or at any age when symptoms occur, for high risk infants as defined above.
 2. Between 30 and 60 minutes of age, at admission, or whenever symptoms occur for
  a. Any infant admitted to the NICU
  b. Any infant of a diabetic mother
 3. When symptoms develop, regardless of risk factors
D. Management:
 For serum glucose measurement less than 40 mg/dL (2.2 mmol/L) or less than 35 mg/dL whole blood:
 1. Asymptomatic infant
  a. Breastfeed, feed expressed breast milk or breast milk substitute immediately po (cup or bottle) or og*
  b. Provide IV glucose if po/og is not tolerated or not given
  c. Repeat serum glucose in 30 minutes
  d. If repeat serum glucose is still low, provide IV glucose; monitor serum glucose serially. Can continue to offer feedings and wean IV glucose as glucose normalizes.
  e. If repeat serum glucose is adequate, monitor serum glucose before next feeding.
 2. Symptomatic infant
  a. Obtain STAT serum glucose and notify doctor

---

*Orogastric (gavage): Some experts consider refusal to po feed as "symptomatic" hypoglycemia: however, infants may not feed for other perinatal reasons.

b. Initiate IV glucose (D10W) immediately

c. Do not rely on po or gavage feeding to correct hypoglycemia

d. Encourage breastfeeding as tolerated

e. If serum glucose is normal, look for other etiology of symptoms

---

REFERENCES

1. American Academy of Pediatrics and American College of Obstetricians and Gynecologists: Guidelines for Perinatal Care, 4th ed., Elk Grove, Ill, American Academy of Pediatrics, 1997, p 161.

2. Cornblath M, Schwartz R: Hypoglycemia in the neonate. J Pediatr Endocrinol 6:113–129, 1993.

3. Srinvasan G, Phildes RS, Cattamanchi G, et al: Plasma glucose values in normal neonates: a new look. J Pediatr 109:114–117, 1986.

4. Hawdon JM, Ward Platt MP, Aynsley-Green A: Patterns of metabolic adaptation for preterm and term neonates in the first postnatal week. Arch Dis Child 67:357–365, 1992.

5. Cornblath M, Reisner SH: Blood glucose in the neonate and its clinical significance. New Engl J Med 273:378–380, 1965.

6. Hawdon JM, Ward Platt MP, Aynsley-Green A: Prevention and management of neonatal hypoglycemia. Arch Dis Child 70:F60–F65, 1994.

7. Lucas A, Bayes S, Bloom SR, Aynsley-Green A: Metabolic and endocrine responses to a milk feed in 6 day old term infants: Differences between breast and cow's milk formula feeding. Acta Paediatr Scand 70:195–200, 1981.

8. Edmond J, Auestad N, Robbins RA, et al: Ketone body metabolism in the neonate: development and the effect of diet. Fed Proc 44:2359–2364, 1985.

9. Yager JY, Heitjan DF, Towfighi J, et al: Effect of insulin-induced and fasting hypoglycemia on perinatal hypoxic-ischemic brain damage. Pediatr Res 31:138–142, 1992.

10. Committee on Fetus and Newborn, American Academy of Pediatrics: Routine evaluation of blood pressure, hematocrit, and glucose in newborns. Pediatrics 92:74–76, 1993.

11. WHO/UNICEF: Protecting, Promoting and Supporting Breast-Feeding: The Special Role of Maternity Services: A Joint WHO/UNICEF Statement. Geneva, World Health Organization, 1989.

12. Durand R, Hodges S, LaRock S, et al: The effect of skin-to-skin breast-feeding in the immediate recovery period on newborn thermoregulation and blood glucose values. Neonatal Intensive Care March–April: 23–29, 1997.

13. Heck LJ, Erenberg A: Serum glucose levels in term neonates during the first 48 hours of life. J Pediatr 110: 119–122, 1987.

14. Hawdon JM: Neonatal hypoglycemia: The consequences of admission to the special care nursery. Child Health 1993; Feb: 48–51

15. Hawdon JM, Ward Platt MP, Aynsley-Green A: Neonatal hypoglycemia—blood glucose monitoring and infant feeding. Midwifery 9:3–6.

16. Cornblath M, Schwartz R: Disorders of Carbohydrate Metabolism in Infancy. Philadelphia, WB Saunders, 1976.

17. American Academy of Pediatrics: Pediatric Nutrition Handbook, Elk Grove Village, Ill, American Academy of Pediatrics, 1992, p 245.

18. Schwartz RP: Neonatal hypoglycemia: How low is too low? editorial. J Pediatr 131:171–173.

19. Cornblath M, Schwartz R, Aynsley-Green A, Lloyd JK: Hypoglycemia in infancy: The need for a rational definition. Pediatrics 92:474–476, 1993.

20. Cornblath M: Metabolism and Endocrinology. In Seidel HM, Rosenstein BT, Pathak A (eds): Primary Care of the Newborn, Johns Hopkins Children's Center, St. Louis, Mosby YearBook, 1993.

21. Williams, Anthony F. Hypoglycaemia of the Newborn: Review of the Literature. Geneva, World Health Organization, 1997 (Download from: www.who.int/chd/pub/imci/bf/hypoglyc/hypoclyc.htm).

Protocol #2: Guidelines for hospital discharge of the breastfeeding term newborn and mother: "Going home protocol"

BACKGROUND

The ultimate success of breastfeeding is measured in the duration of breastfeeding and of exclusive breastfeeding, not solely in the initiation of breast-feeding. Anticipatory attention to the needs of the mother and baby at the time of discharge from the hospital is crucial to ensure successful, long-term breastfeeding. The following principles and practices are recommended for consideration prior to sending a mother and her full-term infant home.

GUIDELINES

1. Formal documented assessment of breastfeeding effectiveness should be performed at least once during the last 8 hours preceding discharge of the mother and baby by a medical professional trained in formal assessment of breastfeeding (in addition to similar assessments performed earlier in the hospitalization). This should include evaluation of positioning, latch, milk transfer, baby's weight, clinical jaundice, and all problems raised by the mother, such as nipple pain or perception of inadequate supply.

2. All problems with breastfeeding, whether observed by hospital staff or raised by the mother, should be attended to and documented in the medical record prior to discharge of mother and baby, with a plan of action that includes follow-up of the problem after discharge.[1]

3. Physicians, nurses, and all other staff should encourage the mother to practice exclusive breastfeeding for the first 6 months of the infant's life and to continue breastfeeding until 1 year of age and beyond, with the addition of complementary food after 6 months of life.[2] Mothers will benefit from education about the rationale for exclusive breastfeeding and why artificial milk supplementation is discouraged. Such education is a regular component of anticipatory guidance that addresses individual beliefs and practices in a culturally sensitive manner. Special counseling is needed for those mothers planning to return to outside employment or school.

4. Families will benefit from appropriate, noncommercial educational materials on breastfeeding (as well as on other aspects of child health care).[3] Discharge packs containing infant formula, pacifiers, commercial advertising materials, and any materials not appropriate for a breastfeeding mother and baby should not be distributed.[2,4-8]

5. Breastfeeding mothers and appropriate others will benefit from anticipatory guidance prior to discharge regarding the next month of breastfeeding (e.g., guidance for engorgement, growth spurts, diminished milk supply). Specific guidance should be provided in written form to all parents regarding assessment of (a) adequacy of stool and urine output, (b) jaundice, and (c) sleep and feeding patterns.

6. Every breastfeeding mother should receive instruction on techniques for expression of milk by hand or by pump so that she can maintain her milk supply and obtain milk for feeding to the infant should she and the infant be separated or the infant be unable to feed directly from the breast.[9]

7. Every breastfeeding mother should be provided with names and phone numbers of individuals and medical services that can provide advice, counseling, and health assessments related to

breastfeeding on a 24 hour-a-day basis, as well as on a less intensive basis.[1,5,10–12]

8. Mothers should be provided with lists of various peer support groups (e.g., La Leche League International) with phone numbers and addresses and encouraged to contact and consider joining one of these groups.[13,14]

9. Prior to discharge, appointments should be made for (a) an office or home visit, within 2 to 3 days, by a physician or a physician-supervised breast-feeding-trained licensed health care provider (infants discharged before 48 hours of age should be seen by 2 to 4 days of age), and (b) the mother's 6-week follow-up visit to the obstetrician or family physician. Additional visits for the mother and infant are recommended until all clinical issues are resolved (e.g., weight gain is well established, jaundice resolving). A routine preventive care visit should occur when the child is 2 to 4 weeks of age.[2,11,12,15,16]

10. If the mother is medically ready for discharge but the infant is not, every effort should be made to allow the mother to remain in the hospital either as a continuing patient or as a "mother-in-residence" with access to the infant for exclusive breastfeeding. Maintenance of a 24-hour rooming-in relationship with the infant is optimal during the infant's extended stay.[17–21]

11. If the mother is discharged from the hospital before the infant is discharged (as in the case of a sick infant), the mother should be encouraged to spend as much time as possible with the infant and to continue regular breastfeeding.[22] During periods when the mother is not in the hospital, she should be encouraged to express and store her milk, bringing it to the hospital for the infant.

REFERENCES

1. Kuan LW, Britto M, Decolongon J, et al: Health system factors contributing to breastfeeding success. Pediatrics 104: 28, 1999.

2. The American Academy of Pediatrics, Work Group on Breastfeeding: Breastfeeding and the use of human milk. Pediatrics 100:1035–1039, 1997.

3. Valaitis RK, Shea E: An evaluation of breastfeeding promotion literature: Does it really promote breastfeeding? Can J Public Health 84:24–27, 1993.

4. Dungy CI, Christensen-Szalanski J, Losch M, Russell D: Effect of discharge samples on duration of breast-feeding. Pediatrics 90:233–237, 1992.

5. Frank DA, Wirtz SJ, Sorenson JR, Heeren T: Commercial discharge packs and breast-feeding counseling: Effects on infant-feeding practices in a randomized trial. Pediatrics 80:845–854, 1987.

6. Bergevin Y, Dougherty C, Kramer M: Do infant formula samples shorten the duration of breast-feeding? Lancet 1(8334)::1148–1151, 1983.

7. Perez-Escamilla R, Pollitt E, Lonnerdal B, Dewey KG: Infant feeding policies in maternity wards and their effect on breast-feeding success: An analytical overview. Am J Public Health 84:89–97, 1994.

8. Aarts C, Hornell A, Kylberg E, Hofvander Y, Gebre-Medhin M: Breastfeeding patterns in relation to thumb sucking and pacifier use. Pediatrics 104:50,1999.

9. World Health Organization, United Nations Children's Fund. Protecting, promoting and supporting breastfeeding: The special role of maternity services (A joint WHO/UNICEF statement). Int J Gynaecol Obstet 31:171–183, 1990.

10. Bloom K, Goldbloom RB, Robinson SC, Stevens FE: Breast versus formula feeding. Acta Paediatr Scand Suppl 300:1–26, 1982.

11. Chen CH: Effects of home visits and telephone contacts on breastfeeding compliance in Taiwan. Matern Child Nurs J21:82–90, 1993.

12. Houston MJ, Howie PW, Cook A, McNeilly AS: Do breast feeding mothers get the home support they need? Health Bull (Edinb) 39:166–172, 1981.

13. Long DG, Funk-Archuleta MA, Geiger CJ, Mozar AJ, Heins JN: Peer counselor program increases breastfeeding rates in Utah Native American WIC population. J Hum Lact 11:279–284, 1995.

14. Kistin N, Abramson R, Dublin P. Effect of peer counselors on breastfeeding initiation, exclusivity, and duration among low-income urban women. J Hum Lact 10:11–15, 1994.

15. Jenner S: The influence of additional information, advice and support on the success of breast feeding in working class primiparas. Child Care, Health Dev 14:319–328, 1988.

16. Jones DA, West RR: Effect of a lactation nurse on the success of breast-feeding: A randomized controlled trial. J Epidemiol Community Health 40:45–49, 1986.

17. Waldenstrom U, Swenson A: Rooming-in at night in the postpartum ward. Midwifery 7:82–89, 1991.

18. Yamauchi Y, Yamanouchi I: The relationship between rooming-in/not rooming-in and breast-feeding variables. Acta Paediatr Scand 79:1017–1022, 1990.
19. Keefe MR: The impact of infant rooming-in on maternal sleep at night. J Obstet Gynecol Neonatal Nurs 17:122–126, 1988.
20. Keefe MR: Comparison of neonatal nighttime sleep-wake patterns in nursery versus rooming-in environments. Nurs Res 36:140–144, 1987.
21. Procianoy RS, Fernandes-Filho PH, Lazaro L, Sartori NC, Drebes S: The influence of rooming-in on breastfeeding. J Trop Pediatr 29:112–114, 1983.
22. Hurst NM, Valentine CJ, Renfro L, Burns P, Ferlic L: Skin-to-skin holding in the neonatal intensive care unit influences maternal milk volume. J Perinatol 17:213–217, 1997.

Protocol #3: Hospital guidelines for the use of supplementary feedings in the healthy term breastfed neonate

DEFINITIONS

Supplementary Feedings: Feedings provided in place of breastfeeding. This may include expressed or banked breast milk. Any foods given prior to 6 months, the recommended duration of exclusive feeding, are thus defined as supplementary.

Complementary Feedings: Feedings provided in addition to breastfeeding. This term is used to describe foods given in addition to breastfeeding after 6 months, a "complement" to breastfeeding needed for adequate nutrition.

BACKGROUND

Given early opportunities to breastfeed, breastfeeding assistance, and instruction, the majority of mothers and babies successfully establish breastfeeding. Some infants may not successfully latch and feed during the first day of life, but they successfully establish breastfeeding with time, appropriate evaluation, and minimal intervention.

Small colostrum feedings are appropriate for the size of the newborn's stomach and are sufficient to prevent hypoglycemia in the healthy, term, appropriate-for-gestational-age infant.[1,16,19] Healthy term infants also have sufficient body water to meet their metabolic needs[11,14,15]; thus, the majority of breastfed infants do not require supplementation. Because some breastfeeding women question the adequacy of colostrum feedings, they may benefit from reassurance, assistance with breastfeeding technique, and education about the physiology of breastfeeding.

Supplementation can prevent the establishment of maternal milk supply, have adverse effects on breastfeeding (e.g., delayed lactogenesis, maternal engorgement), alter infant bowel flora, sensitize the infant to allergens (depending on the content of the feeding and method used), and interfere with maternal-infant bonding.[3] Before supplementary feedings are begun, it is important that a formal evaluation of each mother-baby dyad, including a direct observation of breastfeeding, is completed. The following guidelines address indications for and methods of supplementation for the healthy, term (37–42-week), breastfed infant.

Indications for supplemental feedings

1. Indications for supplementation in term, healthy infants are few[13] (Table P-1).

   A few other clinical situations may arise in which supplemental feedings may be indicated. Table P-2 lists possible indications for the administration of such feedings. The physician

---

TABLE P-1   **Indications for supplementation in term, healthy infants**

1. Hypoglycemia, unresponsive to appropriate frequent breastfeeding[1]
2. Separation
   a) Maternal illness resulting in separation of infant and mother (e.g. psychosis, eclampsia or shock)
   b) Mother not at the same hospital (e.g. maternal death)
3. Infant with inborn error of metabolism (e.g. galactosemia)
4. Infant who is unable to feed at the breast (e.g. congenital malformation, illness)
5. Maternal medications (those contraindicated in breastfeeding)[4]

---

must decide if the clinical benefits outweigh the potential negative consequences of such feedings.

There are common clinical situations in which evaluation and breastfeeding management may be necessary but supplementation is *not* indicated, including the following:

1. The sleepy infant with fewer than 8 to 12 feedings in the first 24 to 48 hours with less than 7% weight loss and no signs of illness.
2. The infant with bilirubin levels less than 20 mg/dL after 72 hours of age, when the baby is feeding well and stooling adequately and weight loss is less than 7%.[2,6]

TABLE P-2   **Possible indications for supplementation in term, healthy infants**

1) Infant indications
   - Hypoglycemia documented by laboratory blood glucose measurement (not bedside screening methods) after infant has had adequate opportunity to breastfeed[1]
   - Clinical evidence of significant dehydration
   - Weight loss of 8% to 10% accompanied by delayed lactogenesis (day 5 or later)
   - Delayed bowel movements or continued meconium stools on day 5
   - Insufficient intake despite an adequate milk supply
   - Hyperbilirubinemia
     - Breastfeeding jaundice where intake is poor despite appropriate intervention
     - Breastmilk jaundice when levels reach >20-25 mg/dL in an otherwise thriving infant and where a diagnostic interruption of breastfeeding may be helpful
   - Low birthweight
     - When sufficient milk is not available
     - When nutrient supplementation is indicated
2) Maternal indications
   - Delayed lactogenesis (day 5 or later) and inadequate intake by infant
   - Intolerable pain during feedings unrelieved by interventions
   - Unavailability of mother due to severe illness or geographic separation
   - Primary glandular insufficiency (primary lactation failure), as evidenced by poor breast growth during pregnancy and minimal indications of lactogenesis, breast pathology or prior breast surgery resulting in poor milk production
   - Delayed lactogenesis
     - Retained placenta (lactogenesis probably will occur after placental fragments are removed)
     - Sheehan syndrome (postpartum hemorrhage followed by absence of lactogenesis)

Adapted from Powers NG, Slusser W: Breastfeeding update. 2: Clinical lactation management. Pediatr Rev 1997; 18:147–161.

3. The infant who is fussy at night or constantly feeding for several hours
4. The sleeping mother.

RECOMMENDATIONS

1. Healthy newborns do not need supplemental feedings for poor feeding for the first 24 to 48 hours, but babies who are too sick to breastfeed or whose mothers are too sick to allow breastfeeding are likely to require supplemental feedings.[13]
2. Supplemental feedings may require a physician's order and informed consent of the mother. When these feedings are not medically indicated, efforts to dissuade maternal requests for them should be documented by the nursing or medical staff. All supplemental feedings should be documented, including the content, volume, method, and medical indication or reason.
3. When supplementary feeding is necessary, the primary goals are to feed the baby and optimize the maternal milk supply while determining the cause of poor feeding or inadequate milk transfer.
4. Whenever possible, it is ideal to have the mother and infant room-in 24 hours per day to enhance opportunities for breastfeeding and lactogenesis.[13]
5. If mother-baby separation is unavoidable, establishment of milk supply is poor or questionable, or the baby is not removing milk from the breast, the mother needs instruction and encouragement to pump or manually express her milk to stimulate production and provide expressed breast milk as necessary for the infant.
6. Optimally, mothers need to express milk each time the baby receives a supplemental feeding, or about every 2 to 3 hours.[7,13] Mothers should be encouraged to start expressing on the first day or as soon as possible. Maternal breast engorgement should be avoided, as it will further compromise the milk supply and may lead to other complications.[13]
7. All infants must be formally evaluated for position, latch, and milk transfer prior to the provision of supplemental feedings.[17] Most babies who remain with their mothers and breastfeed adequately lose less than 7% of their birth weight. Weight loss in excess of 7% may be an indication of inadequate milk transfer or low milk production.[5,12] Weight loss in the range of 8% to10% may be within normal limits, but if all else is going well and the physical exam is normal, it is an indication for careful assessment and possible breastfeeding assistance.
8. The infant's physician should be notified if
   a. The infant exhibits signs of illness in addition to poor feeding.
   b. The mother-infant dyad meets the clinical criteria in Table P-1.
   c. The infant's weight loss is greater than 7%.

Methods of providing supplemental feedings

When supplemental feedings are needed, one of the following techniques may be used: a supplemental nursing device at breast, cup feeding, spoon or dropper feeding, finger-feeding, or bottle feeding.[8–10,17,18] There is little evidence about the safety or efficacy of most alternative feeding methods and their effect on breastfeeding; however, when cleanliness or refrigeration is sub-optimal, cup feeding may be the best choice.[18] Cup feeding has been shown to be safe for term infants and may help preserve breastfeeding duration among those that require multiple supplemental feedings.[8,9]

Choice of feeding

Expressed human milk is the first choice for supplemental feeding,[17] but expressing sufficient colostrum in the first few days may be difficult. The mother may need reassurance and education if such difficulties occur. If the volume of the mother's colostrum does not meet her infant's feeding requirements, pasteurized donor human milk is preferable to other supplements. The physician must weigh the potential risks and benefits of other supplemental fluids, such as standard formula or protein hydrolysate formula, with consideration given to available resources, the family's history for risk factors such as atopy, the infant's age, the amounts needed, and the potential impact on the establishment of breastfeeding.

REFERENCES

1. Academy of Breastfeeding Medicine Protocol Committee. Clinical Protocol Number 1: Guidelines for Glucose Monitoring and Treatment of Hypoglycemia in Breastfed Neonates. ABM News and Views 1999, insert.
2. American Academy of Pediatrics: Practice parameter: management of hyperbilirubinemia in the healthy term newborn. [published erratum appears in Pediatrics 95:58–61, 1995] [see comments]. Pediatrics 94:558–565, 1994.
3. Blomquist HK, Jonsbo F, Serenius F, Persson LA: Supplementary feeding in the maternity ward shortens the duration of breast feeding. Acta Paediatrica 83:1122–1126, 1994.
4. Committee on Drugs, The American Academy of Pediatrics: The transfer of drugs and other chemicals into human milk. Pediatrics 108:776–789, 2001.
5. DeMarzo S, Seacat J, Neifert M: Initial weight loss and return to birth weight criteria for breast-fed infants: Challenging the "rule of thumb." Am J Dis Children 145:402, 1991.
6. Gartner LM, Herschel M: Jaundice and breastfeeding. Pediatr Clin North Am 48:389–400, 2001.
7. Hill PD, Brown LP, Harker TL: Initiation and frequency of breast expression in breastfeeding mothers of LBW and VLBW infants. Nurs Res 44:352–355, 1995.
8. Howard CR, de Blieck EA, ten Hoopen CB, et al: Physiologic stability of newborns during cup- and bottle-feeding. Pediatrics 105:105–107, 1999.
9. Howard CR, Howard FM, Lanphear BP, et al: Complementary feeding methods for breastfed babies. A randomized trial of cup versus bottle and the effect on breastfeeding success. Pediatr Res 49:161A, 2001.
10. Lang S, Lawrence CJ, Orme RL: Cup feeding: An alternative method of infant feeding. Arch Dis Child 71:365–369, 1994.
11. Marchini G, Stock S: Thirst and vasopressin secretion counteract dehydration in newborn infants. J Pediatr 130:736–739, 1997.
12. Muskinja-Montanji G, Molnar-Sabo I, Vekonj-Fajka G: Physiologic neonatal body weight loss in a "baby friendly hospital." [Serbo-Croatian (Roman)]. Medicinski Pregled 52:237–240, 1999.
13. Powers NG, Slusser W: Breastfeeding update. 2: Clinical lactation management. [Review]. Pediatr Rev18:147–161, 1997.
14. Rodriguez G, Ventura P, Samper MP, et al: Changes in body composition during the initial hours of life in breast-fed healthy term newborns. Biol Neonat 77:12–16, 2000.
15. Sachdev HP, Krishna J, Puri RK: Do exclusively breast fed infants need fluid supplementation? Indian Pediatr 29:535–540, 1992.
16. Scammon RE, Doyle LO: Observations on the capacity of the stomach in the first ten days of postnatal life. Am J Dis Child 516–538, 1920.
17. The American Academy of Pediatrics, Work Group on Breastfeeding: Breastfeeding and the use of human milk. Pediatrics 100:1035–1039, 1997.
18. United Nations Children's Fund: Feeding low birth weight babies. UNICEF division of information and public affairs. New York, UNICEF, 1996.
19. Williams AF. Hypoglycemia of the newborn: Review of the literature. Geneva, World Health Organization, 1997; download from www.who.int/chd/pub/imci/bf/hypoglyc/hypoclyc.htm.

Protocol #4: Mastitis

INTRODUCTION

Mastitis is a common condition in lactating women, with an estimated prevalence of 20% in the 6 months postpartum.[1] The majority of cases occur in the first 6 weeks, but mastitis can occur at any time during lactation. There have been few research trials in this area.

DEFINITION AND DIAGNOSIS

The usual clinical definition of mastitis is a tender, hot, swollen, wedge-shaped area of breast associated with fever of 38.5° C or greater, chills, flulike aching, and systemic illness.[2] However, mastitis literally means, and is defined herein, as an inflammation of the breast; this may or may not involve a bacterial infection.[3,4] Redness, pain, and heat may all be present when an area of the breast is engorged or "blocked"/"plugged," but an infection is not necessarily present.

Predisposing factors

The follow factors may predispose a lactating woman to the development of mastitis.[4,5] Other than their being factors that result in milk stasis, the evidence for these associations is inconclusive.

- Infrequent feeds or scheduled frequency or duration of feeds
- Missing feeds
- Poor attachment leading to inefficient removal of milk
- Damaged nipple, especially if colonized with *Staphylococcus aureus*
- Illness in mother or baby
- Oversupply of milk
- Rapid weaning
- Pressure on the breast (e.g., tight bra, car seatbelt)
- White spot on nipple or blocked nipple pore or duct: milk blister, granular material, *Candida*
- Maternal stress and fatigue
- Maternal malnutrition or anemia

INVESTIGATIONS

Laboratory investigations and other diagnostic procedures are not needed and are not performed routinely for mastitis. The WHO publication on mastitis suggests that breast milk culture and sensitivity testing "should be undertaken if there is no response to antibiotics within two days, if the mastitis recurs, if it is hospital-acquired mastitis, or in severe or unusual cases."[4] Breast milk culture may be obtained by collection of a hand-expressed midstream clean-catch sample into a sterile urine container (i.e., a small quantity of the initially expressed milk is discarded to avoid contamination of the sample with skin flora and subsequent milk is expressed into the sterile container taking care not to touch the inside of the container.) Cleansing the nipple prior to collection may further reduce skin contamination and false positive culture results.

MANAGEMENT

Effective milk removal

Because milk stasis is often the initiating factor in mastitis, the most important management step is frequent and effective milk removal. Mothers should be encouraged to breastfeed more frequently, starting on the affected breast. If pain prohibits let-down, feeding may begin on the unaffected breast, switching to the affected breast as soon as let-down is achieved. Positioning the infant at the breast with the chin or nose pointing to the blockage will help drain the area. Massaging the breast during the feed with an edible oil or nontoxic lubricant on the fingers may also be helpful. Massage should be directed from the blocked area moving outward toward the nipple. After the feed, expressing by hand or pump may also augment milk drainage and hasten resolution of the problem.[6]

There is no evidence of risk to the healthy, term infant of continuing breastfeeding.[4] Women who are unable to continue breastfeeding should express the breast by hand or pump, as sudden cessation of breastfeeding leads to a greater risk of abscess development than continuing to feed.[7]

Supportive measures

Rest, adequate fluids and nutrition, and practical help at home are essential measures. Application of heat—for example, a shower or a hot pack—to the breast prior to feeding may help the milk flow. After feeding or expressing, cold packs can be applied to the breast in order to reduce pain and edema.

Hospital admission should be considered in cases in which the woman is extremely ill and does not have supportive care at home. Rooming-in of the baby with the mother is mandatory so that breastfeeding can continue. In some hospitals, rooming-in may require hospital admission of the infant.

Pharmacologic management

Although lactating women are often reluctant to take medications, women with mastitis should be encouraged to take appropriate medications as indicated.

Analgesia

Analgesia may help with the milk ejection reflex and should be encouraged. An antiinflammatory agent such as ibuprofen may be more effective in reducing the symptoms relating to inflammation than a simple analgesic like paracetamol/acetaminophen. Ibuprofen is not detected in breast milk after following doses up to 1.6 g/day and is regarded as compatible with breastfeeding.[8]

Antibiotics

If symptoms of mastitis are mild and have been present for less than 24 hours, conservative management (effective milk removal and supportive measures) may be sufficient. If symptoms are not improving within 12 to 24 hours or if the woman is acutely ill, antibiotics should be started.[4]

The most common pathogen in infective mastitis is penicillin-resistant *S. aureus*.[6,9] Less commonly the organism is a streptococcus or *Escherichia coli*.[6] The preferred antibiotics are usually penicillinase-resistant penicillins,[2] such as dicloxacillin or flucloxacillin 500 mg qid.[10] Cephalexin is usually safe in women with suspected penicillin allergy, but clindamycin is suggested for cases of severe penicillin hypersensitivity.[10] Dicloxacillin appears to have a lower rate of adverse hepatic events than flucloxacillin.[11] It tends to cause phlebitis if given intravenously, however, and so is preferable for oral treatment unless intravenous treatment is necessary.

Many authorities recommend a 10- to 14-day course of antibiotics[12,13]; however this has not been subject to controlled trials.

FOLLOW-UP

Clinical response to the above management is typically rapid and dramatic. If the symptoms of mastitis fail to resolve within several days of appropriate management, including antibiotics, differential diagnoses should be considered. Further investigations may be required to confirm resistant bacteria, abscess formation, an underlying mass, or inflammatory or ductal carcinoma.

More than two or three recurrences in the same location also warrant evaluation to rule out an underlying mass.

COMPLICATIONS

Early cessation of breastfeeding

Mastitis may produce overwhelming acute symptoms that prompt women to consider cessation of breastfeeding. Effective milk removal, however, is the most essential part of treatment.[4] Acute cessation of breastfeeding may exacerbate the mastitis and result in an increased risk of abscess formation; therefore, effective treatment and support from health providers and family are important at this time. Mothers may need reassurance that the antibiotics they are taking are safe to use during breastfeeding.

Abscess

If a well-defined area of the breast remains hard, red, and tender despite appropriate management, then an abscess should be suspected. The initial systemic symptoms and fever may have resolved. A diagnostic breast ultrasound will identify a collection of fluid. The collection can often be drained by needle aspiration, which itself can be diagnostic as well as therapeutic. Serial needle aspirations may be required.[14] Ultrasound guidance for needle aspiration may be necessary in some cases. Surgical drainage may be necessary if the abscess is very large or if there are multiple abscesses. After surgical drainage, breastfeeding should continue. A course of antibiotics should follow drainage of the abscess.

Candida infection

Candidal infection should be considered when a woman develops burning nipple or radiating breast pain after treatment of mastitis.[12] Fungal infection may be either a primary infection or a complication of antibiotic treatment for bacterial mastitis. Diagnosis can be difficult, as the nipples and breasts may look normal on examination and milk culture is not reliable. Antifungal treatment is necessary for both mother and baby.

PREVENTION[5]

Effective management of breast fullness and engorgement

- Mothers should be helped to improve infant's attachment to the breast.
- Feeds should not be restricted.
- Mothers should be taught to hand express if the breasts are too full for the baby to attach or the baby does not relieve breast fullness.

Prompt attention to any signs of milk stasis

- Mothers should be taught to check their breasts for lumps, pain, or redness.
- If the mother notices any signs of milk stasis, she needs to rest, increase the frequency of breast-feeding, apply heat to the breast, and massage any lumpy areas.
- Mothers should seek help from their health care provider if they are not better within 24 hours.

Prompt attention to other difficulties with breastfeeding

Skilled help is needed for mothers with damaged nipples or an unsettled infant or who believe that they have insufficient milk.

Rest

As fatigue is often a precursor to mastitis, health professionals should encourage breastfeeding mothers to obtain adequate rest.

REFERENCES

1. Kinlay JR, O'Connell DL, Kinlay S: Incidence of mastitis in breastfeeding women during the six months after delivery: a prospective cohort study. Med J Aust 169:310–312, 1998.
2. Lawrence RA: The puerperium, breastfeeding, and breast milk. Curr Opin Obstet Gynecol 2:23–30, 1990.
3. Inch S, Renfrew M: Common breastfeeding problems. In Chalmers I, Enkin M, Keirse MJN (eds): Effective Care in Pregnancy and Childbirth. Oxford, Oxford University Press, 1989, pp 1377–1378.
4. World Health Organization. Mastitis: Causes and management. Department of Child and Adolescent Health and Development. WHO/FCH/ CAH/00.13, Geneva, 2000.
5. Walker M: Mastitis in lactating women. Unit 2/Lactation Consultant Series Two. Schaumburg, Ill, La Leche League International, 1999.
6. Thomsen AC, Espersen T, Maigaard S: Course and treatment of milk stasis, noninfectious inflammation of the breast, and infectious mastitis in nursing women. Am J Obstet Gynecol 149:492–495, 1984.
7. Marshall BR, Hepper JK, Zirbel CC: Sporadic puerperal mastitis: an infection that need not interrupt lactation. JAMA 233:1377–1379, 1975.
8. Hale T: Medications and Mother's Milk, 9th ed. Amarillo, TX, Pharmasoft Medical Publishing pp 345–346.
9. Niebyl JR, Spence MR, Parmley TH: Sporadic (nonepidemic) puerperal mastitis. J Reprod Med 20:97–100, 1978.
10. Therapeutic Guidelines: Antibiotics, 10th ed. North Melbourne, Australia: Therapeutics Guidelines Limited, 1998, pp 178–179.
11. Olsson R, Wiholm BE, Sand C et al: Liver damage from flucloxacillin, cloxacillin and dicloxacillin. J Hepatol 15: 154–161, 1992.
12. Lawrence RA, Lawrence RM: Breastfeeding: A Guide for the Medical Profession, 5th ed. St Louis, Mosby, 1999, pp 277–281.
13. Neifert MR: Clinical aspects of lactation: promoting breastfeeding success. Clin Perinatol 26:281–306, 1999.
14. Dixon JM: Repeated aspiration of breast abscesses in lactating women. Br Med J 297:1517–1518, 1988.

Protocol #5: Peripartum breastfeeding management for the healthy mother and infant at term

BACKGROUND

Hospital policies and routines greatly influence breastfeeding success.[1–3] The peripartum hospital experience should include adequate support, instruction, and care to ensure the successful initiation of breastfeeding. Such management is part of a continuum of care and education begun during the prenatal period that promotes breastfeeding as the optimal method of infant feeding and includes information about maternal and infant benefits. The following principles and practices are recommended for care in the peripartum hospital setting.

PRENATAL

All pregnant women must receive education about the benefits and management of breastfeeding to allow an informed decision about infant feeding.[4–6] Prenatal education should include information about the stages of labor, drug-free ways to address labor pain, potential side effects of labor medications, and the benefits to mother and baby of exclusive breastfeeding initiated in the first hour after birth.[4] Educational materials produced by formula manufacturers are inappropriate sources of information about infant feeding.[7]

Maternity care includes an assessment of any medical or physical conditions that could affect a mother's ability to breastfeed her infant. In some cases it may be helpful to obtain a prenatal consultation with the infant's physician or a lactation consultant or specialist and to develop a plan of follow-up to be instituted at the time of delivery.[5] Women will benefit from moderated group discussions or referral to a lay support organization (e.g., La Leche League) prior to delivery.

LABOR AND DELIVERY

Women will benefit from the continuous presence of a close companion (e.g., doula) throughout labor and delivery. The presence of a doula is known to enhance breastfeeding initiation and duration. Many risk factors associated with early breastfeeding termination, including the mean length of labor, the need for surgical intervention, and the use of pain-reducing interventions such as epidurals and other medications, are reduced by the presence of a doula.[8–11]

Immediate postpartum

The healthy newborn can be given directly to the mother for skin-to-skin contact until the first feeding is accomplished. The infant may be dried and assigned Apgar scores and the initial physical assessment performed as the infant is placed with the mother. Such contact provides the infant optimal physiologic stability, warmth, and opportunities for the first feeding.[12,13] Delaying procedures such as weighing, measuring, and administering vitamin K and eye prophylaxis (up to an hour) enhances early parent-infant interaction.

Infants are to be put to the breast as soon after birth as feasible for both mother and infant (within an hour of birth).[14] This is to be initiated in either the delivery room or recovery room, and every mother is to be instructed in proper breastfeeding technique.[4,6,15,16]

Mother-baby rooming-in on a 24-hour basis enhances opportunities for bonding and for optimal breastfeeding initiation. Whenever possible, mothers and infants are to remain together during the hospital stay.[16] To avoid unnecessary separation, infant assessments in the immediate postpartum time period and thereafter are ideally performed in the mother's room. Evidence suggests that mothers get the same amount and quality of sleep whether infants room-in or are sent back to the nursery at night.[17,18]

Education about the benefits of 24-hour rooming-in encourages parents to use it as the standard mode of hospital care for themselves and their baby. Adequate nursing personnel must be available to assess and document the status of the infant and infant feeding while the baby is in the family's room.[4,6,19-21]

Women need help to ensure that they are able to position and attach their babies at the breast. Those delivered by cesarean section may need additional help from nursing staff to attain comfortable positioning.

A trained observer should assess and document the effectiveness of breastfeeding at least once every 8 hours after delivery until mother and infant are discharged. Peripartum care of the couplet should address and document infant positioning, latch, milk transfer, baby's daily weight, clinical jaundice, and all problems raised by the mother, such as nipple pain or the perception of an inadequate breast milk supply. Infants who are breastfeeding well will feed 8 to 12 times or more in 24 hours, for a minimum of 8 feedings every 24 hours. Limiting the time at the breast is not necessary and may be harmful to the establishment of a good milk supply. Infants usually fall asleep or release the breast spontaneously when satiated.

Supplemental feeding should not be given to breastfed infants unless there is a medical indication for such feedings. Supplementation can prevent the establishment of maternal milk supply and have adverse effects on breastfeeding (e.g., delayed lactogenesis, maternal engorgement). Supplements may alter infant bowel flora, sensitize the infant to allergens (depending on the content of the feeding and method used), and interfere with maternal-infant bonding.[22] Before any supplementary feedings are begun, it is important that a formal evaluation of each mother-baby dyad, including a direct observation of breastfeeding, is completed.[23]

In general, acute infectious diseases, undiagnosed fever, and common postpartum infections in the mother are not a contraindication to breastfeeding, if such diseases can be readily controlled and treated. Infants should not be breastfed in the case of maternal HIV infection (in a developed country), untreated active tuberculosis, or herpes simplex when there are breast lesions.[24] Infectious peripartum varicella may require separation of the mother and newborn, limiting direct breastfeeding. The listing of all contraindications is beyond the scope of this document, but reliable sources of information are readily available and include information about medications and radioactive compounds.[24-26]

PROBLEMS AND COMPLICATIONS

Mother-baby couplets at risk for breastfeeding problems benefit from early identification and assistance. Consultation with an expert in lactation management may be helpful in situations including but not limited to the following:

a) Maternal request/anxiety
b) Previous negative breastfeeding experience
c) Mother has flat/inverted nipples
d) Mother has history of breast surgery
e) Multiple births (twins, triplets)
f) Infant is premature (<37 weeks gestation)
g) Infant has congenital anomaly, neurological impairment, or other medical condition that affects the infant's ability to breastfeed
h) Maternal or infant medical condition for which breastfeeding must be temporarily postponed or for which milk expression is required
i) Documentation, after the first few feedings, that there is difficulty in establishing breastfeeding (e.g., poor latch-on, sleepy baby, etc.)

Early discharge from the hospital (<48 hours) of mothers and babies mandates that risks to successful breastfeeding be identified quickly so that the time spent in the hospital is used to maximal benefit.[27] All breastfed infants should be seen by a health care provider within 48 to 72 hours of discharge to evaluate the infant's well being and the successful establishment of breastfeeding.[6,28]

If a neonate needs to be transferred to an intermediate or intensive care area, steps must be taken to maintain lactation in the mother. When possible, transport of the mother to the intermediate or intensive care nursery to continue breastfeeding is optimal. If breastfeeding is not possible, arrangements can be made to continue human milk feeding for the neonate. Mothers must be shown how to maintain lactation through breast pumping or manual expression when they are separated from their infants.[4,6]

If an infant is not consistently feeding at the breast effectively at the time of hospital discharge, the mother should be shown how to maintain lactation through breast pumping or manual expression. The possible need for supplemental feedings for the infant must be addressed, with consideration given to the choice of supplement to be used and the method of feeding. Expressed breast milk should be used if maternal supply is adequate, and cup feeding may help preserve breastfeeding duration among those that require multiple supplemental feedings.[29] The mother-infant dyad will need referral to a professional competent in lactation management for continued assistance and support.

Copyright protected © 2003 The Academy of Breastfeeding Medicine, Inc.
Approved November 16, 2002
The Academy of Breastfeeding Medicine Protocol Committee
Caroline J. Chantry MD, FABM, Co-Chairperson
*Cynthia R. Howard MD, MPH, FABM, Co-Chairperson
*Rosha Champion McCoy MD
Supported in part by a grant from the Maternal and Child Health Bureau, Department of Health and Human Services.

*lead author(s)

REFERENCES

1. Wright A, Rice S, Wells S: Changing hospital practices to increase the duration of breastfeeding. Pediatrics 97:669–675, 1996.

2. World Health Organization: Evidence for the Ten Steps to Successful Breastfeeding, Revised Ed. WHO/CHD/98.9. Geneva, World Health Organization, 1998.

3. Kramer MS, Chalmers B, Hodnett ED, et al: Promotion of breastfeeding intervention trial (PROBIT): A cluster-randomized trial in the republic of Belarus. JAMA 285:4–15, 2001.

4. World Health Organization, United Nations Children's Fund. Protecting, promoting and supporting breastfeeding: The special role of maternity services (A joint WHO/UNICEF statement). Int J Gynecol Obstet 31(suppl 1):171–183, 1990.

5. American College of Obstetricians and Gynecologists, Committees on Health Care for Underserved Women and Obstetric Practice, Queenan JT (ed): Breastfeeding: Maternal and Infant Aspects. Washington, DC, The American College of Obstetricians and Gynecologists. ACOG Educational Bulletin, 2000, 1–15.

6. The American Academy of Pediatrics, Work Group on Breastfeeding: Breastfeeding and the use of human milk. Pediatrics 100:1035–1039, 1997.

7. Howard CR, Howard FM, Lawrence RA, et al: The effect on breastfeeding of physicians' office-based prenatal formula advertising. Obstet Gynecol 95:296–303, 2000.

8. Sosa R, Kennell J, Klaus M, Robertson S, Urrutia J: The effect of a supportive companion on perinatal problems, length of labor, and mother-infant interaction. New Engl J Med 303:597–600, 1980.

9. Klaus MH, Kennell JH: The doula: an essential ingredient of childbirth rediscovered. Acta Paediatr 86:1034–1036, 1997.

10. Zhang J, Bernasko JW, Leybovich E, Fahs M, Hatch MC: Continuous labor support from labor attendant for primiparous women: a meta-analysis. Obstet Gynecol 88(4:Pt 2):1–44, 1996.

11. Kennell J, Klaus M, McGrath S, Robertson S, Hinkley C: Continuous emotional support during labor in a US hospital. A randomized controlled trial [see comments]. JAMA 265:2197–2201, 1991.

12. Christensson K, Siles C, Moreno L, et al: Temperature, metabolic adaptation and crying in healthy full-term newborns cared for skin-to-skin or in a cot. Acta Paediatr 81:488–493, 1992.

13. Varendi H, Christensson K, Porter RH, Winberg J: Soothing effect of amniotic fluid smell in newborn infants. Early Hum Dev 51:47–55, 1998.

14. Righard L, Alade MO: Effect of delivery room routines on success of first breast-feed. Lancet 336(8723):1105–1107, 1990.

15. Righard L, Alade MO: Sucking technique and its effect on success of breastfeeding. Birth 19:185–189, 1992.

16. University of California at San Diego, Wellstart International. Model hospital breastfeeding policies for full-term normal newborn infants. In Woodward-Lopez G, Creer AE (eds): Lactation Management Curriculum: A Faculty Guide for Schools of Medicine, Nursing, and Nutrition. San Diego, CA: Wellstart International, 94 A.D.

17. Keefe MR: The impact of infant rooming-in on maternal sleep at night. J Obstet Gynecol Neonat Nurs 17:122–126, 1988.

18. Waldenstrom U, Swenson A: Rooming-in at night in the postpartum ward. Midwifery 7:82–89, 1991.

19. Perez-Escamilla R, Pollitt E, Lonnerdal B, Dewey KG: Infant feeding policies in maternity wards and their effect on breast-feeding success: An analytical overview. Am J Public Health 84:89–97, 1994.

20. Powers NG, Naylor AJ, Wester RA: Hospital policies: crucial to breastfeeding success. [Review]. Semin Perinatol 18:517–524, 1994.

21. Saadeh R, Akre J: Ten steps to successful breastfeeding: a summary of the rationale and scientific evidence. [Review]. Birth 23:154–160, 1996.

22. Blomquist HK, Jonsbo F, Serenius F, Persson LA: Supplementary feeding in the maternity ward shortens the duration of breast feeding. Acta Paediatr 83:1122–1126, 1994.

23. Protocol Committee Academy of Breastfeeding Medicine: Clinical Protocol #3: Hospital Guidelines for the Use of Supplementary Feedings in the Healthy Term Breastfed Newborn. www.bfmed.org. Academy of Breastfeeding Medicine, 2002.

24. Lawrence RA: A review of the medical benefits and contraindications to breastfeeding in the United States (Maternal and Child Health Technical Information Bulletin). Arlington, Va, National Center for Education in Maternal and Child Health, 1997.

25. Lawrence RA, Lawrence RM: Breastfeeding: A guide for the medical profession, 5th ed. St. Louis: Mosby, 1999.

26. Committee on Drugs, The American Academy of Pediatrics: The transfer of drugs and other chemicals into human milk. Pediatrics 108:776–789, 2001.

27. Naylor A, Wester R: Providing professional lactation management consultation. Clin Perinatol 14:33–38, 1987.

28. Protocol Committee Academy of Breastfeeding Medicine. Clinical Protocol #2: Guidelines for Hospital Discharge of the Breastfeeding Term Infant and Mother, "The Going Home Protocol." www.bfmed.org. Academy of Breastfeeding Medicine, 2002.

29. Howard CR, Howard FM, Lanphear BP, et al: A randomized clinical trial of pacifier use and bottle or cupfeeding and their effect on breastfeeding. Pediatrics 111:511–518, 2003.

Protocol #6: Guideline on co-sleeping and breastfeeding

INTRODUCTION

The Academy of Breastfeeding Medicine is a worldwide organization of physicians dedicated to the promotion, protection, and support of breastfeeding and human lactation. One of the goals of the Academy of Breastfeeding Medicine is the facilitation of optimal breastfeeding practices. This clinical guideline addresses an aspect of parenting that has a significant impact on breastfeeding: infant sleep locations.

BACKGROUND

The term co-sleeping is often used to refer only to the sharing of a sleep surface by an infant and a parent. However, co-sleeping in reality refers to the diverse ways in which infants sleep in close social and/or physical contact with a committed caregiver (usually the mother).[1] This operational definition requires that co-sleepers remain close enough for each to detect and potentially act on the sensory stimuli of the other and includes an infant sleeping alongside a parent on a different piece of furniture or object.

Bed sharing is just one form of co-sleeping. Forms of co-sleeping such as sharing a mat, futon, or the floor are different from bed sharing because the surfaces are different and may not have the same risks as soft mattresses, quilts, water beds, sofas, or couches. In addition, other surfaces such as sofas or couches may have increased risks.[2]

Parent-child co-sleeping provides physical protection for the infant against cold and extends the duration of breastfeeding, thus improving the chances of survival of the slowly developing human infant.[1,3–5] The human infant, relative to other mammals, develops more slowly, requires frequent feedings, and is born neurologically less mature.[1,3–5] In malaria settings, co-sleeping is recommended as the most efficient use of available bednets, and co-sleeping may be necessary in other geographic areas where available bedding or housing is inadequate.

Bed sharing and co-sleeping have received considerable negative comment in the medical literature in recent years as a cause of infant deaths.[6–10] This has led some public health authorities to discourage all parents from bed sharing. The United States Consumer Product Safety Commission (USCPSC) advises parents to "never sleep with your baby" but fails to make important distinctions between the different forms of co-sleeping and safe and unsafe bed sharing.[11]

Bed sharing has long been promoted as a method to enhance parenting behavior or "attachment parenting" and also to facilitate breastfeeding.[12–16] Based on a review of the current literature (see "Justification") the Academy of Breastfeeding Medicine has the following recommendations for health-care providers.

RECOMMENDATIONS

A. Because breastfeeding is the best form of nutrition for infants, any recommendations for infant care that impede its initiation or duration need to be carefully weighed against the many known benefits to infants, their mothers, and society.

B. It should not be assumed that families are practicing only one sleeping arrangement all night every night and during the daytime as well. Health care providers should consider this when obtaining a history on infant sleep practices.[2,22] Parents need to be encouraged to express their views and to seek information and support from their health care providers. Sensitivity to cultural differences is necessary when obtaining sleep histories.

C. There is currently not enough evidence to support routine recommendations against co-sleeping. Parents should be educated about risks and benefits of co-sleeping and unsafe co-sleeping practices and should be allowed to make their own informed decision. Bed sharing is a complex practice. Parental counseling about infant sleep environments should include the following information:

1. Some potentially unsafe practices related to bed sharing/co-sleeping have been identified either in the peer reviewed literature or as a consensus of expert opinion:
   - Environmental smoke exposure and maternal smoking[2,11,17–21]
   - Sharing sofas, couches, or daybeds with infants[2,6,9–11]
   - Sharing waterbeds or the use of soft bedding materials[6,9–11]
   - Sharing beds with adjacent spaces that could trap an infant[6,9–11]
   - Placement of the infant in the adult bed in the prone or side position[6,9–11]
   - The use of alcohol or mind-altering drugs by the adult(s) who is bed sharing[2]

2. Families also should be given all the information that is known about safe sleep environments for their infants, including:
   - Place babies in the supine position for sleep.[23]
   - Use a firm, flat surface and avoid waterbeds, couches, sofas, pillows, soft materials, or loose bedding.[6,9–11,23]
   - Use only a thin blanket to cover the infant. Ensure that the head will not be covered. In a cold room the infant could be kept in an infant sleeper to maintain warmth.[6,9–11,23]
   - Avoid the use of quilts, duvets, comforters, pillows, and stuffed animals in the infant's sleep environment.[6,9–11,23]
   - Never put an infant down to sleep on a pillow or adjacent to a pillow.[6,9–11,23]
   - Never leave an infant alone on an adult bed.[6,9–11,23]
   - Inform families that adult beds have potential risks and are not designed to meet federal safety standards for infants.[6,9–11,23]

- Ensure that there are no spaces between the mattress and headboard, walls, and other surfaces, which may entrap the infant and lead to suffocation.[6,9–11,23]

Placement of a firm mattress directly on the floor away from walls may be a safe alternative. Another alternative to sharing an adult bed or sharing a mattress is the use of an infant bed that attaches to the side of the adult bed and provides proximity and access to the infant but a separate sleep surface. There are currently no peer-reviewed studies of such devices.

JUSTIFICATION

Breastfeeding and bed sharing

A study of bed sharing and breastfeeding found that infants who routinely shared a bed with their mothers breastfed approximately three times longer during the night than infants who routinely slept separately. There was a twofold increase in the number of breastfeeding episodes, and the episodes were 39% longer.[16] Proximity to and sensory contact with the mother during sleep facilitates prompt responses to signs of the infant's readiness to breastfeed and provides psychologic comfort and reassurance to the dependent infant as well as the parents.

A recent large prospective study of more than 10,000 infants in the United State found that up to 22% of 1-month-old infants were bed sharing and that breastfeeding mothers were three times more likely to bed share than mothers who did not breastfeed. Ninety-five percent of infants who shared a bed did so with a parent.[24] Studies in New Zealand and Australia have actually found rates of bed sharing to be greater than 40%.[22,25] A more recent retrospective study in the United States has also shown the rates of co-sleeping to be as high as 45%.[26]

Co-sleeping and infant mortality

SIDS prevention and risk

Several epidemiological studies and a recent meta-analysis have found a significant association between breastfeeding and a lowered SIDS risk, especially when breastfeeding was the exclusive form of feeding during the first four months of life.[27,28] However, there is insufficient evidence at this time to show a causal link between breastfeeding and the prevention of SIDS.

Several studies have also demonstrated an increased risk of SIDS when infants bed share with mothers who smoke cigarettes. Exposure to cigarette smoke as a fetus and in infancy appears to contribute to this risk and is independent of other known risk factors, including social class.[2,17–21,29,30] This has led to the recommendation that infants not bed share with parents who smoke.

Asphyxiation risk

Two studies from the United States Consumer Product Safety Commission using *unverified death certificate* diagnoses concluded that a significant number of infants were asphyxiated as they slept in unsafe sleep environments caused by either accidental entrapment in the sleep surface or overlying by a sleeping adult or older child.[8,10] From these studies the United States Consumer Product Safety Commission (USCPSC) has made recommendations against the use of all types and forms of co-sleeping and advised parents against sleeping with their infants under any circumstances. The USCPSC is concerned about the absence of infant safety standards for adult beds and the hazards that may result from an infant sleeping in an unsafe environment. Two more recent studies done in St. Louis and Cleveland have raised similar concerns,[7,9] yet these studies have flaws similar to those of previous ones. They lack data on the state of intoxication of the co-sleeping adult (drugs or alcohol) and fail to consider the sleep position of the baby at time of death, even though prone sleep position appears to be one of the most significant risk factors for SIDS. They also group all bed sharing into one category, not separating known unsafe sleep environments such as sofas and couches, waterbeds, and upholstered chairs from other, safer sleep surfaces. In these studies there is no assurance of the quality of the data collection, no consistency in the criteria employed in using the term "overlay," and no validation of the conclusions. Bias by medical examiners and coroners may lead them to classify infant deaths that occur in an adult bed, couch, or chair in the presence of an adult as a rollover death even where there is no evidence that an actual overlay occurred. This is especially a problem in the absence of a death scene examination and detailed interviews of those present at the time of death. There is no autopsy method to differentiate between death caused by SIDS versus death from accidental or intentional causes such as infant homicide by pillow smothering. Thus, infant deaths that occur in a crib are usually designated as SIDS, whereas deaths in a couch or adult bed are usually labeled as smothering. Further complicating analyses of infant deaths is the diversity of bed-sharing behaviors. A home visit study of families considered to be at high risk for SIDS because of socioeconomic status found that those bed sharing were more likely to place infants in the prone position and to use softer bed surfaces.[31]

Population-based prospective studies

The only population-based prospective study of bed sharing and SIDS was done in England.[2] The investigators found the following:

- Co-sleeping with an infant on a sofa was associated with particularly high risk of sudden infant death syndrome.
- There was no increased risk associated with bed sharing when the infant was placed back in his or her cot after a period of time and did not spend the whole sleep period in the parent's bed.
- Among infants whose parents do not smoke or infants older than 14 weeks there was no association between infants being found in the parental bed and an increased risk of sudden infant death.
- The risk linked with bed sharing among younger infants seemed to be associated with recent parental consumption of alcohol, overcrowded housing conditions, extreme parental tiredness, and the infant being under a heavy cover such as a quilt.

- Sharing a room with the parents was associated with a lower risk of sudden infant death syndrome.

The authors of this study conclude that "there has been little in the way of direct observation data until recently, but it is becoming clear that sharing a bed both for infants and mothers results in complex interactions that are completely different from isolated sleeping and that need to be understood in detail before application of simplistic labels such as 'safe' or 'unsafe.'" They go on to say, "Perhaps it is not bed sharing per se that is hazardous but rather the particular circumstances in which bed sharing occurs. That some of these circumstances may be modifiable has important implications in terms of social policy and health education."

Ethnic diversity

The rates of SIDS deaths are low in Asian cultures in which co-sleeping is common. However, some argue that co-sleeping in these cultures is different from the bed sharing that occurs in the United States. As Blair and colleagues note in their study, "A baby sleeping at arm's length from the mother on a firm surface, as is often the case in Hong Kong, or a Pacific Island baby sleeping *on* the bed rather than *in* the bed is in a different environment from a baby sleeping in direct contact with the mother on a soft mattress and covered by a thick duvet."[2] A large, prospective study using multivariate analysis of bed sharing found that race or ethnicity appears to have the strongest association with bed sharing at all follow-up periods with black, Asian, and Hispanic mothers four to six times more likely to bed share than white mothers.[24] In a recent study in Alaska, where there is a high rate of co-sleeping among Alaskan Native people, researchers found that almost all SIDS deaths associated with parental bed sharing occurred in conjunction with a history of parental drug use and occasionally in association with prone sleep position or sleeping on surfaces such as couches or waterbeds.[32]

Controlled laboratory studies

McKenna and colleagues have studied bed sharing in the greatest scientific detail in a laboratory setting and have found that infants who shared a bed with the mother had more sleep arousals and spent less time in stage three and four sleep. This may be protective against SIDS since deep sleep and infrequent arousals have been considered as possible risk factors for SIDS.[3,33–36]

Parental factors

The contribution of other parental factors to the risk of bed sharing is unclear. Blair and colleagues found in a multivariate analysis that maternal alcohol consumption of more than 2 drinks (1 drink = 12 oz beer, 5 oz wine or 1½ oz distilled alcohol) and parental tiredness were associated with sudden infant death.[2] A study in New Zealand did not show a clear link with alcohol consumption, however.[20] The role of obesity has been examined in only one study of SIDS cases. They found the mean pregravid weights of bed sharing mothers to be greater than those of non–bed-sharing mothers.[7] If overlying is thought to be the mechanism of infant suffocation, it would seem plausible that the psychologic and physical states of those sharing the bed with an infant could be of importance.

RECOMMENDATIONS FOR FUTURE RESEARCH

A. The Academy of Breastfeeding Medicine urges that more research be undertaken so that the benefits and risks of co-sleeping and bed sharing and their association with breastfeeding can be better understood.

B. The Academy is concerned that co-sleeping and bed sharing are being interdicted based on faulty data collection and erroneous conclusions. If data from medical examiners is to be used in research, medical examiners should develop protocols to investigate unexplained infant deaths using impartial and standardized methods, including detailed site investigations. Data collection must be scientifically sound, verifiable, and include
   • the physical environment of the bed
   • the precise position of the infant in the bed
   • the individual(s) sharing the bed
   • the physical and psychologic status of the adult(s) sharing the bed with the infant, and
   • the medical status of the infant at the time of death

   Complete and critically reviewed autopsies are essential, as are visits by trained unbiased investigators to the site of death

C. Researchers should employ well-designed, impartial, prospective protocols with standardized, well-defined data collection methods. Control data for comparison are an essential part of such research. Studies should be population based, so that actual risk of sudden infant death and overlying smothering due to bed sharing or co-sleeping can be computed. A denominator is needed for calculation of risk and for comparison with a population not practicing co-sleeping or bed sharing. In the final analysis, it is critical that dangerous, modifiable "factors" associated with bed sharing not be considered the same as bed sharing itself. The ethnic diversity of the United States needs to be considered as well.

D. Continuing study of the impact of co-sleeping on infant behavior, SIDS, and breastfeeding is essential.

REFERENCES

1. McKenna JJ, Thoman EB, Anders TF, et al: Infant-parent co-sleeping in an evolutionary perspective: implications for understanding infant sleep development and the sudden infant death syndrome. Sleep 16:263–282, 1993.

2. Blair PS, Fleming PJ, Smith IJ, et al: Babies sleeping with parents: case-control study of factors influencing the risk of the sudden infant death syndrome. CESDI SUDI research group. Br Med J 319:1457–1461, 1999.

3. McKenna JJ: An anthropological perspective on the sudden infant death syndrome (SIDS): the role of parental breathing cues and speech breathing adaptations. Med Anthropol 10:9–92, 1986.

4. McKenna JJ, Mosko S: Evolution and infant sleep: an experimental study of infant-parent co-sleeping and its implications for SIDS. Acta Paediatr 82 (Suppl 389):31–36, 1993.

5. McKenna JJ, Mosko SS: Sleep and arousal, synchrony and independence, among mothers and infants sleeping apart and together (same bed): an experiment in evolutionary medicine. Acta Paediatr Suppl 397:94–102, 1994.

6. Byard RW, Beal S, Bourne AJ: Potentially dangerous sleeping environments and accidental asphyxia in infancy and early childhood. Arch Dis Child 71:497–500, 1994.

7. Carroll-Pankhurst C, Mortimer EA Jr: Sudden infant death syndrome, bedsharing, parental weight, and age at death. Pediatrics 107:530–536, 1994.

8. Drago DA, Dannenberg AL: Infant mechanical suffocation deaths in the United States, 1980–1997. Pediatrics 103:e59, 1999.

9. Kemp JS, Unger B, Wilkins D, et al: Unsafe sleep practices and an analysis of bedsharing among infants dying suddenly and unexpectedly: results of a four-year, population-based, death-scene investigation study of sudden infant death syndrome and related deaths. Pediatrics 106:e41, 2000.

10. Nakamura S, Wind M, Danello MA: Review of hazards associated with children placed in adult beds. Arch Pediatr Adolesc Med 153:1019–1023, 1999.

11. United States Consumer Products Safety Commission: CPSC warns against placing babies in adult beds. SPSC Document #5091. Washington, DC, USCPSC, 1999.

12. Rosenberg KD: Sudden infant death syndrome and co-sleeping. Arch Pediatr Adolesc Med 154:529–530, 2000.

13. Thevenin T: The Family Bed. East Rutherford, NJ, Avery Publishing Group, 1987.

14. Sears W, Sears M: The Baby Book. Boston, Little, Brown and Company, 1993.

15. La Leche League International: The Womanly Art of Breastfeeding, 5th ed. Schaumburg, Ill, LLLI, 1991.

16. McKenna JJ, Mosko SS, Richard CA: Bedsharing promotes breastfeeding. Pediatrics 100(2 Pt 1):214–219, 1997.

17. Mitchell EA, Taylor BJ, Ford RP, et al: Four modifiable and other major risk factors for cot death: the New Zealand study. J Paediatr Child Health 28 Suppl 1:S3–S8, 1992.

18. Mitchell EA, Esmail A, Jones DR, Clements M: Do differences in the prevalence of risk factors explain the higher mortality from sudden infant death syndrome in New Zealand compared with the UK? N Z Med J 109(1030):352–355, 1996.

19. Mitchell EA, Tuohy PG, Brunt JM, et al: Risk factors for sudden infant death syndrome following the prevention campaign in New Zealand: a prospective study. Pediatrics 100(5):835–840, 1997.

20. Scragg R, Mitchell EA, Taylor BJ, et al: Bed sharing, smoking, and alcohol in the sudden infant death syndrome. New Zealand Cot Death Study Group. Br Med J 307(6915): 1312–1318, 1993.

21. Scragg R, Stewart AW, Mitchell EA, Ford RP, Thompson JM: Public health policy on bed sharing and smoking in the sudden infant death syndrome. N Z Med J 108(1001): 218–222, 1995.

22. Rigda RS, McMillen IC, Buckley P: Bed sharing patterns in a cohort of Australian infants during the first six months after birth. J Paediatr Child Health 36(2):117–121, 2000.

23. American Academy of Pediatrics: Changing concepts of sudden infant death syndrome: implications for infant sleeping environment and sleep position. Task Force on Infant Sleep Position and Sudden Infant Death Syndrome. Pediatrics 105(3 Pt 1):650–656, 2000.

24. McCoy RC, Hunt CL, Lesko SM: Population-based study of bedsharing and breastfeeding. Pediatr Res 47:154A. 2000.

25. Tuohy PG, Smale P, Clements M: Ethnic differences in parent/infant co-sleeping practices in New Zealand. N Z Med J 111(1074):364–366, 1998.

26. Willinger M, Ko CW, Hoffman HJ, Kessler RC, Corwin MJ: Trends in infant bed sharing in the United States 1993–2000. The national infant sleep position study. Arch Pediatr Adolesc Med 157:43–49, 2003.

27. Ford RP, Taylor BJ, Mitchell EA, et al: Breastfeeding and the risk of sudden infant death syndrome. Int J Epidemiol 22:885–890, 1993.

28. McVea KL, Turner PD, Peppler DK: The role of breastfeeding in sudden infant death syndrome. J Hum Lact 2000; 16(1):13–20.

29. Mitchell EA, Scragg L, Clements M: Factors related to infants bed sharing. N Z Med J 107(989):466–467, 1994.

30. Scragg RK, Mitchell EA: Side sleeping position and bed sharing in the sudden infant death syndrome. Ann Med 30:345–349, 1998.

31. Flick L, White DK, Vemulapalli C, Stulac BB, Kemp JS: Sleep position and the use of soft bedding during bed sharing among African American infants at increased risk for sudden infant death syndrome. J Pediatr 138:338–343, 2001.

32. Gessner BD, Ives GC, Perham-Hester KA: Association between sudden infant death syndrome and prone sleep position, bed sharing, and sleeping outside an infant crib in Alaska. Pediatrics 108:923–927, 2001.

33. McKenna JJ, Mosko S, Dungy C, McAninch J: Sleep and arousal patterns of co-sleeping human mother/infant pairs: a preliminary physiological study with implications for the study of sudden infant death syndrome (SIDS). Am J Phys Anthropol 83:331–347, 1990.

34. Mosko S, Richard C, McKenna J: Infant arousals during mother-infant bed sharing: implications for infant sleep and sudden infant death syndrome research. Pediatrics 100: 841–849, 1997.

35. McKenna J, Mosko S, Richard C, et al: Experimental studies of infant-parent co-sleeping: mutual physiological and behavioral influences and their relevance to SIDS

(sudden infant death syndrome). Early Hum Dev 38: 187–201, 1994.

36. Mosko S, Richard C, McKenna J, Drummond S, Mukai D: Maternal proximity and infant CO_2 environment during bedsharing and possible implications for SIDS research. Am J Phys Anthropol 103:315–328, 1997.

Copyright protected © 2003 The Academy of Breastfeeding Medicine, Inc
Approved January 20, 2003
The Academy of Breastfeeding Medicine Protocol Committee

Caroline J. Chantry MD, FABM, Co-Chairperson
Lawrence M. Gartner MD
Cynthia R. Howard MD, MPH, FABM, Co-Chairperson
*Rosha Champion McCoy MD
Consultant
James McKenna J. PhD
Supported in part by a grant from the Maternal and Child Health Bureau, Department of Health and Human Services.

*Lead Author(s)

Protocol #7: Model breastfeeding policy

BREASTFEEDING POLICY

"Name of institution" and setting(s)
Policy #:
Issued:
Reviewed/Revised:

PURPOSE

To promote a philosophy of maternal infant care that advocates breastfeeding and supports the normal physiological functions involved in the establishment of this maternal infant process. To assist families choosing to breastfeed with initiating and developing a successful and satisfying experience.

This policy is based on recommendations from the most recent breastfeeding policy statements published by the Office on Women's Health of the U.S. Department of Health and Human Services,[1] the American Academy of Pediatrics,[2] the American College of Obstetrics and Gynecology,[3] the American Academy of Family Physicians,[4] the World Health Organization,[5] the American Dietetic Association,[6] and the Academy of Breastfeeding Medicine,[7] and the UNICEF/WHO evidence-based "Ten Steps to Successful Breastfeeding."[5,8,9]

POLICY STATEMENTS

1. *"Name of institution"* staff will actively support breastfeeding as the preferred method of providing nutrition to infants. A multidisciplinary, culturally appropriate team comprising hospital administrators, physician and nursing staff, lactation consultants and specialists, nutrition staff, parents, and other appropriate staff shall be established and maintained to identify and eliminate institutional barriers to breastfeeding. On a yearly basis, this group will compile and evaluate data relevant to breastfeeding support services and formulate a plan of action to implement needed changes.

2. A written breastfeeding policy will be developed and communicated to all health care staff. The *"name of institution"* breastfeeding policy will be reviewed and updated routinely (biannually) using current research as an evidence-based guide.

3. All pregnant women and their support people as appropriate will be provided with information on breastfeeding and counseled on the benefits of breastfeeding, contraindications to breastfeeding, and risk of formula feeding.

4. The woman's desire to breastfeed will be documented in her medical record.

5. Mothers will be encouraged to exclusively breastfeed unless medically contraindicated. The method of feeding will be documented in the medical record of every infant.
   • Exclusive breastfeeding is defined as providing breast milk as the sole source of nutrition. Exclusively breastfed babies receive no other liquids or solids.

6. At birth or soon thereafter all newborns, if baby and mother are stable, will be placed skin-to-skin with the mother. Skin-to-skin contact involves placing the naked baby prone on the mother's bare chest. Mother-infant couples will be given the opportunity to initiate breastfeeding within 1 hour of birth. Postcesarean-birth babies will be encouraged to breastfeed as soon as possible. The administration of vitamin K and prophylactic antibiotics to prevent ophthalmia neonatorum should be delayed for the first hour after birth to allow uninterrupted mother infant contact and breastfeeding.[10]

7. Breastfeeding mother-infant couples will be encouraged to remain together throughout their hospital stay, including at night (rooming-in). Skin-to-skin contact will be encouraged as much as possible.

8. Breastfeeding assessment, teaching, and documentation will be done on each shift and whenever possible with each staff contact with the mother. After each feeding, staff will document information about the feeding in the infant's medical record. This documentation may include the latch, position, and any problems encountered. For feedings not directly observed, maternal report may be used. Every shift, a direct observation of the baby's position and latch-on during feeding will be performed and documented.

9. Mothers will be encouraged to utilize available breastfeeding resources including classes, written materials, and video presentations, as appropriate. If clinically indicated, the clinician or nurse will make a referral to a lactation consultant or specialist.

10. Breastfeeding mothers will be instructed about
    a. proper positioning and latch on;
    b. nutritive suckling and swallowing;
    c. milk production and release;
    d. frequency of feeding/feeding cues;
    e. expression of breast milk and use of a pump if indicated;
    f. how to assess if infant is adequately nourished; and
    g. reasons for contacting the clinician.
    These skills will be taught to primiparous and multiparous women and reviewed before the mother goes home.

11. Parents will be taught that breastfeeding infants, including cesarean-birth babies, should be put to breast at least 8 to 12 times each 24 hours. Infant feeding cues (such as increased alertness or activity, mouthing, or rooting,) will be used as indicators of the baby's readiness for feeding. Breastfeeding babies will be breastfed at night.

12. Time limits for breastfeeding on each side will be avoided. Infants can be offered both breasts at each feeding but may be interested in feeding only on one side at a feeding during the early days.

13. No supplemental water, glucose water, or formula will be given unless specifically ordered by a physician or nurse practitioner or by the mother's documented and informed request. Prior to nonmedically indicated supplementation, mothers will be informed of the risks of supplementing. The supplement should be fed to the baby by cup if possible and will be no more than 10 to 15 mL in a term baby.[11–13] Alternative feeding methods such as syringe or spoon feeding may also be used; however, these methods have not be shown to be effective in preserving breastfeeding. Bottles will not be placed in a breastfeeding infant's bassinet.

14. This institution does not give group instruction in the use of formula. Those parents who, after appropriate counseling, choose to formula feed their infants will be provided individual instruction.

15. Pacifiers will not be given to normal full-term breastfeeding infants. The pacifier guidelines at *"name of institution"* state that preterm infants in the Neonatal Intensive Care or Special Care Unit or infants with specific medical conditions may be given pacifiers for non-nutritive

sucking. Newborns undergoing painful procedures (circumcision, for example) may be given a pacifier as a method of pain management during the procedure. The infant will not return to the mother with the pacifier. *"Name of institution"* encourages "pain-free newborn care," which may include breastfeeding during the heel stick procedure for the newborn metabolic screening tests.

16. Routine blood glucose monitoring of full term healthy appropriate for gestational age (AGA) infants is not indicated. Assessment for clinical signs of hypoglycemia and dehydration will be ongoing.[14]

17. Antilactation drugs will not be given to any postpartum mother.

18. Routine use of nipple creams, ointments, or other topical preparations will be avoided unless such therapy has been indicated for a dermatological problem. Mothers with sore nipples will be observed for latch-on techniques and will be instructed to apply expressed colostrum or breast milk to the areola after each feeding.

19. Nipple shields or bottle nipples will not be routinely used to cover a mother's nipple to treat latch-on problems or prevent or manage sore or cracked nipples or when a mother has flat or inverted nipples. Nipple shields will be used only in conjunction with a lactation consultation.

20. After 24 hours of life, if the infant has not latched on or fed effectively, the mother will be instructed to begin breast massage and hand expression of colostrum into the baby's mouth during feeding attempts. Skin-to-skin contact will be encouraged. (Parents will be instructed to watch closely for feeding cues and whenever these are observed to awaken and feed the infant.) If the baby continues to feed poorly, pumping with skilled hand expression or a double set-up electric breast pump will be initiated and maintained approximately every 3 hours or a minimum of eight times per day. Any expressed colostrum or mother's milk will be fed to the baby by an alternative method. The mother will be reminded that she may not obtain much milk or even any milk the first few times she pumps her breasts. Until the mother's milk is available, a collaborative decision should be made among the mother, nurse, and clinician regarding the need to supplement the baby. Each day clinicians will be consulted regarding the volume and type of the supplement. Pacifiers will be avoided. In cases of problem feeding, the lactation consultant or specialist will be consulted.[10]

21. If the baby is still not latching on well or feeding well when going home, the feeding/pumping/supplementing plan will be reviewed in addition to routine breastfeeding instructions. A follow-up visit or contact will be scheduled within 24 hours. Depending on the clinical situation it may be appropriate to delay discharge of the couplet to provide further breastfeeding intervention, support, and education.

22. All babies should be seen for follow-up within the first few days postpartum. This visit should be with a pediatrician or other qualified health care practitioner for a formal evaluation of breastfeeding performance, a weight check, assessment of jaundice and age appropriate elimination:
    - For infants discharged at less than 2 days of age (< 48 hours): Follow-up at 2 to 4 days of age
    - For infants discharged at more than 2 days of age (> 48 hours): Follow-up at 4 to 5 days of age
    - All newborns should be seen by 1 month of age.

23. Mothers who are separated from their sick or premature infants will be
    a. instructed on how to use skilled hand expression or the double set up electric breast pump—instructions will include expression at least eight times per day or approximately every 3 hours for 15 minutes (or until milk flow stops, whichever is greater) around the clock and the importance of not missing a pumping session during the night;
    b. encouraged to breastfeed on demand as soon as the infant's condition permits;
    c. taught proper storage and labeling of human milk; and
    d. assisted in learning skilled hand expression or obtaining a double set up electric breast pump prior to going home.

24. Before leaving the hospital,[15] breastfeeding mothers should be able to
    a. position the baby correctly at the breast with no pain during the feeding;
    b. latch the baby to breast properly;
    c. state when the baby is swallowing milk;
    d. state that the baby should be nursed approximately 8 to 12 times every 24 hours until satiety;
    e. state age-appropriate elimination patterns (at least six urinations per day and three to four stools per day by the fourth day of life);
    f. list indications for calling a clinician; and
    g. manually express milk from their breasts.
25. Prior to going home, mothers will be given the names and telephone numbers of community resources to contact for help with breastfeeding, including (the support group or resource recommended by *"name of institution"*).
26. *"Name of institution"* does not accept free formula or free breast milk substitutes. Nursery or NICU discharge bags offered to all mothers will not contain infant formula, coupons for formula, logos of formula companies, or literature with formula company logos.
27. *"Name of institution"* health professionals will attend educational sessions on lactation management and breastfeeding promotion to ensure that correct, current, and consistent information is provided to all mothers wishing to breastfeed.

Application

All breastfeeding patients.

Exceptions

Breastfeeding is contraindicated in the following situations:
- HIV-positive mother in developed countries (e.g., United States, Europe)
- Mother using illicit drugs (for example, cocaine, heroin) unless specifically approved by the infant's health care provider on a case by case basis

- A mother taking certain medications. Although most prescribed and over-the-counter drugs are safe for the breastfeeding infant, some medications may make it necessary to interrupt breastfeeding. These include radioactive isotopes, antimetabolites, cancer chemotherapy, and a small number of other medications. The references used at *"name of institution"* are *Medications and Mothers' Milk* by Thomas Hale,[16] *Breastfeeding: A Guide for the Medical Profession* by R. A. Lawrence and R. M. Lawrence,[17] and the American Academy of Pediatrics Statement on the Transfer of Drugs into Human Milk.[18]
- Mother has active, untreated tuberculosis
- Infant has galactosemia
- Mother has active herpetic lesions on her breast(s) —breastfeeding can be recommended on the unaffected breast (the Infectious Disease Service will be consulted for problematic infectious disease issues)
- Mother with varicella that is determined to be infectious to the infant
- Mother has HTLV1 (human T-cell leukemia virus type 1)

Responsibility

RN, LPN, LC, PNP, MD, CNM

Forms:

- Newborn Flow Sheet
- Maternal Flow Sheet

Other related policies:

Policy #:
Other references/resources[17,19–22]

Initiated by:

Contributing departments:

REFERENCES

1. U.S. Department of Health and Human Services: HHS Blueprint for Action on Breastfeeding. 1–31. Washington, DC, U.S. Department of Health and Human Services, Office on Women's Health, 2000.

2. The American Academy of Pediatrics, Work Group on Breastfeeding: Breastfeeding and the use of human milk. Pediatrics 100:1035–1039, 1997.

3. American College of Obstetricians and Gynecologists and Committees on Health Care for Underserved Women and Obstetric Practice, Queenan, JT (ed): Breastfeeding: Maternal and Infant Aspects. Washington, DC, The American College of Obstetricians and Gynecologists. ACOG Educational Bulletin, 2000, 1–15.

4. The American Academy of Family Physicians. Family Physicians Supporting Breastfeeding: Breastfeeding Position Paper 2002. The American Academy of Family Physicians. Compendium of AAFP positions on selected health issues at http://www.aafp.org/policy/x1641.xml. Kansas City, MO, The American Academy of Family Physicians, 2002.

5. World Health Organization, United Nations Children's Fund: Protecting, promoting and supporting breastfeeding: The special role of maternity services (A joint WHO/UNICEF statement). Int J Gynecol Obstet31:171–183, 1990.

6. Position of the American Dietetic Association: Breaking the barriers to breastfeeding. J Am Diet Assoc101:1213–1220, 2001.

7. Academy of Breastfeeding Medicine Board of Directors. ABM Mission Statement. www.bfmed.org. 2003.

8. WHO/UNICEF Joint Statement. Meeting on Infant and Young Child Feeding. J Nurse-Midwifery25:31–38, 1980.

9. World Health Organization and United Nations Children's Fund: Innocenti Declaration on the Protection, Promotion and Support of Breastfeeding. New York UNICEF, 1990.

10. Protocol Committee Academy of Breastfeeding Medicine, Cordes R, Howard CR: Clinical Protocol #3: Hospital Guidelines for the Use of Supplementary Feedings in the Healthy Term Breastfed Newborn. www.bfmed.org. Academy of Breastfeeding Medicine, 2002.

11. Howard CR, Howard FM, Lanphear B, et al: Randomized clinical trial of pacifier use and bottle-feeding or cupfeeding and their effect on breastfeeding. Pediatrics 111:511–518, 2003.

12. Howard CR, de Blieck EA, ten Hoopen CB, et al: Physiologic stability of newborns during cup- and bottle-feeding. Pediatrics104:1–7, 1999.

13. Marinelli KA, Burke GS, Dodd VL: A comparison of the safety of cup feedings and bottle feedings in premature infants whose mothers intend to breastfeed. J Perinatol 21:350–355, 2001.

14. Protocol Committee Academy of Breastfeeding Medicine, Eidelman AI, Howard CR, Schanler RJ, Wight NE: Clinical Protocol Number 1: Guidelines for Glucose Monitoring and Treatment of Hypoglycemia in Breastfed Neonates. ABM News and Views 5:insert, 1999.

15. Protocol Committee Academy of Breastfeeding Medicine, Gartner L, Howard C R: Clinical Protocol #2: Guidelines for Hospital Discharge of the Breastfeeding Term Infant and Mother, "The Going Home Protocol." www.bfmed.org. Academy of Breastfeeding Medicine, 2002.

16. Hale TW: Medications and Mother's Milk, 10th ed. Amarillo, TX, Pharmasoft Medical Publishing, 2002.

17. Lawrence RA, Lawrence RM: Breastfeeding: A guide for the medical profession, 5th ed. St. Louis, Mosby, 1999.

18. Committee on Drugs, The American Academy of Pediatrics: The transfer of drugs and other chemicals into human milk. Pediatrics108:776–789, 2001.

19. Protocol Committee Academy of Breastfeeding Medicine, Chantry C, Howard CR, McCoy RC: Clinical Protocol #5: Peripartum Breastfeeding Management for the Healthy Mother and Infant at Term. www.bfmed.org. Academy of Breastfeeding Medicine, 2002.

20. Riordan JM, Auerbach KG: Breastfeeding and Human Lactation. Boston, Jones and Bartlett Publishers, 1993.

21. American Academy of Pediatrics. Redbook: 2003 Report of the Committee on Infectious Diseases, 26th ed. Elk Grove, Ill, American Academy of Pediatrics, 2003.

22. Merewood A, Philipp BL: Breastfeeding: Conditions and Diseases. Amarillo, TX, Pharmasoft Publishers, 2001.

THE TEN STEPS TO SUCCESSFUL BREASTFEEDING

1. Have a written breastfeeding policy that is routinely communicated to all health care staff.

2. Train all health care staff in skills necessary to implement this policy.

3. Inform all pregnant women about the benefits and management of breastfeeding.

4. Help mothers initiate breastfeeding within 1 hour of birth.

5. Show mothers how to breastfeed and how to maintain lactation, even if they are separated from their infants.

6. Give newborn infants no food or drink other than breast milk, unless medically indicated.*

---

*A hospital must pay fair market price for all formula and infant feeding supplies that it uses and cannot accept free or heavily discounted formula and supplies.

7. Practice rooming-in—allow mothers and infants to remain together—24 hours a day.
8. Encourage breastfeeding on demand.
9. Give no artificial teats or pacifiers to breast-feeding infants.
10. Foster the establishment of breastfeeding support groups and refer mothers to them, on discharge from the hospital or clinic.

Copyright protected © 2003 The Academy of Breastfeeding Medicine, Inc.

Approved 2/20/04
The Academy of Breastfeeding Medicine Protocol Committee
Caroline J. Chantry, MD, FABM
Cynthia R. Howard, MD, MPH, FABM
*Barbara L. Philipp MD, IBCLC, FABM
Development supported in part by a grant from the Maternal and Child Health Bureau, Department of Health and Human Services

*lead author(s)

Protocol #8: Human milk storage information for home use for healthy full-term infants

STORAGE CONTAINERS

1. Hard-sided containers, such as hard plastic or glass, are the preferred containers for long-term human milk storage. These containers should have an airtight seal.[1]
2. Plastic bags specifically designed for human milk storage can be used for short-term (less than 72 hours) milk storage.[1,2] Use of plastic bags is not recommended for long-term storage as they may spill, leak, or become contaminated more easily than hard-sided containers, and some important milk components may adhere to the soft plastic and be lost.

GENERAL GUIDELINES

1. Hands must be washed prior to expressing or pumping milk.
2. Use containers and pumping equipment that have been washed in hot, soapy water and rinsed. If available, cleaning in a dishwasher is acceptable; dishwashers that additionally heat the water may improve cleanliness. If a dishwasher is not available, boiling the containers after washing is recommended. Boiling is particularly important where the water supply may not be clean.
3. Store in small portions to minimize waste. Most breastfed babies take between 2 and 4 ounces (60–120 mL) of milk when beginning with an alternative feeding method. Storing in 2-ounce (60 mL) amounts and offering additional amounts if the baby is still hungry will prevent having to throw away unfinished milk.
4. Consider storing smaller size portions [1–2 ounces (30–60 mL) each] for unexpected situations. A small amount of milk can keep a baby happy until mom comes to nurse the baby.
5. Several expressions throughout a day may be combined to get the desired volume in a container. Chill the newly expressed milk for at least 1 hour in the main body of the refrigerator or in a cooler with ice or ice packs, and then add it to previously chilled milk expressed on the same day.
6. Do not add warm breast milk to frozen milk because it will partially thaw the frozen milk.
7. Keep milk from one day separate from other days.

8. Do not fill the container; leave some room at the top because breast milk expands as it freezes.

9. Label containers clearly with waterproof labels and ink, if possible.

10. Indicate the date that the milk was expressed and the child's name (for daycare).

11. Expect that the milk will separate during storage because it is not homogenized. The cream will rise to the top of the milk and look thicker and whiter. Before feeding, gently swirling the container of milk will mix the cream back through again. Avoid vigorously shaking the milk.

12. The color of milk may vary from day to day, depending on maternal diet. It may look bluish, yellowish, or brownish. Frozen breast milk may also smell different than fresh breastmilk.[3] There is no reason not to use the milk if the baby accepts it.

Milk storage guidelines

1. Milk may be kept at room temperature (up to 77°F or 25°C) for 6 to 8 hours. Temperatures greater than 77°F (25°C) may not be safe for room temperature storage.[4] Containers should be covered and kept as cool as possible; covering the container with a cool towel may keep milk cooler.

2. Milk may be stored in an insulated cooler bag with ice packs for 24 hours.[5]

3. Milk may be safely refrigerated (39°F or 4°C) for up to 5 days.[6] Store milk in the back of the main body of the refrigerator, where the temperature is the coolest.[7]

4. The type of freezer in which the milk is kept determines timetables for frozen milk. Generally, store milk toward the back of the freezer, where the temperature is most constant.[8] Milk stored for the longer durations in the ranges listed below is safe, but there is some evidence that the lipids in the milk undergo degradation resulting in lower quality.[9]

- Freezer compartment located inside the refrigerator (5°F or −15°C): **2 weeks**
- Refrigerator/freezer with separate doors (0°F or −18°C): **3 to 6 months**
- Chest or upright manual defrost deep freezer that is opened infrequently and maintains ideal temperature (−4°F or −20°C): **6 to 12 months**

5. The above guidelines apply only to healthy, term infants; guidelines are different for hospitalized, sick, or preterm infants.

Thawing or warming milk

1. The oldest milk should be used first.

2. The baby may drink the milk cool, at room temperature, or warmed.

3. Thaw milk by placing it in the refrigerator the night before use or gently rewarm it by placing the container under warm running water or in a bowl of warm water.

4. Do not let the level of water in the bowl or from the tap touch the mouth of the container.

5. Milk may be kept in the refrigerator for 24 hours after it is thawed.

6. Never use a microwave oven or stovetop to heat the milk, as these may cause scald spots and will also destroy antibodies.[10,11]

7. Swirl the container of milk to mix the cream back in, and distribute the heat evenly. Do not stir the milk.

8. Milk left in the feeding container after a feeding should be discarded and not used again.

9. As with all foods, do not re-freeze breast milk once it is thawed or partially thawed.

REFERENCES

1. Garza C, Johnson CA, Harrist R, Nichols BL: Effects of methods of collection and storage on nutrients in human milk. Early Hum Dev 6:295–303, 1982.

2. Williams-Arnold LD: Human Milk Storage for Healthy Infants and Children. Sandwich, MA, Health Education Associates Inc, 2002.

3. Lawrence RA, Lawrence RM: Breastfeeding: A guide for the medical profession, 5th ed. St. Louis, Mosby, 1999, p 698.

4. Hamosh M, Ellis LA, Pollock DR, Henderson TR, Hamosh P: Breastfeeding and the working mother: Effect of time and temperature of short-term storage on proteolysis, lipolysis, and bacterial growth in milk. Pediatrics 97:492–498, 1996.

5. Meek JY: Breastfeeding in the workplace. Pediatr Clin North Am 48:461–474, xvi, 2001.

6. Sosa R, Barness L: Bacterial growth in refrigerated human milk. Am J Dis Child 141:111–112, 1987.

7. Olowe SA, Ahmed I, Lawal SF, Ransome-Kuti S: Bacteriological quality of raw human milk: effect of storage in a refrigerator. Ann Trop Paediatr 7:233–237, 1987.

8. Friend BA, Shahani KM, Long CA, Vaughn LA: The effect of processing and storage on key enzymes, B vitamins, and lipids of mature human milk. I. Evaluation of fresh samples and effects of freezing and frozen storage. Pediatr Res 17:61–64, 1983.

9. Berkow SE, Freed LM, Hamosh M, et al: Lipases and lipids in human milk: effect of freeze-thawing and storage. Pediatr Res 18:257–262, 1984.

10. Quan R, Yang C, Rubinstein S, et al: Effects of microwave radiation on anti-infective factors in human milk. Pediatrics 89(4 Pt 1):667–669, 1992.

11. Sigman M, Burke KI, Swarner OW, Shavlik GW: Effects of microwaving human milk: changes in IgA content and bacterial count. J Am Diet Assoc 89:690–692, 1989.

Copyright protected © 2004 The Academy of Breastfeeding Medicine, Inc.

Approved 3/23/2004

The Academy of Breastfeeding Medicine Protocol Committee

Caroline J. Chantry MD, FABM, Co-Chairperson

*Anne Eglash MD, FABM

Cynthia R. Howard MD, MPH, FABM, Co-Chairperson

Supported in part by a grant from the Maternal and Child Health Bureau, Department of Health and Human Services.

*Lead Author(s)

Protocol #9: Use of galactogogues in initiating or augmenting maternal milk supply

BACKGROUND

Galactogogues (or lactogogues) are medications or other substances believed to assist initiation, maintenance, or augmentation of maternal milk production. Because low milk supply is one of the most common reasons given for discontinuing breastfeeding,[1] both mothers and physicians have sought medicine to address this concern. Breast milk production is a complex physiologic process involving physical and emotional factors and the interaction of multiple hormones, the most important of which is believed to be prolactin. With parturition and expulsion of the placenta, progesterone falls and a full milk supply is initiated (Lactogenesis II).[2] Through interaction with the hypothalamus and anterior pituitary, dopamine agonists inhibit, and dopamine antagonists increase, prolactin secretion and thereby milk production (endocrine control). Thereafter, prolactin levels gradually decrease but milk supply is maintained or increased by local feedback mechanisms (autocrine control).[3] Therefore, an increase in prolactin levels is needed to increase, but not maintain, milk supply. If the breasts are not emptied regularly and thoroughly, milk production declines. Likewise, more frequent and thorough emptying of the breasts typically results in increased milk production. Use of galactogogues for faltering milk supply should generally be reserved for situations after both a thorough evaluation for treatable causes (e.g., maternal hypothyroidism or medication) and increased frequency of breastfeeding or pumping or expression has not been successful.

INDICATIONS FOR GALACTOGOGUES

Common indications for galactogogues are adoptive nursing (induction of lactation in a woman who was not pregnant with the current child), relactation (reestablishing milk supply after weaning), and increasing a faltering milk supply because of maternal or infant illness or separation. Mothers who are not directly breastfeeding but are expressing milk by hand or with a pump often experience a decline in milk production after several weeks. One of the most common indications for galactogogues is to augment a declining milk supply in mothers of preterm or ill infants in the neonatal intensive care unit.

PROCEDURE

1. **Before using any substance to try to increase milk supply, a full evaluation of current maternal milk supply and effectiveness of milk transfer is imperative.** Attention must be directed to the evaluation and augmentation of frequency and thoroughness of milk removal. This can be accomplished through increased frequency and duration of breastfeeding (if the infant has been shown to be effective at emptying the breasts) or pumping. A full-size, automatic cycling breast pump, capable of draining both breasts ("hospital grade") at the same time is recommended, if available. Problems such as inappropriate timing and duration of feedings, inappropriate supplementation, mother-infant separation, ineffective latch, and inadequate milk transfer should be corrected.

2. **Women should be informed of any data (or lack thereof) regarding the efficacy, safety, and timing of use of galactogogues.** With the exception of adoptive nursing, where galactogogues are started *before* the birth of the baby, there is no research to suggest that starting galactogogues within the first week postpartum is efficacious.

3. **Mothers should be screened for contraindications to the chosen medication or substance and informed as to possible side effects.** Although a lactation consultant may recommend the medication or herb, it is the physician's responsibility to prescribe medications and follow the mother and infant.

4. **The physician who prescribes the medication is obligated to follow, or to ensure appropriate follow-up, of both mother and infant regarding milk supply and any side effects.** In practice, many times it is the nurse practitioner, pediatrician, or neonatologist who is asked to prescribe a galactogogue and not the obstetrician-gynecologist. As is commonly found when dealing with lactation, family physicians are ideally situated to manage this issue.

5. **Although short-term use (1–3 weeks) has been evaluated for some of these substances, long-term use has not been studied.** Anecdotal reports suggest no increase in side effects with the most commonly used medications (metoclopramide, domperidone, fenugreek), but long term effects on both mother and infant are unknown.

SPECIFIC GALACTOGOGUES

Many medications, foods, and herbal therapies have been recommended as galactogogues. The medications used often exert their effects through antagonism of dopamine receptors, resulting in increased prolactin. In many cases, the mechanism(s) of action are unknown.

Metoclopramide

Metoclopramide (Reglan) is the most well studied and most commonly used medication for inducing or augmenting lactation in the United States. It promotes lactation by antagonizing the release of dopamine in the central nervous system, thereby increasing prolactin levels.[4] It is an antiemetic and also commonly used for gastroesophageal reflux in infants. Although levels found in breast milk have been measured higher than maternal serum levels, levels in infants have been undetectable or well below infant therapeutic levels with no reported side effects.[5] Metoclopramide does not appear to alter milk composition significantly.[6,7] Many studies have shown its efficacy in the induction and augmentation of milk production.[8–19] However, there is one controlled trial that failed to show efficacy.[20]

Maternal restlessness, drowsiness, fatigue, and diarrhea may occur but usually do not require stopping the medication.[4,15] The drug should be discontinued if any of the rare extrapyramidal side effects of sleeplessness, headache, confusion, dizziness, mental depression, or feelings of anxiety or agitation occur. Acute dystonic reactions are very rare (<.05%) and may require diphenhydramine (Benadryl) treatment. Metoclopramide should not be used if patients have epilepsy or are on anti-seizure medications, have a history of significant depression or are on antidepressant drugs, have a pheochromocytoma or uncontrolled hypertension, have intestinal bleeding or obstruction, or have a known allergy or prior reaction to metoclopramide.[4] Metoclopramide does transfer into the milk, but research has demonstrated no side effects in the infants of mothers taking metoclopramide.[8–19,21]

The usual dose is 30 to 45mg/day in three or four divided doses, with a dose-response effect up to 45 mg daily.[13] It is usually given for 7 to 14 days at full dose with a taper off over 5 to 7 days. Longer periods of use may be associated with an increased incidence of depression. Occasionally a mother's milk supply will falter as the dose is reduced, and the lowest effective dose has been continued for longer periods successfully. Some experts also advise a gradual increase when beginning the dosage.

Domperidone (Motilium)

Domperidone is also a dopamine antagonist that is available outside the United States for the treatment of gastroesophageal reflux and emesis.[22] Because of its drug characteristics it is less likely to cross the maternal blood-brain barrier, resulting in less extrapyramidal side effects than metoclopramide. Domperidone is also less likely than metoclopramide to cross into the breast milk.[11] Administration of domperidone results in significant increases in mean serum prolactin levels in normal women.[24,25] Domperidone is the only galactogogue evaluated in a randomized controlled trial and shown to be safe and effective in increasing breast milk production.[24]

Side effects are very uncommon and include dry mouth, headache (resolved with decreased dosage), and abdominal cramps.[22] Chronic high-dose treatment with domperidone in rodents has been associated with increased numbers of breast tumors. This has not been reported in humans. Domperidone is contraindicated in patients with known sensitivity to the drug and in situations in which gastrointestinal stimulation might be dangerous (e.g., gastrointestinal hemorrhage, mechanical obstruction, or perforation). Despite the fact that domperidone is approved for use in most of the developed world and has been used for many years with an excellent safety record, the U.S. Food and Drug Administration (FDA) issued a warning against its use in the United States based on safety concerns with IV use and risks associated with drug importation.[40] There is no evidence that oral administration is associated with toxicity in either mother or infant.[40]

The usual dosage is 10 to 20 mg three to four times per day taken for 3 to 8 weeks. Most women respond within 3 to 4 days, but some women respond in 24 hours, and some require 2 to 3 weeks to get maximum effect.[25]

Sulpiride (Egonyl) and chlorpromazine (Thorazine)

Sulpiride is an antipsychotic (neuroleptic) medication not available in the United States that acts as a galactogogue by increasing prolactin-releasing hormone from the hypothalamus. Two studies have shown an increase in milk supply over placebo. Maternal side effects may include the extrapyramidal effects listed above for metoclopramide and possibly weight gain. The suggested dosage is 50 mg two or three times daily.[26–28]

Psychiatric practitioners have long noted galactorrhea in both males and females taking chlorpromazine (also a neuroleptic). A dose of 25 mg orally three times daily for 1 week has been shown in case reports to increase milk supply.

As both sulpiride and chlorpromazine increases prolactin levels by blocking dopamine receptors (and therefore the prolactin-inhibiting action of dopamine), extrapyramidal side effects are again possible.[29]

Human growth hormone

One randomized, double-blind, placebo-controlled trial of human growth hormone in a dose of 0.1 IU/kg/day subcutaneously noted a significant increase in milk volume by day 7 in 16 healthy lactating women. There were no documented changes in milk composition or side effects reported in the mothers. The usefulness of this expensive, injectable galactogogue appears limited.[21,30]

Thyrotrophin-releasing hormone

Thyrotrophin-releasing hormone (TRH) is used in the United States to assess thyroid function. It causes the release of both thyroid-stimulating hormone (TSH) and prolactin from the pituitary. The most recent study suggests short-term use is both safe and effective, but long-term use has not been evaluated. Dosage was one spray (1 mg TRH) 4 times daily.[31] Other studies used IV (200 μg) or oral (5 mg) forms.[32] TRH is not commonly used.

Herbal/natural galactogogues

Throughout world history women have used certain herbs or foods to enhance their milk supply. Most of these substances have not been scientifically evaluated but traditional use suggests safety and some efficacy. The mechanisms of action for all are unknown. Herbs commonly mentioned as galactogogues include fenugreek, goat's rue, milk thistle, anise, basil, blessed thistle, fennel seeds, marshmallow, and others. Beer is commonly used in some cultures, but alcohol may actually reduce milk production and there is no evidence to support that the yeasts in beer are effective galactogogues.

It is of note that herbs and dietary supplements were removed by the Federal 1994 Dietary Supplement Act from undergoing the rigorous evaluation by the U.S. Food and Drug Administration that is required for drugs. The composition of herbal and dietary supplements are unknown and have been known to contain toxic substances. This is especially true for herbs from mainland China. There is no standard dosing, preparation, or composition, and fraudulent preparations may be a risk.

Fenugreek (*Trigonella foenum-graecum*) is the most commonly recommended herbal galactogogue, treasured as a spice and medicine throughout India and the Middle East for thousands of years. It is a member of the pea family listed as GRAS (generally regarded as safe) by the U.S. Food and Drug Administration. Usual dose is one to four capsules (580–610 mg) three to four times per day, although as with most herbal remedies there is no standard dosing. The higher of these doses may be required in relactating or adoptive mothers. Alternatively, it can be taken as one cup of strained tea three times per day (1/4 tsp seeds steeped in 8 oz water for 10 minutes).[33] Huggins[34] reported the anecdotal use of fenugreek in at least 1200 women with increased milk supply within 24 to 72 hours. Reported side effects are rare: maple-like odor to sweat, milk, and urine; diarrhea; and increased asthmatic symptoms. Use during pregnancy is not recommended because of its uterine stimulant effects. Fenugreek is known to lower blood glucose, so caution is advised. Two recent preliminary reports suggest effectiveness.[35,36]

Goat's Rue (*Galega officinalis*) is a traditional galactogogue, widely recommended in Europe, based on observations of increased milk supply when fed to cows in the 1900s. No controlled human trials have been done, and no adverse effects have been reported with the following possible exception: Maternal ingestion of a lactation tea containing extracts of licorice (*Glycyrrhiza glabra*), fennel, anise, and goat's rue was linked to drowsiness, hypotonia, lethargy, emesis, and poor suckling in two breastfed neonates. An infection work-up was negative, and symptoms and signs resolved on discontinuation of the tea and a 2-day break from breastfeeding.[37] The tea was not tested for contaminants or adulterants, and there have been no other adverse events reported in Europe or South America, where the herb is also used as a hypoglycemic agent. It is usually used as a tea (1 tsp dried leaves steeped in 8 oz water for 10 minutes) with 1 cup taken three times a day.[33]

Milk thistle *(Silybum marianum)* has been used historically throughout Europe, but there are no randomized controlled trials to validate its use. The plant is still commonly known as St. Mary's thistle in honor of the Virgin Mary. Early Christians believed that the white colored veins in the leaves were symbolic of her breast milk. The American Herbal Products Association gives it a rating of 1, meaning that the herb may be safely consumed when used appropriately and does not contraindicate its use during lactation.[38] It is used as a strained tea (simmer 1 tsp crushed seeds in 8 oz water for 10 minutes) taking two to three cups per day.[33]

CONCLUSIONS

Of the substances used to induce, maintain, or augment milk production, domperidone and metoclopramide appear to be the most clinically useful. Prior to the use of any galactogogue, evaluation and correction of any modifiable factors such as frequency and thoroughness of breast emptying should be addressed. Medication should never replace evaluation and counseling on modifiable factors or reassurance when appropriate. As with any medication given to lactating women, close follow-up of both mother and baby is essential.

REFERENCES

1. Sjolin S, Hofvander Y, Hillervik C: Factors Related to Early termination of Breastfeeding: A Retrospective Study in Sweden. Acta Paediatr Scand 66:505–511, 1977.
2. Neville MC, Morton J, Unemura S: Lactogenesis: Transition from pregnancy to lactation. Ped Clin North Am 48:45–52, 2001.
3. Lawrence RA, Lawrence RM: Breastfeeding: A Guide for the Medical Profession, 5th ed. St. Louis, Mosby, 1999.
4. Murray L (ed): Physicians' Desk Reference, 56th ed. Montvale, NJ, Medical Economics, 2002.
5. Kauppila A, Arvel P, Koivisto M, et al. Metoclopramide and breastfeeding: Transfer into milk and the newborn. Eur J Clin Pharm 25:619–623, 1983.
6. Ertl T, Sulyok E, Ezer E, et al. The influence of metoclopramide on the composition of human breast milk. Acta Paediatr Hung 31:415–422, 1991.
7. deGezelle H, Ooghe W, Thiery M, et al. Metoclopramide and breast milk. Eur J Obstet Gynecol Reprod Biol 15:31–36, 1983.
8. Sousa PLR, Barros FC, Pinheiro GNM, et al: Reestablishment of lactation with metoclopramide. J Trop Pediatr Environ Child Health 21:214, 1975.
9. Guzman V, Toscano G, Canales ES et al: Improvement of defective lactation by using oral metoclopramide. Acta Obstet Gynecol Scand 58:53–55, 1979.
10. Lewis PJ, Devenish C, Kahn C: Contolled trial of metoclopramide in the initiation of breast feeding. Br J Clin Pharmacol 9:217–219, 1980.
11. Tolino A, Tedeschi A, Farace R, et al: The relationship between metoclopramide and milk secretion in puerperium. Clin Exp Obstet Gynecol 8:93–95, 1981.
12. Kauppila A, Kivinen S, Ylikorkala O: Metoclopramide increases prolactin release and milk secretion in puerperium without stimulating the secretion of thyrotropin and thyroid hormones. J Clin Endocrinol Metab 52:436–439, 1981.
13. Kauppila A, Kivinen S, Ylikorkala O: A dose response relation between improved lactation and metoclopramide. Lancet 1(8231):175–157, 1981.
14. deGezelle H, Ooghe W, Thiery M, et al: Metoclopramide and breast milk. Eur J Obstet Gynecol Reprod Biol 15(1):31–36, 1983.
15. Kauppila A, Anunti P, Kivinen S, et al: Metoclopramide and breast feeding: efficacy and anterior pituitary responses of the mother and child. Eur J Obstet Gynecol Reprod Biol 19:19–22, 1985.
16. Gupta AP, Gupta PK: Metoclopramide as a lactogue. Clin Pediatr 24:269–272, 1985.
17. Ehrenkrantz RA, Ackerman BA: Metoclopramide effect on faltering milk production by mothers of premature infants, Pediatrics 78:614, 1986.

18. Liu JH, Lee DW, Markoff E: Differential release of prolactin variants in postpartum and early follicular phase women. J Clin Endocrinol Metab 71:605–610, 1990.

19. Budd SS, Erdman SH, Long DM, et al: Improved Lactation with metoclopramide. A case report. Clin Pediatr 32:53 1993.

20. Lewis PA, Devenish C, Kahn C: Controlled trial of metocloproamide in the initiation of breast feeding. Brit J Clin Pharmacol 9:217–219, 1980.

21. Gabay MP. Galactogogues: Medications that induce lactation. J Hum Lact 18:274–249, 2002.

22. Hutchinson TA, Shahan DR, Anderson ML, eds: DRUGDEX®system, Healthcare Series 121, Englewood, Colo: MICROMEDIX. Edition expires September 30, 2004.

23. Hofmeyr GJ, van Iddekinge B. Domperidone and lactation. Lancet 1983;1(8235):647.

24. daSilva OP, Knoppert DC, Angelini MM, Forret P:. Effect of domperidone on milk production in mothers of premature newborns: a randomized, double-blind, placebo-controlled trial. Can Med Assoc J 164:17–21; 2001.

25. Newman J. Handout #19:Domperidone, January 1998. Retrieved 7/16/04, from http://bflrc.com/newman/lbreastfeeding/domperid.htm

26. Aono T, Ari T, Koike K, et al. Effect of Sulpiride on poor puerperal lactation. Am J Obstet Gynecol 143:927, 1982.

27. Ylikorkali O, Kauppila A, Kivinen S, et al: Sulpiride improves inadequate lactation. Br Med J 285:299, 1982.

28. Ylikorkali O, Kauppila A, Kivinen S, et al: Treatment of inadequate lactation with oral Sulpiride and buccal oxytocin. Obstet Gynecol 63:57, 1984.

29. Brown RE: Relactation: An overview. Pediatrics 60:116, 1977.

30. Caron RW, Janh GA, Deis RP: Lactogenic actions of different growth hormone preparations in pregnant and lactating rats. J Endocrinol 142:535, 1994.

31. Bose CL, D'Ercole J, Lester AG, et al. Relactation by mothers of sick or premature infants. Pediatrics 67:565, 1981.

32. Tyson JE, Perez A, Zanartu J: Human lactational response to oral thyrotropin releasing hormone. J Clin Endocrinol Metab 43:760–776, 1976.

33. Low Dog T: Lactogogues. Presentation at International Lactation Consultants Association (ILCA) Annual Meeting, August 2001.

34. Huggins KE: Fenugreek: One remedy for low milk production. Retrieved 7/16/04 from http://www.breastfeedingonline.com/fenuhugg.shtml

35. Swafford S, Berens P: Effect of fenugreek on breast milk volume. Abstract, 5th International Meeting of the Academy of Breastfeeding Medicine, September 11–13, 2000, Tucson, Ariz.

36. Co MM, Hernandez EA, Co BG: A comparative study on the efficacy of the different galactogogues among mothers with lactational insufficiency. Abstract, AAP Section on Breastfeeding, 2002 NCE, October 21, 2002.

37. Rosti L, Nardini A, Bettinelli ME, Rosti D: Toxic effects of an herbal tea mixture in two newborns. Acta Pediatr 83:683, 1994.

38. McGuffin M, Hobbs C, Upton R, Goldberg A (eds): American Herbal Products Association's Botanical Safety Handbook. Boca Raton, FL, CRC Press, 1997, p 107.

39. U.S. Food and Drug Administration, FDA Talk Paper. June 7, 2004, www.fda.gov/bbs/topics/ANSWERS/2004/ANS01292.html

Copyright protected © 2004 The Academy of Breastfeeding Medicine, Inc Approved July 30, 2004

The Academy of Breastfeeding Medicine Protocol Committee

Caroline J. Chantry MD, FABM, Co-Chairperson

Cynthia R. Howard MD, MPH, FABM, Co-Chairperson

*Anne Montgomery

*Nancy Wight MD, FABM

Supported in part by a grant from the Maternal and Child Health Bureau, Department of Health and Human Services.

*Lead Author(s)

Protocol #10: Breastfeeding the near-term infant (35 to 37 weeks gestation)

GOALS

1. Promote, support, and sustain breastfeeding in the near-term infant
2. Maintain optimal health of infant and mother

PURPOSE

1. Allow infants born at 35 to 37 weeks of gestation to breastfeed and/or breast-milk feed to the greatest extent possible.
2. Heighten awareness of difficulties near-term infants and their mothers may experience with breastfeeding.
3. Offer strategies to anticipate, identify promptly, and manage breastfeeding problems that the near-term infant and mother may experience in the inpatient and outpatient setting.
4. Prevent medical problems such as dehydration, hypoglycemia, hyperbilirubinemia, and failure to thrive in the near-term infant.
5. Maintain awareness of mothers' needs.

DEFINITION

"Near-term infant" refers to infants born between $35^{0/7}$ to $36^{6/7}$ weeks of gestation. **Many problems of the near-term infant are also found in the larger 34- to 35-week preterm infant and the borderline term infant of $37^{0/7}$ to $37^{6/7}$ weeks gestation and, therefore, the following guidelines may be applicable to these infants as well.**

BACKGROUND

The advantages of breast-milk feeding for premature infants appear to be even greater than those for term infants. Establishing breastfeeding in the near-term infant, however, is frequently more problematic than in the full-term infant. Because of their immaturity, near-term infants may be sleepier and have less stamina; more difficulty with latch, suck, and swallow; more difficulty maintaining body temperature; increased vulnerability to infection; greater delays in bilirubin excretion; and more respiratory instability than the full-term infant. The sleepiness and inability to suck vigorously is often misinterpreted as sepsis, leading to unnecessary separation and treatment. Alternatively, the near-term infant may appear deceptively vigorous at first glance. Physically large newborns are often mistaken for being more developmentally mature than their actual gestational age. (Remember the 3.84 kg baby born at 40 weeks was 3.0 kg at 36 weeks of gestation.) Near-term infants are more likely to be separated from their mother as a result of the infant being ill or requiring a screening procedure such as evaluation for sepsis, IV placement for antibiotics, and phototherapy.

Mothers who deliver near, but not at, term are more likely to deliver multiples or have a medical condition such as diabetes, pregnancy-induced hypertension, prolonged rupture of membranes, chorioamnionitis, pitocin induction, or a C-section delivery that may affect the success of breastfeeding. Any one or a combination of these conditions places these mothers and infants at risk for difficulty in establishing successful lactation or for breastfeeding failure.

The potential maternal and infant problems listed above place the near-term breastfeeding infant at increased risk for hypothermia, hypoglycemia, excessive weight loss, dehydration, slow weight gain, failure to thrive, prolonged artificial milk supplementation, exaggerated jaundice, kernicterus, dehydration, fever secondary to dehydration, rehospitalization, and breastfeeding failure. In places where early discharge is the norm, these infants will be sent home soon after delivery. Discussion and parental education become crucial in the proper management of breastfeeding.

Near-term infants have a greater chance of exclusive breastfeeding in hospitals that adhere to the Ten Steps to Successful Breastfeeding. To this end, practitioners should become knowledgeable in the Ten Steps and work with the administration in their maternity hospitals to endorse the guidelines set forth in the Ten Steps (see Protocol #7).

Most of the acute problems encountered in the newborn are managed on the postpartum floor in the first few hours and days after parturition; however, there are times that an infant's condition deteriorates in the interval between discharge and the first office visit. Therefore, timely evaluation of the near-term infant after discharge is critical. Just as many hospitals are becoming breastfeeding friendly, the outpatient office or clinic needs to be not only supportive of the breastfeeding mother, but also able to assist mothers with uncomplicated problems or questions related to breastfeeding. In addition, it is essential to be able to refer mothers and infants in a timely manner to a trained lactation professional for more complicated breastfeeding problems. A lactation referral should be viewed with the same medical urgency as any other acute medical referral.

PRINCIPLES OF CARE

1. Optimal communication
   a. Pathway and order set for breastfeeding the near-term infant
   b. Written feeding plan to follow on hospital discharge
   c. Facilitate communication among physician, nurses, and lactation consultants in the inpatient and outpatient settings
   d. Avoid conflicting advice to mother and family of the near-term infant
2. Assessment/reassessment
   a. Objective assessment of gestational age and associated risk factors

   b. Daily assessment of breastfeeding on the postpartum floor or special care nursery
   c. Careful assessment of breastfeeding issues in the outpatient setting
3. Timely lactation support in the inpatient and outpatient setting
4. Avoid separation of mother and infant
   a. Immediate postpartum period
   b. In cases in which either mother or infant is hospitalized for medical reasons
5. Prevent frequently encountered problems in breastfed near-term infant
   a. Hypoglycemia
   b. Hypothermia
   c. Hyperbilirubinemia
   d. Dehydration or excessive weight loss
6. Education
   a. Ongoing education of staff and care providers of issues specific to breastfeeding the near-term infant in the inpatient and outpatient settings
   b. Have one (or two) outpatient office support person (RN or lactation educator) trained in breastfeeding support, assessment, basic breastfeeding problem solving, and near-term breastfeeding issues
   c. Educate parents about breastfeeding the near-term infant
7. Discharge/follow-up
   a. Develop criteria for discharge readiness
   b. Establish a feeding plan to follow after discharge
   c. Facilitate timely and frequent outpatient follow-up to assure effective breastfeeding after discharge
   d. Careful outpatient monitoring of mother and near-term infant

Inpatient: implementation of principles of care

1. Initial steps:
   a. Communicate the feeding plan through a prewritten order set that can be easily modified.
   b. Encourage immediate and extended skin-to-skin contact to improve postpartum stabiliza-

tion of heart rate, respiratory effort, temperature control, metabolic stability, and early breastfeeding.

c. Assessment of gestational age by obstetrical estimate and Dubowitz scoring. Observe infant closely for 12 to 24 hours to assure physiologic stability (e.g., temperature, apnea, tachypnea, hypoglycemia).

d. Encourage rooming in 24 hours a day. If the infant is physiologically stable and healthy, allow the infant to remain with the mother while receiving IV antibiotics or phototherapy. Depending on the individual situation, use of the bili-blanket during breastfeeds, as well as limiting time outside more intense phototherapy, may be necessary.

e. Allow free access to the breast, encouraging initiation of breastfeeding within 1 hour after birth. Encourage continuous skin-to-skin contact as much as possible.

f. Breastfeeding ad libitum (on demand) should be encouraged. It is very important that the infant be breastfed (or breast-milk fed) *at least* eight times per 24-hour period. Sometimes it may be necessary to wake the baby if he or she does not indicate hunger. A mother may need to express her milk and give it to the baby using a cup or other alternative feeding method. Mothers should be warned that use of bottles at this stage might prevent breastfeeding in some babies.

2. Ongoing care:

a. Communicate daily changes in feeding plan either directly or with use of written bedside tool such as a crib card.

b. Formal evaluation from a lactation consultant or other certified health professional with expertise in lactation management should be completed within 24 hours of delivery.

c. Assess and document breastfeeding at least three times per day by at least two different providers with use of a standardized tool (e.g., LATCH Score,[2] IBFAT,[3] Mother/Baby Assessment Tool.[4]

d. Educate the mother about breastfeeding her infant (e.g., position, latch, duration, early feeding cues, etc.)

e. Monitor vital signs, weight change, stool and urine output, and milk transfer. Pre-post feeding weights where available, may be helpful, especially once lactogenesis II has occurred. Monitor for frequently occurring problems (e.g., obtain bilirubin if jaundiced before discharge, glucose screen before feeds for the first three feeds or until stable if hypoglycemia has occurred [see Protocol #1]). It is recommended to routinely screen for hyperbilirubinemia in near-term infants and to use standardized nomograms to assess risk of hyperbilirubinemia as well as plan for follow-up testing.

f. Avoid excessive weight loss or dehydration. Losses greater than 3% of birth weight by day 1 or greater than 7% by day 3, ineffective milk transfer, or exaggerated jaundice are considered excessive and merit further evaluation and monitoring.

i. The infant may need to be supplemented after breastfeeding with small quantities (5 to 10 mL per feeding on day 1, 10 to 30 cc per feeding thereafter) of expressed breast milk or formula. Mothers may supplement using a supplemental nursing device at the breast, cup feeds, finger feeds, syringe feeds, or bottle depending on clinical situation and mother's preference. Cup feedings have demonstrated safety in both preterm[5] and term infants.[6] Cup feeding may also preserve breastfeeding duration among both preterm[7] and term[8] infants that require multiple supplemental feeds. However, there is little evidence about the safety or efficacy of other alternative feeding methods or their effect on breastfeeding. When cleanliness is suboptimal, cup feeding may be the best choice.[9]

ii. If supplementing, the mother should pump or express milk regularly (use of a hospital grade electric pump is recommended when feasible) during the day (e.g., every 3 hours) until the baby is breastfeeding well or if the mother and infant are separated and unable to breastfeed.

iii. Consider use of an ultrathin silicone nipple shield if there is difficulty with latch or evidence of ineffective milk transfer.[10] The use of nipple shields is controversial and generally requires close supervision of a trained lactation consultant or knowledgeable health care professional. Inappropriate or prolonged nipple shield use can decrease milk supply, and in some situations, nipple shields decrease, rather than increase, milk transfer.

g. Avoid thermal stress by using skin-to-skin (e.g., kangaroo) care or by double wrapping if necessary and by dressing the baby in a shirt and hat. Consider intermittent use of an incubator to maintain temperature. Where it is culturally acceptable, mothers can sleep with their babies to provide warmth.

3. Discharge planning

a. Assess readiness for discharge, including physiologic stability and adequate intake exclusively at breast or with supplements. May use 24-hour test weights, with a scale designed with adequate precision for such weights, for infants with >7% weight loss.[11]

b. Develop discharge-feeding plan. Consider diet, milk intake (mL/kg/day), and method of feeding (breast, bottle, supplemental device, etc.) If supplementing, determine method most acceptable to mother for use after discharge.

c. Make an appointment for follow-up within 48 hours of discharge to recheck weight, feeding adequacy, jaundice.

d. Communicate discharge-feeding plan to pediatric outpatient provider. Written communication is preferred.

Outpatient: implementation of principles of care

1. Initial Visit

a. The first outpatient office or home health visit should be when the infant is 3 to 5 days of life or 1 or 2 days after discharge.

b. Review the inpatient maternal and infant records including prenatal, perinatal, infant and feeding history (e.g., need for supplement in the hospital, problems with latch, need for phototherapy, etc). Gestational age, birth weight, and weight at discharge should be recorded in the outpatient chart.

c. Physician review of breastfeeding since discharge needs to be very specific regarding frequency, approximate duration of feedings, and how baby is being fed (e.g., at breast, expressed breast milk with supplemental device such as supplemental nursing system, finger feeds, or bottle with artificial nipple). Information about stool and urine output, color of stools, baby's state (e.g., crying, not satisfied after a feed, sleepy and difficult to keep awake at the breast during a feed, etc.) should be obtained. If parents have a written feeding record, it should be reviewed.

d. Examination of the infant must include an accurate weight without clothes and calculation of change in weight from birth and discharge, state of alertness, and hydration. Assess for jaundice with cutaneous bilirubin screen and/or serum bilirubin determination if indicated.

e. Assess the mother's breast for nipple shape, pain and trauma, engorgement. and mastitis. The mother's emotional status and degree of fatigue should be considered, especially when considering supplemental feeding routines. Observe the baby feeding at the breast, looking at the latch, suck, and swallow.

2. Problem Solving

a. Poor weight gain (<20 g/day) is most likely the result of inadequate intake. Median daily weight gain of a healthy newborn is 26 to 31 grams per day.[12] The care provider must determine whether the problem is insufficient breast milk production, inability of the infant to transfer enough milk, or a combination of both. The infant who is getting enough breast milk should have six to eight voids and yellow seedy stools daily by day 4, have lost no more than 8% of birth weight, and be satisfied after 20 to 30 minutes of nursing. Consider feeding more frequently or supplementing (preferably with expressed breast milk) after suckling if the mother is not already doing so or increasing the amount of supplement. Consider instituting or increasing frequency of pumping or manual expression. Consider referral to a lactation specialist.

b. For infants with latch difficulties, the baby's mouth should be examined for anatomical abnormalities [e.g., ankyloglossia (tongue-tied),[13] cleft palate], and a digital suck exam performed. A referral to a trained professional lactation specialist or in the case of ankyloglossia a referral to someone trained in frenotomy may be indicated.

c. The jaundiced near-term infant poses more of a problem when considering management of hyperbilirubinemia. Keep in mind all risk factors should be determined, and if the principal factor is lack of milk the primary treatment is to provide milk (preferably through improved breastfeeding or expressed breast milk) to the baby. Institution of phototherapy for breastfeeding jaundice either in the home or in the hospital may actually interfere with the primary treatment of getting increased quantities of milk to the baby.

d. Consider the use of a galactogogue (a medicine or herb that increases breast milk supply) in mothers who have a documented low breast-milk supply (see Protocol #9).

e. The mother's ability to cope and manage the feeding plan needs to be evaluated. If the mother is not coping well, work with her to find help and or modify the feeding plan to something that is more manageable.

3. Follow-up

The near-term infant should have weekly weight checks until 40 weeks postconceptual age or until it is demonstrated that he or she is thriving with no supplements.

a. Babies who are not gaining well and for whom adjustments are being made to the feeding plan may need a visit 2 to 4 days after each adjustment. A home health provider, preferably trained in medical evaluation of the newborn and in lactation support, who reports the weight to the primary care provider could make this visit.

b. Near-term infants have less vitamin D stored at birth, increasing their risk for later deficiency. Depending on sunlight exposure and skin color, vitamin D supplements (200 IU/day) may be indicated if the infant is exclusively breastfed. Strong consideration should be given to starting these supplements earlier than the 2 months of age recommended for term infants in the United States. Consideration should also be given to supplementing the near-term exclusively breastfed infant with iron, as iron stores in these infants are not those of the full-term infant. The American Academy of Pediatrics Committee on Nutrition recommends 2 mg/kg/day of elemental iron for preterm breastfed infants in the form of iron drops from 1 to 12 months of age.

c. After the first week, infants should be monitored for adequate growth and evidence of normal biochemical indices (See Table P-4 from Protocol #12) Weight gain should average more than 20 g/day, and length and head circumference should each increase by an average of more than 0.5 cm/week.

REFERENCES

1. Reynolds A: Breastfeeding and brain development. Pediatr Clin North Am 48:159–171, 2001.
2. Jensen D, Wallace S, Kelsay P: LATCH: a breastfeeding charting system and documentation tool. J Obstet Gynecol Neonatal Nurs 23:27–32, 1994.
3. Matthews MK: Developing an instrument to assess infant breastfeeding behaviour in the early neonatal period. Midwifery 4:154–165, 1988.
4. Mulford C: The mother-baby assessment (MBA): An Apgar "score" for breastfeeding. J Hum Lact 8:79–82, 1992.

5. Marinelli K, Burke G, Dodd V: A comparison of the safety of cup feedings and bottle feedings in premature infants whose mothers intend to breastfeed. J Perinatol 21:350–355, 2001.

6. Howard CR, de Blieck EA, ten Hoopen CB, et al: Physiologic stability of newborns during cup- and bottle-feeding. Pediatrics 104(5 Pt 2):1204–1207, 1999.

7. Collins CT, Ryan P, Crowther CA, et al: Effect of bottles, cups, and dummies on breast feeding in preterm infants: A randomised controlled trial. Br Med J 329:193–198, 2004.

8. Howard, CR, Howard FM, Lanphear B, et al: Randomized clinical trial of pacifier use and bottle-feeding or cupfeeding and their effect on breastfeeding. Pediatrics 111:511–518, 2003.

9. United Nations Children's Fund: Feeding low birth weight babies. UNICEF Division of Information and Public Affairs, 1996.

10. Meier PP, Brown LP, Hurst NM, et al: Nipple shields for preterm infants: Effect on milk transfer and duration of breastfeeding. J Hum Lact 16:106–113, 2000.

11. Meier PP, Engstrom JL, Crichton C, et al: A new scale for in-home test-weighing for mothers of preterm and high-risk infants. J Hum Lact 10:63–68, 1994.

12. National Research Council, Food and Nutrition Board, National Academy of Science: Recommended Daily Allowances, 10th ed. Washington, DC, U.S. Government Printing Office, 1989.

13. Ballard MD, Auer CE, Khoury, JC: Ankyloglossia: Assessment, incidence, and effect of frenuloplasty on the breastfeeding dyad. Pediatrics 110:e63, 2002.

Copyright protected © 2004 The Academy of Breastfeeding Medicine, Inc.

Approved 08/22/04
The Academy of Breastfeeding Medicine Protocol Committee
*Eyla Boies MD
Caroline J. Chantry MD, FABM, Co-Chairperson
Cynthia R. Howard MD, MPH, FABM, Co-Chairperson
*Yvonne Vaucher MD

*lead author(s)

Development supported in part by a grant from the Maternal and Child Health Bureau, Department of Health and Human Services

APPENDIX

Baby friendly hospital initiative steps for successful breastfeeding:

1. Have a written breastfeeding policy.
2. Train all health care staff in the skills necessary to implement the policy.
3. All mothers should be informed of the benefits of breastfeeding.
4. Help mothers initiate breastfeeding within 1 hour of birth.
5. Show mothers how to breastfeed and how to maintain lactation, even if they are be separated from their infant.
6. Give newborn infants no food or drink other than breast milk, unless medically indicated.
7. Practice rooming-in, allow mothers and infants to remain together, 24 hours a day if medically stable.
8. Encourage breastfeeding on demand.
9. Give no artificial teats or pacifiers to breastfeeding infants.
10. Foster the establishment of breastfeeding support groups and refer mothers to them, on discharge form the hospital or clinic.

Protocol # 11: Guidelines for the evaluation and management of neonatal ankyloglossia and its complications in the breastfeeding dyad

DEFINITION

Ankyloglossia, partial: The presence of a sublingual frenulum that changes the appearance or function of the infant's tongue because of its decreased length, lack of elasticity, or attachment too distal beneath the tongue or too close to or onto the gingival ridge. In this document we will refer to partial ankyloglossia as simply "ankyloglossia." "True" or "complete ankyloglossia," extensive fusion of the tongue to the floor of the mouth, is extremely rare and is not within the scope of this discussion.

BACKGROUND

At birth, the infant's tongue is normally able to extend over and past the mandibular gum pad. Significant ankyloglossia prevents an infant from anteriorly extending and elevating the tongue, and many breastfeeding experts believe that these limitations alter the normal peristaltic motion of the tongue during feeding, resulting in the potential for nipple trauma and problems with effective milk transfer and infant weight gain.

Ankyloglossia, commonly known as tongue-tie, occurs in approximately 3.2% to 4.8% of consecutive term infants at birth[1,2] and in 12.8% of infants with breastfeeding problems.[2] The condition has been associated with an increased incidence of breastfeeding difficulties: 25% in affected versus 3% in unaffected infants.[1]

Various methods have been suggested to diagnose and evaluate the severity of ankyloglossia[3,4] and to determine the criteria for intervention.[5,6]

Short- and long-term consequences of ankyloglossia may include feeding and speech difficulties,[7,8] as well as orthodontic and mandibular abnormalities[9–12] and psychological problems.[13]

In the 1990s a number of case reports and observational studies were published that documented an association between ankyloglossia and breastfeeding problems.[14–18] There is considerable controversy regarding the significance of ankyloglossia and its management, both within and among medical specialty groups.[19,20] Both the diagnosis of ankyloglossia and the use of frenotomy, an incision or "snipping" of the frenulum, to treat ankyloglossia vary widely. The frenotomy procedure, carefully performed, has recently been shown to decrease maternal nipple pain to improve infant latch,[2] and to improve milk transfer (personal communication, J. Ballard, July 27, 2004). There is a growing tendency among breastfeeding medicine specialists to favor releasing the tongue of the infant to facilitate breastfeeding and to protect the breastfeeding experience. To date, no randomized trials exist to demonstrate frenotomy for ankyloglossia is effective in treating infant or maternal breastfeeding problems.

ASSESSMENT OF ANKYLOGLOSSIA:

All newborn infants, whether healthy or ill, should have a thorough examination of the oral cavity that assesses function as well as anatomy. This examination should include palpation of the hard and soft palate, gingivae, and sublingual areas in addition to the movements of the tongue, and the length, elasticity, and points of insertion of the sublingual frenulum.

When breastfeeding difficulties are encountered and a short or tight sublingual frenulum is noted, the appearance and function of the tongue may be semi-quantified using a scoring system such as the Hazelbaker[3] (Table P-3). The Hazelbaker scale has been tested for interrater reliability (personal communication, J Ballard, July 27, 2004) and validated in a sample of term neonates.[2] Hazelbaker scores consistent with significant ankyloglossia have been shown to be highly correlated with difficulty with latching the infant onto the breast and maternal complaints of sore nipples.[2] Alternatively, ankyloglossia may be qualified as mild, moderate, or severe by the appearance of the tongue and of the frenulum.

ASSESSMENT OF THE BREASTFEEDING DYAD

Breastfeeding complications caused by ankyloglossia can generally be placed into broad categories of those caused by maternal nipple trauma or failure of the infant to breastfeed effectively. Specific complaints include difficulty latching or sustaining a latch, infant becoming frustrated or falling asleep at breast, prolonged feedings, a dissatisfied baby, gumming or chewing at the breast, poor weight gain, or failure to thrive. Maternal complaints include traumatized nipples, severe unrelenting pain with feeding, inability to let down because of pain, incomplete breast drainage, breast infections, and plugged ducts.

The physician should interview the mother to ascertain her degree of confidence and comfort while breastfeeding. This can be done semi-quantitatively by using a scoring system such as the LATCH score or a similar tool.[21] The LATCH score has been shown to correlate with breastfeeding duration but only due to subscores for breast comfort.[22]

If the mother describes nipple pain, the physician may wish to use a pain scale in order to semi-quantify her perception of the degree of her pain.

This serves to follow trends in the severity of pain, which may help in determining the effectiveness of an intervention.

The infant should be weighed, and the rate of weight gain since birth should be assessed. The physician should observe the mother and infant while breastfeeding to assess the effectiveness of the feeding and provide assistance as appropriate. Problems including an inadequate or nonsustained latch and ineffective feedings should be noted. Test weights may be useful in assessing milk transfer. The infant should be weighed prior to and after breastfeeding without a change in clothing or diaper; the difference between the weights in grams indicates the amount of breast milk consumed in milliliters.

The mother's nipples should be examined carefully for creases, bruises, blisters, cracks, or bleeding. Areolar edema and erythema should be noted as possible signs of nipple infection. A family history of bleeding diatheses should be elicited.

RECOMMENDATIONS

Conservative management of tongue-tie may be sufficient, requiring no intervention beyond breastfeeding assistance, parental education, and reassurance.[19] For partial ankyloglossia, if a tongue-tie release is deemed appropriate, the procedure should be performed by a physician or pedodontist experienced with the procedure; otherwise a referral should be made to an ear, nose, and throat specialist or oral surgeon. Release of the tongue-tie appears to be a minor procedure, but it may be ineffective in solving the immediate clinical problem and may cause complications such as infant pain and distress and postoperative bleeding, infection, or injury to Wharton's duct.[19] Complications are rare, however.[1,2,5,9]

Frenotomy, or simple incision or "snipping," of a tongue-tie is the most common procedure performed for partial ankyloglossia. It should be recognized that postoperative scarring may further limit tongue movement.[19] Excision with lengthening of the ventral surface of the tongue or a z-plasty

TABLE P-3	Hazelbaker assessment tool for lingual frenulum function*

Appearance Items	Function Items

Appearance Items

Appearance of tongue when lifted

2: Round or square
1: Slight cleft in tip apparent
0: Heart- or V-shaped

Elasticity of frenulum

2: Very elastic
1: Moderately elastic
0: Little or no elasticity

Length of lingual frenulum when tongue lifted

2: > 1 cm
1: 1 cm
0: <1 cm

Attachment of lingual frenulum to tongue

2: Posterior to tip
1: At tip
0: Notched tip

Attachment of lingual frenulum to inferior alveolar ridge

2: Attached to floor of mouth or well below ridge
1: Attached just below ridge
0: Attached at ridge

Function Items

Lateralization

2: Complete
1: Body of tongue but not tongue tip
0: None

Lift of tongue

2: Tip to mid-mouth
1: Only edges to mid-mouth
0: Tip stays at lower alveolar ridge or rises to mid-mouth only with jaw closure

Extension of tongue

2: Tip over lower lip
1: Tip over lower gum only
0: Neither of the above, or anterior or mid-tongue humps

Spread of anterior tongue

2: Complete
1: Moderate or partial
0: Little or none

Cupping

2: Entire edge, firm cup
1: Side edges only, moderate cup
0: Poor or no cup

Peristalsis

2: Complete, anterior to posterior
1: Partial, originating posterior to tip
0: None or reverse motion

Snapback

2: None
1: Periodic
0: Frequent or with each suck

*The infant's tongue is assessed using the 5 appearance items and the 7 function items. Significant ankyloglossia is diagnosed when the appearance score total is 8 or less and/or the function score total is 11 or less. (2;3)

Adapted with permission from Hazelbaker AK: The assessment tool for lingual frenulum function (ATLFF): Use in a lactation consultant private practice Masters thesis, Pacific Oaks College, 1993.

release is a procedure with less postoperative scarring, but it carries the additional risks of general anesthesia.[19]

THE FRENOTOMY PROCEDURE

Instruments: Iris scissors and grooved retractor
Supplies: Clean gloves and gauze; gelatin foam.
Method: Parents should be counseled about risks, benefits, and alternatives of the procedure and informed consent should be obtained. This counseling should include a discussion of the possibility that the clinical breastfeeding problem will not improve.

The frenulum may be transilluminated to check for translucency and lack of vasculature. The frenulum is usually a thin, translucent hypovascular membrane, where a simple frenotomy results in an almost bloodless procedure. Rarely, it may be thick and fibrous or muscular and relatively vascular. Thicker frenula are best incised by an otolaryngologist or oral surgeon under controlled conditions.

The frenulum is almost devoid of sensory innervation. Infants under 4 months of age can usually tolerate the frenotomy very well without any local anesthesia. Alternatively, topical anesthetic (e.g., benzocaine gel or paste) may be applied with cotton applicators to both sides of the frenulum in the area to be incised. This, however, may have the undesirable effect of numbing the mouth, such that the baby may not be able to suck effectively after the frenotomy is completed.

The infant is placed supine on the examining table or mother's lap. An assistant holds the baby's elbows firmly against the ears and stabilizes the chin with one index finger. Alternatively, the infant may be swaddled with a receiving blanket to immobilize the arms while the assistant stabilizes the head. Slight extension of the infant's neck allows better visualization of the tongue and frenulum. Using the grooved retractor or physician's fingers, the physician lifts the tongue to expose the frenulum. With the tips of the iris scissors an incision is made in the thinnest portion of the frenulum, close to the retractor and parallel to

the tongue. Care is taken not to incise the tongue, the genioglossus muscle, or the gingival tissue. The incision should extend into the sulcus between the tongue and the genioglossus muscle, just beyond the level of the muscle, carefully avoiding the floor of the mouth. This ensures complete detachment of the tongue from the gingiva, without causing damage to the sublingual mucosa or to the salivary duct (Figure P-1).

The site beneath the tongue is blotted with gauze until little or no blood is seen. In the event of unexpected bleeding beyond 2 to 3 minutes, a strip of gelatin foam may be used to achieve rapid hemostasis. The infant may be returned to the mother immediately to be breastfed. Infant latch and maternal nipple pain should be reassessed at this time. There is no specific aftercare required except for breastfeeding. A small white patch or eschar is seen in some infants for 1 or 2 weeks during the healing process. Infection of the site is exceedingly rare if clean technique is used as described.

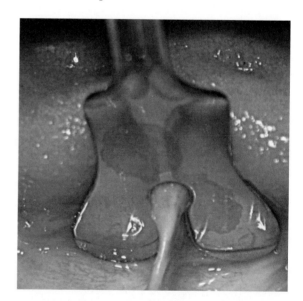

Figure P-1   Using a Lorenz tongue elevator, the lingual frenum is exposed. Pulling upward on the tongue stretches and allows visualization of the frenum and the floor of the mouth. In this infant an 8mm incision was needed to allow sufficient movement of the tongue for effective breastfeeding to occur. (Picture courtesy of Dr. Larry Kotlow.)

Medical equipment used in this procedure should be sterilized or disinfected in accordance with the guidelines of the Centers for Disease Control.[23]

MANAGEMENT OF MATERNAL AND INFANT COMPLICATIONS OF ANKYLOGLOSSIA

If nipple damage or infection is present, a problem-specific treatment program should be instituted. Mastitis and yeast infections should be treated according to established guidelines.[24]

Some mothers may need nipple rest for one to several days to allow healing to occur before reinstituting feedings at the breast. These mothers should be encouraged to express their breast milk in order to maintain their milk supply and to feed their milk to the baby by an alternate method.

Suppressed lactation should be addressed and every attempt made to reestablish the mother's milk supply. Infants who have been gaining weight slowly or failing to thrive may need to receive supplements of expressed breast milk or formula temporarily.

Follow-up for resolution of maternal and infant complications of ankyloglossia should take place by the mother's or infant's primary health care provider within 3 or 4 days of the frenotomy.

FURTHER RESEARCH

This protocol was developed by the Academy of Breastfeeding Medicine to provide clinicians with guidance about the assessment and treatment of ankyloglossia and associated breastfeeding problems. More definitive recommendations await future research in this area. The Academy of Breastfeeding Medicine urges that more research be undertaken so that the benefits and risks of frenotomy for ankyloglossia and its effectiveness in treating breastfeeding concerns can be better understood. We specifically recognize that the Hazelbaker and LATCH instruments cited in this document require further interrater and intrarater reliability and validity testing. We recognize that a critical need exists for clinical tools to assess breastfeeding performance as well as the degree of ankyloglossia and function of the tongue. In addition, a randomized investigator-blinded clinical trial is needed to assess the effectiveness of frenotomy in treating infant and maternal breastfeeding problems associated with ankyloglossia.

Copyright protected © 2004 The Academy of Breastfeeding Medicine, Inc.
Approved August 3, 2004
The Academy of Breastfeeding Medicine Protocol Committee
*Jeanne Ballard, MD
Caroline Chantry MD, FABM, Co-Chairperson
Cynthia R. Howard MD, MPH, FABM, Co-Chairperson
Development supported in part by a grant from the Maternal and Child Health Bureau, Department of Health and Human Services

*lead author(s)

REFERENCES

1. Messner AH, Lalakea ML: Ankyloglossia: controversies in management. Int J Pediatr Otorhinolaryngol 54:123–131, 2000.
2. Ballard JL, Auer CE, Khoury JC: Ankyloglossia: assessment, incidence, and effect of frenuloplasty on the breastfeeding dyad. Pediatrics 110:e63, 2002.
3. Hazelbaker, AK: The assessment tool for lingual frenulum function (ATLFF): Use in a lactation consultant private practice. Master's Thesis, Pacific Oaks College, 1993.
4. Kotlow LA: Ankyloglossia (tongue-tie): a diagnostic and treatment quandary. Quintessence Int 30:259–262, 1999.
5. Masaitis NS, Kaempf JW: Developing a frenotomy policy at one medical center: A case study approach. J Hum Lact 12:229–232, 1996.
6. Sanchez-Ruiz I, Gonzalez Landa G, Perez Gonzalez V, et al: [Section of the sublingual frenulum. Are the indications correct?] [Spanish]. Cir Pediatr 12:161–164, 1999.

7. Garcia Pola MJ, Gonzalez Garcia M, Garcia Martin JM, Gallas M, Seoane Leston J: A study of pathology associated with short lingual frenum. ASDC J Dent Child. 69:59–62, 12, 2002.

8. Messner AH, Lalakea ML: The effect of ankyloglossia on speech in children. Otolaryngol Head Neck Surg 127:539–545, 2002.

9. Wright JE: Tongue-tie. J Paediatr Child Health 31:276–278, 1995.

10. Williams WN, Waldron CM: Assessment of lingual function when ankyloglossia (tongue-tie) is suspected. J Am Dent Assoc 110:353–356, 1985.

11. Yoel J: [Tongue tie and speech disorders]. Trib Odontol (B Aires) 60:195–196, 198, 200, 1976.

12. Hasan N: Tongue tie as a cause of deformity of lower central incisor. J Pediatr Surg8:985, 1973.

13. Ketty N, Sciullo PA: Ankyloglossia with psychological implications. ASDC J Dent Child 41:43–46, 1974.

14. Jain E: Tongue-tie: its impact on breastfeeding. AARN News Lett 1995:18.

15. Notestine GE: The importance of the identification of ankyloglossia (short lingual frenulum) as a cause of breastfeeding problems. J Hum Lact 6:113–115, 1990.

16. Berg KL: Tongue-tie (ankyloglossia) and breastfeeding: A review. J Hum Lact 6:109–112, 1990.

17. Marmet C, Shell E, Marmet R: Neonatal frenotomy may be necessary to correct breastfeeding problems. [Review]. J Hum Lact6:117–121, 1990.

18. Nicholson WL: Tongue-tie (ankyloglossia) associated with breastfeeding problems. J Hum Lact 7: 82–84, 1991.

19. Canadian Paediatric Society, Community Paediatrics Committee: Canadian Paediatric Society Statement: Ankyloglossia and breastfeeding. Paediatr Child Health 7:269–270, 2002.

20. Messner AH, Lalakea ML, Aby J, Macmahon J, Bair E: Ankyloglossia: Incidence and associated feeding difficulties. Arch Otolaryngol Head Neck Surg 126:36–39, 2000.

21. Jensen D, Wallace S, Kelsay P: LATCH: a breastfeeding charting system and documentation tool. J Obstet Gynecol Neonatal Nurs 23:27–32, 1994.

22. Riordan J, Bibb D, Miller M, Rawlins T: Predicting breastfeeding duration using the LATCH breastfeeding assessment tool. J Hum Lact 17:20–23, 2001.

23. Centers for Disease Control: Sterilization or disinfection of medical devices: General principles. www.cdc.gov/ncidod/hip/Sterile/Sterilgp.htm. 8-20-2002.

24. Protocol Committee Academy of Breastfeeding Medicine, Amir LH, Chantry C, Howard C R: Clinical Protocol Number 4: Mastitis. www.bfmed.org. Academy of Breastfeeding Medicine, 2002.

Protocol #12: Transitioning the breastfeeding/breast-milk–fed premature infant from the neonatal intensive care unit to home

I. INTRODUCTION AND BACKGROUND

The practice of breastfeeding or providing expressed mother's milk to premature infants is promoted because of the considerable benefits to their health and well-being.[1,2] Exclusive breastfeeding has been shown to result in adequate postdischarge weight gain even in very-low-birth-weight infants.[3] The following guidelines include recommendations for monitoring and optimizing nutritional support of premature infants after they are discharged from the hospital. These guidelines represent expert opinions and have not been validated experimentally.

This protocol addresses the care of premature infants less than 37 weeks' gestation and less than 2500 g at birth, who are being transitioned from the hospital to home. Depending on the unit, these infants often weigh 1750 to 2000 g at discharge or less if a kangaroo mother care (also known as skin-to-skin) program is practiced, which may allow for more rapid development of feeding skills. Many of the infants weighing 2000 to 2500 g are not admitted to NICU; they may be either in a transitional nursery or in the postnatal ward with their mothers. (Please also refer to Protocol 10) The plan does not distinguish in utero appropriately grown (AGA) from growth restricted (SGA) infants but bases decisions on current nutritional status and body weight.

For infants less than 1500 g at birth, it is recommended that they be fed their mothers' milk fortified with nutrients and calories. Infants 1500 g or more may breastfeed ad libitum as they are able, provided they are supplemented with multivitamins and iron. Near the time of discharge, a decision must be made as to the feeding in the postdischarge period (to 1 year corrected age). Many of these infants do well after discharge with full or partial breastfeeding, or receiving mother's milk by bottle, cup,[4,5] syringe, nasogastric tube, or supplemental nursing (feeding tube) device. Growth faltering, however, has been observed in some premature infants in the postdischarge period if they receive exclusive human milk feedings without nutrient and caloric fortification.[6-11]

Most slow growth in these babies, with the exception of the extremely low-birth-weight infant (ELBW is defined as less than 1000 g at birth), is a function of absolute intake rather than milk composition such that every effort to ensure optimal milk volume should be exhausted prior to switching feedings to formula.

II. PREDISCHARGE: DISCHARGE PLANNING

A. The clinician should work with the mother to devise a feeding plan well before the actual date of discharge. Rooming-in by the mother for a few days prior to discharge during this transition period is strongly recommended. The baby will preferably be on exclusive breast milk, either suckling straight from the breast or by use of expressed breast milk. Less often, the plan may include a combination of breast milk (directly from the breast or expressed) and formula.

B. The following aspects of the current feeding plan should be assessed when making postdischarge plans.
  1. "Type" of feeding: unfortified human milk, fortified human milk, formula, or a combination.
  2. "Amount" of feeding: milk intake (mL/kg/day): this includes either measuring the mothers' pumped milk volume or performing daily test weights[13] for infants who feed at the breast. If the baby is already growing adequately, it is not typically necessary to perform test weights.
  3. "Method" of feeding: oral (breast, bottle, cup, supplemental nursing device, other, or a combination of methods) versus, or in combination with, tube-feeding (nasal or orogastric) or use of a feeding device (e.g., gastrostomy tube).
  4. "Adequacy of growth": in-hospital growth noted as daily rate of weight gain and weekly rate of length gain calculated or plotted on appropriate growth charts (Table P-4).
  5. "Adequacy of nutrition": in-hospital biochemical nutritional status, when feasible (Table P-4).

TABLE P-4   Biochemical* and growth monitoring for premature infants in the postdischarge period

Parameter	Action values
Growth	
Weight gain	<20 g/day
Length increase	<0.5 cm/wk
Head circumference increase	<0.5 cm/wk
Biochemical Markers	
Phosphorus	<4.5 mg/dL
Alkaline phosphatase	>450 IU/L
Blood urea nitrogen	<5 mg/dL

*It is recognized that biochemical monitoring is not feasible in all settings; presence or absence of clinical rickets then becomes a substitute parameter.
Modified from Hall RA: Nutritional follow-up of the breastfeeding premature infant after hospital discharge. Pediatr Clin North Amer 2001; 48: 453–460 and Schanler RJ. Nutrition support of the low birth weight infant. In: Walker WA, Watkins JB; Duggan CP (eds): Nutrition in Pediatrics, 3rd edition, BC Decker, Inc, Hamilton, ON, Canada, 2003, 392–412.

(Note: It is recognized that biochemical monitoring is not feasible in all settings. In such situations, dietary adequacy is based on optimal growth and absence of clinical rickets.)

6. Summary of current nutritional assessment: optimal vs. suboptimal
   a. Optimal status (includes *all* of the following)
      i. Infant can achieve entire intake orally, by breastfeeding or alternate methods.
      ii. Volume of intake is approximately 180 mL/kg/day or more. (Rarely, lower volumes will be adequate if both of the following criteria are met).
      iii. Growth (weight and length) is within normal limits or improving.
      iv. Biochemical indices (phosphorus, alkaline phosphatase, blood urea nitrogen) are within normal limits (Table P-4) or improving.
   b. Suboptimal (includes *any* one or more of the following)
      i. Infant's intake is less than 160 mL/kg/day (with rare exceptions).
      ii. Infant cannot consume all feedings orally.
      iii. Growth is less than adequate (weight gain less than 20 grams/day and/or length gain less than 0.5 cm/week).
      iv. Biochemical indices are abnormal and are not improving.
C. Transition to postdischarge nutrition for infants with "optimal assessment":
   1. If the infant has been receiving fortified human milk with or without preterm formula, the diet may be changed to unfortified human milk ad libitum, by breastfeeding or alternative feeding methods, at least 1 week before anticipated discharge.
      a. Prior to this transition it is necessary to assure that mother's milk supply is appropriate for a trial of breast milk without fortification. This can be done by reviewing the mother's pumping record. Ideally, the mother has been pumping or expressing breast milk regularly. It is recommended that the mother continue pumping or expressing milk at least three times per day in order to have an "oversupply" to facilitate adequate volume consumption by the premature infant at the breast. For some mothers, pumping after each feeding ensures optimal drainage of the breast, optimal milk production, and expression of the highest fat content (hindmilk) for supplemental feedings. This technique of breastfeeding, then feeding previously pumped breast milk, and then pumping any residual volume from the breast is termed "triple feeding." (Note: In many areas manual expression is the norm or only available method for milk expression. Preliminary evidence suggests that greater volumes may be obtained with electric, hospital-grade pumps.[12] Therefore, whenever possible, use of the latter is recommended.)
      b. For infants receiving formula supplements, a trial without formula is appropriate while increasing human milk intake to approximately 180 mL/kg/day, if possible. Use of hindmilk to increase caloric intake for some feedings may be appropriate.
      c. Add iron, 2 mg/kg/day. *If enriched postdischarge formula is used, a decrease in the quantity of iron and multivitamin supplementation is indicated. Generally, if formula constitutes about 50% of the diet, the dose for iron is 1 mg/kg/day and multivitamin preparation is half the doses listed below.*
      d. Add a complete multivitamin preparation. (Dosed to receive at least the following amounts of vitamin A [1500 IU/day], C [20–70 mg/day] and D [400 IU/day]; vitamin C requirements of preterm infants are poorly studied. B vitamins are also necessary for the former preemie receiving unfortified human milk. Typically, appropriate amounts of all vitamins will

be provided by infant multivitamin [MVI] preparations at 1 mL/day). See note under iron above C1.(c) if providing enriched post-discharge formula supplements.

e. Monitor milk intake and growth (weight and length) during this week. Volumes of pumped or expressed milk and daily test weights (for infants fed at the breast) should be recorded during this period.[13]

f. If intake and growth are adequate, continue this diet after discharge

g. If intake and growth are suboptimal, follow D. (d) below

2. If the infant has been receiving unfortified human milk

a. Continue iron (2 mg/kg/day)

b. Continue multivitamin preparation [See dosing above, C.1(c)]

c. Continue this diet after discharge

D. Transition to postdischarge nutrition for infants with "suboptimal assessment":

1. If the infant has been receiving fortified human milk

a. Change the diet to unfortified human milk, with or without preterm formula, ad libitum (by breastfeeding and/or alternative feeding methods) plus a minimum of two to three feedings of enriched post-discharge formula prepared per manufacturer instructions (~22 kcal/oz) at least 1 week before anticipated discharge.

(Note: Many neonatologists and institutions add powdered discharge premature formula to expressed breast milk to provide enriched feeds while still providing the advantages of breast milk. There is no evidence to recommend for or against this practice. This use of powdered premature formula is off-label and the potential for error is great, so be advised to be extremely cautious if using this approach.)

b. Recommend that the mother continue pumping or expressing milk at least three times/ per day [See C.1 (a) above.]

c. Monitor milk intake and growth during this week.

d. Assess adequacy of breastfeeding and address problems or potential problems.

i. Latch

ii. Milk transfer/milk volume. If lactation has been suppressed or the baby is not adequately draining the breast, it may be necessary to intervene to increase volume (i.e., increased pumping after feeds or pumping at some feeds and feeding the expressed milk in lieu or in addition to feeding at the breast.) (Please also see Protocol #9.)

iii. Maternal milk content. Consider the use of hindmilk for some feedings to increase caloric content. This must be considered in conjunction with milk transfer and volume as it may be particularly important if the baby is getting only foremilk and leaving hindmilk.

iv. Frequency of feeds at breast (please note that with "sleepy preemies" subtle feeding cues may be missed).

v. Optimize milk transfer. Suggested techniques may include pumping or expressing to let down before putting baby to breast or using breast compression during feedings.

vi. Maternal satisfaction. Mothers may have preferences regarding timing of feeds, feeding devices, and so on that fit best with the family's needs and can be accommodated without compromising the infant's nutrition.

vii. Consider use of a feeding device.

(A.) Nipple shield to improve milk transfer[15]

(Note: Any mother who is discharged using a nipple shield must be closely monitored by a competent lactation professional to watch for potential associated complications.)

(B.) Supplemental nursing (feeding tube) device while at breast

(C.) May be able to use nipple shield and supplemental nursing device together effectively (e.g., by placing tube inside nipple shield so when baby suckles, the volume of milk available for transfer is increased.

(D.) Test weighing[13]

(I). Monitor milk intake and growth (weight and length) during this week. Record volumes of pumped or expressed milk and daily test weights (for infants fed at the breast) during this period.[13]

(II). If intake and growth are adequate during this week after switching:

(a). Add iron (1–2 mg/kg/day), depending on how much formula is fed

(b). Add multivitamin preparation (half to full dose described above C.1 [c]), depending upon how much formula is fed.

(III). Continue this diet after discharge.

2. If the infant has been receiving unfortified human milk, assess the adequacy of breastfeeding and address problems or potential problems as above, D.1(d).

a. If addressing any existing breastfeeding problems does not result in "optimal assessment," add two to three feedings of enriched postdischarge formula prepared per manufacturer instructions (~22 kcal/oz) [See note under D.1(a) above]. Ensure that the mother is expressing milk to maintain and optimize her milk production. Anticipate at least 1 more week of continued hospitalization before discharge.

i. Monitor milk intake and growth during this week.

ii. Continue iron and multivitamin supplement.

iii. If the feeding assessment continues to be suboptimal after 1 week, increase the number of feedings of enriched postdischarge formula or increase the concentration of enriched formula to 24 to 30 kcal/oz.

III. POSTDISCHARGE ASSESSMENT

A. Nutrition monitoring 1 week after discharge

1. Assess intake

a. History

b. Observation of feeding

c. Consider test weighing if concerns persist[13]

2. Growth—weight and length (Table P-4)

3. Biochemical indices of nutritional status (Table P-4)

4. Reassess nutritional status as "Optimal" vs. "Suboptimal."

a. Infants with an "Optimal" assessment may be reevaluated at 1 month after discharge (See III.B, below).

b. For infants with a "Suboptimal assessment":

i. Assess adequacy of breastfeeding

(A). Latch

(B). Milk transfer/volume

(C). Maternal satisfaction

(D). Milk content—consider hindmilk

(E). Consider use of feeding devices

(I). Nipple shield to improve milk transfer[14]

(II). Test weighing[13] to evaluate milk volume

ii. If addressing any existing breastfeeding problems does not result in an "optimal assessment," add additional feedings of enriched postdischarge formula, prepared as below, per clinical judgment according to the individual infant's assessment.

(A). Prepared per manufacturer instructions (~22 kcal/oz)

(B). Concentrated to 24–30 kcal/oz

(C). Ensure that the mother is expressing milk to maintain and optimize her milk production.

   iii. Frequent follow-up visits for ongoing nutritional monitoring

B. Nutrition monitoring 1 month after discharge

  1. Assess intake

    a. History

    b. Observation of feeding

    c. Consider test weighing if concerns persist[13]

  2. Growth—weight and length (Table P-4)

  3. Biochemical indices of nutritional status (Table P-4)

  4. Reassess nutritional status as "Optimal" vs. "Suboptimal."

    a. Infants with an "Optimal" assessment may be reevaluated at every 2 months to 1 year corrected age.

    b. For infants with a "Suboptimal assessment":

      i. Ensure optimal milk production, breastfeeding

      ii. Add additional feedings of enriched postdischarge formula, individualizing preparation either prepared per manufacturer instructions (~22 kcal/oz) or concentrated to 24–30 kcal/oz.

      iii. Frequent follow-up visits for ongoing nutritional monitoring

C. Once nutrition has been optimized, nutritional monitoring can occur every 2 months until 1 year corrected age.

D. With regard to enriched formula, a few studies have demonstrated a positive effect on growth using enriched formulas for 6 to 9 months. Until more definitive data are available for breastfed former preemies, we recommend continuing an enriched postdischarge formula for a minimum of 6 months.

See Figure P-2 for an algorithm for care of premature infants post discharge.

IV. GENERAL STRATEGIES

A. Enriched postdischarge formula is used because it provides greater nutrient intake than term infant formula. Human milk fortifier usually is not recommended postdischarge because its nutrient content is too great for the infant at the time of discharge and it is expensive and very difficult to prepare according to specifications.

B. Hindmilk, if used, provides extra calories (estimated at 22–24 cal/oz) but no increase in the intake of minerals or protein. (Hindmilk is the fat-rich milk that occurs at the end of the feeding.)

C. It is imperative that the hospital physician communicate with the physician who will provide follow-up care to ensure that the desired plan is carried out and to convey any unique concerns about growth, diet, feeding patterns, and biochemical monitoring.

V. SUPPORT FOR BREASTFEEDING MOTHERS OF PREMATURE INFANTS

A. Support mothers to initiate kangaroo (skin-to-skin) care as early as possible in-hospital.[1,15]

B. Encourage mothers to express their milk soon after delivery and approximately every 3 hours on an ongoing basis. Aim for at least eight pumping sessions in 24 hours, so that if pumping does not occur exactly every 3 hours, sessions will not be missed. Instruct mothers on the use of effective breast pumping methods, either electric rental-grade or effective manual pumps or manual expression. Whenever possible, electric rental-grade pumps should be used for maximal stimulation, particularly for the establishment of milk supply. Skin-to-skin contact, simultaneous milk expression, and

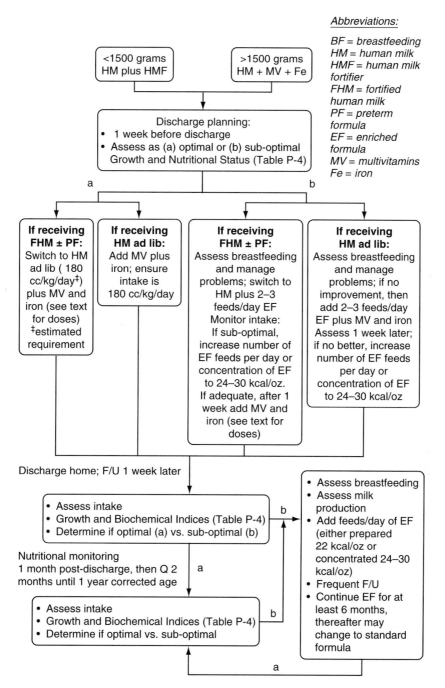

Figure P-2   Algorithm for care of prematures postdischarge by weight (<1500 g or >1500g)

non-nutritive suckling at the breast may facilitate the establishment of the milk supply.

C. Educate mothers that early feeding behaviors emerge during skin-to-skin holding and that mothers can follow the infant's cues for early feeding attempts. Mothers should understand that early feeding attempts are gradual and not expected to result in a full feeding for the infant.

D. Sustained suckling with swallowing for 5 minutes is one indicator that the infant may be ready to transition from nasogastric tube to breast-feeding.[16,17] Other studies suggest that early introduction of oral feeding hastens the development of oral motor skills.[18] Nursing supplementers may provide additional volume.[19]

E. Have trained personnel evaluate breastfeeding (position and latch) on a regular basis. A correct latch is critical for efficient milk removal.

F. Monitor mothers for nipple soreness. If present, this may be an indication of shallow latch.

Temporary use of silicone nipple shields is a helpful adjunct for milk transfer and more efficient latch-on for premature infants with shallow latch.[15]

G. If the infant is achieving partial intake directly at the breast, consider "triple feeding"—put the baby to breast, supplement with expressed breast milk or formula (at breast with the supplemental nursing [tube feeding] device or after the breastfeeding), and then pump or express milk afterward to maintain the milk supply.

H. If the baby is discharged with partial feedings at the breast, consider a scale sensitive enough to distinguish milk intake for home use to help with the transition to total feedings at the breast.

I. Refer and coordinate supportive care services such as community support, visiting nurse, lactation consultant visits, social services, and WIC.

REFERENCES

1. Schanler RJ: Human milk for premature infants. Pediatr Clin North Am 48:207–219, 2001.

2. Bier JAB, Ferguson AE, Morales Y, et al: Breastfeeding infants who were extremely low birth weight. Pediatrics 100:e3, 1997.

3. Slusher T, Slusher I, Biomdo M, et al: Electric breast pump use increases maternal milk volume and decreases time to onset of adequate maternal milk volume in African nurseries. Pediatr Res 55(4, Part 2):445A, 2004.

4. Marinelli K, Burke G, Dodd V: A comparison of the safety of cup feedings and bottle feedings in premature infants whose mothers intend to breastfeed. J Perinatol 21:350–355, 2001.

5. Collins CT, Ryan P, Crowther CA, et al: Effect of bottles, cups, and dummies on breast feeding in preterm infants: A randomised controlled trial. Br Med J 329:193–198, 2004.

6. Lucas A, Bishop NJ, King FJ, Cole TJ: Randomized trial of nutrition for preterm infants after discharge. Arch Dis Child 67:324–327, 1992.

7. Carver JD, Wu PJK, Hall RT, et al: Growth of preterm infants fed nutrient-enriched or term formula after hospital discharge. Pediatrics 107:683–689, 2001.

8. Schanler RJ, Burns PA, Abrams SA, Garza C: Bone mineralization outcomes in human milk-fed preterm infants. Pediatr Res 31:583–586, 1992.

9. Chan GM: Growth and bone status of discharged very low birth weight infants fed different formulas or human milk. J Pediatr 123:439–443, 1993.

10. Greer FR: Feeding the preterm infant after hospital discharge. Pediatr Ann 30:658–665, 2001.

11. Lucas A, Fewtrell MS, Morley R, et al: Randomized trial of nutrient-enriched formulas versus standard formula for post-discharge preterm infants. Pediatrics 108:703–711, 2001.

12. Ramsethu J, Jeyaseelan L, Kirubakaran C: Weight gain in exclusively breastfed preterm infants. J Trop Pediatr 39:152–159, 1993.

13. Meier PP, Engstrom JL, Crichton C, et al: A new scale for in-home test-weighing for mothers of preterm and high-risk infants. J Hum Lact 10:63–68, 1994.

14. Meier PP, Brown LP, Hurst NM, et al: Nipple shields for preterm infants: Effect on milk transfer and duration of breastfeeding. J Hum Lact 16:106–113, 2000.

15. Kirsten GF, Bergman NJ, Hann FM: Kangaroo mother care in the nursery. Pediatr Clin North Am 48:443–452, 2001.

16. Kliethermes PA, Cross ML, Lanese MG, Johnson KM, Simon SD: Transitioning preterm infants with nasogastric tube supplementation: increased likelihood of breastfeeding. J Obstet Gynecol Neonatal Nurs 28:264–273, 1999.

17. Valentine CJ, Hurst NM: A six step feeding strategy for preterm infants. J Hum Lact 11:7–8, 1995.

18. Simpson C, Schanler R, Lau C: Early introduction of oral feeding in preterm infants. Pediatrics 110:517–522, 2002.

19. Meier PP: Breastfeeding in the special care nursery: Prematures and infants with medical problems. Pediatr Clin North Am 48:425–442, 2001.

20. Hall RA: Nutritional follow-up of the breastfeeding premature infant after hospital discharge. Pediatr Clin North Am 48:453–460, 2001.

21. Schanler RJ: Nutrition support of the low birth weight infant. In Walker WA, Watkins JB, Duggan CP (eds): Nutrition in Pediatrics, 3rd ed. Hamilton, ON, Canada, BC Decker, 2003, pp 392–412.

Copyright protected © 2004 The Academy of Breastfeeding Medicine, Inc.
Approved 9/17/04

The Academy of Breastfeeding Medicine Protocol Committee
Caroline J. Chantry, MD, FABM, Co-Chairperson
*Lori Feldman-Winter, MD
Cynthia R. Howard, MD, MPH, FABM, Co-Chairperson
*Richard J. Schanler, MD

Development supported in part by a grant from the Maternal and Child Health Bureau, Department of Health and Human Services

*lead author(s)

$\mathscr{G}$lossary

acinus The tube leading to the smallest lobule of a compound gland; it is characterized by a narrow lumen.

adipose tissue *See* panniculus adiposus.

afferent Conducting inward to, or toward, the center of an organ, gland, or other structure or area. Applies to sensory nerves, arteries, and lymph vessels.

alactogenesis Familial puerperal alactogenesis is genetically transmitted isolated prolactin deficiency.

alveolus A glandular acinus or terminal portion of the alveolar gland where milk is secreted and stored, 0.12 mm in diameter. From 10 to 100 alveoli, or tubulosaccular secretory units, make up a lobulus.

ampulla Elastic portion of the duct, just proximal to the nipple, that expands as milk fills the breast. *See* lactiferous sinuses.

apocrine A term descriptive of a gland cell that loses part of its protoplasmic substance.

Apt test A test, named after its developer, performed on fresh blood to distinguish between adult and fetal hemoglobin. The blood is suspended in saline, and an equal amount of 10% sodium hydroxide (NaOH) is added and mixed; adult hemoglobin turns brown, and fetal hemoglobin remains red. A control sample of known adult blood should also be tested for comparison.

arborization Development of a branched arrangement or structure.

areola mammae Areola. The pigmented area surrounding the papilla mammae, or nipple.

autophagic vacuole Autophagosome. A membrane-bound body within a cell containing degenerating cell organelles.

BALT Bronchus-associated immunocompetent lymphoid tissue, to which the mammary gland may act as an extension. *See* GALT and MALT.

basal lamina The layer of material, 50- to 80-mm thick, that lies adjacent to the plasma membrane of the basal surfaces of epithelial cells. It contains collagen and certain carbohydrates. It is often called the *basement* membrane.

casein A derivative of caseinogen. The fraction of milk protein that forms the tough curd.

colostrum The first milk. This yellow, sticky fluid is secreted during the first few days post partum and provides nutrition and protection against infectious disease. It contains more protein, less sugar, and much less fat than mature breast milk.

columnar secretory cell A type of secretory cell in the shape of a hexagonal prism; it appears rectangular when sectioned across the long axis, the length being considerably greater than the width.

Cooper's ligaments Triangular ligaments stretching between the mammary gland, the skin, the retinacula cutis, the pectineal ligament, and the chorda obliqua. These ligaments underlie the breasts.

corpus mammae The mammary gland; breast mass after freeing breast from deep attachments and removal of skin, subcutaneous connective tissue, and fat.

creamatocrit Measurement for estimating the fat content and therefore the caloric content of a milk sample. A microhematocrit tube is filled with milk (usually a mix of foremilk and hindmilk) and spun in a microcentrifuge for 15 minutes. The layer of fat is measured as a percentage, as one measures a blood hematocrit.

cross nursing   The breastfeeding of a baby that is not her own by a lactating woman, often temporarily, in the role of a child care arrangement.

cuboidal secretory cell   A secretory cell having similar height and breadth measurements.

cytokines   A generic term for nonantibody proteins that are part of the immune system; examples include interferon-γ and interleukin 6.

cytosol   Cell fluid.

doula   An individual who surrounds, interacts with, and aids the mother at any time within the period that includes pregnancy, birth, and lactation; may be a relative, friend, or neighbor and is usually but not necessarily female. One who gives psychological encouragement and physical assistance to a new mother.

efferent   Carrying impulses away from a nerve center.

ejection reflex   A reflex initiated by the suckling of the infant at the breast, which triggers the pituitary gland to release oxytocin into the bloodstream. The oxytocin causes the myoepithelial cells to contract and eject the milk from the collecting ductules. Also called *let-down reflex* or *draught*.

engorgement   The swelling and distention of the breasts, usually in the early days of initiation of lactation, caused by vascular dilatation as well as the arrival of the early milk.

eosinophil   A granular leukocyte possessing large conspicuous granules in the cytoplasm and containing a bilobed nucleus.

finger feeding   Stimulation of an infant's tongue with a finger to initiate sucking. A feeding tube attached to a syringe of milk along the finger will provide milk to the infant when suckling is correct.

foremilk   The first milk obtained at the onset of suckling or expression. Contains less fat than later milk of that feeding (i.e., the hindmilk).

galactocele   A cystic tumor in the ducts of the breast that contains a milky fluid.

galactogogue   A material or action that stimulates the production of milk.

galactopoiesis   The development of milk in the mammary gland. The maintenance of established lactation.

galactorrhea   Abnormal or inappropriate lactation.

galactose   ($C_6H_{12}O_6$). A simple sugar that is a component of the disaccharide lactose, or milk sugar.

galactosemia   A congenital metabolic disorder in which there is an inability to metabolize galactose because of a deficiency of the enzyme galactose-1-phosphate uridyltransferase. It causes failure to thrive, hepatomegaly, and splenomegaly.

GALT   Gut-associated lymphoid tissue to which the mammary gland may act as an extension. *See* BALT and MALT.

gigantomastia   The excessive enlargement of the breast beyond physiologic needs during pregnancy and lactation; usually of unknown cause. When it occurs in association with medications that cause galactorrhea (calcium-channel blockers) it can be reversed by stopping the drug.

Golgi apparatus   A specialized region of the cytoplasm, often close to the nucleus, that is composed of flattened cisternae, numerous vesicles, and some larger vacuoles. In secretory cells it is concerned with packaging the secretory product. It is also probably concerned with the secretion of polysaccharides in some cells, but its full range of functions has not yet been elucidated.

heterophagic vacuole   Heterophagosome. A membrane-bound body within a cell, containing ingested material.

hindmilk   Milk obtained later during the nursing period, that is, the end of the feeding. This milk is usually high in fat and probably controls appetite.

homocystinuria   A rare inborn error of amino acid metabolism characterized by mental deficiency, epilepsy, dislocation of the lens, growth disturbance, thromboses, and defective hair growth.

hyperadenia   The existence of mammary tissue without nipples.

hypergalactia   The excessive, uncontrolled production of milk over and above the needs of a suckling infant.

hyperlactation An oversupply of milk beyond the needs or capacity of the infant.

hypermastia The existence of accessory mammary glands.

hyperthelia The existence of abundant, more or less developed, nipples without accompanying mammary tissue.

immunoglobulin Protein fraction of globulin, which has been demonstrated to have immunologic properties. Immunoglobulins include IgA, IgG, and IgM—factors in breast milk that protect against infection.

induced lactation Process by which a nonpuerperal female (or male) is stimulated to lactate.

kosher Food that is considered ritually fit according to Jewish law (both as to source of food and type of preparation).

lactiferous ducts The main ducts of the mammary gland, which number from 15 to 30 and open onto the nipple. They carry milk to the nipple.

lactiferous sinuses A potential space for milk created by the marked elasticity of the lactiferous ducts as they approach the nipple.

Lactobacillus bifidus Organism of the intestinal tract of breastfed infants.

lactocele Cystic tumor of the breast caused by the dilatation and obstruction of a milk duct usually filled with milk.

lacto-engineering The process of enhancing the nutrient value of human milk by adding nutrients obtained by drying and separating out specific nutrients such as protein from pooled human milk.

lactoferrin An iron-binding protein of external secretions, including human milk. It inhibits the growth of iron-dependent microorganisms in the gut.

lactogenesis Initiation of milk secretion.

let-down reflex *See* ejection reflex.

ligand A low-molecular-weight substance that binds trace elements loosely for ready availability (e.g., zinc ligands in human milk).

lobulus A subunit of the parenchymal structure of the breast made up of 10 to 100 alveoli, or tubulosaccular secretory units. From 20 to 40 lobuli make up a lobus.

lobus A subunit of the parenchymal structure of the breast made up of 20 to 40 lobuli. From 15 to 25 lobi are arranged like the spokes of a wheel with the nipple as the central point.

lymphocyte A mature leukocyte derived through the intermediate stage of lymphoblast from the reticuloendothelium found in lymphatic tissue.

lyophilization The process of rapidly freeze-drying a fluid in a vacuum, resulting in a solid.

MALT Mucosal-associated lymphoid tissue, which includes gut, lung, mammary gland, salivary and lacrimal glands, and genital tract. There is traffic of cells between secretory sites. Immunization at one site may be an effective means of producing immunity at distant sites. *See* GALT and BALT.

mamilla The nipple; any teatlike structure.

mammogenesis Growth of the mammary gland.

mastalgia Painful breasts.

mastitis Inflammation of the breast, including cellulitis, and occasionally abscess formation.

matrescence The state of becoming a mother or motherhood as a new event in an individual's life.

megaloblastic anemia Defective red blood cell formation caused by megaloblastic hyperplasia of the marrow; there are often megaloblasts, or primitive nucleated red blood cells, in the peripheral blood.

merocrine Pertaining to the type of secretion in which the active cell remains intact while forming and discharging the secretory product.

mesencephalon The midbrain.

methylmalonic aciduria The condition of the urine being acidic from an accumulation of methylmalonic acid caused by an inborn error of metabolism.

milk fever A syndrome of fever and general malaise associated with early engorgement of the breasts or with sudden weaning from the breast.

mitogen A substance capable of stimulating cells to enter mitosis.

Montgomery glands Small prominences, sebaceous glands in the areola of the breast, which become more marked in pregnancy. They number 20 to 24 and secrete a fluid that lubricates the nipple and areola.

Morgagni's tubercle   Small sinuses into which the miniature ducts of the Montgomery glands open in the epidermis of the areola.

myoepithelial cell   An epithelial cell, usually around a glandular acinus, in which part of the cytoplasm has contractile properties, serving to empty the sinus of its secretion.

nonnutritive sucking   The act of suckling the breast with little or no secretion of milk. Infant may suckle when distressed or to be calmed or quieted.

nonpuerperal lactation   The production of milk in a woman who has not given birth.

nucleotides   Compounds derived from nucleic acid by hydrolysis and consisting of phosphoric acid combined with a sugar and a purine or pyrimidine derivative. The milk nucleotides are secreted from glandular epithelial cells.

opsonic   Belonging to or characterized by opsonin, a substance in mammalian blood having the power to render microorganisms and blood cells more easily absorbed by phagocytes.

oxytocin   An octapeptide synthesized in the cell bodies of neurons located mainly in the paraventricular nucleus and in smaller amounts in the supraoptic nucleus of the hypothalamus. Oxytocin stimulates the ejection reflex by stimulation of the myoepithelial cells in the mammary gland.

panniculus adiposus   Adipose tissue. The superficial fascia, which contains fatty pellicles.

papilla mammae   Mamilla. The nipple of the breast.

pareve (parve)   Food that does not include any meat or dairy derivatives. This includes milk from any mammal except human. Rabbis have defined human milk as pareve but have prohibited the mixing of human milk with other foods.

perinatal   Around birth. The time from conception through birth, delivery, lactation, and at least 28 days post partum.

plasma cell   Cell derived from the B cell series, which manufactures and secretes antibodies.

prolactin   A hormone present in both male and female and at all ages. During pregnancy it stimulates and prepares the mammary alveolar epithelium for secretory activity. During lactation it stimulates synthesis and secretion of milk. At other ages and in the male it interacts with other steroids.

rachitic   Relating to, characterized by, or affected with rickets.

relactation   Process by which a woman who has given birth but did not initially breastfeed is stimulated to lactate (also applies to reinstituting lactation after it has been discontinued).

squamous epithelium   A sheet of flattened, scalelike epithelium adhering edge to edge.

stroma   The connective tissue basis or framework of an organ.

suck training   A special technique developed to help an infant who cannot coordinate the undulating (peristaltic) motion of the tongue. See *finger feeding.*

switch nursing   Putting the infant to one breast for a short time, usually 5 minutes, moving the infant to the other breast for 5 minutes, and then moving the infant back to the first side in an effort to improve milk production.

tail of Spence   The axillary tail of the breast.

transitional milk   The milk produced early in the postpartum period as the colostrum diminishes and the mature milk develops.

tubuloalveolar   Having both tubular and alveolar qualities.

tubulosaccular   Having both tubular and saccular character.

turgescence   The swelling up of a part. The unusual turgid feeling resulting from swelling with fluid.

whey protein   Protein remaining when the curds of casein have been removed. The mixture of proteins present is complex and includes β-lactoglobulin and α-lactalbumin and enzymes.

witch's milk   Product of neonatal galactorrhea or neonatal breast secretion caused by absorption of placental prolactin.

$\mathscr{I}$ndex

Note: Page numbers followed by b indicate boxes; those followed by f indicate figures; those followed by t indicate tables.